Clinical Mycology

CLINICAL MYCOLOGY

Edited by

WILLIAM E. DISMUKES, M.D.
PETER G. PAPPAS, M.D.
JACK D. SOBEL, M.D.

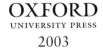

OXFORD
UNIVERSITY PRESS
2003

OXFORD
UNIVERSITY PRESS

Oxford   New York
Auckland   Bangkok   Buenos Aires   Cape Town   Chennai
Dar es Salaam   Delhi   Hong Kong   Istanbul   Karachi   Kolkata
Kuala Lumpar   Madrid   Melbourne   Mexico City   Mumbai
Nairobi   São Paulo   Shanghai   Taipei   Tokyo   Toronto

Copyright © 2003 by Oxford University Press, Inc.

Published by Oxford University Press, Inc.
198 Madison Avenue, New York, New York 10016
http://www.oup-usa.org

Oxford is a registered trademark of Oxford University Press

Library of Congress Cataloging-in-Publication Data
Clinical mycology / edited by William E. Dismukes, Peter G. Pappas, Jack D. Sobel.
p. ; cm.   Includes bibliographical references and index.ISBN 0-19-514809-6 (cloth)
1. Medical mycology.
I. Dismukes, William E. II. Pappas, Peter G. III. Sobel, Jack D.
[DNLM: 1. Mycoses—etiology.
2. Antifungal Agents.
WC 450 C6411 2003]   QR245.C566 2003
616'015—dc21   2002193100

2 4 6 8 9 7 5 3 1
Printed in the United States of America
on acid-free paper

Preface

Systemic fungal infections (systemic mycoses) have progressively emerged over the past 50 years as causes of human disease in normal hosts and, more importantly, in the ever expanding population of immunocompromised hosts. Over this same period of time, much has been learned about the causative fungal organisms, including their molecular biology and ecologic niches. Moreover, we now have a clearer understanding of the epidemiology, pathogenesis, and the broad array of clinical syndromes associated with the various systemic mycoses. Most importantly for our patients, major advances have been achieved in the area of antifungal therapy, namely, development of new classes of drugs with unique fungal targets, (e.g., echinocandins), and modifications of existing classes of drugs to enhance spectrum of activity and improve the therapeutic: toxic ratio (e.g., azoles and polyenes). In addition to the availability of several new drugs, many Phase III and Phase IV clinical trials over the past 25 years have taught us how to use these drugs appropriately to provide more creative and effective management approaches for prophylaxis, empirical therapy, induction and consolidation therapy, and chronic suppressive (maintenance) therapy of systemic fungal diseases. The editors feel there is a need for a comprehensive and up-to-date textbook that not only addresses the many advances alluded to above, but also provides detailed information about the current status of diagnosis and treatment. We believe our book fills this need.

The 32 chapters are written by many of the leading authorities in the field of clinical mycology. These authors, who are distinguished clinicians as well as investigators, both basic and translational, have performed many of the key studies that have transformed our understanding and management of fungal diseases. The book also contains numerous color and black-and-white photos and illustrations, plus tables and algorithms, which help to convey essential information quickly and easily. In addition, the references cited in each chapter represent the latest and most significant publications on each disease, drug, or management strategy.

To facilitate its use, the book is organized into eight distinctive sections. The Introduction (Section I) provides an overview of laboratory aspects of medical mycology, which are pertinent to all fungi. Similarly, an overview of the epidemiology of systemic fungal diseases addresses the complex interactions of the many host and environmental factors that predispose to systemic mycoses.

Systemic Antifungal Drugs (II), which is the largest section in the book and contains 8 chapters, addresses both classes of drugs and specific old and new agents in each class. Drug structure, mechanisms of action, pharmacologic features, drug–drug interactions, adverse events, clinical indications, and major clinical trials are discussed in detail. In addition, two special chapters provide extensive and valuable reviews of important and rapidly evolving areas, namely, resistance to antifungal drugs and adjunctive therapy.

The five sections that follow are organized into the mycotic diseases caused by various type of fungi: Yeasts(III), Moulds(IV), Dimorphic Fungi(V), Skin and Subcutaneous Pathogens(VI), and other mycoses (VII). Within these sections, each chapter on a specific fungal disease consists of comprehensive discussions of pertinent topics including organism, epidemiology, pathogenesis, clinical syndromes, diagnosis and management. The final section—Special Patient Populations (VIII)—addresses those groups at high risk for opportunistic fungal diseases including neutropenic patients, hematopoietic stem cell and bone marrow as well as solid organ transplant recipients, and patients with HIV/AIDS.

The editors express their deep gratitude to the many authors for their scholarly contributions to this book, to Lee Hoke and Windell Ross, our assistants, as well as the staff at Oxford University Press for their invaluable support in the preparation of this work, and to our wives, Pidgie, Alexis, and Audrey, for their continued encouragement and enduring patience. Without these individuals, the existence and timely completion of this book would not have been possible.

Birmingham, Alabama   W.E.D.
Birmingham, Alabama   P.G.P.
Detroit, Michigan   J.D.S.

Contents

Contributors, xi

PART I   INTRODUCTION, 1

1. Laboratory Aspects of Medical Mycology, 3
   Mary E. Brandt and David W. Warnock

2. Epidemiology of Systemic Fungal Diseases: Overview, 23
   Rana A. Hajjeh and David W. Warnock

PART II   SYSTEMIC ANTIFUNGAL DRUGS, 31

3. Amphotericin B, 33
   Stanley W. Chapman, John D. Cleary, and P. David Rogers

4. Liposomal Nystatin, 49
   Richard J. Hamill

5. Flucytosine, 59
   Robert A. Larsen

6. Azole Antifungal Drugs, 64
   Jackson Como and William E. Dismukes

7. Cell Wall Synthesis Inhibitors: Echinocandins and Nikkomycins, 88
   Andreas H. Groll and Thomas J. Walsh

8. Terbinafine, 104
   Peter G. Pappas

9. Resistance to Antifungal Drugs, 111
   Dominique Sanglard

10. Adjunctive Antifungal Therapy, 125
    Emmanuel Roilides, John Dotis, Joanna Filioti, and Elias Anaissie

PART III   MYCOSES CAUSED BY YEASTS, 141

11. Candidiasis, 143
    Jose A. Vazquez and Jack D. Sobel

12. Cryptococcosis, 188
    John W. Baddley and William E. Dismukes

13. *Rhodotorula, Malassezia, Trichosporon*, and Other Yeast-Like Fungi, 206
    Jose A. Vazquez

PART IV   MYCOSES CAUSED BY MOULDS, 219

14. Aspergillosis, 221
    Thomas F. Patterson

15. Zygomycoses, 241
    Ashraf S. Ibrahim, John E. Edwards Jr., and Scott G. Filler

16. Hyalohyphomycoses (other than Aspergillosis and Penicilliosis), 252
    Harrys A. Torres and Dimitrios P. Kontoyiannis

17. Phaeohyphomycoses, 271
    John R. Perfect, Wiley A. Schell, and Gary M. Cox

PART V   MYCOSES CAUSED BY DIMORPHIC FUNGI, 283

18. Histoplasmosis, 285
    Carol A. Kauffman

19. Blastomycosis, 299
    Robert W. Bradsher

20. Coccidioidomycosis, 311
    Neil M. Ampel

21. Paracoccidioidomycosis, 328
    Angela Restrepo-Moreno

22. Sporotrichosis, 346
    Peter G. Pappas

23. Penicilliosis, 355
    Kenrad E. Nelson and Thira Sirisanthana

PART VI   MYCOLOGY INVOLVING SKIN AND SUBCUTANEOUS TISSUES, 365

24. Superficial Cutaneous Fungal Infections, 367
    Jeff Weeks, Stephen A. Moser, and Boni E. Elewski

25. Eumycetoma, 390
    Beatriz Bustamante and Pablo E. Campos

26. Chromoblastomycosis, 399
    John W. Baddley and William E. Dismukes

PART VII   OTHER MYCOSES, 405

27. Pneumocystosis, 407
    Catherine F. Decker and Henry Masur

28. Miscellaneous Fungi, 420
    John W. Baddley and William E. Dismukes

PART VIII   SPECIAL PATIENT POPULATIONS, 425

29. Fungal Infections in Neutropenic Patients, 427
    Juan C. Gea-Banacloche, Andreas H. Groll, and Thomas J. Walsh

30. Fungal Infections in Blood or Marrow Transplant Recipients, 456
    Kieren A. Marr

31. Fungal Infections in Solid Organ Transplant Recipients, 470
    Peter G. Pappas

32. Fungal Infections among Patients with AIDS, 488
    Bertrand Dupont, Peter G. Pappas, and William E. Dismukes

Index, 503

Contributors

NEIL M. AMPEL, MD
Professor of Medicine
Division of Infectious Diseases
University of Arizona School of Medicine and Veterans
 Affairs Medical Center
Tucson, AZ

ELIAS ANAISSIE, MD
Professor of Medicine, Director, Supportive Care
Myeloma Institute for Research and Treatment
The Arkansas Cancer Research Center
University of Arkansas for Medical Sciences
Little Rock AR

JOHN W. BADDLEY, MD
Assistant Professor, Division of Infectious Diseases
Department of Medicine
University of Alabama School of Medicine at Birmingham
Birmingham, AL

ROBERT W. BRADSHER, MD
Richard Ebert Professor of Medicine
Vice Chairman, Department of Medicine
Director, Division of Infectious Diseases
University of Arkansas for Medical Sciences
Central Arkansas Veterans Healthcare System
Little Rock, AR

MARY E. BRANDT, PhD
Research Microbiologist, Mycotic Diseases Branch
National Center for Infectious Diseases
Centers for Disease Control and Prevention
Atlanta, GA

BEATRIZ BUSTAMANTE, MD
Chief of Mycology Laboratory and Associate Researcher
Institute of Tropical Medicine "Alexander von Humboldt"
Peruana Cayetano Heredia University
Lima, Peru

PABLO E. CAMPOS, MD, MPH
Associate Professor
School of Public Health
Institute of Tropical Medicine "Alexander von Humboldt"
Peruana Cayetano Heredia University
Lima, Peru

STANLEY W. CHAPMAN, MD
Director, Division of Infectious Diseases
Professor of Medicine
Department of Medicine and Department of Microbiology
University of Mississippi Medical Center and Department
 of Veterans Affairs Medical Center
Jackson, MS

JOHN D. CLEARY, PharmD
Professor and Vice-Chairman for Research
School of Pharmacy
University of Mississippi Medical Center
Jackson, MS

JACKSON COMO, PharmD
Director, Drug Information
Department of Pharmacy
University of Alabama Hospital
University of Alabama Medical Center
Birmingham, AL

GARY M. COX, MD
Assistant Professor of Medicine
Division of Infectious Diseases
Duke University Medical Center
Durham, NC

CATHERINE F. DECKER, MD
Division of Infectious Diseases
National Naval Medical Center
Bethesda, MD

WILLIAM E. DISMUKES, MD
Professor and Vice-Chairman
Department of Medicine
Director, Division of Infectious Diseases
University of Alabama School of Medicine at Birmingham
Birmingham, AL

JOHN DOTIS, MD
Research Fellow
3rd Department of Pediatrics
Hippokration Hospital
Aristotle University
Thessaloniki, Greece

BERTRAND DUPONT, MD
Professor of Infectious Diseases
University of Paris V, Hospital Necker
Paris, France

JOHN E. EDWARDS, JR.
Director, Division of Infectious Diseases
Professor of Medicine
UCLA School of Medicine
Harbor-UCLA Research and Education Institute
Harbor-UCLA Medical Center
Torrance, CA

BONI E. ELEWSKI, MD
Professor of Dermatology
Department of Dermatology
University of Alabama School of Medicine at Birmingham
Birmingham, AL

SCOTT G. FILLER, MD
Associate Professor of Medicine
UCLA School of Medicine
Division of Infectious Diseases
Harbor UCLA Medical Center
Torrance, CA

JOANNA FILIOTI, MD
Research Fellow
3rd Department of Pediatrics
Hippokration Hospital
Aristotle University
Thessaloniki, Greece

JUAN C. GEA-BANACLOCHE, MD
Experimental Transplantation and Immunology Branch
National Cancer Institute
National Institutes of Health
Bethseda, MD

ANDREAS H. GROLL, MD
Infectious Disease Research Program
Center for Bone Marrow Transplantation and
Department of Pediatric Hematology/Oncology
Wilhelms University Medical Center
Muenster, Germany

RANA A. HAJJEH, MD
Chief, Epidemiology Unit
Mycotic Diseases Branch
Centers for Disease Control and Prevention
Atlanta, GA

RICHARD J. HAMILL, MD
Professor, Departments of Medicine and Molecular
  Virology and Microbiology
Baylor College of Medicine
Staff Physician, Infectious Diseases Section
Veterans Affairs Medical Center
Houston, TX

ASHRAF S. IBRAHIM, PhD
Assistant Professor
UCLA School of Medicine
Los Angeles, CA

CAROL A. KAUFFMAN, MD
Chief, Infectious Diseases Division
Veterans Affairs Ann Arbor Healthcare System
Professor of Internal Medicine
University of Michigan Medical School
Ann Arbor, MI

DIMITRIOS P. KONTOYIANNIS, MD
Associate Professor
Director of Clinical Mycology
The University of Texas M.D. Anderson Cancer Center
Department of Infectious Diseases, Infection Control and
  Employee Health
Adjunct Associate Professor University of Houston College
  of Pharmacy
Houston, TX

ROBERT A. LARSEN, MD
Associate Professor of Medicine
Division of Infectious Diseases
University of Southern California School of Medicine
Los Angeles, CA

KIEREN A. MARR, MD
Assistant Member
Program in Infectious Diseases
Fred Hutchinson Cancer Research Center
Seattle, WA

HENRY MASUR, MD
Chief, Critical Care Medicine Department
Warren Magnuson Clinical Center
National Institutes of Health
Bethesda, MD

STEPHEN A. MOSER, PhD
Associate Professor of Pathology and Microbiology
University of Alabama School of Medicine at Birmingham
Birmingham, AL

KENRAD E. NELSON, MD
Professor, Department of Epidemiology
Bloomberg School of Public Health
Johns Hopkins University
Baltimore, MD

PETER G. PAPPAS, MD
Professor of Medicine
Division of Infectious Diseases
University of Alabama School of Medicine at Birmingham
Birmingham, AL

THOMAS F. PATTERSON, MD
Professor of Medicine
Division of Infectious Diseases
University of Texas Health Sciences Center
San Antonio, TX

JOHN R. PERFECT, MD
Director, Duke University Mycology Research Unit
Professor of Medicine
Duke University Medical Center
Durham, NC

ANGELA RESTREPO-MORENO, PhD
Senior Researcher, Corporación para Investigaciones
  Biológicas
Medellin, Colombia

P. DAVID ROGERS, PharmD, PhD
Assistant Professor of Pharmacy
Pharmaceutical Sciences and Pediatrics
Colleges of Pharmacy and Medicine
University of Tennessee Health Sciences Center
Memphis, TN

EMMANUEL ROILIDES, MD, PhD
Assistant Professor
3rd Department of Pediatrics
Hippokration Hospital
Aristotle University
Thessaloniki, Greece

DOMINIQUE SANGLARD, PD, MER
Institute of Microbiology
University Hospital Lausanne
Lausanne, Switzerland

WILEY A. SCHELL, MS
Associate in Research
Department of Medicine
Division of Infectious Diseases
Duke University Medical Center
Durham, NC

THIRA SIRISANTHANA, MD
Professor of Medicine
Research Institute for Health Sciences
Chiang Mai University
Chiang Mai, Thailand

JACK D. SOBEL, MD
Professor of Internal Medicine
Director, Division of Infectious Diseases
Wayne State University School of Medicine
Detroit, MI

HARRYS A. TORRES, MD
Post Doctoral Research Fellow
The University of Texas M.D. Anderson Cancer Center
Department of Infectious Diseases, Infection Control and
  Employee Health
Houston, TX

JOSE A. VAZQUEZ, MD
Associate Professor of Medicine
Division of Infectious Diseases
Wayne State University School of Medicine
Detroit, MI

THOMAS J. WALSH, MD
Chief, Immunocompromised Host Section
Pediatric Oncology Branch
National Cancer Institute
National Institutes of Health
Bethesda, MD

DAVID W. WARNOCK, PhD, FRC, PATH
Chief, Mycotic Diseases Branch
National Center for Infectious Diseases
Centers for Disease Control and Prevention
Atlanta, GA

JEFF WEEKS, MD
Resident in Dermatology
Department of Dermatology
University of Alabama School of Medicine at Birmingham
Birmingham, AL

I

INTRODUCTION

1

Laboratory aspects of medical mycology

MARY E. BRANDT AND DAVID W. WARNOCK

Over the course of time, more than 100,000 species of fungi have been recognized and described. However, fewer than 500 of these species have been associated with human disease, and no more than 100 are capable of causing infection in otherwise normal individuals. The remainder are only able to produce disease in hosts that are debilitated or immunocompromised.

WHAT ARE FUNGI?

Fungi are not plants. Fungi form a separate group of higher organisms, distinct from both plants and animals, which differ from other groups of organisms in several major respects. First, fungal cells are encased within a rigid cell wall, mostly composed of chitin and glucan. These features contrast with animals, which have no cell walls, and plants, which have cellulose as the major cell wall component.

Second, fungi are heterotrophic. This means that they are lacking in chlorophyll and cannot make their organic food as plants can, through photosynthesis. Fungi live embedded in a food source or medium, and obtain their nourishment by secreting enzymes for external digestion and by absorbing the nutrients that are released from the medium. The recognition that fungi possess a fundamentally different form of nutrition was one of the characteristics that led to their being placed in a separate kingdom.

Third, fungi are simpler in structure than plants or animals. There is no division of cells into organs or tissues. The basic structural unit of fungi is either a chain of tubular, filament-like cells, termed a hypha or hyphae (plural) or an independent single cell. Fungal cell differentiation is no less sophisticated than is found in plants or animals, but it is different. Many fungal pathogens of humans and animals change their growth form during the process of tissue invasion. These dimorphic pathogens usually change from a multicellular hyphal form in the natural environment to a budding, single-celled form in tissue.

In most multicellular fungi the vegetative stage consists of a mass of branching hyphae, termed a mycelium. Each individual hypha has a rigid cell wall and increases in length as a result of apical growth. In the more primitive fungi, the hyphae remain aseptate (without cross-walls). In the more advanced groups, however, the hyphae are septate, with more or less frequent cross-walls. Fungi that exist in the form of microscopic multicellular mycelium are often called moulds.

Many fungi that exist in the form of independent single cells propagate by budding out similar cells from their surface. The bud may become detached from the parent cell, or it may remain attached and itself produce another bud. In this way, a chain of cells may be produced. Fungi that do not produce hyphae, but just consist of a loose arrangement of budding cells are called yeasts. Under certain conditions, continued elongation of the parent cell before it buds results in a chain of elongated cells, termed a pseudohypha.

Fourth, fungi reproduce by means of microscopic propagules called spores. Many fungi produce spores that result from an asexual process. Except for the occasional mutation, these spores are identical to the parent. Asexual spores are generally short-lived propagules that are produced in enormous numbers to ensure dispersion to new habitats. Many fungi are also capable of sexual reproduction. Some species are homothallic and able to form sexual structures within individual colonies. Most, however, are heterothallic and do not form their sexual structures unless two different mating strains come into contact. Meiosis then leads to the production of the sexual spores. In some species the sexual spores are borne singly on specialized generative cells and the whole structure is microscopic in size. In other cases, however, the spores are produced in millions in "fruiting bodies" such as mushrooms and puffballs. In current mycological parlance, the sexual stage of a fungus is known as the teleomorph, and the asexual stage as the anamorph.

CLASSIFICATION OF FUNGI

Mycologists are interested in the structure of the reproductive bodies of fungi and the manner in which these are produced because these features form the basis for the classification and naming of fungi. Most recently the kingdom Fungi has been divided into four lesser groups, termed divisions, based on differences in their reproductive structures, as follows.

Chytridiomycota

This division consists of a single class with approximately 100 genera and 1000 species, none of which are pathogenic to humans. Most species live in an aqueous environment. Sexual reproduction, if it occurs, consists of fusion of compatible nuclei. Meiosis then occurs and motile (swimming) spores, termed zoospores, are produced.

Zygomycota

This division consists of about 175 genera and 1000 species. The thallus (vegetative body of a fungus) is aseptate. The asexual spores, or sporangiospores, are nonmotile and are produced inside a closed sac, termed a sporangium, the wall of which ruptures to release them. Sexual reproduction consists of fusion of nuclei from compatible colonies, followed by the formation of a single large zygospore with a thickened wall. Meiosis occurs on germination and haploid mycelium then develops.

This division contains two orders of medical importance, the Entomophthorales and the Mucorales. The former includes the genera *Basidiobolus* and *Conidiobolus*, and the latter includes the genera *Absidia*, *Mucor*, *Rhizomucor*, and *Rhizopus*.

Ascomycota

This division contains at least 3200 genera and approximately 32,000 species. The thallus is septate. Asexual reproduction consists of the production of spores, termed conidia, from a generative or conidiogenous cell. In some species the conidiogenous cell is not different from the rest of the mycelium. In others, the conidiogenous cell is contained in a specialized hyphal structure, termed a conidiophore. Sexual reproduction results from fusion of nuclei from compatible colonies. After meiosis, haploid spores, termed ascospores, are produced in a sac-like structure, termed an ascus. The Ascomycota show a gradual transition from primitive forms that produce single asci to species that produce large structures, termed ascocarps, containing numerous asci.

This division includes the genus *Ajellomyces*, the main teleomorph genus of dimorphic systemic fungal pathogens. Anamorph genera are *Blastomyces*, *Emmonsia*, and *Histoplasma*. The Ascomycota also include the genus *Pseudallescheria*, the teleomorph of the anamorph genus *Scedosporium*. This division also includes the ascomycetous yeasts, many of which have an anamorph stage belonging to the genus *Candida*.

Basidiomycota

This division contains approximately 22,000 species. The thallus is septate. Asexual reproduction is variable, with some species producing conidia like those of the Ascomycota, but many others are not known to produce conidia at all. Sexual reproduction is by fusion of nuclei from compatible colonies, followed by meiosis and production of basidiospores on the outside of a generative cell, termed a basidium. The basidia are often produced in macroscopic structures, termed basidiocarps, and the spores are often forcibly discharged.

Only a few members of this large division are of medical importance. The most prominent are the basidiomycetous yeasts of the genera *Cryptococcus*, *Malassezia*, and *Trichosporon*. Filamentous basidiomycetes of clinical importance include the genus *Schizophyllum*.

CLASSIFICATION OF ANAMORPHIC FUNGI

In many fungi asexual reproduction has proved so successful that the sexual stage (the teleomorph) has disappeared, or at least, has not been discovered. Most of these anamorphic fungi are presumed to have (or to have had) a teleomorph that belonged to the division Ascomycota; some are presumed to belong to the division Basidiomycota. Even in the absence of the teleomorph it is now often possible to assign these fungi to one or other of these divisions on the basis of ultrastructural or molecular genetic characteristics. In the past, however, these anamorphic fungi were termed the Fungi Imperfecti and were divided into three artificial classes according to their form of growth and production of asexual reproductive structures. Many current mycological texts still employ this system of classification.

Hyphomycetes

The mycelium is septate. The conidia are produced directly on the hyphae or on special hyphal branches termed conidiophores. This class contains a large number of anamorphic fungi of medical importance, including the genera *Aspergillus*, *Cladophialophora*, *Fusarium*, *Microsporum*, *Phialophora*, *Scedosporium*, and *Trichophyton*.

Coelomycetes

The mycelium is septate. The conidia are produced in structures that are either spherical with an apical opening (termed pycnidia), or flat and cup-shaped (termed acervuli). Only a few members of this class are of medical importance. These include the genera *Lasiodiplodia*, and *Pyrenochaeta*.

Blastomycetes

The thallus consists of loose budding single cells or a pseudomycelium. These organisms are identified on the basis of their physiologic rather than their morphologic characteristics. This class contains the yeasts of the anamorphic genus *Candida*. Most of the so-called black yeasts are able to produce true mycelium and are therefore classified under the Hyphomycetes.

NOMENCLATURE OF FUNGI AND FUNGAL DISEASES

As Odds has commented, there are few things more frustrating to the clinician than changes in the names of diseases or disease agents, particularly when the diseases concerned are not very common ones (Odds, 1996). The scientific names of fungi are subject to the International Botanical Code of Nomenclature. In general the correct name for any organism is the earliest (first) name published in line with the requirements of the Code of Nomenclature. To avoid confusion, however, the Code allows for certain exceptions. The most significant of these is when an earlier generic name has been overlooked, a later name is in general use, and a reversion to the earlier name would cause much confusion.

There are two main reasons for renaming. The first is reclassification of a fungus in the light of more detailed investigation of its characteristics. The second is the discovery of the teleomorph (sexual stage) of a previously anamorphic fungus. Many fungi bear two names, one designating their sexual stage and the other their asexual stage. Often there are two names because the anamorphic and teleomorphic stages were described and named at different times without the connection between them being recognized. Both names are valid under the Code of Nomenclature, but that of the teleomorph should take precedence. In practice, however, it is more common (and correct) to refer to a fungus by its asexual designation because this is the stage that is usually obtained in culture.

Unlike the names of fungi, disease names are not subject to strict international control. Their usage tends to reflect local practice. One popular method has been to derive disease names from the generic names of the causal organisms: for example, aspergillosis, candidiasis, sporotrichosis, etc. However, if the fungus changes its name, then the disease name has to be changed as well. For example, moniliasis has become candidiasis or candidosis, and pseudallescheriasis has been variously designated monosporiosis, petriellidiosis, allescheriasis and now scedosporiosis to match the changing name of the pathogen. In 1992 a subcommittee of the International Society for Human and Animal Mycology recommended that the practice of forming disease names from the names of their causes should be avoided, and that, whenever possible individual diseases should be named in the form "pathology A due

to (or caused by) fungus B" (Odds et al, 1992). This recommendation was not intended to apply to long-established disease names, such as aspergillosis; rather it was intended to offer a more flexible approach to nomenclature.

There is also much to be said for the practice of grouping together mycotic diseases of similar origins under single headings. One of the broadest and most useful of these collective names is the term *phaeohyphomycosis*, which is used to refer to a range of subcutaneous and deep-seated infections caused by brown-pigmented moulds that adopt a septate hyphal form in tissue (Ajello, 1975). The number of organisms implicated as etiologic agents of phaeohyphomycosis has increased from 16 in 1975 to more than 100 at the present time (Matsumoto and Ajello, 1998). Often these fungi have been given different names at different times and the use of the collective disease name has helped to reduce the confusion in the literature.

The term *hyalohyphomycosis* is another collective name that is increasing in usage. This term is used to refer to infections caused by colorless (hyaline) moulds that adopt a septate hyphal form in tissue (Ajello, 1986). To date, more than 70 different organisms have been implicated. The disease name is reserved as a general name for those infections that are caused by less common moulds, such as species of *Fusarium*, that are not the cause of otherwise-named infections, such as aspergillosis.

LABORATORY PROCEDURES FOR THE DIAGNOSIS OF FUNGAL INFECTION

As with other microbial infections, the diagnosis of fungal infection relies upon a combination of clinical observation and laboratory investigation. Superficial and subcutaneous fungal infections often produce characteristic lesions that suggest the diagnosis, but laboratory input can aid the diagnostic process where this is not the case, either because several microorganisms and/or noninfectious processes produce similar clinical pictures, or because the appearance of the lesions has been rendered atypical by previous treatment. In many situations where systemic fungal infection is entertained as a diagnosis, the clinical presentation is nonspecific and can be caused by a wide range of infections, underlying illnesses, or complications of treatment. The definitive diagnosis of these infections is based almost entirely on the results of laboratory investigation.

The successful laboratory diagnosis of fungal infection depends in major part on the collection of adequate clinical specimens for investigation. Inappropriate collection or storage of specimens can result in a missed diagnosis. Moreover, to ensure that the most appropriate laboratory tests are performed, it is essential for the clinician to indicate that a fungal infection is suspected and to provide sufficient background information. In addition to specifying the source of the specimen, the clinician should provide information on any underlying illness, recent travel or previous residence abroad, and the patient's occupation. This information will help the laboratory to anticipate which pathogens are most likely to be involved and permit the selection of the most appropriate test procedures. These differ from one mycotic disease to another, and depend on the site of infection as well as the presenting symptoms and clinical signs. Interpretation of the results of laboratory investigations can sometimes be made with confidence, but at times the findings may be helpful or even misleading.

Laboratory methods for the diagnosis of fungal infections remain based on three broad approaches: the microscopical detection of the etiologic agent in clinical material; isolation and identification of the pathogen in culture; and the detection of a serologic response to the pathogen or some other marker of its presence, such as a fungal cell constituent or metabolic product. New diagnostic procedures, based on the detection of fungal DNA in clinical material, are presently being developed, but have not yet had a significant impact in clinical laboratories. In the sections that follow, the value and limitations of current diagnostic procedures for fungal infections are reviewed.

Direct Microscopic Examination of Clinical Specimens

In many instances, the tentative or definitive diagnosis of fungal infection can be made by the direct microscopic detection of fungal elements in clinical material. Microscopic examination of skin scrapings or other superficial material can reveal a fungal organism in a matter of minutes. This examination is very helpful to guide treatment decisions, to determine whether an organism recovered later in culture is a contaminant or a pathogen, and to assist the laboratory in selecting the most appropriate culture conditions to recover organisms visualized on direct smear. Because direct microscopic examination is less sensitive than culture, the latter procedure should generally always be performed on clinical materials.

Keratinized tissues require pretreatment to dissolve the material and more readily reveal fungal elements. Skin scrapings and other dermatological specimens, sputum and other lower respiratory tract specimens, and minced tissue samples can be examined after treatment with warm 10%–20% potassium hydroxide (KOH). These samples can then be examined directly, without stain, as a wet preparation (See Color Figs. 1–1 and 1–2 in separate color insert). Alternatively, a drop of lactophenol cotton blue, methylene blue, or other

fungal stain can be mixed with the sample on the microscope slide. Another useful tool is the chemical brightener, calcofluor white, a compound that stains the fungal cell wall. The preparation is stained with calcofluor white, with or without KOH, and then read with a fluorescence microscope. The fungal elements appear brightly staining against a dark background.

India ink is useful for negative staining of cerebrospinal fluid (CSF) sediment to reveal encapsulated *Cryptococcus neoformans* cells. Gram staining can be helpful in revealing yeasts in various fluids and secretions. Both Giemsa stain and Wright's stain can be used to detect *Histoplasma capsulatum* in bone marrow preparations or blood smears. The Papanicolaou stain can be used on sputum or other respiratory tract samples to detect fungal elements.

It is necessary to appreciate that both false-positive and false-negative results do occur with direct microscopic examination. The results may vary with the quality and age of the specimen, the extent of the disease process, the nature of the tissue being examined, and the experience of the microscopist.

Histopathologic Studies

Histopathologic examination of tissue sections is one of the most reliable methods of establishing the diagnosis of subcutaneous and systemic fungal infections. However, the ease with which a fungal pathogen can be recognized in tissue is dependent not only on its abundance, but also on the distinctiveness of its appearance. Many fungi stain poorly with hematoxylin and eosin and this method alone may be insufficient to reveal fungal elements in tissue. There are a number of special stains for detecting and highlighting fungal organisms and the clinician should request these if a mycotic disease is suspected. Methenamine-silver (Grocott or Gomori) and periodic acid-Schiff staining are among the most widely used procedures for specific staining of the fungal cell wall. Mucicarmine can be used to stain the capsule of *C. neoformans*.

It should be appreciated that these staining methods, although useful at revealing the presence of fungal elements in tissue, seldom permit the precise fungal genus involved to be identified. For example, the detection of nonpigmented branching, septate hyphae is typical of *Aspergillus* infection, but it is also characteristic of a large number of less common organisms, including species of *Fusarium* and *Scedosporium*. Likewise, the detection of small, budding fungal cells seldom permits a specific diagnosis. Tissue-form cells of *H. capsulatum* and *Blastomyces dermatitidis*, for instance, can appear similar, and can be confused with nonencapsulated cells of *C. neoformans*. To overcome this problem, a number of methods have been developed on a research basis for identifying various fungal organisms specifically in tissue. Immunoperoxidase and immunofluorescent staining reagents, both monoclonal and polyclonal, are available for some fungal agents (Arrese-Estrada et al, 1990; Kaufman et al, 1997). Immunochemical staining can facilitate the identification of atypical fungal elements and the detection of small numbers of organisms. For example, an IgG1 monoclonal antibody 3H8 has been described that specifically recognizes *Candida albicans* in tissue sections using either immunofluorescent or immunohistochemical staining formats (Marcilla et al, 1999). Currently under investigation are a number of techniques that involve specific binding of DNA probes to the nucleic acid of the fungal agent either directly on the slide (in situ hybridization) or in a test tube (Lischewski et al, 1997; Zimmerman et al, 2000).

Culture

Isolation in culture will permit most pathogenic fungi to be identified. Most of these organisms are not fastidious in their nutritional requirements and will grow on the media used for bacterial isolation from clinical material. However, growth on these media can be slow and development of the spores and other structures used in fungal identification can be poor. For these reasons, most laboratories use several different culture media and incubation conditions for recovery of fungal agents. However, a variety of additional incubation conditions and media may be required for growth of particular organisms in culture. The laboratory should be made aware of the particular fungal agent(s) that are suspected in a given sample so that the most appropriate media can be included.

Most laboratories use a medium, such as the Emmons modification of Sabouraud's dextrose agar or malt agar that will recover most common fungi. However, many fastidious organisms such as yeast-phase *H. capsulatum* will not grow on these substrates, and require the use of richer media, such as brain heart infusion agar. CHROMagar Candida medium (CHROMagar Co., Paris, France) is a chromogenic agar that incorporates multiple chemical dyes in a solid medium. The medically important *Candida* species appear as different colored colonies due to differential uptake of these chromogenic compounds. After incubation for 48–72 hours *C. albicans* produces green colonies, while *C. tropicalis* produces blue colonies, *C. glabrata* produces dark pink colonies, and *C. parapsilosis* produces cream to pale pink colonies. CHROMagar can be helpful in detecting the presence of mixed cultures, as well as providing a preliminary species identification.

Many clinical specimens submitted for fungal culture are contaminated with bacteria and it is essential to add antibacterial antibiotics to fungal culture media. Media containing chloramphenicol are commercially available. However, gentamicin, vancomycin, and other antimicrobial agents are increasingly being used to suppress growth of bacteria resistant to older agents. If dermatophytes or dimorphic fungi are being isolated, cycloheximide (actidione) should be added to the medium, to prevent overgrowth by faster-growing fungi.

The optimum growth temperature for most pathogenic fungi is around 30°C. Material from patients with a suspected superficial infection should be incubated at 25°C–30°C, because most dermatophytes will not grow at higher temperatures. Material from subcutaneous or deep sites should be incubated at two temperatures, 25°C–30°C and 37°C, because a number of important pathogens, including *H. capsulatum*, *B. dermatitidis* and *Sporothrix schenckii*, are dimorphic and the change in their growth form, depending on the incubation conditions, is useful in identification. At 25°C–30°C these organisms develop as moulds on Sabouraud's dextrose agar, but at higher temperatures on an enriched medium, such as brain–heart infusion agar, these organisms grow as budding yeasts. Many pathogenic fungi grow slowly in culture and require plates to be held for up to 4 weeks, before being discarded as negative. However, some common pathogenic fungi, such as *Aspergillus fumigatus* and *C. albicans*, will produce identifiable colonies within 1 to 3 days. Cultures should be examined at frequent intervals (at least three times weekly) and appropriate subcultures made, particularly from blood-enriched media on which fungi often fail to sporulate.

It is important to appreciate that growth of an organism in culture does not necessarily establish its role as a pathogen. When organisms such as *H. capsulatum* or *Trichophyton rubrum* are isolated, the diagnosis can be established unequivocally. If, however, an opportunistic organism such as *A. fumigatus* or *C. albicans* is recovered, its isolation may have no clinical relevance unless there is additional evidence of its involvement in a pathogenic process. In these cases, culture results should be compared with those of microscopic examination. Isolation of opportunistic fungal pathogens from sterile sites, such as blood or cerebrospinal fluid, often provides reliable evidence of deep-seated infection, but their isolation from material such as pus, sputum or urine must be interpreted with care. Attention should be paid to the amount of fungus isolated and further investigations undertaken.

Many unfamiliar moulds have been reported as occasional causes of lethal systemic infection in immunocompromised patients. No isolate should be dismissed as a contaminant without careful consideration of the clinical condition of the patient, the site of isolation, the method of specimen collection, and the likelihood of contamination. It is, however, notable that, in a recent study only 24% of 135 unusual moulds isolated from sterile body sites were shown to be responsible for significant clinical disease (Rees et al, 1998). In another recent report, only 245 of 1209 isolates of *Aspergillus* species collected from hospitalized patients represented cases of clinical aspergillosis (Perfect et al, 2001). In addition to demonstrating that not every fungal isolate represents a pathogen, these studies also make a case that laboratories should investigate the clinical significance of fungal isolates before indiscriminately identifying to species level every isolate that is recovered from a patient sample.

Although culture often permits the definitive diagnosis of a fungal infection, it has some important limitations. In particular, the failure to recover an organism does not rule out the diagnosis, as a negative culture may be due to inadequate specimen collection or improper or delayed transport of specimens. Incorrect isolation procedures and inadequate periods of incubation are other important factors.

Blood Culture

In general, *Candida* species are more readily recovered from blood than are dimorphic fungi and moulds. Isolation rates are higher when the medium is vented and aerated, and biphasic media incorporating both agar and broth phases are more effective than broth. The chances of successful isolation are increased if multiple samples of blood are collected, and larger volumes are cultured. The lysis-centrifugation method (Isolator, Wampole Laboratories, Cranbury, NJ) is currently the most reliable procedure for isolation of fungi from blood, but it is more labor-intensive than other methods, precluding its routine use in some laboratories. With this procedure, 10 milliliters of blood are collected into a tube that contains chemicals that lyse blood cells and inactivate antimicrobial substances present in blood. The tube is centrifuged and the sediment is then inoculated onto appropriate culture media. With this method, fungi are recovered at a higher rate and much faster than with other blood culture methods (Elder and Roberts, 1986). Recent improvements in the formulation of blood culture media, together with the development of improved automated blood culture systems, have made the recovery of *Candida* species from blood culture bottles almost as effective as that from lysis centrifugation tubes (Wilson et al, 1993). However, lysis centrifugation remains superior to other systems for recovery of *C. neoformans*, dimorphic fungi and moulds (Reimer et al, 1997).

Fungal Identification

Most fungi can be identified after growth in culture. Classical phenotypic identification methods for moulds are based on a combination of macroscopic and microscopic morphologic characteristics. Macroscopic characteristics, such as colonial form, surface color and pigmentation, are often helpful in mould identification, but it is essential to examine slide preparations of the culture under a microscope. If well prepared these will often give sufficient information on the form and arrangement of the spores and spore-bearing structures to allow identification of the fungus. Because identification is usually dependent on visualization of the particular structures an organism produces when it is sporulating, identification is usually dependent on the ability of the organism to sporulate (See Color Figs. 1–3 and 1–4 in separate color insert). For "difficult" organisms, much laboratory time is spent attempting to induce sporulation on various media so that these structures can be studied. Moulds often grow best on rich media, such as Sabouraud's dextrose agar, but overproduction of mycelium often results in loss of sporulation. If a mould isolate fails to produce spores or other recognizable structures after two weeks, it should be subcultured to a less-rich medium to encourage sporulation. Media such as cornmeal, oatmeal, and potato-sucrose agars can be used for this purpose. The use of DNA-based identification methods may eliminate this requirement in future.

With some moulds, such as species of *Aspergillus*, the characteristic spore-bearing structures can be easily identified after a small portion of the growth is removed from the culture plate, mounted in a suitable stain (such as lactofuchsin) on a microscope slide and examined. However, it is sometimes essential to prepare a slide culture in order to identify an isolate. In this technique, a thin square block of a suitable agar is placed on a sterile microscope slide, inoculated with a small amount of the fungal culture, covered with a sterile cover slip, and incubated for up to 2 weeks. The cover slip and agar block are then removed, mounting fluid is added, and a clean cover slip applied to the slide. The fungal growth on the slide is then examined for the presence of spores and other characteristic structures.

Historically, dimorphic fungi such as *Coccidioides immitis*, *H. capsulatum*, and *B. dermatitidis* were identified by observing the conversion of mycelial growth at 25°C to yeast-like growth at 37°C. However, development of DNA probe-based tests (Accuprobe, Gen-Probe Inc., San Diego, CA) has enabled these pathogens to be identified using only a small amount of mycelial material.

Yeasts are usually identified on the basis of their morphologic and biochemical characteristics. Useful morphologic characteristics include the color of the colonies, the size and shape of the cells, the presence of a capsule around the cells, the production of hyphae or pseudohyphae, and the production of chlamydospores. Useful biochemical tests include the assimilation and fermentation of sugars, and the assimilation of nitrate and urea. Most yeasts associated with human infections can be identified using one of the numerous commercial identification systems, such as API 20C AUX (bioMerieux-Vitek Inc., Hazelwood, MO), that are based on the differential assimilation of various carbon compounds. However, it is important to remember that morphologic examination of Dalmau plate cultures on cornmeal agar is essential to avoid confusion between organisms with identical biochemical profiles. A number of simple rapid tests have been devised for the presumptive identification of some of the most important human pathogens. Foremost among these is the serum germ tube test for *C. albicans*, which can be performed in less than 3 hours, and the urease test for *C. neoformans*. In recent years a number of rapid commercial tests have been developed. These include the RapID Yeast Plus system (Innovative Diagnostic Systems, Norcross, GA) that contains conventional and chromogenic substrates and requires 4 hours to perform. Most of these rapid test systems are more accurate in the identification of the common rather than unusual yeast pathogens (Espinel-Ingroff et al, 1998).

Molecular Methods for Identification of Fungi

The use of molecular methods to identify organisms relies on the assumption that strains belonging to the same species will demonstrate less genetic variation than organisms that are less closely related. Identification of unknown fungal isolates can be made by comparing a partial DNA sequence of that organism with sequences in a central database such as GenBank, operated by the National Library of Medicine [www.ncbi.nlm.nih.gov/BLAST], or European Molecular Biology Laboratory (EMBL). The preparation of high molecular weight DNA and determination of the sequence of a DNA fragment have become much easier in recent years with the advent of commercial kits and the utilization of the polymerase chain reaction (PCR) in sequencing. Refinements in the GenBank Internet website interface have also made it faster and easier for users to conduct searches and to deposit novel DNA sequences.

Two of the regions of DNA more commonly used in fungal identification are portions of ribosomal DNA, such as the intervening transcribed spacers (ITS) region located between the small and large ribosomal subunits, and the D1/D2 region of the large (26S) ribosomal subunit. These regions contain sufficient sequence heterogeneity to provide differences at the species level. In general, strains of the same species have fewer than 1% nucleotide substitutions in the region of interest, whereas strains that are separate species have more than this number of substitutions (Kurtzman, 1994; Valente et al, 1999). DNA sequencing offers a method for identifying organisms that fail to sporulate or are otherwise refractory to conventional identification methods. The reliability of the molecular identification is, of course, related to the reliability of the database with which comparisons are made. An extensive GenBank database of large ribosomal subunit sequences exists for ascomycetous and basidiomycetous yeasts, as well as for black yeasts (Kurtzman and Robnett, 1998; Fell et al, 2000). Many ITS sequencing studies are also contributing to an expansion of the GenBank database (Chen et al, 2000; Chen et al, 2001).

The last decade has seen a massive expansion of research into the phylogenetics of pathogenic fungi (Guarro et al, 1999). Analysis of aligned ribosomal, mitochondrial, and other nuclear DNA sequences has been used to determine degrees of genetic relatedness among many groups of fungi. One outcome of this work has been the demonstration of close genetic relationships between several anamorphic (asexual) fungi and organisms with teleomorphs (sexual stages) that belong to the Ascomycota or Basidiomycota (Gené et al, 1996). Phylogenetics research has led to the deposition in international databases of large numbers of DNA sequences for many groups of fungi, both pathogenic and saprophytic. The availability of this sequence information and increased understanding of phylogenetic relatedness have proven enormously helpful in the development of DNA-based diagnostics for fungal infections.

At this time the GenProbe system is the only commercial nucleic acid-based test for fungal identification approved for diagnostic use in the United States. However, many new systems are being developed and validated for rapid DNA-based identification of pathogenic fungi. One of the earliest methods was the restriction fragment length polymorphism (RFLP) procedure. In RFLP, fungal DNA is digested with a restriction enzyme, which cuts the DNA at prescribed regions to generate a family of fragments. These fragments are separated on an agarose gel and stained with ethidium bromide to reveal their relative sizes. Identification of various *Candida* species has been reported based on the analysis of RFLPs within the ribosomal DNA repeat (genes encoding rRNA) of these species (Scherer and Stevens, 1987). Members of the same species shared common fragments, or common RFLP patterns, where members of different species showed fragments of different sizes. The sensitivity of this method has been improved by reacting the DNA fragments with specific isotopically or chemically labeled DNA probes in Southern blots that reveal patterns, or DNA fingerprints, for that organism (Riggsby, 1989).

Newer and more commonly used methods of species identification have exploited the enormous resolving power of PCR. With PCR, as little as a few picograms of input DNA can be amplified so that, after 30–40 cycles, the resulting product can be easily visualized on an agarose gel. Furthermore, amplification occurs in a specific manner that is determined by the temperature selected for the primer annealing step and by the sequence of the complementary primers. These are short DNA segments that initiate the PCR elongation step upon binding (annealing) to the input DNA. Current methods utilize the PCR primed with short oligonucleotides that will amplify only DNA of a particular genus or species, generating a species-specific DNA product or family of products. These assays have been shown to distinguish between related species of filamentous fungi and yeasts (Niesters et al, 1993; Sandhu et al, 1995; Thanos et al, 1996; Mannarelli and Kurtzmann, 1998).

The sensitivity and specificity of these assays has been improved by performing nested PCR. In this technique a DNA product of broad specificity (for example, the ITS region) is amplified in the first round, and then this product is reacted with species-specific internal primers in a second round of PCR (Zhao et al, 2001). The product that is generated after the second round is specific for the intended target from the species of interest only. In another method, PCR with arbitrary primers has proven useful for species identification of fungal isolates. This technique of randomly amplified polymorphic DNA (RAPD) analysis was developed in 1990 (Williams et al, 1990; Welsh and McClelland, 1991). This procedure uses random ten-mer oligonucleotide primers to amplify DNA. The advantage of this method is that no prior knowledge of the genome or DNA sequences of interest is required. Species-specific patterns and/or fragments can be demonstrated using appropriate primer sets (Berg et al, 1994). Microsatellite primers have also been used to generate species-specific fingerprints for 26 species of *Candida* and eight other fungal species (Thanos et al, 1996). Oligonucleotide primers that are complementary to intron splice sites have been used to show polymorphisms between isolates of different species (de Barros Lopes et al, 1998). More recently, fluorescence capillary electrophoresis has been used to speciate pathogenic yeasts by measuring size differences (length polymorphisms) within amplified ITS 1 and ITS 2 regions. A PCR is used to amplify products from these regions, where two species can differ by only 1–2 nucleotides in the length of the sequence. These length differences can be distinguished with great precision using capillary electrophoresis, thus using the length of the ITS regions to discriminate among isolates of different species (Chen et al, 2000; Chen et al, 2001).

Differences in the electrophoretic karyotype, the pattern of migration shown by chromosomes placed in an electric field, have also been used to some extent to distinguish different species of yeasts (Magee and Magee, 1987). However, this technique requires considerable technical expertise and has not been widely used as a primary means of fungal speciation.

Other systems have utilized binding of a specific DNA probe to a complementary sequence within the DNA or RNA of the organism of interest. In these approaches differences in the DNA sequence of different species (sequence polymorphisms) are exploited, rather than differences in sizes or patterns of DNA fragments. A universal DNA target, such as the ITS region, is amplified and then that target molecule is reacted with a number of species-specific probes until specific binding is achieved. Specific binding of a particular probe enables an unknown DNA sample to be identified as that species. Earlier generations of probes were labeled with peroxidase or phosphatase, and specific binding was demonstrated by a color change that could be observed visually [PCR-EIA] (Fujita et al, 1995; Elie et al, 1998). Other studies have used slot blot hybridization, line-probe assays, or single-strand conformational polymorphism (SSCP) gels to detect specific binding of probes to DNA targets (Hui et al, 2000; Loeffler et al, 2000a; Martin et al, 2000). Newer generations of probes use fluorescent labels, where complementary binding leads to a release of energy that can be detected by laser-containing instruments such as TaqMan (Perkin-Elmer Applied Biosystems Inc., Foster City, CA) (Brandt et al, 1998; Guiver et al, 2001) or Light Cycler (Roche Molecular Biochemicals Inc., Indianapolis, IN) (Loeffler et al, 2000b). At this time, the newest tools are microarrays, where many thousands of probe-to-target sequence binding reactions can be performed on the surface of a microchip and then be rapidly detected and analyzed by computer (Lucchini et al, 2001).

Many techniques have been described in the literature for the DNA-based identification of fungal cultures. In general, these procedures have not been validated using large representative populations of the species of interest. Furthermore, most of these methods are not commercially available and require expertise usually found only in research laboratories. Their interlaboratory reproducibility is also generally unknown. With continued use of these tools will come more knowledge about them and better understanding of their role in the mycology laboratory. However, it is important to note that, as has been stated earlier, many fungal isolates recovered from clinical samples do not represent significant disease. Hence, it is wasteful to devote resources to the molecular identification of fungal isolates without a corresponding understanding of their clinical relevance. The identification of fungal pathogens requires input from both the clinician and the laboratorian for the diagnostic process to be successful and productive.

Molecular Subtyping of Fungi

Molecular subtyping is the process of assessing the genetic relatedness of a group of isolates of the same species. Molecular subtyping may be performed in the context of an epidemiologic investigation where particular isolates are being assessed as the potential source of an outbreak. In a broader sense, molecular subtyping data can also be used to determine the relationship between colonization and infection, to trace the emergence of drug-resistant strains in a population, or to address questions regarding the role of relapse versus reinfection in recurrent disease. In a global sense, molecular subtyping data can be used to trace the spread of virulent clones throughout a particular geographic region, or around the world.

Various methods can be used for subtyping of fungi. In general, phenotype-based methods have proved irreproducible and are no longer used for this purpose. Furthermore, *C. albicans* and related species have been shown to undergo high-frequency switching among a number of phenotypes, thus altering a number of phenotypic traits with each activation-deactivation of the switch phenotype (Soll, 1992).

Strain typing methods for pathogenic fungi are now based on procedures that measure genetic relatedness. To be successful, DNA fingerprinting methods should meet several criteria: they should not be affected by changes in the environment, and they should provide, insofar as this is possible, an effective measure of genetic distance between any two isolates in the population. In addition, typing methods should assess DNA sequences that are fairly stable over time, i.e., do not undergo recombination, gene exchange, or genomic switching events at high frequencies. The ability to store data electronically and to retrieve data rapidly is also helpful as it enables results of different studies to be compared over time (Soll, 2000).

In interpreting subtyping data, it is important to understand that every genome contains segments that evolve at different rates. Thus, it is important to assess the resolution of the subtyping probe, i.e., which "speed" of the molecular clock is being measured by the chosen probe. It is also important to decide the epidemiologic question being asked prior to choosing molecular subtyping probes, important because different probes may be more or less useful for different circumstances. For example, a study examining serial patient isolates collected over a period of years may require a distinction to be made between bands that change as a result of microevolution (undergo recombination at extremely high frequency) and bands that change less rapidly. Thus when any two isolates are examined, it can be determined whether band changes are due to microevolution within a single isolate, or due to the appearance of a second unrelated fungal strain. The ideal subtyping probe for this type of study may be different from that chosen for an analysis of a hospital outbreak, where isolates collected at one point in time are to be studied.

Multilocus enzyme electrophoresis (MEE) has been used to assess cellular isoenzymes or allozymes. A cell extract is electrophoresed through a nondenaturing gel and then replicate gel slices are stained with specific substrates to detect enzyme activity. The enzyme activities are directly related to the alleles of the genes coding for these enzymes, so that by comparing allelic differences within a series of isolates their genetic relatedness can be directly assessed. Multilocus enzyme electrophoresis detects enzymes in both haploid (one band of enzymatic activity) and diploid (one or two bands) organisms. If enough enzymes are assessed, MEE is extremely useful in developing genetic similarity data for a group of organisms. However, MEE is time-consuming and requires a high level of technical expertise.

Restriction fragment length polymorphism analysis, as described earlier, was one of the earliest methods used to assess genetic relatedness among fungal isolates. For DNA fingerprinting, the classical RFLP method suffers from a lack of sensitivity. Generally, only bands of high staining intensity can be resolved, and these bands do not provide sufficient information to resolve a series of isolates. Sensitivity may be improved by transferring the DNA to a membrane and hybridizing with a labeled DNA probe. The resolution of single-copy probes, which generate one or two bands per sample, is usually not sufficient for most epidemiologic studies. When mitochondrial or ribosomal DNA probes are used, the pattern can vary sufficiently to distinguish among unrelated strains of fungi. However, these methods have not been used in broad epidemiologic studies of pathogenic fungi.

One of the most commonly used probes has been the repetitive element or complex probe, which is a DNA fragment containing sequences that are dispersed throughout the genome of the organism. Repetitive element probes, which have been described for *A. fumigatus, C. albicans, C. glabrata, C. parapsilosis, C. tropicalis,* and *C. dubliniensis* (Soll, 2000), are useful because they provide fingerprints of sufficient complexity so that genetic variability can be analyzed at multiple levels. These fingerprint patterns contain bands that arise as a result of microevolution (most variable), as well as bands of moderate variability, and low or no variability. Repeat sequences have also been used to develop probes for *C. neoformans* (Spitzer and Spitzer, 1992) and *A. flavus* (Monod et al, 1990).

Microsatellite regions of the genome have been used as fingerprinting probes. In this approach, Southern blots are probed with poly (G-T), $(CT)_8$, or other repeat sequences (Meyer et al, 1993; Metzgar et al, 1998). Molecular subtyping has also been performed by analysis of minisatellite, microsatellite, and nuclear gene polymorphic markers determined by direct sequencing of amplified target sequences (Lott and Effat, 2001).

Another popular method for DNA fingerprinting is RAPD analysis, also described earlier. Randomly amplified polymorphic DNA has been used in DNA fingerprinting of many organisms including *C. albicans*, *C. glabrata*, *C. parapsilosis*, *C. tropicalis*, *C. lusitaniae*, *A. fumigatus*, *A. flavus*, *C. neoformans*, *B. dermatitidis*, and *H. capsulatum* (Soll, 2000). One reason for the popularity of the RAPD is that no prior information about the genome of the organism is required. However, a number of problems have been identified in obtaining intra- and interlaboratory reproducibility of this method (Meunier and Grimont, 1993).

Electrophoretic karyotyping has also been used for DNA fingerprinting analysis. Karyotyping has been used to fingerprint a number of *Candida* species, as well as *C. neoformans*, *A. nidulans*, *H. capsulatum*, and *C. immitis* (Soll, 2000). Karyotyping appears to be able to discriminate among unrelated strains. However, the phenomenon of high-frequency switching in *C. albicans* may make karyotyping unsuitable for studying moderately related isolates.

Serologic Testing

Serologic testing often provides the most rapid means of diagnosing a fungal infection. The majority of tests are based on the detection of antibodies to specific fungal pathogens, although tests for fungal antigens are now becoming more widely available. At their best, individual serologic tests can be diagnostic, e.g., tests for antigenemia in cryptococcosis and histoplasmosis. In general, however, the results of serologic testing are seldom more than suggestive or supportive of a fungal diagnosis. These tests must be interpreted with caution and considered alongside the results of other clinical and laboratory investigations.

Tests for antibodies have proved useful in diagnosing endemic fungal diseases, such as histoplasmosis and coccidioidomycosis, in immunocompetent persons. In these individuals, the interval between exposure and the development of symptoms (2–6 weeks) is usually sufficient for a humoral response to develop. Tests for fungal antibodies are most helpful when paired serum specimens (acute and convalescent) are obtained, so that it can be determined whether titers are rising or falling.

Tests for detection of antibodies are much less useful in immunocompromised persons, many of whom are incapable of mounting a detectable humoral response to infection.

In this situation, tests for detecting fungal antigens can be helpful. Antigen detection is an established procedure for the diagnosis of cryptococcosis and histoplasmosis, and similar tests are currently being evaluated for aspergillosis and candidiasis. Antigen detection methods are complicated by several important factors. First, antigen is often released in minute amounts from fungal cells necessitating the use of highly sensitive test procedures to detect low amounts of circulating antigen in serum. Second, fungal antigen is often cleared very rapidly from the circulation necessitating frequent collection of samples (Jones, 1980). Third, antigen is often bound to circulating IgG, even in immunocompromised individuals, and therefore steps must be taken to dissociate these complexes before antigen can be detected (Reiss et al, 1982).

Numerous methods are available for the detection of antibodies in persons with fungal diseases. Immunodiffusion (ID) is a simple, specific and inexpensive method, but is insensitive, thereby reducing its usefulness as a screening test. Complement fixation (CF) is more sensitive, but more difficult to perform and interpret than ID. However, CF remains an important test for a number of fungal diseases, including histoplasmosis and coccidioidomycosis. Latex agglutination (LA) is a simple, but insensitive method that can be used for detection of antibodies or antigens, and has proved most useful for detection of the polysaccharide capsular antigens of *C. neoformans* that are released in large amounts in most patients with cryptococcosis. More sensitive procedures, such as radioimmunoassay (RIA) and enzyme-linked immunosorbent assay (ELISA) have also been developed and evaluated for the diagnosis of a number of fungal diseases.

Serologic testing is a valuable adjunct to the diagnosis of histoplasmosis. At this time the CF and ID tests are the principal methods used to detect antibodies in individuals with this disease (Wheat, 2001; Reiss et al, 2002). The CF test is more sensitive, but less specific than ID. Approximately 95% of patients with histoplasmosis are positive by CF, but 25% of these are positive only at titers of 1:8 or 1:16. CF titers of at least 1:32 or rising titers in serial samples are considered to be strong presumptive evidence of infection. Because low titers of CF antibodies can persist for years following acute histoplasmosis, and because cross-reactions can occur in patients with other fungal infections, care must be taken to exclude these diseases if the clinical signs and symptoms are not typical of histoplasmosis. The ID test is more specific, but less sensitive than CF and can be used to assess the significance of weakly positive CF results. Using histoplasmin as antigen, two major precipitin bands can be detected with the ID test. The M band can be detected in up to 75% of patients with acute histoplasmosis, but may also be found in nearly all individuals with a past infection, as well as in those who have undergone a recent skin test with histoplasmin. The H band is specific for active disease, but only occurs in 10%–20% of proven cases. Attempts to improve the serologic diagnosis of histoplasmosis by replacing the CF test with more sensitive procedures, such as RIA or ELISA, have largely proved unsuccessful, due to the presence of cross-reactive moieties associated with the H and M antigens.

Antigen detection has proved a useful method for the rapid diagnosis of histoplasmosis in patients presenting with acute disease, as well as in those with disseminated infection. In acute disease, antigen can be detected within the first month after exposure before antibodies appear. Several test formats have been developed including a solid-phase RIA (Wheat et al, 1986) and a sandwich ELISA (Durkin et al, 1997). Histoplasma polysaccharide antigen has been detected in serum, urine, CSF, and bronchoalveolar lavage fluid. The test has proved particularly successful in detecting antigen in urine from HIV-infected individuals with disseminated histoplasmosis. Antigen usually disappears with effective treatment, and its reappearance can be used to diagnose relapse (Wheat, 2001).

Serologic testing is also invaluable in the diagnosis and management of patients with coccidioidomycosis. The immunodiffusion tube precipitin (IDTP) test, using heated coccidioidin as antigen, detects IgM antibodies to C. immitis and is most useful for diagnosing recent infection. These antibodies can be found within 1–3 weeks after the onset of symptoms, but disappear within a few months of self-limited disease (Pappagianis and Zimmer, 1990). The sensitivity of the IDTP test is improved by concentration of serum prior to performing the test. A LA test is also available for the detection of IgM antibodies. This test is faster to perform and more sensitive than the IDTP test. However, LA has a false-positive rate of at least 5% (Huppert et al, 1968) and the results should be confirmed using the ID method.

The CF test measures IgG antibodies against C. immitis (Pappagiannis and Zimmer, 1990). These antibodies do not appear until 4–12 weeks after infection, but may persist for long periods in patients with chronic pulmonary or disseminated disease, thus providing useful diagnostic information. Low CF titers of 1:2 to 1:8 are commonly found in individuals without coccidioidomycosis, but high or rising titers of CF antibodies are consistent with spread of disease beyond the respiratory tract. More than 60% of patients with dis-

seminated coccidioidomycosis have CF titers of >1:32. However, titer alone should not be used as the basis for diagnosis of dissemination, but should be considered alongside the results of other clinical and laboratory investigations.

A commercial ELISA test is available for measurement of IgM and IgG antibodies to C. immitis (Premier EIA, Meridian Diagnostics, Cincinnati, OH). Published evaluations suggest this test has acceptable sensitivity and specificity (Kaufman et al, 1995; Martins et al, 1995).

Tests for Aspergillus antibodies have been extensively evaluated for the rapid diagnosis of invasive aspergillosis, but their role remains uncertain. Tests for detection of antibodies include ID, indirect hemagglutination, and ELISA. The ID test is simple to perform and has proved valuable for the diagnosis of aspergilloma and allergic bronchopulmonary aspergillosis in immunocompetent individuals (Reiss et al, 2002). Tests for Aspergillus antibodies have, however, seldom been helpful in diagnosis of invasive or disseminated infection in immunocompromised patients.

Tests for the detection of Aspergillus antigens in blood and other body fluids offer a rapid means of diagnosing aspergillosis in these individuals. Low concentrations of galactomannan, a major cell wall component of Aspergillus species, have been detected in serum, urine and bronchoalveolar lavage fluid from infected patients. However, galactomannan is rapidly cleared from the blood and tests for its detection are helpful in management only if performed on a regular basis.

Two tests to detect circulating Aspergillus galactomannan antigen are commercially available in a number of countries. Both utilize the same monoclonal, EB-A2, in either an LA or sandwich ELISA format. The LA test was the first to be developed (Pastorex Aspergillus, Sanofi Diagnostics Pasteur, Paris, France) but, despite its ease of use, it is relatively insensitive (Verweij et al, 1995a). The sandwich ELISA (Platelia Aspergillus, Sanofi Diagnostics Pasteur) is more sensitive than the LA test and can detect galactomannan in serum at an earlier stage of infection (Verweij et al, 1995b; Sulahian et al, 1996; Maertens et al, 1999).

Tests for Candida antibodies have been extensively evaluated but remain of limited usefulness in the diagnosis of invasive forms of candidiasis. These tests are complicated by false-positive results in patients with mucosal colonization or superficial infection, and by false-negative results in immunocompromised individuals (Buckley et al, 1992; De Repentigny et al, 1994). In an attempt to reduce false-positive results, efforts have been made to identify antigens of Candida species which are associated with invasive infection rather than colonization (Ponton et al, 2002). However, despite the numerous methods and reagents which have been devised for *Candida* antibody detection, none of them has found widespread clinical use.

Antigen detection tests have also been extensively evaluated for the rapid diagnosis of invasive forms of candidiasis. Numerous circulating antigens have been studied as potential targets, including mannan (a heat-stable cell wall component), enolase, proteinase, and other immunodominant cytoplasmic antigens (Ponton et al, 2002). Test formats that have been investigated include LA, ELISA, and dot immunoassay. Several LA tests are commercially available for detection of mannan (LA-Candida Antigen Detection System, Immuno-Mycologics, Norman, OK; Pastorex Candida, Sanofi Diagnostics Pasteur), but these have been found to be relatively insensitive (Herent et al, 1992; Mitsutake et al, 1996).

The CAND-TEC test (Ramco Laboratories Inc., Houston, TX) is based on the work of Gentry et al (1983) who developed a LA test using serum from rabbits immunized with whole, heat-killed *C. albicans* cells to detect an uncharacterized heat-sensitive antigen of *C. albicans*. The antigen does not contain mannan and it has been suggested that the test may detect a neo-antigen derived from *C. albicans* after host processing, or it may be a host component that is cross-reactive with an antigen of *C. albicans* (Jones, 1990). Although there is an extensive literature on the CAND-TEC test (Ponton et al, 2002), there is no consensus about its value in the diagnosis of invasive candidiasis because of the highly variable results reported in different studies. In general, recent evaluations have concluded that, despite its ease of performance, the test is not acceptable for diagnostic use.

The LA test for *C. neoformans* polysaccharide antigen in serum and CSF is invaluable in the diagnosis of meningeal and disseminated forms of cryptococcosis (Reiss et al, 2002). The test is sensitive and specific, giving positive results with CSF specimens from well over 90% of infected patients. In general, CSF and serum antigen titers are higher in persons with acquired immunodeficiency syndrome (AIDS) than in other immunocompromised individuals. In the CSF, high or rising titers in general indicate progression of infection, while falling titers indicate regression of disease and response to treatment. Changes in serum titers are less indicative of disease activity and response to therapy. Occasional false-positive results have been caused by infection with other organisms, such as *Trichosporon asahii* (*T. beigelii*), that share cross-reacting antigens with *C. neoformans* (McManus and Jones, 1985), or by nonspecific interference from rheumatoid factor, which can be eliminated by prior treatment of the sample with pronase (Stockman and Roberts, 1983). False-

negative results can occur if the organism load is low, or if the organisms are not well encapsulated. False-negative results have also been reported with the LA test owing to a prozone effect, but this can be corrected by dilution of the sample (Stamm and Polt, 1980).

In general, tests for antibodies to *C. neoformans* are of little diagnostic usefulness. Antibodies may be detected during the early stages of cryptococcosis or in patients with localized infection, but they are rapidly eliminated by the large amounts of capsular antigen released during evolution of the infection. Antibodies may subsequently reappear after successful treatment.

Molecular Diagnostics
At this time, no DNA-based tests are commercially available for the detection of fungal agents in clinical samples. Many assays have been developed and are currently being evaluated in individual research laboratories. Methods have been described for the detection of fungal DNA in blood, CSF, respiratory tract fluids, ocular materials, and dermatologic samples. Most molecular diagnostic assays are PCR-based, to take advantage of the increase in sensitivity offered by the many-fold amplification of PCR targets as well as the specificity offered by appropriate primer/probe design. Either nested or panfungal PCR formats have generally been used. Nested PCR has been described earlier. In panfungal PCR, amplification with generic fungal primers (usually targeting ribosomal DNA) generates a product that is then hybridized with various short species-specific DNA probes until a positive reaction is achieved. Quantitative real-time PCR with the TaqMan system has also been used in the diagnosis of invasive pulmonary aspergillosis (Kami et al, 2001).

One of the most active areas of current research is in the development of assays to detect and identify *Aspergillus* and *Candida* species in blood. In general, these tests are designed to facilitate prospective monitoring of immunosuppressed patients at risk for difficult-to-diagnose fungal diseases, particularly invasive pulmonary or disseminated aspergillosis and hepatosplenic (chronic disseminated) candidiasis. Investigators described a PCR designed to amplify a fungal-specific 18S ribosomal sequence and then to identify the fungal pathogen using species-specific hybridization (Einsele et al, 1997). In a later report, these same investigators showed that, in neutropenic patients, a panfungal PCR, performed prospectively once weekly on a blood sample, enabled identification of patients at high risk for invasive fungal infections (Hebart et al, 2000). More recently, the same group described a nucleic acid sequence-based amplification (NASBA) assay for the detection and identification of *Aspergillus* species in blood (Loeffler et al, 2001). In this protocol, *Aspergillus* genus-specific RNA sequences are specifically amplified by using T7 RNA polymerase. Results could be obtained within 6 hours with a detection limit of 1 colony forming unit (CFU). Other authors have described the detection of *Fusarium* species DNA in spiked human blood samples (Hue et al, 1999).

A two-step PCR has been used to detect *Aspergillus* species DNA in bronchoalveolar lavage samples (Skladny et al, 1999; Buchheidt et al, 2002). *Aspergillus* DNA was detected 4 days prior to culture in a patient with *A. fumigatus* meningitis (Verweij et al, 1999). A panfungal PCR was used to diagnose disseminated zygomycosis using a blood sample from a patient infected with *Cunninghamella bertholletiae* (Rickerts et al, 2001). In this case the causative agent was identified by a positive hybridization of the amplicon with a probe detecting several different *Cunninghamella* species.

Several reports have described the use of PCR to detect fungal agents in corneal tissue, vitreous fluids, and other ocular samples (Okhravi et al, 2000). In one representative study, nested PCR was used for detection and identification of *A. fumigatus*, *C. albicans*, and *Fusarium solani* (Jaeger et al, 2000). The authors noted that one patient sample was PCR-positive but culture-negative, suggesting that molecular testing may permit a diagnosis to be made even when organisms cannot be grown from the sample.

Using a panfungal PCR that was designed for the detection and identification of fungal DNA in deep tissue specimens, DNA from any of eight organisms (*A. flavus*, *A. fumigatus*, *C. albicans*, *C. krusei*, *C. glabrata*, *C. parapsilosis*, *C. tropicalis*, and *C. neoformans*) could be detected in 20 tissue samples (Hendolin et al, 2000). In addition, a nested PCR has been described that detects DNA from *Trichophyton* and *Microsporum* species in dermatologic samples (Turin et al, 2000). DNA could be detected even in the presence of bacterial contamination. DNA from various *Malassezia* species has been detected in dressings applied to skin lesions of affected patients (Sugita et al, 2001).

Molecular diagnostics offer great hope for the rapid detection and identification of difficult-to-culture organisms, for detection of antifungal drug resistance, and for rapid diagnosis directly from host tissues and fluids. At this time, many research laboratories offer in-house procedures for molecular identification of fungal isolates from culture plates, from tissue, or from body fluids. Their sensitivity, specificity, predictive value, and clinical relevance have not always been rigorously investigated. Hopefully, in the future the relevance of these assays will be demonstrated and these assays will become available to a much broader group of clinical microbiology laboratories.

Antifungal Drug Susceptibility Testing

As with antibacterial compounds, tests designed to ascertain the minimum amount of drug needed to inhibit the growth of fungal isolates in culture (minimum inhibitory concentration or MIC) are often assumed to be the most dependable means of determining the relative effectiveness of different antifungal agents, and of detecting the development of drug-resistant strains. In addition, it is often assumed that the clinical outcome of treatment can be predicted from the results of in vitro testing of a patient's isolate against a panel of potentially useful agents. Such an approach to the selection of antifungal agents has become more reasonable with the development of a reliable and reproducible reference procedure for in vitro testing of *Candida* species against azole antifungal agents (particularly fluconazole) and the demonstration of correlations with clinical outcome for some forms of candidiasis. However, the pitfalls of assuming a correlation between the results of susceptibility testing of other antifungal drugs and organisms in vitro and outcome in vivo should not be underestimated. Nevertheless, with drug resistance demonstrated among such diverse fungi as *A. fumigatus*, *A. terreus*, *C. neoformans*, *H. capsulatum*, and *S. apiospermum* (Walsh et al, 1995; Denning et al, 1997b; Wheat et al, 1997; Perfect and Cox, 1999; Sutton et al, 1999; Walsh et al, 1995; Wheat et al, 1997), clearly the need for meaningful methods of in vitro testing of both new and established agents is increasing.

In 1997, the National Committee for Clinical Laboratory Standards (NCCLS) published an approved reference method (document M27-A) for the in vitro testing of five antifungal agents (amphotericin B, flucytosine, fluconazole, itraconazole, and ketoconazole) against *Candida* species and *C. neoformans* (National Committee for Clinical Laboratory Standards, 1997). Although imperfect, the method is a reproducible procedure that has facilitated the establishment of interpretive breakpoints for *Candida* species and fluconazole and itraconazole. The M27-A document describes a broth macrodilution method and its microdilution modifications. The latter has become the method of choice because of its less cumbersome nature. The M27-A document specifies a defined test medium (RPMI-1640 broth buffered to pH 7.0 with MOPS), as well as an inoculum standardized by spectrophotometric reading to approximately 1000 cells per ml, and visual determination of the MIC endpoint after incubation at 35°C for 48 hours (*Candida* species) or 72 hours (*C. neoformans*).

The M27-A method continues to be augmented and a second edition of the document (M27-A2) has been published (National Committee for Clinical Laboratory Standards, 2002a). The original document provides quality control (QC) limits at 48 hours for amphotericin B, flucytosine, fluconazole, itraconazole and ketoconazole. These QC data have now been expanded to include 24-hour QC limits for these agents (Barry et al, 2000). In addition, QC limits at 24 and 48 hours have been provided for anidulafungin, caspofungin, posaconazole, ravuconazole, and voriconazole (Barry et al, 2000). However, and as subsequently discussed, interpretive breakpoints have been established for fluconazole, itraconazole, and flucytosine against *Candida* species only after 48 hours of incubation.

Although the M27-A reference method has permitted much greater standardization of the in vitro testing of antifungal agents, several problems remain unresolved. These include the poor performance of the recommended culture medium in tests with some organisms and with amphotericin B, the method of endpoint determination, and the proper interpretation of trailing growth in tests with azole agents.

The defined culture medium described in the NCCLS reference procedure (RPMI-1640 broth buffered to pH 7.0 with MOPS) has proved less than ideal for the testing of some *Candida* species and *C. neoformans*; thus, it is not surprising that papers documenting potentially useful modifications have appeared. Increasing the glucose concentration of the medium from 0.2% to 2% results in better growth of most isolates of *Candida* species, making the visual determination of endpoints easier without significantly altering the observed MICs of amphotericin B, flucytosine, fluconazole, or ketoconazole (Cuenca-Estrella et al, 2001; Rodriguez-Tudela and Martinez-Suarez, 1995). Another modification that appears to be helpful is the use of yeast nitrogen base medium in tests with *C. neoformans* (Sanati et al, 1996).

It has become evident that the use of the M27-A method to test *Candida* spp. against amphotericin B results in a restricted range of MICs. Given these results, there has been concern that the reference procedure might not detect resistance to amphotericin B. The difference in amphotericin B MICs between susceptible and resistant strains is more pronounced when antibiotic medium 3 (AM3) is used instead of standard RPMI-1640 medium (Rex et al, 1995). However, complete separation of resistant from susceptible isolates has not been achieved by using AM3 medium. In addition, AM3 is a nonstandardized medium and lot-to-lot variation is a limiting factor to its use (Lozano-Chiu et al, 1997). It is recommended that laboratories that use this alternative medium introduce susceptible and resistant strains of *Candida* species with known amphotericin B MICs as controls.

The M27-A procedure relies upon the visual determination of MIC endpoints. However, the recommended endpoints differ for different antifungal agents.

For amphotericin B, the endpoint is defined as the lowest concentration at which there is complete inhibition of growth. The end point for azoles for both macro- and microdilution testing has been defined as the point at which there is a prominent reduction in growth. For macrodilution testing, prominent reduction in growth has been shown to correspond to an 80% reduction in growth relative to that observed in the growth control. However, when the microdilution format is utilized and read with a spectrophotometer, the specified prominent visual reduction in growth best corresponds to a 50% spectrophotometric growth inhibition endpoint (Odds et al, 1995; Pfaller et al, 1995).

The M27-A document recommends an endpoint reading at 48 hours for tests with *Candida* species. However, recent work has begun to include 24-hour readings because MICs can often be determined at this time, and because readings taken at 24 hours may be more relevant for some isolates. Isolates for which the earlier reading is important show a dramatic rise in drug MIC between 24 hours and 48 hours due to "trailing" growth. The term "trailing" has been used to describe the reduced but persistent growth which some isolates of *Candida* species exhibit over an extended range of azole drug concentrations, making interpretation of the MIC endpoint difficult (Revankar et al, 1998; Rex et al, 1998). Estimated as occurring in about 5% of isolates (Arthington-Skaggs et al, 2000), this trailing growth can be so great as to make an isolate that appears to be susceptible after 24 hours appear completely resistant at 48 hours. Two independent in vivo investigations of this phenomenon that employed murine models of disseminated candidiasis (Rex et al, 1998; Arthington-Skaggs et al, 2000) have shown that trailing isolates should be classed as susceptible rather than resistant. This concept has been corroborated by the clinical demonstration that most episodes of oropharyngeal candidiasis due to trailing *Candida* isolates respond to low doses of fluconazole, the same doses used to treat susceptible isolates (Revankar et al, 1998).

The inclusion of a colorimetric indicator into the culture medium has been found to produce much clearer visual endpoints in tests with azole antifungal agents, and to generate MICs that are in close agreement with those obtained using the standard broth dilution procedures (Pfaller et al, 1994; To et al, 1995). Commercial colorimetric microdilution plate panels for the in vitro testing of antifungal agents are now available for diagnostic use in the United States. Comparisons of the Sensititre Yeast One Colorimetric Antifungal Panel (Trek Diagnostics Systems Inc., Westlake, OH), which incorporates alamar blue as the colorimetric indicator with the M27-A reference procedure have demonstrated good agreement between the methods (Pfaller et al, 1998; Davey et al, 1998; Espinel-Ingroff et al, 1999). In addition to clearer endpoints, other benefits include reduced incubation times.

Following the principles established for testing *Candida* species and *C. neoformans*, the NCCLS subcommittee on antifungal susceptibility testing has developed an approved reference procedure (document M38-A) for broth microdilution susceptibility testing of conidium-forming filamentous fungi (National Committee for Clinical Laboratory Standards, 2002b). The essential features of this method include the use of a broth microdilution format, a defined test medium (RPMI-1640 broth buffered to pH 7.0 with MOPS), as well as an inoculum standardized by spectrophotometric reading to around 10,000 colony forming units per ml, and visual determination of the MIC endpoint after incubation at 35°C for 24–72 hours. This procedure was developed using isolates of *Aspergillus* species, *Fusarium* species, *S. apiospermum*, and *Sporothrix schenckii*. The methods of inoculum preparation, choice of inoculum size, time of reading, and endpoint selection have all been evaluated in a series of multicenter investigations (Espinel-Ingroff et al, 1995; Espinel-Ingroff et al, 1997). Nongerminated conidia are used because, at least with *Aspergillus* species, similar results have been obtained for germinated and nongerminated conidia (Manavathu et al, 1999; Espinel-Ingroff, 2001a).

Although the M27-A reference procedure served as the starting point for the M38 document, there are several significant differences between the two methods. The inoculum is about 10 times higher than for yeasts and requires a different method of preparation. Because of the differences in the size and light-scattering properties of the spores produced by these fungi, the M38-A document specifies different optical densities for each genus. Careful preparation of the inoculum is essential, since a concentration outside the specified range will result in an altered MIC to most antifungal agents (Gehrt et al, 1995).

The endpoint definition is another point of difference between the M38 and M27 procedures. In M27, azoles are read at a partial inhibition endpoint (defined as the lowest drug concentration producing a prominent reduction in growth). While this wording was used in the M38-P document for the azoles (National Committee for Clinical Laboratory Standards, 1998), more recent work suggests that reading the endpoint at 100% inhibition (no growth) better detects resistance of *Aspergillus* species to itraconazole and the newer triazoles (Denning et al, 1997a; Espinel Ingroff et al, 2001b). This modification has been incorporated into the M38-A document.

The development of the M27 and M38 reference procedures for in vitro testing has provided an essential standard against which possible alternative methods can be evaluated. Microdilution procedures are time-consuming and labor-intensive, and there is a need for simpler and more economical methods of antifungal susceptibility testing for routine clinical use. Among the simpler methods that are now being evaluated are the Etest and agar disc diffusion tests.

The Etest (AB Biodisk, Solna, Sweden), a patented commercial method for the quantitative determination of MICs, is set up in a manner similar to a disc diffusion test, but the disc is replaced with a calibrated plastic strip impregnated with a continuous concentration gradient of the antimicrobial agent. Following incubation, the MIC is determined from the point of intersection of the growth inhibition zone with the calibrated strip. Both nonuniform growth of the fungal lawn and the presence of a trailing growth edge can make endpoint determination difficult. However, with experience and standardized procedures, the correlation between the Etest and the M27-A reference procedure has been acceptable for most *Candida* species and the azole antifungal agents (Colombo et al, 1995; Pfaller et al, 1996; Warnock et al, 1998). For many moulds, including *Aspergillus* species, good correlations with amphotericin B and itraconazole Etest and MICs by the M38 method have been reported (Szekely et al, 1999; Pfaller et al, 2000). The Etest has proved useful for the determination of amphotericin B MICs and represents one of the more reliable ways to detect resistant isolates (Wanger et al, 1995; Clancy and Nguyen, 1999; Peyron et al, 2001). Quality control Etest limits for the two M27 QC isolates against amphotericin B, flucytosine, fluconazole, itraconazole, and ketoconazole have been proposed (Pfaller et al, 1996).

Although agar disc diffusion has seen widespread use for antibacterial drug testing, this method has had limited application in antifungal drug susceptibility testing. It has proved useful for in vitro testing of flucytosine, but early attempts to develop a standardized method for fluconazole were complicated by the lack of a reference method with which the results of the disc diffusion test could be compared (Pfaller et al, 1992). More recently, several investigations have demonstrated good correlations between agar disc diffusion results for fluconazole and MICs by the M27-A method (Barry and Brown, 1996; Meis et al, 2000). Clearly, disc diffusion has the potential to provide a simpler means of performing in vitro tests with fluconazole and other antifungal agents, but more work is needed.

As Rex and coworkers have commented, the ability to generate an MIC is of little value without the corresponding ability to interpret its clinical meaning (Rex et al, 2001). However, this process is far from straightforward for a number of reasons. First, MICs are not a physical measurement. Second, host factors play a critical role in determining clinical outcome. Third, susceptibility in vitro does not uniformly predict therapeutic success in vivo. Fourth, resistance in vitro will often, but not always, correlate with treatment failure (Rex et al, 1997).

The original M27-A document (National Committee for Clinical Laboratory Standards, 1997) included interpretive breakpoints for *Candida* species when tested against fluconazole, itraconazole, and flucytosine. The data for each drug had different strengths and weaknesses for determining these breakpoints, but one weakness that applied to all the data sets was the small amount of information that was available on isolates for which the MICs were elevated. A second limitation was that all (itraconazole) or most (fluconazole) of the MIC-clinical outcome correlation data were derived from studies of mucosal candidiasis. There are fewer data for invasive forms of candidiasis. Despite these limitations, the general level of clinical correlation achieved to date has been similar to that seen with antibacterial agents (Rex et al, 2001).

The incidence of invasive mould infections is too low to permit large-scale prospective comparisons of antifungal drug MICs with the clinical outcome of treatment. For this reason, several groups of investigators have sought to confirm the relevance of in vitro test results in animal models of infection. One group tested nine mould isolates (two *Aspergillus* species, three *Fusarium* species, two *S. apiospermum* isolates, and two *Rhizopus arrhizus* isolates), but found that amphotericin B and itraconazole MICs determined by the M38-P reference method provided few clues to the likelihood of in vivo response (Odds et al, 1998). A second group conducted in vitro and in vivo tests with six *A. fumigatus* isolates, two of which were collected from patients who did not respond to itraconazole treatment (Denning et al, 1997a). These isolates were resistant to itraconazole in a murine model of invasive aspergillosis and had elevated itraconazole MICs. However, the choice of in vitro test conditions was critical in the detection of these elevated MICs. In further work, this group conducted in vitro and in vivo tests with an isolate of *A. fumigatus* from a patient who responded incompletely to amphotericin B and an isolate of the intrinsically amphotericin B-resistant species *A. terreus* (Johnson et al, 2000). Both isolates were unresponsive to amphotericin B in a murine model of invasive aspergillosis, but only the *A. terreus* isolate tested resistant in vitro. A wide range of media and test conditions failed to distinguish the resistant *A. fumigatus* isolate from two isolates that were susceptible in vivo. In contrast, using a straightforward adaptation of the M27 procedure, Lass-Florl and coworkers demonstrated a good correlation between amphotericin B MICs of ≥ 2 μg/ml and an increased likelihood of clinical failure in patients with aspergillosis (Lass-Florl et al, 1998).

These reports of an association between MICs and clinical outcome are encouraging, but further studies with animals and patients will be required for a more definitive evaluation. At present, it would appear that testing of *A. fumigatus* isolates against azole antifungal agents has significant potential value. Testing of amphotericin B is, however, more problematic.

In summary, antifungal drug susceptibility testing has become a useful clinical tool, but its original application remains uncertain in many circumstances. It is not an infallible guide to the treatment of fungal infections. Testing is most helpful for isolates of *Candida* species (especially for species other than *C. albicans*) from deep sites. Testing of oropharyngeal isolates of *Candida* species from patients who have failed to respond to standard azole treatment can help to distinguish failures due to drug resistance from other causes. Susceptibility testing for other fungi or settings is of unclear value. At present, testing of mould isolates should not be done on a routine basis. However, clinically important mould isolates should be identified to the species level as speciation can potentially provide useful therapeutic information.

REFERENCES

Ajello L. Phaeohyphomycosis: definition and etiology. In: *Proceedings of the Third International Conference on the Mycoses*. Scientific Publication 304. Washington DC: Pan American Health Organization, 126–133, 1975

Ajello L. Hyalohyphomycosis and phaeohyphomycosis: two global disease entities of public health importance. *Eur J Epidemiol* 2: 243–251, 1986

Arrese-Estrada J A, Stynen D, Goris A, Pierard G E. Identification immunohistochimique des Aspergillus par l'anticorps monclonal EB-A1. *Ann Pathol* 10: 198–200, 1990.

Arthington-Skaggs B A, Warnock D W, Morrison C J. Quantitation of *Candida albicans* ergosterol content improves the correlation between in vitro antifungal susceptibility test results and in vivo outcome after fluconazole treatment in a murine model of invasive candidiasis. *Antimicrob Agents Chemother* 44: 2081–2085, 2000.

Barry A L, Brown S D. Fluconazole disk diffusion procedure for determining susceptibility of *Candida* species. *J Clin Microbiol* 34: 2154–2157, 1996.

Barry A L, Pfaller M A, Brown S D, Espinel-Ingroff A, Ghannoum M A, Knapp C, Rennie R P, Rex J H, Rinaldi M G. Quality control limits for broth microdilution susceptibility tests of ten antifungal agents. *J Clin Microbiol* 38: 3457–3459, 2000.

Berg D E, Akopyants N S, Kersulyte D. Fingerprinting microbial genomes using the RAPD or AP-PCR method. *Meth Mol Cell Biol* 5: 13–24, 1994.

Brandt M E, Padhye A A, Mayer L W, Holloway B P. Utility of random amplified polymorphic DNA PCR and TaqMan automated detection in molecular identification of *Aspergillus fumigatus*. *J Clin Microbiol* 36: 2057–2062, 1998.

Buchheidt D, Baust C, Skladny H, Baldus M, Brauninger S, Hehlmann R. Clinical evaluation of a polymerase chain reaction assay to detect *Aspergillus* species in bronchoalveolar lavage samples of neutropenic patients. *Br J Haematol* 116: 803–811, 2002.

Buckley H R, Richardson M D, Evans E G V, Wheat L J. Immunodiagnosis of invasive fungal infection. *J Med Vet Mycol* 30 (suppl. 1): 249–260, 1992.

Chen Y C, Eisner J D, Kattar M M, Rassoulian-Barrett S L, Lafe K, Yarfitz S L, Limaye A P, Cookson B T. Identification of medically important yeasts using PCR-based detection of DNA sequence polymorphisms in the internal transcribed spacer 2 region of the rRNA genes. *J Clin Microbiol* 38: 2302–2310, 2000.

Chen Y C, Eisner J D, Kattar M M, Rassoulian-Barrett S L, Lafe K, Bui U, Limaye A P, and Cookson B T. Polymorphic internal spacer region 1 DNA sequences identify medically important yeasts. *J Clin Microbiol* 39: 4042–4051, 2001.

Clancy C J, Nguyen M H. Correlation between in vitro susceptibility determined by E test and response to therapy with amphotericin B: results from a multicenter prospective study of candidemia. *Antimicrob Agents Chemother* 43: 1289–1290, 1999.

Colombo A L, Barchiesi F, McGough D A, Rinaldi M G. Comparison of E test and National Committee for Clinical Laboratory Standards broth macrodilution method for azole antifungal susceptibility testing. *J Clin Microbiol* 33: 535–540, 1995.

Cuenca Estrella M, Diaz-Guerra T M, Mellado E, Rodriguez-Tudela J L. Influence of glucose supplementation and inoculum size on growth kinetics and antifungal susceptibility testing of *Candida* spp. *J Clin Microbiol* 39: 525–532, 2001.

Davey K G, Szekely A, Johnson E M, Warnock D W. Comparison of a new commercial colorimetric microdilution method with a standard method for in-vitro susceptibility testing of *Candida* spp. and *Cryptococcus neoformans*. *J Antimicrob Chemother* 42: 439–444, 1998.

de Barros Lopes M, Soden A, Martens A L, Henschke P A, Langridge P. Differentiation and species identification of yeasts using PCR. *Int J System Bacteriol* 48: 279–286, 1998.

De Repentigny L, Kaufman L, Cole G T, Kruse D, Latge J P, Matthews R C. Immunodiagnosis of invasive fungal infections. *J Med Vet Mycol* 32 (suppl. 1): 239–252, 1994.

Denning D W, Radford S A, Oakley K L, Hall L, Johnson E M, Warnock D W. Correlation between in vitro susceptibility testing to itraconazole and in-vivo outcome of *Aspergillus fumigatus* infection. *J Antimicrob Chemother* 40: 401–414, 1997a.

Denning D W, Venkateswarlu K, Oakley K L, Anderson M J, Manning N J, Stevens D A, Warnock D W, Kelly S L. Itraconazole resistance in *Aspergillus fumigatus*. *Antimicrob Agents Chemother* 41: 1364–1368, 1997b.

Durkin M M, Connolly P A, Wheat L J. Comparison of radioimmunoassay and enzyme-linked immunoassay methods for detection of *Histoplasma capsulatum* var. *capsulatum* antigen. *J Clin Microbiol* 35: 2252–2255, 1997.

Einsele H, Hebart H, Roller G, Loffler J, Rothenhofer I, Muller C A, Bowden R A, van Burik J, Engelhard D, Kanz L, Schumacher U. Detection and identification of fungal pathogens in blood by using molecular probes. *J Clin Microbiol* 35: 1353–1360, 1997.

Elder B L, Roberts G D. Rapid methods for the diagnosis of fungal infections. *Lab Med* 17: 591–596, 1986.

Elie C M, Lott T J, Burns B M, Reiss E, Morrison C J. Rapid identification of *Candida* species using species-specific DNA probes. *J Clin Microbiol* 36: 3260–3265, 1998.

Espinel-Ingroff A, Dawson K, Pfaller M, Anaissie E, Breslin B, Dixon D, Fothergill A, Paetznick V, Peter J, Rinaldi M, Walsh T. Comparative and collaborative evaluation of standardization of antifungal susceptibility testing for filamentous fungi. *Antimicrob Agents Chemother* 39: 314–319, 1995.

Espinel-Ingroff A, Bartlett M, Bowden R, Chin N X, Cooper C, Fothergill A, McGinnis M R, Menezes P, Messer S A, Nelson P W, Odds F C, Pasarell L, Peter J, Pfaller M A, Rex J H, Rinaldi M G, Shankland G S, Walsh T J, Weitzman I. Multicenter evaluation of proposed standardized procedure for antifungal sus-

ceptibility testing of filamentous fungi. *J Clin Microbiol* 35: 139–143, 1997.

Espinel-Ingroff A, Stockman L, Roberts G, Pincus D, Pollack J, Marler J. Comparison of RapID Yeast Plus system with API 20C system for identification of common, new, and emerging yeast pathogens. *J Clin Microbiol* 36: 883–886, 1998.

Espinel-Ingroff A, Pfaller M, Messer S A, Knapp C C, Killian S, Norris H A, Ghannoum M A. Multicenter comparison of the Sensititre Yeast One Colorimetric Antifungal Panel with the National Committee for Clinical Laboratory Standards M27-A reference method for testing clinical isolates of common and emerging *Candida* spp., *Cryptococcus* spp., and other yeasts and yeast-like organisms. *J Clin Microbiol* 37: 591–595, 1999.

Espinel-Ingroff A. Germinated and nongerminated conidial suspensions for testing of susceptibilities of *Aspergillus* spp. to amphotericin B, itraconazole, posaconazole, ravuconazole, and voriconazole. *Antimicrob Agents Chemother* 45: 605–607, 2001a.

Espinel-Ingroff A, Bartlett M, Chaturvedi V, Ghannoum M, Hazen K C, Pfaller M A, Rinaldi M, Walsh T J. Optimal susceptibility testing conditions for detection of azole resistance in *Aspergillus* spp.: NCCLS collaborative evaluation. *Antimicrob Agents Chemother* 45: 1828–1835, 2001b.

Fell J W, Boekhout T, Fonseca A, Scorzetti G, Statzell-Tallman A. Biodiversity and systematics of basidiomycetous yeasts as determined by large-subunit rDNA D1/D2 domain sequence analysis. *Int J System Evolut Microbiol* 50: 1351–1371, 2000.

Fujita S-I, Lasker B A, Lott T J, Reiss E, Morrison C J. Microtitration plate enzyme immunoassay to detect PCR-amplified DNA from *Candida* species in blood. *J Clin Microbiol* 33: 962–967, 1995.

Gehrt A, Peter J, Pizzo P A, Walsh T J. Effect of increasing inoculum sizes of pathogenic filamentous fungi on MICs of antifungal agents by broth microdilution method. *J Clin Microbiol* 33: 1302–1307, 1995.

Gené J, Guillamon J M, Guarro J, Pujol J, Ulfig K. Molecular characterization, relatedness, and antifungal susceptibility of the basidiomycetous *Hormographiella* species and *Coprinus cinereus* from clinical and environmental sources. *Antonie Leeuwenhoek Int J Genet* 70: 49–57, 1996.

Gentry L O, Wilkinson I D, Lea A S, Price M F. Latex agglutination test for detection of Candida antigenemia in patients with disseminated disease. *Eur J Clin Microbiol* 2: 122–128, 1983.

Guarro J, Gené J, Stchigel A M. Developments in fungal taxonomy. *Clin Microbiol Rev* 12: 454–500, 1999.

Guiver M, Levi K, Oppenheim B A. Rapid identification of *Candida* species by TaqMan PCR. *J Clin Pathol* 54: 362–366, 2001.

Hebart H, Loeffler J, Reitze H, Engal A, Schumacher U, Klingebiel T, Bader P, Böhme A, Martin H, Bunjes D, Kern W V, Kanz L, Einsele H. Prospective screening by a panfungal polymerase chain reaction assay in patients at risk for fungal infections: implications for the management of febrile neutropenia. *Br J Haematol* 111: 635–640, 2000.

Hendolin P H, Paulin L, Koukila-Kahkola P, Anttila V-J, Malmberg H, Richardson M, Ylikoski J. Panfungal PCR and multiplex liquid hybridization for detection of fungi in tissue specimens. *J Clin Microbiol* 38: 4186–4192, 2000.

Herent P, Stynen D, Hernando F, Fruit J, Poulain D. Retrospective evaluation of two latex agglutination tests for detection of circulating antigen during invasive candidosis. *J Clin Microbiol* 30: 2158–2164, 1992.

Hue F X, Huerre M, Rouffault M A, de Bievre C. Specific detection of *Fusarium* species in blood and tissues by a PCR technique. *J Clin Microbiol* 37: 2434–2438, 1999.

Hui M, Ip M, Chan P K S, Chin M L, Cheng A F B. Rapid identification of medically important *Candida* to species level by polymerase chain reaction and single-strand conformational polymorphism. *Diagn Microbiol Infect Dis* 38: 95–99, 2000.

Huppert M, Peterson E T, Sun S H, Chitjian P A, Derrevere W J. Evaluation of a latex particle agglutination test for coccidioidomycosis. *Am J Clin Pathol* 49: 96–102, 1968.

Jaeger E E M, Carroll N M, Choudhury S, Dunlop A A S, Towler H M A, Matheson M M, Adamson P, Okhravi N, Lightman S. Rapid detection and identification of *Candida*, *Aspergillus*, and *Fusarium* species in ocular samples using nested PCR. *J Clin Microbiol* 38: 2902–2908, 2000.

Johnson E M, Oakley K L, Radford S A, Moore C B, Warn P, Warnock D W, Denning D W. Lack of correlation of in vitro amphotericin B susceptibility testing with outcome in a murine model of Aspergillus infection. *J Antimicrob Chemother* 45: 85–93, 2000.

Jones J M. Kinetics of antibody responses to cell wall mannan and a major cytoplasmic antigen of *Candida albicans* in rabbits and humans. *J Lab Clin Med* 96: 845–860, 1980.

Jones J M, Laboratory diagnosis of invasive candidiasis. *Clin Microbiol Rev* 3: 32–45, 1990.

Kami M, Fukui T, Ogawa S, Kazuyama Y, Machida U, Tanaka Y, Kanda Y, Kashima T, Yamazaki Y, Hamaki T, Mori S, Akiyama H, Mutou Y, Sakamaki H, Osumi K, Kimura S, Hirai H. Use of real-time PCR on blood samples for diagnosis of invasive aspergillosis. *Clin Infect Dis* 33: 1504–1512, 2001.

Kaufman L, Sekhon A S, Moledina N, Jalbert M, Pappagianis D. Comparative evaluation of commercial Premier EIA and microimmunodiffusion and complement fixation tests for *Coccidioides immitis* antibodies. *J Clin Microbiol* 33: 618–619, 1995.

Kaufman L, Standard P G, Jalbert M, Kraft D E. Immunohistologic identification of *Aspergillus* spp. and other hyaline fungi by using polyclonal fluorescent antibodies. *J Clin Microbiol* 35: 2206–2209, 1997.

Kurtzman C P. Molecular taxonomy of the yeasts. *Yeast* 10: 1727–1740, 1994.

Kurtzman C P, Robnett C J. Identification and phylogeny of ascomycetous yeasts from analysis of nuclear large subunit (26S) ribosomal DNA partial sequences. *Antonie van Leeuwenhoek* 73: 331–371, 1998.

Lass-Florl C, Kofler G, Kropshofer G, Hermans J, Kreczy A, Dierich M P, Niederwieser D. In-vitro testing of susceptibility to amphotericin B is a reliable predictor of clinical outcome in invasive aspergillosis. *J Antimicrob Chemother* 42: 497–502, 1998.

Lischewski A, Kretschmar M, Hof H, Amann R, Hacker J, Morschhauser J. Detection and identification of *Candida* species in experimentally infected tissue and human blood by rRNA-specific fluorescent in situ hybridization. *J Clin Microbiol* 35: 2943–2948, 1997.

Loeffler J, Hebart H, Magga S, Schmidt D, Klingspor L, Tollemar J, Schumacher U, Einsele H. Identification of rare *Candida* species and other yeasts by polymerase chain reaction and slot blot hybridization. *Diagn Microbiol Infect Dis* 38: 207–212, 2000a.

Loeffler J, Henke N, Hebart H, Schmidt D, Hagmeyer L, Schumacher U, Einsele H. Quantification of fungal DNA by using fluorescence resonance energy transfer and the light cycler system. *J Clin Microbiol* 38: 586–590, 2000b.

Loeffler J, Hebart H, Cox P, Flues N, Schumacher U, Einsele H. Nucleic acid sequence-based amplification of Aspergillus RNA in blood samples. *J Clin Microbiol* 39: 1626–1629, 2001.

Lott T, Effat M. Evidence for a more recently evolved clade within a *Candida albicans* North American population. *Microbiology* 147: 1687–1692, 2001.

Lozano-Chiu M, Nelson P W, Lancaster M, Pfaller M A, Rex J H. Lot-to-lot variability of antibiotic medium 3 used for testing susceptibility of Candida isolates to amphotericin B. *J Clin Microbiol* 35: 270–272, 1997.

Lucchini S, Thompson A, Hinton J C D. Microarrays for microbiologists. *Microbiology* 147: 1403–1414, 2001.

Maertens J, Verhaegen J, Demuynck H. Autopsy-controlled prospective evaluation of serial screening for circulating galactomannan by a sandwich enzyme-linked immunosorbent assay for hematological patients at risk for invasive aspergillosis. *J Clin Microbiol* 37: 3223–3228, 1999.

Magee B B, Magee P T. Electrophoretic karyotypes and chromosome numbers in *Candida* species. *J Gen Microbiol* 133: 425–430, 1987.

Manavathu E K, Cutright J, Chandrasekar P H. Comparative study of susceptibilities of germinated and ungerminated conidia of *Aspergillus fumigatus* to various antifungal agents. *J Clin Microbiol* 37: 858–861, 1999.

Mannarelli B M, Kurtzman C P. Rapid identification of *Candida albicans* and other human pathogenic yeasts by using short oligonucleotides in a PCR. *J Clin Microbiol* 36: 1634–1641, 1998.

Marcilla A, C Monteagudo, S Mormeneo, R Sentandreu. Monoclonal antibody 3H8: a useful tool in the diagnosis of candidiasis. *Microbiology* 145: 695–701, 1999.

Martin C, Roberts D, van der Weide M, Rossau R, Jannes G, Smith T, Maher M. Development of a PCR-based line probe assay for identification of fungal pathogens. *J Clin Microbiol* 38: 3735–3742, 2000.

Martins T B, Jaskowski T D, Mouritsen C L, Hill H R. Comparison of commercially available enzyme immunoassay with traditional serological tests for detection of antibodies to *Coccidioides immitis*. *J Clin Microbiol* 33: 940–943, 1995.

Matsumoto T, Ajello L. Agents of phaeohyphomycosis. In: Collier L, Balows A, Sussman M, eds. *Topley and Wilson's Microbiology and Microbial Infections*, 9th ed. Vol 4 Medical Mycology. New York: Oxford University Press, 503–524, 1998.

McManus E J, Jones J M. Detection of a *Trichosporon beigelii* antigen cross-reactive with *Cryptococcus neoformans* capsular polysaccharide in serum from a patient with disseminated trichosporon infection. *J Clin Microbiol* 21: 681–685, 1985.

Meis J, Petrou M, Bille J, Ellis D, Gibbs D. A global evaluation of the susceptibility of *Candida* species to fluconazole by disk diffusion. *Diagn Microbiol Infect Dis* 36: 215–223, 2000.

Metzgar D, van Belkum A, Field D, Haubrich R, Wills C. Random amplification of polymorphic DNA and microsatellite gentyping of pre- and post-treatment isolates of *Candida* spp. from human immunodeficiency virus-infected patients on different fluconazole regimens. *J Clin Microbiol* 36: 2308–2313, 1998.

Meunier J-R, Grimont P A D. Factors affecting reproducibility of random amplified polymorphic DNA fingerprinting. *Res Microbiol* 144: 373–379, 1993.

Meyer W, Lieckfeldt E, Kuhls K, Freedman E Z, Borner T, Mitchell T G. DNA- and PCR-fingerprinting in fungi. In: Pena SDJ, Chakrabarty R, Epplen JT, Jeffreys AJ, eds. *DNA Fingerprinting: State of the Science*. Basel: Birkhauser Verlag, 311–320, 1993.

Mitsutake K, Miyazaki T, Tashiro T, Yamamoto Y, Kakeya H, Otsubo T, Kawamura S, Hossain M A, Noda T, Hirakata Y, Kohno S. Enolase antigen, mannan antigen, Cand-Tec antigen, and β-glucan in patients with candidemia. *J Clin Microbiol* 34: 1918–1921, 1996.

Monod M, Porchet S, Baudraz-Rosselet F, Frenk E. The identification of pathogenic yeast strains by electrophoretic analysis of their chromosomes. *J Med Microbiol* 32: 123–129, 1990.

National Committee for Clinical Laboratory Standards. Reference method for broth dilution antifungal susceptibility testing of yeasts. Approved standard. Document M27-A. Wayne, PA: National Committee for Clinical Laboratory Standards, 1997.

National Committee for Clinical Laboratory Standards. Reference method for broth dilution antifungal susceptibility testing of conidium-forming filamentous fungi. Proposed standard. Document

M38-P. Wayne, PA: National Committee for Clinical Laboratory Standards, 1998.

National Committee for Clinical Laboratory Standards. Reference method for broth dilution antifungal susceptibility testing of yeasts. Approved standard: second edition. Document M27-A2. Wayne, PA: National Committee for Clinical Laboratory Standards, 2002a.

National Committee for Clinical Laboratory Standards. Reference method for broth dilution antifungal susceptibility testing of filamentous fungi. Approved standard. Document M38-A. Wayne, PA: National Committee for Clinical Laboratory Standards, 2002b.

Niesters H G M, Goessens W H F, Meis J F M G, Quint, W G V. Rapid, polymerase chain reaction-based identification assays for *Candida* species. *J Clin Microbiol* 31: 904–910, 1993.

Odds F C. The fungal kingdom: essentials of mycology. In: Kibbler CC, Mackenzie DWR, Odds FC, eds. *Principles and Practice of Clinical Mycology*, Chichester: John Wiley & Sons, 1–6, 1996.

Odds F C, Arai T, Disalvo A F, Evans E G V, Hay R J, Randhawa H S, Rinaldi M G, Walsh T J. Nomenclature of fungal diseases: a report and recommendations from a sub-committee of the International Society for Human and Animal Mycology (ISHAM). *J Med Vet Mycol* 30: 1–10, 1992.

Odds F C, Vranckx L, Woestenborghs F. Antifungal susceptibility testing of yeasts: evaluation of technical variables for test automation. *Antimicrob Agents Chemother* 39: 2051–2060, 1995.

Odds F C, van Gerven F, Espinel-Ingroff A, Bartlett M S, Ghannoum M A, Lancaster M V, Pfaller M A, Rex J H, Rinaldi M G, Walsh T J. Evaluation of possible correlations between antifungal susceptibilities of filamentous fungi in vitro and antifungal treatment outcomes in animal infection models. *Antimicrob Agents Chemother* 42: 282–288, 1998.

Okhravi N, Adamson P, Lightman S. Use of PCR in endophthalmitis. *Ocul Immunol Inflamm* 8: 189–200, 2000.

Pappagiannis D, Zimmer B L. Serology of coccidioidomycosis. *Clin Microbiol Rev* 3: 247–268, 1990.

Perfect J R, Cox G M. Drug resistance in *Cryptococcus neoformans*. *Drug Resist Updates* 2: 259–269, 1999.

Perfect J R, Cox G M, Lee J Y, Kauffman C A, deRepetigny L, Chapman S W, Morrison V A, Pappas P, Hiemenz J W, Stevens D A. The impact of culture isolation of *Aspergillus* species: a hospital-based survey of aspergillosis. *Clin Infect Dis* 33: 1924–1833, 2001.

Peyron F, Favel A, Michel-Nguyen A, Gilly M, Regli P, Bolmstrom A. Improved detection of amphotericin B-resistant isolates of *Candida lusitaniae* by Etest. *J Clin Microbiol* 39: 339–342, 2001.

Pfaller M A, Dupont B, Kobayashi G S, Muller J, Rinaldi M G, Espinel-Ingroff A, Shadomy S., Troke P F, Walsh T J, Warnock D W. Standardized susceptibility testing of fluconazole: an international collaborative study. *Antimicrob Agents Chemother* 36: 1805–1809, 1992.

Pfaller M A, Vu Q, Lancaster M, Espinel-Ingroff A, Fothergill A, Grant C, McGinnis M R, Pasarell L, Rinaldi M G, Steele-Moore L. Multisite reproducibility of colorimetric broth microdilution method for antifungal susceptibility testing of yeast isolates. *J Clin Microbiol* 32: 1625–1628, 1994.

Pfaller M A, Messer S A, Coffmann S. Comparison of visual and spectrophotometric methods of MIC endpoint determinations by using broth microdilution methods to test five antifungal agents, including the new triazole, D0870. *J Clin Microbiol* 33: 1094–1097, 1995.

Pfaller M A, Messer S A, Bolmstrom A, Odds F C, Rex J H. Multisite reproducibility of the E test method for antifungal susceptibility of yeast isolates. *J Clin Microbiol* 34: 1691–1693, 1996.

Pfaller M A, Messer S A, Hollis R J, Espinel-Ingroff A, Ghannoum M A, Plavan H, Killian S B, Knapp C C. Multisite reproducibility of MIC results by the Sensititre Yeast One colorimetric antifungal susceptibility panel. *Diagn Microbiol Infect Dis* 31: 543–547, 1998.

Pfaller M A, Messer S A, Mills K, Bolmstrom A. In vitro susceptibility testing of filamentous fungi: comparison of Etest and reference microdilution methods for determining itraconazole MICs. *J Clin Microbiol* 38: 3359–3361, 2000.

Ponton J, Moragues M D, Quindos G. Non-culture-based diagnostics. In: Calderone RA, ed. *Candida and Candidiasis*. Washington, DC: ASM Press, 395–425, 2002.

Rees J R, Pinner R W, Hajjeh R A, Brandt M E, Reingold A L. The epidemiological features of invasive mycotic infections in the San Francisco Bay area 1992–1993: results of population-based active surveillance. *Clin Infect Dis* 27: 1138–1147, 1998.

Reimer L G, Wilson M L, Weinstein M P. Update on detection of bacteremia and fungemia. *Clin Microbiol Rev* 10: 444–465, 1997.

Reiss E, Stockman L, Kuykendall R S, Smith S J. Dissociation of mannan-serum complexes and detection of *Candida albicans* mannan by enzyme immunoassay variations. *Clin Chem* 28: 306–310, 1982.

Reiss E, Kaufman L, Kovacs J A, Lindsley M D. Clinical immunomycology. In: Rose NR, Hamilton RG, Detrick B, eds. *Manual of Clinical Laboratory Immunology*, 6th ed. Washington DC: ASM Press, 559–583, 2002.

Revankar S G, Kirkpatrick W R, McAtee R K, Fothergill A W, Redding S W, Rinaldi M G, Patterson T F. Interpretation of trailing endpoints in antifungal susceptibility testing by the National Committee for Clinical Laboratory Standards method. *J Clin Microbiol* 36: 153–156, 1998.

Rex J H, Cooper C R, Merz W G, Galgiani J N, Anaissie E J. Detection of amphotericin B-resistant *Candida* isolates in a broth-based system. *Antimicrob Agents Chemother* 39: 906–909, 1995.

Rex J H, Pfaller M A, Galgiani J N, Bartlett M S, Espinel-Ingroff A, Ghannoum M A, Lancaster M, Odds F C, Rinaldi M G, Walsh T J, Barry A L. Development of interpretive breakpoints for antifungal susceptibility testing: conceptual framework and analysis of in vitro—in vivo correlation data for fluconazole, itraconazole, and Candida infections. *Clin Infect Dis* 24: 235–247, 1997.

Rex J H, Nelson P W, Paetznick V L, Lozano-Chiu M, Espinel-Ingroff A, Anaissie E J. Optimizing the correlation between results of testing in vitro and therapeutic outcome in vivo for fluconazole by testing critical isolates in a murine model of invasive candidiasis. *Antimicrob Agents Chemother* 42: 129–134, 1998.

Rex J H, Pfaller M A, Walsh T J, Chaturvedi V, Espinel-Ingroff A, Ghannoum M A, Gosey L L, Odds F C, Rinaldi M G, Sheehan D J, Warnock D W. Antifungal susceptibility testing: practical aspects and current challenges. *Clin Microbiol Rev* 14: 643–658, 2001.

Rickerts V, Loeffler J, Böhme A, Einsele H, Just-Nübling G. Diagnosis of disseminated zygomycosis using a polymerase chain reaction assay. *Eur J Clin Microbiol Infect Dis* 20: 744–745, 2001.

Riggsby W S. DNA probes for medically important yeasts. In: Swaminathan B, Prakash G, eds. *Nucleic Acid and Monoclonal Antibody Probes-Applications in Diagnostic Microbiology*. New York: Marcel Dekker, 277–304, 1989.

Rodriguez-Tudela J L, Martinez-Suarez J V. Defining conditions for microbroth antifungal susceptibility tests: influence of RPMI and RPMI-2% glucose on the selection of endpoint criteria. *J Antimicrob Chemother* 35: 739–749, 1995.

Sanati H, Messer S A, Pfaller M, Witt M, Larsen R, Espinel-Ingroff A, Ghannoum M. Multi-center evaluation of broth microdilution method for susceptibility testing of *Cryptococcus neoformans* against fluconazole. *J Clin Microbiol* 34: 1280–1282, 1996.

Sandhu G S, Kline B C, Stockman L, Roberts G D. Molecular probes for diagnosis of fungal infections. *J Clin Microbiol* 33: 2913–2919, 1995.

Scherer S, Stevens D A. Application of DNA typing methods to epidemiology and taxonomy of *Candida* species. *J Clin Microbiol* 25: 675–679, 1987.

Skladny H, Buchheidt D, Baust C, Krieg-Schneider F, Seifarth W, Leib-Mosch C, Hehlmann R. Specific detection of *Aspergillus* species in blood and bronchoalveolar lavage samples of immuinocompromised patients by two-step PCR. *J Clin Microbiol* 37: 3865–3871, 1999.

Soll D R. High-frequency switching in *Candida albicans*. *Clin Microbiol Rev* 5: 183–203, 1992.

Soll D R. The ins and outs of DNA fingerprinting the infectious fungi. *Clin Microbiol Rev* 13: 332–370, 2000.

Spitzer E D, Spitzer S G. Use of a dispersed repetitive DNA element to distinguish clinical isolates of *Cryptococcus neoformans*. *J Clin Microbiol* 30: 1094–1097, 1992.

Stamm A M, Polt S S. False-negative cryptococcal antigen test. *JAMA* 244: 1359, 1980.

Stockman L, Roberts G D. Corrected version. Specificity of the latex test for cryptococcal antigen: a rapid, simple method for eliminating interference factors. *J Clin Microbiol* 17: 945–947, 1983

Sugita T, Suto H, Unno T, Tsuboi R, Ogawa H, Shinoda T, Nishikawa A. Molecular analysis of *Malassezia* microflora on the skin of atopic dermatitis patients and healthy subjects. *J Clin Microbiol* 39: 3486–3490, 2001.

Sulahian A, Tabouret M, Ribaud P, Sarfati J, Gluckman E, Latge J P, Derouin F. Comparison of an enzyme immunoassay and latex agglutination test for detection of galactomannan in the diagnosis of invasive aspergillosis. *Eur J Clin Microbiol Infect Dis* 15: 139–145, 1996.

Sutton D A, Sanche S E, Revankar S G, Fothergill A W, Rinaldi M G. In vitro amphotericin B resistance in clinical isolates of *Aspergillus terreus*, with a head-to-head comparison to voriconazole. *J Clin Microbiol* 37: 2343–2345, 1999.

Szekely A, Johnson E M, Warnock D W. Comparison of E-test and broth microdilution methods for antifungal drug susceptibility testing of molds. *J Clin Microbiol* 37: 1480–1483, 1999.

Thanos M, Schönian G, Meyer W, Schweynoch C, Graser Y, Mitchell T G, Presber W, Tietz H J. Rapid identification of *Candida* species by DNA fingerprinting with PCR. *J Clin Microbiol* 34: 615–621, 1996.

To W K, Fothergill A W, Rinaldi M G. Comparative evaluation of macrodilution and alamar colorimetric microdilution broth methods for antifungal susceptibility testing of yeast isolates. *J Clin Microbiol* 33: 2660–2664, 1995.

Turin L, Riva F, Galbiati G, Cainelli T. Fast, simple and highly sensitive double-rounded polymerase chain reaction assay to detect medically relevant fungi in dermatological specimens. *Eur J Clin Invest* 30: 511–518, 2000.

Valente P, Ramos J P, Leoncini O. Sequencing as a tool in yeast molecular taxonomy. *Can J Microbiol* 45: 949–958, 1999.

Verweij P E, Rijs A J, De Pauw B E, Horrevorts A M, Hoogkamp-Korstanje J A, Meis J F. Clinical evaluation and reproducibility of the Pastorex Aspergillus antigen latex agglutination test for diagnosing invasive aspergillosis. *J Clin Pathol* 48: 474–476, 1995a.

Verweij P E, Stynen D, Rijs A J, De Pauw B E, Hoogkamp-Korstanje J A A, Meis J F. Sandwich enzyme-linked immunosorbent assay compared with Pastorex latex agglutination test for diagnosing invasive aspergillosis in immunocompromised patients. *J Clin Microbiol* 33: 1912–1914, 1995b.

Verweij P E, Brinkman K, Kremer H P, Kullberg B J, Meis J F. Aspergillus meningitis: diagnosis by non culture-based microbiological methods and management. *J Clin Microbiol* 37: 1186–1189, 1999.

Walsh T J, Peter J, McGough D A, Fothergill A W, Rinaldi M G, Pizzo P A. Activities of amphotericin B and antifungal azoles alone and in combination against *Pseudallescheria boydii*. *Antimicrob Agents Chemother* 39: 1361–1364, 1995.

Wanger A, Mills K, Nelson P W, Rex J H. Comparison of Etest and National Committee for Clinical Laboratory Standards broth macrodilution method for antifungal susceptibility testing: enhanced ability to detect amphotericin B-resistant *Candida* isolates. *Antimicrob Agents Chemother* 39: 2520–2522, 1995.

Warnock D W, Johnson E M, Rogers T R F. Multi-centre evaluation of the Etest method for antifungal drug susceptibility testing of *Candida* spp. and *Cryptococcus neoformans*. *J Antimicrob Chemother* 42: 321–331, 1998.

Welsh J, McClelland M. Genomic fingerprinting using arbitrarily primed PCR and a matrix of pairwise combinations of primers. *Nucl Acids Res* 19: 5275–5279, 1991.

Wheat L J, Kohler R B, Tewari R P. Diagnosis of disseminated histoplasmosis by detection of *Histoplasma capsulatum* antigen in serum and urine specimens. *N Engl J Med* 314: 83–88, 1986.

Wheat J, Marichal P, Vanden Bossche H, Monte AL, Connolly P. Hypothesis on the mechanisms of resistance to fluconazole in *Histoplasma capsulatum*. *Antimicrob Agents Chemother* 41: 410–414, 1997.

Wheat L J. Laboratory diagnosis of histoplasmosis: update 2000. *Semin Resp Infect* 16: 131–140, 2001.

Williams J G K, Kubelik A R, Livak K J, Rafalski J A, Tingey S V. DNA polymorphisms amplified by arbitrary primers are useful as genetic markers. *Nucl Acids Res* 18: 6531, 1990.

Wilson M L, Davis T E, Mirrett S, Reynolds J, Fuller D, Allen S D, Flint K K, Koontz F, Reller L B. Controlled comparison of the BACTEC high-blood-volume fungal medium, BACTEC Plus 26 aerobic blood culture bottle, and 10-milliliter Isolator blood culture system for detection of fungemia and bacteremia. *J Clin Microbiol* 31: 865–871, 1993.

Zhao J, Kong F, Li R, Wang X, Wan Z, Wang, D. Identification of *Aspergillus fumigatus* and related species by nested PCR targeting ribosomal DNA internal transcribed spacer regions. *J Clin Microbiol* 39: 2261–2266, 2001.

Zimmerman R L, Montone K T, Fogt F, Norris A H. Ultra fast identification of *Aspergillus* species in pulmonary cytology specimens by in situ hybridization. *Int J Molec Med* 5: 427–429, 2000.

2

Epidemiology of systemic
fungal diseases: overview

RANA A. HAJJEH AND DAVID W. WARNOCK

The last 2 decades have seen unprecedented changes in the pattern of systemic fungal diseases in humans. These infections have assumed a much greater importance, largely as a result of major advances in health care that have made possible the improved support of transplant recipients, critical-care patients, and other immunosuppressed individuals for longer periods of time. In developed countries, changing demographic patterns, in particular an aging population with a higher incidence of chronic illness and debilitation, have also resulted in an increase in the size of the population at risk for fungal infections. In addition to infections acquired in hospitals and other health-care settings, another significant development has been an increase in the occurrence of several of the endemic mycoses, in particular histoplasmosis and coccidioidomycosis, among previously healthy persons (Ampel et al, 1998; Cano and Hajjeh, 2001). Urban development, migration of populations, and natural disasters are among the factors that have contributed to this trend.

The AIDS epidemic is one of the most important factors that have contributed to the rising incidence of fungal diseases. Prior to the widespread usage of highly active antiretroviral therapy (HAART) in developed countries, up to 80% of human immunodeficiency virus (HIV)-infected persons developed mucosal candidiasis, while others developed cryptococcosis, histoplasmosis, or coccidioidomycosis during the course of their disease. In this population, these infections are frequently disseminated and often life threatening. In many developing countries, the HIV epidemic is continuing to escalate, and has led to dramatic increases in the incidence of diseases previously considered rare, such as cryptococcosis and disseminated histoplasmosis. In many parts of Africa, the prevalence of cryptococcosis has risen to more than 30% of persons living with AIDS. In Southeast Asia, cryptococcosis and *Penicillium marneffei* infection are now among the most common opportunistic infections in these individuals.

Analysis of U.S. National Center for Heath Statistics (NCHS) death records showed that fungal infections were the seventh most common cause of infectious disease-related mortality in 1992, and that mycotic

disease-related fatalities had increased more than three-fold since 1980 (Pinner et al, 1996). Additional analysis revealed that candidiasis and aspergillosis were the two specific diseases that accounted for most of these deaths (McNeil et al, 2001). The NCHS data also showed that, in 1994, fungal diseases resulted in 30,000 hospitalizations, and accounted for the fourth highest annual percentage increase (10%) since 1980 (Simonsen et al, 1998).

As invasive fungal infections have become more common among the growing number of immunocompromised and other susceptible individuals in the population, physicians are now faced with managing more of these infections, whether they are health-care–related, or acquired in the community. A better understanding of the epidemiologic features of these diseases will enable physicians to implement better management strategies and prevention measures.

SURVEILLANCE

Fungal infections are under diagnosed and underreported. Surveillance is important to measure the true magnitude and health-care costs of fungal diseases, to detect new pathogens, and to evaluate quality of care in hospitals. Surveillance is also essential to measure the effectiveness of interventions, such as prevention guidelines. Epidemiologic surveillance (which should be distinguished from microbiologic surveillance) consists of the systematic collection, analysis and interpretation of outcome-specific data for use in public health practice. Various surveillance systems have been used to investigate fungal diseases.

Sentinel systems, such as the SENTRY antimicrobial surveillance program (Pfaller et al, 1998a, 2002), SCOPE (Surveillance and Control of Pathogens of Epidemiologic Importance) (Pfaller et al, 1998b) and NEMIS (National Epidemiology of Mycoses Study) programs (Pfaller et al, 1998c; Rangel-Frausto et al, 1999), that focus on particular infections or hospitals, have proved very useful to monitor the emergence of non-*albicans Candida* species as causes of nosocomial bloodstream infection, and to follow trends in azole antifungal drug resistance among bloodstream isolates. Data from the National Nosocomial Infections Surveillance (NNIS) system, a sentinel surveillance system of U.S. hospitals established by the Centers for Disease Control and Prevention (CDC) in 1970 (http://www.cdc.gov/ncidod/hip/NNIS), demonstrated that the rate of hospital-acquired *Candida* bloodstream infections increased by almost 500% in large teaching hospitals during the 1980s, and by 219% to 370% in small teaching hospitals and large nonteaching hospitals respectively (Banerjee et al, 1991). This trend continued into the early 1990s, at which time *Candida* spp. were the sixth most common hospital-acquired pathogen overall (Emori and Gaynes, 1993). *Candida* spp. were the fourth most common bloodstream pathogens in NNIS hospitals during 1990–1992, accounting for 8%–10% of all hospital-acquired bloodstream infections.

Although *C. albicans* remained the most common cause of *Candida* bloodstream infections and disseminated candidiasis throughout the 1980s, 30%–50% of these infections were due to other *Candida* spp. (Banerjee et al, 1991; Beck-Sague and Jarvis, 1993). However, a recent analysis of NNIS data for *Candida* bloodstream infections in intensive care units found a significant decrease in the incidence of these infections overall among intensive care unit patients between 1989 and 1999 (Trick et al, 2002). Furthermore, the same analysis revealed a significant increase in the incidence of *C. glabrata* bloodstream infections.

Many U.S. hospitals have participated, or currently participate, in NNIS, or maintain their own surveillance system. Physicians need to consult with their infection control personnel at regular intervals to be aware of the baseline incidence rates of different fungal infections in their individual hospitals, as well as the incidence of antifungal resistance among organisms such as *Candida* spp., whenever these data are available. Although national sentinel surveillance systems provide extremely valuable data, the published information may not always be representative of the general population, especially when the institutions involved are mostly large academic or tertiary care referral centers.

Passive surveillance systems are not ideal for fungal infections. Because these diseases are not notifiable and not usually transmissible, there is minimal incentive to report cases. In the United States, some endemic mycoses are reportable, in particular histoplasmosis and coccidioidomycosis, but usually only in states where they are endemic. Coccidioidomycosis is the only fungal disease reportable nationally (Centers for Disease Control and Prevention, 1997a). Efficient reporting of these diseases to local and state health departments helps public health personnel to detect outbreaks at an earlier stage, and serves to alert physicians. In addition,

better surveillance and adequate reporting allow physicians to identify which diseases are common in their areas and assist in developing a differential diagnosis.

Active surveillance for fungal diseases is expensive and often difficult to conduct, but it has enabled accurate population-based incidence rates to be determined for the first time for several invasive fungal infections, including *Candida* bloodstream infections and cryptococcosis, (Rees et al, 1998; Kao et al, 1999; Hajjeh et al, 1999; Hajjeh et al, 2001). It has also permitted a more representative description of the epidemiology of these diseases. As an example, population-based active surveillance for *Candida* bloodstream infections, conducted at different sites in the United States during 1992–1994 (Kao et al, 1999), and again during 1998–2000 (Hajjeh et al, 2001), showed that the incidence of these infections is approximately 8–10 per 100,000 population. These data provide a clear indication of the public health importance of this common mycotic infection, when compared to many other infectious diseases. In addition, these surveillance studies revealed that the incidence of fluconazole resistance among *C. albicans* isolates, a problem that many clinicians feared might significantly affect treatment of *Candida* bloodstream infections, remains very low (about 1%) and has not changed over time.

The various surveillance systems mentioned above have also been crucial in documenting epidemiologic trends. For example, the proportion of infections caused by non-*albicans Candida* spp. has increased during the 1990s and these organisms now account for more than 50% of all *Candida* bloodstream infections (Pfaller et al, 2000; Hajjeh et al, 2001). This trend has obvious clinical implications, because many non-*albicans Candida* spp. (except for *C. parapsilosis*) are usually less susceptible to azole drugs than *C. albicans*, and may require different management.

Whatever surveillance system is chosen, the quality of the data generated is heavily dependent on several key components: a defined population, a clear case definition, a mechanism for reporting, and a sufficient incentive for all participants to conduct the surveillance. The collaboration of physicians with their hospital infection control personnel, as well as with their local public health personnel, is crucial to ensure the collection of adequate and reliable surveillance data.

UNDERSTANDING EXPOSURE AND TRANSMISSION

Many fungal diseases are usually acquired by inhalation of airborne spores from an environmental reservoir, e.g., aspergillosis and the endemic mycoses. In contrast, some fungi, such as *Candida* and *Malassezia* spp., are normal commensal residents of humans, and infection is endogenous in origin or transmitted from person to person. These yeast infections can also be spread via medical devices and fomites, particularly in health-care settings. An adequate understanding of the mechanisms of transmission of these infections has important implications for decisions on prevention measures, ranging from the need for specific containment and environmental measures to the consideration of antifungal drug prophylaxis. In addition, host factors play an important role in predisposing persons to invasive fungal infections.

Aspergillosis

Invasive aspergillosis usually occurs in patients who are neutropenic following treatment for hematologic and other malignancies, in hematopoietic stem cell transplant (HSCT) and solid organ transplant recipients, and in patients with neutrophil deficiencies (such as acquired marrow failure or congenital neutropenia) or dysfunction, e.g., chronic granulomatous disease (Warnock et al, 2001). Invasive aspergillosis can be acquired following a wide range of exposures inside or outside the hospital environment. Because the majority of cases of invasive aspergillosis either start in, or are confined to, the lungs and because *Aspergillus* spores are commonly found in the indoor and outdoor air, inhalation is thought to be the usual route of infection. Possible environmental sources of these spores include the soil, decomposing plant matter, household dust, building materials, ornamental plants, flower arrangements, items of food, and water. The relative importance of these various sources is very difficult to determine, particularly for sporadic cases of *Aspergillus* infection (Hajjeh and Warnock, 2001). Furthermore, the mechanisms of transmission during outbreaks of aspergillosis may be very different from those involved in sporadic disease.

The best evidence for the role of contaminated air as a source of *Aspergillus* infection comes from the temporal association between some hospital-based outbreaks of invasive aspergillosis and periods of construction or renovation in or near the wards in which infected patients were housed (Arnow et al, 1978; Krasinski et al, 1985; Weems et al, 1987b; Barnes and Rogers, 1989). Further support for this hypothesis comes from reports of reduced rates of infection in hospitals following the opening of new facilities with improved air handling systems. In addition, housing high-risk patients in rooms supplied with HEPA-filtered air has helped to prevent the acquisition of *Aspergillus* infection within the hospital (Sherertz et al, 1987; Barnes and Rogers, 1989; Rhame et al, 1991; Cornet et al, 1999).

Hospital water has been suggested as another possible source of *Aspergillus* infection in hospitals (Anaissie and Costa, 2001; Anaissie et al, 2002). Although *As-*

pergillus spp. have been recovered from hospital and municipal water in several countries (Arvanitidou et al, 1999; Anaissie and Costa, 2001; Warris et al, 2002), there is currently no definitive proof that water is an important source of human infection. To date, the clearest published evidence to support this hypothesis is a single case report of a patient who died of aspergillosis. An isolate of *A. fumigatus* from this patient had an identical RAPD profile to those of isolates obtained from the patient's hospital room water, but differed from those of other environmental isolates obtained during the same period from other locations (Anaissie et al, 2002). Although hospital water is a feasible environmental reservoir for *Aspergillus* infection, and has a precedent in nosocomial legionellosis, further epidemiologic studies are needed to confirm transmission from water, and the proportion of cases it accounts for. In addition to hospital-based investigations, it will clearly be essential to conduct epidemiologic studies, with molecular typing of *Aspergillus* isolates, to look for potential sources of water-borne infection in the home environment.

Regardless of the environmental reservoir of *Aspergillus*, most cases of aspergillosis in hospitalized patients are not outbreak-related. It seems probable that some individuals are colonized before their admission to the hospital and develop invasive disease when rendered neutropenic. Indeed, estimates are that up to 70% of cases of aspergillosis diagnosed over a 3-year period of surveillance during construction in one North American hospital were community-acquired (Patterson et al, 1997). Although the major risk period for aspergillosis is during the profound neutropenia, which follows conditioning for transplantation, HSCT recipients who develop graft-versus-host disease often develop aspergillosis some time after transplantation, following their discharge from hospital. In several recent series, such patients have formed the majority of HSCT recipients with aspergillosis. Clearly, it is important to ascertain whether this disease is predominantly a hospital- or community-acquired infection, because hospital infection control measures will not prevent community-acquired cases. Other control and prevention measures should be considered in these patients, such as home environmental control for at-risk patients and prophylactic treatment with antifungal agents.

Candida Bloodstream Infections

Candida spp. are normal commensals of humans, being commonly found on the skin, in the gastrointestinal (GI) tract, and in the female genital tract (Odds, 1988). Most cases of *Candida* bloodstream infections occur sporadically, and are usually due to endogenous transmission, i.e., the strain causing bloodstream infection was derived from the individual's normal flora.

However, many outbreaks of *Candida* bloodstream infections have been reported in the literature, and these have significantly increased our understanding of the epidemiology of the disease. Outbreaks are usually due to transmission within the hospital environment, either from health-care personnel or as a consequence of various procedures that facilitate entry of the organisms intravascularly.

The GI tract has long been known to be a source of entry of *Candida* organisms into the bloodstream (Krause et al, 1969). Recently, as part of the NEMIS study, a large collection of isolates was subtyped, using a variety of molecular typing methods (pulse field gel electrophoresis, restriction enzyme analysis, and electrokaryotyping) (Pfaller et al, 1998c). Most isolates had a unique DNA type, supporting the concept of endogenous infection. While the role of catheters in transmission of candidemia has been a subject of controversy (Nucci and Anaissie, 2001; Nucci and Anaissie 2002), clearly, catheters serve as an important route of entry for the organisms intravascularly. Recent literature also suggests that local thrombophlebitis at the skin site of catheter entry may be the cause of *Candida* bloodstream infection in some cases (Benoit et al, 1998).

Various factors have been associated with increased risk of *Candida* bloodstream infections. These can be divided into host factors, such as immunosuppression due to various underlying conditions, and hospitalization-related factors, such as central venous catheters, excessive antibiotic use, and surgical procedures. The widespread use of antibiotics, leading to overgrowth of *Candida* organisms in the GI tract, and intravascular devices, including catheters and presssure monitoring devices, are major predisposing factors. Other risk factors include cytotoxic therapy leading to neutropenia, other immunosuppressive conditions, loss of integrity of the GI tract, and abdominal surgery. Previous colonization with *Candida* spp. has been found to be independently associated with increased risk of *Candida* bloodstream infection in many studies (Wey et al, 1988; Pittet et al, 1994b; Marr et al, 2000). The intensity of colonization, when expressed as the number of sites colonized, has been helpful in predicting invasive *Candida* infections in critically ill surgical patients (Pittet et al, 1994a).

Risk factors for *Candida* bloodstream infections may also differ by species. For example, although central venous catheters and hyperalimentation have been associated with increased risk for *Candida* bloodstream infections in general, they are particularly important for infections with *C. parapsilosis* (Solomon et al, 1984, 1986; Weems et al, 1987a). This association may be due to the propensity of this species to proliferate in high concentrations of glucose and lipids and to adhere to prosthetic devices (Weems, 1992). Risk factors also differ by patient population. A recent subanalysis of data from the NEMIS study examined risk factors for *Candida* bloodstream infections among infants in neonatal intensive care units (Saiman et al, 2000), and found that, in addition to some common risk factors (such as central venous catheters, parenteral nutrition and shock), other factors, including low gestational age, H2 blockers, and low Apgar scores were also associated with increased risk of infection.

OUTBREAK INVESTIGATIONS

Outbreak investigations are an important and challenging component of public health practice. Careful investigation of outbreaks has increased our understanding of fungal diseases, their sources and modes of transmission, and risk factors for infection, and in so doing has assisted in the design of improved control measures for these infections. Investigations of hospital-based outbreaks of aspergillosis and candidiasis have led to the development of more effective strategies for prevention and control of these infections in hospitals. Investigations of outbreaks have also provided much useful information about the transmission and risk factors for the endemic fungal infections, such as histoplasmosis, blastomycosis, and coccidioidomycosis, thus helping to reduce the overall burden of these diseases.

Outbreak investigations are usually necessary in order to prevent others from being infected (if the outbreak is ongoing) or to prevent similar outbreaks in the future. Investigating an outbreak consists of multiple steps, including first confirming that the outbreak is real, deciding on a case definition, defining the size of the outbreak, generating and testing hypotheses for the reasons and source (s) behind the outbreak, conducting an environmental investigation, and implementing control measures (Reingold, 1998).

Investigations of outbreaks of fungal diseases can present major challenges. These include limited sample size, difficulties with the case definition, exposures that are ubiquitous or too restricted, and the fact that molecular subtyping methodologies for fungi are often unavailable or less than ideal. In many outbreaks, the number of cases is limited and, therefore, the statistical power of the investigation is limited, making it difficult to identify the source of the infection (by detecting significant differences in exposure between cases and controls). If, as is often the case with outbreaks of fungal infection, detection of the outbreak is delayed, important clinical and environmental samples may be difficult to obtain.

Once it is clear that a suspected outbreak is not the result of laboratory error (e.g., due to specimen contamination) (Laurel et al, 1999), the next step is to establish whether the observed number of cases is in excess of the usual number (i.e., that an outbreak has occurred), and to find all the cases in a given population over a certain period. A knowledge of the background rate of a disease either in the hospital or in the community is essential. For fungal diseases, establishing the background rate in a hospital can be done by reviewing the preexisting surveillance data if available, or by reviewing other records, such as laboratory summaries, pathology results, or hospital discharge records. In the community, baseline rates of disease can sometimes be determined by consulting with local health departments. This approach may be more difficult for diseases like the endemic mycoses since reporting is often incomplete. Among other factors, changes in the population at risk can affect the background rate of a disease. For example, an increase in the number of patients undergoing HSCT, or a change in the proportion undergoing bronchoscopy for diagnosis, may result in an increase in the number of cases of aspergillosis in a particular hospital unit. Therefore, it is always important to calculate rates of disease when an outbreak is suspected, rather than relying only on the number of cases.

In some outbreaks, formulating the case definition and exclusion criteria is straightforward; in others, the case definition and exclusion criteria are complex, particularly if the disease is new or if the range of clinical manifestations is very broad. In many investigations of outbreaks of fungal infection (e.g., aspergillosis), multiple case definitions are needed (e.g., laboratory-confirmed case, clinical case, proven case, probable case, possible case) and the resulting data are analyzed by using different case definitions.

By collecting detailed patient data, case-finding provides important information about the descriptive epidemiologic features of an outbreak. By reviewing the times of onset of the cases, and by examining the characteristics (e.g., age, sex, residence, occupation, recent travel) of those affected, epidemiologists can often generate hypotheses about the cause and source of the outbreak. For example, careful investigation of a large outbreak of blastomycosis in Wisconsin during 1984 enabled the incubation period for the infection to be determined, and the risk factors for human disease to be identified, as well as leading to a much clearer understanding of the natural habitat of the fungus and the sources of human infection (Klein et al, 1986). Likewise, bird roosts and bat guano have been clearly implicated in outbreaks of histoplasmosis (Sarosi et al, 1971), and archaeological digs and construction work in endemic regions are among the factors that have been implicated in outbreaks of coccidioidomycosis (Werner et al, 1972; Cairns et al, 2000). It is notable that, for those fungal infections that have never been associated with outbreaks (e.g., cryptococcosis), information about the precise source(s) of human infection and the incubation period remains very limited. Once hypotheses explaining the occurrence of an outbreak are generated, an analytic epidemiologic study to test these hypotheses is usually the next step. In many instances, a case-control study is used, but in others a retrospective cohort or cross-sectional study may be more appropriate.

Environmental specimens can support epidemiologic findings. However, these need to be collected as soon as possible, either before they are no longer available, as in the case of contaminated parenteral nutrition fluids, etc., or before environmental interventions are implemented, as in the case of repairing a malfunctioning air-filtration unit. Finding or not finding the causative organism in environmental samples is often perceived as powerful evidence implicating or exonerating an environmental source; however, both positive and negative findings can be misleading. For example, finding a ubiquitous organism such as *Aspergillus fumigatus* in an item of hospital food does not prove that the food (rather than some other source) is responsible for an outbreak of aspergillosis. Likewise, not finding the causative organism in an environmental sample does not conclusively rule out a source as the cause of the problem. This is especially true for difficult-to-culture organisms, such as *Blastomyces dermatitidis*.

Central to any outbreak investigation is the implementation of appropriate control measures to minimize further illness and death. For example, although most cases of *Candida* bloodstream infections are endogenous in origin, investigation of outbreaks in neonatal and surgical intensive care units has demonstrated that carriage of organisms on the hands of health-care providers is a common cause of transmission in hospitals (Burnie et al, 1985; Finkelstein et al, 1993). In turn, this finding has facilitated the development of rational preventive measures, such as rigorous hand washing before and between all patient contacts in units dealing with high-risk patients. Investigation of hospital-based outbreaks of *Aspergillus* infection has also contributed to the development of measures for the control and prevention of this devastating disease.

Finally, outbreak investigations have provided much useful information that has enabled prevention guidelines to be formulated (see PREVENTION). In addition, outbreak investigations have offered excellent opportunities to develop new molecular sub-typing methods, and to evaluate and validate existing ones.

PREVENTION

Developing effective prevention measures for fungal infections is the ultimate goal of all epidemiologic studies. However, unlike other diseases of public health importance, prevention of fungal diseases has proved to be difficult for many reasons. These include the nature of the population at risk (many of whom are hospitalized immunocompromised patients) because only a few risk factors are preventable or potentially modifiable. In addition, the ubiquitous occurrence of many opportunistic molds in the environment, and the ecology of others, such as the endemic pathogens *Histoplasma capsulatum* and *Coccidioides immitis*, makes it difficult to prevent exposure. Prevention of fungal diseases to date has focused on two areas: environmental control measures, either in the community or in the health-care environment, and antifungal drug chemoprophylaxis.

With the continuing increase in the number of immunocompromised patients, the prevention of opportunistic fungal infections, such as aspergillosis, has become an issue of major importance in the management of all at-risk groups. Environmental control measures, designed to protect high-risk patients from exposure to mold spores at home or in the hospital, are difficult. Housing these individuals in rooms supplied with HEPA-filtered air has helped to prevent the acquisition of *Aspergillus* infection within the hospital (Sherertz et al, 1987; Barnes and Rogers, 1989). The CDC, in collaboration with the Hospital Infection Control Practices Advisory Committee (HICPAC), has published guidelines for prevention of aspergillosis in the hospital environment (Centers for Disease Control and Prevention, 1997b), describing all these environmental measures. These guidelines are currently being updated and can be obtained from the following Web site: http://www.cdc.gov/ncidod/hip/pneumonia/pneu_mmw.htm.

In the case of *Candida* bloodstream infections, evidence from outbreak investigations has implicated carriage of organisms on the hands of health-care providers as a major cause of transmission in hospitals. As a result, guidelines have been developed by the CDC and the Association for Professionals in Infection Control and Epidemiology (APIC) (http://www.cdc.gov/ncidod/hip/guide/handwash_pre.htm) to enforce rigorous hand washing before and between all patient contacts, especially when dealing with high-risk patients.

Guidelines have also been developed for protection against some community-acquired infections in special risk groups. Examples include prevention of histoplasmosis among workers (Lenhart et al, 1997; http://www.cdc.gov/niosh/tc97146.html), and prevention of opportunistic fungal infections in persons with AIDS, developed in collaboration with the Infectious Diseases Society of America (Centers for Disease Control, 2002; http://www.cdc.gov/mmwr/preview/mmwrhtml/rr5108a1.htm).

Currently, prophylactic regimens with fluconazole are only recommended for use among selected leukemia or bone marrow transplant patients (Goodman et al, 1992; Rex et al, 2000). However, fluconazole chemoprophylaxis also appears to be effective in some critically ill, nonneutropenic patients. A recent study found prophylaxis with fluconazole (400 mg/d) to be effective in selected patients, such as those with recurrent gastrointestinal perforations or anastomotic leakages (Eggiman et al, 1999). Another study found that a similar regimen of fluconazole prophylaxis decreased the incidence of fungal infections in high-risk patients in surgical intensive care units (Pelz et al, 2001). These patients, however, tended to be older and had a higher incidence of recent surgeries and chronic conditions, such as diabetes and liver dysfunction.

Chemoprophylaxis has been employed to prevent invasive aspergillosis, but few large comparative trials have been conducted and its usefulness remains controversial (Warnock et al, 2001). The results of three large randomized, controlled trials of itraconazole as prophylaxis in patients receiving chemotherapy or HSCT for hematologic malignancies have recently been published (Menichetti et al, 1999; Morgenstern et al, 1999; Harousseau et al, 2000). Because the efficacy of prophylaxis against invasive aspergillosis has not been clearly established, chemoprophylaxis of all immunocompromised patients does not appear to be justified. The high incidence of infection, coupled with a high mortality rate, supports the use of prophylaxis against invasive aspergillosis in allogeneic HSCT recipients, as well as in liver and lung transplant recipients (Singh, 2000). Given the much lower incidence of the disease in autologous HSCT recipients and other solid organ transplant recipients, routine antifungal prophylaxis may not be indicated. Other promising therapeutic approaches that deserve further evaluation include specific strategies designed to boost the immunological response of the host.

Since chemoprophylaxis may be associated with development of antifungal drug resistance, as well as with side effects related to drug toxicity, clinicians should be careful about extending such measures to other critically ill patients in intensive care units, unless further studies identify additional risk factors that better define patients who might benefit from such an approach.

REFERENCES

Ampel N A, Mosley D G, England B E, Vertz D P, Komatsu K, Hajjeh R A. Coccidioidomycosis in Arizona: increase in incidence from 1990–95. *Clin Infect Dis* 27:1528–1530, 1998.

Anaissie E J, Costa S F. Nosocomial aspergillosis is waterborne. *Clin Infect Dis* 33: 1546–1548, 2001.

Anaissie E J, Stratton S L, Dignani M C, Summerbell R C, Rex J H, Monson T P, Spencer T, Kasai M, Francesconi A, Walsh T J. Pathogenic *Aspergillus* species recovered from a hospital water system: a 3-year prospective study. *Clin Infect Dis* 34:780–789, 2002.

Arnow P M, Anderson R I, Mainous P D, Smith E J. Pulmonary aspergillosis during hospital renovation. *Am Rev Respir Dis* 118: 49–53, 1978.

Arvanitidou M, Kanellou K, Constantinides T C, Katsouyannopoulos V. The occurrence of fungi in hospital and community potable waters. *Lett Appl Microbiol* 29:81–84, 1999.

Banerjee S N, Emori T G, Culver D H, Gaynes R P, Jarvis W R, Horan T, Edwards J R, Tolson J, Henderson T, Martone W J. Secular trends in nosocomial primary bloodstream infections in the United States, 1980–1989. National Nosocomial Infections Surveillance System. *Am J Med* 91:86S–89S, 1991.

Barnes R A, Rogers T R. Control of an outbreak of nosocomial aspergillosis by laminar air-flow isolation. *J Hosp Infect* 14:89–94, 1989.

Beck-Sague C, Jarvis W R. Secular trends in the epidemiology of nosocomial fungal infections in the United States, 1980–1990. *J Infect Dis* 167:247–1251, 1993.

Benoit D, Decruyenaere J, Vandewoude K, Roosens C, Hoste E, Poelaert J, Vermassen F, Colardyn F. Management of candidal thrombophlebitis of the central veins: case report and review. *Clin Infect Dis* 26:393–397, 1998.

Burnie J P, Odds F C, Lee W, Webster C, Williams J D. Outbreak of systemic *Candida albicans* in an intensive care unit caused by cross infection. *BMJ* 290:746–748, 1985.

Cairns L, Blythe D, Kao A, Pappagianis D, Kaufman L, Kobayashi J, Hajjeh R. Outbreak of coccidioidomycosis in Washington State residents returning from Mexico. *Clin Infect Dis* 30:61–64, 2000.

Cano M, Hajjeh R A. The epidemiology of histoplasmosis, a review. *Semin Respir Infect* 16:109–118, 2001.

Centers for Disease Control and Prevention. Case Definitions for Infectious Conditions under Public Health Surveillance. *MMWR* 46:(No.RR-10), 1997a.

Centers for Disease Control and Prevention. Guidelines for Prevention of Nosocomial Pneumonia. *MMWR* 46 (No. RR-01), 1997b.

Centers for Disease Control and Prevention. Guidelines for Preventing Opportunistic Infections Among HIV-Infected Persons: Recommendations of the U.S. Public Health Service and the Infectious Diseases Society of America. *MMWR* 51:(No. RR-08), 2002.

Cornet M, Levy V, Fleury L, Lortholary J, Barquins S, Coureul M H, Deliere E, Zittoun R, Brucker G, Bouvet A. Efficacy of prevention by high-efficiency particulate air filtration or laminar airflow against Aspergillus airborne contamination during hospital renovation. *Infect Control Hosp Epidemiol* 20:508–513, 1999.

Eggimann P, Francioli P, Bille J, Schneider R, Wu M M, Chapuis G, Chiolero R, Pannatier A, Schilling J, Geroulanos S, Glauser M P, Calandra T. Fluconazole prophylaxis prevents intra-abdominal candidiasis in high-risk surgical patients *Crit Care Med* 27:1066–1072, 1999.

Emori T G, Gaynes R P. An overview of nosocomial infections, including the role of the microbiology laboratory. *Clin Microbiol Rev* 6:428–442, 1993.

Finkelstein R, Reinhartz G, Hashman N, Merzbach D. Outbreak of *Candida tropicalis* fungemia in a neonatal intensive care unit. *Infect Control Hosp Epidemiol* 14: 587–590, 1993.

Goodman J L, Winston D J, Greenfield R A, Chandrasekar P H, Fox B, Kaizer H, Shadduck R K, Shea T C, Stiff P, Friedman D J, Powderly W G, Silber J L, Horowitz H, Lichtin A, Wolff S N, Mangan S F, Silver S M, Weisdorf D, Ho W G, Gilbert G, Buell D. A controlled trial of fluconazole to prevent fungal infections in patients undergoing bone marrow transplantation *N Eng J Med* 326: 845–851, 1992.

Hajjeh R A, Conn L A, Stephens D S, Baughman W, Hamil R, Graviss E, Pappas P G, Thomas C, Reingold A, Rothrock G, Hutwagner

L C, Schuchat A, Brandt M E, Pinner R W. Cryptococcosis in the United States: population-based multistate active surveillance and risk factors in HIV-infected persons. *J Infect Dis* 179: 449–454, 1999.

Hajjeh R A, Sofair A, Harrison L. Fluconazole resistance among Candida bloodstream isolates: incidence and correlation with outcome from a population-based study. Abstracts of the 39th Annual Meeting of the Infectious Diseases Society of America. San Francisco, CA. Abstract 641, 2001.

Hajjeh R A, Warnock D W. Invasive aspergillosis and the environment: rethinking our approach to prevention. *Clin Infect Dis* 33:1549–1552, 2001.

Harousseau J L, Dekker A W, Stamatoullas-Bastard A, Fassa A, Linkesch W, Gouvia J, Bock R D, Rovira M, Seifert W, Joosen H, Peeters M, Beule K D. Itraconazole oral solution for primary prophylaxis of fungal infections in patients with hematological malignancy and profound neutropenia: a randomized double-blind, double-placebo, multicenter trial comparing itraconazole and amphotericin B. *Antimicrob Agents Chemother* 44:1887–1893, 2000.

Kao A S, Brandt M E, Pruitt W R, Conn L A, Perkins B, Stephens D S, Baughman W S, Reingold A L, Rothrock G A, Pfaller M, Pinner R W, Hajjeh R A. The epidemiology of candidemia in 2 U.S. cities: results of a population-based active surveillance. *Clin Infect Dis* 29:1164–1170, 1999.

Klein B S, Vergeront J M, Weeks R J, Kumar U N, Matha G, Varkey B, Kaufman L, Bradsher R W, Stoebig J F, Davis J P. Isolation of *Blastomyces dermatitidis* in soil associated with a large outbreak of blastomycosis in Wisconsin. *N Engl J Med* 314:529–534, 1986.

Krasinski K, Holzman RS, Hanna B, Greco M A, Graff M, Bhogal M. Nosocomial fungal infection during hospital renovation. *Infect Control* 6:278–282, 1985.

Krause W, Matheis H, Wulf K. Fungaemia and funguria after oral administration of *Candida albicans*. Lancet 1:598–599, 1969.

Laurel VL, Meier PA, Astorga A, Dolan D, Brockett R, Rinaldi MG. Pseudoepidemic of *Aspergillus niger* infections traced to specimen contamination in the microbiology laboratory. J Clin Microbiol 37: 1612–1616, 1999.

Lenhart SW, Schafer MP, Singal M, Hajjeh RA. Histoplasmosis: protecting workers at risk. DHHS (NIOSH) Publication No. 97–146. National Institute for Occupational safety and Health, Cincinnati, Ohio, 1997.

Marr KA, Seidel K, White TC, Bowden RA. Candidemia in allogeneic blood and marrow transplant recipients: evolution of risk factors after the adoption of prophylactic fluconazole. *J Infect Dis* 181:309–316, 2000.

McNeil MM, Nash SL, Hajjeh RA, Phelan M A, Conn L A, Plikaytis B D, Warnock D W. Trends in mortality due to invasive mycotic diseases in the United States, 1980–1997. *Clin Infect Dis* 33: 641–647, 2001.

Menichetti F, Del Favero A, Martino P, Bucaneve G, Micozzi A, Girmenia C, Barbabietola G, Pagano L, Leoni P, Specchia G, Caiozzo A, Raimondi R, Mandelli F, and the GIMEMA Infection Program. Itraconazole oral solution as prophylaxis for fungal infections in neutropenic patients with hematologic malignancies: a randomized, placebo-controlled, double-blind, multicenter trial. *Clin Infect Dis* 28:250–255, 1999.

Morgenstern G R, Prentice A G, Prentice H G, Ropner J, Schey S, Warnock D. A randomized controlled trial of itraconazole versus fluconazole for the prevention of fungal infections in patients with haematological malignancies. *Br J Haematol* 105:901–911, 1999.

Nucci M, Anaissie E. Revisiting the source of candidemia: skin or gut? *Clin Infect Dis* 33:1959–1967, 2001.

Nucci M, Anaissie E. Should vascular catheters be removed from all patients with candidemia? An evidence-based review. *Clin Infect Dis* 34:591–599, 2002.

Odds FC. Candida and candidosis. Bailliere Tindall, London, 1988.

Patterson J E, Zidouh A, Miniter P, Andriole V T, Patterson T F. Hospital epidemiologic surveillance for invasive aspergillosis: patient demographics and the utility of antigen detection. *Infect Control Hosp Epidemiol* 18:104–108, 1997.

Pelz R K, Hendrix C W, Swoboda S M, Merz W G, Lipsett P A. A double-blind placebo controlled trial of prophylactic fluconazole to prevent Candida infections in critically ill surgical patients. *Ann Surg* 233:542–548, 2001.

Pfaller M A, Jones R N, Doern G V, Sader H S, Hollis R J, Messer S A. International surveillance of bloodstream infections due to *Candida* species: frequency of occurrence and antifungal susceptibilities of isolates collected in 1997 in the United States, Canada, and South America for the SENTRY Program. The Sentry Participant Group. *J Clin Microbiol* 36:1886–1889, 1998a.

Pfaller M A, Jones R N, Messer S A, Edmond M B, Wenzel R P. National surveillance of nosocomial blood stream infection due to *Candida albicans*: frequency of occurrence and antifungal susceptibility in the SCOPE Program. *Diagn Microbiol Infect Dis* 31:327–332, 1998b.

Pfaller M A, Messer S A, Houston A, Rangel-Frausto M S, Wiblin T, Blumberg H M, Edwards J E, Jarvis W, Martin M A, Neu H C, Saiman L, Patterson J E, Dibb J C, Roldan D M, Rinaldi M G, Wenzel R P. National epidemiology of mycoses survey: a multicenter study of strain variation and antifungal susceptibility among isolates of *Candida* species. *Diagn Microbiol Infect Dis* 31:289–296, 1998c.

Pfaller M A, Jones R N, Doern GV, Sader H S, Messer S A, Houston A, Coffman S, Hollis R J. Bloodstream infections due to *Candida* species: SENTRY antimicrobial surveillance program in North America and Latin America, 1997–1998. *Antimicrob Agents Chemother* 44:747–751, 2000.

Pfaller M A, Diekema D J, Jones R N, Messer S A, Hollis R J, and the SENTRY Participants Group. Trends in antifungal susceptibility of *Candida* spp. isolated from pediatric and adult patients with bloodstream infections: SENTRY antimicrobial surveillance program, 1997 to 2000. *J Clin Microbiol* 40:852–856, 2002.

Pinner R W, Teutsch S M, Simonsen L, Klug L A, Graber J M, Clarke M J, Berkelman R L. Trends in infectious diseases mortality in the Unites States. *JAMA* 275: 189–193, 1996.

Pittet D, Monod M, Suter P M, Frenk E, Auckenthaler R. Candida colonization and subsequent infections in critically ill surgical patients. *Ann Surg* 220:751–758, 1994a.

Pittet D, Tarara D, Wenzel R P. Nosocomial bloodstream infection in critically ill patients. Excess length of stay, extra costs, and attributable mortality. *JAMA* 271: 1598–1601, 1994b.

Rangel-Frausto M S, Wiblin T, Blumberg H M, Saiman L, Patterson J, Rinaldi M, Pfaller M, Edwards J E, Jarvis W, Dawson J, Wenzel R P, and the NEMIS Study Group. National epidemiology of mycoses survey (NEMIS): variations in rates of bloodstream infections due to *Candida* species in seven surgical intensive care units and six neonatal intensive care units. *Clin Infect Dis* 29:253–258, 1999.

Rees J R, Pinner R W, Hajjeh R A, Brandt M E, Reingold A L. The epidemiologic features of invasive mycotic infections in the San Francisco Bay Area 1992–1993: results of population-based laboratory active surveillance. *Clin Infect Dis* 27: 1138–1147, 1998.

Reingold, A L. Outbreak investigations—a perspective. *Emerg Infect Dis* 4:21–7, 1998.

Rex J H, Walsh T J, Sobel J D, Filler S, Pappas P, Dismukes W, Edwards J. Practice guidelines for the treatment of candidiasis. Infectious Diseases Society of America. *Clin Infect Dis* 30:662–678, 2000.

Rhame F S. Prevention of nosocomial aspergillosis. *J Hosp Infect* 18 (suppl A):466–472, 1991.

Saiman L, Ludington E, Pfaller M, Rangel-Frausto S, Wiblin R, Dawson J, Blumberg H, Patterson J, Rinaldi M, Edwards J, Wenzel R, Jarvis W. Risk factors for candidemia in neonatal intensive care unit patients. The National Epidemiology of Mycosis Survey study group. *Pediatr Infect Dis J* 19: 319–324, 2000.

Sarosi G A, Parker J D, Tosh F E. Histoplasmosis outbreaks: their patterns. In: Ajello L, Chick EW, Furcolow ML, eds. Histoplasmosis. Proceedings of the Second National Conference. Springfield, Illinois: Charles C Thomas, 123–128, 1971.

Sherertz R J, Belani A, Kramer B S, Elfenbein G J, Weiner R S, Sullivan M L, Thomas R G, Samsa G P. Impact of air filtration on nosocomial aspergillus infections. Unique risk of bone marrow transplant recipients. *Am J Med* 83:709–718, 1987.

Simonsen L, Conn L A, Pinner R W, Teutsch S. Trends in infectious disease hospitalizations in the United States, 1980–1994. *Arch Intern Med* 158: 1923–1928, 1998.

Singh N: Antifungal prophylaxis for solid organ transplant recipients: seeking clarity amidst controversy. *Clin Infect Dis* 31: 545–553, 2000.

Solomon S L, Alexander H, Eley J W, Anderson R L, Goodpasture H C, Smart S, Furman R M, Martone W J. Nosocomial fungemia in neonates associated with intravascular pressure-monitoring devices. *Pediatr Infect Dis* 5:680–685, 1986.

Solomon S L, Khabbaz R F, Parker R H, Anderson R L, Geraghty A, Furman R M, Martone W J. An outbreak of *Candida parapsilosis* bloodstream infections in patients receiving parenteral nutrition. *J Infect Dis* 149:98–102, 1984.

Trick W E, Fridkin S K, Edwards J R, Hajjeh R A, Gaynes R P, and the National Nosocomial Infections Surveillance system hospitals. Secular trend of hospital-acquired candidemia among intensive care unit patients in the United States during 1989–1999. *Clin Infect Dis* 35: 627–630, 2002.

Warnock D W, Hajjeh R A, Lasker B A. Epidemiology and prevention of invasive aspergillosis. *Curr Infect Dis Rep* 3:507–516, 2001.

Warris A, Voss A, Abrahamsen T G, Verweij P E. Contamination of hospital water with *Aspergillus fumigatus* and other molds. *Clin Infect Dis* 34:1159–1160, 2002.

Weems J J Jr. *Candida parapsilosis*: epidemiology, pathogenicity, clinical manifestations, and antimicrobial susceptibility. *Clin Infect Dis* 14:756–766, 1992.

Weems J J Jr, Chamberland M E, Ward J, Willy M, Padhye A A, Solomon S L. *Candida parapsilosis* fungemia associated with parenteral nutrition and contaminated blood pressure transducers. *J Clin Microbiol* 25:1029–1032, 1987a.

Weems J J, Davis B J, Tablan O C, Kaufman L, Martone W J. Construction activity: an independent risk factor for invasive aspergillosis and zygomycosis in patients with hematologic malignancy. *Infect Control* 8:71–75, 1987b.

Werner S B, Pappagianis D, Heindl I, Mickel A. An epidemic of coccidioidomycosis among archeology students in northern California. *N Engl J Med* 286:507–512, 1972.

Wey S B, Mori M, Pfaller M A, Woolson R F, Wenzel R P. Hospital-acquired candidemia. The attributable mortality and excess length of stay. *Arch Intern Med* 148:2642–2645, 1988.

II

SYSTEMIC ANTIFUNGAL DRUGS

3

Amphotericin B

STANLEY W. CHAPMAN, JOHN D. CLEARY, AND P. DAVID ROGERS

Amphotericin B has been the cornerstone of antifungal therapy for almost 50 years. Discovered in the late 1950s, it was approved for human use as an antimycotic in 1960. Initial formulations of amphotericin B were plagued with impurities. Allergic responses, presumably secondary to these impurities, and endotoxinlike infusion-related reactions were common. Although improvements in purification and fermentation over the last 30 years have enhanced tolerability, infusion-related reactions and renal dysfunction are still commonplace with the use of the deoxycholate solubilized formulation. Formulations using a lipid carrier have significantly improved tolerability. Safety aside, amphotericin B remains the most effective, broad-spectrum, fungicidal agent with the greatest experience for the treatment of systemic mycoses. Both intrinsic and acquired resistance are limited. The treatment failures seen with amphotericin B are multifaceted. These can be attributed to delays in diagnosis of invasive mycoses, the immune compromised state of the patient being treated, the unique pharmacokinetic/pharmacodynamic properties of the different formulations, and dose limitations related to toxicity. In an effort to enhance antifungal efficacy and reduce toxicity, amphotericin B has been combined with other agents (e.g., flucytosine, azoles, and terbinafine) with promising results. It is the authors' opinion that combination therapy will be used increasingly for the treatment of systemic mycoses.

This chapter discusses amphotericin B deoxycholate and the lipid preparations of amphotericin separately. Where appropriate we compare and contrast these different formulations with an emphasis on unique pharmacologic properties or clinically relevant differences in toxicity or outcome that favor one preparation over another. Table 3–1 presents a summary of the indications, chemistry, pharmacology, efficacy, and toxicities of each of these formulations.

AMPHOTERICIN B DEOXYCHOLATE

Chemistry

Amphotericin B is a polyene antifungal that, along with amphotericin A, is produced by the soil actinomycete *Streptomyces nodosus*. The amphotericin B molecule is a heptaene macrolide consisting of seven conjugated double bonds within the main ring, a connecting mycosamine through a glycoside side chain, and a connecting free carboxyl group (Fig. 3–1). Amphotericin B is relatively insoluble in water and derives its name from its amphoteric property to form methanol soluble salts under both basic and acidic conditions (Gallis et al, 1990; Lyman and Walsh, 1992).

Amphotericin B is available as an intravenous preparation formulated by combination with sodium deoxycholate, which results in formation of a micellar dispersion upon reconstitution in 5% dextrose or water (Gallis et al, 1990; Patel, 1998). Alternative formulations of amphotericin B have been devised in an effort to improve the therapeutic index of this agent. A water-soluble methyl ester preparation showed promise initially as higher doses of the drug could be administered without associated nephrotoxicity. Unfortunately several patients developed leukoencephalopathy in clinical trials and the product was abandoned (Schmitt, 1993).

Recently three lipid-based preparations of amphotericin B have been developed. Despite their significant cost, many institutions preferentially utilize these formulations owing to reduced adverse reactions. These amphotericin B lipid preparations are discussed in detail later in this chapter under LIPID PREPARATIONS OF AMPHOTERICIN B.

Mechanisms of Action

The primary antifungal activity of amphotericin B is mediated by its preferential binding to ergosterol in the fungal cell membrane. This interaction results in the formation of pores consisting of eight amphotericin B molecules in the membrane, allowing leakage of potassium and other cellular components that ultimately leads to cell death (Brajtburg et al, 1990). Although amphotericin B has a greater affinity for the fungal ergosterol, it still has some affinity for binding to the cholesterol of mammalian cell membranes. The latter probably plays an important role in its associated toxicity (Abu-Salah, 1996).

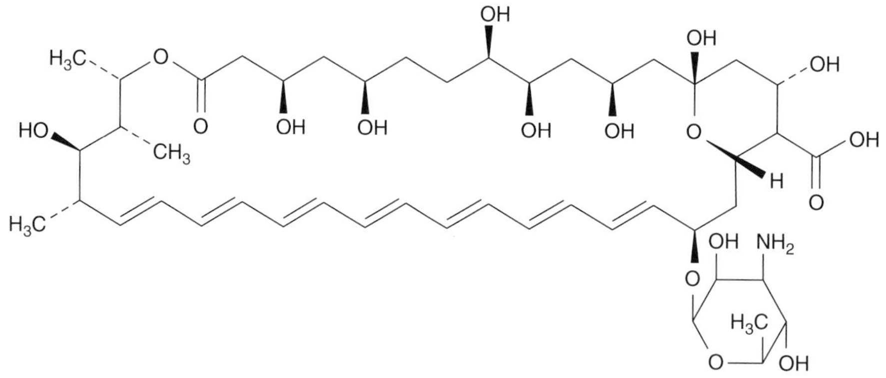

FIGURE 3–1. Amphotericin B polyene structure. The molecular formula of the drug is $C_{47}H_{73}NO_{17}$; its molecular weight is 924.10.

There is also evidence to suggest that amphotericin B-mediated cell killing may be due in part to the oxidizing properties of the drug that results in the production of reactive oxygen species and lipid peroxidation of fungal cell membrane (Brajtburg et al, 1990). In support of oxidative cell injury, Sokol-Anderson and colleagues have shown that amphotericin B-mediated lysis of *C. albicans* protoplasts and whole cells is reduced, independent of potassium leakage, in the absence of oxygen and in the presence of exogenous catalase and superoxide dismutase (Sokol-Anderson et al, 1986). The presence of seven conjugated double bonds in the chemical structure of amphotericin B renders it prone to auto-oxidation (Sokol-Anderson et al, 1986; Osaka et al, 1997), leading some investigators to speculate that amphotericin B may also act as an antioxidant, although clinical data to support this hypothesis are lacking. Finally, amphotericin B also has been shown to inhibit the respiration of actively metabolizing *Aspergillus fumigatus* (Sandhu, 1979).

Amphotericin B may indirectly modulate antifungal efficacy by its ability to alter immune function. The immunomodulatory effects of amphotericin B have been found to be diverse and contradictory. The reported differences in amphotericin B-induced immunomodulation may be the result of a number of factors including the concentration of drug, the in vitro conditions, or the animal model used. Amphotericin B has been shown to act as an immunoadjuvant by stimulating cell proliferation and cell mediated immunity in murine models (Bistoni et al, 1985). Amphotericin B has also been shown to enhance the phagocytic and antibacterial activity of macrophages and to increase colony-stimulating factor concentrations in mice (Lin et al, 1977). Chapman and coworkers found that amphotericin B enhances macrophage tumoricidal activity that was independent of its ionophoretic properties (Chapman and Hibbs, 1978). Amphotericin B induces production of IL-1β, TNF-α, and IL-1Rα in murine and human monocytes and macrophages (Gelfand et al, 1988; Chia

and Pollack, 1989; Cleary et al, 1992; Rogers et al, 1998), and increases nitric oxide synthesis in human monocytes (Mozaffarian et al, 1997). It has also been shown to increase both IL-12 and IFN-gamma levels in mice with gastrointestinal or systemic *Candida* infection (Cenci et al, 1997).

In contrast, amphotericin B has been shown to inhibit the chemotactic responsiveness, phagocytic capacity, and killing by human neutrophils (Bjorksten et al, 1976; Marmer et al, 1981). Inhibition of both spontaneous and antigen-induced transformation, as well as antibody-dependent cellular toxicity of human lymphocytes has been reported with amphotericin B (Roselle and Kauffman, 1978; Nair and Schwartz, 1982). It has also been reported to diminish hPBMC and T-cell responses to phytohemagglutinin (Stewart et al, 1981) and to impair NK cell activity (Nair and Schwartz, 1982; Hauser and Remington, 1983).

Taken collectively, these data suggest that amphotericin B exerts its direct antifungal activity through three mechanisms of action: pore formation, oxidative damage, and inhibition of metabolic activity. While the direct antifungal activity of amphotericin B has been extensively validated, the in vivo role of its immunomodulatory properties has not been sufficiently defined.

Spectrum of Activity

Amphotericin B is active against most of the common yeasts, moulds, and dimorphic fungi causing human infection including: *Candida* species, *Cryptococcus neoformans*, *Blastomyces dermatitidis*, *Histoplasma capsulatum*, *Coccidioides immitis*, *Paracoccidioides brasiliensis*, *Sporothrix schenckii*, *Aspergillus* species, and the agents of mucormycosis. This polyene also has some degree of activity against the protozoa *Leishmania brasiliensis*, and *Naegleria fowleri* (Gallis et al, 1990; Patel, 1998).

Relatively few organisms manifest intrinsic resistance to amphotericin B. *Scedosporium apiospermum*

(*Pseudallescheria boydii*), *Candida lusitaniae*, *Candida guilliermondii*, *Scopulariopsis* species, and *Fusarium* species generally are considered intrinsically resistant to amphotericin B (Speeleveld et al, 1996; Patel, 1998). Acquired resistance to amphotericin B, whether through selective laboratory techniques or after clinical usage, appears to be uncommon. Recently, however, resistant isolates of *C. albicans*, *C. glabrata*, *C. tropicalis*, and *Cryptococcus neoformans* have been isolated from patients with AIDS (Powderly et al, 1992; Le et al, 1996; Kelly et al, 1997).

Studies of resistant clinical isolates of *C. albicans* and *C. neoformans* suggest that resistance occurs through alterations of the genes encoding $\alpha^{8,7}$-isomerase or $\alpha^{5,6}$-desaturase within the sterol biosynthesis pathway. These isolates accumulate alternative sterols, allowing the organism to evade the activity of amphotericin B (Georgopapadakou and Walsh, 1996; Le et al, 1996; Kelly et al, 1997). Others have suggested that resistance to amphotericin B in yeasts may occur through increased catalase activity, impairing amphotericin B-induced oxidative damage (Georgopapadakou and Walsh, 1996).

Susceptibility Testing

Routine susceptibility testing for amphotericin B is problematic. Interpretive break points that correlate in vitro activity with clinical outcomes are limited (Vanden Bossche et al, 1998; White et al, 1998a; Ghannoum and Rice, 1999). The use of in vitro susceptibility studies is further complicated owing to the variable results seen for many different technical reasons (i.e., media, temperature, pH, cation content etc). The recent efforts of the National Committee of Clinical Laboratory Standards (NCCLS) have been instrumental in the development of standardized methodology for antifungal susceptibility testing. Despite these improvements, the routine use of susceptibility testing of clinical isolates to amphotericin B is not recommended. Susceptibility testing of clinical isolates may be helpful for patients who are failing amphotericin B. For example, clinical failure using amphotericin B to treat serious candidal and cryptococcal infections has been associated with MICs of ≥ 1.0 ug/ml (Powderly et al, 1988; Powderly et al, 1992). It should be noted, however, that clinical failure in amphotericin-treated patients is not necessarily indicative of fungal resistance, but is often related to the underlying immunodeficiency of the patient. Susceptibility testing may also be clinically useful in guiding treatment of rare pathogens where resistance is likely or unpredictable. When patient samples can be processed in a clinically relevant time frame and stronger clinical correlations are developed, routine susceptibility testing will need to be reevaluated. For a more complete discussion, see Chapter 1.

Pharmacology and Pharmacokinetics (Table 3–1)

Amphotericin B is poorly absorbed after oral administration (less than 5%), hence the requirement of an intravenous formulation for the treatment of systemic mycoses. Following an intravenous infusion, amphotericin B is bound primarily to lipoproteins, cholesterol, and erythrocytes. Peak serum concentrations of approximately 1–3 ug/mL are achieved during the first hour following a 4 to 6–hour amphotericin B infusion at a dose of 0.6 mg/kg. Serum concentrations rapidly fall to a prolonged plateau phase with measured amphotericin B concentrations of 0.2–0.5 ug/mL. Following an initial half-life of 24–48 hours, there is a terminal elimination half-life of approximately 15 days. This terminal elimination phase most likely represents the slow release of amphotericin B from the tissues (Table 3–1).

Amphotericin B is distributed to many tissues including the lungs, spleen, liver, and kidneys (Collette et al, 1989). The volume of distribution is 4 liters/kg and appears to follow a three-compartment model of distribution. Amphotericin B, however, does not distribute into adipose tissue, supporting the premise that dosage should be based on lean body mass. Unfortunately, the measurement of lean body mass is not always practical. Hence dosing of amphotericin B in obese patients should be based on calculated ideal body weight. Amphotericin B is bound extensively in tissues and can be detected in the liver, spleen, and kidney for months after treatment has been terminated (Christiansen et al, 1985). Despite this extensive and prolonged tissue binding, the relationship of serum vs. tissue concentration and clinical efficacy or toxicity has not been clearly established.

Amphotericin B concentrations in peritoneal, pleural, and synovial fluids are less than half of the simultaneous serum concentrations. Although clinical efficacy of amphotericin B has been repeatedly documented for the treatment of central nervous system fungal infections (e.g., cryptococcal meningitis), cerebrospinal fluid levels are low, usually less than 5% even in the presence of inflamed meninges. This enhanced clinical efficacy may reflect higher levels of amphotericin B in the meninges as compared to the cerebrospinal fluid that has been documented in animal models of meningitis (Gallis et al, 1990).

Despite almost 50 years of clinical experience, little is known about the metabolism of amphotericin B. No metabolites have yet been identified. Less than 5% of the administered dose is excreted in the urine and bile. Serum concentrations, as such, are not changed and accumulation of amphotericin B does not occur in patients with hepatic or renal failure. Likewise, hemodialysis or peritoneal dialysis does not influence serum levels (Bindschlader and Bennett, 1969; Atkin-

TABLE 3–1. *Amphotericin B Characteristics*

Category	Amphotericin B [AmB; Fungizone®] Apothecon	Amphotericin B Lipid Complex [ABLC; Abelcet] Enzon Inc.	Amphotericin B Colloidal Dispersion [ABCD; Amphotec®] InterMune Inc.	Liposomal Amphotericin B [LAmB; AmBisome®] Fujisawa Healthcare Inc.	Amphotericin B in Lipid Emulsion [ABLE] No Manufacturer
Primary Reference	Janknegt et al, 1992 Christiansen et al, 1985	Package Insert	Package Insert	Package Insert	Ayestaran et al, 1996 Villani et al, 1996
FDA Approved Indication	Life-threatening fungal infections Visceral leishmaniasis	Refractory/intolerant to AmB	Invasive aspergillosis in patients refractory/intolerant to AmB	Empirical therapy in neutropenic FUO Refractory/intolerant to AmB Visceral leishmaniasis	NA
Formulation	MICELLE	RIBBONS/SHEETS	LIPID DISK	UNILAMELLAR VESICLES	Safflower and Soybean Oils
Sterol	None	None	Cholesteryl Sulfate	Cholesterol Sulfate (5)*	10–20 g/100 mL
Phospholipid	None	DMPC & DMPG (7:3)*	None	EPC & DSPG (10:4)*	EPC > 2.21 g/100 mL Glycerin > 258 g/100 mL
Size (nm)	< 10	1600–11,000	122 (±48)	80–120	333–500
Stability	1 week at 2°C–8°C or 24 hours at 27°C	15 hours at 2°C–8°C or 6 hours at 27°C	24 hours at 2°C–8°C	24 hours at 2°C–8°C	Unstable
FDA Approved Dosage & Rate	0.3–1.0 mg/kg/day over 1–6 hours	5.0 mg/kg/day at 2.5 mg/kg/hour	3.0–6.0 mg/kg/day over 2 hours	3.0–5.0 mg/kg/day over 2 hours	Investigational: 1.0 mg/kg/day over 1–8 hours
Lethal Dose 50%	3.3 mg/kg	10–25 mg/kg	68 mg/kg	175 mg/kg	Unknown
Pharmacokinetic Dose Administered	0.5 mg/kg	5.0 mg/kg × 7 days	5.0 mg/kg × 7 days	5 mg/kg × 7 days	0.8 mg/kg/day × 13 days
Serum Concentrations					
Peak	1.2 μg/mL	1.7 μg/mL	3.1 μg/mL	83.0 μg/mL	2.13–2.83 μg/mL
Trough	0.5 μg/mL	0.7 μg/mL		4.0 μg/mL	0.42 μg/mL
Half-life (Beta)	91.1 hours	173.4 hours	28.5 hours	6.8 hours	7.75–15.23 hours
Area Under the Curve (0–24)	14 μg/mL · hour	17 μg/mL · hour	43.0 μg/mL · hour	555 μg/mL · hour	26.37–37 μg/mL · hour
Volume of Distribution	3–5.0 L/kg	131.0 L/kg	4.3 L/kg	0.10 L/kg	0.45–0.56 L/kg
Protein Binding (%)	< 10%	ND	ND	ND	ND
Adipose**	0.12 (ND)	ND	ND	ND	ND
Brain**	1.02 (0.3)	1.6 (ND)	ND	0.56 (0.1)	ND
CSF/Serum (%)	2–4 (40–90 in neonates)	9.7	ND	ND	ND
Heart**	1.73 (0.4)	5 (ND)	ND	4.3 (0.1)	ND
Kidney**	10.4–18.9 (0.8–1.5)	6.9 (ND)	ND	22.8 (0.3)	ND
Liver**	45.9–93.2 (26.2–27.5)	196 (ND)	ND	175.7 (18.3)	ND
Lung**	5.29–12.9 (3.1–3.2)	222 (ND)	ND	16.8 (0.6)	ND
Pancreas**	7.6 (0.2)	ND	ND	ND	ND
Spleen**	28.7–59.3 (1–5.2)	290 (ND)	ND	201.5	ND
Clearance	38.0 mL/hour/kg	436.0 mL/hour/kg	0.117 mL/hour/kg	11.0 mL/hour/kg	37.0 mL/hour/kg
Urine (%)	2%–5% in 24 hours				
Feces (%)	ND				

EPC, Egg phosphatidylcholine; DSPG, Distearolyphosphatidylglycerol; DMPC, Dimyristoyl phosphatidylcholine; DMPG, Dimyristoyl phosphatidyl glycerol; ND, not done.

* Molar ratio of each component, respectively.

** Amount in tissue (ug/g) then in parenthesis (%) of total dose.

son and Bennett, 1978; Daneshmend and Warnock, 1983; Gallis et al, 1990; Patel, 1998; Gussak et al, 2001).

Several pharmacokinetic parameters of amphotericin B are different in children as compared to adults (Starke et al, 1987; Benson and Nahata, 1989). For instance, children have a smaller volume of distribution and a larger clearance compared to adults. When equivalent weight-based doses of amphotericin B are administered, peak serum concentrations in children are approximately one-half of those obtained in adults. The increased clearance of amphotericin B in children may, in part, explain the clinical finding that higher doses are better tolerated in children as compared to adults. Despite the lower serum concentrations seen in children, cerebrospinal fluid concentrations of amphotericin B treated neonates are higher than those noted in adults.

Pharmacodynamics

Pharmacodynamics involves the integration of several pharmacologic measurements made in vitro (e.g., susceptibility studies, time-kill studies, dynamic models, viability, postantibiotic effect [PAE], etc.) and in vivo (drug concentrations, toxicity, efficacy, etc.). In bacteriology, several variables have been assigned quantitative limits that are predictive of therapeutic success and include the time that the serum drug concentration exceeds MIC [T > MIC]; the ratio of maximum serum drug concentration to MIC [C_{max}:MIC]; and the ratio of the area under the concentration–time curve during a 24-hour dosing period to MIC [AUC_{0-24}:MIC] (Gunderson et al, 2001). These parameters have proven useful in classifying antibiotics as either concentration-dependent or time-dependent in their bactericidal activity. These parameters have also been instrumental in selecting the optimal anti-infective treatment regimens for bacterial infections.

Pharmacodynamic parameters are less clearly defined for the antimycotic drugs. Amphotericin B has traditionally been portrayed as a concentration-dependent antifungal agent. Concentration-dependence is characterized by a long PAE and therapeutic success when the C_{max}:MIC ratio is high. Determination of C_{max}:MIC ratios of amphotericin B and their relationship to clinical outcome in human infections is incomplete. The lack of standardized antifungal susceptibility testing has also hindered studies exploring amphotericin B pharmacodynamics. The recent efforts of the NCCLS to standardize antifungal testing should facilitate future studies dealing with amphotericin B and other antifungals. Additional studies are required to evaluate the predictive value and clinical usefulness of these pharmacodynamic parameters in optimizing therapy of human infections.

Initial studies evaluating amphotericin B pharmacodynamic models in vitro and in vivo have been contradictory. For example the PAE of amphotericin B for *Candida* species was prolonged when studied in vivo. In a study of neutropenic mice infected with *Candida*, the antimycotic effects of amphotericin B were observed for 23–30 hours (Andes, 1999). In contrast, several in vitro studies have shown a shorter duration of antimycotic effect (0–10.6 hours) dependent on the MIC of the organism and the length of drug exposure (Carver, 1993; Turnidge et al, 1994; Ernst et al, 2000). The longer PAE noted in vivo might be due to the immunomodulatory properties of amphotericin B and/or the slow release of amphotericin from tissue. Also confounding pharmacodynamic studies is the issue dealing with determination of the PAE, which is the composite result of drug concentration at the site of infection, the MIC of the organism, and the density of organisms at the site of infection. Data on these important parameters affecting antimycotic pharmacodynamics and clinical outcome have not been adequately defined.

Despite the limitations discussed above, some studies have begun to define clinically relevant pharmacodynamic parameters of antifungals that affect clinical outcome. Drutz and colleagues reported improved clinical outcomes when amphotericin B serum concentrations are maintained at a level greater than twice the MIC of the fungus (Drutz et al, 1968). Animal models of infection have further demonstrated that high peaks relative to the MIC are correlated with improved survival and decreased fungal burden, as defined by CFU per gram of tissue in a variety of organs (Andes, 1999; Lewis et al, 1999; Groll et al, 2000). When studied in a neutropenic mouse model of infection, a serum C_{max}:MIC ratio ~10:1 was associated with the greatest decrease in kidney fungal burden. Additionally, using non-linear regression, a strong relationship was also found for the length of time the serum concentration remained above the MIC. This latter pharmacodynamic property is characteristic of a nonconcentration-dependent (i.e., time-dependent) antimycotic drug such as an azole (Andes, 1999; Groll et al, 2000). A reasonable hypothesis in reconciling these results involves the enhanced tissue binding of amphotericin B. Specifically, the enhanced tissue storage and long elimination rates of amphotericin B confound traditional dynamic estimates and the release of free drug from tissue sites is difficult to discriminate from the residual effects of inhibitory antifungal concentrations.

Adverse Effects

The utility of amphotericin B is hindered by significant toxicity. Although amphotericin B has a greater affinity for ergosterol, its affinity for cholesterol in the mammalian cell membrane likely plays a role in its toxicity

(Abu-Salah, 1996). The resulting, nonselective disruption of mammalian cells is believed to be the underlying cause of most of the adverse effects associated with this drug (Andreoli, 1973; Hsuchen and Feingold, 1973). Reversible renal impairment occurs within 2 weeks of therapy in more than 80% of amphotericin B treated patients (Butler et al, 1964). Infusion-related fever and chills are observed in over half of the patients receiving amphotericin B. The clinical consequences can be significant in certain patient populations such as the elderly and critically ill. Other adverse effects include thrombophlebitis, nausea, vomiting, headaches, myalgias, and arthralgias. Less frequently, cardiac arrhythmias and pulmonary toxicities have been reported.

It is clinically useful to classify these reactions as infusion-related, dose-related, or idiosyncratic reactions. Infusion-related reactions include a symptom complex of fever, chills, nausea, vomiting, headache, and hypotension. Cardiac arrhythmias may occur when high concentrations are rapidly infused, especially in patients with heart disease, patients with renal failure and those receiving an accidental drug overdosage (Cleary et al, 1993). Caution is also recommended for patients receiving the drug by a central venous catheter. Dose-related reactions occur with longer courses of treatment and are related to total dose. Examples include renal dysfunction with secondary electrolyte imbalances and anemia. Idiosyncratic reactions are unpredictable and include anaphylaxis, liver failure, hypertension, and respiratory failure.

Infusion-related fever and chills are observed in over half the patients receiving amphotericin B. Our clinical experience is that patients having severe infusion reactions often have undiagnosed adrenal insufficiency (especially those with disseminated histoplasmosis); consequently, adrenal function should be evaluated in these individuals. These infusion-related effects are believed to be due to the production of proinflammatory mediators by monocytes and macrophages in response to amphotericin B (Gigliotti et al, 1987; Chia and Pollack, 1989; Cleary et al, 1992). Amphotericin B has been shown to up-regulate a number of genes encoding pro-inflammatory molecules such as IL-1α, IL-1β, TNFα, IL-8, MIP-1α, MIP-1β, and MCP-1 (Rogers et al, 1998; Rogers et al, 2000, Rogers et al, 2002). Production of these respective gene products, along with release of PGE$_2$ from endothelial cells, likely mediates the infusion-related toxicity of amphotericin B. The patient to patient variability of amphotericin B infusion-related toxicity may correlate with quantitative differences in cytokine production in vivo (Gelfand et al, 1988).

The clinical manifestations of amphotericin B-induced nephrotoxicity include decreased glomerular filtration, decreased renal blood flow, and renal tubular acidosis. Secondary consequences such as hypokalemia and hypomagnesemia are common. Additionally, normochromic, normocytic anemia is frequently observed, likely in response to decreased erythropoietin production (Lin et al, 1990). Calcium deposits have been found in the renal tubule lumen, tubule cells, and interstitium upon histopathologic examination of renal tissue specimens obtained from patients treated with amphotericin B (Sabra and Branch, 1990; Carlson and Condon, 1994).

Onset of nephrotoxicity often occurs before laboratory or clinical signs and symptoms are evident. Many clinicians accept an endpoint at which some intervention is required as a rise in serum creatinine of greater than 0.5 mg/dL for patients with baseline values less than 3.0 mg/dL. For patients with a serum creatinine above 3.0 mg/dL, a rise of greater than 1.0 mg/dL is considered an appropriate endpoint. The action taken is variable and ranges from amphotericin B discontinuation or dosage reduction, stopping concurrent nephrotoxic drugs, changing to an alternate day infusion schedule and pretreating patients with normal saline. There are no clinical trials that identify the optimal therapeutic option.

The mechanism of amphotericin B-induced nephrotoxicity is multifaceted. Animal studies have demonstrated the vasoconstrictive properties of amphotericin B, particularly with regard to the afferent arteriole (Sawaya et al, 1991). Increased tubule permeability has also been demonstrated (Cheng et al, 1982). Other studies suggest that amphotericin B inhibits sodium-potassium ATPases and affects proton exchange, which could contribute to renal tubular acidosis. Conversely, damage to the medullary thick ascending limb by amphotericin B was ameliorated by ouabain in a rat kidney model, suggesting an alternative role for this pump in amphotericin B-induced nephrotoxicity. Others have suggested a role for amphotericin B-induced release of prostaglandins and leukotrienes as well as oxidative injury in this process (Carlson and Condon, 1994).

The tubuloglomerular feedback mechanism normally involved in renal homeostasis also plays a prominent role in the pathogenesis of amphotericin B-induced nephrotoxicity (Branch et al, 1987). This feedback process is believed to be activated by transport of sodium chloride across the macula densa cells into the distal nephron, resulting in constriction of the afferent arteriole, possibly mediated by adenosine, and subsequent impairment of glomerular filtration (Sabra and Branch, 1990). Dehydration and sodium depletion accentuate this response and exacerbate amphotericin-induced renal failure. Sodium loading with intravenous administration of 500 mL to 1000 mL of normal saline prior to initiation of amphotericin B, when tolerated by the patient, is recommended in order to decrease the likelihood of renal toxicity (Branch, 1988).

Drug Interactions

Drugs that interact with amphotericin B are best categorized by the effect they have on a clinical outcome of amphotericin treatment. It is useful to classify these agents as *(1)* those that alter therapeutic outcome, *(2)* those that alter toxicity, and *(3)* those that have miscellaneous outcomes. Agents that alter therapeutic outcome include those that exert a direct synergistic or antagonistic effect on the microbiologic activity of amphotericin B and those that improve therapeutic outcome indirectly by enhancing the patient's immunity. Agents that are synergistic with amphotericin (e.g., flucytosine) and cytokines that enhance antifungal immunity (e.g., colony stimulating factors) are discussed in more detail in a separate section of this chapter—see under Combination Therapy.

Corticosteroids and nonsteroidal antiinflammatory drugs (NSAIDs) are the agents most frequently used to prevent infusion-related toxicities (Goodwin et al, 1995). Controversy exists concerning the risk:benefit ratio of corticosteroids for prevention of infusion-related reactions. Clinical experience overwhelmingly supports the therapeutic benefit of administering hydrocortisone to patients suffering infusion-related reactions. However, circumstantial evidence suggests that administration of this immunosuppressant could be detrimental to the therapeutic success of amphotericin B (North 1971; Snyder and Unanue, 1982; Tatro, 1998). Although further investigation of this therapeutic issue is required, it seems prudent to limit the dose and duration of corticosteroids by a therapeutic taper once infusion-related reactions are ameliorated. Likewise, routine use of NSAIDs for premedication should be avoided owing to their potential to enhance amphotericin-induced renal insufficiency. Intravenous meperidine has proven useful in abrogating infusion-related rigors (Burks et al, 1980).

Enhanced nephrotoxicity associated with amphotericin B administration has been observed with cyclosporine or tacrolimus (Tatro, 1998), diuretics, NSAIDs, pentamidine (Antoniskis and Larsen, 1990) and other nephrotoxic agents such as aminoglycosides or radioopaque dyes (Tatro, 1998). Diligent monitoring of renal function is warranted in patients treated concurrently with these nephrotoxic agents.

A variety of other therapeutic agents may result in amphotericin B-associated adverse events that require diligent monitoring. Pulmonary leukostasis and respiratory failure associated with concomitant leukocyte transfusions or indium-labeled leukocyte scanning can be life-threatening (Wright et al, 1981; Dutcher et al, 1989). However, the incidence of this reaction has markedly decreased with less frequent use of autoinfusion of leukocytes. Skeletal muscle relaxants and neuromuscular blocking agents have been reported to enhance curariform effects related to the hypokalemia (Tatro, 1998). Amphotericin B-induced hypokalemia can also enhance the cardiac effects of digitalis glycosides (Tatro, 1998). In these cases, patients suffered cardiac dysfunction that would be difficult to differentiate from the direct effects of amphotericin B on the myocardial tissue (Cleary et al, 1993). Amiloride has been suggested for concomitant administration to decrease the hypokalemia in patients receiving digitalis glycosides. However, the effect is difficult to predict and requires further study. Cyclophosphamide and doxorubicin appear to penetrate cells more effectively when administered with amphotericin B and this results in enhanced toxicity (Present et al, 1977).

Drug interactions also encompass incompatibilities of pharmaceuticals in solution. Amphotericin B deoxycholate and the amphotericin B lipid formulations are incompatible in solutions with high saline content, including lactated Ringer's or sodium chloride. In addition, the infusion of amphotericin B formulations concomitantly with other antiinfectives (amikacin, ampicillin, aztreonam, carbenicillin, clindamycin, cotrimoxazole, fluconazole, gentamicin, linezolid, nitrofurantoin, penicillin G, and pipercillin) may induce precipitation of either agent.

Combination Therapy

One potentially exciting approach to improving the activity and/or toxicity profile of amphotericin B is its administration in combination with another antifungal or pharmacologic agent. Animal data and anecdotal experience suggest that colony stimulating factors, rifampin or macrolides may be effective adjuvants. Antitumor necrosis factor or interleukin-1 beta antibodies appear to have a detrimental effect. A more traditional approach would be to use another antimycotic in combination with amphotericin B. While many in vitro studies of antifungal combinations with amphotericin B have been performed, the results of these have not been consistent. For example, pretreatment with an imidazole prior to the administration of amphotericin B has been reported to be antagonistic (Sugar, 1995). Other studies, however, have documented additive or synergistic activity when triazoles were combined with amphotericin B (Peacock et al., 1993). Owing to these differing results, the routine use of an azole with amphotericin B has not been recommended. This caveat may be reexamined in light of the completion of a recent trial comparing amphotericin B in combination with fluconazole to amphotericin alone for the initial treatment of candidemia (Rex et al, 2003). In contrast to studies with the azoles, the clinical benefit of using amphotericin B in combination with flucytosine for the treatment of cryptococcal meningitis has been clearly documented in both AIDS and non-AIDS patients (Bennett et al, 1979; Dismukes et al, 1987; van der Horst et al, 1997). In addition, smaller cohorts of patients with candidemia and other serious candidal infections have been treated successfully with amphotericin B combined with flucytosine. Unfortunately, clinical studies evaluating the efficacy of other antifungal combinations are relatively few (Lewis and Kontoyiannis, 2001).

In a seminal study of the treatment of cryptococcal meningitis in non-AIDS patients, amphotericin B deoxycholate (0.3 mg/kg/day) combined with flucytosine (150 mg/kg/day) given for 6 weeks was superior to 10 weeks of amphotericin B alone (0.4 mg/kg/day). Patients who received the amphotericin B-flucytosine combination had fewer failures and relapses, and experienced a shorter time to sterilization of the cerebrospinal fluid (Bennett et al, 1979). A subsequent study evaluated the same combination given for either 4 weeks or 6 weeks. The shorter course of treatment had similar efficacy in nonimmunocompromised patients and good prognostic findings (Dismukes et al, 1987).

Several studies have also evaluated the treatment of cryptococcal meningitis in AIDS patients. A recent large multicenter study compared amphotericin (0.7 mg/kg/day) with or without flucytosine (100 mg/kg/day) for the first 2 weeks of therapy (van der Horst et al, 1997). Those patients who received combination therapy had a lower mortality and more rapid sterilization of the CSF during the first 2 weeks of treatment. Based on these findings, combination therapy of cryptococcal meningitis is recommended for the initial 2 weeks, or until the patient's clinical status improves or stabilizes (van der Horst et al, 1997). Following this induction therapy, patients can be changed to fluconazole for another 8 to 10 weeks. For more information about the treatment of cryptococcal meningitis, see Chapter 12.

Amphotericin B has also been combined with fluconazole in the treatment of candidemia. A large, multicenter, randomized trial was recently completed that compared fluconazole (12 mg/kg/day) to fluconazole plus amphotericin B deoxycholate (0.7 mg/kg/day) for the initial therapy of candidemia in nonneutropenic adults (Rex et al, 2003). Despite randomization, the treatment groups were not equivalent for disease severity based on APACHE score. The group of patients who received only fluconazole were more severely ill than those who received combination therapy. Although the interpretation of this study was limited by this randomization bias, the trial did demonstrate that, in nonneutropenic patients, the combination of fluconazole plus amphotericin B was not antagonistic and treatment outcomes trended towards improved success even though statistical significance was not achieved. As in

previous studies, vascular catheter removal reduced the time to clearance of Candida from the bloodstream (Rex et al, 2001).

Administration

There are no well-controlled trials that delineate the optimal dosing regimen for amphotericin B. The daily dose has traditionally ranged from 0.3 mg/kg up to 1.5 mg/kg depending on the specific mycosis and severity of disease. The duration of therapy for most systemic fungal infections has varied from 4 to 12 weeks, although courses of many months have been reported. The availability of the triazoles, however, has resulted in amphotericin B being used for shorter treatment courses, usually until clinical improvement is evident, before step-down therapy is initiated with a less toxic azole.

Specific administration and dosing recommendations are as variable as the number of institutions that utilize this antifungal polyene. Selection of dosing regimens, including premedications, is often based on clinicians' fears of toxicity rather than achievement of efficacy. Dosing recommendations that have been approved by the Food and Drug Administration are outlined in Table 3–1. Specific recommendations for the administration of amphotericin B deoxycholate (based on the authors' clinical experience) are outlined in Table 3–2. Clinical trials supporting these recommendations are needed but most likely will never be performed.

The practice of administering a 1 mg test dose of amphotericin B prior to the initial dose, while recommended by the manufacturer, is controversial among clinicians (Griswold et al, 1998). The dose is administered as 1 mg amphotericin B in 50 mL of D5W administered over 30 to 60 minutes. Alternatively, the test dose may be given as part of the initial dose, which in turn is then given in full if no adverse effects are observed. The test dose is designed to identify patients who will experience immediate type hypersensitivity reactions or pronounced infusion-related reactions. While evidence supporting this practice is sparse, many experienced clinicians continue to use this approach. Others argue that immediate type hypersensitivity would be observed with the test dose, whereas the amphotericin B concentration provided by a test dose would be insufficient to produce the proinflammatory response responsible for fever and chills. Also of concern is the potential delay in therapy that may occur with the use of an initial test dose (Griswold et al, 1998). The authors do not recommend a test dose (Table 3–2).

A second controversy centers around the length of infusions, e.g., short vs. long. Several studies have explored toxicity and tolerability of standard infusion

TABLE 3–2. *Amphotericin B Infusion Protocol*

Administration and Dosing

Dilute amphotericin B in D5W, the final concentration not exceeding 0.1 mg/mL. Initial dosing (0.25 mg/kg based on lean body mass) should not exceed 30 mg. Infuse the dose over 0.75–4 hours immediately after a meal. Record temperature, pulse rate and blood pressure every 30 min for 4 hours. If patient develops significant chills, fever, respiratory distress and hypotension, administer adjunctive medication prior to next infusion. If initial dose is tolerated, advance to maximum dose by the third to the fifth day. Consult an INFECTIOUS DISEASES CLINICIAN for any questions concerning maximum daily dose, total dose, and duration of therapy.

Adjunctive Medications

1. Heparin 1000 units may diminish thrombophlebitis for peripheral lines. Observe the contraindications to the use of heparin, such as thrombocytopenia, increased risk of hemorrhage, and concomitant anticoagulation.
2. Administration of 500–1000 mL of normal saline, as tolerated, prior to amphotericin B may help decrease renal dysfunction.
3. Acetaminophen administered 30 minutes prior to amphotericin B infusion may ameliorate the fever.
4. Hydrocortisone 0.7 mg/kg (Solu-Cortef) can be added to the amphotericin B infusion. Hydrocortisone is given to decrease the infusion-related reactions. This should only be used for significant fever (> 2.0°F elevation from baseline) and chills with infusions and should be discontinued as soon as possible (3–5 days). It is not necessary to add hydrocortisone if the patient is receiving supraphysiologic doses of adrenal corticosteroids.
5. Meperidine hydrochloride 25–50 mg parenterally in adults may be utilized to prevent or ameliorate chills.

Monitoring

1. At least twice weekly for the first 4 weeks, then weekly: hematocrit, reticulocyte count, magnesium, potassium, BUN, creatinine, bicarbonate, urinalysis. The GFR may fall 40% before stabilizing in these patients. DISCONTINUE FOR 2–5 DAYS IF RENAL FUNCTION CONTINUES TO DETERIORATE AND REINSTATE AFTER IMPROVEMENT. Hematocrit frequently falls 22%–35% of the starting level.
2. Monitor closely for hypokalemia and hypomagnesemia.

Caveats and Patients Requiring Closer Monitoring

1. Electrolytes: Addition of an electrolyte to the amphotericin B solution causes the colloid to aggregate and probably gives a suboptimal therapeutic effect. This includes IV piggyback medications containing electrolytes.
2. Filtering: The colloidal solution is partially retained by 0.22 micron pore membrane filter; do not use filters routinely.
3. The infusion bottle need not be light-shielded.
4. Patients with adrenal insufficiency tolerate infusion poorly. Treatment with corticosteroids improves patient tolerance.
5. Patients should not receive granulocyte transfusion (including Indium scanning).
6. Patients with anuria or previous cardiac history may have an increased risk of arrhythmias and slower infusions are recommended.

times (4 to 6 hours) vs. more rapid infusions of 2 to 4 hours and even less than an hour (Cleary et al, 1988). The results of these studies indicate that rapid infusion times are equally well tolerated and have similar rates of adverse events as compared to infusions given over 4 to 6 hours. Due to the risk of cardiac arrhythmias, rapid infusions should not be used in patients with renal failure, heart disease, history of cardiac arrhythmias and in those receiving amphotericin B through a central venous catheter (Craven and Gremillion, 1985; Bowler et al, 1992). A recent study reported less toxicity, including nephrotoxicity, in febrile neutropenic patients treated with continuous infusion amphotericin B when compared to patients treated with 4-hour infusions (Eriksson et al, 2001). However, clinical experience with continuous infusion of amphotericin B is limited and, until safety and efficacy are better documented, continuous infusion cannot be recommended at this time.

Other routes of administration for amphotericin B are used when therapeutic goals are not or cannot be achieved with intravenous dosing (Gallis et al, 1990; Peacock et al, 1993; Patel, 1998). Topical preparations (3% lotion, creams or ointments, 10 mg lozenges or oral suspension, 100 mg/mL) may be compounded as needed for the treatment of superficial or cutaneous yeast infections. Intrathecal or intraventricular routes have been used in refractory cases of fungal meningitis, most frequently coccidioidal meningitis (Gallis et al, 1990; Wen et al, 1992; Peacock et al, 1993). Intrathecal administration is problematic due to the poor distribution and the development of arachnoiditis at the injection site. Intraventricular administration is preferred. Long-term administration should be performed using a subcutaneous Ommaya reservoir. The amphotericin B dose should be mixed with the patient's cerebrospinal fluid or sterile water to a final concentration of 250 μg/mL. Initial dosing (25–50 μg) is then escalated up to dose of 250 μg/day or 500 μg to 1000 μg every other day depending on the mycosis being treated and patient tolerance. This route of administration is often limited by local reactions (radicular pain, headache, vomiting, and arachnoiditis). More severe neurological complications include ventricular hemorrhage and bacterial superinfection (Wen et al, 1992).

Ocular administration of amphotericin B is frequently used for the treatment of fungal eye infections (Lesar and Fiscella, 1985; Gallis et al, 1990). Topical ophthalmic application (0.25%–1.5% solution) or sub-conjunctival injection (0.1–0.2 mg/0.5 mL) is appropriate for most superficial infections; however, little medication penetrates into the vitreous fluid. Intravitreal injection (0.005 mg/0.1 mL) or an approximate concentration added to vitrectomy solutions during the procedure is often used (Lesar and Fiscella, 1985).

The therapeutic benefit and optimal dose of other routes of administration are not well established and local inflammatory responses specific to the sites of administration are common and are frequently dose limiting (Gallis et al, 1990; Peacock et al, 1993). Intraperitoneal administration for the prevention or treatment of peritoneal dialysis-associated *Candida* infections can be achieved by administering amphotericin B within the dialysate (1–4 ug/mL dialysate) or intraperitoneally (25 mg every 48 hours). Intraarticular doses (5–15 mg) administered for fungal arthritis or joint infection and irrigation of a body cavity has been common practice. Bladder instillation/irrigation with an amphotericin B solution (50 ug/mL) by continuous infusion through a triple lumen catheter for 5 days has been used for candidal cystitis and candiduria (Fan-Havard et al, 1995). Amphotericin B (2 mg/mL; 10 mg twice a day [bid]) has been administered via nebulization for prevention of pulmonary aspergillosis in neutropenic patients (O'Riordan and Faris, 1999; Diot et al, 2001). Specific adverse reactions with aerosolized amphotericin B include dyguesia, gastrointestinal distress, and respiratory distress (dyspnea, cough). Less frequently, intracavitary irrigation (50 mg/day; 500–800 mg total dose) is used for treatment of pulmonary aspergilloma.

Use in Pregnancy

Amphotericin B is the antifungal agent with which there has been the most experience in pregnancy (King et al, 1998; Sobel, 2000). Both the deoxycholate and lipid-based formulations are assigned to risk category B by their manufacturers. While the pharmacokinetics of amphotericin B in pregnancy have not been studied, the drug appears to cross the placenta and enter the fetal circulation (King et al, 1998). Among case reports of amphotericin B use in pregnancy, azotemia was the most common maternal adverse drug reaction reported, followed by anemia, hypokalemia, acute nephrotoxicity, fever, chills, headache, nausea, and vomiting. Individual cases of possible fetal toxicity include transient acidosis with azotemia, anemia, transient maculopapular rash, and respiratory failure requiring mechanical ventilation. Only a single case of congenital malformation (microcephaly with a pilonidal dimple) has been associated with amphotericin B. To date there have been no reports of animal teratogenesis attributed to amphotericin B (King et al, 1998; Sobel, 2000).

LIPID PREPARATIONS OF AMPHOTERICIN B

Three lipid-based products are currently available in the United States: amphotericin B colloidal dispersion (ABCD), liposomal amphotericin B (L-AmB), and amphotericin B lipid complex (ABLC) (Color Fig. 3–2 in separate color insert). In addition to these commercial formulations, lipid-based preparations have been admixed by individual institutions by combining amphotericin B deoxycholate and 20% lipid emulsion (Caillot et al, 1993; Ayestaran et al, 1996). While amphotericin B lipid emulsion is attractive from the standpoint of cost, several concerns have been raised, encompassing the stability of the emulsion, the need for filtration, and the possibility of fat overload syndrome. One pharmaceutical company pursued development of this formulation for several years, but a stable suspension was not achieved. Administration of this formulation is, therefore, not recommended (Cleary, 1996).

Chemistry (Table 3–1)

The commercial lipid formulations are distinct as regards their phospholipid content, particle size and shape, electrostatic charge, and bilayer rigidity (Slain, 1999). These biochemical/biophysical properties have a profound effect on the pharmacology of these lipid formulations (Table 3–1). For example, the smaller liposomes (L-AmB) are not as readily taken up by the macrophages. As such, L-AmB achieves higher serum concentrations and a greater area under the curve (AUC) in blood compared to conventional amphotericin B or the other lipid preparations. On the other hand, the larger lipid formulation, ABLC, is more readily taken up by the tissues and has the greatest volume of distribution. For a more detailed discussion, see section on Pharmacology and Pharmacokinetics.

Liposomal amphotericin B is formulated as a unilamellar spherical vesicle with a single lipid bilayer comprised of hydrogenated phosphatidylcholine, cholesterol, and distearoyl phosphatidylglycerol in a 2:1:0.8 ratio. Amphotericin is located on the inside and outside of the vesicle. Liposomal amphotericin B has the smallest particle size. Amphotericin B colloidal dispersion was developed by complexing amphotericin B with cholesteryl sulfate in a 1:1 molar ratio. These complexes form tetramers that have a hydrophobic and a hydrophilic portion. The tetramers aggregate to form disk-like structures that are larger in size than L-AmB. Amphotericin B lipid complex consists of nonliposomal amphotericin B-complexed ribbon structures and was originally derived from multilaminar liposomes prepared by mixing two phospholipids, dimyristoyl phosphatidylcholine (DMPC) and dimyristoyl phosphatidylglycerol (DMPG) in a 7:3 molar ratio. Amphotericin B lipid complex is much larger in size than the other two formulations (Janknergt et al, 1992; Slain, 1999; Robinson and Nahata, 1999) (Table 3–1; See Color Fig. 3–2 in separate color insert).

Proposed Mechanisms for Enhanced Therapeutic Index

Although the lipid formulations have been shown to have an improved therapeutic index as compared to amphotericin B deoxycholate, the mechanism(s) by which this occurs has not been adequately defined. Several mechanisms have been proposed. The unifying concept in all of these proposals involves the ability of lipid formulations to prevent binding to the kidney and the selective distribution of lipid-bound amphotericin to other tissues (Slain, 1999).

The first mechanism involves the rapid endocytic uptake of lipid-associated amphotericin by macrophages in tissues, often at the sites of infection. Following this targeted delivery, amphotericin B is then slowly released into the tissues and the circulation. In addition to this selective tissue targeting, macrophage uptake of amphotericin B also limits the amount of free drug (and presumably also LDL-bound drug) in the circulation capable of binding to human cells. The second mechanism involves the selective transfer of amphotericin from the lipid carrier to the fungal cell membrane. In this instance, the amphotericin B has a stronger affinity for the lipid carrier than for the cholesterol in mammalian cells. On the other hand, the affinity of amphotericin B for ergosterol in the fungal cell is stronger than its affinity for either the lipid carrier or the cholesterol. A third mechanism proposes that the lipid-based formulations are less nephrotoxic by limiting the amount of free drug in the blood and by preventing amphotericin B binding to circulating LDL. Free amphotericin and LDL-bound amphotericin B are considered more nephrotoxic than either HDL or lipid-bound amphotericin B. The fourth mechanism proposes that the lipid-based formulations elicit a reduced cytokine (i.e., TNF-alpha, IL-1, etc.) response from human cells as compared to amphotericin B deoxycholate. These proinflammatory cytokines are putative mediators for infusion-related reactions and nephrotoxicity. This fourth hypothesis is supported primarily by in vitro data. The last purported mechanism involves the action of extracellular phospholipases produced by yeasts and moulds in releasing the lipid-bound amphotericin B at the site of infection. As such, more amphotericin B is released in the infected tissues. The phospholipid carrier of ABLC is especially susceptible to these fungal phospholipases.

Therapeutic Indications

In general, all three lipid formulations are indicated for the treatment of systemic fungal infection in patients refractory to or intolerant to therapy with amphotericin B deoxycholate (Table 3–1; Robinson and Nahata, 1999; Slain, 1999). Liposomal amphotericin B has also been approved for the empiric therapy of presumed fungal infection in febrile neutropenic patients (Walsh et al, 1999). In routine clinical practice, however, lipid formulations are frequently used as primary therapy for patients with baseline renal insufficiency and in patients at high risk for renal failure (e.g., transplant recipients and patients receiving concurrent treatment with other nephrotoxic agents). Lipid preparations, however, should not be used as primary therapy for dialysis-dependent patients unless they fail conventional amphotericin B. Some authors consider the lipid formulations, due to their high concentrations in the liver and spleen, to be ideal for the treatment of patients with chronic disseminated candidiasis (Walsh et al, 1997). Finally, many infectious disease physicians experienced in treating fungal infections consider lipid formulations of amphotericin B to be superior to amphotericin B deoxycholate for the treatment of patients with aggressive mould diseases such as invasive aspergillosis and zygomycosis. The data supporting this use are anecdotal and comparative trials documenting the superiority of lipid formulations for these infections are lacking at present.

Pharmacology and Pharmacokinetics (See Table 3–1)

Comparative data on the pharmacokinetic parameters of the lipid formulations, either compared to each other or to amphotericin B deoxycholate, are limited. However, profound differences in some of the parameters have been documented and have led to unique therapeutic options (Table 3–1; Janknergt et al, 1992; Villani et al, 1996). For example, peak serum concentrations and AUC are much greater for L-AmB as compared to amphotericin B deoxycholate and the other two lipid preparations. The increases in peak serum concentrations of L-AmB are most likely secondary to decreases in the volume of distribution and clearance from the blood. In contrast, the tissue distribution and the volume of distribution are significantly greater for ABLC than for either of the other preparations. This tissue saturation also results in increased drug clearance from the serum (Caillot et al, 1993). Whether any of these pharmacologic differences significantly affect clinical outcome or toxicity has not adequately been studied.

Pharmacodynamics

Owing to a variety of confounding variables, the pharmacodynamic information obtained with amphotericin B deoxycholate cannot be directly extrapolated to the lipid formulations. In general, studies utilizing amphotericin B lipid formulations have revealed a poor correlation between pharmacodynamic parameters and outcome (Groll et al, 2000). Measurement of free amphotericin B has been hypothesized to potentially resolve these discrepancies. However, the ability to accurately measure or predict free amphotericin B is difficult (Walsh et al, 1997).

As mentioned earlier, L-AmB achieves serum concentrations many fold higher than the other lipid formulations of amphotericin B, leading to a tremendously increased area under the serum concentration versus time curve that in turn impacts all pharmacodynamic calculations. Using traditional calculations, L-AmB would not be predicted to be an effective therapy for central nervous system infections. To the contrary, L-AmB proved effective in animal studies (Groll et al, 2000) and in 2 clinical trials of patients with AIDS-associated cryptococcal meningitis (Leenders et al, 1997; Hamill et al, 1999). Although cerebrospinal fluid levels were low or undetectable, brain tissue concentrations exceeded expectations and, in the animal studies, were higher than either conventional amphotericin B or the other lipid formulations. Brain tissue concentrations (mean amount = 0.56 μg/g) in patients receiving L-AmB were not as high as those documented in the animal studies (Leenders et al, 1997; Groll et al, 2000).

Disproportionate distribution into the reticuloendothelial system has been observed for two lipid formulations, ABLC and L-AmB. As a result, very high tissue concentrations of these agents are detected in the liver and spleen relative to serum. These high tissue levels have been hypothesized to be a therapeutic advantage for these agents in treating patients with chronic disseminated candidiasis (Walsh et al, 1997). In support of this theory, clearance of *C. albicans* from the liver was superior in mice treated with L-AmB (1.5 mg/kg) compared to mice treated with conventional amphotericin B at equal doses (Kretschmar et al, 1996). In contrast, clearance of yeasts from lung was not enhanced in LAmB treated mice. High concentrations of ABLC were detected in lung tissue, suggesting that this fomulation may be optimal for the treatment of pulmonary mycoses.

Adverse Events

All three lipid-based preparations currently available in the United States exhibit less nephrotoxicity than amphotericin B deoxycholate (Slain, 1999; Wingard et al, 2000). However, infusion-related toxicities similar to amphotericin B deoxycholate are still seen with ABLC and ABCD (White et al, 1997; White et al, 1998a; Wingard et al, 2000), whereas other studies demonstrated significantly fewer infusion-related adverse events associated with L-AmB compared to ampho-

tericin B deoxycholate (Slain, 1999; Walsh et al, 1999). Although uncommon, acute respiratory events have been associated with administration of amphotericin B and are typically characterized by tachypnea, dyspnea, and wheezing. Recently, there have also been reports of chest discomfort and altered pulmonary function associated with the lipid-based preparations of amphotericin B (Johnson et al, 1998; Collazos et al, 2001). The mechanisms causing these reactions are unclear, but may be related to the ability of amphotericin B to elicit chemokine production from monocytes (Rogers et al, 1998; Rogers et al, 2000). The ability of IL-8 to recruit neutrophils could then mediate the pulmonary toxicity occasionally observed during administration of this agent. The lipid formulations of amphotericin B deliver higher amounts of drug to the pulmonary tissue (Johnson et al, 1998). Thus, it is conceivable that enhanced pulmonary neutrophil recruitment in response to elevated local concentrations of IL-8 could lead to pulmonary leukostasis, and thereby explain in part the pulmonary toxicity associated with amphotericin B preparations. Indeed, studies in animal models have demonstrated that amphotericin B pulmonary toxicity involves neutrophil recruitment to the lungs (McDonnell et al, 1988; Hardie et al, 1992). Another possibility is that the lipid component of these preparations may itself contribute to these physiologic effects. Irrespective of the cause of the pulmonary toxicity, it seems prudent to administer the initial dose of any of the amphotericin B lipid formulations under close observation and to reduce the rate of infusion in instances where these effects are observed (Johnson et al, 1998; Collazos et al, 2001).

Other adverse events reported with the lipid preparations include headache, hypotension, hypertension, diarrhea, nausea, vomiting, and rashes. Laboratory abnormalities reported include hypokalemia, hypomagnesemia, hypocalcemia, elevated liver function tests, and thrombocytopenia (Slain, 1999). Regarding frequency of infusion-related adverse events of available amphotericin B preparations, data suggest the following rank order by greatest to least frequency: amphotericin B deoxycholate = ABCD > ABLC > L-AmB.

Comparative Trials

Comparative trials between the lipid amphotericin B preparations and the deoxycholate formulation are enlightening. Empiric therapy for febrile neutropenic patients has received the most attention. In two different studies, ABCD (4 mg/kg/day) and L-AmB (3 mg/kg/day) were each compared to standard therapy with amphotericin deoxycholate (0.6–0.8 mg/kg/day) (White et al, 1998b; Walsh et al, 1999). In both studies, patients treated with the lipid preparations had a more rapid defervescence and lower death rate; although in neither study were these clinical differences statistically significant. In contrast, patients receiving either of the lipid preparations had statistically superior outcomes compared to patients treated with conventional amphotericin B for *(1)* the time to onset and rates of renal dysfunction; *(2)* rates of infusion-related reactions; and *(3)* prevention of breakthrough invasive fungal infections (White et al, 1998b; Walsh et al, 1999). Another study of therapy for febrile neutropenic patients compared two different doses of L-AmB (3 mg/kg/day and 5 mg/kg/day) to ABLC (5 mg/kg/day). Clinical outcomes were equivalent for all patient groups, except that the rates of renal dysfunction were significantly less for either dose of L-AmB compared to the ABLC formulation (Wingard et al, 2000).

Comparative studies of the different amphotericin B formulations in the treatment of documented infections have been primarily nonblinded and limited in number. Amphotericin B colloidal dispersion (0.5–8 mg/kg/day), L-AmB (4 mg/kg/day) and ABLC (1.2–5 mg/kg/day) have been compared to amphotericin B deoxycholate (0.1–1.5 mg/kg/day) for the treatment of invasive aspergillosis (White et al, 1997; Bowden et al, 2002) and cryptococcal meningitis (Sharkey et al, 1996; Leenders et al, 1997). Patients with proven or probable aspergillosis who received ABCD experienced higher response rates (~50%) compared to a historical control group treated with conventional amphotericin B (White et al, 1997). However, in the only prospective, double-blind trial reported to date, ABCD showed equal but no better efficacy than conventional amphotericin B as therapy for invasive aspergillosis (52% vs. 51%) (Bowden et al, 2002). In two open label, randomized trials comparing a lipid formulation for the treatment of AIDS-associated cryptococcal meningitis, the clinical and microbiologic responses rates favored the lipid preparations (Sharkey et al, 1996; Leenders et al, 1997). In a third trial, a randomized comparison of L-AmB vs. amphotericin B deoxycholate, the clinical and microbiologic responses were equivalent (Hamill et al, 1999). Of note, in these studies, significantly lower rates of nephrotoxicity were observed in patients treated with the lipid formulations.

Administration and Dosage
The approved daily dose and rate of administration for each lipid formulation are somewhat different. Other than for ABCD, the maximal daily dose that can be safely administered in humans has not been adequately defined. More interestingly, the equivalent dose of the individual lipid formulations that compares to the recommended dose of amphotericin B deoxycholate for a particular fungal infection has not been established.

The recommended initial dose of L-AmB is 3 mg/kg/day for empiric therapy and 3 to 5 mg/kg/day for

documented systemic fungal infections. The drug is usually infused over 2 hours but may be increased to 1 hour if tolerated. The currently approved daily dose of ABLC is 5 mg/kg and this is infused at a rate of 2.5 mg/kg/hour. Daily doses of L-AmB and ABLC have been titrated considerably higher than the recommended daily doses and well tolerated in selected patients with treatment-refractory diseases. Treatment with ABCD should be initiated with a daily dose of 3 to 4 mg/kg. The dose can then be escalated to 6 mg/kg/day based on patient tolerance and clinical response. The recommended maximal daily dose is 7.5 mg/kg. Infusion related toxicities with ABCD become clinically significant with doses of 8 mg/kg or greater.

Costs
A major consideration about the lipid-based formulations of amphotericin B is their high cost in comparison to conventional amphotericin B deoxycholate. Data indicate that the lipid formulations range from 10- to 50-fold higher in acquisition cost per dose (Rex and Walsh, 1999). Although these agents are less nephrotoxic than conventional amphotericin B and their overall therapeutic:toxic ratio is clearly improved over that of the parent drug, superiority in clinical efficacy has not been definitively established in head-to-head comparative trials. Consequently, well-done pharmacoeconomic studies are needed to justify the higher cost of the lipid formulations.

REFERENCES

Abu-Salah K M. Amphotericin B: An update. *Br J Biomed Sci* 53:122–133, 1996.

Andes D. In vivo pharmacodynamics of amphotericin B against C. *albicans.* In: Abstracts of the 39th Interscience Conference on Antimicrobial Agents and Chemotherapy. San Francisco, CA. American Society for Microbiology, Abstract # 1002, 1999.

Andreoli T E. On the anatomy of amphotericin B-cholesterol pores in lipid bilayer membranes. *Kidney Int* 4:337–345, 1973.

Antoniskis D, Larsen R A. Acute, rapidly progressive renal failure with simultaneous use of amphotericin B and pentamidine. *Antimicrob Agents Chemother* 34:470–472, 1990.

Atkinson A J Jr, Bennett J E. Amphotericin B pharmacokinetics in humans. *Antimicrob Agents Chemother* 13: 271–276, 1978.

Ayestaran A, Lopez R M, Montoro J B, Estibalez A, Pou L, Julia A, Lopez A, Pascual B. Pharmacokinetics of conventional formulation versus fat emulsion formulation of amphotericin B in a group of patients with neutropenia. *Antimicrob Agents Chemother* 40:609–612, 1996.

Bennett J E, Dismukes W E, Duma R J, Medoff G, Sande M A, Gallis H, Leonard J, Fields B T, Bradshaw M, Haywood H, McGee Z A, Cate T R, Cobbs C G, Warner J F, Alling D W. A comparison of amphotericin B alone and combined with flucytosine in the treatment of cryptococcal meningitis. *N Engl J Med* 301:126–131, 1979.

Benson J M, Nahata M C. Pharmacokinetics of amphotericin B in children. *Antimicrob Agents Chemother* 33:1989–1993, 1989.

Bindschladler D D, Bennett J E. A pharmacologic guide to the clinical use of amphotericin B. *J Infect Dis* 120:427–436, 1969.

Bistoni F, Vecchiarelli A, Mazzolla R, Puccetti P, Marconi P, Garaci E. Immunoadjuvant activity of amphotericin B as displayed in mice infected with *Candida albicans. Antimicrob Agents Chemother* 27: 625–631, 1985.

Bjorksten B, Ray C, Quie P G. Inhibition of human neutrophil chemotaxis and chemiluminescence by amphotericin B. *Infect Immun* 14:315–317, 1976.

Bowden R, Chandrasekar P, White M H, Li X, Pietrelli L, Gurwith M, van Burik J, Laverdiere M, Safrin S, Wingard J R. A double-blind, randomized, controlled trial of amphotericin B colloidal dispersion for treatment of invasive aspergillosis in immunocompromised patients. *Clin Infect Dis* 35: 359–366, 2002.

Bowler W A, Weiss P J, Hill H E, Hoffmeister K A, Fleck R P, Blackey A R, Oldfield E C 3rd. Risk of ventricular dysrythmias during one hour infusions of amphotericin B in patients with preserved renal function. *Antimicrob Agents Chemother* 36:2542–2543, 1992.

Brajtburg J, Powderly W G, Kobayashi G S, Medoff G. Amphotericin B: Current understanding of mechanisms of action. *Antimicrob Agents Chemother* 34:183–188, 1990.

Branch R A, Jackson E K, Jacqz E, Stein R, Ray W A, Ohnhaus E E, Mensers P, Heidemann H. Amphotericin B nephrotoxicity in humans decreased by sodium supplements with coadministration of ticarcillin or intravenous saline. *Klin Wochenschr* 65:500–506, 1987.

Branch R A. Prevention of amphotericin B-induced renal impairment: a review of the use of sodium supplementation. *Arch Intern Med* 148:2389–2394, 1988.

Burks, L C, Aisner, J, Fortner, C L, Wiernik, P H. Meperidine for the treatment of shaking chills and fever. *Arch Intern Med* 140: 483–484, 1980.

Butler W T, Bennet J E, Alling D W, Wertlake P T, Utz J P, Hill G J, II. Nephrotoxicity of amphotericin B. Early and late effects in 81 patients. *Ann Intern Med* 61:175–187, 1964.

Caillot D, Casasnovas O, Solary E, Chavanet P, Bonnotte B, Reny G, Entezam F, Lopez J, Bonnin A, Guy H. Efficacy and tolerance of an amphotericin B lipid (Intralipid) emulsion in the treatment of candidemia in neutropenic patients. *J Antimicrob Chemother* 31:161–169, 1993.

Carlson M A, Condon R E. Nephrotoxicity of amphotericin B. *J Am Coll Surg* 179:361–381, 1994.

Carver P. Effect of pH, concentration and time of exposure on the postantibiotic effect (PAE) of combinations of antifungal agents. In: Abstracts of the 33rd Interscience Conference on Antimicrobial Agents and Chemotherapy. New Orleans, LA. American Society for Microbiology. Abstract # 659, 1993.

Cenci E, Mencacci A, Del Sero G, Bistoni F, Romani L. Induction of protective Th1 responses to *Candida albicans* by antifungal therapy alone or in combination with an interleukin-4 antagonist. *J Infect Dis* 176:217–226, 1997.

Chapman H A, Hibbs J B. Modulation of macrophage tumoricidal capability by polyene antibiotics: Support for membrane lipid as a regulatory determinant of macrophage function. *Proc Natl Acad Sci USA* 75:4349–4353, 1978.

Cheng J T, Witty R T, Robinson R R, Yarger W E. Amphotericin B nephrotoxicity: increased renal resistance and tubule permeability. *Kidney Int* 22:626–633, 1982.

Chia J K, Pollack M. Amphotericin B induces tumor necrosis factor production by murine macrophages. *J Infect Dis* 159:113–116, 1989.

Christiansen K J, Bernard E M, Gold J W M, Armstrong D. Distribution and activity of amphotericin B in humans. *J Infect Dis* 152:1037–43, 1985.

Cleary J D, Weisdorf D, Fletcher C V. Effect of infusion rate on amphotericin B-associated febrile reactions. *Drug Intell Clin Pharm* 22:769–772, 1988.

Cleary J D, Chapman S W, Nolan R L. Pharmacologic modulation of interleukin-1 expression by amphotericin B-stimulated human mononuclear cells. *Antimicrob Agents Chemother* 36:977–981, 1992.

Cleary J D, Hayman J, Sherwood J, Lasala G P, Piazza-Hepp T. Amphotericin B overdose in pediatric patients with associated cardiac arrest. *Ann Pharmacother* 27:715–718, 1993.

Cleary J D. Amphotericin B formulated in a lipid emulsion. *Ann Pharmacotherapy* 30: 409–412, 1996.

Collazos J, Martinez E, Mayo J, Ibarra S. Pulmonary reactions during treatment with amphotericin B: review of published cases and guidelines for management. *Clin Infect Dis* 33:E75–E82, 2001.

Collette N, van der Auwera P, Lopez A P, Heymans C, Meunier F. Tissue concentrations and bioactivity of amphotericin B in cancer patients treated with amphotericin B-deoxycholate. *Antimicrob Agents Chemother*. 33:362–368, 1989.

Craven, P C, Gremillion, D H. Risk factors for ventricular fibrillation during rapid amphotericin B infusion. *Antimicrob Agents Chemother* 27:868–871, 1985.

Daneshmend T K, Warnock D W. Clinical pharmacokinetics of systemic antifungal drugs. *Clin Pharmacokinet* 8: 17–42, 1983.

Diot P, Dequin P F, Rivoire B, Gagnadoux F, Faurisson F, Diot E, Boissinot E, Le Pape A, Palmer L, Lemarie E. Aerosols and anti-infectious agents. *J Aerosol Med* 14:55–64, 2001.

Dismukes W E, Cloud G, Gallis H A, Kerkering T M, Medoff G, Craven P C, Kaplowitz L G, Fisher J F, Gregg C R, Bowles C A, Shadomy S, Stamm A M, Diasio R B, Kaufman L, Soong S-J, Blackwelder W C, and the National Institute of Allergy and Infectious Diseases Mycoses Study Group. Treatment of cryptococcal meningitis with combination amphotericin B and flucytosine for four as compared with six weeks. *N Engl J Med* 317:334–341, 1987.

Drutz D J, Spickard A, Rogers D E, Koenig M G. Treatment of disseminated mycotic infections. A new approach to amphotericin B therapy. *Am J Med* 45: 405–18, 1968.

Dutcher J P, Kendall J, Norris D, Schiffer C, Aisner J, Wiernik P H. Granulocyte transfusion therapy and amphotericin B adverse reactions? *Am J Hematol* 31:102–108, 1989.

Eriksson U, Seifert B, Schaffner A. Comparison of effects of amphotericin B deoxycholate infused over 4 or 24 hours: randomized controlled trial. *Br Med J* 322:579–582, 2001.

Ernst E, Klepser M E, Pfaller M A. Post-antifungal effects of echinocandin, azole, and polyene antifungal agents against *Candida albicans* and *Cryptococcus neoformans. Antimicrob Agents Chemother* 44:1108–1111, 2000.

Fan-Havard P, Odonovan C, Smith S M, Oh J, Bamberger M, Eng R H K. Oral fluconazole versus amphotericin B bladder irrigation for treatment of candidal funguria. *Clin Infect Dis* 21:960–965, 1995.

Gallis H A, Drew R H, Pickard W W. Amphotericin B: 30 years of clinical experience. *Rev Infect Dis* 12:308–329, 1990.

Gelfand J A, Kimball K, Burke J K, Dinarello C A. Amphotericin B treatment of human mononuclear cells in vitro results in secretion of tumor necrosis factor and interleukin-1. *Clin Res* 36:456A, 1988.

Georgopapadakou, N H, Walsh, T J. Antifungal agents: chemotherapeutic targets and immunologic stratagies. *Antimicrob Agents Chemother* 40:279–291, 1996.

Ghannoum M A, Rice L B. Antifungal agents: mode of action, mechanisms of resistance, and correlation of these mechanisms with bacterial resistance. *Clin Microbiol Rev* 12:501–517, 1999.

Gigliotti F, Shenep J L, Lott L, Thornton D. Induction of prostaglandin synthesis as the mechanism responsible for the chills and fever produced by infusing amphotericin B. *J Infect Dis* 156: 784–789, 1987.

Goodwin S D, Cleary J D, Walawander C A, Taylor J W, Grasela

T H. Pretreatment regimens for adverse events related to infusion of amphotericin B. *Clin Infect Dis* 20:755–761, 1995.

Griswold M W, Briceland L L, Stein D S. Is amphotericin B test dosing needed? *Ann Pharmacother* 32:475–477, 1998.

Groll A H, Giri N, Petraitis V, Petraitiene R, Candelario M, Bacher J S, Piscitelli S C, Walsh T J. Comparative efficacy and distribution of lipid formulations of amphotericin B in experimental *Candida albicans* infection of the central nervous system. *J Infect Dis* 182:274–282, 2000.

Gunderson, B W, Ross G H, Ibrahim K H, Rotschafer J C. What do we really know about antibiotic pharmacodynamics? *Pharmacother* 21(11 Pt 2):302S-318S, 2001.

Gussak H M, Rahman S, Bastani B. Administration and clearance of amphotericin B during high-efficiency or high-efficiency/high-flux dialysis. *Am J Kidney Dis* 37:E45, 2001.

Hamill R J, Sobel J, El-Sadr W, Johnson W, Graybill J R, Javaly K, Barker D. Randomized, double-blind trial of AmBisome (liposomal amphotericin B) and amphotericin B in acute cryptococcal meningitis in AIDS patients. In: Abstracts of the 39th Annual Interscience Conference on Antimicrobial Agents and Chemotherapy. San Francisco, CA. American Society for Microbiology, Abstract # 1161, 1999.

Hardie W D, Wheeler A P, Wright P W, Swindell B B, Bernard G R. Effect of cyclooxygenase inhibition on amphotericin B-induced lung injury in awake sheep. *J Infect Dis* 166:134–138, 1992.

Hauser W E, Remington J S. Effects of amphotericin B on natural killer cell activity in vitro. *J Antimicrob Chemother* 11:257–262, 1983.

Hsuchen C C, Feingold D S. Selective membrane toxicity of the polyene antibiotics: studies on natural membranes. *Antimicrob Agents Chemother* 4:316–319, 1973.

Janknegrt R, de Marie S, Bakker-Woudenberg I A J M, Crommelin D J A. Liposomal and lipid formulations of amphotericin B: Clinical pharmacokinetics. *Clin Pharmacokinet* 23: 279–291, 1992.

Johnson M D, Drew R H, Perfect J R. Chest discomfort associated with liposomal amphotericin B: report of three cases and review of the literature. *Pharmacother* 18:1053–61, 1998.

Kelly, S L, Lamb, D C, Kelly, D E, Manning, N J, Loeffler, J, Hebart H, Schumacker U, Einsele H. Resistance to fluconazole and cross resistance to amphotericin B in *Candida albicans* from AIDS patients caused by defective sterol delta 5,6-desaturation. *FEBS Lett* 400:80–82, 1997.

King C T, Rogers P D, Cleary J D, Chapman, S W. Antifungal therapy during pregnancy. *Clin Infect Dis* 27:1151–1160, 1998.

Kretschmar M, Nichterlein T, Hannak D, Hof H. Effects of amphotericin B incorporated into liposomes and in lipid suspensions in the treatment of murine candidiasis. *Arzneimittelforschung (Drug Research).* 46:711–715, 1996.

Le T P, Tuazoncu, Levine M, Vorumm, Rollhauser, C. Resistance to fluconazole and amphotericin B in patients with AIDS who are being treated for candidal esophagitis. *Clin Infect Dis* 23:649–650, 1996.

Leenders A C, Reiss P, Portegies P, Clezy K, Hop W C, Hoy J, Borleffs J C, Allworth T, Kauffmann R H, Jones P, Kroon F P, Verbrugh H A, de Marie S. Liposomal amphotericin B (AmBisome) compared with amphotericin B both followed by oral fluconazole in the treatment of AIDS-associated cryptococcal meningitis. *AIDS* 11:1463–1471, 1997.

Lesar T S, Fiscella R G. Antimicrobial drug delivery to the eye. *Drug Intelligence Clin Pharm* 19:642–654, 1985.

Lewis R E, Klepser M E, Piscitelli S C, Groll A, De Lallo V C, Quintiliani R, Ernst E J, Walsh T J, Pfaller M A. In vivo activity of high-dose liposomal amphotericin B (AmBisome) in a neutropenic murine candidal thigh infection model. In: Program and abstracts of the 39th Interscience Conference on Antimicrobial Agents and

Chemotherapy, San Francisco, CA. American Society for Microbiology, Abstract #1001, 1999.

Lewis R E, Kontoyiannis D P. Rationale for combination antifungal therapy. *Pharmacother* 21:149S-164S, 2001.

Lin A C, Goldwasser E, Bernard E M, Chapman S W. Amphotericin B blunts erythropoietin response to anemia. *J Infect Dis* 161: 348–351, 1990.

Lin H, Medoff G, Kobayashi G S. Effects of amphotericin B on macrophages and their precursor cells. *Antimicrob Agents Chemother* 11:154–160, 1977.

Lyman C A, Walsh T J. Systemically administered antifungal agents. A review of their clinical pharmacology and therapeutic applications. *Drugs* 44:9–35, 1992.

Marmer D J, Fields B T, France G L, Steele R W. Ketoconazole, amphotericin B, and amphotericin B methyl ester: Comparative in vitro and in vivo toxicological effects on neutrophil function. *Antimicrob Agents Chemother* 20:660–665, 1981.

McDonnell T J, Chang S W, Westcott J Y, Voelkel N F. Role of oxidants, eicosanoids, and neutrophils in amphotericin B lung injury in rats. *J Appl Physiol* 65:2195–2206, 1988.

Mozaffarian N, Berman J W, Casadevall A. Enhancement of nitric oxide synthesis by macrophages represents an additional mechanism of action for amphotericin B. *Antimicrob Agents Chemother* 41:1825–1829, 1997.

Nair M P N, Schwartz S A. Immunomodulatory effects of amphotericin-B on cellular cytotoxicity of normal human lymphocytes. *Cell Immunol* 70:287–300, 1982.

North R J. The action of cortisone acetate on cell-mediated immunity to infection: Suppression of host cell proliferation and alteration of cellular composition of infective foci. *J Exp Med* 134: 1485–1500, 1971.

O'Riordan T, Faris M. Inhaled antimicrobial therapy. *Respir Care Clin N Am* 5:617–631, 1999.

Osaka K, Ritov V B, Bernardo J F, Branch R A, Kagan V E. Amphotericin B protects cis-parinaric acid against peroxyl radical-induced oxidation: amphotericin B as an antioxidant. *Antimicrob Agents Chemother* 41:743–747, 1997.

Patel, R. Antifungal Agents. Part I. Amphotericin preparations and flucytosine. *Mayo Clin Proc* 1973:1205–1225, 1998.

Peacock J E Jr., Herrington D A, Cruz J M. Amphotericin B therapy: Past, present, future. *Infect Dis Clin Pract* 2:81–93, 1993.

Powderly W G, Kobayashi G S, Herzig G P, Medof G. Amphotericin B-resistant yeast infection in severely immunocompromised patients. *Am J Med* 84:826–832, 1988.

Powderly W G, Keath E J, Sokol-Anderson M, Robinson K, Kitzd, Little J R. Amphotericin B resistant *Cryptococcus neoformans* in a patient with AIDS. *Infect Dis Clin Pract* 1:314–316, 1992.

Present C A, Klahr C, Santala R. Amphotericin B induction of sensitivity to adriamycin, 1, 3-bis (2-chloroethyl)-1 nitrosourea (BCNU) plus cyclophosphamide in human neoplasia. *Ann Intern Med* 86:47–49, 1977.

Rex J H, Walsh T J. Editorial response: estimating the true cost of amphotericin B. *Clin Infect Dis* 29: 1408–1410, 1999.

Rex J H, Pappas P G, Karchmer A W, Sobel J, Edwards J E, Hadley S, Brass C, Vazquez J A, Chapman S W, Horowitz H W, Zervos M, Lee J, for the National Institute of Allergy and Infectious Diseases Mycoses Study Group. A randomized, blinded, multicenter trial of high dose fluconazole plus placebo versus fluconazole plus amphotericin B as therapy of candidemia in non-neutropenic patients. In press, *Clin Infect Dis*, 2003.

Robinson R F, Nahata M C. A comparative review of conventional and lipid formulations of amphotericin B. *J Clin Pharm Ther* 24:249–257, 1999.

Rogers P D, Jenkins J K, Chapman S W, Ndebele K, Chapman B A, Cleary J D. Amphotericin B activation of human genes encoding for cytokines. *J Infect Dis* 178:1726–1733, 1998.

Rogers P D, Stiles J K, Chapman S W, Cleary J D. Amphotericin B induces expression of genes encoding chemokines and cell adhesion molecules in the human monocytic cell line THP-1. *J Infect Dis* 182:1280–1283, 2000.

Rogers P D, Perason M M, Cleary J D, Chapman S W, Sullivan D C. Differential expression of genes encoding for immunodulatory proteins in response to amphotericin B in the human monocytic cell line THP-1 identified by cDNA array analysis. *J Antimicrob Chemother* 50:811–817, 2002.

Roselle G A, Kauffman C A. Amphotericin B and 5-fluorocytosine: In vitro effects on lymphocyte function. *Antimicrob Agents Chemother* 14:398–402, 1978.

Sabra R, Branch R A. Amphotericin B nephrotoxicity. *Drug Saf* 5: 94–108, 1990.

Sandhu D K. Effect of amphotericin B on the metabolism of *Aspergillus fumigatus*. *Mycopathologia* 68:23–29, 1979.

Sawaya, B P, Weihprech T H, Campbell W R, Lorenz J N, Webb R C, Briggs J P, Schnermann J. Direct basal vasoconstriction as a possible cause for amphotericin B nephrotoxicity in rats. *J Clin Infect* 87:2097–2107, 1991.

Schmitt H J. New methods of delivery of amphotericin B. *Clin Infect Dis* 17 (Suppl 2):S501–S506, 1993.

Sharkey P K, Graybill J R, Johnson E S, Hausrath S G, Pollard R B, Kolokathis A, Mildvan D, Fan-Havard P, Eng R H, Patterson T F, Pottage J C Jr, Simberkoff M S, Wolf J, Meyer R D, Gupta R, Lee L W, Gordon D S. Amphotericin B lipid complex compared with amphotericin B in the treatment of cryptococcal meningitis in patients with AIDS. *Clin Infect Dis* 22:329–330, 1996.

Slain D. Lipid-based amphotericin B for the treatment of fungal infections. *Pharmacother* 19:306–323, 1999.

Snyder D S, Unanue E R. Corticosteroids inhibit murine macrophage Ia expression and interleukin 1 production. *J Immun* 129:1803–1805, 1982.

Sobel J D. Use of antifungal drugs in pregnancy: a focus on safety. *Drug Safety* 23:77–85, 2000.

Sokol-Anderson M L, Brajtburg J, Medoff G. Amphotericin B-induced oxidative damage and killing of *Candida albicans*. *J Infect Dis* 154:76–83, 1986.

Speeleveld E, Gordts B, Van Landuyt H W, De Vroey C, Raes-Wuytack C. Susceptibility of clinical isolates *Fusarium* to antifungal drugs. *Mycoses* 39:37–40, 1996.

Starke J R, Mason E O Jr., Kramer W G, Kaplan S L. Pharmacokinetics of amphotericin B in infants and children. *J Infect Dis* 155: 766–774, 1987.

Stewart, S J, Spagnuolo P J, Ellner J J. Generation of suppressor T lymphocytes and monocytes by amphotericin B. *J Immunol* 127: 135–139, 1981.

Sugar A M. Use of amphotericin B with azoles with antifungal drugs: what are we doing? *Antimicrob Agents Chemother* 39:1907–1912, 1995.

Tatro D S (ed.). Drug Interaction Facts. Facts and Comparisons, St. Louis, MO, 1998.

Turnidge J D, Gudmondsson S, Vogelman B, Craig W A. The postantibiotic effect of antifungal agents against common pathogenic yeast. *J Antimicrob Chemother* 34: 83–92, 1994.

Van der Horst C M, Saag M S, Cloud G A, Hamill R J, Graybill J R, Sobel J D, Johnson P C, Tuazon C U, Kerkering T, Moskovitz B L, Powderly W G, Dismukes W E, National Institute of Allergy and Infectious Diseases Mycoses Study Group and AIDS Clinical Trials Group. Treatment of cryptococcal meningitis associated with the acquired immunodeficiency syndrome. *N Engl J Med* 337:15–21, 1997.

Vanden Bossche H, Dromer F, Improvisi I, Lozano-Chiu M, Rex J H, Sangland D. Antifungal drug resistance in pathogenic fungi. *Med Mycol* 36(Suppl 1):119–128, 1998.

Villani R, Regazzi M B, Maserati R, Viale P, Alberici F, Giacchino R. Clinical and pharmacokinetic evaluation of a new lipid-based delivery system of amphotericin B in AIDS patients. *Arzneimittelforschung* (Drug Research) 46:445–449, 1996.

Walsh T J, Whitcomb P, Piscitelli S, Figg W D, Hill S, Chanock S J, Jarosinski P, Gupta R, Pizzo P A. Safety, tolerance, and pharmacokinetics of amphotericin B lipid complex in children with hepatosplenic candidiasis. Antimicrob Agents Chemother 41:1944–1948, 1997.

Walsh T J, Finberg R W, Arndt C, Hiemenz J, Schwartz C, Bodensteiner D, Pappas P, Seibel N, Greenberg R N, Dummer S, Schuster M, Holcenberg J S, National Institute of Allergy and Infectious Diseases Mycoses Study Group. Liposomal amphotericin B for empirical therapy in patients with persistent fever and neutropenia. *N Engl J Med* 340:764–771, 1999.

Wen D Y, Bottini A G, Hall W A, Haines S J. Infections in neurologic surgery. The intraventricular use of antibiotics. *Neurosurg Clin N Am* 3:343–354, 1992.

White M H, Anaissie E J, Kusne S, Wingard J R, Hiemenz J W, Cantor A, Gurwith M, Du Mond C, Mamelok R D, Bowden R A. Amphotericin B colloidal dispersion vs. amphotericin B as therapy for invasive aspergillosis. *Clin Infect Dis* 24:635–642, 1997.

White T C, Marr K A, Bowden R A. Clinical, cellular, and molecular factors that contribute to antifungal drug resistance. *Clin Microbiol Rev* 11:382–402, 1998a.

White M H, Bowden R A, Sandler E S, Graham M L, Noskin G A, Wingard J R, Goldman M, van Burik J A, McCabe A, Lin J S, Gurwith M, Miller C B. Randomized, double-blind clinical trial of amphotericin B colloidal dispersion vs. amphotericin B in the empirical treatment of fever and neutropenia. *Clin Infect Dis* 27: 296–302, 1998b.

Wingard J R, White M H, Anaissie E, Raffalli J, Goodman J, Arrieta A. L Amph/ ABLC Collaborative Study Group. A randomized, double-blind comparative trial evaluating the safety of liposomal amphotericin B versus amphotericin B lipid complex in the empirical treatment of febrile neutropenia. *Clin Infect Dis* 31:1155–1163, 2000.

Wright D G, Robichaud K J, Pizzo PA, Deisseroth A B. Lethal pulmonary reactions associated with the combination use of amphotericin B and leukocyte transfusions. *N Engl J Med* 304:1185–1189, 1981.

4

Liposomal nystatin

RICHARD J. HAMILL

Nystatin, the first successful antifungal agent, was isolated and subsequently developed through the collaborative efforts of Rachel Fuller Brown, a biochemist employed by the New York State Department of Health in Albany, and Elizabeth Lee Hazen, a microbiologist working in New York City. In a soil sample obtained from a dairy farm in Virginia, Hazen isolated a *Streptomyces* species, later identified as *Streptomyces noursei*. This organism produced two antifungal substances; one was later found to be too toxic for subsequent development. A second compound was present in the alcohol extracts from surface growth in liquid media of 5–7 day-old cultures. This material had a broad spectrum of antifungal activity and prolonged the life of mice infected with *Cryptococcus neoformans* and *Histoplasma capsulatum* (Hazen and Brown, 1950). Hazen and Brown originally called this agent fungicidin (Hazen and Brown, 1951), but later changed the name to nystatin after the New York State Department of Health Laboratories. They presented their discovery at the 1950 meeting of the National Academy of Sciences (Hazen and Brown, 1951), and were subsequently awarded a patent on June 25, 1957. E.R. Squibb & Sons received the license for the patent and began marketing the drug as Mycostatin® in 1954.

Because of its hydrophobic nature, parenteral preparations of nystatin were difficult to prepare. Furthermore, initial human studies with intravenous nystatin preparations were complicated by substantial adverse reactions including phlebitis, fevers, chills, and nausea (Lehan et al, 1957). Although nystatin demonstrated clinical activity and toxicities similar to amphotericin B in these early human studies, further development of intravenous nystatin did not occur.

Despite its toxicity when administered parenterally, nystatin possesses several properties that make it an attractive antifungal agent, including a broad spectrum of antifungal activity, even against some amphotericin B resistant isolates and proven antifungal activity in animals and humans (Campbell et al, 1955). Consequently, in the 1980s, based on their previous successful experiences with liposomal formulations of amphotericin B, Lopez-Berestein and colleagues at the University of Texas MD Anderson Cancer Center developed a liposomal formulation of nystatin (Mehta et al, 1987a). In vitro, liposomal nystatin was as active or more active than free nystatin (Mehta et al, 1987a). Liposomal encapsulation substantially reduced the toxicity of nystatin and demonstrated therapeutic activity in experimental models of systemic candidiasis (Mehta et al, 1987b).

CHEMISTRY OF NYSTATIN

Nystatin is a tetraene diene macrolide polyene with the molecular formula of $C_{47}H_{75}NO_{17}$ and a molecular weight of 926.13. Because, in all of its properties except UV absorption, nystatin behaves as a heptaene, like amphotericin B, nystatin is sometimes referred to as a degenerate heptaene (Hammond, 1977). The macrolide ring contains 37 carbons with a series of double bonds and has an attached hexosamine sugar, mycosamine, which imparts amphoteric properties on the molecule due to the presence of both basic (hexosamine) and acidic (carboxyl) residues (Fig. 4–1).

The relative insolubility of nystatin is determined by the unsaturated chromophore, and is limited in water or nonpolar organic solvents like most alcohols. Commercial preparations of nystatin contain a single, highly pure chromatographic peak (A1) when suspended in organic solvents (Ostrosky-Zeichner et al, 2001). However, in biologic fluids such as human plasma or culture medium, chromatographic analysis reveals a second peak (A2); formation of the second peak is accelerated at pH values > 7.0. Peaks A1 and A2 are quite similar by mass spectrometry and nuclear magnetic resonance analysis, and are probably structural isomers of each other. Nystatin A1 is considerably more stable and predominates. Antifungal activity of the compound probably resides wholly within nystatin A1 (Ostrosky-Zeichner et al, 2001).

Recently, the complete set of genes in *S. noursei* responsible for biosynthesis of nystatin have been cloned and analyzed (Brautaset et al, 2000). The DNA sequence contains 6 genes encoding a modular polyketide synthase, genes for thioesterase, deoxysugar biosynthesis,

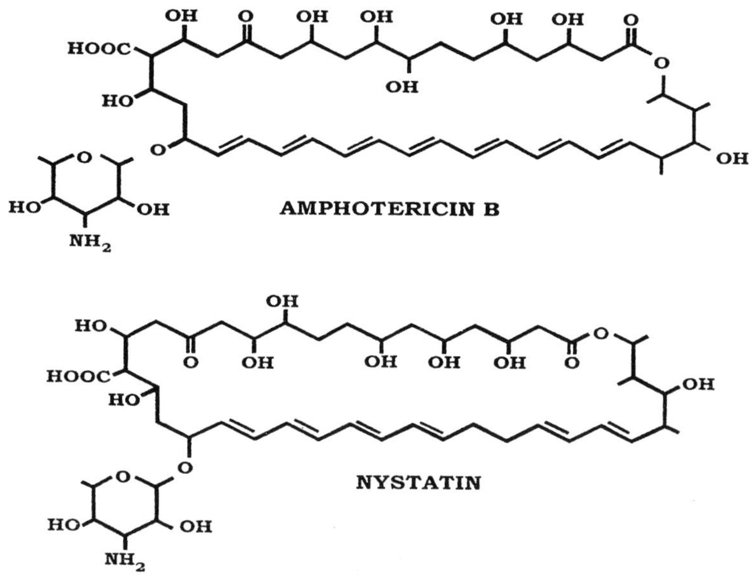

FIGURE 4–1. Comparison of the structures of amphotericin B and nystatin. Note the absence of the double bond between the tetraene and diene chromophores within the macrolide ring of nystatin.

modification, transport, and regulatory proteins. The polyketide synthases are responsible, in a manner similar to fatty acid biosynthesis, for producing an extended polyketide chain beginning with acetyl-CoA, proceeding through a condensation step using 3 methyl-malonyl-CoAs and 15 malonyl CoA extender units. Thioesterase is responsible for release of this polyketide chain from the polyketide synthase and probably also for cyclization and modification of the macrolactone ring. The coding of the genes of *S. noursei* and subsequent studies represent the first example of the complete DNA sequence analysis of a polyene antibiotic and may facilitate future development of other polyenes (Brautaset et al, 2002).

LIPOSOMAL NYSTATIN

Liposomal nystatin is very similar to liposomal amphotericin B in composition and consists of multilamellar spherical liposomes 0.1–3 μm in diameter that contain dimyristoylphosphatidylcholine and dimyristoylphosphatidyglycerol in a 7:3 molar ratio (Mehta et al, 1987a). The nystatin component makes up 7 mol%. Antigenics, Inc. currently holds the license for development of liposomal nystatin.

MECHANISM OF ACTION

Although the exact mechanism of action of the polyene antibiotics is somewhat controversial, several lines of evidence support the hypothesis that an irreversible interaction with sterols, particularly ergosterol, in the plasma membrane is important (Lampen et al, 1962):

(1) organisms that lack sterols in the plasma membrane are not susceptible to nystatin; *(2)* the antifungal activity of nystatin is inhibited by the exogenous addition of sterols, particularly those with a 3β-hydroxyl group, a planar sterol nucleus and a long C_{17} side chain; *(3)* membranes that are extracted with organic solvents to remove sterols fail to bind nystatin; *(4)* sterol complexing agents (e.g., digitonin) interfere with nystatin activity and can release a significant portion of bound nystatin; and *(5)* limited spectroscopic evidence suggests a direct interaction of sterols with polyenes.

The structure of nystatin is very closely related to that of amphotericin B, except that in the nystatin molecule the double bond system is interrupted by saturation of the bond separating the tetraene and diene chromophores (Fig. 4–1). Presumably, this allows for greater flexibility of an otherwise rigid structure. The structural similarities of amphotericin B and nystatin suggest that a similar mechanism of activity should exist for the 2 drugs. Microarray measurements of differential gene expression in *Saccharomyces cerevisiae* exposed to amphotericin B or nystatin supports this supposition (Zhang et al, 2002). A similar configuration to that of amphotericin B-sterol pores has been proposed for nystatin in artificial sterol-lecithin bilayers (Kleinberg and Finkelstein, 1984). The permeability characteristics of nystatin pores closely resemble those of amphotericin B pores, and in artificial membranes, mixed pores containing both drugs can be produced. In order to assemble functioning pores, certain requirements are necessary: *(1)* intact polyene molecules are necessary; *(2)* permeability changes are dependent on the antibiotic concentration; for amphotericin B, between 5 and 10 molecules/pore of amphotericin B are required and, presumably, a similar number for nystatin; *(3)* the polyene-sterol interaction is hydrophobic and the interaction occurs in such a way that the membrane sterols are pulled away from interactions with other membrane lipids. All of this results in dynamic aqueous pores that coalesce and reform in a continuous fashion. Amphotericin B pores have a Stokes-Einstein radius of 7–10 Å, while those of nystatin are somewhat smaller at 4–7 Å (Finkelstein and Holz, 1973). The water and nonelectrolyte permeability induced in thin lipid membranes by the polyene antibiotics, as well as space-filling molecular models of amphotericin B, suggest that the channel that is formed consists of 2 "barrels" hydrogen-bonded end-to-end, with each barrel consisting of 8–10 polyene monomers arranged circumferentially as staves of this barrel. All of this results in selective intracellular K^+ leakage, which occurs within 2 minutes of antibiotic application and a subsequent change in intracellular ADP/ATP ratios, due to the dependence of the intracellular glycolytic pathway on K^+. Potassium loss is followed at a later time by loss of Mg^{++}, acidification of the fungal cell and precipitation of cytoplasmic components (Hammond, 1977). However, K^+ release in and of itself does not completely account for killing activity of nystatin; potassium leakage is greater with nystatin, but fungal death is faster with amphotericin B (Chen et al, 1978).

Presumably, liposomal encapsulation of nystatin results in localization of the drug within cells of the reticuloendothelial system, such as macrophages, and possible concentration in inflammatory foci. The mechanism by which nystatin is transferred to fungal cells from liposomes has not been elucidated.

Pharmacokinetics

When liposomal nystatin is incubated in human plasma, disruption of the liposomal structure ensues within 5 minutes (Wasan et al, 1997). Most of the nystatin, however, remains lipid associated, suggesting that lipid-drug complexes form. These then fuse rapidly with lipoproteins with approximately 13% associated with the LDL fraction, 44% in the HDL fraction and 42% in the lipoprotein-deficient plasma, principally associated with albumin and α-1-glycoprotein (Wasan et al, 1997). The association of liposomal nystatin with the HDL portion probably results from the attraction of the dimyristoylphosphatidylglycerol component to apoproteins AI and AII. As the protein content of the HDL increases, so does the amount of nystatin found associated with the HDL fraction (Cassidy et al, 1998). It has been hypothesized that the reduced association of liposomal nystatin with the LDL fraction may account for its decreased frequency of nephrotoxicity, as renal tubular uptake of polyene antibiotics appears to be dependent on the presence of LDL receptors on the renal tubular cell surface (Wasan et al, 1994).

Single-dose pharmacokinetics of liposomal nystatin were evaluated in 17 patients with HIV infection (Rios et al, 1993). Four patient groups were studied, each at doses of 0.25, 0.5, 0.75, and 1 mg/kg (Table 4–1). After intravenous administration, initial clearance is rapid with a terminal half-life of approximately 5 hours. The drug approximately distributes into the whole blood volume. At doses of 0.25 to 0.75 mg/kg, the area under the concentration-time curve appeared to increase in direct proportion to the administered dose; at higher doses, the AUC did not increase, suggesting saturation of drug clearance mechanisms. Saturation of these clearance mechanisms was also supported by the observation that the terminal half-life continued to increase as the dose was increased. These results suggest that there is increasing tissue exposure of the drug with higher doses, most likely resulting in increased intracellular concentrations.

Multiple dose pharmacokinetics were also evaluated in patients with HIV infection (Cossum et al, 1996) at doses of 2, 3, 4, 5, and 7 mg/kg given every other day. Therapeutic blood levels were achieved, and maintained for several hours, even at the lowest dose administered. The concentration at the end of the infusion and AUC continued to increase with increasing

TABLE 4–1. *Single-Dose Pharmacokinetic Parameters of Liposomal Nystatin*

Parameter	Liposomal Nystatin Dose (mg/kg)			
	0.25	0.5	0.75	1.0
Initial clearance (min)	9.1 ± 1	12 ± 4.8	10.2 ± 4.2	7.3 ± 3
Secondary half-life (min)	—	—		42.6 ± 16
Terminal-phase half-life (min)	155 ± 62	207 ± 79	255 ± 55	331 ± 113
Initial blood concentration (μg/mL)	3.7 ± 6.3	5.9 ± 0.8	6.5 ± 0.5	9 ± 0.6
Area under concentration-time curve (μg/mL/min)	452 ± 86	732 ± 172	1274 ± 483	1263 ± 301
Volume of distribution (L)	5.2 ± 0.7	7.6 ± 1.5	10 ± 0.8	9.1 ± 1.6
Clearance rate from blood (mL/kg/min)	0.6 ± 0.1	0.8 ± 0.2	0.9 ± 0.2	1.0 ± 0.4

Source: Table modified, with permission, from Rios et al, 1993.

doses, with maximal blood concentrations increasing from 4.8 to 24.1 μg/mL for doses of 2 and 5 mg/kg, respectively. The volume of distribution and terminal half-life did not increase with increasing doses.

Plasma pharmacokinetics for liposomal nystatin after intravenous infusions in rabbits are comparable to those in the blood for humans, supporting the use of rabbits as an experimental model (Groll et al, 2000b). The drug exhibits nonlinear, dose dependent pharmacokinetics over a dosage range of 2 to 6 mg/kg/day. Peak plasma levels that are several fold higher than the MICs of susceptible fungi can be achieved. The drug is rapidly distributed after infusion and eliminated relatively slowly with an elimination half-life of 1 to 2 hours. After administration of multiple doses for 15 days, the highest concentrations of nystatin were found in the lungs, liver, and spleen, followed by the kidney. Levels in the cerebrospinal fluid at 2, 4, or 6 mg/kg/day were too low to quantitate.

The urinary pharmacokinetics and disposition of liposomal nystatin have not been studied in humans, but have been investigated in rabbits, whose serum pharmacokinetics qualitatively approximate those of humans (Groll et al, 2000a). After administration of single intravenous doses of 2, 4, or 6 mg/kg, maximal urinary concentrations of nystatin were obtained that were at least 10-fold higher and AUC values at least 4-fold higher than those obtained with amphotericin B deoxycholate given at a dose of 1 mg/kg. At the 2 mg/kg dose of liposomal nystatin, the C_{max} in the urine was 16.83 μg/mL, suggesting a potential role for liposomal nystatin for treatment of urinary tract infections due to susceptible fungi.

Unlike amphotericin B, murine pharmacokinetics for liposomal nystatin do not reflect those of the human. Mice exhibit lower peak concentration values and area under the curve than those found in humans, suggesting that nystatin may be less efficacious in mice than in humans (Arikan et al, 1998).

ADVERSE EFFECTS

Although nystatin binds to fungal membrane ergosterol with greater affinity, binding to human cell membranes containing cholesterol also occurs and is likely responsible for many of the adverse effects of the drug through the production of pores in human cells (Zager, 2000). Sodium influx is a dominant consequence. As a result, the human cells compensate by utilizing Na^+, K^+-adenosine triphosphatase-driven sodium extrusion that causes increased ATP utilization. To maintain the intracellular levels of ATP, dose-dependent increases in mitochondrial respiration, and consequently, oxygen consumption result. As the energy demand outstrips

ATP production, energy depletion occurs along with free radical generation and overload of intracellular calcium. The ultimate consequence is cellular death. Nystatin appears to be less toxic to renal tubular cells than amphotericin B as evidenced by substantially less impairment of cellular energetics. Liposomal nystatin also produces decreases in the ATP/ADP ratio; however, at about 1/16th the toxicity of free nystatin. Based on in vitro data, liposomal nystatin has similar cellular toxicity as liposomal amphotericin B and amphotericin B lipid complex.

In addition to effects on cellular energetics, the polyenes also demonstrate hemolytic activity. Nystatin has been previously demonstrated to be markedly less toxic to mammalian cells in vitro than amphotericin B (Kinsky, 1963; Thomas, 1986); the capacity of nystatin to induce K^+ leakage from yeast cells surpasses its ability to induce K^+ leakage from human RBCs by almost 300-fold (Kotler-Brajtburg et al, 1979). Furthermore, liposomal encapsulation of nystatin protected erythrocytes from the hemolytic toxicity of free nystatin (Mehta et al, 1987a).

Liposomal incorporation of nystatin substantially decreases the toxicity of free nystatin in vivo. In a murine model of systemic candidiasis, the maximal tolerated dose of free nystatin was 4 mg/kg of body weight; at that dose, there was no beneficial microbiological effect of the drug. On the other hand, the maximal tolerated dose of liposomal nystatin was 16 mg/kg of body weight, a dose that was associated with a significant improvement in the survival of the animals (Mehta et al, 1987b).

The predominant toxicity seen upon the intravenous administration of liposomal nystatin is nephrotoxicity, as demonstrated in rats and dogs by elevations in blood urea nitrogen and creatinine, and histopathologic changes in the kidneys. Liposomal nystatin appears to be much more toxic in rats and dogs than in humans. In dogs, large increases in serum blood urea nitrogen and creatinine occur after single intravenous doses of 1 mg//kg. However, tolerance appears to develop with repeated doses.

The most frequent adverse events reported in patients receiving multiple doses of liposomal nystatin in human trials included chills (17%), hypokalemia (16%), elevated creatinine (16%), fever (14%), headache (14%), pain (13%), nausea (13%), dyspnea (13%), rash (13%), abdominal pain (10%), and asthenia (10%).

A phase I study performed in refractory febrile neutropenic patients with hematological malignancies to determine the maximum tolerated dose of liposomal nystatin could not demonstrate a clear association between dose and drug-related toxicity (Boutati et al, 1995) Patients that developed nephrotoxicity had received the higher doses of liposomal nystatin (6 and

8 mg/kg), suggesting that nephrotoxicity may be the dose-limiting toxicity.

IN VITRO ACTIVITY

Nystatin has broad antifungal activity and is effective in vitro against most clinically important yeast and mould isolates. Unlike the situation that exists with amphotericin B, where the lipid formulations tend to produce higher MIC values, liposomal nystatin generally exhibits somewhat better activity in vitro than free nystatin (Mehta et al, 1987a; Johnson et al, 1998; Oakley et al, 1999; Quindós et al, 2000b; Arikan et al, 2002). However, the optimum testing methods and conditions, and the relevance of in vitro tests using liposomal nystatin remain unknown. Composition of test media and incubation time have been shown to substantially influence the determination of MIC values for both nystatin and liposomal nystatin for several *Candida* species (Arikan et al, 2002).

Typical minimal inhibitory concentrations for nystatin, liposomal nystatin and amphotericin B are shown in Table 4–2 for various clinically relevant fungi. At the therapeutic doses of 2–4 mg/kg of liposomal nystatin used in clinical trials to date, serum levels of nystatin that can be achieved are in excess of the MIC values for the majority of species that have been studied.

In an in vitro study comparing the relative activities of free nystatin, liposomal nystatin, amphotericin B deoxycholate, liposomal amphotericin B, amphotericin B colloidal dispersion and amphotericin B lipid complex against clinical isolates of *Aspergillus*, *Candida* and *C. neoformans*, liposomal nystatin was as active as free nystatin with MICs and MLCs that were similar to or lower than, those of free nystatin (Johnson et al, 1998). Neither formulation was as active as amphotericin B deoxycholate or amphotericin B lipid complex, with the MIC_{90} and MLC_{90} values for the latter drugs being 2–8-fold lower. The activities of both free and liposomal nystatin were similar to amphotericin B colloidal dispersion, but more effective in vitro than liposomal amphotericin B. Another study that examined the in vitro activity of conventional nystatin, liposomal nystatin, amphotericin B, liposomal amphotericin B, amphotericin B lipid complex, amphotericin B colloidal dispersion and itraconazole against 60 clinical *Aspergillus* isolates demonstrated that liposomal nystatin had acceptable MICs and MLCs for all strains tested (Oakley et al, 1999). Liposomal nystatin MICs were significantly higher, however, for strains of *A. terreus* compared to other *Aspergillus* species.

The effect of different test media and incubation periods on susceptibilities of several *Candida* species was evaluated and demonstrated that antibiotic medium 3 supplemented with 2% glucose produced MIC results for liposomal nystatin that were lower than those achieved with conventional medium (Arikan et al, 2002). Liposomal nystatin was active against the majority of strains in this study, even most amphotericin B resistant isolates. A few strains with dissociation between MIC values for nystatin and liposomal nystatin

TABLE 4–2. *Comparative In Vitro Susceptibility of Selected Fungi to Nystatin, Liposomal Nystatin, and Amphotericin B.*

Organism	Minimal Inhibitory Concentration Ranges (µg/mL)		
	Nystatin	Liposomal Nystatin	Amphotericin B
Candida albicans	0.78–10	0.31–2.5	0.04–2.5
Candida dubliniensis	—	0.25–1.0	0.5–1.0
Candida glabrata	0.15–2.5	0.62–5.0	0.15–2.0
Candida guilliermondii	2.0	1.0–2.0	0.25–1.0
Candida kefyr	2–8	1.0–4.0	1.0
Candida krusei	0.15–> 16	0.05–4.0	0.31–2.0
Candida lipolytica	1.0	2.0	—
Candida lusitaniae	0.03–2.0	0.5–2.0	0.06–1.0
Candida parapsilosis	0.15–4.0	0.62–4.0	0.31–2.0
Candida tropicalis	0.56–4.0	0.01–2.0	0.08–2.0
Cryptococcus neoformans	0.02–8.0	0.12–4.0	0.04–0.62
Trichosporon beigelii	0.5–1.0	0.5–1.0	0.12–1.0
Coccidioides immitis	2.0–8.0	2.0–4.0	0.25–0.5
Sporothrix schenckii	2.0	1.0	0.5–16
Fusarium sp.	4.0	2.0	1–2
Aspergillus flavus	2.0–8.0	1.0–4.0	0.5–4.0
Aspergillus fumigatus	2–> 8	1.0–4.0	0.5–2.0
Aspergillus niger	2.0–4.0	1.0–4.0	0.25–1.0
Scedosporium apiospermum	2.0–> 16	2.0–> 16	2.0–16
Scedosporium prolificans	8.0–> 16	4.0–> 16	1.0–> 16

Source: Data compiled from Johnson et al, 1998; Carillo-Muñoz et al, 1999; Oakley et al, 1999; Jessup et al, 2000; Quinidós et al, 2000a; Quindós et al, 2000b; Arikan et al, 2002; Meletiadis et al, 2002.

were identified; liposomal nystatin MICs were lower for these strains. For isolates of *C. krusei* with high amphotericin B MICs, liposomal nystatin had relatively low MICs and may offer an alternative for treatment of clinically significant infections due to this organism.

Clinical strains of *C. dubliniensis*, some of which were resistant to the various azole agents, were uniformly susceptible to liposomal nystatin, as well as to the other polyene agents (Quindós et al, 2000a). Liposomal nystatin was shown to have activity against *Coccidioides immitis*, regardless of what saprobic stage was tested in vitro (González et al, 2002). In vitro activity of liposomal nystatin was poor against 55 clinical isolates of *Scedosporium prolificans* and 13 isolates of *S. apiospermum*, but approximately paralleled the activity of amphotericin B (Meletiadis et al, 2002).

Only one study has evaluated the in vitro interaction of liposomal nystatin with other antifungal agents (Jessup et al, 2000). In combination with amphotericin B, liposomal nystatin was synergistic against 2 of 3 strains of *C. glabrata* tested and additive against the remaining isolate. In combination with itraconazole or flucytosine, liposomal nystatin was additive against 3 *C. krusei* isolates and was also additive in combination with amphotericin B against 2 of 3 *Aspergillus fumigatus* isolates tested. Several other fungi demonstrated additive activity; no combinations, however, exhibited antagonism. These results suggest that in the appropriate clinical situation, combination therapy that includes liposomal nystatin may be feasible.

RESISTANCE

Clinically significant resistance to nystatin, like amphotericin B, is very unusual. In vitro, it is possible to select for resistance by serial transfer of isolates on media containing increasing concentrations of nystatin (Athar and Winner, 1971). Emergence of resistance to nystatin in vivo has been described in individuals who have received amphotericin B therapy (Drutz and Lehrer, 1978; Merz and Sandford, 1979; Dick et al, 1980) and oral nystatin (Safe et al, 1977), but has not yet been described in patients who have received liposomal nystatin. Resistance to nystatin does not confer resistance to nonpolyene antifungal agents; however, there is considerable, but not invariable, cross-resistance between nystatin and amphotericin B (Athar and Winner, 1971; Broughton et al, 1991; Arikan et al, 2002). Multiple potential mechanisms of resistance to nystatin have been described (Wallace and Lopez-Berestein, 1999), although most cases have been associated with qualitative or quantitative changes in the sterol component of the fungal cell membrane (Hammond, 1977). In those situations where sterol analyses have been performed, the abnormalities tend to fall into 3 groups, which are not necessarily exclusive: *(1)* either

a decrease in ergosterol content compared to the wild type strain or complete absence of ergosterol; *(2)* replacement of ergosterol by another sterol, with the replacement sterol having a lower affinity for nystatin than ergosterol; and *(3)* an absolute increase in the amount of ergosterol in the membrane.

In vitro isolates resistant to nystatin have been selected by plating on increasing concentrations of the agent (Athar and Winner, 1971; Bard, 1972; Molzahn and Woods, 1971). Compared with their polyene-susceptible parent isolates, some of these mutants demonstrated decreased growth rate, reduced production of germ tubes, slower production of chlamydospores and reduced pathogenicity (Athar and Winner, 1971). In vivo emergence of resistance to nystatin due to a decrease or the absence of cell membrane ergosterol has been described in patients receiving oral nystatin (Safe et al, 1977) and amphotericin B (Woods et al, 1974; Drutz and Lehrer, 1978; Merz and Sandford, 1979; Dick et al, 1980). Several different species of *Candida* were affected, including *C. krusei*, *C. parapsilosis*, *C. tropicalis*, *C. albicans* and *C. glabrata*. In a study that demonstrated that 7.4% of 747 isolates from oncology patients were resistant, the rate of resistance among the different *Candida* species roughly paralleled the frequency of isolation of these species from the population (Dick et al, 1980). Factors predisposing to colonization or infection by a resistant strain included extended lengths of hospitalization, receipt of cytotoxic chemotherapy, periods of granulocytopenia and receipt of prolonged courses of antibiotics, including amphotericin B and oral nonabsorbable nystatin.

The second mechanism of resistance relates to replacement of ergosterol by another sterol, with the replacement sterol having a lower affinity for nystatin than ergosterol. The replacement sterol may be novel, and not normally found in the synthetic ergosterol pathway, e.g., $\Delta^{8,22}$-ergostadien-3β-ol found in nystatin-resistant strains of *S. cerevisiae* isolated in vitro (Molzahn and Woods; 1972). Even in isolates that contain some ergosterol, the presence of a new sterol with low affinity for nystatin may result in resistance (Woods, 1971). The third mechanism of resistance is related to an absolute increase in the amount of ergosterol in the membrane. This situation has been described in vitro by production of *C. albicans* mutants resistant to nystatin after exposure to the mutagenic agent, N′-methyl-N′-nitrosoguanidine (Hamilton-Miller, 1972). Presumably, the ergosterol is masked or reoriented in such a manner that it is not available for binding with the polyene.

POSTANTIFUNGAL EFFECT

The postantifungal effect (PAFE) of nystatin has been investigated for different species of *Candida*. Significant intraspecies variations in the duration of the postantifungal effect have been obtained; therefore, the results from a single isolate should not be extrapolated to define the postantifungal effect for an individual species of *Candida*. In addition, substantial interspecies variations also occur. For *C. albicans*, the mean PAFE has varied from 5.9 to 12.3 hours (Ellepola and Samaranayake, 1999; Egusa et al, 2000; Gunderson et al, 2000; Anil et al, 2001); for *C. tropicalis* from 5 to 14.8 hours (Ellepola and Samaranayake, 1999; Gunderson et al, 2000; Anil et al, 2001); for *C. glabrata* from 5 to 8.5 hours (Ellepola and Samaranayake, 1999; Gunderson et al, 2000); for *C. krusei* from 6.5 to 11.5 hours (Ellepola and Samaranayake, 1999; Gunderson et al, 2000); and for *C. parapsilosis* approximately 15.1 hours (Ellepola and Samaranayake, 1999). One study found a highly positive significant correlation between the MIC and PAFE for individual isolates of *Candida* (Gunderson et al, 2000). Despite the inconsistencies in the absolute length of the postantifungal effect, the relatively extended duration of the PAFE for *Candida* suggests that prolonged dosing intervals with liposomal nystatin are feasible.

AMIMAL MODELS OF INFECTION

In a neutropenic mouse model of disseminated *A. fumigatus* infection, doses of liposomal nystatin as low as 2 mg/kg/day protected mice against *Aspergillus*-induced death in a statistically significant manner. Liposomal nystatin was effective in clearing multiple organs, including the lungs, spleen, pancreas, kidney, and liver, although amphotericin B was significantly better (Wallace et al, 1997).

The activity of liposomal nystatin was investigated in persistently neutropenic rabbits with invasive pulmonary aspergillosis (Groll et al, 1999a). Liposomal nystatin was administered at doses of 1, 2, and 4 mg/kg daily and compared to amphotericin B 1.0 mg/kg/day given along with saline loading. At a dose of 1 mg/kg, liposomal nystatin was effective in reducing fungal tissue burden. Liposomal nystatin at 2 mg/kg/day or 4 mg/kg/day prolonged survival and reduced fungus-mediated tissue injury as well as excess lung weight similar to the results obtained with amphotericin B. Amphotericin B was more effective at clearing infected pulmonary tissues. Resolution of pulmonary lesions was demonstrated by ultrafast computed tomography in both the liposomal nystatin and amphotericin B-treated animals to a similar degree. Liposomal nystatin was well tolerated by the animals; mild elevations of blood urea nitrogen and creatinine values occurred to a degree similar to that in animals that received amphotericin B with saline loading. Survival was somewhat better in the liposomal nystatin-treated animals and potassium loss was less.

In a neutropenic guinea pig model of disseminated candidiasis, liposomal nystatin 3 mg/kg/day was compared to amphotericin B deoxycholate at 0.75 mg/kg/day (Reyes et al, 2000). Liposomal nystatin significantly reduced death and resulted in a significant reduction of fungal burden in the kidneys. Furthermore, liposomal nystatin was significantly better than amphotericin B in clearing the kidneys of *C. albicans*.

In a model of persistently neutropenic rabbits with subacute disseminated candidiasis, liposomal nystatin at doses or 2 mg/kg/day or 4 mg/kg/day were compared to amphotericin B deoxycholate 1 mg/kg/day and fluconazole 10 mg/kg/day with regards to the ability of the drugs to clear organisms from blood and tissues (Groll et al, 1999b). A significant dose dependent response to treatment was seen with liposomal nystatin. Activity of liposomal nystatin was similar to amphotericin B and fluconazole in terms of clearance of residual burden of *C. albicans* from kidney, liver, spleen, lung, and brain. Mean serum blood urea nitrogen and creatinine levels were significantly lower in animals that received either dose of liposomal nystatin compared to amphotericin B.

The CNS antifungal activity of liposomal nystatin was evaluated in a nonimmunocompromised rabbit model of disseminated candidiasis (Groll et al, 2001). Liposomal nystatin was given as either 2.5 mg/kg twice daily or 5.0 mg/kg once daily in rabbits with systemic candidiasis and compared to amphotericin B deoxycholate at 1 mg/kg daily or liposomal amphotericin B 5.0 mg/kg daily. Both liposomal nystatin regimens had similar efficacy to the two amphotericin B regimens in clearing extracerebral tissues. However, both doses of liposomal nystatin were significantly less active in the central nervous system. Furthermore, animals that had received the 5 mg/kg once daily dose had a significantly reduced survival due to CNS candidiasis. The reduced activity in the CNS correlated with cerebral tissue concentrations below the MIC of the infecting *Candida* isolate.

In a neutropenic mouse model that compared the activity of liposomal nystatin to amphotericin B deoxycholate, liposomal amphotericin B, and amphotericin B lipid complex in the treatment of systemic infection due to an isolate of *A. fumigatus* with reduced susceptibility to amphotericin B, liposomal nystatin at 5 mg/kg was significantly better in clearing tissues of the organism (Denning and Warn, 1999). Doses of liposomal nystatin as high as 10 mg/kg were toxic to animals and resulted in fits and respiratory arrest.

As a result of these animal studies, several conclusions regarding liposomal nystatin appear warranted: *(1)* there is a dose-dependent response to therapy that exists for *Candida* and *Aspergillus* species; doses in the range of 2–5 mg/kg prolong survival and result in clearance of the fungal burden from most tissues. However, at least in mice, the maximal tolerated dose is approximately 10 mg/kg; *(2)* the drug does not appear to be effective for treatment of central nervous system infections at the doses tested, probably because insufficient nystatin levels are achieved in cerebral tissues; and *(3)* renal toxicity and urinary potassium loss are less severe with liposomal nystatin than with amphotericin B.

HUMAN CLINICAL STUDIES

Data are available from only a few human clinical trials that have utilized liposomal nystatin. In a historical comparison of 43 nonneutropenic patients with candidemia that received liposomal nystatin 2 mg/kg/day and 109 patients reported earlier that had been treated with amphotericin B 0.5 mg/kg/day (Rex et al, 1994), the success rate with both regimens was 67%; 23% of patients that received liposomal nystatin died compared to 40% that received amphotericin B (Gordon et al, 1997). Renal toxicity, as defined by a doubling of serum creatinine, occurred in 14% of liposomal nystatin recipients and 37% of amphotericin B recipients, a difference that was not statistically significant.

In a multicenter study designed to evaluate two doses of liposomal nystatin in 109 nonneutropenic patients with candidemia, subjects received either 2 mg/kg/day or 4 mg/kg/day of liposomal nystatin (Williams and Moore, 1999). The response rate was 82.8% in the low dose group and 85.7% in the higher dose group. Twenty-five patients died, 2 possibly related to liposomal nystatin. Eighty-six adverse events were reported in 57 patients, but only 6 of the events were thought to be related to the study drug, although 29.4% of the patients developed hypokalemia.

In a multicenter trial of empiric antifungal therapy in 538 patients with neutropenic fever and presumed fungal infection, liposomal nystatin 2 mg/kg/day was compared to amphotericin 0.6–0.8 mg/kg/day (Powles et al, 1999). In the modified intent to treat population, 36% (65/180) of the evaluable patients who received liposomal nystatin were successfully treated compared to 39% (66/168) of the evaluable patients who received amphotericin B; these differences were not significant. Patients who received amphotericin B had significantly more renal adverse events, including BUN elevation ($p = 0.0009$), creatinine elevation ($p = 0.0001$), and hypokalemia ($p = 0.0007$), compared to those who received liposomal nystatin.

In 75 nonneutropenic patients with candidemia refractory to conventional agents, clinical success with liposomal nystatin at 2 mg/kg/day or 4 mg/kg/day was achieved in 60% of treated patients and mycological success was achieved in 55% (Rolston et al, 1999). No patient required discontinuation of nystatin therapy due to adverse events.

The efficacy of liposomal nystatin in 24 patients with invasive aspergillus who were refractory to (21 patients) or intolerant of (3 patients) amphotericin B was evaluated in a phase II trial (Offner et al, 2000). Objective responses were seen in 6 of these patients. Liposomal nystatin was discontinued in 2 patients because of severe rigors, chills, and hypotension. Liposomal nystatin also was evaluated in another small group of oncology patients with invasive aspergillosis who were unresponsive to or intolerant of conventional agents (Krupova et al, 2001). Five patients were given 4 mg/kg/day; 4 of the 5 obtained a cure of their infection and 1 patient died due to progression of invasive aspergillosis. All patients had developed creatinine elevations when treated previously with amphotericin B; these elevations resolved while receiving liposomal nystatin. One patient required pretreatment with corticosteroids due to clinically significant infusion-related reactions.

CONCLUSIONS

Liposomal encapsulation of nystatin results in a formulation that has some potential advantages over conventional antifungal agents like amphotericin B. Limited animal and human studies suggest that liposomal nystatin has substantially less renal toxicity than amphotericin B, and appears to have activity in vitro against some amphotericin B resistant fungi. In addition, it may be possible to successfully combine liposomal nystatin with other antifungal drugs with additive or synergistic effects. However, at the present time, the plan for further development of liposomal nystatin remains somewhat uncertain, making the future of liposomal nystatin unclear.

REFERENCES

Anil S, Ellepola A N B, Samaranayake L P. Post-antifungal effect of polyene, azole and DNA-analogue agents against oral *Candida albicans* and *Candida tropicalis* isolates in HIV disease. *J Oral Pathol Med* 30:481–488, 2001.

Arikan S, Paetznick V L, Arizmendi A, Lal L, Khyne T A, Lozano-Chiu M, Wallace T, Bazemore S, Rex J H. Comparative murine pharmacokinetics of polyene antifungal agents. Program and Abstracts of the 38th Interscience Conference on Antimicrobial Agents and Chemotherapy, American Society for Microbiology, San Diego, CA, Abstract #J-79, 1998.

Arikan S, Ostrosky-Zeichner L, Lozano-Chiu M, Paetznick V, Gordon D, Wallace T, Rex J H. In vitro activity of nystatin compared with those of liposomal nystatin, amphotericin B, and fluconazole against clinical *Candida* isolates. *J Clin Microbiol* 40:1406–1412, 2002.

Athar M A, Winner H I. The development of resistance by *Candida* species to polyene antibiotics in vitro. *J Med Microbiol* 4:505–517, 1971.

Bard M. Biochemical and genetic aspects of nystatin resistance in *Saccharomyces cerevisiae*. *J Bacteriol* 111:649–657, 1972.

Boutati E I, Maltezour H C, Lopez-Berestein G, Vartivarian S E,

Anaissie E J. Phase I study of maximum tolerated dose of intravenous liposomal nystatin (L-NYST) for the treatment of refractory febrile neutropenia (FRN) in patients with hematological malignancies. Program and Abstracts of the 35th Interscience Conference on Antimicrobial Agents and Chemotherapy. American Society for Microbiology, San Francisco, CA, Abstract #LM22, 1995.

Brautaset T, Bruheim P, Sletta H, Hagen L, Ellingsen T E, Strøm A R, Valla S, Zotchev SB. Hexaene derivatives of nystatin produced as a result of an induced rearrangement within the nysC polyketide synthase gene in *S. noursei* ATCC 11455. *Chem Biol* 9:367–373, 2002.

Brautaset T, Sekurova O N, Sletta H, Ellingsen T E, Strøm A R, Valla S, Zotchev S B. Biosynthesis of the polyene antifungal antibiotic nystatin in *Streptomyces noursei* ATCC 11455: analysis of the gene cluster and deduction of the biosynthetic pathway. *Chem Biol* 7:395–403, 2000.

Broughton M C, Bard M, Lees N D. Polyene resistance in ergosterol producing strains of *Candida albicans*. *Mycoses* 34:75–83, 1991.

Campbell C C, O'Dell E T, Hill G B. Therapeutic activity of nystatin in experimental systemic mycotic infections. *Antibiot Annu* 1954–1955:858–862, 1955.

Carrillo-Muñoz A J, Quindós G, Tur C, Ruesga M T, Miranda Y, del Valle O, Cossum P A, Wallace T L. In vitro antifungal activity of liposomal nystatin in comparison with nystatin, amphotericin B cholesteryl sulphate, liposomal amphotericin B, amphotericin B lipid complex, amphotericin B deoxycholate, fluconazole and itraconazole. *J Antimicrob Chemother* 44:397–401, 1999.

Cassidy S M, Strobel F W, Wasan K M. Plasma lipoprotein distribution of liposomal nystatin is influenced by protein content of high-density lipoproteins. *Antimicrob Agents Chemother* 42:1878–1888, 1998.

Chen W C, Chou D-L, Feingold D S. Dissociation between ion permeability and the lethal action of polyene antibiotics on *Candida albicans*. *Antimicrob Agents Chemother* 13:914–917, 1978.

Cossum P A, Wyse J, Simmons V, Wallace T L, Rios A. Pharmacokinetics of Nyotran (liposomal nystatin) in human patients. Program and Abstracts of the 36th Interscience Conference on Antimicrobial Agents and Chemotherapy. American Society for Microbiology, New Orleans, LA, Abstract #A88, 1996.

Denning D W, Warn P. Dose range evaluation of liposomal nystatin and comparisons with amphotericin B and amphotericin B lipid complex in temporarily neutropenic mice infected with an isolate of *Aspergillus fumigatus* with reduced susceptibility to amphotericin B. *Antimicrob Agents Chemother* 43:2592–2599, 1999.

Dick J D, Merz W G, Saral R. Incidence of polyene-resistant yeasts recovered from clinical specimens. *Antimicrob Agents Chemother* 18:158–163, 1980.

Drutz D, Lehrer R I. Development of amphotericin B-resistant *Candida tropicalis* in a patient with defective leukocyte function. *Am J Med Sci* 276:77–92, 1978.

Egusa H, Ellepola A N, Nikawa H, Hamada T, Samaranayake L P. Sub-therapeutic exposure to polyene antimycotics elicits a postantifungal effect (PAFE) and depresses the cell surface hydrophobicity of oral *Candida albicans* isolates. *J Oral Pathol Med* 29:206–213, 2000.

Ellepola A N B, Samaranayake L P. The in vitro post-antifungal effect of nystatin on *Candida* species of oral origin. *J Oral Pathol Med* 28:112–116, 1999.

Finkelstein A, Holz R. Aqueous pores created in thin lipid membranes by the polyene antibiotics nystatin and amphotericin B. In: Eisenman G (ed): *Membranes, Lipid Bilayers and Antibiotics*. Vol. II. Marcel Dekker, New York, 1973, pp. 377–408.

González G M, Tijerina R, Sutton D A, Graybill J R, Rinaldi M G. In vitro activities of free and lipid formulations of amphotericin B and nystatin against clinical isolates of *Coccidioides immitis* at various saprobic stages. *Antimicrob Agents Chemother* 46:1583–1585, 2002.

Gordon D, Baird I, Darouiche R, Fainstein V, Jaregui L, Levy C, Lewis P. Liposomal nystatin (LNY) vs. amphotericin B (AMB) for candidemia in non-neutropenic patients: a historical comparison. 35th Annual Meeting of the Infectious Diseases Society of America, San Francisco, CA, Abstract #144, 1997.

Groll A H, Gonzalez C E, Giri N, Kligys K, Love W, Peter J, Feuerstein E, Bacher J, Piscitelli S C, Walsh T J. Liposomal nystatin against experimental pulmonary aspergillosis in persistently neutropenic rabbits: efficacy, safety, and non-compartmental pharmacokinetics. *J Antimicrob Chemother* 43:95–103, 1999a.

Groll A H, Petraitis V, Petraitiene R, Field-Ridley A, Calendario M, Bacher J, Piscitelli S C, Walsh T J. Safety and antifungal efficacy of multilamellar liposomal nystatin against disseminated candidiasis in persistently neutropenic rabbits. *Antimicrob Agents Chemother* 43:2463–2467, 1999b.

Groll A H, Mickiene D, Petraitis V, Petraitiene R, King C, Hoyler S L, Piscitelli S C, Walsh T J. Comparative urinary pharmacokinetics and drug disposition of multilamellar liposomal nystatin and amphotericin B. Program and Abstracts of the 40th Interscience Conference on Antimicrobial Agents and Chemotherapy. American Society for Microbiology. Toronto, Ontario, Abstract #1680, 2000a.

Groll A H, Mickiene D, Werner K, Petraitiene R, Petraitis V, Calendario M, Field-Ridley A, Crisp J, Piscitelli S C, Walsh T J. Compartmental pharmacokinetics and tissue distribution of multilamellar liposomal nystatin in rabbits. *Antimicrob Agents Chemother* 44:950–957, 2000b.

Groll A H, Mickiene D, Petraitis V, Petraitiene R, Hemmings M, Roussillon K, Bacher J S, Walsh T J. Pharmacodynamics of multilamellar liposomal nystatin against experimental disseminated candidiasis. Program and Abstracts of the 41st Interscience Conference on Antimicrobial Agents and Chemotherapy. American Society for Microbiology. Chicago, IL, Abstract #J-1606, 2001.

Gunderson S M, Hoffman H, Ernst E J, Pfaller M A, Klepser M E. In vitro pharmacodynamic characteristics of nystatin including time-kill and postantifungal effect. *Antimicrob Agents Chemother* 44:2887–2890, 2000.

Hamilton-Miller J M T. Physiological properties of mutagen-induced variants of *Candida albicans* resistant to polyene antibiotics. *J Med Microbiol* 5:425–440, 1972.

Hammond S M. Biological activity of polyene antibiotics. *Prog Med Chem* 14:103–116, 1977.

Hazen E L, Brown R. Two antifungal agents produced by a soil actinomycete. *Science* 112:423, 1950.

Hazen E L, Brown R. Fungicidin, an antibiotic produced by a soil actinomycete. *Proc Soc Exp Biol Med* 76:93–97, 1951.

Jessup C, Wallace T, Ghannoum M. An in vitro interaction study with Nyotran (liposomal nystatin) and conventional antifungals, antibiotics, antivirals, and immunosuppressive drugs against common fungal pathogens. Program and Abstracts of the 39th Interscience Conference on Antimicrobial Agents and Chemotherapy, American Society for Microbiology, San Francisco, CA, Abstract #163, 2000.

Johnson E M, Ojwang J O, Szekely A, Wallace T L, Warnock D W. Comparison of in vitro antifungal activities of free and liposome-encapsulated nystatin with those of four amphotericin B formulations. *Antimicrob Agents Chemother* 42:1412–1416, 1998.

Kinsky S C. Comparative responses of mammalian erythrocytes and microbial protoplasts to polyene antibiotics and vitamin A. *Arch Biochem* 102:180–188, 1963.

Kleinberg M E, Finkelstein A. Single-length and double-length channels formed by nystatin in lipid bilayer membranes. *J Membr Biol* 80:257–269, 1984.

Kotler-Brajtburg J, Medoff G, Kobayashi G S, Boggs S, Schlessinger D, Pandey R C, Rinehart K L Jr. Classification of polyene antibiotics according to chemical structure and biological effects. *Antimicrob Agents Chemother* 15:716–722, 1979.

Krupova Y, Mistrik M, Bojitarova E, Sejnova D, Ilavska I, Krcmery V Jr. Liposomal nystatin (L-NYS) in therapy of pulmonary aspergillosis refractory to conventional amphotericin B in cancer patients. *Support Care Cancer* 9:209–210, 2001.

Lampen J O, Arnow P M, Borowska Z, Laskin A I. Location and role of sterol at nystatin-binding sites. *J Bacteriol* 84:1152–1160, 1962.

Lehan P H, Yates J L, Brasher C A, Larsh H W, Furcolow M L. Experiences with the therapy of sixty cases of deep mycotic infections. *Dis Chest* 32:597–614, 1957.

Mehta R T, Hopfer R L, Gunner L A, Juliano R L, Lopez-Berestein G. Formulation, toxicity, and antifungal activity in vitro of liposome-encapsulated nystatin as therapeutic agent for systemic candidiasis. *Antimicrob Agents Chemother* 31:1897–1900, 1987a.

Mehta R T, Hopfer R L, McQueen T, Juliano R L, Lopez-Berestein G. Toxicity and therapeutic effects in mice of liposome-encapsulated nystatin for systemic fungal infections. *Antimicrob Agents Chemother* 31:1901–1903, 1987b.

Meletiadis J, Jacques F G M M, Mouton J W, Rodriquez-Tudela J L, Donnelly J P, Verweij P E, & the EUROFUNG Network. In vitro activity of new and conventional antifungal agents against clinical *Scedosporium* isolates. *Chemother* 46:62–68, 2002.

Merz W G, Sandford G R. Isolation and characterization of a polyene-resistant variant of *Candida tropicalis. J Clin Microbiol* 9:677–680, 1979.

Molzahn S W, Woods R A. Polyene resistance and the isolation of sterol mutants of *Saccharomyces cerevisiae. J Gen Microbiol* 72:339–348, 1972.

Oakley K L, Moore C B, Denning D W. Comparison of in vitro activity of liposomal nystatin against *Aspergillus* species, with those of nystatin; amphotericin B (AB) deoxycholate, AB colloidal dispersion, liposomal AB, AB lipid complex, and itraconazole. *Antimicrob Agents Chemother* 5:1264–1266, 1999.

Offner F C J, Herbrecht R, Engelhard D, Guiot H F L, Samonis G, Marinus A, Roberts R J, De Pauw B E. EORTC-IFCG phase II study on liposomal nystatin in patients with invasive *Aspergillus* (IA) infections, refractory or intolerant to conventional/lipid ampho B (AB). Program and Abstracts of the 40th Interscience Conference on Antimicrobial Agents and Chemotherapy. American Society for Microbiology. Toronto, Ontario, Abstract #1102, 2000.

Ostrosky-Zeichner L, Bazemore S, Paetznick V L, Rodriguez J R, Chen E, Wallace T, Cossum P, Rex J H. Differential antifungal activity of isomeric forms of nystatin. *Antimicrob Agents Chemother* 45:2781–2786, 2001.

Powles R, Mawhorter S, Williams T. Liposomal nystatin (Nyotran®) vs. amphotericin B (Fungizone®) in empiric treatment of presumed fungal infections in neutropenic patients. Program and Abstracts of the 39th Interscience Conference on Antimicrobial Agents and Chemotherapy, American Society for Microbiology. San Francisco, CA, Abstract #LB-4, 1999.

Quindós G, Carrillo-Muñoz A J, Arévalo M P, Salgado J, Alonso-Vargas R, Rodrigo J M, Ruesga M T, Valverde A, Pemán J, Cantón E, Martin-Mazuelos E, Pontón J. In vitro susceptibility of *Candida dubliniensis* to current and new antifungal agents. *Chemotherapy* 46:395–401, 2000a.

Quindós G, Carrillo-Muñoz A J, Ruesga M T, Alonso-Vargas R, Miranda Y, Tur-Tur C, Rubio M, Wallace T L, Cossum P A, Martin-Mazuelos E, Cisterna R, Pontón J. In vitro activity of a new liposomal nystatin formulation against opportunistic fungal pathogens. *Eur J Clin Microbiol Infect Dis* 19:645–648, 2000b.

Rex J H, Bennett J E, Sugar A M, Pappas P G, van der Horst C M, Edwards J E, Washburn R G, Scheld W M, Karchmer A W, Dine A P, Levenstein M J, Webb C D, the Candidemia Study Group and the NIAID Mycoses Study Group. A randomized trial comparing fluconazole with amphotericin B for the treatment of candidemia in patients without neutropenia. *N Engl J Med* 331:1325–1330, 1994.

Reyes G H, Long L A, Florentino F, Ghannoum M A. Efficacy of Nyotran™ (liposomal nystatin) in the treatment of disseminated candidiasis in a neutropenic guinea pig model. Program and Abstracts of the 40th Interscience Conference on Antimicrobial Agents and Chemotherapy, American Society for Microbiology, Toronto, Ontario, Abstract #1676, 2000.

Rios A, Rosenblum M, Crofoot G, Lenk R P, Hayman A, Lopez-Berestein G. Phamacokinetics of liposomal nystatin in patients with human immunodeficiency virus infection. *J Infect Dis* 168:253–254, 1993.

Rolston K, Baird I, Graham D R, Jauregui L. Treatment of refractory candidemia in non-neutropenic patient with liposomal nystatin (Nyotran®). Program and Abstracts of the 38th Interscience Conference on Antimicrobial Agents and Chemotherapy, American Society for Microbiology. San Diego, CA, Abstract #LB-1, 1999.

Safe, L M, Safe S H, Subden R E, Morris D C. Sterol content and polyene antibiotic resistance in isolates of *Candida krusei, Candida parakrusei,* and *Candida tropicalis. Can J Microbiol* 23:398–401, 1977.

Thomas A H. Suggested mechanism for the antimycotic activity of the polyene antibiotics and the N-substituted imidazoles. *J Antimicrob Chemother* 17:269–279, 1986.

Wallace T L, Paetznick V, Cossum P A, Lopez-Berestein G, Rex J H, Anaissie E. Activity of liposomal nystatin against disseminated *Aspergillus fumigatus* infection in neutropenic mice. *Antimicrob Agents Chemother* 41:2238–2243, 1997.

Wallace T L, Lopez-Berestein G. Nystatin. In: Yu V L, Merigan T C Jr., Barriere S L (eds): *Antimicrobial Therapy and Vaccines.* Williams & Wilkins, Baltimore, 1999, pp. 1185–1191.

Wasan K M, Rosenblum M G, Cheung L, Lopez-Berestein G. Influence of lipoproteins on renal cytotoxicity and antifungal activity of amphotericin B. *Antimicrob Agents Chemother* 38:223–227, 1994.

Wasan K M, Ramaswamy M, Cassidy S M, Kazemi M, Strobel F W, Thies R L. Physical characteristics and lipoprotein distribution of liposomal nystatin in human plasma. *Antimicrob Agents Chemother* 41:1871–1875, 1997.

Williams A H, Moore J E. Multicenter study to evaluate the safety and efficacy of various doses of liposomal-encapsulated nystatin in non-neutropenic patients with candidemia. Program and Abstracts of the 39th Interscience Conference on Antimicrobial Agents and Chemotherapy, American Society for Microbiology. San Francisco, CA, Abstract #1420, 1999.

Woods R A. Nystatin-resistant mutants of yeast: alterations in sterol content. *J Bacteriol* 108:69–73, 1971.

Woods R A, Bard M, Jackson I E, Drutz D J. Resistance to polyene antibiotics and correlated sterol changes in two isolates of *Candida tropicalis* from a patient with amphotericin B-resistant funguria. *J Infect Dis* 129:53–58, 1974.

Zager R A. Polyene antibiotics: relative degrees of in vitro cytotoxicity and potential effects on tubule phospholipid and ceramide content. *Am J Kidney Dis* 36:238–249, 2000.

Zhang L, Zhang Y, Zhou Y, An S, Zhou Y, Cheng J. Response of gene expression in *Saccharomyces cerevisiae* to amphotericin B and nystatin measured by microarrays. *J Antimicrob Chemother* 49:905–915, 2002.

5

Flucytosine

ROBERT A. LARSEN

Flucytosine (5-fluorocytosine; 5-flucytosine; 5-FC) is one of the oldest antifungal agents in use (Utz, 1972). It was initially synthesized in 1957, but was not discovered to possess significant antifungal properties until 1964, when activity against *Cryptococcus neoformans* and *Candida* species was shown (Grunmberg et al, 1964). Human clinical trials were initiated in the late 1960s for both cryptococcal meningitis and disseminated candidiasis (Tassel and Madoff, 1968; Utz et al, 1968). The rapid emergence of flucytosine resistance was observed, particularly among *C. neoformans* isolates, limiting its utility as single agent therapy (Normark and Schönebeck, 1972; Block et al, 1973; Hospenthal and Bennett, 1998). Presently, flucytosine is utilized as single agent therapy in only a limited number of settings including urinary candidiasis and chromoblastomycosis (Graybill and Craven, 1983). The seminal studies of combination therapy of flucytosine with amphotericin B for patients with cryptococcal meningitis were the first to firmly establish a role for combination antifungal therapy in a well defined invasive fungal infection (Bennett et al, 1979; Dismukes et al, 1987).

MECHANISM OF ACTION

Flucytosine is taken up by fungal cells by a unique fungal-specific cytosine permease. Two important and independent pathways for fungal cell injury occur: one leading to protein synthesis inhibition, and the other resulting in DNA synthesis inhibition. Flucytosine is converted by intracellular deamination to 5-fluorouracil and ultimately processed into 5-fluorourindine triphosphate, which is incorporated into fungal RNA. This results in miscoding during translation from RNA into amino acid sequencing, causing structural abnormalities during protein synthesis (Bennett, 1977; Diasio et al, 1978). The second mechanism of action is characterized by the conversion of 5-fluorouracil to 5-fluorodeoxyuridine monophosphate, which inhibits thymidylate synthetase and subsequently DNA biosynthesis (Polak and Scholer, 1980; Waldorf and Polak, 1983). Resistance to flucytosine may arise from mutations that affect the production of three key enzymes, uridine monophosphate pyrophosphorylase, cytosine permease, and cytosine deaminase, or through increased production of pyrimidines (Francis and Walsh, 1992).

PHARMACOLOGY

Both intravenous and oral formulations of flucytosine have been developed and are in clinical use. However, in the United States, only the oral formulation of flucytosine is available and comes in 250 mg and 500 mg capsules. Following oral administration, 78%–89% of the drug is absorbed with peak concentrations achieved in approximately 2 hours (Cutler et al, 1978). Food, antacids, and renal insufficiency can impair absorption. Over 90% of the drug is eliminated by urinary excretion unchanged (Schönebeck et al, 1973). As such, impaired renal function leads to drug accumulation and dramatically alters the serum half-life from approximately 4 hours in those with normal renal function (range 2.4 to 4.8 hours) to over 85 hours in those with severe renal impairment (Daneshmend and Warnock, 1983). Consequently, the daily dose must be adjusted for patients with renal dysfunction (Stamm et al, 1987). Hemodialysis, hemofiltration, and peritoneal dialysis reduce plasma flucytosine levels (Lau and Kronfol, 1995). Flucytosine demonstrates only limited protein binding (approximately 3%–4%). The penetration of flucytosine into cerebrospinal, peritoneal, and synovial fluids is approximately 75% of simultaneous plasma concentrations (Bennett et al, 1979).

Following oral administration of 2.0 grams of flucytosine in subjects with normal renal function, peak serum levels reach 30–40 mcg/mL. Repeated dosing every 6 hours results in peak concentrations of 70–80 mcg/mL. Serum concentrations of greater than 100 mcg/mL are associated with increased toxicity and can rapidly be achieved in the setting of renal failure, particularly that caused by concomitant amphotericin B administration (Stamm et al, 1987). For these reasons, it is important to monitor renal function closely among all patients receiving flucytosine. Additionally, many experts recommend serial measurement of serum flucytosine levels. Alternatively, these levels can be accurately predicted based upon known population pharmacokinetic studies (Vermes et al, 2000a). In addition, a nomogram for flucytosine dosing in the setting of impaired renal function is available (Stamm et al, 1987).

DOSAGE AND ADMINISTRATION

The current standard daily dose of flucytosine is 100 mg/kg daily given in four divided doses in persons with normal renal function. Doses ranging between 50 and 150 mg/kg daily have been utilized successfully among patients with established fungal infection.

Early studies among patients with cryptococcal meningitis used flucytosine doses of 150 mg/kg daily, but in these studies, serum levels were monitored carefully and adjustments in dosing were made based on these determinations. Recent studies have employed lower dose regimens of flucytosine (100 mg/kg daily) for shorter periods (2 weeks) and have relied much less on monitoring serum levels (van der Horst, 1997).

Serum flucytosine levels are not universally available, and delays in obtaining test results often render these data less useful. When available, flucytosine levels can be a helpful adjunct to monitoring therapy and preventing hematologic toxicities. Some have advocated frequent monitoring of total leukocyte and platelet counts as a means of monitoring toxicity without measuring flucytosine levels. Gastrointestinal complaints are probably not related to serum levels. When monitored, serum levels should be maintained between 50–100 mcg/mL, although lower levels may be effective (Francis and Walsh, 1992; Walsh and Lyman, 1995).

CLINICAL INDICATIONS

Flucytosine is indicated for patients with cryptococcosis, various forms of candidiasis, and chromoblastomycosis. Development of drug resistance is more common in patients treated with flucytosine alone. The most common use of flucytosine is in the management of serious infections caused by *Cryptococcus neoformans* (Bennett et al, 1979; Graybill and Craven, 1983; Dismukes et al, 1987; Larsen et al, 1990; de Gans et al, 1992; Larsen et al, 1994; Mayanja-Kizza et al, 1998; Saag et al, 2000; Pappas et al, 2001). In this setting, flucytosine is usually combined with amphotericin B or fluconazole, and occasionally with itraconazole. A number of recent studies in Thailand have demonstrated successful initial therapy for AIDS-associated cryptococcal meningitis with the combination of flucytosine and itraconazole (Chotmongkol and Jitpimolmard, 1994; Chotmongkol and Jitpimolmard, 1995; Riantawan and Ponglertnapakorn, 1996; Chotmongkol et al, 1997). However, the combination of flucytosine with either amphotericin B or fluconazole has been most intensively investigated. Such combinations have

been shown to result in more rapid culture conversion of the cerebrospinal fluid from positive to negative and to improved clinical outcomes when compared to single agent therapy. For a detailed discussion of combination therapy utilizing flucytosine as therapy for cryptococcal meningitis, see Chapter 12.

Flucytosine can be employed as a single agent or in combination with amphotericin B against organisms responsible for chromoblastomycosis, e.g., *Fonsecaea* and *Cladosporium* species, with moderate success (Lopes et al, 1978; Silber et al, 1983; Restrepo, 1994). A recent large evaluation of in vitro activity of flucytosine (using National Committee for Clinical Laboratory Standards methodology) against over 8500 clinical isolates of *Candida* species showed that primary resistance to flucytosine was very uncommon among all species with the exception of *C. krusei* (only 5% susceptible) (Pfaller et al, 2002). Even though most *Candida* species are susceptible to flucytosine, most invasive *Candida* infections are not treated with flucytosine alone. Given the availability of effective alternative agents, such as the azoles (fluconazole, itraconazole, and voriconazole) and the echinocandins (caspofungin), flucytosine alone or as part of combination therapy with amphotericin B is an increasingly uncommon approach to serious *Candida* infections. However, some authorities still recommend flucytosine in combination with amphotericin B for selected patients with central nervous system candidiasis, *Candida* endocarditis, hepatosplenic (multiorgan) candidiasis, and other seriously ill patients with life-threatening candidiasis (Record et al, 1971; Smego et al, 1984; Francis and Walsh, 1992; Kujath et al, 1993; Walsh and Lyman, 1995; Abele-Horn et al, 1996). In addition, flucytosine alone is sometimes used to treat urinary candidiasis (Wise et al, 1980), although less toxic agents are available.

Aspergillus species may respond to the combination of amphotericin B and flucytosine, but the benefit of adding flucytosine is not well established by limited clinical trials (Denning et al, 1998; Pogliani and Clini, 1994; Denning and Stevens, 1990; Yu et al, 1980). *Histoplasma capsulatum*, *Coccidioides immitis*, *Blastomyces dermatitidis*, *Sporothrix schenckii*, and *Scedosporium apiospermum* are not susceptible to flucytosine and therefore this drug has no role in these fungal infections. Although *Penicillium marneffei* is inhibited in vitro by flucytosine (Supparatpinyo et al, 1993), the therapeutic utility of flucytosine for penicilliosis is not established.

ADVERSE EFFECTS

The most common adverse effects associated with flucytosine use are gastrointestinal complaints of nausea, vomiting, and diarrhea (Benson and Nahata, 1988). These events are rarely serious, and can often be ameliorated by taking the medication over 15–30 minutes. Hepatic toxicities, including elevated transaminase and alkaline phosphatase levels, have been reported in 0%–25% of subjects taking flucytosine. Rarely, hyperbilirubinemia occurs with flucytosine administration, but bilirubin levels usually decline once the drug is stopped (Scholer, 1980). Clinically significant hepatitis is rare, but deaths have been attributed to flucytosine-induced hepatic disease. None of the gastrointestinal or hepatic side effects have been demonstrated to be dose dependent (Vermes et al, 2000b). Although the mechanism of gastrointestinal toxicity is not well established, it is postulated to result from 5-fluorouracil accumulation from intestinal microflora metabolism of flucytosine (Harris et al, 1986; Malet-Marino et al, 1991).

Serious adverse effects usually arise from bone marrow injury (Kauffman and Diasio, 1977; Stamm et al, 1987). Thrombocytopenia, granulocytopenia and anemia (least common) may arise at any time during the course of therapy, particularly if flucytosine drug levels accumulate because of decreased renal clearance associated with concomitant amphotericin B administration. Bone marrow toxicity has been observed in 60% of subjects with flucytosine serum levels greater than 100 mcg/mL, whereas only 12% developed bone marrow toxicity when serum levels were less than 100 mcg/mL (Kauffman and Diasio, 1977). Although flucytosine-induced blood dyscrasias are usually reversible on discontinuation of drug, fatal bone marrow suppression has been reported. Prior radiation therapy appears to exacerbate the potential for bone marrow toxicity.

Therapeutic monitoring of serum flucytosine levels, where timely reporting is available, followed by adjustment of flucytosine dose may reduce the frequency of severe bone marrow toxicity. A complete blood and platelet count provides a good indication of flucytosine toxicity when serum levels are unavailable. Gastrointestinal and hepatic toxicity are not easily predicted based on serum flucytosine levels. Thus, flucytosine may be safely employed in settings with limited ability to monitor drug levels. Careful observation of renal function is critical, as drug levels may change rapidly if renal function changes.

Drug Interactions

Cytosine arabinoside has been reported to inactivate flucytosine (Holt, 1978). No other significant drug–drug interactions are known.

PRECAUTIONS

Flucytosine should be used with care during pregnancy. Teratogenic effects have been observed in rats and rabbits (spinal fusion, cleft lip and palate, and microg-

nathia); thus, this agent is assigned pregnancy category C by the U.S. Food and Drug Administration. However, flucytosine has been employed during pregnancy with success (Ely et al, 1998; Chen and Wong, 1996). Flucytosine has not been approved for use in children, but there has been considerable experience in this age group, particularly for treatment of central nervous system and urinary infections due to *Candida* species (Stamos and Rowley, 1995; Rowen and Tate, 1998). Nursing mothers should avoid flucytosine as it may be excreted in breast milk.

SUMMARY

Flucytosine, a fluorine analogue of cytosine, a normal body constituent, remains a useful antifungal drug, primarily in combination with amphotericin B or fluconazole for primary therapy of cryptococcal meningitis. Flucytosine is also used in combination with amphotericin B for therapy of complicated *Candida* syndromes (e.g., endocarditis and meningitis), and is occasionally given as single drug therapy for chromoblastomycosis. Limitations of the drug include its potential to cause serious adverse events including gastrointestinal, hepatic, and bone marrow toxicities and its association with emergence of primary or secondary drug resistance. Moreover, the availability of newer broad spectrum antifungal agents, such as the azoles, has narrowed the therapeutic indications for flucytosine. Importantly, this drug is not generally available in the developing world.

REFERENCES

Abele-Horn M, Kopp A, Sternberg U, Ohly A, Dauber A, Russwurm W, Buchinger W, Nagengast O, Emmerling P. A randomized study comparing fluconazole with amphotericin B/5-flucytosine for the treatment of systemic *Candida* infections in intensive care patients. *Infection* 24:426-432, 1996.

Bennett J E. Flucytosine. *Ann Intern Med* 86:319–321, 1977.

Bennett J E, Dismukes W E, Duma R J, Medoff G, Sande M A, Gallis H A, Leonard J, Fields B T, Bradshaw M, Haywood H B, McGee Z A, Cate T R, Cobbs C G, Warner J F, Alling D A. A comparison of amphotericin B alone and combined with flucytosine in the treatment of cryptococcal meningitis. *N Engl J Med* 301:126–131, 1979.

Benson J M, Nahata M C. Clinical use of systemic antifungal agents. *Clin Pharm* 7:424–438, 1988.

Block E R, Jennings A E, Bennett J E. Experimental therapy of cladosporiosis and sporotrichosis with 5-fluorocytosine. *Antimicrob Agents Chemother* 3:95–99, 1973.

Chen C P, Wang K G. Cryptococcal meningitis in pregnancy. *Am J Perinatol* 13:35–36, 1996.

Chotmongkol V, Jitpimolmard S. Treatment of cryptococcal meningitis with combination itraconazole and flucytosine. *J Med Assoc Thai* 77:253–256, 1994.

Chotmongkol V. Jitpimolmard S. Treatment of cryptococcal meningitis with triple combination of amphotericin B, flucytosine and itraconazole. *Southeast Asian J Trop Med Pub Health* 26:381–383, 1995.

Chotmongkol V. Sukeepaisarncharoen W. Thavornpitak Y. Comparison of amphotericin B, flucytosine and itraconazole with amphotericin B and flucytosine in the treatment of cryptococcal meningitis in AIDS. *J Med Assoc Thai* 80:416-425, 1997.

Cutler R E, Blair A D, Kelly M R. Flucytosine kinetics in subjects with normal and impaired renal function. *Clin Pharmacol Ther* 24:333–341, 1978.

Daneshmend T K, Warnock D W. Clinical pharmacokinetics of systemic antifungal drugs. *Clin Pharmacokinet* 8:17–42, 1983.

de Gans J, Portegies P, Tiessens G, Eeftinck Schattenkerk J K, van Boxtel C J, van Ketel R J, Stam J. Itraconazole compared with amphotericin B plus flucytosine in AIDS patients with cryptococcal meningitis. *AIDS* 6:185–190, 1992.

Denning D W, Stevens D A. Antifungal and surgical treatment of invasive aspergillosis: review of 2,121 published cases. [erratum appears in *Rev Infect Dis* 13:345, 1991.]. *Rev Infect Dis* 12:1147–1201, 1990.

Denning D W, Marinus A. Cohen J, Spence D, Herbrecht R, Pagano L, Kibbler C, Kcrmery V, Offner F, Cordonnier C, Jehn U, Ellis M, Collette L, Sylvester R. An EORTC multicentre prospective survey of invasive aspergillosis in haematological patients: diagnosis and therapeutic outcome. EORTC Invasive Fungal Infections Cooperative Group. *J Infect* 37:173–180, 1998.

Diasio R B, Bennett J E, Myers C E. Mode of action of 5–fluorocytosine. *Biochem Pharmacol* 27:703–707, 1978.

Dismukes W E, Cloud G, Gallis H A, Kerkering T M, Medoff G, Craven P C, Kaplowitz L G, Fisher J F, Gregg C R, Bowles C A, Shadomy S, Stamm A M, Diasio R B, Kaufman L, Soong S-J, Blackwelder W C, the National Institute of Allergy and Infectious Diseases Mycoses Study Group. Treatment of cryptococcal meningitis with combination amphotericin B and flucytosine for four as compared with six weeks. *N Engl J Med* 317:334–341, 1987.

Ely E W, Peacock J E Jr., Haponik E F, Washburn R G. Cryptococcal pneumonia complicating pregnancy. *Medicine* 77:153–167, 1998.

Francis P, Walsh T J. Evolving role of flucytosine in immunocompromised patients: new insights into safety, pharmacokinetics, and antifungal therapy. *Clin Infect Dis* 15:1003–1018, 1992.

Graybill J R, Craven P C. Antifungal agents used in systemic mycoses. Activity and therapeutic use. *Drugs* 25:41–62, 1983.

Grunmberg E, Titsworth E, Bennett M. Chemotherapeutic activity of 5-fluorocytosine. *Antimicrob Agents Chemother* 3:566–568, 1964.

Harris B E, Manning W B, Federle T W, Diasio R B. Conversion of 5-fluorocytosine to 5-fluorouracil by human intestinal microflora. *Antimicrob Agents Chemother* 29:44–48, 1986.

Holt R J. Clinical problems with 5-fluorocytosine. *Mykosen* 21:363–369, 1978.

Hospenthal D R, Bennett J E. Flucytosine monotherapy for cryptococcosis. *Clin Infect Dis* 27:260–264, 1998.

Kauffman C A, Diasio R B. Bone marrow toxicity associated with 5-fluorocytosine therapy. *Antimicrob Agents Chemother* 11:244–247, 1977.

Kujath P, Lerch K, Kochendorfer P, Boos C. Comparative study of the efficacy of fluconazole versus amphotericin B/flucytosine in surgical patients with systemic mycoses. *Infection* 21:376-382, 1993.

Larsen R A, Leal M A, Chan L S. Fluconazole compared to amphotericin B plus flucytosine for cryptococcal meningitis in AIDS. A randomized trial. *Ann Intern Med* 113:183–187, 1990.

Larsen R A, Bozzette S A, Jones B E, Haghighat D, Leal M A, Forthal D, Bauer M, Tilles J G, McCutchen J A, Leedom J M. Fluconazole combined with flucytosine for treatment of cryptococcal meningitis in patients with AIDS. *Clin Infect Dis* 19:741–745, 1994.

Lau A H, Kronfol N O. Elimination of flucytosine by continuous hemofiltration. *Am J Nephrol* 15:327–331, 1995.

Lopes C F, Alvarenga R J, Cispalpino E O, Resende M A, Oliveira L G. Six years experience in treatment of chromomycosis with 5-fluorocytosine. *Int J Dermatol* 17:414–418, 1978.

Malet-Marino M C, Martino R. deForni M, Andremont A, Hartman O, Armand J P. Flucytosine conversion to fluorouracil in humans: does a correlation with gut flora status exist? *Infection* 19:178–180, 1991.

Mayanja-Kizza H, Oishi K, Mitarai S, Yamashita H, Nelongo K, Watanabe K, Izumi T, Ococi-Jungale, Augustine K, Mugerwa R, Nagatake T, Matsumoto K. Combination therapy with fluconazole and flucytosine for cryptococcal meningitis in Ugandan patients with AIDS. *Clin Infect Dis* 26:1362–1366, 1998.

Normark S, Schönebeck J. *In vitro* studies of 5-flucytosine resistance in *Candida albicans* and *Torulopsis glabrata*. *Antimicrob Agents Chemother* 2:114–121, 1972.

Pappas P G, Perfect J R, Cloud G A, Larsen R A, Pankey G A, Lancaster D J, Henderson H, Kauffman C A, Haas D W, Saccente M, Hamill R J, Holloway M S, Warren R M, Dismukes W E. Cryptococcosis in human immunodeficiency virus-negative patients in the era of effective azole therapy. *Clin Infect Dis* 33:690–699, 2001.

Pfaller M A, Messer S A, Boyken L, Huynh H, Hollis R J, Diekema D J, In vitro activities of 5-fluorocytosine against 8,803 clinical isolates of *Candida* spp.: global assessment of primary resistance using National Committee for Clinical Laboratory Standards Susceptibility Testing Methods. *Antimicrob Agents Chemother* 46:3518–3521, 2002.

Pogliani E. Clini E. Association therapy as a prognostic factor in deep fungal infection complicating oncohaematological diseases. *Supportive Care Cancer* 2:385–388, 1994.

Polak A, Scholer H J. Mode of action of 5-fluorocytosine. *Rev Inst Pasteur Lyon* 13:233–244, 1980.

Record C O, Skinner J M, Sleight P, Speller D C. *Candida* endocarditis treated with 5-fluorocytosine. *Brit Med J* 1:262–264, 1971.

Restrepo A. Treatment of tropical mycoses. *J Am Acad Dermatol* 31: S91–S102, 1994.

Riantawan P, Ponglertnapakorn P. Clinical efficacy of itraconazole with initial flucytosine in AIDS-related cryptococcal meningitis: a preliminary study. *J Med Assoc Thai* 79:429–433, 1996.

Rowen J L, Tate J M. Management of neonatal candidiasis. Neonatal Candidiasis Study Group. *Pediat Infect Dis J* 17:1007–1011, 1998.

Saag M S, Graybill R J, Larsen R A, Pappas P G, Perfect J R, Powderly W G, Sobel J D, Dismukes W E for the Mycoses Study Group Cryptococcal Subproject. Practice guidelines for the management of cryptococcal disease. Infectious Diseases Society of America. *Clin Infect Dis* 30:710–718, 2000.

Scholer H J. Flucytosine. In: Speller D C E (ed.), *Antifungal Chemotherapy*. Wiley, Chichester pp 35–106, 1980.

Schönebeck J, Polak A, Fernex M, Scholer H J. Pharmacokinetic studies on the oral antimycotic agent 5-fluorocytosine in individuals with normal and impaired kidney function. *Chemother* 18:321–336, 1973.

Silber J G, Gombert M E, Green K M, Shalita A R. Treatment of chromomycosis with ketoconazole and 5-fluorocytosine. *J Am Acad Dermatol* 8:236–238, 1983.

Smego R A Jr., Perfect J R, Durack D T. Combined therapy with amphotericin B and 5-fluorocytosine for *Candida* meningitis. *Rev Infect Dis* 6:791–801, 1984.

Stamm A M, Diasio R B, Dismukes W E, Shadomy S, Cloud G A, Bowles C A, Karam G H, Espinel-Ingroff A. Toxicity of amphotericin B plus flucytosine in 194 patients with cryptococcal meningitis. *Am J Med* 83:236–242, 1987.

Stamos J K, Rowley A H. Candidemia in a pediatric population. *Clin Infect Dis* 20:571–575, 1995.

Supparatpinyo K, Nelson K E, Merz W G, Breslin B J, Cooper C R, Jr., Kamwan C, Sirisanthana T. Response to antifungal therapy by human immunodeficiency virus-infected patients with disseminated *Penicillium marneffei* infections and in vitro susceptibilities of isolates from clinical specimens. *Antimicrob Agents Chemother* 37:2407–2411, 1993.

Tassel D, Madoff M A. Treatment of *Candida* species and *Cryptococcus* meningitis with 5-fluorocytosine. A new antifungal agent. *JAMA* 206:830–832, 1968.

Utz J P, Tynes B S, Shadomy H J, Duma R J, Kannan M M, Mason K N. 5-fluorocytosine in human cryptococcosis. *Antimicrob Agents Chemother* 8:344–346, 1968.

Utz J P. Flucytosine. *N Engl J Med* 286:777–778, 1972.

van der Horst C M, Saag M S, Cloud G A, Hamil R J, Graybill J R, Sobel J D, Johnson P C, Tuazon C U, Kerkering T, Moskovitz B, Powderly W G, Dismukes W E, and the National Institute of Allergy and Infectious Diseases Mycoses Study Group and AIDS Clinical Trials Group. Treatment of cryptococcal meningitis associated with the acquired immunodeficiency syndrome. *N Engl J Med* 337:15–21, 1997.

Vermes A, Mathot R A A, ven der Sijs I H, Dankert J, Guchelaar H J. Population pharmacokinetics of flucytosine: comparison and validation of three models using STS, NPEM, and NONMEM. *Therapeutic Drug Monitor* 6:676–687, 2000a.

Vermes A, van der Sijs I H, Guchelaar H J. Flucytosine: correlation between toxicity and pharmacokinetic parameters. *Chemother* 46:86–94, 2000b.

Waldorf A R, Polak A. Mechanisms of action of 5-fluorocytosine. *Antimicrob Agents Chemother* 23:79–85, 1983.

Walsh T J, Lyman C A. New antifungal compounds and strategies for treatment of invasive fungal infections in patients with neoplastic diseases. *Cancer Treat Res* 79:113–148, 1995.

Wise G J, Kozinn P J, Goldberg P. Flucytosine in the management of genitourinary candidiasis: 5 years experience. *J Urol* 124:70–72, 1980.

Yu V L. Wagner G E, Shadomy S. Sino-orbital aspergillosis treated with combination antifungal therapy. Successful therapy after failure with amphotericin B and surgery. *JAMA* 244:814–815,1980.

6

Azole antifungal drugs

JACKSON COMO AND WILLIAM E. DISMUKES

The introduction of the azole class of antifungal drugs with the licensing of miconazole in 1979 marked the beginning of a new era in therapy for systemic fungal diseases. Although miconazole, an intravenous formulation associated with significant toxicity, is no longer commercially available, it set the stage for the development and subsequent licensing of three oral azole drugs, ketoconazole, fluconazole, and itraconazole. For many systemic mycoses, these drugs have been effective and safe alternatives to the older antifungal drugs, amphotericin B, a member of the polyene class and for years the so-called "gold standard" of therapy, and flucytosine, a fluorinated pyrimidine. Ketoconazole introduced in 1981, fluconazole (1990), and itraconazole (1992) have been attractive agents because of their excellent spectrum of activity against *Candida* species and the endemic fungi (e.g., *Histoplasma capsulatum* and *Coccidioides immitis)*, overall efficacy, safety, and ease of oral administration. However, these drugs for the most part lack significant activity against mould pathogens, the important group of emerging opportunistic fungi. Consequently, the past several years have witnessed the development of an exciting group of second generation triazole drugs (see under CHEMISTRY), which possess an expanded spectrum of activity, especially against various moulds and resistant *Candida* species. Voriconazole, approved in 2002, is the first of these to become commercially available; posaconazole (SCH 56592) and ravuconazole (BMS 207147) are the two other triazoles that are far along in development but not yet licensed. Our purpose in this chapter is to compare and contrast the pharmacologic properties of the older oral azoles and the newer triazoles and to provide perspective on the clinical indications for these agents.

CHEMISTRY

Chemical structures for the commercially available (ketoconazole, fluconazole, itraconazole, and voriconazole) and selected investigational (posaconazole and ravuconazole) azole drugs are shown in the Figure 6–1. The antifungal azoles are classified chemically as imidazoles or triazoles based on the number of nitrogen atoms (two or three, respectively) in the azole ring (Saag and Dismukes, 1988). Among the azoles shown in Figure 6–1, the only imidazole compound is ketoconazole; miconazole, also an imidazole, is no longer commercially available. These azole drugs can also be distinguished by their relative molecular size and aqueous solubility. Ketoconazole, itraconazole, posaconazole and ravuconazole are poorly soluble or insoluble in water at physiologic pH, thereby reducing their oral bioavailability and complicating the development of a suitable parenteral dosage form. Different approaches have been taken to assure efficient and safe delivery of these lipophilic compounds into the systemic circulation. As one example, the recently introduced oral solution and parenteral formulations of itraconazole have incorporated the azole in a carrier complex of hydroxypropyl-β-cyclodextrin, a large ring of substituted glucose molecules with a hydrophilic outer surface and a cylindrical hydrophobic inner core (DeBeule and Van Gestel, 2001). In contrast, the manufacturers of posaconazole and ravuconazole are conducting investigations with water-soluble prodrugs, SCH-59884 and BMS-379224, respectively (Nomier et al, 1999; Loebenberg et al, 1999; Ueda et al, 2002). Experiments in animals given SCH-59884 intravenously indicate this compound is dephosphorylated in vivo to an ester intermediate, which is subsequently hydrolyzed to posaconazole.

Fluconazole is unique among the antifungal azoles owing to its relatively small molecular size and high aqueous solubility. Voriconazole, a second-generation triazole, was developed via systematic chemical manipulation of fluconazole to produce a compound with enhanced potency and spectrum of activity. Specific changes include the addition of a methyl group to the three-member carbon backbone and replacement of one of the triazole rings with a fluoropyrimidine moiety. These modifications increase voriconazole's affinity for the target enzyme in *Aspergillus fumigatus* by 10-fold over that of fluconazole (Sabo and Abdel-Rahman, 2000). The primary physicochemical consequence of these changes was a decrease in aqueous solubility. As

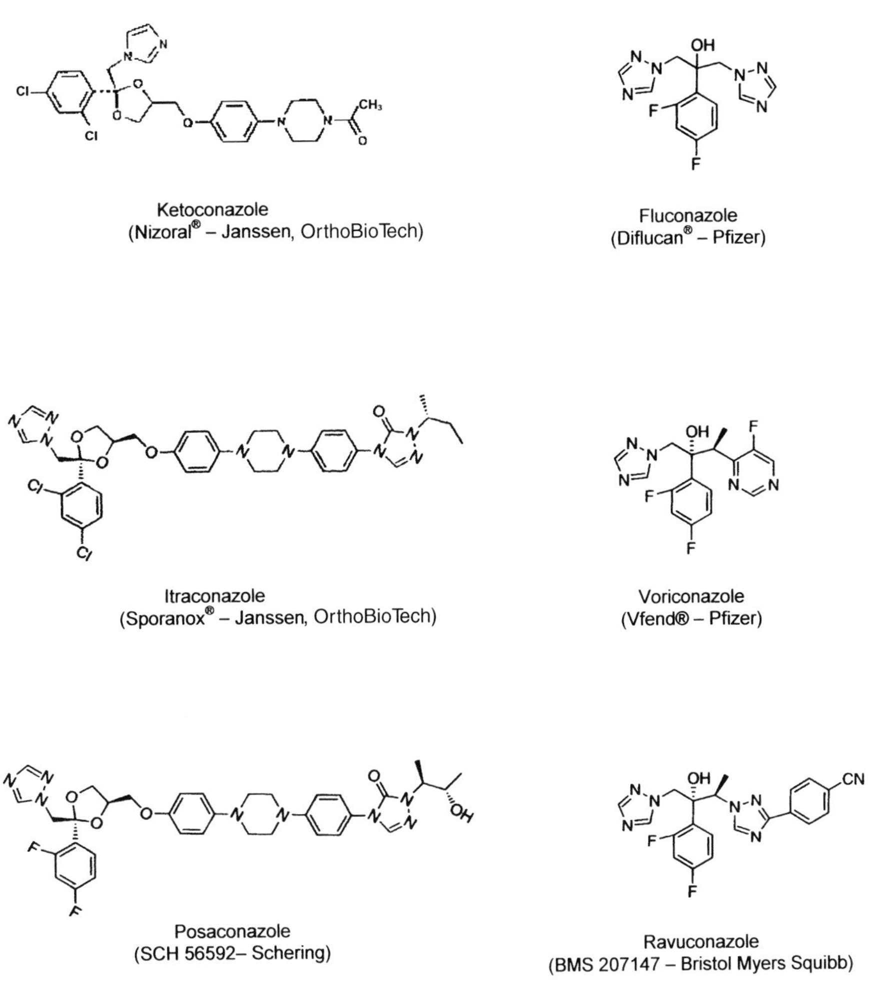

FIGURE 6–1. Chemical structures of antifungal azoles.

a result, the parenteral formulation of voriconazole contains a cyclodextrin-based solubilizing agent similar to the compound used with itraconazole (Voriconazole package insert, 2002). Ravuconazole, another second-generation triazole with marked structural similarity to fluconazole, is in early stages of clinical development as a broad-spectrum antifungal agent (Hoffman et al, 2000). Little published information is available regarding the physicochemical properties of ravuconazole.

MECHANISM OF ACTION

The primary antifungal effect of the azoles occurs via inhibition of a fungal cytochrome P-450 enzyme involved in the synthesis of ergosterol, the major sterol in the fungal cell membrane (Como and Dismukes, 1994; Sanati et al, 1997). On a molecular level, binding of the free azole nitrogen with the heme moiety of fungal C-14α demethylase inhibits demethylation of lanosterol, thereby depriving the cell of ergosterol and

allowing accumulation of various 14α methylsterols. The net result is a disruption of normal structure and function of the cell membrane and ultimately, the inhibition of cell growth and morphogenesis. Earlier studies with imidazole compounds suggested several additional antifungal effects including the inhibition of endogenous respiration, a toxic interaction with membrane phospholipids and a disruption in chitin synthesis (Sud et al, 1979; De Brabander et al, 1980; Van den Bossche et al, 1983). More recent experiments with newer azoles have concluded the antifungal activities of the triazole derivatives are due to the inhibition of 14α demethylase exclusively (Sanati et al, 1997; Hitchcock and Whittle, 1993).

Azoles are generally recognized as fungistatic agents at clinically achievable concentrations. However, recent in vitro studies with itraconazole and voriconazole demonstrated fungicidal activity against conidial suspensions of *Aspergillus fumigatus* and several other *Aspergillus* spp. at concentrations below those attained with recommended dosages (Manavathu et al, 1998).

TABLE 6–1. *Pharmacokinetic Parameters of Antifungal Azoles*

Parameter	Ketoconazole	Fluconazole	Itraconazole	Voriconazole	Posaconazole	Ravuconazole
Bioavailability (%) Fasting	75*	> 90	55–> 90**	≥ 90	8–47***	48–74***
Effect of Food on Bioavailability	Variable	No effect	See text	Decreases	Increases	NA
Time to Peak Concentration (hours)	1–4	1–2	4–5 [6–9]†	1–3	3	NA
Peak Concentration (mcg/ml) at Steady State: IV (Dosage)	NA	3.86–4.96 (100 mg daily)	2.9 [1.9]† (200 mg bid × 2, then 200 mg daily ×5)	3.0 3 mg/kg bid)	NA	NA
Oral (Dosage)	1–4 (400 mg daily)	4.1–8.1 (400 mg × 1)	2.0–2.3 [2.1–2.6] (200 mg bid)	1.9 (200 mg bid)	1.1 (200 mg bid)	3.9 (200 mg bid)
Volume of Distribution (L/kg)	0.87***	0.7–1	10.7	4.6	7–15	NA
Tissue Penetration (% simultaneous serum) CSF	< 10	50–94	< 1	42–67	NA	NA
Lung	—	100	100	NA	NA	> 100***
Protein Binding (%)	99	11–12	99.8 [99.5]†	58	NA	NA
Elimination Half-life (hours)	7–10††	22–31	38–64†† [27–56]†	6††	24	103–115
% Unchanged Drug in Urine	2–4	80	< 1	< 5	Minimal	NA
References:	Como and Dismukes, 1994.	Grant and Clissold, 1990	Como and Dismukes, 1994; Haria et al, 1996; Barone et al, 1998; Stevens, 1999	Sabo and Abdel-Rahman, 2000; Voriconazole package insert, 2002; Hoffman et al 2000; Schwartz et al, 1997; Johnson and Kauffman, 2003	Hoffman et al, 2000; Ernst, 2001; Ezzet et al, 2001	Hoffman et al, 2000; Grasela et al, 2000; Ernst, 2001

CSF, cerebrospinal fluid. NA, Data not available.

*Absolute oral bioavailability is not known due to absence of parenteral dosage form. Value represents bioavailability relative to oral solution.

**Oral bioavailability is dependent on dosage form. Higher values represent data from commercially available oral solution when given to healthy volunteers.

***Human data not currently available. Values represent data from animal studies.

†Values in brackets are parameters for hydroxyitraconazole.

††Dose dependent elimination has been reported. Values may be higher or lower depending on dosage.

Other interesting experimental observations that merit further study are the existence of a postantifungal effect after exposure of yeasts to therapeutic concentrations of second-generation triazoles (Garcia et al, 1999) and enhanced killing of *Candida* spp. by immune effector cells after exposure to combinations of azoles and colony-stimulating factors or gamma-interferon (Vora et al, 1998; Baltch et al, 2001).

PHARMACOKINETICS

The major pharmacokinetic parameters of the antifungal azoles are presented in Table 6–1. With the exception of itraconazole capsules, the azoles are sufficiently absorbed after oral administration to permit oral use in most medically stable patients. Fluconazole is unique among current agents in that food does not appreciably influence its absorption. In contrast, the presence of food, especially a high-fat meal, significantly increases absorption of posaconazole and the capsule formulation of itraconazole (Barone et al, 1993; DeBeule and Van Gestel, 2001; Courtney et al, 2002a). Conversely, when given with meals, the bioavailability of itraconazole (cyclodextrin-based oral solution) and voriconazole is decreased by 40% and 24%, respectively (Barone et al, 1998; Voriconazole package insert, 2002). No data are currently available regarding the influence of food or other factors on the absorption of ravuconazole.

Peak plasma concentrations of azoles are typically reached within 2–3 hours after administration. With fluconazole, ravuconazole, and posaconazole (up to 800 mg/day), peak concentrations are proportional to the dose administered (Como and Dismukes, 1994;

Grasela et al, 2000; Ernst, 2001; Ezzet et al, 2001). In contrast, peak serum levels of voriconazole and itraconazole increase disproportionately with larger doses, suggesting the presence of saturable first-pass metabolism (Haria et al, 1996; DeBeule and Van Gestel, 2001; Voriconazole package insert, 2002). Plasma concentrations of itraconazole and voriconazole at steady state (typically 7–14 days) are two- to several-fold higher than after single doses. Initiation of therapy with the parenteral formulation and/or the administration of a loading regimen is necessary to assure rapid attainment of therapeutic concentrations (Como and Dismukes, 1994; Poirier and Cheymol, 1998; Grasela et al, 2000; DeBeule and Van Gestel, 2001; Voriconazole package insert, 2002; Johnson and Kauffman, 2003).

Once absorbed into the systemic circulation, the portion of an azole drug not bound to plasma proteins distributes readily to body tissues and fluids. Due to its high aqueous solubility and low protein binding, fluconazole attains relatively high concentrations in CSF, sputum, saliva, and other body fluids (Grant and Clissold, 1990; Thaler et al, 1995). Limited experience with voriconazole suggests it also distributes extensively to extravascular tissues. Cerebrospinal fluid concentrations of voriconazole in a patient with central nervous system (CNS) aspergillosis were 42%–67% of simultaneous serum concentrations (Schwartz et al, 1997). Continuous administration of highly lipophilic azoles, such as itraconazole, effects relatively high concentrations of the drug in many tissues including bone, adipose tissue, and lung (Haria et al, 1996). Similarly, concentrations of itraconazole in brain tissue are high; however, the CSF concentration of itraconazole is very low, compared with that of fluconazole and voriconazole. In addition, concentrations of itraconazole in keratinous tissues are exceptionally high (up to 19-fold higher than plasma), thereby allowing intermittent or pulse therapy for infections localized to the skin and nails (Haria et al, 1996; DeBeule and Van Gestel, 2001). Although data on the newer agents are limited, fluconazole appears to be the only azole that reliably attains therapeutic concentrations in urine (Grant and Clissold, 1990).

With the exception of fluconazole, which is eliminated largely as unchanged drug in urine, the azoles undergo extensive hepatic metabolism via cytochrome P-450 enzymes and are eliminated in urine or bile as inactive metabolites (Grant and Clissold, 1990; Como and Dismukes, 1994; Haria et al, 1996; Hoffman et al, 2000; Sabo and Abdel-Rahman, 2000; DeBeule and Gestel, 2001; Ernst, 2001; Voriconazole package insert, 2002). Itraconazole is unique because its major metabolite, hydroxyitraconazole, possesses antifungal activity that approaches that of the parent compound (Haria et al, 1996; Ernst, 2001). Studies in rodents in-

dicate that posaconazole undergoes significant enterohepatic circulation and is eliminated almost entirely in bile and feces (Hoffman et al, 2000). Metabolism of voriconazole and itraconazole is saturable within the range of clinically effective dosages and plasma clearance of these agents is significantly reduced (elimination half-life is prolonged) as doses approach 400 mg. Pharmacokinetic data for ravuconazole and posaconazole in special patient populations are not yet published.

An earlier study with itraconazole (Haria, et al, 1996) and recent investigations with voriconazole (Tan et al, 2001) indicate clearance of these agents may be reduced significantly in patients with impaired hepatic function; therefore, dosage reduction is warranted in patients with mild to moderate cirrhosis of the liver (Child-Pugh Classes A and B). Clearance of fluconazole declines with increasing degrees of renal impairment and dosages of this agent should be reduced accordingly. Standard hemodialysis and some forms of continuous hemofiltration remove significant amounts of fluconazole from plasma (Grant and Clissold, 1990; Valtonen et al, 1997; Muhl et al, 2000). Supplemental dosing and/or administration of higher dosages may be necessary to maintain therapeutic concentrations in patients undergoing these interventions. The solubilizing agent (hydroxypropyl-β-cyclodextrin) used in the parenteral formulation of itraconazole is cleared almost exclusively via the kidneys (Stevens, 1999). Intravenous itraconazole should not be used in patients with a creatinine clearance less than 30 ml/minute due to accumulation of hydroxypropyl-β-cyclodextrin (Itraconazole package insert, 2001). Similar cautions are warranted with voriconazole in patients with moderate to severe renal impairment due to accumulation of the carrier compound (Voriconazole package insert, 2002).

DRUG INTERACTIONS

Clinical use of the antifungal azoles is problematic in some patients because of the potential for significant interactions with coadministered drugs (Grant and Clissold, 1990; Como and Dismukes, 1994; Lomaestro and Piatek, 1998; Venkatakrishnon et al, 2000; Piscitelli and Gallicano, 2001; Voriconazole package insert, 2002; Johnson and Kauffman, 2003). These interactions can be broadly categorized in two major types: those that result in decreased serum concentrations of the azoles, and those interactions in which the azoles produce increased plasma concentrations and/or clinical effect of another agent. Specific interactions reported with individual azoles are provided in Table 6–2.

Due to the possibility of serious adverse cardiovascular events with concomitant use, all systemic azoles are contraindicated in patients receiving cisapride. In

TABLE 6–2. *Drug Interactions Involving Antifungal Azoles*

Effect of Interaction	Ketoconazole	Fluconazole	Itraconazole	Voriconazole	Posaconazole (SCH 56592)
Decreased Absorption of Azoles	Antacids H2 receptor antagonists Proton pump inhibitors Didanosine Sucralfate		Antacids* H2 receptor antagonists* Proton pump inhibitors* Didanosine*		H2 receptor antagonists Proton pump inhibitors
Decreased Plasma Concentration of Azole Due to metabolism	Rifampin Rifabutin Phentyoin Isoniazid ? Carbamazepine	Rifampin	Rifampin Rifabutin Phenytoin Isoniazid Carbamazepine Nevirapine Phenobarbital	Rifampin Rifabutin Phenytoin Carbamazepine Phenobarbital	Rifampin ? Rifabutin Phenytoin
Increased Plasma Concentration of Coadministered Drug	Warfarin ? Sulfonylureas Cyclosporine Tacrolimus Midazolam Triazolam Alprazolam Corticosteroids ? Digoxin ? Ritonavir Calcium channel antagonists*** Quinidine Vinca alkaloids ? Indinavir ? Saquinavir Chlordiazepoxide Carbamazepine Amprenavir Nelfinavir ? Zolpidem	Warfarin Sulfonylureas ? Cyclosporine Tacrolimus Phenytoin Midazolam Triazolam Rifabutin Diazepam Theophylline ? Zidovudine Amitriptyline Nortriptyline Losartan Irbesartan Sulfamethoxazole Methadone Cyclophosphamide	Warfarin ? Sulfonylureas Cyclosporine Tacrolimus Midazolam Triazolam Alprazolam Corticosteroids ? Digoxin Rifabutin Ritonavir Calcium channel antagonists*** Quinidine Vinca alkaloids Indinavir ? Saquinavir Verapamil Pimozide Statins** Bupivacaine ? Buspirone Busulfan Sildenafil Dofetilide	Warfarin Cyclosporine Tacrolimus Phenytoin Midazolam Triazolam Alprazolam Rifabutin Calcium channel antagonists*** Quinidine Omeprazole Sirolimus Pimozide Ergotamine Dihydroergotamine Statins*** NNRTI****	Sulfonylureas Cyclosporine Phenytoin Rifabutin ? Ritonavir

*Applies only to itraconazole capsule formulation.

**Includes lovastatin, simvastatin, and atorvastatin.

***Includes felodipine, nifedipine, isradipine and nisoldipine.

****Non nucleoside reverse transcriptase inhibitors.

?, Interaction of questionable clinical significance and/or more likely only with higher dosages of the interacting agents.

addition, the following combinations are contraindicated on the basis of serious drug–drug interactions: voriconazole with pimozide, quinidine, ergot alkaloids, sirolimus, rifabutin, rifampin, carbamazepine, or long-acting barbiturates; itraconazole with pimozide, quinidine, dofetilide, oral midazolam or triazolam, lovastatin or simvastatin; and ketoconazole with oral triazolam (Ketoconazole package insert, 1998; Fluconazole package insert, 1998; Itraconazole package insert, 2001; Voriconazole package insert, 2002; Johnson and Kauffman, 2003).

Drug interactions that result in decreased concentrations of the azole occur via two primary mechanisms. In the first type, solubilization and subsequent absorption of weakly basic, highly lipophilic azoles is impaired by agents that decrease gastric acidity. The agents most affected are ketoconazole and itraconazole, although a preliminary study with a tablet formulation of posaconazole found a 40% reduction in oral bioavailability of this azole when it was coadministered with cimetidine (Courtney et al, 2002b). Since posaconazole is being developed for oral use as a suspension, the condition of a low gastric pH for optimal absorption will no longer be necessary. Similarly, administration of itraconazole as an oral solution assures adequate absorption, irrespective of gastric pH (Terrell, 1999). In situations where the oral solid-dosage form of ketoconazole or itraconazole is used in patients receiving antisecretory therapy, administration of the azole with an acidic beverage, e.g., Classic Coca-Cola® or Pepsi®, is recommended (Gepta et al, 1999).

The second mechanism by which serum concentrations of the azole are reduced is via induction of azole metabolism by agents that increase hepatic cytochrome P-450 activity (Venkatakrishnon et al, 2000). All azoles are affected, although the clinical significance of these interactions with fluconazole is typically minimal since hepatic metabolism plays only a minor role in clearance of this drug. In contrast, the impact on other agents, especially itraconazole, is substantial and therapeutic failures are possible in patients receiving itraconazole with enzyme-inducing agents (Haria et al, 1996; Venkatakrishnon et al, 2000). Whenever possible, concomitant therapy with azoles and these inducing agents should be avoided.

The drug interactions involving azoles that have received the most attention are those in which the azole inhibits the metabolism of the coadministered drug. The ability to predict these interactions has increased in parallel with an expanded understanding of the various CYP450 isoforms involved in the biotransformation of different drugs and the interaction of the azoles with specific CYP450 isoenzymes (Venkatakrishnon et al, 2000). Current experimental and clinical evidence indicates that the extent of the interaction is dependent on several factors, including the relative affinity of the azole and the object drug for a specific isoenzyme, the concentration of the agents in hepatic cells, and the extent to which the coadministered drug depends on CYP450 enzymes for total body clearance (Albengres et al, 1998). The interaction of these factors can vary substantially among patients, thus making the clinical impact in any given patient difficult to predict. Careful monitoring of patient response and determination of serum concentrations, when available, should guide dosages of the coadministered drug.

Of the antifungal azoles, ketoconazole has the most broad ranging and potent inhibitory effects on CYP450 enzymes. Specific CYP450 isoenzymes inhibited include CYP1A1, CPY1A2, CYP2A6, CYP2C9/2C19, CYP2D6, and CYP3A4 (Venkatakrishnon et al, 2000). Of these, the CYP3A4 isoenzyme is most susceptible to ketoconazole inhibition. Itraconazole and posaconazole share the inhibitory effects of ketoconazole on CYP3A4, although the affinity of the triazoles for this enzyme is manyfold lower than that of imidazoles (Venkatakrishnon et al, 2000; Wexler et al, 2002). Even so, clinically important interactions with itraconazole (and possibly posaconazole) and CYP3A4 substrates are possible due to higher concentrations of these lipophilic triazoles in hepatic tissues.

Fluconazole and voriconazole are potent inhibitors of the closely related CYP2C9/2C19 isoenzyme families (Venkatakrishnon et al, 2000; Voriconazole package insert, 2002). Significant interactions reported with fluconazole and warfarin, phenytoin, or oral hypoglycemic agents (tolbutamide) occur via inhibition of these enzymes. Preliminary data from interaction studies with voriconazole indicate that a similar spectrum of interaction is possible with this fluconazole derivative (Ghahramani et al, 2000; Wood et al, 2001; Voriconazole package insert, 2002). Although fluconazole exhibits only weak inhibitory effects on CYP3A4 isoenzymes, significant interactions with some agents (e.g., cyclosporine) have been reported, especially when fluconazole was given in higher daily dosages (≥ 400 mg) (Como and Dismukes, 1994; Terrell, 1999; Venkatakrishnon et al, 2000). The inhibitory profile of voriconazole and ravuconazole on CYP3A4 enzymes remains to be fully explored.

Another mechanism, via which antifungal azoles may increase plasma concentrations and/or the effect of coadministered agents, involves inhibition of P-glycoprotein, an ATP-dependent plasma membrane transporter involved in intestinal absorption, brain penetration, and renal secretion of a number of chemically diverse agents (Venkatakrishnon et al, 2000). Of the available azoles, itraconazole and ketoconazole have the highest potential to interact with P-glycoprotein. Inhibition of this transporter is thought to be the primary mechanism by which itraconazole enhances the neurotoxicity of vincristine (Böhme et al, 1995) and decreases renal clearance (increases serum concentration) of digoxin (Ito and Koren, 1997). Further investigation is necessary to determine the extent to which the newer triazole derivatives interact with P-glycoprotein.

SPECTRUM OF ACTIVITY

As a class, the azoles possess a broad spectrum of activity that includes most of the fungal pathogens associated with systemic infections (Table 6–3) (Grant and Clissold, 1990; Como and Dismukes, 1994; Haria et al, 1996; Espinel-Ingroff, 1998; Fung-Tomc et al, 1998; Nguyen and Yu, 1998; Pfaller et al, 1998; Saag and Dismukes, 1988; Cuenca-Estrella et al, 1999a; Pfaller et al, 1999; Terrell, 1999; Cuenca-Estrella et al, 1999b; Abraham et al, 1999; Sutton et al, 1999; Cacciapuoti et al, 2000; Hoffman et al, 2000; Li et al, 2000; Manavathu et al, 2000; Yamazumi et al, 2000; Carrillo and Guarro, 2001; Espinel-Ingroff, 2001a; Espinel-Ingroff, 2001b; Huczko et al, 2001; Pfaller et al, 2001; Uchida et al, 2001; Pfaller et al, 2002; Sun et al, 2002a; Voriconazole package insert, 2002; Cuenca-Estrella et al, 2002; Espinel-Ingroff et al, 2002; Sutton et al, 2002; Paphitou et al, 2002).

Against the dimorphic fungi, the older azoles, ketoconazole and itraconazole have better activity than flu-

TABLE 6–3. *Spectrum of Activity of Antifungal Azoles Against Selected Pathogenic Fungi*

Organism	Ketoconazole	Fluconazole	Itraconazole	Voriconazole	Posaconazole (SCH 56592)	Ravuconazole (BMS 207147)
Yeasts						
C. albicans	+	++	++	++	++	++
Flu/Itra resistant	—/+	—	—/+	+	+	+
C. glabrata	+	—/+	—/+	+	+	+
C. krusei	++	—	—/+	++	++	++
C. tropicalis	+/++	+	++	++	++	++
C. parapsilosis	+/++	++	++	++	++	++
C. lusitaniae	+/++	++	++	++	++	+
Cryptococcus neoformans	+/++	++	+/++	++	++	++
Trichosporon ashaii	NA	+/++	++	++	++	++
Dimorphic fungi						
Blastomyces dermatitidis	+/++	+	++	+/++	++	++
Histoplasma capsulatum	+	+	++	++	++	++
Coccidiodes immitis	+	+	+	+	+	+
Sporothrix schenckii	+	+	++	+	++	+
Paracoccidiodes brasiliensis	++	+	++	NA	++	NA
Moulds						
Aspergillus fumigatus	—/+	—	+	++	++	++
Aspergillus flavus	—/+	—	++	++	++	++
Aspergillus terreus	—/+	—	++	+	++	++
Fusarium solani	NA	—	—	—/+	—/+	—/+
Rhizopus sp.	—	—	—/+	—	+	+
Mucor sp.	—	—	—/+	—	—	—
Scedosporium apiospermum	—	+	+	+/++	+/++	—/+
Scedosporium prolificans	—	—	—	—/+	—	—
Dematiaceous fungi	NA	—	+/++	+/++	+/++	+

+Moderate activity in vitro and/or in animal models.
++Excellent activity in vitro and/or in animal models.
—, No clinically useful activity.
NA, not available.

conazole. Voriconazole and posaconazole, the new triazoles, are also quite active against this group of organisms. Similarly, all of the azole drugs exhibit moderate to excellent activity against *Cryptococcus neoformans*. Fluconazole possesses the narrowest in vitro spectrum in that it exhibits relatively poor activity against the common moulds or filamentous organisms and only moderate activity against dimorphic fungi. *Candida krusei* and many strains of *C. glabrata* are also resistant in vitro to fluconazole in clinically achievable concentrations (Saag and Dismukes, 1988; Grant and Clissold, 1990; Como and Dismukes, 1994). Many *Candida* spp. resistant to first generation triazoles are susceptible to the newer second generation agents, although MICs are typically several-fold higher than for fluconazole- or itraconazole-susceptible isolates (Espinel-Ingroff, 1998; Fung-Tomc et al, 1998; Marco et al, 1998; Nguyen and Yu, 1998; Pfaller et al, 1998; Chavez et al, 1999; Cuenca-Estrella et al, 1999a; Ernst, 2001). In addition, when compared with fluconazole, the second generation triazoles exhibit significantly enhanced in vitro activity against *Aspergillus*

spp and variable activity against *Scedosporium* species, *Fusarium* species and the dematiaceous fungi (Clancy and Nguyen, 1998; Fung-Tomc et al, 1998; Arikan et al, 1999; Cuenca-Estrella et al, 1999b; Espinel-Ingroff, 2001a; Espinel-Ingroff, 2001b; Pfaller et al, 2002). Voriconazole is not active in vitro against Zygomycetes (Gomez-Lopez et al, 2001; Pfaller et al, 2002; Sun et al, 2002a), whereas posaconazole and ravuconazole do show promising activity against some Zygomycetes, especially *Rhizopus* species (Pfaller et al, 2002; Sun et al, 2002a). Limited in vitro data suggest that posaconazole may also possess clinically useful activity against voriconazole-resistant strains of *Aspergillus fumigatus* (Manavathu et al, 2000; Manavathu et al, 2001).

Clinical activity in humans for the newer triazoles, especially posaconazole and ravuconazole, against many organisms remains to be confirmed. However, studies with voriconazole and posaconazole in animal models of invasive aspergillosis have demonstrated activity comparable, or superior, to that of itraconazole (Martin et al, 1997; Murphy et al, 1997; Graybill et al, 1998; Cacciapuoti et al, 2000; Kirkpatrick et al,

2000; Petraitiene et al, 2001). In addition, promising activity has been shown for voriconazole in a variety of other experimental animal in vivo models including hematogenous *Candida krusei* infections (Ghannoum et al, 1999), fusariosis (Reyes et al, 2001), and pulmonary blastomycosis (Sugar and Liu, 2001); for posaconazole, animal in vivo infections with *Fusarium* spp (Lozano-Chiu et al, 1999), *Scedosporium apiospermum* (Gonzalez et al, 2001), *Histoplasma capsulatum* (Connolly et al, 2000), and Zygomycetes (Sun et al, 2002b); and for ravuconazole, in vivo infections with *H. capsulatum* (Clemons et al, 2002) and Zygomycetes (Dannaoui et al, 2002).

IN VITRO SUSCEPTIBILITY TESTING

Until recently, in vitro antifungal susceptibility testing has been considered to be of limited clinical value due to the poor correlation between in vitro test results and outcomes of infection (Como and Dismukes, 1994; Terrell, 1999). In 1997, the National Committee for Clinical Laboratory Standards (NCCLS) published reference guidelines (M27-A Method) for conducting in vitro susceptibility testing of *Candida* spp. and *Cryptococcus neoformans*. These guidelines have recently been updated to the essentially identical M27-A2 methodology (National Committee for Clinical Laboratory Standards, 2002a). In addition to specifying conditions for performing the tests, the guidelines also provide antifungal concentration breakpoints for interpreting results of tests with fluconazole and itraconazole. Based on the NCCLS data, isolates of *Candida* spp. with a MIC ≤ 8 mcg/ml are considered susceptible to fluconazole and isolates with a MIC > 32 mcg/ml are considered resistant. Fluconazole MICs of 16–32 mcg/ml are reported as susceptible-dose dependent (S-DD), implying that positive outcomes are more likely with higher dosages. Itraconazole breakpoints for categories of susceptible, S-DD, and resistant correspond to MICs of ≤ 0.125 mcg/ml, 0.25–0.5 mcg/ml, and > 0.5 mcg/ml respectively. Standards for performing susceptibility tests with filamentous fungi have also been approved (NCCLS document M38-P), but studies to determine the correlation with clinical outcomes are ongoing (National Committee for Clinical Laboratory Standards, 2002b; Espinel-Ingroff et al, 2001c).

Optimal use of in vitro susceptibility tests with azoles requires an understanding of their origin and potential limitations in clinical application (Rex et al, 2000). At present, clinical confirmation of the breakpoints for fluconazole has been obtained only in patients with mucosal (oropharyngeal and esophageal) or systemic (invasive) candidiasis, the latter group of infections consisting primarily of catheter-related candidemia in non-

neutropenic patients (Rex et al, 1995; Rex et al, 1997). Breakpoints for itraconazole were derived in smaller numbers of patients with oropharyngeal candidiasis (Rex et al, 1997). Extrapolation of these breakpoints to patients with deep-seated *Candida* infections or mucosal infections in nonimmunocompromised patients should be done with caution, if at all. Similarly, extrapolation of MICs determined by methods other than those delineated in the reference method (broth macrodilution or microdilution) should be avoided, since even small variations in methodology can produce significantly different test results (Rex et al, 2000). Several more convenient and/or less time consuming methods for performing antifungal susceptibility tests have shown reasonably good interlaboratory and intralaboratory reproducibility, and if high correlation with the reference method is confirmed, may provide more economical alternatives for use in the clinical laboratory (Hoffman and Pfaller, 2001). For a more detailed discussion of in vitro susceptibility testing of fungi, see Chapter 1.

IN VITRO RESISTANCE

Two types of in vitro resistance to azoles have been described. Primary or "intrinsic" resistance results from the natural interaction between an organism and the antifungal agent and is independent of previous drug exposure (Vazquez and Sobel, 1997; Klepser, 2001). The most notable example of intrinsic resistance involving azoles is the universal resistance to fluconazole among isolates of *C. krusei*. Since primary resistance is usually predictable, it rarely presents a problem in patient management if clinicians are aware of the differences in susceptibility to the azoles for the organism(s) causing the infection. The more problematic clinical issue related to primary resistance is the selection of resistant organisms during azole therapy for a more susceptible pathogen. For example, the emergence of *C. krusei* or *C. glabrata* during fluconazole prophylaxis or therapy for *C. albicans* is now a well-recognized phenomenon in HIV-infected patients (Sangeorzan et al, 1994; Sobel et al, 2001) and other immunosuppressed patients after organ transplantation or chemotherapy (Wingard et al, 1991; Wingard et al, 1993; Nguyen et al, 1996; Abi-Said et al, 1997). Increases in the frequency of isolation of resistant *Candida* spp. have also been attributed to extensive use of triazoles in a specific institution or local geographic region (Sangeorzan et al, 1994; Nguyen et al, 1996; Safdar et al, 2001). Clinicians should be aware of location-specific resistant frequencies when selecting empiric antifungal therapy.

Secondary or "acquired" resistance to the azoles remains uncommon except in immunocompromised patients (primarily those with HIV infection) who are receiving prolonged and/or frequent courses of therapy (Redding et al, 1994; Espinel-Ingroff et al, 1996; Quart et al, 1996; Vazquez and Sobel, 1997; Goldman et al, 2000; Klepser, 2001; Marr et al, 2001). Extensive laboratory investigation with *Candida* spp. has revealed several potential mechanisms via which these organisms express resistance after exposure to the azoles (Vazquez and Sobel, 1997; Graybill et al, 1998a; Klepser, 2001). The most common mechanisms include alteration or overexpression of the fungal target enzyme (C-14α demethylase) of azole drugs, exclusion of drug from fungal cells, and reduction or loss of function of Δ5,6 desaturase, thereby preventing intracellular accumulation of toxic 14-methoxysterols (Sanglard et al, 1997; Graybill et al, 1998a; Marr et al, 1998; Miyazaki et al, 1998; Abraham et al, 2001; Klepser, 2001; Sanglard et al, 2001). Of these mechanisms, prevention of drug entry or extrusion of the azole via activation of energy-dependent drug-efflux pumps is thought to be the most common (Graybill et al, 1998a).

Two families of multidrug efflux pumps have been identified in clinical isolates: the major facilitators, which are encoded by the *MDR1* (*BEN'*) gene, and the ATP-binding cassette transporters (ABCT), which are expressed by *CDR1* and *CDR2* genes in *Candida* spp. All azoles, including ketoconazole, are substrates for ABCT efflux pumps, but current data suggest that only fluconazole and ravuconazole are substrates for the major facilitator transport system (Klepser, 2001; Sanglard et al, 2002). Reports of cross resistance to itraconazole and other azoles in isolates of *Candida* spp. with acquired resistance to fluconazole are at least partially explained by the upregulation of CDR1 genes (Sanglard et al, 1997; Abraham et al, 2001). The extent to which acquired resistance and/or cross-resistance will compromise the therapeutic utility of the second-generation

triazoles remains to be determined. However, fluconazole- and itraconazole-resistant isolates of *C. albicans* that exhibit cross-resistance to voriconazole have already been recovered in HIV-infected children (Muller et al, 2000). For a detailed discussion of resistance to azoles, see Chapter 9.

ADVERSE EFFECTS

The clinical attractiveness of the antifungal azoles is due in part to their low potential for serious adverse effects (Table 6–4), especially compared with polyene agents (nystatin and amphotericin B). The most common patient complaints about azole drugs are directed at the GI tract and consist primarily of anorexia, nausea, vomiting, diarrhea, and abdominal pain. Fortunately, rates of discontinuation due to GI side effects range from only 1%–6% when daily dosages are 400 mg or lower (Terrell, 1999; Voriconazole package insert, 2002). Another shared adverse effect is the potential of antifungal azoles to cause disturbances in hepatic function. All available azoles may transiently increase transaminase levels; therefore, baseline and periodic monitoring of hepatic enzymes is warranted in any patient receiving an azole for more than a few days (Como and Dismukes, 1994; Terrell, 1999; Voriconazole package insert, 2002). Rare instances of severe, and sometimes fatal, hepatic failure associated with ketoconazole, fluconazole, itraconazole, and voriconazole indicate practitioners should be more vigilant in monitoring hepatic function in patients receiving these agents (Como and Dismukes, 1994; Itraconazole package insert, 2001; Voriconazole package insert, 2002). A third common side effect of the azoles is development of a generalized erythematous rash, with or without pruritus (Como and Dismukes, 1994; Terrell, 1999;

TABLE 6–4. *Adverse Effects of Currently Available Antifungal Azoles*

	Ketoconazole	Fluconazole	Itraconazole	Voriconazole
Gastrointestinal tract	Abdominal pain, anorexia, nausea, vomiting	Anorexia, nausea, vomiting	Anorexia, nausea, vomiting	Anorexia, nausea, vomiting
Skin	Pruritus ± rash	Rash	Rash	Rash, photosensitivity
Liver	Hepatitis*	Hepatitis*	Hepatitis, liver failure	Hepatitis*
Endocrine	Decreased libido, impotence, oligospermia, gynecomastia, menstrual irregularities			
Other	Photophobia, somnolence, headache	Alopecia, teratogenicity	Hypokalemia, pedal edema, hypertension, heart failure, teratogenicity	Visual disturbances, e.g., blurred vision
References:	Como and Dismukes, 1994; Terrell, 1999	Como and Dismukes, 1994; Terrell, 1999	Como and Dismukes, 1994; Terrell, 1999; Itraconazole package insert, 2001	Hoffman and Rathburn, 2002; Herbrecht et al, 2002; Voriconazole package insert, 2002; Johnson and Kauffman, 2003

*Usually asymptomatic elevations of transaminases.

Hoffman and Rathburn, 2002). More severe cutaneous reactions, such as Stevens-Johnson syndrome and toxic epidermal necrolysis, have been associated with voriconazole and fluconazole, typically in patients with serious underlying disease who are also receiving other medications (Como and Dismukes, 1994; Hoffman and Rathburn, 2002; Voriconazole package insert, 2002). The appearance of an erythematous rash in patients receiving these agents warrants a reevaluation of therapy. Voriconazole has also been associated with photosensitivity-induced erythema/desquamation of exposed skin and blistering of lips. Therefore, patients should be instructed to avoid strong, direct sunlight while receiving voriconazole (Voriconazole package insert, 2002).

In addition to these common, shared adverse effects, each of the commercially available azoles is associated with unique reactions that merit physician awareness. Most notable among these are: endocrine disturbances secondary to ketoconazole, reversible alopecia with fluconazole, and negative inotropic effects leading rarely to congestive heart failure associated with itraconazole (Como and Dismukes, 1994; Terrell, 1999; Itraconazole package insert, 2001; Hoffman and Rathburn, 2002). All of these effects are dose-related and are usually reversible after discontinuation of the azole.

For most practitioners, the most likely unique azole-specific side effect that will be encountered in clinical practice is visual disturbance with voriconazole (Voriconazole package insert, 2002; Herbrecht et al, 2002). Approximately 30% of subjects receiving this azole experience altered visual perception, blurred vision, and/or photophobia. Fortunately, these effects are mild, transient and appear to be fully reversible after discontinuation of therapy. Onset is commonly within 30 minutes after administration, and duration is typically 30 minutes or less (Hoffman and Rathburn, 2002). Patients receiving voriconazole should be warned about these visual effects and the potential hazards of driving or operating equipment. The mechanism of this voriconazole-associated visual disturbance is unknown; no permanent sequelae have been reported.

CLINICAL INDICATIONS

Candidiasis

For an in-depth discussion of the treatment approaches, including use of azole drugs, for the various *Candida* syndromes, see Chapter 11. In addition, in this chapter, are provided two separate tables accompanied by key references. Table 6–5 addresses azole therapy of selected mucocutaneous *Candida* syndromes, including oropharyngeal candidiasis (thrush), esophageal candidiasis, *Candida* vaginitis, *Candida* cystitis, and *Candida* onychomycosis. Note that every mucocutaneous

TABLE 6–5. *Azole Therapy of Selected Mucocutaneous Candida Syndromes*

Syndrome and Recommended Azole Drugs	References
Oropharyngeal candidiasis (OPC)	
• Clotrimazole troche 10 mg 5× per day	Schectman et al, 1984 Koletar et al, 1990 Pons et al, 1993
• Fluconazole tablet or oral suspension 100 mg/day for 7–14 days. Higher doses (200–800 mg/day) may be required in AIDS patients with recurrent or fluconazole-resistant OPC	Koletar et al, 1990 De Wit et al, 1989 Hay, 1990
• Itraconazole oral solution 200 mg (200 mg/day) for 7–14 days. Especially useful in patients with fluconazole-refractory OPC	Graybill et al, 1996 Phillips et al, 1998 Saag et al, 1999a
Esophageal candidiasis	
• Fluconazole tablet or oral suspension 100–400 mg/day (depending on severity of disease) for 14–21 days	Wilcox et al, 1996 Laine et al, 1992 Barbaro et al, 1996 Eichel et al, 1996 Wilcox et al, 1997
• Itraconazole oral solution 200 mg/ day for 14–21 days	
Candida vaginitis	
• Topical azole, e.g., clotrimazole, miconazole, butoconazole, tioconazole, terconazole	Reef et al, 1995 Sobel et al, 1998
• Fluconazole tablet 150 mg/day × 1 dose	Brammer and Feczko, 1988 Reef et al, 1995 Sobel et al, 1998
• Itraconazole capsule 200 mg bid × 1 day or 200 mg qd × 3 days	Stein and Mummaw, 1993 Reef et al, 1995
• Recurrent or complicated vaginitis requires ≥ 7 days of therapy	Sobel, 1992
Candida cystitis	
• Fluconazole 200 mg/day × 7–14 day	Jacobs et al, 1996 Sobel et al, 2000
Candida onychomycosis	
• Itraconazole 200 mg bid for one week/month or 200 mg q day–3 months for toenails and 2 months for fingernails	de Doncker et al, 1995 Scher, 1999
• Fluconazole 150–450 mg once weekly for 6 months for toenails and 3 months for fingernails	Scher et al, 1998

Candida syndrome, e.g., *Candida intertrigo* and chronic mucocutaneous candidiasis, is not addressed here.

The advent of the AIDS epidemic in the early 1980s brought new focus to the management of oropharyngeal candidiasis (OPC). Physicians quickly recognized that many patients with OPC failed therapy with topical agents including nystatin swish and swallow, clotrimazole troches, and oral amphotericin B (Schectman et al, 1984; Koletar et al, 1990; Pons et al, 1993). Consequently, much attention shifted to evaluation of the efficacy and safety of oral azoles, especially fluconazole and itraconazole, for treatment of OPC. Multiple studies showed that the clinical responses of OPC are excellent to both fluconazole (DeWit et al, 1989; Hay, 1990; Koletar et al, 1990) and itraconazole (Graybill et al, 1998b; Phillips et al, 1998) and both drugs are well tolerated (Table 6–5). Itraconazole oral solution is more effective than itraconazole capsule. Ketoconazole, the original oral azole, is less effective for OPC than fluconazole and itraconazole and less well tolerated. In the mid 1990s, concerns developed about emergence of resistance of *Candida* species, particularly *C. albicans*, to the azole drugs, especially fluconazole, in patients with low CD4 cell counts (< 50–100/mm^3), and those receiving prolonged courses of azoles (Maenza et al, 1996; Revanker et al, 1996). In such patients with recurrent or fluconazole-resistant OPC, alternative treatment strategies have evolved, including high-dose fluconazole (400–800 mg daily), switch to another azole, e.g., itraconazole oral solution (Saag et al, 1999a), or voriconazole (Hegener et al, 1998), or switch to another class of drug, e.g., a polyene such as amphotericin B or an echinocandin such as caspofungin. To date, the incidence of fluconazole-resistant *Candida* species causing OPC appears to have leveled off in the 5% range.

Esophageal candidiasis (EC), regardless of the host, usually cannot be successfully treated with a topical agent such as nystatin or clotrimazole. Consequently, fluconazole or itraconazole is the initial drug of choice for EC (Table 6–5). Both oral azoles are effective in most patients, providing the infecting *Candida* species is susceptible to the azole and the patient does not have advanced AIDS. The recommended doses are fluconazole tablet or suspension, 100–400 mg/day for 14–21 days (Barbaro et al, 1996; Laine et al, 1992; Wilcox et al, 1996) and itraconazole oral solution, 200 mg/day for 14–21 days (Eichel et al, 1996; Wilcox et al, 1997). A recent blinded trial compared voriconazole and fluconazole as therapy of EC in immunocompromised patients (Ally et al, 2001). Both treatment arms showed similar high success rates (> 95%) and patient tolerability. In those few EC patients who fail azole therapy, treatment with intravenous amphotericin B or caspofungin is warranted.

Topical azole drugs, such as clotrimazole or miconazole, or nonazole topical agents, such as nystatin or tolnaftate, as therapy of *Candida* vaginitis have long been associated with high rates of success, especially in immunocompetent patients with infrequent episodes. However, these topical agents are messy, inconvenient to use, and not always effective. Increasingly, women are utilizing short course, oral azole therapy for treatment of *Candida* vaginitis (Table 6–5). Oral fluconazole and itraconazole are both highly effective in women without complicated disease or advanced immunosuppression (Brammer and Feczko, 1988; Stein and Mummaw, 1993; Reef et al, 1995; Sobel et al, 1998). Therapy of recurrent or complicated *Candida* vaginitis requires at least 7 days of oral azole therapy (Sobel et al, 1992).

Asymptomatic colonization of the bladder by *Candida* species in a patient with an indwelling Foley catheter rarely requires treatment (Kauffman et al, 2000a). In such a patient, treatment will not eradicate *Candida* from the bladder as long as the catheter remains in place. Within a few days after stopping therapy, the urine will again become colonized with *Candida*. For those occasional patients who have symptomatic *Candida* cystitis and no indwelling catheter, fluconazole is the azole of choice and an effective therapy, owing to the high concentration of active drug (≥ 80%) in the urine (Jacobs et al, 1996; Sobel et al, 2000) (Table 6–5).

Candida onychomycosis, a less frequent occurrence than dermatophyte onychomycosis and frequently associated with *Candida* paronychia, is most effectively treated with an oral azole, either itraconazole or fluconazole (Table 6–5). Most patients are treated with itraconazole, utilizing a so-called "pulse regimen," 1 week per month for 3 months or a daily regimen for 3 months (de Doncker et al, 1995; Scher, 1999). Fluconazole is also administered in a variant of the itraconazole pulse regimen (Scher, 1999; Scher et al, 1998). Both drugs are associated with remission rates in the 60% range and both are well tolerated. Griseofulvin, frequently used in the past to treat dermatophyte onychomycosis, is not active in vitro against *Candida* species.

Among the various forms of systemic or invasive candidiasis, the syndrome of candidemia is the most common and lends itself best to comparative clinical trials for evaluation of management strategies. Table 6–6 provides data on the five large clinical trials reported to date dealing with azole treatment of candidemia. In these trials, amphotericin B and fluconazole were the two comparators. Three of the trials were randomized multicenter studies in nonneutropenic patients; among these, two were nonblinded (Rex et al, 1994; Phillips et al, 1997) and one was blinded (Rex et al, in press, 2003). The fourth study was a prospective observational trial in nonneutropenic patients (Nguyen et al, 1995) and the fifth study was a matched cohort trial in cancer patients (including a few patients with neutropenia)(Anaissie et al, 1996). For detailed outcomes data, see Table 6–6.

Several important findings emerged from these trials. One, in all trials, fluconazole was associated with less toxicity than amphotericin B, irrespective of the different doses of study drugs. Two, the success rates were

TABLE 6–6. *Azole Therapy of Candidemia*

Type of Study (Reference)	Treatment Regimen**	Efficacy % Success	Mortality Rate***	Persisten Candidemia Rate
Randomized, nonblinded nonneutropenic patients. (Rex et al, 1994)	FLU 400 mg/day × 18 days vs. AMB 0.5–0.6 mg/kg/day × 17 days	70% (72/103) vs. 79% (81/103) p = 0.27	33% vs. p = 0.20 40%	15% vs. 12%
Randomized, nonblinded, nonneutropenic patients. (Phillips et al, 1997)	FLU 400 mg/day × 4 weeks vs. AMB 0.6 mg/kg/day × 4 weeks	57% (24/42) vs. 62% (26/42) p = 0.66	38% vs. p = 0.82 34%	16% vs. 10%
Observational, prospective* (Nguyen et al, 1995)	FLU median daily dose 200 mg vs. AMB "low dose" – total dose < 500 mg and AMB "high dose" – total dose > 500 mg	NA NA NA	~40% vs. p = N.S. ~35%	10% vs. 14%
Randomized, blinded nonneutropenic patients (Rex et al, in press, 2003)	FLU 800 mg/day + placebo for median, 13 days vs. FLU 800 mg/day + AMB 0.7 mg/kg/day for median,13 days	56% (60/107) vs. 69% (77/112) p = 0.043	39% vs. p = NS 40%	17% vs. p = 0.02 6%
Matched cohort study, nonrandomized, cancer patients* (Anaissie et al, 1996)	FLU 200–600 mg/day median duration, 13 days vs. AMB 0.3–1.2 mg/kg/day median duration, 10 days	73% (33/45) vs. 71% (32/45) p = 0.55	13% vs. p = NS 22%	29% vs. p = NS 26%

FLU = fluconazole; AMB = amphotericin B; NA = nonavailable; NS = nonsignificant

*Only a small percent of patients in this study were neutropenic at time of episode of candidemia.

**In all five studies, FLU was less toxic than AMB.

***Duration of follow-up varies by study: Rex et al, 1994 (~60 days); Phillips et al, 1997 (60 days); Nguyen et al, 1995 (30 days); Rex et al, in press, 2003 (90 days); Anaissie et al, 1966 (end of therapy).

comparable in the two randomized trials that used similar doses of fluconazole, 400 mg/day, and amphotericin B, 0.5–0.6 mg/day (Rex et al 1994; Phillips et al, 1997) and the matched cohort study (Anaissie et al, 1996). Third, significant differences were observed in two measures of outcome only in the blinded trial, which compared combination amphotericin B and high-dose fluconazole, 800 mg/day, to high-dose fluconazole alone, with success rates of 69% and 56%, respectively, and persistent candidemia rates of 6% and 17%, respectively (Rex et al, in press, 2003). The 6% rate of persistent candidemia for the combination treatment arm was lower than the rates of persistent candidemia for all treatment arms in the prior studies. Also of note in this study, the baseline APACHE II scores were higher in the fluconazole treatment group. While the mortality rates in both treatment groups were similar, the toxicity rate was significantly higher in the combination treatment arm. Fourth, in this same study, the combination of amphotericin B and fluconazole was not microbiologically antagonistic compared to fluconazole alone (Rex et al, in press, 2003). Fifth, in all studies, removal of vascular catheters reduced time to clearance of the candidemia. The collective results of these five trials establish that fluconazole and ampho-

tericin B are equally effective therapies for candidemia, especially in nonneutropenic patients; and fluconazole is better tolerated and less toxic than amphotericin B. Combination fluconazole and amphotericin B may have a role in selected patients with candidemia, e.g., critically ill and neutropenic patients. A metaanalysis of published results of all candidemia trials arrives at similar conclusions (Kontoyiannis et al, 2001).

Although data are not shown here, fluconazole has been used successfully for other forms of systemic or invasive candidiasis including endophthalmitis, peritonitis, bone/joint disease, hepatosplenic disease, renal parenchymal disease, and endocarditis (Rex et al, 2000). While itraconazole is active in the laboratory against most *Candida* species, the clinical efficacy of itraconazole therapy for candidemia and other forms of systemic candidiasis has not been adequately studied. Finally, a large multicenter study to compare the efficacy and safety of voriconazole versus amphotericin B as therapy of candidemia is currently ongoing.

Cryptococcosis

Azole drugs have greatly impacted the management of cryptococcosis over the past several years. While amphotericin B and flucytosine remain key drugs for this disease, fluconazole and, to a lesser extent, itraconazole, have a definite role, especially in the management of AIDS-associated cryptococcosis. Cryptococcal meningitis is the most common form of fungal meningitis in both normal and immunocompromised hosts. Moreover, fluconazole is the most attractive of the available azoles for therapy of fungal meningitis because of its excellent penetration into the CSF (Table 6–1). Although the measurable concentrations in CSF of itraconazole are low, this drug does show moderate efficacy in treatment of cryptococcal meningitis, owing in part to its high lipophilicity.

Fluconazole and itraconazole have been used as treatment approaches for different clinical manifestations of cryptococcosis; however, most of the experience has been in therapy of cryptococcal meningitis. Many authorities agree that optimal primary therapy consists of two parts, an induction regimen for 2–3 weeks with amphotericin B and flucytosine, followed by a consolidation regimen for 8–10 weeks with an azole, preferably fluconazole (Saag et al, 2000). The definitive study in AIDS patients of this treatment approach showed the following: *(1)* after 2 weeks of induction therapy, CSF cultures were negative in 60% of patients who received the combination regimen vs. 51% of patients who received amphotericin B alone ($p = 0.06$); *(2)* at the conclusion of the 10-week induction/consolidation treatment regimen, clinical responses were similar, 68% in the fluconazole-treated patients and 70% in the itraconazole-treated patients; *(3)* CSF cultures were negative in 72% of patients in the fluconazole group, and 60% of the itraconazole group (Van der Horst et al, 1997). Although this important study was performed in AIDS patients, the results have been extrapolated to the management of cryptococcal meningitis in non-AIDS patients.

Another important indication for fluconazole relates to maintenance therapy in AIDS patients with cryptococcal meningitis. Once primary therapy is completed and successful, maintenance therapy is required to prevent relapse, which occurs in approximately 15% of patients (Bozzette et al, 1991). Two large randomized trials demonstrated the efficacy of fluconazole in this setting. An initial trial compared oral fluconazole, 200 mg daily, to intravenous amphotericin B, 1 mg/kg/week. The relapse rate in the fluconazole-treated group was only 2% vs. 18% in the amphotericin B-treated group (Powderly et al, 1992). A subsequent trial compared two azoles, fluconazole, 200 mg daily, vs. itraconazole, 200 mg daily. Again fluconazole was superior, showing a 4% relapse rate compared with a 23% relapse rate in the itraconazole group (Saag et al, 1999b). Accordingly, fluconazole is the recommended maintenance therapy in AIDS patients who have successfully completed primary therapy for cryptococcal meningitis (Saag et al, 2000). Recent evidence supports discontinuation of maintenance therapy in patients who have no symptoms of cryptococcosis and have achieved immune reconstitution with HAART therapy (Masur et al, 2002).

Azole therapy, especially fluconazole, has also been utilized for nonmeningeal forms of cryptococcosis in AIDS and non-AIDS patients including pulmonary disease, bone disease, skin disease, and isolated cryptococcemia (Dromer et al, 1996; Yamaguchi et al, 1996; Denning et al, 1989; Pappas et al, 2001). For a more detailed discussion about azole therapy of cryptococcosis, the reader is referred to the Infectious Diseases Society of America (IDSA) consensus guidelines (Saag et al, 2000).

Endemic Mycoses (Blastomycosis, Coccidioidomycosis, Histoplasmosis, Penicilliosis, Paracoccidioidomycosis, and Sporotrichosis)

These endemic mycoses, as a rule, tend to be chronic, indolent illnesses. Exceptions are coccidioidomycosis, which often causes potentially devastating fungal meningitis, and histoplasmosis and penicilliosis, which may cause other forms of life-threatening disseminated disease. In addition, these same endemic, mycoses, namely, coccidioidomycosis, histoplasmosis and penicillosis, are opportunistic in nature and associated with more serious disease in immunocompromised hosts, such as HIV/AIDS patients, transplant recipients and those receiving corticosteroid therapy. Since the introduction of ketoconazole in 1981, the older oral antifungal azoles have played an important role in the therapy of the endemic mycoses (Table 6–7). For those patients with serious life-threatening endemic fungal diseases, amphotericin B is usually given as an initial therapy; after the patient is stabilized, an azole drug is usually employed. Here, data on azole treatment of each mycosis are summarized briefly. More detailed information on the key treatment studies for each endemic mycosis, except penicilliosis, is provided in Table 6–7.

Both ketoconazole and itraconazole are highly effective in the majority of patients with blastomycosis. Early on, several studies established the efficacy (70%–100%) and relative safety of ketoconazole (Dismukes et al, 1983; NIAID-Mycoses Study Group, 1985; Bradsher et al, 1985). Subsequently, a large open-label study demonstrated similar efficacy (90%–95% of patients) with itraconazole and fewer adverse events compared with ketoconazole (Dismukes et al, 1992). The dose of itraconazole is lower, 200–400 mg daily, compared to ketoconazole, 400–800 mg daily. Fluconazole is less active in vitro against *Blastomyces dermatitidis*; consequently, high daily doses are required (Pappas et al, 1995; Pappas et al, 1997). Voriconazole, the newest

TABLE 6–7. *Azole Therapy of Endemic Mycoses*

Disease	Ketoconazole	Itraconazole	Fluconazole
Blastomycosis	Highly effective. Dose: 400–800 mg/day for 3–6 months.	Azole of choice. Dose: 200–400 mg/day for 3–6 months. 200 mg/day usually sufficient.	Efficacy similar to ketoconazole. Dose: 400–800 mg/day for 6–9 months.
References	Dismukes et al, 1983 NIAID-MSG, 1985 Bradsher et al, 1985 Chapman et al, 2000	Dismukes et al, 1992 Chapman et al, 2000	Pappas et al, 1995 Pappas et al, 1997 Chapman et al, 2000
Histoplasmosis	Moderately effective, 70–85%, but high relapse rates. Dose: 400–800 mg/day for 6–24 months.	Azole of choice in both non-HIV and AIDS patients. Dose: 200–400 mg/day for 6–24 months. In patients with AIDS, chronic suppressive therapy, 200 mg/day is recommended.	Less effective than itraconazole or ketoconazole. Dose: 400–800 mg/day for 12–24 months.
References	Negroni et al, 1980 Dismukes et al, 1983 Slama, 1983 NIAID-MSG, 1985 Wheat, 2000	Negroni et al, 1987 Dismukes et al, 1992 Wheat et al, 1993 Wheat et al, 1995 Wheat et al, 2000	Diaz et al, 1992 McKinsey et al, 1996 Wheat et al, 1997 Wheat et al, 2000
Sporotrichosis	Only modest efficacy; consequently, not recommended.	Azole of choice with 90%–100% efficacy. Dose: 100–200 mg/day for 3–6 months.	Moderate efficacy. Reserve for patients who do not tolerate itraconazole. Dose: 400–800 mg/day for 3–9 months.
References	Dismukes et al, 1983 Calhoun et al, 1991 Kauffman et al, 2000b	Restrepo et al, 1986 Sharkey-Mathis et al, 1993 Winn et al, 1993 Kauffman et al, 2000b	Diaz et al, 1992 Kauffman et al, 1996 Kauffman et al, 2000b
Coccidioidomycosis	Second-line drug. High relapse rate in initial responders. Not recommended for patients with coccidioidal meningitis. Dose: 400–800 mg/day for prolonged duration.	Moderate efficacy, 63%–75%. Preferred azole drug for patients with coccidioidal skeletal disease. Dose: 400 mg/day for prolonged duration.	Moderate efficacy, 50%–67%. Preferred azole for patients with coccidioidal meningitis. Dose: 400 mg/day for prolonged duration.
References	Defelice et al, 1982 Catanzaro et al, 1982 Galgiani et al, 1988 Galgiani et al, 2000b	Graybill et al, 1990 Tucker et al, 1990 Galgiani et al, 2000a Galgiani et al, 2000b	Diaz et al, 1992 Galgiani et al, 1993 Catanzaro et al, 1995 Dewsnup et al, 1996 Galgiani et al, 2000a Galgiani et al, 2000b
Paracoccidioidomycosis	Highly effective, 85%–95%. Less expensive than itraconazole. Dose: 200–400 mg/day for 6–18 months.	Azole of choice, 90–95% efficacy. Dose: 50–100 mg/day for ~6 months.	Effective, but limited clinical experience. Dose: 200 mg/day for ~6 months. Most expensive azole.
References	Negroni et al, 1980 Restrepo et al, 1983 Restrepo et al, 1994	Negroni et al, 1987 Naranjo et al, 1990 Restrepo, 1994	Diaz et al, 1992

triazole, is active in vitro (Li et al, 2000) and in animals (Sugar and Liu, 2001) but this drug has not been used to treat blastomycosis in humans. Consensus guidelines by the IDSA indicate that itraconazole is currently the antifungal azole of choice for the majority of patients with blastomycosis, especially since it is better tolerated than ketoconazole (Chapman et al, 2000).

Over the years, coccidioidomycosis has been considered one of the most difficult to treat systemic mycoses. Formerly, intravenous amphotericin B and miconazole, to a lesser extent, were the mainstays of therapy. Nowa-

days, itraconazole and fluconazole are the principal antifungal drugs for this disease, owing in large part to their efficacy, ease of administration by either the oral or intravenous routes, and relatively low toxicity profiles (Graybill et al, 1990; Tucker et al, 1990; Diaz et al, 1992; Galgiani et al, 1993; Catanzaro et al, 1995; Dewsnup et al, 1996) when compared to amphotericin B and miconazole. A recent large, comparative trial of itraconazole and fluconazole in patients with progressive, nonmeningeal coccidioidomycosis confirmed the efficacy of these drugs (Galgiani et al, 2000a). Cure or improvement was achieved in 63% (61/97) of itraconazole recipients and in 50% (47/94) of fluconazole recipients (absolute difference, 13%, 95% CI, −2 to 28). In addition, itraconazole tended to be more effective in patients with coccidioidal skeletal disease. Both drugs were well tolerated. Serious adverse events occurred in 6% of itraconazole patients and 8% of fluconazole patients. While initial studies with oral ketoconazole demonstrated moderate efficacy, the high daily doses (400–800 mg) to achieve efficacy were poorly tolerated (Defelice et al, 1982; Catanzaro et al, 1982; Galgiani et al, 1988). In addition, ketoconazole, because of its poor penetration into CSF, is not recommended for coccidioidal meningitis (Graybill et al, 1988). Voriconazole has good in vitro activity against *C. immitis* (Li et al, 2000) and good penetration into CSF, but no clinical experience with this new drug in coccidioidomycosis has been reported. IDSA consensus guidelines emphasize the important role of the antifungal azoles in the management of coccidioidomycosis and indicate that both itraconazole and fluconazole provide attractive options as initial therapy for most patients with this disease (Galgiani et al, 2000b). Fluconazole is the treatment of choice for patients with coccidioidal meningitis and must be continued for life in most patients (Galgiani et al, 1993; Dewsnup et al, 1996).

Azole drugs have also significantly altered the approach to therapy of histoplamosis. Formerly, amphotericin B was the treatment of choice for this disease, with clinical response rates ranging from 57% to 100% in patients with chronic pulmonary disease and 71%–88% in patients with disseminated disease, but amphotericin B was poorly tolerated (NIAID-MSG, 1985). Ketoconazole was the first azole drug to prove effective in patients with both forms of histoplasmosis, but relapse rates were high and drug associated toxicity was problematic (Negroni et al, 1980; Dismukes et al, 1983; Slama, 1983; NIAID-MSG, 1985). Later studies with itraconazole established this azole as the treatment of choice, initially in non-HIV infected patients and subsequently in AIDS patients with disseminated histoplasmosis (Negroni et al, 1987; Dismukes et al, 1992; Wheat et al, 1993; Wheat et al, 1995). Itraconazole is clearly more effective than ketoconazole in AIDS-associated histoplasmosis. Utilizing a regimen of a loading dose of 600 mg daily for 3 days, followed by a daily dose of 400 mg, itraconazole was effective in 85% (50 of 59) patients with AIDS-associated indolent disseminated disease (Wheat et al, 1995). In a second study, maintenance therapy with itraconazole, 200 mg daily, prevented relapse of histoplasmosis in 85% of AIDS patients (Wheat et al, 1993). Fluconazole is a less effective therapy of histoplasmosis than either ketoconazole or itraconazole (McKinsey et al, 1996; Wheat et

al, 1997), as is the case with blastomycosis and coccidioidomycosis. Voriconazole shows good in vitro activity against *H. capsulatum* (Li et al, 2000), but no data from human studies are available. Consensus guidelines by the IDSA indicate that itraconazole is the first choice therapy for the majority of non-AIDS patients with chronic indolent forms of histoplasmosis; ketoconazole is an acceptable alternative and less expensive (Wheat et al, 2000). For most AIDS patients with disseminated histoplasmosis, itraconazole is the drug of choice for both primary and maintenance therapy (Wheat et al, 2000). As noted earlier, for patients with serious life-threatening disseminated histoplasmosis, amphotericin B is the preferred initial treatment.

The therapy of paracoccidioidomycosis, which is highly endemic in selected areas of Mexico and Central and South America, has also benefited from the advent of azole drugs. For years, sulfonamides and amphotericin B were the mainstays of treatment for this chronic, multiorgan mycosis. Studies with ketoconazole, 200–400 mg daily, showed high efficacy rates, 85%–95%, but prolonged duration of therapy was required (Negroni et al, 1980; Restrepo et al, 1983). Subsequent studies with itraconazole, 50%–100 mg daily, showed even higher efficacy rates, 90%–95%, with duration of therapy in the 6-month range (Negroni et al, 1987; Naranjo et al, 1990). Both drugs, at the doses employed, are generally well tolerated. While limited data suggest that fluconazole is also effective (Diaz et al, 1992), this azole is more expensive than the other oral azoles. In vitro activity of voriconazole against *P. brasiliensis* has been shown, but no experience in humans has been reported. Authorities agree that itraconazole is the azole drug of choice for paracoccidioidomycosis on the basis of its superior efficacy, low daily dose, low frequency of adverse events, and relatively short duration of therapy (Restrepo, 1994). However, ketoconazole is an excellent option and less expensive.

Itraconazole has largely replaced saturated solution of potassium iodide (SSKI) as the drug of choice for lymphocutaneous sporotrichosis (Kauffman et al, 2000b). Several open-label trials have shown superior efficacy of itraconazole, 100–200 mg daily for 3 to 6 months, and fewer side effects of this azole compared with SSKI (Restrepo et al, 1986; Sharkey-Mathis et al, 1993; Winn et al, 1993). Earlier experiences with ketoconazole as treatment for sporotrichosis were disappointing (Dismukes et al, 1983; Calhoun et al, 1991). Similarly, fluconazole at high doses, 400–800 mg daily, was only moderately effective (Diaz et al, 1992; Kauffman et al, 1996). Voriconazole shows in vitro activity against *S. schenckii*, but no human data are available. Although itraconazole has become the treatment of choice for most patients with sporotrichosis, primary therapy with amphotericin B should be initiated in those rare patients with disseminated or severe pulmonary sporotrichosis (Kauffman et al, 2000b).

Finally, recent studies have demonstrated the efficacy of azole therapy, namely itraconazole, for patients with disseminated penicilliosis. This opportunistic mycosis, which is endemic in Southeast Asia, especially northern Thailand, has been a significant cause of morbidity and mortality in HIV/AIDS patients in that geographic area. While both amphotericin B and itraconazole have been utilized as primary therapy of penicilliosis in these patients, data indicate that combination therapy with amphotericin B and itraconazole is more effective primary therapy than either drug alone (Sirisanthana et al, 1998). After completion of successful primary therapy, maintenance therapy is required and itraconazole, the drug of choice, is associated with a very low rate of relapse (Supparatpinyo et al, 1998). Moreover, in Thailand where the incidences of penicilliosis, cryptococcosis and histoplasmosis are high, primary prophylaxis with itraconazole is significantly effective (Chariyalertsak et al, 2002). No large clinical trials have evaluated ketoconazole, fluconazole, or the newer triazoles as therapy or prevention of penicilliosis.

Mould Diseases

Mould fungi have emerged as an important group of pathogens in compromised hosts, especially heart and lung transplant recipients, AIDS patients, and patients with neutropenia secondary to chemotherapy or bone marrow transplantation. Whereas *Aspergillus* species remain the most common opportunistic mould organisms, other opportunistic moulds are increasingly recognized, including *Fusarium* species, *Scedosporium apiospermum* (*Pseudallescheria boydii*), *Scedosporium prolificans*, and dematiaceous fungi such as *Alternaria* species, *Bipolaris* species and *Cladophialophora* species. Among the older azoles, only itraconazole exhibits moderately good in vitro activity against *Aspergillus* species, *F. solani*, *S. apiospermum*, and some dematiaceous fungi (Table 6–3). By contrast, the newer triazoles have more promising in vitro activity against these same mould organisms. Of note, neither itraconazole nor voriconazole show significant activity against Zygomycetes. However, the two investigational triazoles, posaconazole and ravuconazole, appear to be moderately actively against *Rhizopus* species. For detailed discussion of in vivo animal studies with the new triazoles against mould pathogens, see SPECTRUM OF ACTIVITY.

Invasive aspergillosis is notoriously refractory to treatment, especially in the face of persistent immunocompromise, such as persistent neutropenia or prolonged high-dose corticosteroid therapy. Standard therapy for invasive aspergillosis has been amphotericin B deoxycholate, although responses are suboptimal (less than 40%) (Stevens et al, 2000). Newer treatment approaches have been tried, including lipid formulations of amphotericin B, itraconazole (both oral and intravenous formulations), combination antifungal drugs, and immunotherapy, without significant improvement in outcome. Several studies have evaluated itraconazole therapy of invasive aspergillosis and reported cure/improvement rates ranging from 39% to 63% (Dupont, 1990; Denning et al, 1994; Stevens and Lee, 1997). However, several problems with itraconazole are encountered including patient intolerance of the drug, inadequate absorption of the oral capsules, and significant itraconazole-drug interactions. Some authorities have advocated itraconazole as a consolidation regimen following initial therapy with amphotericin B (Stevens et al, 2000).

A recently completed randomized multicenter trial compared voriconazole versus amphotericin B as primary therapy of invasive aspergillosis (Herbrecht et al, 2002). Patients were allowed to switch from the initial study drug to other licensed antifungal treatment if the initial therapy failed or if the patient was intolerant to the initial drug. Successful outcomes (complete or partial responses) were noted in 53% of the voriconazole group and 32% of the amphotericin B group (absolute difference 21%, 95% C.I., 10.4–32.9). The survival rate was also higher in the voriconazole group, 71% vs. 58%, and voriconazole-treated patients had significantly fewer severe drug-related adverse events. An earlier open, noncomparative multicenter trial of voriconazole therapy for invasive aspergillosis in immunocompromised patients showed similarly good outcomes (Denning et al, 2002). Taken together, the results of these two studies are extremely encouraging and, for the first time, indicate that an azole drug may be a more effective therapy for invasive aspergillosis than the "gold standard," amphotericin B (Johnson and Kauffman, 2003). Of note, voriconazole was approved by both the U.S. and European drug regulatory groups as primary therapy for invasive aspergillosis, largely on the basis of the results of these two studies. Another promising approach to treatment of invasive aspergillosis is to combine a new triazole and an echinocandin, based on results in vitro and in animal models (Kirkpatrick et al, 2002; Petraitiene et al, 2002; Perea et al, 2002).

With regard to azole therapy of non-*Aspergillus* mould diseases, experience, until recently, has been primarily with itraconazole. This older triazole has mainly been used to treat phaeohyphomycosis (Sharkey et al, 1990; Whittle and Koninis, 1995) and scedosporiosis (Goldberg et al, 1993). However, no large trials have been performed, reports consist of only one to a few cases, and only moderate success has been observed.

Given the promising in vitro activity of voriconazole against many non-*Aspergillus* moulds, this new triazole has been given to a limited number of patients on a compassionate basis and encouraging results have been noted. For example, among 24 patients with disease caused by *S. apiospermum*, success was reported in 15 (63%). Three of these relapsed within 4 weeks of stopping voriconazole. Among 10 patients with scedosporiosis of the CNS, 6 had a successful outcome although one of these later relapsed (Voriconazole package insert, 2002; Johnson and Kauffman, 2003). Case reports of clinical responses to voriconazole in patients with disseminated and CNS scedosporiosis are beginning to emerge (Munoz et al, 2000; Nesky et al, 2000). Another 21 patients have received voriconazole for treatment of fusariosis; 9 (43%) were considered successes and 2 of these later relapsed (Voriconazole package insert, 2002). A recent case report also describes successful outcome of posaconazole therapy in a patient with a brain abscess caused by *S. apiospermum* (Mellinghoff et al, 2002).

Voriconazole has also been evaluated as empirical therapy in persistently febrile neutropenic patients, a population at high risk for invasive mould diseases. In a large (849 patients), randomized, multicenter trial, voriconazole was compared to liposomal amphotericin B (L-AmB) (Walsh et al, 2002). The composite success rates were 26% for the voriconazole-treated patients and 31% for the L-AmB-treated patients (95% C.I. for difference in percentages −10.6%–1.6%). Voriconazole patients experienced fewer breakthrough invasive fungal infections, fewer infusion-related reactions, and less nephrotoxicity. These results led the investigators to conclude that voriconazole is a suitable alternative to amphotericin B formulations for empirical antifungal therapy in persistently neutropenic patients.

Prophylaxis

Azole drugs have been used extensively as prophylaxis in various non-AIDS patient population groups at risk for systemic fungal diseases; these groups include neutropenic patients, bone marrow transplant recipients, selected solid organ (e.g., liver and lung) transplant recipients, and intensive care unit and burn patients. This chapter does not address further this important but somewhat controversial area. Rather, see discussions on the topic in Chapters 11, 29, 30, and 31. In addition, the reader is referred to a recent provocative perspective on prophylactic antifungal therapy in the intensive care unit (Rex and Sobel, 2001).

SUMMARY

As a class, the azole drugs represent a major advance in antifungal therapy since their introduction over 30 years ago. Fluconazole has proven extremely useful in

the therapy of *(1)* the many different *Candida* syndromes, including both mucosal and invasive disease, and *(2)* cryptococcal disease, especially meningitis. In addition, itraconazole has become the treatment of choice for most patients with endemic mycoses, including blastomycosis, histoplasmosis, paracoccidioidomycosis, sporotrichosis, and penicilliosis. Both fluconazole and itraconazole are effective therapy for coccidioidomycosis. The past few years have witnessed the development of the second generation–extended spectrum triazoles including voriconazole (licensed) and posaconazole and ravuconazole (currently investigational). These newer drugs have moderate to excellent activity not only against *Candida* species, including fluconazole-resistant species, but also against many of the increasingly important mould pathogens that cause aspergillosis, fusariosis, scedosporiosis, and the phaeohyphomycoses. A second attractive feature of all azoles is their relatively benign toxicity profiles (especially compared to the polyenes). Finally, the newer triazoles hold great promise for use in a combination regimen with an echinocandin or amphotericin B preparation against selected, difficult to treat diseases such as aspergillosis or fusariosis in persistently compromised patients.

REFERENCES

Abi-Said D, Anaissie E, Uzun O, Raad I, Pinzcowski H, Vartivarian S. The epidemiology of hematogenous candidiasis caused by different *Candida* species. *Clin Infect Dis* 24:1122–1128, 1997.

Abraham O C, Manavathu E K, Cutright J L, Chandrasekar P H. In vitro susceptibilities of *Aspergillus species* to voriconazole, itraconazole, and amphotericin B. *Diagn Microbiol Infect Dis* 33:7–11, 1999.

Abraham C J, Park S, Koll B, Raucher B, Motyl M, Safdar V, Chaturvedi V, Perlin D S. Azole resistance in *Candida glabrata*. 41st Interscience Conference on Antimicrobial Agents and Chemotherapy. Chicago, IL. American Society for Microbiology, Abstract J-824, 2001.

Albengres E, Louet H L, Tillement J P. Systemic antifungal agents: drug interactions of clinical significance. *Drug Safety* 18:83–97, 1998.

Ally R, Schurmann D, Kreisel W, Carosi G, Aguirrebengoa K, Dupont B, Hodges M, Troke P, Romero A J. A randomized double-blind, double-dummy, multicenter trial of voriconazole and fluconazole in the treatment of esophageal candidiasis in immunocompromised patients. *Clin Infect Dis* 33:1447–1454, 2001.

Anaissie E J, Vartivarian S E, Abi-Said D, Uzon O, Pinczowski H, Kontoyiannis D P, Khoury P, Papadakis K, Gardner A, Raad II, Gilbreath J, Bodey G P. Fluconazole versus amphotericin B in the treatment of hematogenous candidiasis: a matched cohort study. *Am J Med* 101:170–176, 1996.

Arikan S, Lozano-Chiu M, Paetznick V, Nangia S, Rex J H. Microdilution susceptibility testing of amphotericin B, itraconazole, and voriconazole against clinical isolates of *Aspergillus* and *Fusarium* species. *J Clin Microbiol* 37:3946–3951, 1999.

Baltch A L, Smith R P, Franke M A, Ritz W J, Michelsen P B, Bopp L H. Effects of cytokines and fluconazole on the activity of human monocytes against *Candida albicans*. *Antimicrob Agents Chemother* 45:96–104, 2001.

Barbaro G, Barbarini G, Calderon W, Grisorio B, Alcini P, Di Lorenzo G. Fluconazole versus itraconazole for *Candida* esophagitis in acquired-immunodeficiency syndrome. *Gastroenterol* 111:1169–1177, 1996.

Barone J A, Koh J G, Bierman R H, Colaizzi J L, Swanson K A, Gaffar M C, Moskovitz B L, Mechlinski W, Van de Velde V. Food interaction and steady state pharmacokinetics of itraconazole capsules in healthy male volunteers. *Antimicrob Agents Chemother* 37:778–784, 1993.

Barone J A, Moskovitz B L, Guarnieri J, Hassel A E, Colaizzi J L, Bierman R H, Jessen L. Food interaction and steady-state pharmacokinetics of itraconazole oral solution in healthy volunteers. *Pharmacotherapy* 18:295–301, 1998.

Böhme A, Ganser A, Hoelzer D. Aggravation of vincristine-induced neurotoxicity by itraconazole in the treatment of adult ALL. *Am Haematol* 71:311–312, 1995.

Bozzette S A, Larsen R A, Chiu J, Leal M A E, Jacobsen J, Rothman P, Robinson P, Gilbert G, McCutchan J A, Tilles J, Leedom J M, Richman D D, The California Collaborative Treatment Group. A placebo-controlled trial of maintenance therapy with fluconazole after treatment of cryptococcal meningitis in the acquired immunodeficiency syndrome. *N Engl J Med* 324:580–584, 1991.

Bradsher R W, Rice D C, Abernathy R S. Ketoconazole therapy for endemic blastomycosis. *Ann Intern Med* 103:872–879, 1985.

Brammer K W, Feczko J M. Single-dose oral fluconazole in the treatment of vaginal candidiasis. *Ann NY Acad Sci* 544:561–563, 1988.

Cacciapuoti A, Loebenberg D, Corcoran E, Menzel F, Moss E L, Norris C, Michalski M, Raynor K, Halpern J, Mendrick C, Arnold B, Antonacci B, Parmegiani R, Yarosh-Tomaine T, Miller G H, Hare R S. In vitro and in vivo activities of SCH 56592 (posaconazole), a new triazole antifungal agent, against *Aspergillus* and *Candida*. *Antimicrob Agents Chemother* 44:2017–2022, 2000.

Calhoun D L, Waskin H, White M P, Bonner J R, Mulholland J H, Rummans L W, Stevens D A, Galgiani J N. Treatment of systemic sporotrichosis with ketoconazole. *Rev Infect Dis* 13:47–51, 1991.

Carrillo A J, Guarro J. In vitro activities of four novel triazoles against *Scedosporium spp*. *Antimicrob Agents Chemother* 45:2151–2153, 2001.

Catanzaro A, Einstein H, Levine B, Burr-Ross J, Schillaci R, Fierer J, Friedman P J. Ketoconazole for treatment of disseminated coccidioidomycosis. *Ann Intern Med* 96:436–440, 1982.

Catanzaro A, Galgiani J N, Levine B E, Sharkey-Mathis P K, Fierer J, Stevens D A, Chapman S W, Cloud G, and others in the NIAID Mycoses Study Group. Fluconazole in the treatment of chronic pulmonary and non-meningeal disseminated coccidioidomycosis. *Am J Med* 98:249–256, 1995.

Chapman S W, Bradsher R W, Campbell G D, Pappas P G, Kauffman C A. Practice guidelines for the management of patients with blastomycosis. *Clin Infect Dis* 30:679–683, 2000.

Chariyalertsak S, Supparatpinyo K, Sirisanthana T, Nelson K E. A controlled trial of itraconazole as primary prophylaxis for systemic fungus infections in patients with advanced immunodeficiency virus infection in Thailand. *Clin Infect Dis* 34:277–284, 2002.

Chavez M, Bernal S, Valverde A, Gutierrez M J, Quindos G., Mazuelos E M. In vitro activity of voriconazole (UK-109,496), LY 303366 and other antifungal agents against oral *Candida spp*. isolates from HIV-infected patients. *J Antimicrob Chemother* 44:697–700, 1999.

Clancy C J, Nguyen M H. In vitro efficacy and fungicidal activity of voriconazole against *Aspergillus* and *Fusarium* species. *J Clin Microbiol Infect Dis* 17:573–575, 1998.

Clemons K V, Martinez M, Calderon L, Stevens D A. Efficacy of ravuconazole in treatment of systemic murine histoplasmosis. *Antimicrob Agents Chemother* 46:922–924, 2002.

Como J A, Dismukes W E. Oral azole drugs as systemic antifungal therapy. *N Engl J Med* 334:263–272, 1994.

Connolly P, Wheat L J, Schnizlein-Bick C, Durkin M, Kohler S, Smedem M, Goldberg J, Brizendine E, Loebenberg D. Comparison of a new triazole, posaconazole, with itraconazole and amphotericin B for treatment of histoplasmosis following pulmonary challenge in immunocompromised mice. *Antimicrob Agents Chemother* 44:2604–2608, 2000.

Courtney R, Statkevich P, Lim J, Laughlin M, Batra V. Effect of food and antacid on the pharmacokinetics of posaconazole in healthy volunteers. 42nd Interscience Conference on Antimicrobial Agents and Chemotherapy, San Diego, CA. American Society for Microbiology, Abstract A-1837, 2002a.

Courtney R, Wexler D, Statkevich P, Lim J, Batra V, Laughlin M. Effect of cimetidine on the pharmacokinetics of posaconazole in healthy volunteers. 42nd Interscience Conference on Antimicrobial Agents and Chemotherapy, San Diego, CA. American Society for Microbiology, Abstract A-1838, 2002b.

Cuenca-Estrella M, Díaz-Guerra T M, Mellado E, Monzon A, Rodriguez-Tudela J L. Comparative in vitro activity of voriconazole and itraconazole against fluconazole-susceptible and fluconazole-resistant clinical isolates of *Candida species* from Spain. *Eur J Clin Microbiol Infect Dis* 18:432–435, 1999a.

Cuenca-Estrella M, Ruiz-Diez B, Martinez-Suarez J V, Monzon A, Rodriguez-Tudela J L. Comparative in vitro activity of voriconazole (UK-109,496) and six other antifungal agents against clinical isolates of *Scedosporium prolificans* and *Scedosporium apiospermum*. *J Antimicrob Chemother* 43:149–151, 1999b.

Cuenca-Estrella M, Mellado E, Gomez-Lopez A, Monzon A, Rodriguez-Tudella J L. Activity in vitro of ravuconazole against Spanish clinical isolates of yeasts and filamentous fungi. 42nd Interscience Conference on Antimicrobial Agents and Chemotherapy, San Diego, CA. American Society for Microbiology, Abstract M-1514, 2002.

Dannaoui E, Meis J F G, Loebenberg D, Verweij P E. In vivo activity of posaconazole in a murine model of disseminated zygomycosis. 42nd Interscience Conference on Antimicrobial Agents and Chemotherapy, San Diego, CA. American Society for Microbiology, Abstract M-193, 2002.

De Brabander M, Aerts F, van Cutsem J, van den Bossche H, Borgers M. The activity of ketoconazole in mixed cultures of leukocytes and *Candida albicans*. *Sabouraudia* 28:197–210, 1980.

De Doncker P, van Lint J, Dockx P, Roseeuw D. Pulse therapy with one-week itraconazole monthly for three or four months in the treatment of onychomycosis. *Cutis* 56:180–183, 1995.

De Wit S, Weerts D, Goossens H, Clumeck N. Comparison of fluconazole and ketoconazole for oropharyngeal candidiasis in AIDS. *Lancet* 1:746–748, 1989.

DeBeule K, Van Gestel J. Pharmacology of itraconazole. *Drugs* 61(Supp 1):26–37, 2001.

Defelice R, Galgiani J N, Campbell S C, Palpant S D, Friedman B A, Dodge R R, Weinberg M G, Lincoln L J, Tennican P O, Barbee R A. Ketoconazole treatment of primary coccidioidomyosis: evaluation of 60 patients during three years of study. *Am J Med* 72:681–687, 1982.

Denning D W, Tucker R M, Hanson L H, Hamillton J R, Stevens D A. Itraconazole therapy for cryptococcal meningitis and cryptococcosis. *Arch Intern Med* 149:2301–2308, 1989.

Denning D W, Lee J Y, Hostetler J S, Pappas P, Kauffman C A, Dewsnup D H, Galgiani J N, Graybill J R, Sugar A M, Catanzaro A, Gallis H, Perfect J R, Dockery B, Dismukes W E, Stevens DA. NIAID Mycoses Study Group multicenter trial of oral itraconazole therapy for invasive aspergillosis. *Am J Med* 97:135–144, 1994.

Denning D W, Ribaud P, Milpied N, Caillot D, Herbrecht R, Thiel

E, Haas A, Ruhnke M, Lode H. Efficacy and safety of voriconazole in the treatment of acute invasive aspergillosis. *Clin Infect Dis* 34:563–71, 2002.

Dewsnup D H, Galgiani J N, Graybill J R, Diaz M, Rendon A, Cloud G A, Stevens, D A. Is it ever safe to stop azole therapy for *Coccidioides immitis* meningitis? *Ann Intern Med* 124:305–310, 1996.

Diaz M, Negroni R, Montero-Gei F, Castro L G, Sampaio S A, Borelli D, Restrepo A, Franco L, Bran J L, Arathoon E G, Stevens D A, and other investigators of the Fluconazole Pan-American Study Group. A Pan-American 5 year study of fluconazole therapy for deep mycoses in the immunocompetent host. *Clin Infect Dis* 14(Suppl 1):S68–S76, 1992.

Dismukes W E, Stamm A, Graybill J R, Craven P C, Stevens D A, Stiller R L, Sarosi G A, Medoff G, Gregg C R, Gallis H A, Fields B T Jr, Marier R L, Kerkering T A, Kaplowitz L G, Cloud G A, Bowles C, Shadomy S. Treatment of systemic mycoses with ketoconazole: emphasis on toxicity and clinical response in 52 patients. *Ann Intern Med* 98:13–20, 1983.

Dismukes W E, Bradsher R W, Cloud G C, Kauffman C A, Chapman S W, George R B, Stevens D A, Girard W M, Saag M, Bowles-Patton C, and others in the NIAID Mycoses Study Group. Itraconazole therapy of blastomycosis and histoplasmosis. *Am J Med* 93:489–497, 1992.

Dromer F, Mathoulin S, Dupont B, Brugiere O, Letenneur L, the French Cryptococcosis Study Group. Comparison of the efficacy of amphotericin B and fluconazole in the treatment of cryptococcosis in human immunodeficiency virus-negative patients: retrospective analysis of 83 cases. *Clin Infect Dis* 22(Suppl 2):S154–S160, 1996.

Dupont B. Itraconazole therapy in aspergillosis: Study in 49 patients. *J Am Acad Dermatol* 23:607–614, 1990.

Eichel M, Just-Nubling G, Helm E B, Stille W. Itraconazole suspension in the treatment of HIV-infected patients with fluconazole-resistant oropharyngeal candidiasis and esophagitis. *Mycoses* 39(Suppl 1):102–106, 1996.

Ernst E J. Investigational antifungal agents. *Pharmacotherapy* 21 (Suppl):165–174, 2001.

Espinel-Ingroff A, Quart A, Steele-Moore L, Metcheva I, Buck G A, Bruzzese V L, Reich D. Molecular karyotyping of multiple yeast species isolated from nine patients with AIDS during prolonged fluconazole therapy. *J Med Vet Mycol* 34:111–116, 1996.

Espinel-Ingroff A. In vitro activity of the new triazole voriconazole (UK-109,496)) against opportunistic filamentous and dimorphic fungi and common and emerging yeast pathogens. *J Clin Microbiol* 36:198–202, 1998.

Espinel-Ingroff A. Germinated and nongerminated conidial suspensions for testing of susceptibilities of *Aspergillus spp.* to amphotericin B, itraconazole, posaconazole, ravuconazole, and voriconazole. *Antimicrob Agents Chemother* 45:605–607, 2001a.

Espinel-Ingroff A. In vitro fungicidal activities of voriconazole, itraconazole, and amphotericin B against opportunistic moniliaceous and dematiaceous fungi. *J Clin Microbiol* 39:954–958, 2001b.

Espinel-Ingroff A, Bartlett M, Chaturvedi V, Ghannoum M, Hazen K C, Pfaller M A, Rinaldi M, Walsh T J. Optimal susceptibility testing conditions for detection of azole resistance in *Aspergillus spp.*: NCCLS collaborative evaluation. *Antimicrob Agents Chemother* 45:1828–1835, 2001c.

Espinel-Ingroff A, Johnson E, Troke P. Activity of voriconazole, itraconazole and amphotericin B in vitro against 577 molds from the Voriconazole Phase III clinical studies. 42nd Interscience on Antimicrobial Agents and Chemotherapy, San Diego, CA. American Society for Microbiology, Abstract M-1518, 2002.

Ezzet F, Wexler D, Courtney R, Laughlin M, Lim J, Clement R, Batra V, Anaissie E. The pharmacokinetics of posaconazole in neutropenic oncology patients. *41st Interscience Conference on Antimicrobial Agents and Chemotherapy*. Chicago, IL. American Society for Microbiology, Abstract A-26, 2001.

Fluconazole package insert, 1998.

Fung-Tomc J C, Huczko E, Minassian B, Bonner D P. In vitro activity of a new oral triazole, BMS-207147 (ER-30346). *Antimicrob Agents Chemother* 42:313–318, 1998.

Galgiani J N, Stevens D A, Graybill J R, Dismukes W, Cloud G, others in the NIAID Mycoses Study Group. Ketoconazole therapy of progressive coccidioidomycosis: comparison of 400 and 800 mg doses and observations at higher doses. *Am J Med* 84:603–610, 1988.

Galgiani J N, Catanzaro A, Cloud G A, Higgs J, Friedman B A, Larsen R A, Graybill J R, the NIAID Mycoses Study Group. Fluconazole therapy for coccidioidal meningitis. *Ann Intern Med* 119:28–35, 1993.

Galgiani J N, Catanzaro A, Cloud G A, Johnson R H, Williams P L, Mirels L F, Nassar F, Lutz J, Stevens D A, Sharkey P K, Singh V R, Larsen R A, Delgado K L, Flanigan C, Rinaldi M G, the NIAID Mycoses Study Group. Comparison of oral fluconazole and itraconazole for progressive nonmeningeal coccidioidomycosis. *Ann Intern Med* 133:676–686, 2000a.

Galgiani J N, Ampel N M, Catanzaro A, Johnson R H, Stevens D A, Williams P L. Practice guidelines for the treatment of coccidioidomycosis. *Clin Infect Dis* 30:658–661, 2000b.

Garcia M T, Llorente M T, Lima E, Minguez F, Dei Moral F, Prieto J. Activity of voriconazole: post antifungal effect, effects of low concentrations and of pretreatment on the susceptibility of *Candida albicans* to leukocytes. *Scand J Infect Dis* 31:501–504, 1999.

Gepta A K, Katz H I, Shear N H. Drug interactions with itraconazole, fluconazole and terbinafine and their management. *J Am Acad Dermatol* 41:237–249, 1999.

Ghahramani P, Purkins L, Kleinermans D, Nichols D J. Voriconazole potentiates warfarin-induced prolongation of prothrombin time. 40th Interscience Conference on Antimicrobial Agents and Chemotherapy. Toronto, Ontario, Canada. American Society for Microbiology, Abstract 846, 2000.

Ghannoum M A, Okogbule-Wonodi I, Bhat N, Sanati H. Antifungal activity of voriconazole (UK-109,496), fluconazole and amphotericin B against hematogenous *Candida krusei* infection in neutropenic guinea pig model. *J Chemother* 11:34–39, 1999.

Goldberg S L, Geha D J, Marshall W F, Inwards D J, Hoagland H C. Successful treatment of simultaneous pulmonary *Pseudallescheria boydii* and *Aspergillus terreus* infection with oral itraconazole. *Clin Infect Dis* 16:803–805, 1993.

Goldman M, Cloud G A, Smedema M, LeMonte A, Connolly P, McKinsey D S, Kauffman C A, Moskovitz B, Wheat L J, and National Institute of Allergy and Infectious Diseases Mycoses Study Group. Does long-term itraconazole prophylaxis result in in vitro azole resistance in mucosal *Candida albicans* isolates from persons with advanced human immunodeficiency virus infection? *Antimicrob Agents Chemother* 44:1585–1587, 2000.

Gomez-Lopez A, Cuenca-Estrella VA, Monzon A, Rodriquez-Tudela J L. In vitro susceptibility of clinical isolates of Zygomycota to amphotericin B, flucytosine, itraconazole, and voriconazole. *J Antimicrob Chemother* 48:919–921, 2001.

Gonzalez G, Tijerina R, Najvar L, Bocanegra R, Rinaldi M, Loebenberg D, Graybill J. Therapeutic efficacy of posaconazole (POSA) in a murine *Pseudallescheria boydii* infection. 41st Interscience Conference on Antimicrobial Agents and Chemotherapy. Chicago, IL. American Society for Microbiology, Abstract J-1615, 2001.

Grant S M, Clissold S P. Fluconazole: a review of its pharmacodynamic and pharmacokinetic properties, and therapeutic potential in superficial and systemic mycoses. *Drugs* 39:877–916, 1990.

Grasela D M, Olsen S J, Mummaneni V, Rolan P, Christopher L, Norton J, Hadjilambris O W, Marino M R. Ravuconazole: multiple ascending oral dose study in healthy subjects. 40th Interscience Conference on Antimicrobial Agents and Chemotherapy. Toronto, Ontario, Canada. American Society for Microbiology, Abstract 839, 2000.

Graybill J R, Stevens D A, Galgiani J N, Sugar A M, Craven P C, Gregg C, Huppert M, Cloud G, Dismukes W E, the NIAID Mycoses Study Group. Ketoconazole treatment of coccidioidal meningitis. *Ann New York Acad Sci* 544:488–496, 1988.

Graybill J R, Stevens D A, Galgiani J N, Dismukes W E, Cloud G A, the NIAID Mycoses Study Group. Itraconazole treatment of coccidioidomycosis. *Am J Med* 89:282–290, 1990.

Graybill J R, Montalbo E, Kirkpatrick W R, Luther M F, Revankar S G, Patterson T F. Fluconazole versus *Candida albicans*: a complex relationship. *Antimicrob Agents Chemother* 42:2938–2942, 1998a.

Graybill J R, Vazquez J, Darouiche R O, Morhart R, Greenspan D, Tuazon C, Wheat L J, Carey L, Leviton I, Hewitt R G, MacGregor R R, Valenti W, Restrepo A, Moskovitz B L. Randomized trial of itraconazole oral solution for oropharyngeal candidiasis in HIV/AIDS patients. *Am J Med* 104:33–39, 1998b.

Graybill J R, Bocanegra R, Najvar L K, Luther M F, Loebenberg D. SCH56592 treatment of murine invasive aspergillosis. *J Antimicrob Chemother* 42:539–542, 1998.

Haria M, Bryson H M, Goa K L. Itraconazole, a reappraisal of its pharmacological properties and therapeutic use in the management of superficial fungal infections. *Drugs* 51:585–620, 1996.

Hay R J. Overview of studies of fluconazole in oropharyngeal candidiasis. *Rev Infect Dis* 3(Suppl 3):334–337, 1990.

Hegener P, Troke P F, Fatkenheuer G, Diehl V, Ruhnke M. Treatment of fluconazole-resistant candidiasis with voriconazole in patients with AIDS. *AIDS* 12:2227–2228, 1998.

Herbrecht R, Denning D W, Patterson T F, Bennett J E, Greene R E, Oestmann J-W, Kern W V, Marr K A, Ribaud P, Lortholary O, Sylvester R, Rubin R H, Wingard, J R, Stark P, Durand C, Caillot D, Thiel E, Chandrasekar P H, Hodges M R, Schlamm H T, Troke P F, de Pauw B, for the Invasive Fungal Infections Group of the European Organisation for Research and Treatment of Cancer and the Global Aspergillus Study Group. Voriconazole versus amphotericin B for primary therapy of invasive aspergillosis. *N Engl J Med* 347:408–415, 2002.

Hitchcock C A, Whittle P J. Chemistry and mode of action of fluconazole. In: W Rippon and R A Fromtling, eds. *Cutaneous antifungal agents: selected compounds in clinical practice and development.* Marcel Dekker, Inc. New York, NY, pp.183–197, 1993.

Hoffman H L, Ernst E J, Klepser M E. Novel triazole antifungal agents. *Exp Opin Invest Drugs* 9:593–605, 2000.

Hoffman H L, Pfaller M A. In vitro antifungal susceptibility testing. *Pharmacother* 21:111S-123S, 2001.

Hoffman H L, Rathbun R C. Review of the safety and efficacy of voriconazole. *Exp Opin Invest Drugs* 11:409–429, 2002

Huczko E, Minassian B, Washo T, Bonner D, Fung-Tomc J. In vitro activity of ravuconazole against Zygomycetes, *Scedosporium* and *Fusarium* isolates. 41st Interscience Conference on Antimicrobial Agents and Chemotherapy. Chicago, IL. American Society for Microbiology, USA. Abstract J-810, 2001.

Ito S, Koren G. Comment: possible mechanism of digoxin-itraconazole interaction. *Ann Pharmacother* 31:1091–1092, 1997.

Itraconazole package insert, 2001.

Jacobs L G, Skidmore E A, Freeman K, Lipshultz D, Fox N. Oral fluconazole compared with bladder irrigation with amphotericin B for treatment of fungal urinary tract infections in elderly patients. *Clin Infect Dis* 22:30–35, 1996.

Johnson LB, Kauffman CA. Voriconazole: A new triazole antifungal agent (Review). *Clin Infect Dis* 36:630–637, 2003.

Kauffman C A, Pappas P G, McKinsey D S, Greenfield R A, Perfect J R, Cloud G A, Thomas C J, Dismukes W E, NIAID Mycoses Study Group. Treatment of lymphocutaneous and visceral sporotrichosis with fluconazole. *Clin Infect Dis* 22:44–50, 1996.

Kauffman C A, Vazquez J A, Sobel J D, Gallis H A, McKinsey D S, Karchmer A W, Sugar A M, Sharkey P K, Wise G J, Mangi R, Mosher A, Lee J Y, Dismukes W E, the NIAID Mycoses Study Group. Prospective multicenter surveillance study of funguria in hospitalized patients. *Clin Infect Dis* 30:14–18, 2000a.

Kauffman C A, Hajjeh R, Chapman S W for the Mycoses Study Group. Practice guidelines for the management of patients with sporotrichosis. *Clin Infect Dis* 30:684–687, 2000b.

Ketoconazole package insert, 1998.

Kirkpatrick W R, McAtee R K, Fothergill A, Rinaldi M G, Patterson T F. Efficacy of voriconazole in a guinea pig model of disseminated invasive aspergillosis. *Antimicrob Agents Chemother* 44:2865–2868, 2000.

Kirkpatrick W R, Perea S, Coco B J, Patterson T F. Efficacy of caspofungin alone and in combination with voriconazole in a guinea pig model of invasive aspergillosis. *Antimicrob Agents Chemother* 46:2564–2568, 2002.

Klepser M E. Antifungal resistance among *Candida species. Pharmacother* 21:124S–132S, 2001.

Koletar S L, Russell J A, Fass R J, Plouffe J F. Comparison of oral fluconazole and clotrimazole troches as treatment for oral candidiasis in patients infected with human immunodeficiency virus. *Antimicrob Agents Chemother* 34:2267–2268, 1990.

Kontoyiannis D P, Bodey G P, Mantzoros C S. Fluconazole vs amphotericin B for the management of candidemia in adults: a meta-analysis. *Mycoses* 44:125–135, 2001.

Laine L, Dretler R H, Conteas C N, Tuazon C, Koster F M, Sattler F, Squires K, Islam M Z. Fluconazole compared with ketoconazole for the treatment of *Candida* esophagitis in AIDS: a randomized trial. *Ann Intern Med* 117:655–660, 1992.

Li R K, Ciblak M A, Nordoff N, Pasarell L, Warnock D W, McGinnis M R. In vitro activities of voriconazole, itraconazole, and amphotericin B against *Blastomyces dermatitidis, Coccidioides immitis,* and *Histoplasma capsulatum. Antimicrob Agents Chemother* 44:1734–1736, 2000.

Loebenberg D, Menzel F, Corcoran E, Mendrick C, Raynor K, Cacciapuoti A F, Hare R S. SCH 59884, the intravenous prodrug of the antifungal triazole SCH 56592. 39th Interscience Conference on Antimicrobial Agents and Chemotherapy. San Francisco, CA. American Society for Microbiology, Abstract 1933, 1999.

Lomaestro B M, Piatek M A. Update on drug interactions with azole antifungal agents. *Am Pharmacother* 32:915–928, 1998.

Lozano-Chiu M, Arikan S, Paetznick V L, Anaissie E J, Loebenberg D, Rex J H. Treatment of murine fusariosis with SCH56592. *Antimicrob Agents Chemother* 43:589–591, 1999.

Maenza J R, Keruly J C, Moore R D, Chaisson R E, Merz W G, Gallant J E. Risk factors for fluconazole resistant candidiasis in human immunodeficiency virus-infected patients. *J Infect Dis* 173:219–225, 1996.

Manavathu E K, Cutright J L, Chandrasekar P H. Organism-dependent fungicidal activities of azoles. *Antimicrob Agents Chemother* 43:3018–3021, 1998.

Manavathu E K, Cutright J L, Loebenberg D, Chandrasekar P H. A comparative study of the in vitro susceptibilities of clinical and laboratory-selected resistant isolates of *Aspergillus spp.* to amphotericin B, itraconazole, voriconazole and posaconazole (SCH 56592). *J Antimicrob Chemother* 46:229–234, 2000.

Manavathu E K, Abraham O C, Chandrasekar P H. Isolation and in vitro susceptibility to amphotericin B, itraconazole and posaconazole of voriconazole-resistant laboratory isolates of *Aspergillus fumigatus. Clin Microbiol Infect* 7:130–137, 2001.

Marco F, Pfaller M A, Messer S, Jones R N. In vitro activities of voriconazole (UK-104,496) and four other antifungal agents against 394 clinical isolates of *Candida* spp. *Antimicrob Agents Chemother* 42:161–163, 1998.

Marr K A, Lyons C N, Rustad T R, Bowden R A, White T C, Rustad T. Rapid, transient fluconazole resistance in *Candida albicans* is associated with increased mRNA levels of *CDR*. *Antimicrob Agents Chemother* 42:2584–2589, 1998.

Marr K A, Lyons C N, Ha K, Rustad T R, White T C. Inducible azole resistance associated with heterogeneous phenotype in *Candida albicans*. *Antimicrob Agents Chemother* 45:52–59, 2001.

Martin M V, Yates J, Hitchcock C A. Comparison of voriconazole (UK-109,496) and itraconazole in prevention and treatment of *Aspergillus fumigatus* endocarditis in guinea pigs. *Antimicrob Agents Chemother* 41:13–16, 1997.

Masur H, Kaplan J E, Holmes K K. Recommendationis of the U.S. Public Health Service and the Infectious Diseases Society of America. Guidelines for preventing opportunistic infections among HIV-infected persons—2002. *Ann Intern Med* 137, Supp. No. 5 (Part 2): 435–477, 2002.

McKinsey D S, Kauffman C A, Pappas P G, Cloud G A, Girard W M, Sharkey-Mathis P K, Hamill R J, Thomas C J, Dismukes W E, the NIAID Mycoses Study Group. Fluconazole therapy for histoplasmosis. *Clin Infect Dis* 23:996–1001, 1996.

Mellinghoff I K, Winston D J, Mukwaya G, Schiller G J. Treatment of *Scedosporium apiospermum* brain abscesses with posaconazole. *Clin Infect Dis* 34:1648–1650, 2002.

Miyazaki H, Miyazaki Y, Geber A, Parkinson T, Hitchcock C, Falconer D J, Ward D J, Marsden K, Bennett J E. Fluconazole resistance associated with drug efflux and increased transcription of a drug transporter gene, PDH1, in *Candida glabrata*. *Antimicrob Agents Chemother* 42:1695–1701, 1998.

Muhl E, Martens T, Iven H, Rob P, Bruch H P. Influence of continuous veno-venous haemodiafiltration and continuous venovenous haemofiltration on the pharmacokinetics of fluconazole. *Eur J Clin Pharmacol* 56:671–678, 2000.

Muller F-M C, Weig M, Peter J, Walsh T J. Azole cross-resistance to ketoconazole, fluconazole, itraconazole and voriconazole in clinical *Candida albicans* isolates from HIV-infected children with oropharyngeal candidosis. *J Antimicrob Chemother* 46:338–341, 2000.

Munoz P, Marin M, Tornero P, Martin-Rabadan P, Rodriguez-Creixems M, Bonza E. Successful outcome of *Scedosporium apiospermum* disseminated infection treated with voriconazole in a patient receiving corticosteroid therapy. *Clin Infect Dis* 31:1501–1503, 2000.

Murphy M, Bernard E M, Ishimaru T, Armstrong D. Activity of voriconazole (UK-109,496) against clinical isolates of *Aspergillus* species and its effectiveness in an experimental model of invasive aspergillosis. *Antimicrob Agents Chemother* 41:496–498, 1997.

Naranjo M S, Trujillo M, Munera M I, Restrepo P, Gomez I, Restrepo A. Treatment of paracoccidioidomycosis with itraconazole. *J Med Vet Mycol* 28:67–76, 1990.

National Committee for Clinical Laboratory Standards. Reference method for broth dilution antifungal susceptibility testing of yeasts: approved standard NCCLS document M27-A2. Wayne, PA: National Committee for Clinical Laboratory Standards, 2002a.

National Committee for Clinical Laboratory Standards. Reference method for broth dilution antifungal susceptibility testing of filamentous fungi. Approved standard. Document M38-A. Wayne, PA: National Committee for Clinical Laboratory Standards, 2002b.

National Institute of Allergy and Infectious Diseases Mycoses Study Group. Treatment of blastomycosis and histoplasmosis with ketoconazole: results of a prospective randomized clinical trial. *Ann Intern Med* 103:861–872, 1985.

Negroni R, Palmieri O, Koren F, Tiraboschi I N, Galimberti R L.

Oral treatment of paracoccidiomycosis and histoplasmosis with itraconazole in humans. *Rev Infect Dis* 9(Suppl 1):S47–S50, 1987.

Negroni R, Robles A M, Arechavala A, Tuculet M A, Galimberti R. Ketoconazole in the treatment of paracoccidioidomycosis and histoplasmosis. *Rev Infect Dis* 2:643–649, 1980.

Nesky M A, McDougal E C, Peacock J E. *Pseudallescheria boydii* brain abscess successfully treated with voriconazole and surgical drainage: case report and literature review of central nervous system pseudallescheriasis. *Clin Infect Dis* 31:673–77, 2000.

Nguyen M H, Peacock J E Jr, Tanner D C, Morris A J, Nguyen M L, Snydman D R, Wagener M M, Yu V L. Therapeutic approaches in patients with candidemia. *Arch Intern Med* 155:2429–2435, 1995.

Nguyen M H, Peacock J E, Jr, Morris A J, Tanner D C, Nguyen M L, Snydman D R, Wagener M M, Rinaldi M G, Yu V L. The changing face of candidemia: emergence of non-*Candida albicans* species and antifungal resistance. *Am J Med* 100:617–623, 1996.

Nguyen M H, Yu C Y. Voriconazole against fluconazole-susceptible and resistant *Candida* isolates: in vitro efficacy compared with that of itraconazole and ketoconazole. *J Antimicrob Chemother* 42:253–256, 1998.

Nomier A A, Kumari P, Gupta S, Loebenberg D, Cacciapuoti A, Hare R, Lin C C, Cayen M N. Pharmacokinetics of SCH 59884, an IV prodrug for the oral antifungal SCH 56592 in animals and its conversion to SCH 59592 by human tissues. 39th Interscience Conference on Antimicrobial Agents and Chemotherapy. San Francisco, CA. American Society for Microbiology, Abstract 1934, 1999.

Paphitou N I, Ostrosky-Zeichner L, Paetznick V L, Rodriguez J R, Chen E, Rex J H. In vitro antifungal susceptibilities of *Trichosporon* species. *Antimicrob Agents Chemother* 46:1144–1146, 2002.

Pappas P G, Bradsher R W, Chapman S W, Kauffman C A, Dine A, Cloud G A, Dismukes W E, and the NIAID Mycoses Study Group. Treatment of blastomycosis with fluconazole. *Clin Infect Dis* 20:267–71, 1995.

Pappas P G, Bradsher R W, Kauffman C A, Cloud G A, Thomas C T, Campbell, G D Jr., Chapman S W, Newman C, Dismukes W E, the NIAID Mycoses Study Group. Treatment of blastomycosis with higher dose fluconazole. *Clin Infect Dis* 25:200–205, 1997.

Pappas P G, Perfect J R, Cloud G A, Larsen R A, Pankey G A, Lancaster D J, Henderson H. Kauffman C A, Haas D W, Saccente M, Hamill R J, Holloway M S, Warren R M, Dismukes W E. Cryptococcosis in human immunodeficiency virus-negative patients in the era of effective azole therapy. *Clin Infect Dis* 33:690–699, 2001.

Perea S, Gonzalez G, Fothergill A W, Kirkpatrick W R, Rinaldi M G, Patterson T F. In vitro interaction of caspofungin acetate with voriconazole against clinical isolates of *Aspergillus* spp. *Antimicrob Agents Chemother* 46:3039–3041, 2002.

Petraitiene R, Petraitis V, Groll A H, Sein T, Piscatelli S, Candelario M, Field-Ridley A, Avila N, Bacher J, Walsh T W. Antifungal activity and pharmacokinetics of posaconazole (SCH 56592) in treatment and prevention of experimental invasive pulmonary aspergillosis: correlation with galactomannan antigenemia. *Antimicrob Agents Chemother* 45:857–869, 2001.

Petraitiene R, Petraitis V, Sarafandi A, Kelaher A, Lyman C A, Sein T, Groll A H, Mickiene D, Bacher J, Walsh T J. Synergistic activity between ravuconazole and the echinocandin micafungin in treatment of experimental pulmonary aspergillosis. 42nd Interscience Conference on Antimicrobial Agents and Chemotherapy, San Diego, CA. American Society for Microbiology, Abstract M-857, 2002.

Pfaller M A, Messer S A, Hollis R J, Jones R N, Doern G V, Brandt M E, Hajjeh R A. In vitro susceptibilties of *Candida* bloodstream isolates to the new triazole antifungal agents BMS-207147, SCH 56592, and voriconazole. *Antimicrob Agents Chemother* 42: 3242–3244, 1998.

Pfaller M A, Zhang J, Messer S A, Brandt M E, Hajjeh R A, Jessup C J, Tumberland M, Mbidde E K, Ghannoum, M A. In vitro activities of voriconazole, fluconazole, and itraconazole against 566 clinical isolates of *Cryptococcus neoformans* from the United States and Africa. *Antimicrob Agents Chemother* 43:169–171, 1999.

Pfaller M A, Messer S A, Hollis R J, Jones R N. In vitro activities of posaconazole (SCH 56592) compared with those of itraconazole and fluconazole against 3,685 clinical isolates of *Candida* spp. and *Cryptococcus neoformans*. *Antimicrob Agents Chemother* 45:2862–2864, 2001.

Pfaller M A, Messer S A, Hollis R J, Jones R N. Sentry Participants Group. Antifungal activities of posaconazole, ravuconazole and voriconazole compared to those of amphotericin B against 239 clinical isolates of *Aspergillus* spp and other filamentous fungi: report from the Sentry Antimicrobial Surveillance Program, 2000. *Antimicrob Agents Chemother* 46:1032–1037, 2002.

Phillips P, Shafran S, Garber G, Rotstein C, Smaill F, Fong I, Salit I, Miller M, Williams K, Conly J M, Singer J, Ioannou S, the Canadian Candidemia Study Group. Multicenter randomized trial of fluconazole versus amphotericin B for treatment of candidemia in non-neutropenic patients. *Eur J Clin Microbiol Infect Dis* 16:337–345, 1997.

Phillips P, DeBeulle K, Frechette G, Tchamouroff S, Vandercam B, Weitner L, Hoepelman A, Stingl G, Clotet B. A double-blind comparison of itraconazole oral solution and fluconazole capsules for the treatment of orpharyngeal candidiasis in patients with AIDS. *Clin Infect Dis* 26:1368–1373, 1998.

Piscitelli S C, Gallicano K D. Interactions among drugs for HIV and opportunistic infections. *N Engl J Med* 344:984–996, 2001.

Poirier J M, Cheymol G. Optimisation of itraconazole therapy using target drug concentrations. *Clin Pharmacokinet* 35:461–473, 1998.

Pons V G, Greenspan D, Debruin M, the Multicenter Study Group. Therapy for oropharyngeal candidiasis in HIV-infected patients: a randomized study of oral fluconazole versus clotrimazole troches. *J Acquir Immune Defic Syndr* 6:1311–1316, 1993.

Powderly W G, Saag M S, Cloud G A, Robinson P, Meyer R D, Jacobson J M, Graybill J R, Sugar A M, McAuliffe V J, Follansbee S E, Tuazon C U, Stern J J, Feinberg J, Hafner R, Dismukes W E, the NIAID AIDS Clinical Trials Group and the NIAID Mycoses Study Group. A controlled trial of fluconazole or amphotericin B to prevent relapse of cryptococcal meningitis in patients with the acquired immunodeficiency syndrome. *N Engl J Med* 326:793–798, 1992.

Quart A M, Espinel-Ingroff A, Steele-Moore L, Reich D. Evaluation of fluconazole in the treatment of oropharyngeal candidiasis in patients with AIDS. *Infect Med* 13:708–713, 1996.

Redding S, Smith J, Farinacci G, Rinaldi M, Fothergill A, Rhine-Chalberg J, Pfaller M. Resistance of *Candida albicans* to fluconazole during treatment of oropharyngeal candidiasis in a patient with AIDS: documentation by in vitro susceptibility testing and DNA subtype analysis. *Clin Infect Dis* 18:240–242, 1994.

Reef S E, Levine W C, McNeill M M, Fisher-Hochs, Hohnberg S D, Duerr A, Smith D, Sobel J D, Pinner R W. Treatment options for vulvovaginal candidiasis. Background paper for development of 1993 STD treatment recommendations. *Clin Infect Dis* 20(Suppl 1):S80–S90, 1995.

Restrepo A, Gomez I, Cano L E, Arango M D, Gutierrez F, Sanin A, Robledo M A. Treatment of paracoccidioidomycosis with ketoconazole: a three-year experience. *Am J Med* 74 (Suppl 1B):48–52, 1983.

Restrepo A, Robledo J, Gomez I, Tabares A M, Gutierrez R. Itra-

conazole therapy in lymphangitic and cutaneous sporotrichosis. *Arch Dermatol* 122:413–417, 1986.

Restrepo A. Treatment of tropical mycoses. *J Am Acad Dermatol* 31(Suppl):S91–S102, 1994.

Revankar S G, Kirkpatrick W R, McAtee R K, Dib O P, Fothergill A W, Redding S W, Rinaldi M G, Patterson T F. Detection and significance of fluconazole resistance in oropharyngeal candidiasis in human immunodeficiency virus infected patients. *J Infect Dis* 174:821–827, 1996.

Rex J H, Bennett J E, Sugar A M, Pappas P G, van der Horst C M, Edwards J E, Washburn R G, Scheld W M, Karchmer A W, Dine A P, Levenstein M J, Webb C B, for the Candidemia Study Group and the National Institute of Allergy and Infectious Diseases Mycoses Study Group. A randomized trial comparing fluconazole with amphotericin B for the treatment of candidemia in patients without neutropenia. *N Engl J Med* 331:1325–1330, 1994.

Rex J H, Pfaller M A, Barry A L, Nelson P W, Webb C D. Antifungal susceptibility testing of isolates from a randomized, multicenter trial of fluconazole versus amphotericin B as treatment of nonneutropenic patients with candidemia. NIAID Mycoses Study Group and the Candidemia Study Group. *Antimicrob Agents Chemother* 39:40–44, 1995.

Rex J H, Pfaller M A, Galgiani J N, Bartlett M S, Espinel-Ingroff A, Ghannoum M A, Lancaster M, Odds F C, Rinaldi M G, Walsh T J, Barry A L, for the Subcommittee on Antifungal Susceptible Testing of the National Committee for Clinical Laboratory Standards. Development of interpretive breakpoints for antifungal susceptibility testing: conceptual framework and analysis of in vitro in vivo correlation data for fluconazole, itraconazole, and *Candida* infections. *Clin Infect Dis* 24:235–247, 1997.

Rex J H, Walsh T J, Sobel J D, Filler S G, Pappas P G, Dismukes W E, Edwards J E. Practice guidelines for the treatment of candidiasis. *Clin Infect Dis* 30:662–678, 2000.

Rex J H, Sobel J D. Prophylactic antifungal therapy in the intensive care unit. *Clin Infect Dis* 32:1191–1200, 2001.

Rex J H, Pappas P G, Karchmer A W, Sobel J, Edwards J E, Hadley S, Brass C, Vazquez J A, Chapman S W, Horowitz H W, Zervos M, Lee J, for the National Institute of Allergy and Infectious Diseases Mycoses Study Group. A randomized, blinded, multicenter trial of high dose fluconazole plus placebo versus fluconazole plus amphotericin B as therapy of candidemia in non-neutropenic patients. In Press, *Clin Infect Dis*, 2003.

Reyes G H, Long L, Hossain M., Ghannoum M A. Evaluation of voriconazole efficacy in the treatment of murine fusariosis. 41st Interscience Conference on Antimicrobial Agents and Chemotherapy. Chicago, IL. American Society for Microbiology, USA. Abstract J-1604, 2001.

Saag M S, Dismukes W E. Azole antifungal agents: emphasis on new triazoles. *Antimicrob Agents Chemother* 32:1–8, 1988.

Saag M S, Fessel W J, Kaufman C, Merrill K W, Ward D J, Moskovitz B L, Thomas C, Oleka N, Guarnieri J A, Lee J, Brenner-Gati L, Klausner M. Treatment of fluconazole-refractory oropharyngeal candidiasis with itraconazole oral solution in HIV-positive patients. *AIDS Res Human Retrovir* 15:1413–1417, 1999a.

Saag M S, Cloud G A, Graybill J R, Sobel J D, Tuazon C U, Johnson P C, Fessel J Y, Moskovitz B L, Weisinger B, Cosmatos D, Riser L, Thomas C, Hafner R, Dismukes W E, the NIAID Mycoses Study Group. A comparison of itraconazole versus fluconazole as maintenance therapy for AIDS-associated cryptococcal meningitis. *Clin Infect Dis* 28:291–296, 1999b.

Saag M S, Graybill R J, Larsen R A, Pappas P G, Perfect J R, Powderly W G, Sobel J D, Dismukes W E. Practice guidelines for the management of cryptococcal disease. *Clin Infect Dis* 30:710–718, 2000.

Sabo J, Abdel-Rahman S M. Voriconazole: a new triazole antifungal. *Ann Pharmacother* 34:1032–1043, 2000.

Safdar A, Chaturvedi V, Cross E W, Park S, Bernard E M, Armstrong D, Perlin D S. Prospective study of *Candida* species in patients at a comprehensive cancer center. *Antimicrob Agents Chemother* 45:2129–2133, 2001.

Sanati H, Belanger P, Fratti R, Ghannoum M. A new triazole, voriconazole (UK-109,496) blocks sterol biosynthesis in *Candida albicans* and *Candida krusei*. *Antimicrob Agents Chemother* 41:2492–2467, 1997.

Sangeorzan J A, Bradley S F, He X, Zarins L T, Ridenour G L, Tiballi R n, Kauffman C A. Epidemiology of oral candidiasis in HIV-infected patients: colonization, infection, treatment, and emergence of fluconazole resistance. *Am J Med* 97:339–346, 1994.

Sanglard D, Ischer F, Monod M, Bille J. Cloning of *Candida albicans* genes conferring resistance to azole antifungal agents: Characterization of *CDR2*, a new multidrug ABC transporter gene. *Microbiol* 143:405–416, 1997.

Sanglard D, Ischer F, Bille J. Role of ATP-binding-cassette transporter genes in high-frequency acquisition of resistance to azole antifungals in *Candida glabrata*. *Antimicrob Agents Chemother* 45:1174–1183, 2001.

Sanglard D, Ischer F, Bille J. Interactions of ravuconazole with yeast multidrug efflux transporters and different cytochrome P450 mutant forms. 42nd Interscience Conference on Antimicrobial Agents and Chemotherapy, San Diego, CA. American Society for Microbiology, Abstract M-221, 2002.

Schectman L B, Funaro L, Robin T, Bottone E J, Cuttner J. Clotrimazole treatment of oral candidiasis in patients with neoplastic disease. *Am J Med* 76:91–94, 1984.

Scher R K, Breneman D, Rich P, Savin R C, Feingold D S, Konnikov N, Shupack J L, Pinnel S, Levine N, Lowe N J, Aly R, Odom R B, Greer D L, Mormon M R, Bucko A D, Tschen E H, Elewski B E, Smith E B. Once weekly fluconazole (150,300 or 450mg) in the treatment of distal subungual onychomycosis of the toenail. *J Am Acad Dermatol* 38:S77–S86, 1998.

Scher R K. Onychomycosis: therapeutic update. *J Am Acad Dermatol* 40:521–526, 1999.

Schwartz S, Milatovic D, Thiel E. Successful treatment of cerebral aspergillosis with a novel triazole (voriconazole) in a patient with acute leukemia. *Br J Haematol* 97:663–665, 1997.

Sharkey P K, Graybill J R, Rinaldi M G, Stevens D A, Tucker R M, Peterie J D, Hoeprich P D, Greer D L, Frenkel L, Counts G W. Itraconazole treatment of phaeohyphomycosis. *J Am Acad Dermatol* 23:577–586, 1990.

Sharkey-Mathis P K, Kauffman C A, Graybill J R, Stevens D A, Hostetler J S, Dismukes W E, the NIAID Mycoses Study Group. Treatment of sporotrichosis with itraconazole. *Am J Med* 95:279–285, 1993.

Sirisanthana T, Supparatpinyo K, Perriens T, Nelson K E. Amphotericin B and itraconazole for treatment of disseminated *Penicillium marneffei* infection in human immunodeficiency virus-infected patients. *Clin Infect Dis* 26:1107–1110, 1998.

Slama T G. Treatment of disseminated and progressive cavitary histoplasmosis with ketoconazole. *Am J Med* 74(Suppl 1B):70–73, 1983.

Sobel J D. Pathogenesis and treatment of recurrent vulvovaginal candidiasis. *Clin Infect Dis* 14(Suppl 1):S148–S153, 1992.

Sobel J D, Faro S, Force R W, Foxman B, Ledger W J, Nyirjesy P R, Reed B D, Summers P R. Vulvovaginal candidiasis: epidemiologic, diagnostic, and therapeutic considerations. *Am J Obstet Gynecol* 178:203–221, 1998.

Sobel J D, Kauffman C A, McKinsey D, Zervos M, Vazquez J A, Karchmer A W, Lee J, Thomas C. Candiduria: a randomized, double blind study of treatment with fluconazole and placebo. *Clin Infect Dis* 30:19–24, 2000.

Sobel J D, Ohmit S E, Schuman P, Klein R S, Mayer K, Duerr A, Vazquez J A, Rompalo A for the HIV Epidemiology Research Study Group. The evolution of *Candida species* and fluconazole susceptibility among oral and vaginal isolates recovered from human immunodeficiency virus (HIV)-seropositive and at-risk HIV-seronegative women. *J Infect Dis* 183:286–93, 2001.

Stein G E, Mummaw N. Placebo controlled trial of itraconazole for treatment of acute vaginal candidiasis. *Antimicrob Agents Chemother* 37:89–92, 1993.

Stevens D A, Lee J Y. Analysis of compassionate use itraconazole therapy of invasive aspergillosis by the NIAID Mycoses Study Group criteria. *Arch Intern Med* 157:1857–1862, 1997.

Stevens D A. Itraconazole in cyclodextrin solution. *Pharmacotherapy* 19:603–611, 1999.

Stevens D A, Kan V L, Judson M A, Morrison V A, Dummer S, Denning D W, Bennett J E, Walsh T J, Patterson T F, Pankey G A. Practice guidelines for diseases caused by *Aspergillus*. *Clin Infect Dis* 30:696–709, 2000.

Sud I J, Chou D L, Feingold D S. Effect of free fatty acids on liposome susceptibility to imidazole antifungals. *Antimicrob Agents Chemother* 16:660–663, 1979.

Sugar A M, Liu X P. Efficacy of voriconazole in treatment of murine pulmonary blastomycosis. *Antimicrob Agents Chemother* 45:601–604, 2001.

Sun Q N, Fothergill A W, McCarthy D C, Rinaldi M G, Graybill J R. In vitro activities of posaconazole, itraconazole, voriconazole, amphotericin B and fluconazole against 37 clinical isolates of Zygomycetes. *Antimicrob Agents Chemother* 46:1581–1582, 2002a.

Sun Q N, Najvar L K, Bocanegra R, Loebenberg D, Graybill J R. In vivo activity of posaconazole against *Mucor* spp in an immunosuppressed-mouse model. *Antimicrob Agents Chemother* 46:2310–2312, 2002b.

Supparatpinyo K, Perriens J, Nelson K E, Sirisanthana T. A controlled trial of itraconazole to prevent relapse of *Penicillium marneffei* infection in patients infected with the human immunodeficiency virus. *N Engl J Med* 339:1739–1744, 1998.

Sutton D A, Sanche S E, Revankar S G, Fothergill A W, Rinaldi M G. In vitro amphotericin B resistance in clinical isolates of *Aspergillus terreus*, with a head-to-head comparison to voriconazole. *J Clin Microbiol* 37:2343–2345, 1999.

Sutton D A, Fothergill A W, McCarthy D, Rinaldi M G. In vitro activity of voriconazole against 71 clinical isolates of dematiaceous filamentous fungi. 42nd Interscience Conference on Antimicrobial Agents and Chemotherapy, San Diego, CA. American Society for Microbiology, Abstract M-1516, 2002.

Tan K K C, Wood N, Weil A. Multiple dose pharmacokinetics of voriconazole in chronic hepatic impairment. 41st Interscience Conference on Antimicrobial Agents and Chemotherapy. Chicago, IL. American Society for Microbiology, Abstract A-16, 2001.

Terrell C L. Antifungal agents. Part II. The azoles. *Mayo Clin Proc* 74:78–100, 1999.

Thaler F, Bernard B, Tod M, Jedynak C P, Petitjean O, Derome P, Loirat P. Fluconazole penetration in cerebral parenchyma in humans at steady state. *Antimicrob Agents Chemother* 39:1154–1156, 1995.

Tucker R M, Denning D W, Dupont B, Stevens D A. Itraconazole therapy for chronic coccidioidal meningitis. *Ann Intern Med* 112:108–112, 1990.

Uchida K, Yokota N, Yamaguchi H. In vitro antifungal activity of posaconazole against various pathogenic fungi. *Int J Antimicrob Agents* 18:167–172, 2001.

Ueda Y, Barbour N, Bronson J J, Connolly T P, Dali M, Gao Q, Golik J, Huang S, Hudyma T W, Kang S, Knipe J, Mathew M, Matiskella J D, Mosure K, Tejwani R, Varia S, Venkatesh S, Zheng M. BMS-379, 224, a water-soluble proding of ravuconazole. 42nd Interscience Conference on Antimicrobial Agents and Chemotherapy, San Diego, CA. American Society for Microbiology, Abstract F-817, 2002.

Valtonen M, Tiula E, Neuvonen P J. Effect of continuous venovenous haemofiltration and haemodiafiltration on the elimination of fluconazole in patients with acute renal failure. *J Antimicrob Chemother* 40:695–700, 1997.

Van den Bossche H, Willemsens G, Cools W. Marichal P, Lauwers W. Hypothesis on the molecular basis of the antifungal activity of N-substituted imidazoles and triazoles. *Biochem Soc Trans* 11:665–667, 1983.

Van der Horst C, Saag M S, Cloud G A, Hamill R J, Graybill J R, Sobel J D, Johnson P C, Tuazon C U, Kerkering T, Moskovitz B L, Powderly W G, Dismukes W E, the National Institute of Allergy and Infectious Diseases Mycoses Study Group and AIDS Clinical Trials Group. Treatment of cryptococcal meningitis associated with the acquired immunodeficiency syndrome. *N Engl J Med* 337:15–21, 1997.

Vazquez J A, Sobel J D. Epidemiologic overview of resistance to oral antifungal agents in the immunocompromised host. In: *Opportunistic Infections in the Immunocompromised Host*. Elsevier Sciences BV, Amsterdam, p. 1–11, 1997.

Venkatakrishnon K, von Moltke L L, Greenblatt D J. Effects of the antifungal agents on oxidative drug metabolism. *Clin Pharmacokinet* 38:111–180, 2000.

Vora S, Purimetta N, Brummer E, Stevens D A. Activity of voriconazole, a new triazole, combined with neutrophils or monocytes against *Candida albicans*: effect of granulocyte colony-stimulating factor and granulocyte-macrophage colony-stimulating factor. *Antimicrob Agents Chemother* 42:907–910, 1998.

Voriconazole package insert, 2002.

Walsh T J, Pappas P, Winston D, Blumer J, Finn P, Raffalli J, Yanovich S, Stiff P, Greenberg R, Donowitz G, Lee J, Schuster M, Reboli A, Wingard J, Arndt C, Reinhardt J, Hadley S, Finberg R, Laverdiere M, Perfect J, Garber G, Fioritoni G, Anaissie E, for the NIAID Mycoses Study Group. Voriconazole versus liposomal amphotericin B for empirical antifungal therapy in persistently febrile neutropenic patients: a prospective, randomized, multicenter, international trial. *N Engl J Med* 346:225–334, 2002.

Wexler D, Laughlin M, Courtney R, Lim J, Batra V. Effect of posaconazole on drug metabolizing enzymes. 42nd Interscience Conference on Antimicrobial Agents and Chemotherapy, San Diego, CA. American Society for Microbiology, Abstract A-1839, 2002.

Wheat J, Hafner R, Wulfsohn M, Spencer P, Squires K, Powderly W, Wong B, Rinaldi M, Saag M, Hamill R, Murphy R, Connolly-Stringfield P, Briggs N, Owens S, Johnson J, Relue J, Lengendre R, the NIAID AIDS Clinical Trials Group and Mycoses Study Group collaborators. Prevention of relapse of histoplasmosis with itraconazole in patients with the acquired immunodeficiency syndrome. *Ann Intern Med* 118:610–616, 1993.

Wheat J, Hafner R, Korzun A H, Limos M T, Spencer P, Larsen R A, Hecht F M, Powderly W. Itraconazole treatment of disseminated histoplasmosis in patients with the acquired immunodeficiency syndrome. *Am J Med* 98:336–342, 1995.

Wheat J, MaWhinney S, Hafner R, McKinsey D, Chen D, Korzun A, Shakan K J, Johnson P, Hamill R, Bamberger D, Pappas P, Stansell J, Koletar S, Squires K, Larsen R A, Cheung T, Hyslop N, Lai KK, Schneider D, Kauffman C, Saag M, Dismukes W, Powderly W for the National Institute of Allergy and Infectious Diseases AIDS Clinical Trials Group and Mycoses Study Group. Treatment of histoplasmosis with fluconazole in patients with acquired immunodeficiency syndrome. *Am J Med* 103:223–232, 1997.

Wheat J, Sarosi G, McKinsey D, Hamill R, Bradsher R, Johnson P, Loyd J, Kauffman C. Practice guidelines for the management of patients with histoplasmosis. *Clin Infect Dis* 30:688–695, 2000.

Whittle D L, Koninis S. Use of Itraconazole for treating subcutaneous phaeohyphomycosis caused by *Exophila jeanselmei*. *Clin Infect Dis* 21:1068, 1995.

Wilcox C M, Alexander L N, Clark W S, Thompson S E III. Fluconazole compared with endoscopy for human immunodeficiency virus-infected patients with esophageal symptoms. *Gastroenterol* 110:1803–1809, 1996.

Wilcox C M, Darouiche R O, Laine L, Moskovitz B L, Mallegol I, Wu J. A randomized double-blinded comparison of itraconazole oral solution and fluconazole tablets in the treatment of esophageal candidiasis. *J Infect Dis* 176:227–232, 1997.

Winn R E, Anderson J, Piper J, Aronson N E, Pluss J. Systemic sporotrichosis treated with itraconazole. *Clin Infect Dis* 17:210–217, 1993.

Wingard J R, Merz W G, Rinaldi M G, Johnson T R, Karp J E, Saral R. Increase in *Candida krusei* infection among patients with bone marrow transplantation and neutropenia treated prophylactically with fluconazole. *N Engl J Med* 325:1274–1277, 1991.

Wingard J R, Merz W G, Rinaldi M G, Miller C B, Karp J E, Saral R. Association of *Torulopsis glabrata* infections with fluconazole prophylaxis in neutropenic bone marrow transplant patients. *Antimicrob Agents Chemother* 37:1847–1849, 1993.

Wood N, Tan K, Allen R, Fielding A, Nichols DJ. Effect of voriconazole on the pharmacokinetics of omeprazole. 41st Interscience Conference on Antimicrobial Agents and Chemotherapy. Chicago, IL. American Society for Microbiology, Abstract A-19, 2001.

Yamaguchi H, Ikemoto H, Watanabe K, Ito A, Hara K, Kohno S. Fluconazole monotherapy for cryptococcosis in non-AIDS patients. *Eur J Clin Microbiol Infect Dis* 15:787–792, 1996.

Yamazumi T, Pfaller M A, Messer S A, Houston A, Hollis R J, Jones R N. In vitro activities of ravuconazole (BMS-207147) against 541 clinical isolates of *Cryptococcus neoformans*. *Antimicrob Agents Chemother* 44:2883–2886, 2000.

7

Cell wall synthesis inhibitors: echinocandins and nikkomycins

ANDREAS H. GROLL AND THOMAS J. WALSH

Ever since the discovery that penicillin inhibits bacterial cell wall synthesis, developing equivalent agents to target the fungal cell wall has been a focus in antifungal drug development. Because the cell wall is essential to the vitality of fungal organisms and because its components are absent in the mammalian host, the fungal cell wall represents an ideal target for antifungal compounds.

With considerable variation among different species, the gross macromolecular components of the cell wall of most fungi include chitin, alpha- or beta-linked glucans and a variety of mannoproteins. The dynamics of the fungal cell wall are closely coordinated with cell growth and cell division, and its predominant function is to control the internal turgor pressure of the cell. Disruption of the cell wall structure leads to osmotic instability, and may ultimately result in the lysis of the fungal cell.

Systemic antifungal agents directed against or involving the major constituents of the fungal cell wall include the new class of echinocandin lipopeptides and the nucleoside-peptide antibiotic nikkomycin Z.

GLUCAN-SYNTHESIS INHIBITORS: ECHINOCANDIN ANALOGUES

The echinocandins are a novel class of semisynthetic amphiphilic lipopeptides that are composed of a cyclic hexapeptide core linked to a variably configured lipid side chain. The first compound of this class undergoing major preclinical evaluation was cilofungin (LY 121019), a semisynthetic echinocandin B derivative with activity limited to *Candida* spp. However, clinical development was abandoned in early stages due to toxicity concerns associated with the intravenous polyethylene glycol formulation vehicle (Hector, 1993; Debono and Gordee, 1994; Groll et al, 1998). Over the past few years, a second generation of semisynthetic echinocandins with extended antifungal spectrum, fa-

vorable safety profile, and pharmacokinetic characteristics have entered clinical development: anidulafungin (VER-002, formerly LY303366; Versicor Inc, Freemont, CA), caspofungin (MK-0991; Merck & Co., Inc., Rahway, NJ), and micafungin (FK463; Fujisawa Inc., Deerfield, IL) (Fig. 7–1). Current data indicate that these agents are similar with respect to their pharmacokinetic and pharmacodynamic properties. One of the three agents, caspofungin, has received limited approval in the United States and the European community for second line treatment of invasive aspergillosis.

Mechanism of Action

The echinocandins act by noncompetitive inhibition of the synthesis of 1,3-beta-glucan, a polysaccharide in the cell wall of many pathogenic fungi (Fig. 7–2). Together with chitin, the rope-like glucan fibrils are responsible for the strength and shape of the cell wall. They are important in maintaining the osmotic integrity of the fungal cell and play a key role in cell division and cell growth (Hector, 1993; Debono and Gordee, 1994; Groll et al, 1998). The proposed molecular target of the echinocandins, glucan synthase, is a heteromeric enzyme complex composed of at least one large integral membrane protein encoded by the FKS genes that bind the substrate (UDP-glucose), and one small regulatory subunit, Rho1p, a GTP-binding protein. Additional, yet unidentified components may also be involved (Kurtz and Douglas, 1997; Thompson et al, 1999).

Antifungal Activity In Vitro

The current echinocandins have potent and broad spectrum in vitro activity against *Candida* and *Aspergillus* spp. and also have demonstrated efficacy against invasive infections by these organisms in various animal models. The mode of antifungal action against *Candida* and *Aspergillus* spp., however, appears species-dependent. While similarly potent activity at the target enzyme has been demonstrated in membrane preparations of *Candida* and *Aspergillus* spp., whole cell in

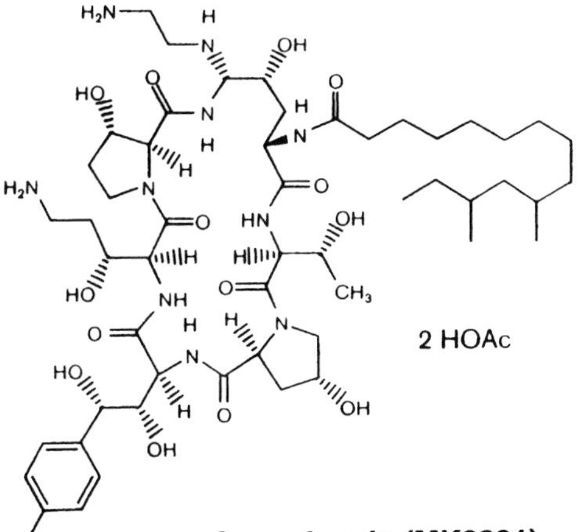

Caspofungin (MK0991)

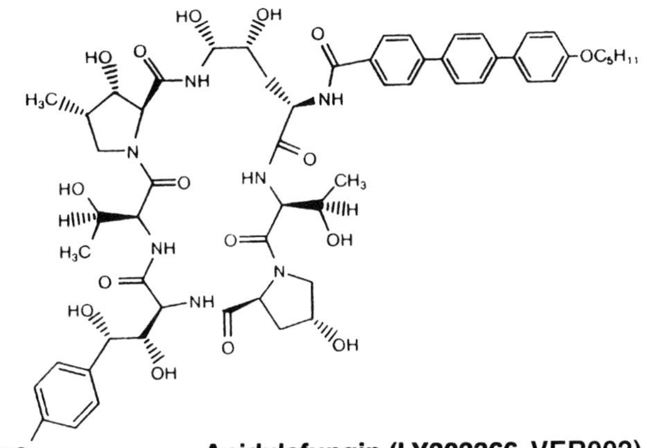

2 HOAc

Anidulafungin (LY303366, VER002)

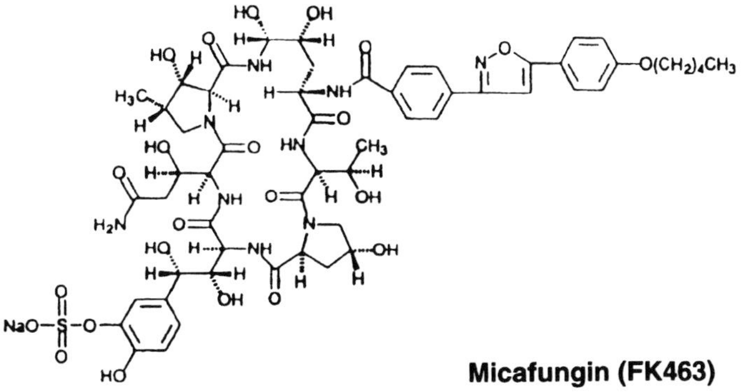

Micafungin (FK463)

FIGURE 7–1. Structural formulas of anidulafungin, caspofungin, and micafungin. The echinocandins are composed of a cyclic hexapep-tide core that is attached to an individually configured acyl side chain.

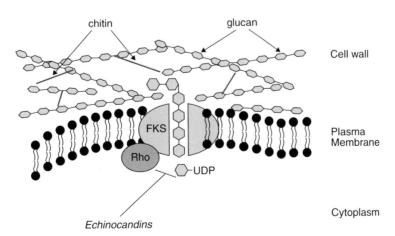

FIGURE 7–2. Schematic of the proposed mechanism of action of echinocandin lipopeptides. Echinocandins inhibit the synthesis of cell wall 1,3-beta glucan at the level of the cell membrane. Fks is the pro-posed catalytic subunit, and Rho the proposed regulatory subunit of the glucan synthase complex. Modified from Kurtz and Douglas, 1997, by permission of the publisher.

vitro assays reveal fungicidal activity against most *Candida* spp. but not against *Aspergillus* spp. (Tang et al, 1993; Bartizal et al, 1997). Microscopic examination of exposed organisms shows a dose-dependent formation of microcolonies with progressively truncated, swollen hyphal elements that appear to be cell-wall deficient, but are able to regain their cell walls upon subculture in the absence of drug (Kurtz et al, 1994; Rennie et al, 1997; Oakley et al, 1998; Douglas et al, 2000). These observations indicate differences in functional target sensitivity in both species that are not understood fully (Groll et al, 2001d).

The current echinocandins have variable activity against dematiaceous and endemic moulds, but are inactive against most hyalohyphomycetes, zygomycetes, *Cryptococcus neoformans*, and *Trichosporon asahii* (*beigelii*). Of note, all echinocandins have demonstrated preventive and therapeutic activity in animal models of *Pneumocystis carinii* pneumonia (Hawser, 1999; Groll and Walsh, 2000; Groll and Walsh, 2001e).

As expected from their mechanism of action, the echinocandins show no cross-resistance to amphotericin B and fluconazole resistant *Candida* isolates. Inherited resistance to echinocandins in otherwise susceptible fungal yeast species is rare; most mutations conferring resistance have been mapped to the FKS gene (Kurtz and Douglas, 1997). Results from studies with caspofungin demonstrate a low potential for induced resistance in *Candida* spp. (Bartizal et al, 1997). The frequency of primary echinocandin resistance among clinical isolates of *Aspergillus* spp. and induction of secondary resistance in vitro have not been studied thus far.

Pharmacokinetics

The echinocandins, which are currently only available for intravenous use, exhibit dose-proportional plasma pharmacokinetics with a triexponential elimination pattern. Their beta half–life is between 10 and 15 hours, allowing for once daily dosing without major accumulation after multiple dosing. All echinocandins are highly (> 95%) protein bound and distribute into all major organ sites including the brain; however, concentrations in uninfected CSF are low. The echinocandins are metabolized by the liver and slowly excreted into urine and feces; only small fractions (< 2%) of a dose are excreted into urine in unchanged form (Hawser, 1999; Groll and Walsh, 2000; Groll and Walsh, 2001e). The echinocandins, as a class, appear to have no significant potential for drug interactions mediated by the CYP450 cytochrome enzyme system. Whether differences in individual pharmacokinetic parameters such as AUC, peak plasma levels, volume of distribution, and clearance of the echinocandins, are of clinical significance remains to be elucidated.

Safety and Tolerance

At their currently investigated dosages, all echinocandins are generally well-tolerated, and only a small fraction of patients (< 5%) enrolled on the various clinical trials discontinued echinocandin therapy due to drug-related adverse events (Brown et al, 2000b; Maertens et al, 2000; Pettengel et al, 2000; Villanueva et al, 2001a; Arathoon et al, 2002). Detailed safety data, however, have been published for caspofungin only.

ANIDULAFUNGIN

Antifungal Activity In Vitro

Anidulafungin has potent and broad-spectrum in vitro antifungal activity against most *Candida* spp. (with lower activity against *C. parapsilosis* and *C. guilliermondii*), *Aspergillus* spp., and against both the trophic and cystic forms of *P. carinii*. As expected, anidulafungin is active against both fluconazole-sensitive and fluconazole-resistant strains of *Candida* spp. Although to a lesser extent, anidulafungin has activity against individual phaeohyphomycetes and against *Blastomyces dermatitidis*, *Histoplasma capsulatum*, and *Sporothrix schenckii*. Notable omissions in the spectrum of activity of this agent are *C. neoformans*, *T. asahii*, *Fusarium* spp., and the Zygomycetes (Pfaller et al, 1989; Zhanel et al, 1997; Espinel-Ingroff, 1998; Marco et al, 1998; Oakley et al, 1998; Pfaller et al, 1997; Karlowsky et al, 1999) (Table 7–1 and Table 7–2).

Anidulafungin displays prolonged antifungal effects of up to 12 hours and rapid concentration- and time-dependent fungicidal dynamics against *Candida* spp. (Ernst et al, 1996; Karlowsky et al, 1997; Ernst et al, 2000).

TABLE 7–1. *In Vitro Susceptibilities of Clinical Yeast Isolates to Anidulafungin*

Organism (No. of Isolates)	MIC Range (μg/mL)	MIC 90 (μg/mL)
C. albicans (10)*	< 0.03–0.25	0.25
C. albicans (10)**	< 0.03–0.25	0.06
C. glabrata (12)	0.06–0.25	0.25
C. guilliermondii (8)	0.25–4.0	ND
C. krusei (13)	0.12–1.0	1.0
C. lusitaniae (12)	0.25–2.0	2.0
C. parapsilosis (12)	0.5–2.0	2.0
C. tropicalis (12)	0.12–0.5	0.5
Cr. neoformans (10)	> 16	> 16
T. beigelii (5)	> 16	ND

Antifungal susceptibility assays were determined according the NCCLS M27-A broth microdilution method for yeasts.
*fluconazole MIC > 16 μg/mL.
**fluconazole MIC ≤ 1 μg/mL.
MIC, minimum inhibitory concentration; ND, not obtained.
Source: Modified from Espinel-Ingroff, 1998.

TABLE 7–2. *In Vitro Susceptibilities of Clinical Mould Isolates to Anidulafungin*

Organism (No. of Isolates)	MIC Range (μg/mL)	Geometric Mean MIC (μg/mL)
Aspergillus fumigatus (13)	0.06	0.06
Aspergillus flavus (11)	< 0.03–0.12	0.08
Aspergillus terreus (2)	< 0.03	ND
Bipolaris spp. (6)	1.0–4.0	2.7
Cladophialophora bantiana (5)	1.0–4.0	2.0
Fusarium oxysporum (6)	16–> 16	> 16
Fusarium solani (6)	> 16	> 16
Phialophora spp. (5)	1.0–> 16	9
Pseudallescheria boydii (6)	2.0–4.0	2.5
Rhizopus arrhizus (5)	> 16	> 16
Scedosporium prolificans (2)	4.0	ND
Blastomyces dermatitidis (5)	2.0–8.0	4
Histoplasma capsulatum (5)	2.0–4.0	3.6

MICs were determined by following a procedure under evaluation by the National Committee for Clinical Laboratory Standards (NC-CLS) for broth microdilution testing of the filamentous fungi.

MIC, minimum inhibitory concentration; ND, not obtained.

Source: modified from Espinel-Ingroff, 1998.

Antimicrobial Interactions

In combination with fluconazole, anidulafungin was indifferent against *Candida* spp. and *C. neoformans* in vitro; in combination with nikkomycin, however, anidulafungin showed synergistic activity against *Aspergillus fumigatus* (Stevens, 2000; Roling et al, 2002; Chiou et al, 2001).

Efficacy in Animal Models

Anidulafungin has demonstrated efficacy in several murine models of superficial and disseminated candidiasis, disseminated aspergillosis and *P. carinii* pneumonia in both normal and immunocompromised animals (Current et al, 1993; Zeckner et al, 1993a; Zeckner et al, 1993b; Zeckner et al, 1994; Roberts et al, 2000). The compound was effective against esophageal and oropharyngeal candidiasis caused by fluconazole-resistant strains of *C. albicans* in immuno-compromised rabbits (Petraitis et al, 2001). In persistently neutropenic rabbits, anidulafungin showed dose-dependent clearance of all organs in experimental subacute disseminated candidiasis (Petraitiene et al, 1999) and it prolonged survival in invasive pulmonary aspergillosis (Petraitis et al, 1998). Pharmacodynamic modeling showed highly predictable pharmacokinetic–pharmacodynamic relationships in experimental disseminated candidiasis; however, no concentration-effect relationships were observed against experimental pulmonary aspergillosis using survival and the residual fungal tissue burden as endpoints of antifungal efficacy (Groll et al, 2001b).

Preclinical Pharmacokinetics and Tissue Distribution

The plasma pharmacokinetics of anidulafungin have been studied in rabbits, rats, and dogs (Zornes et al, 1993; Groll et al, 2001b). In normal rabbits, anidulafungin exhibited linear, time-independent plasma pharmacokinetics over a dosage range of 0.1 to 20 mg/kg (Groll et al, 2001b). Plasma concentration data fitted to a three-compartment open pharmacokinetic model with a terminal elimination half-life of up to 30 hours. Tissue concentrations at trough after multiple dosing were highest in lung and liver, followed by spleen and kidney. Measurable concentrations in brain tissue were noted at dosages of ≥ 0.5 mg/kg. No differences were observed in comparison to the plasma pharmacokinetics in other animal species (Zornes et al, 1993). Notably, however, in rabbits with experimental invasive fungal infections, the mean plasma clearance was significantly slower along with a trend towards higher AUC values, higher plasma concentrations at the end of the dosing interval, and a smaller volume of distribution (Groll et al, 2001b).

Clinical Pharmacokinetics and Metabolism

Dosages of 35, 50, 70, and 100 mg, given by the intravenous route to healthy volunteers, revealed linear, time-independent pharmacokinetics of anidulafungin with mean peak plasma levels ranging from 1.71 to 3.82 μg/mL, and mean $AUC_{0-\infty}$ values from 37.46 to 104.81 μg · h/mL. The mean volume of distribution was between 0.72 and 0.90 L/kg, and the terminal half-life was approximately 40 hours (Table 7–3) (Rajman et al, 1997).

In human volunteers with mild to moderate hepatic impairment, a single dose of 50 mg anidulafungin did not cause clinically significant changes in the pharma-

TABLE 7–3. *Plasma Pharmacokinetics of IV Anidulafungin in Healthy Volunteers*

Dose (mg)	C_{max} (μg/mL)	$AUC_{0-\infty}$ (μg · hr/mL)	VD_{ss} (L/kg)	$T_{1/2}$* (hours)
35	1.719	37.46	0.81	42.0
50	2.516	53.32	0.72	39.3
70	2.906	69.35	0.90	45.6
100	3.825	104.81	0.78	42.3

Pharmacokinetic parameters represent mean values of a single-dose cross-over dose-escalation pharmacokinetic study in healthy male and female volunteers. Doses up to 35 mg were administered IV over 20 minutes, and doses of 50 mg and above were administered IV at a constant rate of 1.1 mg/minute. C_{max}, peak plasma concentration: $AUC_{0-\infty}$, area under the concentration-vs.-time curve from zero to infinity: VD_{ss}, estimated volume of distribution at steady state; $T_{1/2}$, half life

*gamma half–life

Source: modified from Rajman et al, 1997.

cokinetics in comparison to healthy subjects (Thye et al, 2001a).

Clinical Efficacy

The antifungal efficacy of anidulafungin has been investigated in a phase II, randomized, open label study comparing two dosage regimens in the treatment of esophageal candidiasis (Brown et al, 2000b). A total of 36 predominantly HIV-infected patients received a 50 mg loading dose on day 1, followed by 25 mg daily, or a 70 mg loading dose, followed by 35 mg daily for a total of 14 to 21 days. The endoscopic response in the 29 evaluable patients was 81% and 85%, respectively, and the clinical response 69% and 82%. No serious drug-related side effects were noted in both cohorts. A phase II open label, dose-ranging trial of anidulafungin for patients with candidemia has been completed recently but results are not yet available.

Safety and Tolerance

Two dose-optimization studies have been conducted. Healthy volunteers received a loading dose on day 1, followed by a daily maintenance dose on days 2 to 10. Investigated dosages included 100 mg loading dose/ 70 mg daily dose, 140 mg/100 mg (8 subjects each), and 150 mg/75 mg, 200 mg/100 mg, and 260 mg/130 mg (10 subjects each), respectively. In these studies, anidulafungin was well-tolerated without dose limiting toxicities. Two subjects in the 140/100 mg regimen had grade II toxicity (epigastric pain, nausea, and headache), and three subjects in the 260/130 mg regimen experienced transient elevations of hepatic transaminases that exceeded twice the upper limit of normal. In both studies, anidulafungin exhibited linear, time-independent pharmacokinetics (Brown et al, 2000a; Thye et al, 2001b).

Drug Interactions

In vitro, in concentrations of up to 30ug/mL, anidulafungin had no effect on the CYP3A4 mediated metabolism of cyclosporin A (White and Thye, 2001).

Status of Clinical Development

Anidulafungin is not yet licensed for prevention or treatment of fungal infections in humans. Currently, the drug is being studied in a phase III, randomized, comparative trial for treatment of Candida esophagitis and a phase III comparative trial for treatment of invasive candidiasis and/or candidemia.

CASPOFUNGIN

Antifungal Activity In Vitro

Similar to anidulafungin and micafungin, caspofungin has potent and broad-spectrum activity against clini-

TABLE 7–4. *In Vitro Susceptibilities of Clinical Yeast Isolates to Caspofungin*

Organism (No. of Isolates)	MIC Range (µg/mL)	MIC 90 (µg/mL)
C. albicans (10)*	0.25–2.0	1.0
C. albicans (10)**	0.25–2.0	1.0
C. glabrata (12)	0.5–2.0	1.0
C. guilliermondii (8)	> 16	ND
C. krusei (13)	0.5–4.0	2.0
C. lusitaniae (12)	1.0–4.0	2.0
C. parapsilosis (12)	0.5–2.0	2.0
C. tropicalis (12)	0.5–2.0	1.0
Cr. neoformans (10)	16–> 16	> 16
T.beigelii (5)	16–> 16	ND

Antifungal susceptibility assays were determined according to the NCCLS M27-A broth microdilution method for yeasts.
*fluconazole MIC > 16 µg/mL
**fluconazole MIC ≤ 1 µg/mL
MIC, minimum inhibitory concentration; ND, not obtained.
Source: modified from Espinel-Ingroff, 1998.

cally relevant *Candida* spp. with somewhat higher MICs for *C. parapsilosis* and *C. guilliermondii*. As expected, caspofungin shows no cross-resistance to amphotericin B and fluconazole resistant *Candida* clinical isolates (Table 7–4) (Bartizal et al, 1997; Espinel-Ingroff, 1998; Marco et al, 1998). Caspofungin showed prolonged concentration-dependent postantifungal effects against *C. albicans* for up to 12 hours and longer, and exhibited strain and species dependent, predominantly concentration-dependent fungicidal activity against *Candida* spp. in time-kill experiments (Bartizal et al, 1997; Ernst et al, 1999; Ernst et al, 2000). Caspofungin is active against *Saccharomyces cerevisiae*, but has virtually no in vitro activity (MICs $\geq$ 16 µg/mL) against *T. asahii* and *C. neoformans* (Espinel-Ingroff, 1998; Groll and Walsh, 2001). Results from studies demonstrate a low potential for induction of resistance. Repeat exposure of *C. albicans* to subinhibitory concentrations of caspofungin did not significantly alter MICs and minimum fungicidal concentrations (MFCs) after 40 passages (Bartizal et al, 1997).

Caspofungin also has broad-spectrum in vitro activity against *Aspergillus* spp. as determined by reduction in turbidity (MIC) and the occurrence of morphological changes (minimum effective concentration, MEC) (Kurtz et al, 1994; Espinel-Ingroff, 1998; Pfaller et al, 1998) (Table 7–5). The frequency of resistance among clinical isolates of *Aspergillus* species is unknown and induction of resistance in *Aspergillus* species has not been studied yet. Caspofungin has essentially no intrinsic in vitro activity against *Fusarium* spp., the Zygomycetes and dermatophytes. The in vitro susceptibility of dematiaceous fungi appears variable (Groll and Walsh, 2001e).

Caspofungin is active in vitro against dimorphic fungi, including *H. capsulatum*, *B. dermatitidis*, *Coccidioides immitis*, and *S. schenckii*, although variable

TABLE 7–5. *In Vitro Susceptibilities of Clinical Mould Isolates to Caspofungin*

Organism (No. of Isolates)	MIC range (μg/mL)	Geometric Mean MIC (μg/mL)
Aspergillus fumigatus (13)	0.5–> 16	2.15
Aspergillus flavus (11)	0.5	0.5
Aspergillus terreus (2)	0.5	ND
Bipolaris spp. (6)	1.0–2.0	1.7
Cladophialophora bantiana (5)	2.0–8.0	3.6
Fusarium oxysporum (6)	> 16	> 16
Fusarium solani (6)	16–> 16	> 16
Phialophora spp. (5)	1.0–16	2.8
Pseudallescheria boydii (6)	0.5–4.0	1.3
Rhizopus arrhizus (5)	> 16	> 16
Scedosporium prolificans (2)	4.0–8.0	ND
Blastomyces dermatitidis (5)	0.5–8.0	2
Histoplasma capsulatum (5)	0.5–4.0	1.3

MICs were determined by following a procedure under evaluation by the National Committee for Clinical Laboratory Standards (NC-CLS) for broth microdilution testing of the filamentous fuingi.

MIC, minimum inhibitory concentration; ND, not obtained.

Source: modified from Espinel-Ingroff, 1998.

and at considerably higher concentrations than reported for *Candida* and *Aspergillus* spp. (Espinel-Ingroff, 1998; Pfaller et al, 1998; Groll and Walsh, 2001e) (Table 7–5).

Antimicrobial Interactions

In vitro studies using checkerboard methodologies have consistently shown no antagonism in vitro between caspofungin and other antifungal agents (Groll and Walsh, 2001e). The combination with amphotericin B was additive to synergistic against *A. fumigatus* and *C. neoformans* but indifferent against *C. albicans* (Bartizal et al, 1997). Against *C. neoformans*, subinhibitory concentrations of caspofungin were synergistic with amphotericin B, and showed synergy, additivity, or autonomy in combination with fluconazole (Franzot and Casadevall, 1997). Other investigators found synergistic interactions in vitro with caspofungin in combination with amphotericin B or itraconazole against *Aspergillus* spp. (Manavathu et al, 2000; Arikan et al, 2000) and *Fusarium* isolates (Arikan et al, 2000). In coculture with monocytes and macrophages, caspofungin had significantly increased antifungal activity against germlings of *A. fumigatus* as compared to either modality alone (Chiller et al, 2001). These data suggest potentially increased efficacy of caspofungin in vivo as it combines with host defenses against *A. fumigatus*.

Efficacy in Animal Models

In both immunocompetent and immunocompromised murine models of disseminated candidiasis, caspofungin prolonged survival and led to a significant reduction in the residual burden of *Candida* spp. in kidney tissue (Abruzzo et al, 1997; Abruzzo et al, 2000; Groll and Walsh, 2001e). Consistent with the in vitro data, caspofungin alone was ineffective in improving survival and reducing residual fungal burden in brain and spleen in a mouse model of disseminated cryptococcosis (Abruzzo et al, 1997).

Caspofungin significantly prolonged survival in immunocompetent and transiently neutropenic mouse models of disseminated aspergillosis in a manner comparable to amphotericin B (Abruzzo et al, 1997; Abruzzo et al, 2000; Groll and Walsh, 2001e). Caspofungin also had similar preventive and therapeutic activity as amphotericin B in conferring survival in a corticosteroid-immunosuppressed rat model of pulmonary aspergillosis (Bernard et al, 1993). In persistently neutropenic rabbits with invasive pulmonary aspergillosis, caspofungin prolonged survival and reduced pulmonary tissue damage (Petraitiene et al, 2002).

Caspofungin demonstrated efficacy in murine models of disseminated and pulmonary histoplasmosis (Graybill et al, 1998b; Kohler et al, 2000), and disseminated coccidioidomycosis (Gonzalez et al, 2001), and was effective as a preventive and therapeutic modality against *P. carinii* pneumonia, and selectively eliminated the cyst forms of the organism from lung tissue. When caspofungin was used as prophylaxis, neither stage of *P. carinii* was found (Powles et al, 1998).

Preclinical Pharmacokinetics and Tissue Distribution

Studies performed in mice, rats, rhesus monkeys, and chimpanzees after single intravenous dosages of 0.5 to 5.0 mg/kg exhibited constant pharmacokinetic parameters across all investigated species. Clearance ranged from 0.26 to 0.51 mL/minute/kg; half-life ranged from 5.2 to 7.6 hours, and the volume of distribution was 0.11 to 0.27 L/kg (Hajdu et al, 1997). In normal rabbits, following intravenous administration of doses of 1 to 6 mg/kg, caspofungin displayed dose-independent plasma pharmacokinetics that fitted to a three-compartment open pharmacokinetic model. Following multiple daily dosing over 7 days, the apparent volume of distribution at steady state ranged from 0.299 to 0.351 L/kg; clearance ranged from 0.086 to 0.043 L/kg/hour, and the mean terminal half-life was between 30 and 34 hours. Caspofungin achieved sustained concentrations in plasma that were multiple times in excess of reported MIC values for susceptible opportunistic fungi without significant accumulation in plasma after multiple daily dosing (Groll et al, 2001a). Tissue distribution studies in mice after a single dose of 1 mg/kg of radiolabeled caspofungin intraperitoneally revealed preferential exposure of liver, kidney, and large intestine, whereas exposure for small intestine, lung and spleen was equivalent to that for plasma.

Organs with lower level of exposure included the heart, thigh, and brain (Hajdu et al, 1997).

Clinical Pharmacokinetics and Metabolism

Caspofungin is extensively bound to serum albumin (97%), and distribution into red blood cells is minimal. The compound is slowly metabolized by peptide hydrolysis and N-acetylation; only a small fraction (~1.4% of dose) is excreted unchanged in urine, and renal clearance is low (0.15 mL/minute) (Balani et al, 2000; Stone et al, 2002).

After infusion of single dosages ranging from 5 to 100 mg, caspofungin exhibited dose-proportional pharmacokinetics with a beta half-life of 9–10 hours and an average plasma clearance of 10 to 12 mL/minute (Table 7–6). At higher dosages, an additional, longer gamma half-life of 40–50 hours was evident. Multiple dose studies at dosages of 15, 35, and 70 mg daily for 2 weeks (all regimens) and 3 weeks (70 mg/day regimen only) revealed dose-dependent accumulation of drug in plasma of up to 50%. The 70 mg/day-dosing regimen achieved mean peak plasma levels of approximately 10 μg/mL and maintained mean trough plasma levels above 1 μg/mL from day 1 onward, which is above the reported MIC values for most susceptible fungi. Similarly, a loading dose of 70 mg, followed by 50 mg/day, maintained plasma concentrations above this target, while concentrations fell below 1 μg/mL if the loading dose was not given (Stone et al, 2002).

Dosage adjustment is not necessary for patients with impaired renal function and end-stage renal insufficiency. Following single 70 mg doses, exposure to caspofungin in dialysis-dependent patients with a creatinine clearance < 10 mL/minute was only moderately increased (130% to 149%) as measured by the $AUC_{0-\infty}$. While patients with mild hepatic insufficiency (Child-Pugh score 5 to 6) do not require a dosage adjustment, a dosage of 35 mg daily after the initial 70 mg loading dose is recommended for patients with moderate hepatic insufficiency (Child-Pugh score 7 to 9) due to

an average increase of 76% in AUC. There is no clinical experience in patients with severe hepatic insufficiency (Child-Pugh score > 9). Studies in human volunteers revealed no necessity of dosage adjustment based on gender, advanced age, or race. Thus far, pharmacokinetics, safety, and efficacy of caspofungin in pediatric patients (< 18 years of age) are not available. Caspofungin has been shown to cross the placental barrier and to be embryotoxic in rats and rabbits (Package circular: Cancidas®, 2001) (Groll and Walsh, 2001e). Adequate data in pregnant women do not exist.

Clinical Efficacy

Two separate, randomized, double-blind, multicenter trials have been published that compared caspofungin at dosages of 35, 50, and 70 mg/day given for 7 to 14 days with conventional amphotericin B (0.5 mg/kg for the same duration) in the treatment of esophageal or oropharyngeal candidiasis in a total of 268, mostly HIV-infected individuals (Villanueva et al, 2001b; Arathoon et al, 2002). Efficacy was assessed by clinical symptoms and residual endoscopic lesions at the completion of treatment and 14 days post therapy. A favorable response was noted in 74% to 91% of patients in the caspofungin groups compared to 63% in the amphotericin B group. Caspofungin was well-tolerated without serious adverse events. In another multicenter, randomized, double-blind study comparing caspofungin (50 mg daily) and fluconazole (200 mg daily) for treatment of esophageal candidiasis in 175 mostly HIV-infected patients, response rates were similar for both cohorts, 82% vs. 85%. Both interventions were similarly well-tolerated (Villanueva et al, 2001a).

The efficacy of caspofungin as primary treatment of invasive *Candida* infections has been investigated in a multicenter, randomized, double-blind phase III clinical trial in neutropenic and nonneutropenic patients (Mora-Duarte et al, 2002). Patients were randomized to intravenous caspofungin (70 mg loading dose on the first day, followed by 50 mg once daily) or intravenous amphotericin B deoxycholate (0.6 to 1.0 mg/kg/day). Patients were treated for 14 days after the last positive culture, but could be switched to fluconazole after 10 days of intravenous therapy. Success required both symptom resolution and microbiological clearance. At study entry, 13% of patients were neutropenic; the majority had candidemia (83%). The predominant organism was *C. albicans* (45%), followed by *C. parapsilosis* (19%), *C. tropicalis* (16%), and *C. glabrata* (11%). Among patients receiving ≥ one dose of study drug, 73% (80/109) of the caspofungin cohort and 61.7% (71/115) of the amphotericin B cohort were classified as therapeutic success at the end of intravenous therapy; among patients who received ≥ 5 doses of study drug, the response rates were 80.7% (71/88) and 64.9% (63/97), respectively. At 6 to 8

TABLE 7–6. *Plasma Pharmacokinetics of Caspofungin in Healthy Volunteers*

Dose (mg)	C_{max} (μg/mL)	$AUC_{0-\infty}$ (μg · hour/mL)	C_{24hour} (μg/mL)	$T_{1/2}$* (hours)
20	3.06	30.97	0.36	10.72
40	6.17	55.60	0.57	9.64
70	12.04	118.45	1.42	9.29
100	14.03	134.11	1.47	8.61

Pharmacokinetic parameters represent mean values of a single-dose dose-escalation pharmacokinetic study in healthy male volunteers. Caspofungin was administered IV over 1 hour.

C_{max}, peak plasma concentration; $AUC_{0-\infty}$, area under the concentration-vs.-time curve from zero to infinity; C_{24hour}, plasma concentration 24 hours after the start of the infusion: $T_{1/2}$, half life; *beta half–life

Source: modified from Stone et al, 2002.

weeks follow-up, there was no difference in relapse or survival. Significantly fewer patients in the caspofungin cohort had drug-related clinical or laboratory adverse events. This trial provides evidence of an important advance in the treatment of invasive candidiasis (Walsh, 2002).

The clinical efficacy of caspofungin against *invasive aspergillosis* has been studied in a multicenter, open-label, noncomparative phase II trial in patients with definite or probable invasive aspergillosis refractory to or intolerant of standard therapies (Maertens et al, 2000). Caspofungin was administered at a dose of 70 mg on day 1, followed by 50 mg once daily. Clinical efficacy was assessed at end of therapy and 4 weeks after discontinuation of study drug. A total of 63 patients (neutropenic, 22%; treated with steroids, 37%) received caspofungin for a mean duration of 33.7 days (range, 1 to 162 days). The majority (66%) had hematological malignancies or had undergone bone marrow transplantation, and most had refractory *Aspergillus* infections (84%). A complete resolution or clinically meaningful improvement of all signs and symptoms and attributable radiographic findings was achieved in 41% (26/63) of patients receiving at least one dose of caspofungin; in patients receiving the drug for > 7 days, a favorable response was seen in 50% (26/52).

Safety and Tolerance

Caspofungin appears generally well tolerated. In the five clinical trials discussed in detail earlier, less than 5% of patients discontinued caspofungin prematurely due to drug-related clinical adverse experiences. Of note, there was no apparent dose-dependency of adverse events over the investigated dosage range of 35 to 70 mg/day (Sable et al, 2001).

The most commonly reported possibly, probably, or definitely drug-related clinical adverse experiences occurring in ≥ 5% of 228 patients in 3 active control studies included fever (3.6% to 26%), phlebitis (1.5% to 15.7%), nausea (2.5% to 6%), and headache (6.0% to 11.3%) (Package circular: Cancidas®, 2001). Symptoms such as rash, facial swelling, pruritus, or sensation of warmth (which could potentially have been mediated through endogenous histamine release), have been reported in isolated cases; a reversible anaphylactic reaction occurred in 1 patient during initial administration of caspofungin (Sable et al, 2001).

Laboratory abnormalities occurred in ≥ 5% of patients and included increased liver transaminases (10.6 to 13%), decreased serum albumin (4.6%–8.6%), increased serum alkaline phosphatase (7.7%–10.5%), decreased serum potassium (3.7%–10.8%), decreased hemoglobin (3.1%–12.3%), decreased white blood cell count (4.6%–6.2%) and increased urine white blood cell count (0%–7.7%) (Package circular:Cancidas®, 2001).

Drug Interactions

Caspofungin is not a substrate of P-glycoprotein and is a poor substrate of cytochrome P-450 enzymes and a weak cytochrome P-450 enzyme inhibitor (Balani et al, 2000). In healthy volunteers, no pharmacokinetic interactions were observed between caspofungin and itraconazole, amphotericin B deoxycholate, and mycophenolate mofetil. While tacrolimus has no effect on the plasma pharmacokinetics of caspofungin, chronic dosing of caspofungin reduced the AUC of tacrolimus by approximately 20%. In turn, cyclosporine increased the AUC of caspofungin by approximately 35%; however, caspofungin did not increase the plasma levels of cyclosporine. Because of transient elevations of hepatic transaminases not exceeding 2 to 3 times the upper limit of normal in single-dose interaction studies, the concomitant use of caspofungin with cyclosporine is presently not recommended (Package circular: Cancidas®, 2001; Groll and Walsh, 2001e).

Coadministration of inducers of drug clearance and/or mixed inducer/inhibitors, namely efavirenz, nelfinavir, nevirapine, phenytoin, rifampin, dexamethasone, and carbamazepine with caspofungin may result in clinically meaningful reductions in caspofungin concentrations. Accordingly, the manufacturer recommends an increase in the dosage of caspofungin to 70 mg daily in patients who are concurrently receiving any of the drugs listed above and not clinically responding (Package circular: Cancidas®, 2001; Groll and Walsh, 2001e). The safety and efficacy of doses above 70 mg daily have not been adequately studied.

Status of Clinical Development

Caspofungin currently is approved for the treatment of invasive aspergillosis in patients who are refractory to or intolerant of other therapies. Based on the recently completed trial of caspofungin for invasive candidiasis with encouraging outcome data, an indication for first-line treatment of invasive candidiasis and esophageal candidiasis is expected. A phase III study for empirical antifungal therapy in persistently febrile neutropenic patients has recently been completed, and a phase I/II clinical pharmacology study in pediatric patients is ongoing.

MICAFUNGIN

Antifungal Activity In Vitro

Micafungin has potent and broad spectrum in vitro activity against *Candida* spp. with somewhat higher MIC_{90} values for *C. parapsilosis* and *C. guilliermondii* and no cross-resistance to fluconazole-resistant clinical isolates (Table 7–7). Micafungin produces a strain- and species-dependent postantifungal effect against *Can*-

TABLE 7-7. *In Vitro Susceptibilities of Clinical Yeast Isolates to Micafungin*

Organism (No. of Isolates)	MIC Range (µg/mL)	MIC 90 (µg/mL)
Candida albicans (37)	< 0.003–0.015	0.0156
Candida albicans, FLCZ resistant (4)	0.015–0.031	0.0313
Candida tropicalis (20)	0.015–0.031	0.0313
Candida glabrata (20)	0.007–0.015	0.0156
Candida krusei (11)	0.125–0.250	0.125
Candida parapsilosis (17)	0.5–2.0	1
Candida guilliermondii (12)	0.25–2.0	2
Cryptococcus neoformans (5)	> 64	> 64
Trichosporon cutaneum (5)	> 64	> 64

Antifungal susceptibility assays were performed according to current NCCLS guidelines.
Source: modified from Tawara et al, 2000

dida spp. of up to 19 hours duration (Ernst et al, 2001). Negligible changes in MIC values after repeated exposure of *C. albicans* to subinhibitory concentrations of micafungin suggest a low potential for resistance induction. Similar to anidulafungin and caspofungin, micafungin has virtually no in vitro activity against *C. neoformans* and is inactive against *T. cutaneum* (Maki et al, 1998; Tomishima et al, 1999; Mikamo et al, 2000; Tawara et al, 2000; Muller et al, 2001; Ostrosky-Zeichner et al, 2000).

Micafungin also has potent in vitro activity against *Aspergillus* spp. but was inactive (i.e., MIC values of ≥ 64 µg/mL) against *Fusarium* spp., *Scedosporum apiospermum* (*Pseudallescheria boydii*), and Zygomycetes (Table 7-8). Moderate activity was found against dematiaceous fungi such as *Cladosporium trichoides*, *Exophiala* spp., and *Fonsecaea pedrosi* (MIC values of 0.5 to 2.0 µg/mL). In vitro activity against *H. capsulatum*, *B. dermatitidis*, and *C. immitis* was limited to the mycelial forms of these organisms (Maki et al, 1998; Nakai et al, 2002; Tomishima et al, 1999; Tawara et al, 2000).

Antimicrobial Interactions

Combination of micafungin with amphotericin B was neither synergistic nor antagonistic in vitro and in vivo against various clinical *Aspergillus* isolates (Petraitis et al, 1999; Stevens, 1999). Analysis of the in vitro activity of the combination of micafungin and nikkomycin Z against opportunistic moulds revealed synergy against *A. fumigatus*, additive effects against *Rhizopus oryzae*, and indifference against *A. flavus*, *A. terreus*, *A. niger*, and *F. solani* (Chiou et al, 2001).

Efficacy in Animal Models

The antifungal efficacy of micafungin against disseminated candidiasis has been documented in immunocompetent, transiently neutropenic, and corticosteroid-immunosuppressed murine screening models. Treatment with micafungin resulted in a dose-dependent, statisti-

cally significant prolongation of survival and a dose-dependent reduction in the residual fungal kidney burden comparable to amphotericin B (Matsumoto et al, 1998; Ikeda et al, 2000; Maesaki et al, 2000). In persistently neutropenic rabbits with subacute nonlethal disseminated candidiasis, micafungin (0.25 to 1 mg/kg/d) demonstrated dosage dependent clearance of *C. albicans* from tissues. Time-kill curves revealed time- and concentration-dependent fungicidal activity of micafungin that correlated with the in vivo results (Petraitis et al, 2002).

Micafungin also prolonged the survival of transiently neutropenic mice intravenously infected with *A. fumigatus* in a dose-dependent manner (Ikeda et al, 2000). In mouse models of pulmonary aspergillosis (Wakai et al, 1998; Matsumoto et al, 2000), micafungin significantly prolonged the survival of transiently neutropenic animals, and in corticosteroid-immunosuppressed animals, a dose-dependent reduction in the residual burden of *A. fumigatus* in lung tissue was demonstrated when the drug was administered as continuous infusion. In a rigorous persistently neutropenic rabbit model of invasive pulmonary aspergillosis, micafungin prolonged the survival and led to a significant decrease of organism-mediated pulmonary injury (Petraitis et al, 2002). In less stringent immunocompromised murine models of pulmonary aspergillosis, enhanced activity of the combination of micafungin and amphotericin B was noted using survival, residual fungal burden (Kohno et al, 2000) and histopathological evaluation of pulmonary infection (Nakajima et al, 2000) as endpoints of efficacy.

Micafungin was also highly effective for prevention of *P. carinii* pneumonia in SCID mice leading to a complete absence of cyst forms of *P. carinii* and only minor injury to alveolar cells at the termination of the experiments (Ito et al, 2000).

TABLE 7-8. *In Vitro Susceptibilities of Clinical Mould Isolates to Micafungin*

Organism (No. of Isolates)	MIC range (µg/mL)	MIC 90 (µg/mL)
Aspergillus fumigatus (29)	0.007–0.031	0.0156
Aspergillus niger (15)	0.003–0.015	0.0078
Aspergillus flavus (13)	0.007–0.015	0.0156
Aspergillus terreus (7)	0.003–0.007	0.0078
Cladosporium trichoides (5)	0.125–0.5	ND
Exophiala dermatitidis (6)	1–> 64	ND
Exophiala spinifera (6)	0.125–2.0	ND
Fonseca pedrosei (6)	0.5–8.0	ND
Absidia corymbifera (1)	> 64	ND
Cunninghamella elegans (1)	> 64	ND
Rhizopus oryzae (1)	> 64	ND
Fusarium solani (1)	> 64	ND
Pseudallescheria boydii (1)	> 64	ND

Antifungal susceptibility assays were performed according to current NCCLS guidelines.
MIC, minimum inhibitory concentration.
Source: modified from Tawara et al, 2000 and Nakai et al, 2002.

Pharmacokinetics

Preclinical Pharmacokinetics and Tissue Distribution. In mice, rats, and dogs, follwing intravenous bolus administration of dosages of 0.32, 1, and 3.2 mg/kg (Suzuki et al, 1998), and in rabbits following administration of 0.5, 1, and 2 mg/kg (Groll et al, 2001c), micafungin displayed linear pharmacokinetics without fundamental interspecies differences. Plasma concentrations declined in a biexponential fashion with a half-life in the range of 3 to 6 hours. Total clearance ranged from 0.59 to 1.50 mL/minute/kg, and the volume of distribution was 0.23 to 0.56 L/kg. In the rabbit, at the end of the initial distributive phase following the last of eight daily dosages of 0.5, 1, or 2 mg/kg, tissue concentrations ranged from 1.5 to 11 μg/g and were highest in the lung, liver, spleen, and kidney. Micafungin was undetectable in cerebrospinal fluid, but brain tissue concentrations exceeded the MIC90 and MEC90 values for most susceptible fungi (Groll et al, 2001c). After bolus administration of ^{14}C-micafungin into rats and dogs, approximately 15% of radioactivity was excreted in the urine with the remainder being excreted in the feces (Suzuki et al, 1998).

Clinical Pharmacokinetics and Metabolism. In healthy volunteers receiving micafungin as a 2-hour intravenous infusion at dosages of 2.5, 5, 12.5, 25, or 50 mg, plasma concentrations after completion of the infusion declined in a biexponential pattern. The half-life ranged from 11.6 to 15.2 hours, total clearance ranged from 0.192 to 0.225 mL/minute/kg, and the volume of distribution ranged from 0.215 to 0.242, respectively. A dose-proportional increase in $AUC_{0-\infty}$ hour indicated linear plasma pharmacokinetics. Following multiple dosing at 25 mg once daily for a total of 7 days, steady state was achieved by day 4 after approximately 1.5 fold accumulation. The mean peak plasma level at day 7 was 2.46 ± 0.27 μg/mL, $AUC_{0-\infty}$ 29.6 ± 4.6 μg · hour/mL, half-life 14.6 ± 1.5 hours, and total clearance 0.222 ± 0.027 mL/minute/kg, respectively (Table 7–9). Less than 1% of drug was found in the urine in unchanged form (Azuma et al, 1998). At least six metabolites have been detected in both animals and humans to date; similar to caspofungin and anidulafungin, micafungin is not metabolized to a significant extent through the cytochrome P450 enzyme system (Groll and Walsh, 2000).

No differences in drug disposition were noted in older patients, aged 66–78 years (Mukai et al, 2001). In febrile neutropenic pediatric patients who received the compound for a mean of 8 days (range, 1–14 days) at dosages ranging from 0.5 to 3 mg/kg, micafungin displayed linear disposition with a mean half-life of 12 to 13 hours on day 1 and day 4 for 0.5 mg/kg dose and on day 1 for 1.0 mg/kg dose. The half-life at day

TABLE 7–9. *Plasma Pharmacokinetics of Micafungin in Healthy Volunteers*

Dose (mg)	C_{max} (μg/mL)	$AUC_{0-\infty}$ (μg · hour/mL)	VD_{SS} (L/K)	$T_{1/2}$* (hours)
12.5	0.94	17.11	0.24	15.2
25	1.86	32.26	0.23	14.8
50	3.36	60.93	0.23	15.2

Pharmacokinetic parameters represent mean values of a single-dose pharmacokinetic study in healthy male volunteers. Micafungin was administered IV over 2 hours.

C_{max}, peak plasma concentration: $AUC_{0-\infty}$, area under the concentration-vs.-time curve from zero to infinity: VD_{SS}, estimated volume of distribution at steady state; $T_{1/2}$, half life.

*beta-half life.

Source: Modified from Azuma et al, 1998.

4 for 1 mg/kg dose was variable resulting in a mean of 20.8 hours (Seibel et al, 2000).

Clinical Efficacy

In an open label, multicenter, dose de-escalation study in 74 HIV-infected patients with endoscopically documented *Candida* esophagitis, micafungin was administered at dosages of 50, 25, and 12.5 per day as 1-hour infusion for a mean of 12 days (range, 1–21 days). In patients who received the drug for at least 8 days, resolution or improvement of clinical signs and symptoms was observed at end of therapy in 21/21 (100%) receiving 50 mg, 18/20 (90%) receiving 25 mg, and 17/21 (81%) receiving 12.5 mg (Pettengell et al, 1999). Further dose escalation to a daily dosage of 75 and 100 mg and endpoint evaluation by endoscopy demonstrated consistent results with clearance or improvement of endoscopic lesions in 35/36 (97.2%) of patients receiving at least 10 days of therapy (Pettengell et al, 2000).

In an open-label, multicenter trial conducted in Japan, 70 patients, with proven or presumed infections caused by *Aspergillus* or *Candida* spp., received micafungin at dosages ranging from 12.5 to 150 mg once daily for 7 to 56 days (Kohno et al, 2001). Among patients evaluable for efficacy, 6/10 patients with invasive pulmonary aspergillosis, 6/9 with chronic necrotizing pulmonary aspergillosis, 12/22 with aspergilloma, 6/6 with candidemia, and 5/7 with esophageal candidiasis responded to therapy with micafungin.

Among 14 cancer patients, of whom 6 were neutropenic at the start of treatment, 8 had a complete and 3 had a partial response to micafungin therapy. In this study, micafungin was given as monotherapy ($n = 7$) or in combination with other antifungal agents at dosages ranging from 50 to 150 mg/day for a median duration of 15 days (range, 4–26 days) (Kontoyiannis et al, 2001). In all four studies, micafungin appeared well-tolerated without dose-limiting adverse events.

The largest phase III clinical trial to date involving micafungin has been completed and preliminary results are very promising. A double-blind study compared micafungin and fluconazole as prophylaxis against fungal infections in 889 patients undergoing a hematopoietic stem cell transplant (van Burik et al, 2002). Success was defined as (1) absence of a proven or probable fungal infection during the period of prophylaxis and during the 4 weeks after stopping study drug; and (2) no discontinuation of study drug due to toxicity. Among 425 micafungin-treated patients, success was noted in 80%, compared with success in 73.5% of 457 fluconazole-treated patients, 95% C.I. (0.9%–12.0%) around the difference between the success rates, suggesting superiority of micafungin. There were 7 breakthrough fungal infections in the micafungin group (aspergillosis, 1; candidiasis, 4; and other, 2) and 11 breakthrough fungal infections in the fluconazole group (aspergillosis, 7; candidiasis, 2; and other, 2). Survival was the same in both groups and both micafungin and fluconazole were very well tolerated.

Safety and Tolerance

In healthy volunteers receiving single dosages of 2.5, 5, 12.5, 25, or 50 mg, and multiple dosages of 25 mg once daily for a total of 7 days, micafungin was well tolerated (Azuma et al, 1998). In febrile neutropenic pediatric patients who received the drug for a mean of 8 days (range, 1 to 14 days) at dosages ranging from 0.5 to 3 mg/kg, no evidence for differences in safety were noted in these children compared to adults (Seibel et al, 2000).

In 74 HIV-infected patients with endoscopically documented *Candida* esophagitis receiving 50, 25, and 12.5 mg per day for a mean of 12 days, 3 patients discontinued micafungin due to possible adverse events, and 1 discontinued due to lack of efficacy (12.5 mg). There was one serious adverse event (diarrhea and dehydration) that was assessed as possibly related to micafungin. Infusion-related toxicity or reactions attributable to histamine release were not reported, and nephro- or hepatotoxicity was not observed (Pettengell et al, 1999). Further dose escalation to a daily dosage of 75 and 100 mg in 36 patients revealed no additional safety issues (Pettengell et al, 2000).

A phase I, randomized, blinded, sequential group, dose-escalation tolerance study investigated micafungin plus fluconazole 400 mg/day vs. normal saline plus fluconazole 400 mg/day given as prophylaxis in 74 adult hematopoietic stem cell transplant patients. The drug regimens were administered from the time of transplant until neutrophil recovery (Hiemenz et al, 1999). Seven dosage-levels of micafungin were studied: 12.5, 25, 50, 75, 100, 150, and 200 mg/day. At least 10 patients were enrolled per dosage group, with 8 patients/group

randomized to the micafungin-fluconazole regimen, and 2 patients/group to the control regimen. The average length of dosing was 10 days (range, 1–27 days). Micafungin was well-tolerated; two patients (3.2%) discontinued due to a possibly or probably related adverse event. No histamine-like reactions or infusion-related toxicity was noted. Overall, there were no changes from baseline to end of therapy in serum creatinine or liver function tests.

The maximum tolerated dosage of micafungin was further investigated in a formal dosage escalation study in another group of hematopoietic stem cell transplant patients, who were given micafungin as antifungal prophylaxis (Powles et al, 2001). Sequential cohorts of 10 patients received micafungin at 3 and 4 mg/kg once daily for a median of 16.5 (range, 13–28 days) and 18.5 days (range, 8–28 days), respectively. In the first cohort, grade I and II toxicities consisted of 1 patient with vomiting, cellulitis, diarrhea, fever, and somnolence; 1 patient with generalized edema, fever, and albuminuria, and 1 patient with hypocalcemia. In the 4 mg/kg cohort, two patients had phlebitis and one dyspepsia. There were no treatment-related grade III and IV toxicities. After completed study of the 2 cohorts, the maximum-tolerated dosage was not reached.

Drug Interactions

No formal interaction studies have been reported thus far.

Status of Clinical Development

Micafungin is not yet licensed for prevention or treatment of fungal infections in humans, but licensing is expected on the basis of the results of the large phase III, randomized, comparative prophylaxis trial in patients receiving hematopoietic stem cell transplants (van Burik et al, 2002). Other studies with micafungin ongoing or planned include treatment trials for invasive candidiasis and invasive aspergillosis.

CHITIN-SYNTHESIS INHIBITORS: NIKKOMYCINS

The nikkomycins, which are antifungal antibiotics produced by *Streptomyces tender*, were discovered in the 1970s through programs searching for new fungicides and insecticides for agricultural use (Hector, 1993). These compounds are pyrimidine nucleosides that are linked to a di- or tripeptide moiety (Fig. 7–3), and are structurally similar to UDP-N-acetylglucosamine, the precursor substrate for chitin, a linear polymer of b-(1–4)-linked N-acetylglucosamine residues.

The nikkomycins act as competitive inhibitors of chitin synthesis, leading to inhibition of septation, chaining, and osmotic swelling of the fungal cell (Hec-

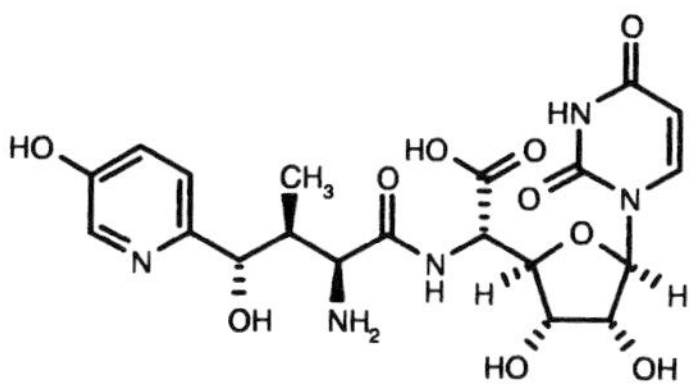

FIGURE 7–3. Structural formula of nikkomycin Z.

tor, 1993; Debono and Gordee, 1994). In *Candida albicans*, three different membrane-bound isoenzymes of chitin-synthase have been described. Although the absence of all three isoenzymes is uniformely lethal, no single one is essential, and each enzyme may be inhibited to different degrees by different compounds. Of note, the nikkomycins are required to be transported into the cell via one or more permeases. This transport system, however, is subject to antagonism by extracellular peptides. In addition, various proteases can inactivate the nucleoside-peptide compounds, resulting in a wide range of susceptibility of intact fungi to nikkomycins, even though their isolated enzyme preparations are uniformly susceptible (Hector, 1993; Debono and Gordee, 1994; Groll et al, 1998).

To date, only nikkomycin Z has been investigated to a significant extent. Nevertheless, natural peptidyl nucleoside leads continue to be investigated for development of new antifungal agents.

Nikkomycin Z

Nikkomycin Z has been shown to have particularly good activity both in vitro and in vivo against the chitinous dimorphic fungi, *C. immitis* and *B. dermatitidis* (Hector et al, 1990b; Clemons and Stevens, 1997). In vitro activity against *H. capsulatum*, *C. albicans*, and *C. neoformans* is only moderate; and nonalbicans *Candida* spp. and filamentous fungi are essentially resistant (Hector and Yee, 1990a). However, nikkomycin Z has inhibitory activity in murine models of both systemic candidiasis and histoplasmosis (Hector and Schaller, 1992; Graybill et al, 1998a; Goldberg et al, 2000).

Notably, synergy between nikkomycin Z and antifungal triazoles against *C. albicans*, *C. neoformans*, and *A. fumigatus* has been observed in vitro (Milewski et al, 1991; Hector and Schaller, 1992; Li and Rinaldi, 1999). Synergy with fluconazole was also demonstrated in a mouse model of systemic candidiasis (Hector and Schaller, 1992). Whereas synergy of nikkomycins with glucan synthesis inhibitors against *C. albicans* in vitro was described early on (Hector and Braun, 1986; Pfaller et al, 1989), more recent in vitro and in vivo studies also provided strong evidence for an additive or synergistic cooperation between nikkomycin Z and

echinocandin against *Aspergillus fumigatus* and, more variably, against other filamentous fungi (Stevens, 2000; Capilla-Luque et al, 2001; Chiou et al, 2001).

A phase I study of safety and pharmacokinetics of single oral doses of nikkomycin Z 0.25 to 2.0 mg/kg has been performed in human volunteers. Phase II studies of nikkomycin Z are under consideration for patients with nonlife–threatening and nonmeningeal coccidioidomycosis.

Nikkomycin Z may prove useful for therapy of other mycoses as well, particularly in combination with antifungal drugs such as triazoles and echinocandins. Thus, nikkomycin Z remains a candidate for further clinical development.

REFERENCES

Abruzzo G K, Flattery A M, Gill C J, Kong L, Smith J G, Pikounis V B, Balkovec J M, Bouffard A F, Dropinski J F, Rosen H, Kropp H, Bartizal K. Evaluation of the echinocandin antifungal MK-0991 (L-743,872): efficacies in mouse models of disseminated aspergillosis, candidiasis, and cryptococcosis. *Antimicrob Agents Chemother* 41:2333–2338, 1997.

Abruzzo G K, Gill C J, Flattery A M, Kong L, Leighton C, Smith J G, Pikounis V B, Bartizal K, Rosen H. Efficacy of the echinocandin caspofungin against disseminated aspergillosis and candidiasis in cyclophosphamide-induced immunosuppressed mice. *Antimicrob Agents Chemother* 44:2310–2318, 2000.

Arathoon E G, Gotuzzo E, Noriega L M, Berman R S, DiNubile M J, Sable C A. Randomized, double-blind, multicenter study of caspofungin versus amphotericin B for treatment of oropharyngeal and esophageal candidiasis. *Antimicrob Agents Chemother* 46:451–457, 2002.

Arikan S, Lozano-Chiou M, Paetznick V, Rex J H. In vitro synergy studies with caspofungin and amphotericin B against *Aspergillus* and *Fusarium* species. In: Program and Abstracts of the 40th Interscience Conference on Antimicrobial Agents and Chemotherapy, Toronto, Canada. American Society for Microbiology, Washington, DC: abstr.932, p.368, 2000.

Azuma J, Yamamoto I, Ogura M, Mukai T, Suematsu H, Kageyama H, Nakahara K, Yoshida K, Takaya T. Phase I study of FK463, a new antifungal agent, in healthy adult male volunteers. In: Program and Abstracts of the 38th Interscience Conference on Antimicrobial Agents and Chemotherapy, San Diego, CA. American Society for Microbiology, Washington, DC: abstr.F-146, p.269, 1998.

Balani S K, Xu X, Arison B H, Silva M V, Gries A, DeLuna F A, Cui D, Kari P H, Ly T, Hop C E, Singh R, Wallace M A, Dean D C, Lin J H, Pearson P G, Baillie T A. Metabolites of caspofungin acetate, a potent antifungal agent, in human plasma and urine. *Drug Metab Dispos* 28:1274–1278, 2000.

Bartizal K, Gill C J, Abruzzo G K, Flattery A M, Kong L, Scott P M, Smith J G, Leighton C E, Bouffard A, Dropinski J F, Balkovec J. In vitro preclinical evaluation studies with the echinocandin antifungal MK-0991 (L-743,872). *Antimicrob Agents Chemother* 41:2326–2332, 1997.

Bernard E M, Ishimaru T, Armstrong D: Low doses of the pneumocandin, L-743,872, are effective for prevention and treatment in an animal model of pulmonary aspergillosis. In: Program and Abstracts of the 36st Interscience Conference on Antimicrobial Agents and Chemotherapy, New Orleans, LA. American Society for Microbiology, Washington, DC: abst. F39, p. 106, 1993.

Brown G L, White R J, Turik M. Phase I dose optimization study for V-echinocandin. In: Abstracts of the 40th Interscience Conference on Antimicrobial Agents and Chemotherapy, Toronto, Canada. American Society for Microbiology, Washington, DC: abstr.1105, p.371, 2000a.

Brown G L, White R J, Turik M: Phase II, randomized, open label study of two intravenous dosing regimens of V-echinocandin in the treatment of esophageal candidiasis. In: Abstracts of the 40st Interscience Conference on Antimicrobial Agents and Chemotherapy, Toronto, Canada. American Society for Microbiology, Washington, DC: abstr.1106, p.371, 2000b.

Capilla-Luque J, Clemons K V, Stevens D A. Efficacy of FK-463 alone and in combination against systemic murine aspergillosis. In: Abstracts of the 41st Interscience Conference on Antimicrobial Agents and Chemotherapy, Chicago, IL. American Society for Microbiology, Washington, DC: abstr.J-1834, p.397, 2001.

Chiller T, Farrokhshad K, Brummer E, Stevens D A: The interaction of human monocytes, monocyte-derived macrophages, and polymorphonuclear neutrophils with caspofungin (MK-0991), an echinocandin, for antifungal activity against *Aspergillus fumigatus. Diagn Microbiol Infect Dis* 39:99–103, 2001.

Chiou C C, Mavrogiorgos N, Tillem J, Hector R, Walsh T J. Synergy, pharmacodynamics, and time-sequenced ultrastructural changes of the interaction between nikkomycin Z and the echinocandin FK463 against *Aspergillus fumigatus. Antimicrob Agents Chemother* 45:3310–3321, 2001.

Clemons K V, Stevens D A. Efficacy of nikkomycin Z against experimental pulmonary blastomycosis. *Antimicrob Agents Chemother* 41:2026–2028, 1997.

Current W L, Boylan C J, Rabb P P. Anti-pneumocystis activity of LY 303366 and other echinocandin B analogues. In: Program and Abstracts of the 33th Interscience Conference on Antimicrobial Agents and Chemotherapy, New Orleans, LA. American Society for Microbiology, Washington, DC: abstr.368, p.186, 1993.

Debono M, Gordee R S. Antibiotics that inhibit fungal cell wall development *Ann Rev Microbiol* 48:471–497, 1994.

Douglas C M, Bowman J C, Abruzzo G K et al. The glucan synthesis inhibitor caspofungin acetate (Cancidas™, MK-0991, L-743872) kills *Aspergillus fumigatus* hyphal tips in vitro and is efficacious against disseminated aspergillosis in cyclophosphamide induced chronically leukopenic mice. In: Program and abstracts of the 40th Interscience Conference on Antimicrobal Agents and Chemotherapy, Toronto, Canada. American Society for Microbiology, Washington, DC: abstr.1683, p.387, 2000.

Ernst M E, Klepser M E, Wolfe E J, Pfaller M A. Antifungal dynamics of LY 303366, an investigational echinocandin B analog, against *Candida* spp. *Diagn Microbiol Infect Dis* 26:125–131, 1996.

Ernst E J, Klepser M E, Ernst M E, Messer S A, Pfaller M A. In vitro pharmacodynamic properties of MK-0991 determined by time-kill methods. *Diagn Microbiol Infect Dis* 33:75–80, 1999.

Ernst E J, Klepser M E, Pfaller M A. Postantifungal effects of echinocandin, azole, and polyene antifungal agents against *Candida albicans* and *Cryptococcus neoformans. Antimicrob Agents Chemother* 44:1108–1111, 2000.

Ernst E J, Roling E E, Petzold C R, Keele D J, Klepser M E. In vitro activity of micafungin (FK-463) against *Candida* spp.: microdilution, time-kill, and postantifungal-effect studies. *Antimicrob Agents Chemother* 46:3846–3853, 2002.

Espinel-Ingroff A. Comparison of in vitro activities of the new triazole SCH56592 and the echinocandins MK-0991 (L-743,872) and LY303366 against opportunistic filamentous and dimorphic fungi and yeasts. *J Clin Microbiol* 36:2950–2956, 1998.

Franzot S P, Casadevall A. Pneumocandin L-743,872 enhances the activities of amphotericin B and fluconazole against *Cryptococcus neoformans* in vitro. *Antimicrob Agents Chemother* 41:331–336, 1997.

Goldberg J, Connolly P, Schnizlein-Bick C, Durkin M, Kohler S,

Smedema M, Brizendine E, Hector R, Wheat J. Comparison of nikkomycin Z with amphotericin B and itraconazole for treatment of histoplasmosis in a murine model. *Antimicrob Agents Chemother* 44:1624–1629, 2000.

Gonzalez G M, Tijerina R, Najvar L K, Bocanegra R, Luther M, Rinaldi M G, Graybill J R. Correlation between antifungal susceptibilities of *Coccidioides immitis* in vitro and antifungal treatment with caspofungin in a mouse model. *Antimicrob Agents Chemother* 45:1854–1859, 2001.

Graybill J R, Najvar L K, Bocanegra R. Efficacy of nikkomycin Z in the treatment of murine histoplasmosis. *Antimicrob Agents Chemother* 42:2371–2374, 1998a.

Graybill J R, Najvar L K, Montalbo E M, Barchiesi F J, Luther M F, Rinaldi M G. Treatment of histoplasmosis with MK-991 (L-743,872). *Antimicrob Agents Chemother* 42:151–153, 1998b.

Groll A H, Piscitelli S C, Walsh T J. Clinical pharmacology of systemic antifungal agents: a comprehensive review of agents in clinical use, current investigational compounds, and putative targets for antifungal drug development. *Adv Pharmacol* 44:343–500, 1998.

Groll A H, Walsh T J. FK-463. *Curr Opin Antiinfect Drugs* 2:405–412, 2000.

Groll A H, Gullick B M, Petraitiene R, Petraitis V, Candelario M, Piscitelli S C, Walsh T J. Compartmental plasma pharmacokinetics of the antifungal echinocandin MK-0991 in rabbits. *Antimicrobial Agents Chemother* 45:596–600, 2001a.

Groll A H, Mickiene D, Petraitiene R, Petraitis V, Field-Ridley A, Candelario M, Piscitelli S C, Walsh T J. Pharmacokinetic and pharmacodynamic modeling of anidulafungin (LY303366): Reappraisal of its efficacy in neutropenic animal models of opportunistic mycoses using optimal plasma sampling. *Antimicrob Agents Chemother* 45:2845–2855, 2001b.

Groll A H, Mickiene D, Petraitis V, Petraitiene R, Alfaro R, Ibrahim K H, Piscitelli S C, Walsh T J. Compartmental pharmacokinetics and tissue distribution of the antifungal echinocandin-like lipopeptide FK463 in rabbits. *Antimicrob Agents Chemother* 45:3322–3327, 2001c.

Groll A H, Piscitelli S C, Walsh T J. Antifungal pharmacodynamics. Concentration-effect relationships in vitro and in vivo. *Pharmacother* 21:133S–148S, 2001d.

Groll A H, Walsh T J. Caspofungin: Pharmacology, safety, and therapeutic potential in superficial and invasive fungal infections. *Exp Opin Invest Drugs* 10:1545–1558, 2001e.

Hajdu R, Thompson R, Sundelof J G, Pelak B A, Bouffard F A, Dropinski J F, Kropp H. Preliminary animal pharmacokinetics of the parenteral antifungal agent MK-0991 (L-743,872). *Antimicrob Agents Chemother* 41:2339–2344, 1997.

Hawser S: LY-303366. *Curr Opin Anti-infect Investig Drugs* 1:353–360, 1999.

Hector R F, Braun P C. Synergistic action of nikkomycin X and Z with papulacandin B on whole cells and regenerating protoplasts of *Candida albicans. Antimicrob Agents Chemother* 29:389–394, 1986.

Hector R F, Yee E. Evaluation of Bay R 3783 in rodent models of superficial and systemic candidiasis, meningeal cryptococcosis, and pulmonary aspergillosis. *Antimicrob Agents Chemother* 34:448–454, 1990a.

Hector R F, Zimmer B L, Pappagianis D. Evaluation of nikkomycin X and Z in murine models of coccidiodomycosis, histoplasmosis, and blastomycosis. *Antimicrob Agents Chemother* 34:587–593, 1990b.

Hector R F, Schaller K, Positive interaction of nikkomycins and azoles against *Candida albicans* in vitro and in vivo. *Antimicrob Agents Chemother* 36:1284–1289, 1992.

Hector, R F: Compounds active against cell walls of medically important fungi. *Clin Microbiol Rev* 6:1–21, 1993.

Hiemenz J, Cagnoni P, Simpson D, Devine S, Chao N. Maximum

tolerated dose and pharmacokinetics of FK463 in combination with fluconazole for the prophylaxis of fungal infections in adult bone marrow or peripheral stem cell transplant patients. In: Program and Abstracts of the 39th Interscience Conference on Antimicrobial Agents and Chemotherapy, San Francisco, CA. American Society for Microbiology, Washington, DC: abstr. 1648, p. 576, 1999.

Ikeda F, Wakai Y, Matsumoto S, Maki K, Watabe E, Tawara S, Goto T, Watanabe Y, Matsumoto F, Kuwahara S. Efficacy of FK463, a new lipopeptide antifungal agent, in mouse models of disseminated candidiasis and aspergillosis. *Antimicrob Agents Chemother* 44:614–618, 2000.

Ito M, Nozu R, Kuramochi T, Eguchi N, Suzuki S, Hioki K, Itoh T, Ikeda F. Prophylactic effect of FK463, a novel antifungal lipopeptide, against *Pneumocystis carinii* infection in mice. *Antimicrob Agents Chemother* 44:2259–2262, 2000.

Karlowsky J A, Harding G A, Zelenitsky S A, Hoban D J, Kabani A, Balko T V, Turik M, Zhanel G G. In vitro kill curves of a new semisynthetic echinocandin, LY-303366, against fluconazole-sensitive and -resistant *Candida* species. *Antimicrob Agents Chemother* 41:2576–2578, 1997.

Kohler S, Wheat L J, Connolly P, Schnizlein-Bick C, Durkin M, Smedema M, Goldberg J, Brizendine E. Comparison of the echinocandin caspofungin with amphotericin B for treatment of histoplasmosis following pulmonary challenge in a murine model. *Antimicrob Agents Chemother* 44:1850–1854, 2000.

Kohno S, Maesaki S, Iwakawa J, Miyazaki Y, Nakamura K, Kakeya H, Yanagihara K, Ohno H, Higashiyama Y, Tashiro T. Synergistic effects of combination of FK463 with amphotericin: Enhanced efficacy in a murine model of invasive pulmonary aspergillosis. In: Program and Abstracts of the 40st Interscience Conference on Antimicrobial Agents and Chemotherapy, Toronto, Canada. American Society for Microbiology, Washington, DC: abstr.1686, p.388, 2000.

Kohno S, Masaoka T, Yamaguchi H. A multicentre, open-label clinical study of FK463 in patients with deep mycoses in Japan. In: Abstracts of the 41st Interscience Conference on Antimicrobial Agents and Chemotherapy, Chicago, IL. American Society for Microbiology, Washington, DC: abstr. J-834, p.384, 2001.

Kontoyiannis D P, Buell D, Frisbee-Hume S. Initial experience with FK463 for the treatment of candidemia in cancer patients. In: Abstracts of the 41st Interscience Conference on Antimicrobial Agents and Chemotherapy, Chicago, IL. American Society for Microbiology, Washington, DC: abstr. J-1629, p. 394, 2001.

Kurtz M B, Heath I B, Marrinan J, Dreikorn S, Onishi J, Douglas C M. Morphological effects of lipopeptides against *Aspergillus fumigatus* correlate with activities against (1,3)-beta-D-glucan synthase. *Antimicrob Agents Chemother* 38:1480–1489, 1994.

Kurtz M B, Douglas C M: Lipopeptide inhibitors of fungal glucan synthase. *J Med Vet Mycol* 35:79–86, 1997.

Li R K, Rinaldi M G. In vitro antifungal activity of nikkomycin Z in combination with fluconazole or itraconazole. *Antimicrob Agents Chemother* 43:1401–1405, 1999.

Maertens J, Raad I, Sable C A, Ngai A, Berman R, Patterson T F, Denning D, Walsh T J. Multicenter, noncomparative study to evaluate safety and efficacy of caspofungin in adults with invasive aspergillosis refractory or intolerant to amphotericin B, amphotericin B lipid formulations, or azoles. In: Abstracts of the 40th International Conference on Antimicrobial Agents and Chemotherapy, Toronto, Canada. American Society for Microbiology, Washington, DC: abstr.1103, p.371, 2000.

Maesaki S, Hossain M A, Miyazaki Y, Tomono K, Tashiro T, Kohno S. Efficacy of FK463, a (1,3)-beta-D-glucan synthase inhibitor, in disseminated azole-resistant *Candida albicans* infection in mice. *Antimicrob Agents Chemother* 44:1728–1730, 2000.

Maki K, Morishita Y, Iguchi Y, Watabe E, Otomo K, Teratani M, Watanabe Y, Ikeda F, Tawara S, Goto T, Tomishima M, et al.

In vitro antifungal activity of FK463, a novel water-soluble echinocandin-like lipopeptide. In: Program and Abstracts of the 38th Interscience Conference on Antimicrobial Agents and Chemotherapy, San Diego, CA. American Society for Microbiology, Washington, DC: abstr. F-141,p.268, 1998.

Manavathu E K, Krishnan S, Cutright J L, Chandrasakar P H: A comparative study of the in vitro susceptibility of *Aspergillus fumigatus* to antifungal agents individually and in combination by the fractional inhibitory concentration index, tetrazolium reduction, and radiometric assay. In: Program and Abstracts of the 40th Interscience Conference on Antimicrobial Agents and Chemotherapy, Toronto, Canada. American Society for Microbiology, Washington, DC: abstr.931, p.368, 2000.

Marco F, Pfaller M A, Messer S A, Jones R N: Activity of MK-0991 (L-743,872), a new echinocandin, compared with those of LY303366 and four other antifungal agents tested against blood stream isolates of *Candida* spp. *Diagn Microbiol Infect Dis* 32:33–37, 1998.

Matsumoto S, Wakai Y, Maki K, Watabe E, Ushitani T, Otomo K, Nakai T, Watanabe Y, Ikeda F, Tawara S, Goto T et al. Efficacy of FK463, a novel water-soluble echinocandin-like lipopeptide, in murine models of disseminated candidiasis. In: Program and Abstracts of the 38th Interscience Conference on Antimicrobial Agents and Chemotherapy, San Diego, CA. American Society for Microbiology, Washington, DC: abstr. F-142, p.268, 1998.

Matsumoto S, Wakai Y, Nakai T, Hatano K, Ushitani T, Ikeda F, Tawara S, Goto T, Matsumoto F, Kuwahara S. Efficacy of FK463, a new lipopeptide antifungal agent, in mouse models of pulmonary aspergillosis. *Antimicrob Agents Chemother* 44:619–621, 2000.

Mikamo H, Sato Y, Tamaya T. In vitro antifungal activity of FK463, a new water-soluble echinocandin-like lipopeptide. *J Antimicrob Chemother* 46:485–487, 2000.

Milewski S, Mignini F, Borowski E. Synergistic action of nikkomycin X/Z with azole antifungals on *Candida albicans*. *J Gen Microbiol* 137:2155–2161, 1991.

Mora-Durate J, Betts R, Rotstein C, Columbo AL, Thompson-Moya L, Smietana J, Lupinacci R, Sable C, Kartsonis N, Perfect J for the Caspofungin Invasive Candidiasis Study Group. Comparison of caspofungin and amphotericin B for invasive candidiasis. *N Engl J Med* 347:2020–2029, 2002.

Muller F M, Kurzai O, Hacker J, Frosch M, Muhlschlegel F. Effect of the growth medium on the in vitro antifungal activity of micafungin (FK-463) against clinical isolates of *Candida dubliniensis*. *J Antimicrob Chemother* 48:713–715, 2001.

Mukai T, Ohkuma T, Nakahara K, Takaya T, Uematsu T, Azuma J. Pharmacokinetics of FK463, a novel echinocandin analogue, in elderly and non-elderly subjects. In: Program and Abstracts of the 41st Interscience Conference on Antimicrobial Agents and Chemotherapy, Chicago, IL. American Society for Microbiology, Washington, DC: abstr. A-30, p. 5, 2001.

Nakai T, Uno J, Otomo K, Ikeda F, Tawara S, Goto T, Nishimura K, Miyaji M. In vitro activity of FK463, a novel lipopeptide antifungal agent, against a variety of clinically important molds. *Chemotherapy* 48:78–81, 2002.

Nakajima M, Tamada S, Yoshida K, Wakai Y, Nakai T, Ikeda F, Goto T, Niki Y, Matsushima T. Pathological findings in a murine pulmonary aspergillosis model: treatment with FK463, amphotericin B and a combination of FK463 and amphotericin B. In: Program and Abstracts of the 40th Interscience Conference on Antimicrobial Agents and Chemotherapy, Toronto, Canada. American Society for Microbiology, Washington, DC: abstr. 1685, p.387, 2000.

Oakley K L, Moore C B, Denning D W: In vitro activity of the echinocandin antifungal agent LY303,366 in comparison with itraconazole and amphotericin B against *Aspergillus* spp. *Antimicrob Agents Chemother* 42:2726–2730, 1998.

Ostrosky-Zeichner L, Paetznick V L, Mohr J, Rodriguez J R, Chen E, Sancak B, Rex J H. In vitro antifungal activity of FK463 against *Candida* spp. In: Program and Abstracts of the 40th Interscience Conference on Antimicrobial Agents and Chemotherapy, Toronto, Canada. American Society for Microbiology, Washington, DC: abstr.197, p.352, 2000.

Package Circular: Cancidas® (caspofungin acetate for injection). January 2001.

Petraitiene R, Petraitis V, Groll A H, Candelario M, Sein T, Bell A, Peter J, Lyman C A, Schaufele R L, McMillian C L, Bacher J, Walsh T J. Antifungal efficacy, safety, and single-dose pharmacokinetics of LY303366, a novel echinocandin, in experimental disseminated candidiasis in persistently neutropenic rabbits. *Antimicrob Agents Chemother* 43:2148–2155, 1999.

Petraitiene R, Petraitis V, Groll A H, Sein T, Schaufele R, Francesconi A, Avila N, Bacher J, Walsh T J. Antifungal efficacy of caspofungin (MK-0991) in experimental pulmonary aspergillosis in persistently neutropenic rabbits: Pharmacokinetics, drug disposition, and relationship to galactomannan-antigenemia. *Antimicrob Agents Chemother* 46:12–23, 2002.

Petraitis V, Petraitiene R, Groll A H, Bell A, Callender D P, Candelario M, Lyman C A, Bacher J, Walsh T J. Efficacy of LY-303366 against invasive pulmonary aspergillosis. *Antimicrob Agents Chemother* 42:2898–2905, 1998.

Petraitis V, Petraitiene R, Leguit R J, Candelario M, Sein T, Peter J, Field-Ridley A, Irwin R, Groll A, Walsh T J. Combination antifungal therapy with FK463 plus amphotericin B in treatment of experimental pulmonary aspergillosis. In: Program and Abstracts of the 39th Interscience Conference on Antimicrobial Agents and Chemotherapy, San Francisco, CA. American Society for Microbiology, Washington, DC: abstr. 2003, p. 581, 1999.

Petraitis V, Petraitiene R, Groll A H, Sein T, Schaufele R L, Lyman C A, Francesconi A, Bacher J, Piscitelli S, Walsh T J. Dose-dependent antifungal efficacy of the echinocandin VER-002 (LY-303366) against experimental oropharyngeal and esophageal candidiasis. *Antimicrob Agents Chemother* 45:45:471–479, 2001.

Petraitis V, Petraitiene R, Groll A H, Sein T, Schaufele R L, Bacher J, Walsh T J. Comparative antifungal activity of the echinocandin micafungin against disseminated candidiasis and invasive pulmonary aspergillosis in persistently neutropenic rabbits. *Antimicrob Agents Chemother* 46:1857–1869, 2002.

Pettengell K, Mynhardt J, Kluyts T, Soni P. A multicenter study to determine the minimal effective dose of FK463 for the treatment of esophageal candidiasis in HIV-positive patients. In: Program and Abstracts of the 39th Interscience Conference on Antimicrobial Agents and Chemotherapy, San Francisco, CA. American Society for Microbiology, Washington, DC: abstr. 1421, p. 567, 1999.

Pettengell K, Mynhardt J, Kluyts T, Simjee A, Baraldi E: A multicenter study of the echinocandin antifungal FK463 for the treatment of esophageal candidiasis in HIV positive patients, In: Program and Abstracts of the 40th Interscience Conference on Antimicrobial Agents and Chemotherapy, Toronto, Canada. American Society for Microbiology, Washington, DC: abstr. 1104, p. 371, 2000.

Pfaller M A, Wey S, Gerarden T, Houston A, Wenzel R P. Susceptibility of nosocomial isolates of *Candida* species to LY121019 and other antifungal agents. *Diagn Microbiol Infect Dis* 12:1–4, 1989.

Pfaller M A, Messer S A, Coffman S. In vitro susceptibilities of clinical yeasts isolates to a new echinocandin derivative, LY 303366, and other antifungal agents. *Antimicrob Agents Chemother* 41:763–766, 1997.

Pfaller M A, Marco F, Messer S A, Jones R N. In vitro activity of two echinocandin derivatives, LY 303366 and MK-0991 (L-743,792), against clinical isolates of *Aspergillus, Fusarium,*

Rhizopus, and other filamentous fungi. *Diagn Microbiol Infect Dis* 30:251–255, 1998.

Powles M A, Liberator P, Anderson J, Karkhanis Y, Dropinski J F, Bouffard F A, Balkovec J M, Fujioka H, Aikawa M, McFadden D, Schmatz D. Efficacy of MK-991 (L-743,872), a semisynthetic pneumocandin, in murine models of *Pneumocystis carinii. Antimicrob Agents Chemother* 42:1985–1989, 1998.

Powles R, Sirohi B, Chopra R, Russel N, Prentice H G. Assessment of maximum tolerated dose (MTD) of FK-463 in cancer patients undergoing hematopoietic stem cell transplantation. In: Program and Abstracts of the 41st Interscience Conference on Antimicrobial Agents and Chemotherapy, Chicago, IL. American Society for Microbiology, Washington, DC: abstr. J-676, p. 376, 2001.

Rajman I, Desante K, Hatcher B, Hemmingway J, Lachno R, Brooks S, Turik M. LY303366 single intravenous dose pharmacokinetics and safety in healthy volunteers. In: Program and Abstracts of the 37th Interscience Conference on Antimicrobial Agents and Chemotherapy, Toronto, Canada. American Society for Microbiology, Washington, DC: abstr. F-74, p.158, 1997.

Rennie R, Sand C, Sherburne R. Electron microscopic evidence of the effect of LY303366 on *Aspergillus fumigatus*. In: Abstracts of the 13th Meeting of the International Society for Human and Animal Mycology, abstr. P451, p.191, 1997.

Roberts J, Schock K, Marino S, Andriole V T. Efficacies of two new antifungal agents, the triazole ravuconazole and the echinocandin LY-303366, in an experimental model of invasive aspergillosis. *Antimicrob Agents Chemother* 44:3381–3388, 2000.

Roling E E, Klepser M E, Wasson A, Lewis R E, Ernst E J, Pfaller M A. Antifungal activities of fluconazole, caspofungin (MK0991), and anidulafungin (LY 303366) alone and in combination against *Candida* spp. and *Crytococcus neoformans* via time-kill methods. *Diagn Microbiol Infect Dis* 43:13–17, 2002.

Sable C A, Nguyen B Y, Chodakewitz J A, DeStefano M, Berman R S, DiNubile M J: Safety of caspofungin acetate in the treatment of fungal infections. In: Abstracts of Focus on Fungal Infections 11: 21, 2001.

Seibel N, Schwartz C, Arrieta A, Flynn P, Shad A, Albano E, Walsh T J. A phase I study to determine the safety and pharmacokinetics of FK463 in febrile neutropenic pediatric patients. In: Program and Abstracts of the 40th Interscience Conference on Antimicrobial Agents and Chemotherapy, Toronto, Canada. American Society for Microbiology, Washington, DC: abstr. 18, p. 1, 2000.

Stevens D A. Drug interaction in vitro between a polyene (AmBisome) and an echinocandin (FK463) vs. *Aspergillus* species. In: Program and Abstracts of the 39th Interscience Conference on Antimicrobial Agents and Chemotherapy, San Francisco, CA. American Society for Microbiology, Washington, DC: abstr. 151, p. 543, 1999.

Stevens D A. Drug interaction studies of a glucan synthase inhibitor (LY 303366) and a chitin synthase inhibitor (Nikkomycin Z) for inhibition and killing of fungal pathogens. *Antimicrob Agents Chemother* 44:2547–2548, 2000.

Stone J A, Holland S D, Wickersham P J, Sterrett A, Schwartz M, Bonfiglio C, Hesney M, Winchell G A, Deutsch P J, Greenberg H, Hunt T L, Waldman S A. Single- and multiple-dose pharmacokinetics of caspofungin in healthy men. *Antimicrob Agents Chemother* 46:739–745, 2002.

Suzuki S, Terakawa M, Yokobayashi F, Fujiwara F, Hata T. Pharmacokinetics of FK463, a novel water-soluble echinocandin-like lipopeptide, in animals. In: Program and Abstracts of the 38th Interscience Conference on Antimicrobial Agents and Chemotherapy, San Francisco, CA. American Society for Microbiology, Washington, DC: abstr. F-144, p. 269, 1998.

Tang T R, Parr T R, Turner W, Debono M, LaGrandeur L, Burkhardt F, Rodriquez M, Zweifel M, Nissen J, Clingerman K. LY-303366: A non-competitive inhibitor of (1,3)-b-D glucan synthases from

Candida albicans and *Aspergillus fumigatus*. In: Program and Abstracts of the 33rd Interscience Conference on Antimicrobial Agents and Chemotherapy, New Orleans, LA. American Society for Microbiology, Washington, DC: abstr. 367, p. 186, 1993.

Tawara S, Ikeda F, Maki K, Morishita Y, Otomo K, Teratani N, Goto T, Tomishima M, Ohki H, Yamada A, Kawabata K, Takasugi H, Sakane K, Tanaka H, Matsumoto F, Kuwahara S. In vitro activities of a new lipopeptide antifungal agent, FK463, against a variety of clinically important fungi. *Antimicrob Agents Chemother* 44:57–62, 2000.

Thompson J R, Douglas C M, Li W, Jue C K, Pramanik B, Yuan X, Rude T H, Toffaletti D L, Perfect J R, Kurtz M. A glucan synthase FKS1 homolog in *Cryptococcus neoformans* is single copy and encodes an essential function. *J Bacteriol* 181: 444–453, 1999.

Thye D, Kilfoil T, White R J, Lasseter K. Anidulafungin: Pharmacokinetics in subjects with mild to moderate hepatic impairment. In: Program and Abstracts of the 41st Interscience Conference on Antimicrobial Agents and Chemotherapy, Chicago, IL. American Society for Microbiology, Washington, DC: abstr. A-34, p. 6, 2001a.

Thye D, Shepherd B, White R J, Weston I E, Henkel T. Anidulafungin: a phase I study to identify the maximum tolerated dose in healthy volunteers. In: Program and Abstracts of the 41st Interscience Conference on Antimicrobial Agents and Chemotherapy, Chicago, IL. American Society for Microbiology, Washington, DC: abstr. A-36, p. 6, 2001b.

Tomishima M, Ohki H, Yamada A, Takasugi H, Maki H, Tawara S, Tanaka A. FK463, a novel water-soluble echinocandin lipopeptide: synthesis and antifungal activity. *J Antibiot* 52: 674–676, 1999.

van Burik J, Ratanatharathorn V, Lipton J, Miller C, Bunin N, Walsh T. Randomized double-blind trial of micafungin vs fluconazole for prophylaxis of invasive fungal infections in patients undergoing hematopoietic stem cell transplant (HSCT). In: Program and Abstracts of the 42nd Interscience Conference on Antimicrobial Agents and Chemotherapy, San Diego, CA. American Society of Microbiology, Washington, DC, abstract M-1238, 2002.

Villanueva A, Gotuzzo E, Arathoon E, Noriega L M, Kartsonis N, Lupoinacci R, Smietana J, Berman R S, Dinubile N J, Sable C A. The efficacy, safety, and tolerability of caspofungin versus fluconazole in the treatment of esophageal candidiasis. In: Program and Abstracts of the 41st Interscience Conference on Antimicrobial Agents and Chemotherapy, Chicago, IL. American Society for Microbiology, Washington, DC: abstr. J-675, p. 676, 2001a.

Villanueva A, Arathoon E G, Gotuzzo E, Berman R S, DiNubile M J, Sable C A. A randomized double-blind study of caspofungin versus amphotericin for the treatment of candidal esophagitis. *Clin Infect Dis* 33:1529–1535, 2001b.

Wakai Y, Matsumoto S, Maki K, Watabe E, Otomo K, Nakai T, Hatano K, Watanabe Y, Ikeda F, Tawara S, Goto T, Matsumoto F, Kuwahara S. Efficacy of FK463, a novel water-soluble echinocandin-like lipopeptide, in murine models of pulmonary aspergillosis. In: Program and Abstracts of the 38th Interscience Conference on Antimicrobial Agents and Chemotherapy, San Diego, CA. American Society for Microbiology, Washington, DC: abstr F-143, p. 268, 1998.

Walsh T J. Echinocandins: an important advance in the primary treatment of invasive candidiasis. *N Engl J Med* 347:2070–2072, 2002.

White R J, Thye D. Anidulafungin does not affect the metabolism of cyclosporin by human hepatic microsomes. In: Program and Abstracts of the 41st Interscience Conference on Antimicrobial Agents and Chemotherapy, Chicago, IL. American Society for Microbiology, Washington, DC: abstr. A-35, p.6, 2001.

Zeckner D, Butler T, Boylan C, Boyll B, Lin Y, Raab P, Schmidtke J, Current W. LY303366 activity against systemic aspergillosis and histoplasmosis in murine models. In: Program and Abstracts of the 33rd Interscience Conference on Antimicrobial Agents and Chemotherapy, New Orleans, LA. American Society for Microbiology, Washington, DC: abstr. 364, p. 186, 1993a.

Zeckner D, Butler T, Boylan C, Boyll B, Lin Y, Raab P, Schmidtke J, Current W. LY303366, activity in a murine systemic candidiasis model. In: Program and Abstracts of the 33rd Interscience Conference on Antimicrobial Agents and Chemotherapy, New Orleans, LA. American Society for Microbiology, Washington, DC: abstr. 365, p. 186, 1993b.

Zeckner D, Butler T, Boylan C, Boyll B, Raab P, Current W. LY303366, Activity in a rat mucocutaneous vaginal candidiasis model. In: Program and Abstracts of the 34th Interscience Conference on Antimicrobial Agents and Chemotherapy, Orlando, FL. American Society for Microbiology, Washington, DC: abstr. F-169, p. 252, 1994.

Zhanel G G, Karlowsky J A, Harding G A, Balko T V, Zelenitsky S A, Friesen M, Kabani A, Turik M, Hoban D J. In vitro activity of a new semisynthetic echinocandin, LY 303366, against systemic isolates of *Candida species*, *Cryptococcus neoformans*, *Blastomyces dermatitidis*, and *Aspergillus* species. *Antimicrob Agents Chemother* 41:863–865, 1997.

Zornes L, Stratford R, Novilla M, Turner D, Boylan C, Boyll B, Butler T, Lin Y, Zeckner W, Turner W, Current W. Single dose IV bolus and oral administration pharmacokinetics of LY303366, a new lipopeptide antifungal agent related to echinocandin B, in female Lewis rats and Beagle dogs. In: Program and Abstracts of the 33rd Interscience Conference on Antimicrobial Agents and Chemotherapy, New Orleans, LA. American Society for Microbiology, Washington, DC: abst. 370, p. 187, 1993.

8

Terbinafine

PETER G. PAPPAS

Terbinafine is a newly developed oral and topical antifungal agent in the allylamine class of antifungal compounds (Petranyi et al, 1984). Discovered in 1983, it is closely related to naftifine. Terbinafine became available in Europe in 1991, and in 1996 in the United States. Terbinafine is the only oral allylamine available in the United States and is used largely for the treatment of superficial fungal infections, especially those due to dermatophytes. There has been significant interest in developing the drug for the treatment of deep mycoses, either alone or in combination, for disorders such as cryptococcosis, invasive aspergillosis, and other mould infections, but there are only scant clinical data evaluating its efficacy in these settings. Terbinafine is a very valuable antifungal drug for the treatment of superficial fungal infections, and has potential as an adjunctive agent in the treatment of selected deep mycoses.

PHARMACODYNAMICS

Mechanism of Action

Terbinafine has a unique mechanism of action among the antifungal agents (Petranyi et al, 1984; Balfour and Faulds, 1992), inhibiting the synthesis of ergosterol, a key sterol component in the plasma membrane of the fungal cell. Terbinafine inhibits squalene epoxidase, the enzyme which catalyzes the conversion of squalene to squalene-2,3 epoxide, a precursor of lanosterol, which in turn is a direct precursor of ergosterol (Ryder and Dupont 1985; Birnbaum, 1990). A deficiency of ergosterol is detrimental to the integrity of the cell membrane resulting in a fungistatic effect similar to that seen with the azole antifungal compounds. In addition to this action, terbinafine also causes excessive intracellular accumulation of squalene, which is believed to exert a further toxic effect on susceptible fungal cells, thereby exerting a fungicidal effect (Ryder, 1992). In this regard, the mechanism of action of terbinafine is distinct from that of the azoles even though both compounds inhibit ergosterol biosynthesis through interruption of the synthesis of its precursors. Terbinafine has a strong affinity for fungal cell enzymes, but unlike the azoles, terbinafine has a very low affinity for the human cytochrome P-450 family of enzymes (Schuster, 1985; Katz, 1999). This low affinity for the mammalian P-450 enzymes probably accounts for the favorable adverse event profile of terbenafine and the relatively few drug–drug interactions.

Antifungal Spectrum

Terbinafine is a very broad spectrum antifungal agent, exhibiting the best activity against the dermatophytes of all the antifungal agents (Petranyi et al, 1987; Rinaldi, 1993; Ryder and Favre, 1997; Arzeni et al, 1998). Terbinafine also demonstrates reasonable in vitro activity against many *Aspergillus* species including *A. fumigatus*, *A. flavus*, *A. niger*, and *A. ustus* (Schmitt et al, 1987; Ryder and Leitner, 1996; Schiraldi and Columbo, 1997; Ryder and Favre, 1997). Other moulds that appear susceptible based on in vitro testing include many of the dematiaceous fungi such as *Fonsecaea* and *Cladophialophora* species (Shadomy et al, 1985) and the agents of eumycetoma (Venugopal et al, 1993). Selected case reports of successful therapy with terbinafine in a patient with disseminated *Phialophora parasitica* (Wong et al, 1989) and another patient with *Curvularia lunata* endocarditis (Bryan et al, 1993) suggest clinically relevant antifungal activity against these dematiaceous pathogens. Terbinafine does not consistently demonstrate significant in vitro activity against the hyaline moulds such *Fusarium* species and *Scedosporium apiospermum* (*Pseudoallescheria boydii*) and the Zygomycetes. The in vitro activity of terbinafine versus selected dermatophytes and moulds is demonstrated in Tables 8–1, 8–2, 8–3.

Terbinafine demonstrates good in vitro activity against *C. neoformans* (Shadomy et al, 1985; Hiratani et al, 1991), but it has relatively poor activity against other yeasts including many *Candida* species with the

TABLE 8–1. *Minimum Inhibitory Concentrations of Terbinafine Against Selected Dermatophytes*

Organism	MIC range (ug/ml)
Epidermophyton floccosum	0.001–0.05
Microsporum audouinii	0.001–< 0.04
Microsporum canis	0.0001–0.1
Microsporum gypseum	0.003–< 0.04
Microsporum persicolor	0.002–0.003
Trichophyton mentagrophytes	0.0001–0.05
Trichophyton mentagrophytes var. *interdigitale*	0.002–0.005
Trichophyton rubrum	0.001–0.15
Trichophyton simii	0.1–0.25
Trichophyton tonsurans	0.003–0.25
Trichophyton violaceum	0.001–0.1
Trichophyton verrucosum	0.001–0.006

MIC, minimum inhibitory concentration.
Source: Adapted from Ryder and Favre, 1997.

TABLE 8–3. *Minimum Inhibitory Concentrations of Terbinafine Against Selected Dematiaceous Fungi*

Organism	MIC Range (ug/ml)
Alternaria alternata	0.6–5
Cladophialophora bantianum	0.012–1
Cladophialophora carrionii	< 0.04–1.25
Curvularia lunata	0.2–2
Curvularia fallax	0.25–0.5
Dactylaria constricta	0.01–0.03
Drechslera rostrata	10
Exophilia jeanselmei	< 0.06–2.5
Fonsecaea compacta	< 0.04
Fonsecaea pedrosi	< 0.04–0.13
Madurella mycetomatis	< 0.01–1
Madurella grisea	< 0.01–2.5
Madurella spp.	1–4
Phaeoannellomyces werneckii	0.04–4
Phialophora verrucosa	< 0.04–0.13
Phialophora parasitica	0.1
Wangiella dermatitidis	0.001–0.08

MIC, minimum inhibitory concentration.
Source: adapted from Ryder and Favre, 1997.

exception of *C. parapsilosis* (Ryder et al, 1998; Jessup et al, 2000). Moreover, terbinafine is fungistatic against all of the *Candida* spp. Table 8–4 summarizes the in vitro activity against selected yeasts.

Terbinafine demonstrates excellent activity against some of the dimorphic fungi, including *Sporothrix schenckii*, against which it exhibits MICs comparable to some of the azole antifungal compounds, including itraconazole (Shadomy et al, 1985; Petranyi et al, 1987). In vitro activity against other dimorphic fungi such as *Blastomyces dermatitidis*, *Histoplasma capsulatum*, and *Coccidioides immitis* is good (Shadomy et al, 1985; Ryder and Favre, 1997). There are little in vitro or clinical data concerning the use of terbinafine against other dimorphic fungi including *Penicillium marneffii* and *Paracoccidioides brasiliensis*. The in vitro susceptibility data for these dimorphic pathogens are shown in Table 8–5.

PHARMACOKINETICS

Oral

The pharmacokinetics of terbinafine have been reviewed recently (Jensen, 1989; Faergemann, 1997). Terbinafine for systemic use is only formulated for oral administration. There is no intravenous formulation in part due to the drug's significant lipophilicity. Terbinafine is well-absorbed following oral dosing with at least 80% bioavailability (Jensen, 1989). The drug demonstrates linear kinetics over a broad range of therapeutic doses with a proportional increase in the area under the curve (AUC) with increasing dose. Peak serum concentrations are achieved within 2 hours following oral administration in both adults and children, although at similar doses, peak concentrations are

TABLE 8–2. *Minimum Inhibitory Concentrations of Terbinafine Against Selected Filamentous Fungi*

Organism	MIC range (ug/ml)
Acremonium spp.	0.25–8
Aspergillus flavus	0.01–1
Aspergillus fumigatus	0.02–5
Aspergillus nidulans	0.02–0.5
Aspergillus niger	0.005–2.5
Aspergillus terreus	< 0.04–5
Aspergillus ustus	0.1–0.5
Fusarium moniliforme	0.5–10
Fusarium oxysporum	0.25–20
Fusarium solani	1–> 128
Mucor spp.	64–> 128
Paecilomyces spp.	1–64
Penicillium spp.	1–5
Pseudallescheria boydii	10–> 64
Rhizopus spp.	64–> 100
Scopulariopsis brevicaulis	0.5–8

MIC, minimum inhibitory concentrations.
Source: adapted from Ryder and Favre, 1997.

TABLE 8–4. *Minimum Inhibitory Concentrations of Terbinafine Against Selected Yeasts*

Organism	MIC Range (ug/ml)
Candida albicans	0.03–> 128
Candida glabrata	10–> 128
Candida guilliermondii	0.8–> 128
Candida humicola	1
Candida kefyr	0.5–50
Candida krusei	10–100
Candida parapsilosis	0.03–10
Candida tropicalis	1.2–> 128
Cryptococcus laurentii	0.08–0.6
Cryptococcus neoformans	0.06–2
Malassezia furfur	0.06–80
Rhodototula rubra	2.5–5
Trichosporon asahii	0.5–> 128

MIC, minimum inhibitory concentration.
Source: adapted from Ryder and Favre, 1997.

TABLE 8–5. *Minimum Inhibitory Concentrations of Terbinafine Against Selected Dimorphic Fungi*

Organism	MIC Range (ug/ml)
Blastomyces dermatitidis	< 0.04–1.25
Coccidioides immitis	0.3–0.6
Histoplasma capsulatum	< 0.04–0.2
Paracoccidiodes brasiliensis	0.04–0.16
Sporothrix schenckii	< 0.05–2

MIC, minimum inhibitory concentration.
Source: adapted from Ryder and Favre, 1997.

somewhat higher in adults than in children (Nejjam et al, 1995). Peak concentrations in adults following a 125 mg (2 mg/kg) dose range from 0.3 to 0.9 μg/ml, whereas the same dose in children (125 mg or 5 mg/kg) yields peak concentrations ranging between 0.4 and 1.0 μg/ml (Nejjam et al, 1995). Absorption does not appear to be influenced by coadministration of food, antacids, most H-2 receptor antagonists, or proton pump inhibitors. Coadministration with rifampin may, however, significantly increase clearance, and cimetidine can cause a 33% decrease in clearance of terbinafine (Katz, 1999).

Terbinafine, a lipophilic compound highly bound to plasma proteins (> 95%), is found in highest concentrations in adipose tissue and the keratinous tissues of the skin, nails, hair, and in sebum (Faergemann et al, 1993). Concentrations in these tissues may be 10-fold higher than simultaneous levels found in plasma.

Terbinafine is metabolized extensively by the liver and at least 15 metabolites have been identified, although none of these demonstrate significant antifungal activity (Humbert et al, 1995). Approximately 80%–85% of terbinafine metabolites are excreted in the urine and 15%–20% are excreted in the bile. The elimination half-life in normal adults is approximately 26 hours (Zehender et al, 1994). Among patients with significant renal or hepatic dysfunction, drug elimination may be delayed (Nejjam et al, 1995). Accordingly, it has been suggested that the dosing amount be reduced by 50% without altering frequency of administration among patients with either significant renal or hepatic dysfunction.

Because of the unique affinity of terbinafine for keratinous tissue, therapeutic levels can be found in stratum corneum, hair, and nails for up to 12 weeks following discontinuation of therapy. Moreover, measurable concentrations of terbinafine may be found in nail clippings up to 10 months following discontinuation of a limited course (1 to 4 weeks) of terbinafine (Faergemann et al, 1993; 1994). Among the antifungal agents, only itraconazole possesses this unique affinity for keratinous tissue and demonstrates similarly prolonged levels in skin and nails.

Topical

Topical terbinafine is widely available as an over-the-counter preparation for milder forms of dermatomycosis and onychomycosis. It is not absorbed systemically in any measurable quantity, but significant levels are achieved in the stratum corneum and the nails, although these levels do not approach those achieved with oral terbinafine (Hill et al, 1992; Faergemann et al, 1995a).

DOSING AND ADMINISTRATION

Terbinafine is available in 250 mg tablets and in a topical 1% ointment. There is no parenteral form available. Because of its extended half-life with oral administration (approximately 26 hours), the drug can be dosed once daily. When higher doses (≥ 1000 mg per day) are given, it is recommended to split the daily dose to limit gastrointestinal disturbances. Topical therapy is administered twice daily. Duration of therapy for oral terbinafine is dependant on the condition being treated. For most cases of onychomycosis, courses of 3 months may be successful, although courses from 6 to 12 months may be necessary to achieve a lasting response (Roberts, 1997). For sporotrichosis, courses of 3 to 12 months have been used successfully for patients with uncomplicated cutaneous disease (Hull and Vismer, 1997; Pappas et al, 2001). For other invasive mycoses, little data are available concerning length of oral therapy.

CLINICAL USES

Onychomycosis

The term *tinea unguium* refers to nail infections caused by typical dermatophytes whereas *onychomycosis* refers to the broader category of nail infections that also includes nondermatophytic fungi and yeast (see Chapter 24). There is considerable clinical overlap in these two entities, and few clinical clues to distinguish from among the wide assortment of causative agents (Weitzman and Summerbell, 1995).

Several open-label and placebo-controlled studies have been performed to evaluate oral terbinafine for the treatment of onychomycosis (Arenas et al, 1995; Roberts, 1997). Mycologic response rates for toenail infections treated with terbinafine 250 mg daily range between 82% and 92% among patients given 3 to 6 months of therapy (Hofmann et al, 1995; Abdel-Rahman and Nahata, 1997). Clinical cure rates are slightly less than mycologic response rates. For fingernail infections, response rates of 70% at 3 months of therapy, and 100% at 6 months have been achieved (Zaias and Serrano, 1989; Baudraz-Rosselet et al, 1992;

Goodfield et al, 1997). Surgical or chemical removal of the nail in conjunction with oral terbinafine does not appear to enhance the efficacy of terbinafine alone for onychomycosis (Albanese et al, 1995).

Based on results of comparative trials, terbinafine demonstrates greater efficacy than griseofulvin for both fingernail and toenail onychomycosis (Faergemann et al, 1995b; Haneke et al, 1995; Roberts, 1997; Abdel-Rahman and Nahata, 1997). Given the availability of safe and more effective preparations such as terbinafine and itraconazole, griseofulvin has largely fallen into disuse, having been superceded by these two newer oral antifungal agents.

Studies comparing itraconazole 200 mg daily and terbinafine 250 mg daily given for 3 months suggest similar efficacy. These compounds are associated with mycologic cure rates ranging from 67% to 92%, and clinical cure rates from 63% to 80% (Arenas et al, 1995; Brautigam et al, 1995; Roberts, 1997).

Tinea Capitis

Tinea capitis, usually caused by *Trichophyton tonsurans*, is unique among the dermatophytoses in that it does not typically respond to topical antifungal therapy. Accordingly, oral terbinafine has been evaluated for the treatment of children with tinea capitis, effecting clinical cure rates of 80% to 100% and mycologic cure rates between 90% to 100% (Haroon et al, 1992; Nejjam et al, 1995). Compared to griseofulvin in randomized, double-blind studies, clinical cure rates are generally higher with terbinafine (90% vs. 80%). Mycologic cure rates are similar (Roberts, 1997).

Other Superficial Mycoses

For other superficial dermatophyte infections such as tinea corporis, tinea cruris, tinea imbricata, and tinea pedis due to a variety of dermatophytes including *Trichophyton rubrum*, *T. mentagrophytes*, *Microsporum canis*, and *Epidermophyton floccosum*, oral terbinafine is quite effective, but for most patients with these conditions, topical therapy can be used with excellent results. Ordinarily, for patients with superficial mycoses not involving nails and/or scalp, topical therapy with terbinafine is an appropriate alternative to systemic antifungal therapy with terbinafine or itraconazole.

Sporotrichosis

Among the deep mycoses, there has been a modest experience with terbinafine for the treatment of sporotrichosis, and there have been limited reports of success with terbinafine at daily doses from as low as 125 mg per day for 3 to 18 months (Hull and Vismer, 1992; Hull and Vismer, 1997; Kudoh et al, 1996). A recently completed randomized double-blind trial compared two doses of terbinafine, either 500 mg or 1000 mg daily, administered for up to 24 weeks among patients with cutaneous or lymphocutaneous sporotrichosis (Pappas et al, 2001). Mycologic and clinical response rates approached 90% in higher dose (1000 mg/day) recipients. This success rate is not surprising given the significant concentration of terbinafine in the skin as well as excellent in vitro activity against *S. schenckii*. These response rates with terbinafine are similar to those with itraconazole for the treatment of cutaneous sporotrichosis (Restrepo et al, 1986).

Chromomycosis (Chromoblastomycosis)

Chromomycosis is a tropical fungal disease characterized by dense dermal fibrosis associated with organized granulomata. The agents of chromomycosis are typically dematiaceous (pigmented) fungi, and include such organisms as *Fonsecea pedrosi* and *Cladophialophora carrionii*. There has been sporadic use of terbinafine for patients with chromomycosis (Esterre et al, 1997). In the largest study to date, 42 patients from Madagascar with chromomycosis received terbinafine 500 mg daily for up to 1 year, and experienced 12-month mycologic and clinical cure rates of 85% and 74%, respectively (Esterre et al, 1998). While other experience with terbinafine for this disorder is limited to a small series of case reports, terbinafine appears to be a promising agent among patients with this very difficult to treat disease.

Fungal Mycetoma

There are at least 16 different fungal organisms that can cause fungal mycetoma. Terbinafine has been used sporadically at doses of 500 or 1000 mg daily with some encouraging results (Hay, 1999). For most cases of fungal mycetoma, a combined surgical and antifungal approach is necessary to achieve optimum response. No randomized and controlled studies for this disorder have been performed. For more information about eumycetoma, see Chapter 25.

Other Endemic Mycoses

Terbinafine demonstrates excellent in vitro activity vs. *H. capsulatum* and *B. dermatitidis*, but there have been no clinical trials of terbinafine therapy for these disorders. A few patients have received terbinafine for treatment of blastomycosis and histoplasmosis, generally with encouraging results (Hay, 1999). Taken together with the encouraging in vitro data, terbinafine might be considered as potential salvage therapy among patients unable to tolerate any azole drug or amphotericin B. However, given the availability and excellent efficacy of azole compounds for these conditions, it is very unlikely that terbinafine will be studied prospectively for treatment of these mycoses.

Combination Therapy for Other Deep Mycoses

One potential use of terbinafine is for combination therapy with other approved antifungal agents among patients with deep mycoses including cryptococcosis and invasive mould infections, especially invasive aspergillosis. In vitro data supporting the activity of terbinafine against *C. neoformans* led to the use of terbinafine combined with fluconazole or amphotericin B in selected patients with acute CNS cryptococcosis (Andrews et al, 1999). No significant drug–drug interactions have been observed and this combined therapeutic approach appears to be well tolerated. While prospective data assessing this approach have been not well documented, combination therapy utilizing terbinafine and fluconazole is commonly administered to patients with acute CNS cryptococcosis in Australia.

Among patients with invasive mould disease, especially invasive aspergillosis, terbinafine has been an attractive potential agent for combination therapy with either amphotericin B or a triazole such as itraconazole or voriconazole. No prospective randomized studies have been done, but small series and sporadic case reports suggest a favorable response among highly selected patients (Schiraldi and Colombo, 1997; Harari et al, 1997). For example, a group of four lung transplant patients with *Aspergillus* bronchitis were treated effectively with terbinafine 250–500 mg daily in combination with liposomal amphotericin B. Other reports of successful combination therapy among immunocompromised patients with invasive pulmonary aspergillosis have also been documented. Up to 2000 mg per day of terbinafine has been given successfully with stable clinical outcome and has been well tolerated (Schiraldi et al, 1996; Hay, 1999).

ADVERSE EFFECTS

Oral terbinafine appears to be well tolerated in the vast majority of patients and few drug–drug interactions occur. In the largest study of its kind, adverse effects were assessed in a postmarketing study involving 25,884 patients who had received terbinafine (Hall et al, 1997). Findings showed that 10.5% of patients experienced a drug-associated adverse event. Among these, the most common side effects were gastrointestinal tract symptoms including nausea, diarrhea, abdominal pain, and dyspepsia, which occurred in about 5% of patients. Skin disorders were the second most common adverse event, effecting fewer than 3% of patients. Most of the skin findings are benign rashes; however, at least 4 patients have developed psoriasis on terbinafine (Gupta et al, 1997), 2 developed significant erythema multiforme (Hall et al, 1997) and 1 a generalized pustular eruption (Bennett et al, 1999). Hepatobiliary adverse events have been reported in fewer than 1% of patients and include cholestatic jaundice with mild to moderate hepatocellular dysfunction (Gupta et al, 1998a; Fernandes et al, 1998; Conjeevaram et at, 2001). Less commonly reported adverse events include neutropenia (Gupta et al, 1998b; Shapiro et al, 1999), thrombocytopenia (Kovacs et al, 1994; Amichai and Gruhwald, 1998), toxic epidermal necrolysis (Carstens et al, 1994) and angioedema (Hall et al, 1997). No deaths have been attributed directly to terbinafine.

Despite the frequent concomitant use of other medications, including immunosuppressive agents as well as any other systemic antifungal compounds, terbinafine is an unusual cause of significant drug–drug interaction (Balfour and Faulds, 1992; Katz, 1999). The lack of interaction of terbinafine with the mammalian cytochrome P-450 enzyme system is believed to be responsible for this important characteristic. Unlike the azole antifungal compounds, terbenafine does not appear to significantly alter the metabolism of cyclosporine, tacrolimus, or sirolimus.

SUMMARY

Terbinafine is a broad spectrum oral and topical antifungal agent that possesses a unique mechanism of activity distinct from other available systemic antifungal agents. Most clinical experience with this antifungal has been in the treatment of onychomycosis and other superficial fungal infections, but there is a growing body of experience with terbinafine for the treatment of deeper mycoses, especially cutaneous and lymphocutaneous sporotrichosis. The potential for use of terbinafine as a combination agent with another antifungal drug for the treatment of cryptococcosis and invasive mould disease is exciting. However, prospectively designed studies to address this question have not been performed; thus, this potential remains largely unexplored.

REFERENCES

Abdel-Rahman S M, Nahata M C. Oral terbinafine: a new antifungal agent. *Ann Pharmacother* 31:445–456, 1997.
Albanese G, DiCintio R, Martini C, Nocoletti A. Short therapy for tinea unguium with terbinafine: four different courses of treatment. *Mycoses* 38:211–214, 1995.
Amichai B, Grunwald M H. Adverse drug reactions of the new oral antifungal agents–terbinafine, fluconazole, and itraconazole. *Int J Dermatol* 37: 410–415, 1998.
Andrews A, Pfeiffer T, Bell J, Ellis D. In vitro activity of terbinafine and fluconazole against 205 clinical and environmental isolates of *Cryptococcus neoformans*. Programme and Abstracts 4th Annual International Conference on Cryptococcus and Cryptococcosis, September 12–16, London, England, Abstract #PC 30, p. 197, 1999.
Arenas R, Dominguez-Cherit J, Fernandez L M. Open randomized comparison of itraconazole versus terbinafine in onychomycosis. *Int J Dermatol* 34:138–143, 1995.
Arzeni D, Barchiesi F, Compagnuci P, Cellini A, Simonetti O, Offi-

dani A M, Scalisi G. In vitro activity of terbinafine against clinical isolates of dermatophytes. *Med Mycol* 36:235–237, 1998.

Balfour J A, Faulds D. Terbinafine: a review of its pharmacodynamic and pharmacokinetic properties, and therapeutic potential in superficial mycoses. *Drugs* 43:259–284, 1992.

Baudraz-Rosselet F, Rakosi T, Wili P B, Kenzelmann R. Treatment of onychomycosis with terbinafine. *Br J Dermatol* 126(suppl 39):40–46, 1992.

Bennett M L, Jorizzo J L, White W L. Generalized pustular eruptions associated with oral terbinafine. *Int J Dermatol* 38:596–600, 1999.

Birnbaum J E. Pharmacology of allylamines. *J Am Acad Dermatol* 23:782–785, 1990.

Brautigam M, Nolting S, Schopf R E, Weidinger G. Randomized double-blind comparison of terbinafine and itraconazole for the treatment of toenail tinea infections. *Br Med J* 311:919–922, 1995.

Bryan C S, Smith C W, Berg D E, Karp R B. *Curvularia lunata* endocarditis treated with terbinafine: case report. *Clin Infect Dis* 16:30–32, 1993.

Carstens J, Wendelboe P, Sogaard H, Thestrup-Pederson K. Toxic epidermal necrolysis and erythema multiforme following therapy with terbinafine. *Acta Dermatol Venereol* 74:391–392, 1994.

Conjeevaram G, Vongthavaravat V, Summer R, Koff R S. Terbinafine-induced hepatitis and pancytopenia. *Dig Dis Sci* 46:1714–1716, 2001.

Esterre P, Ratsioharana M, Roig P. Potential use of terbinafine in the treatment of chromoblastomycosis. *Rev Contemp Pharmacother* 8:357–362, 1997.

Esterre P, Intani C, Ratsioharana M, Andriantsmahavandy A. A multicenter trial of terbinafine in patients with chromoblastomycosis: effect on clinical and biologic criteria. *J Dermatol Treat* 9:529–534, 1998.

Faergemann J, Zehender H, Denouel J, Hilarious L. Levels of terbinafine in plasma, stratum corneum, dermis-epidermis (without stratum corneum), sebum, hair, and nails during and after 250 mg terbinafine orally once per day for four weeks. *Acta Dermatol Venereol* 73:305–309, 1993.

Faergemann J, Zehender H, Denouel J, Hilarious L. Levels of terbinafine in plasma, stratum corneum, dermis-epidermis without stratum corneum), sebum, hair, and nails during and after 250 mg terbinafine orally once daily for 7 and 14 days. *Clin Exp Dermatol* 19:121–126, 1994.

Faergemann J, Zehender H, Boukhabza A, Ganslandt J, Jones T C. Comparison of terbinafine levels in stratum corneum and dermis-epidermis (without stratum corneum) after topical or topical combined with oral therapy in healthy volunteers. *J Eur Acad Dermatol Venereol* 5(Suppl 1):S94, 1995a.

Faergemann J, Anderson C, Hersle K, Hradil E, Nordin P, Kaaman T, Molin L, Petterson A. Double-blind, parallel-group comparison of terbinafine and griseofulvin in the treatment of toenail onychomycosis. *J Am Acad Dermatol* 32:750–753, 1995b.

Faergemann J. Pharmacokinetics of terbinafine. *Rev Contemp Pharmacother* 8:289–297, 1997.

Fernandes N F, Geller S A, Fong T L. Terbinafine hepatotoxicity: case report and review of the literature. *Am J Gastroenterol* 93:459–460, 1998.

Goodfield M J, Andrew L, Evans E G. Short-term treatment of dermatophyte onychomycosis with terbinafine. *Br Med J* 304:1151–1154, 1992.

Gupta A K, Sibbald R G, Knowles S R, Lynde C W, Shear N H. Terbinafine therapy may be associated with the development of psoriasis de novo or its exacerbation: four case reports and a review of drug-induced psoriasis. *J Am Acad Dermatol* 36:858–862, 1997.

Gupta A K, Del Rosso J Q, Lynde C W, Brown G H, Shear N H. Hepatitis associated with terbinafine therapy: three case reports and a review of the literature. *Clin Exp Dermatol* 23:64–67, 1998a.

Gupta A K, Soori G S, Del Rossa J Q, Bartos P B, Shear N H. Severe neutropenia associated with oral terbinafine therapy. *J Am Acad Dermatol* 38:765–767, 1998b.

Hall M, Monka C, Krupp P, O'Sullivan D. Safety of oral terbinafine: results of a post marketing surveillance study in 25,884 patients. *Arch Dermatol* 133:1213–1219, 1997.

Haneke E, Tausch I, Brautigam M, Weidinger G, Welzel D. Short-duration treatment of fingernail dermatophytosis: a randomized, double-blind study with terbinafine and griseofulvin. *J Am Acad Dermatol* 32:72–77, 1995.

Harari S, Schiraldi G F, de Juli E, Gronda E. Relapsing *Aspergillus* bronchitis in a double lung transplant patient, successfully treated with a new oral antimycotic agent [Letter] *Chest* 111:835–836, 1997.

Haroon T S, Hussain I, Mahmood A, Nagi A H, Ahman D, Zahid M. An open clinical pilot study of the efficacy and safety of oral terbinafine in dry non-inflammatory tinea capitis. *Br J Dermatol* 126(Suppl 39):47–50, 1992.

Hay R J. Therapeutic potential of terbinafine in subcutaneous and systemic mycoses. *Br J Dermatol* 141(Suppl. 56):36–40, 1999.

Hill S, Thomas R, Smith S G. An investigation of the pharmacokinetics of topical terbinafine 1% cream. *Br J Dermatol* 127:396–400, 1992.

Hiratani T, Asagi Y, Yamaguchi H. Evaluation of in vitro antimycotic activity of terbinafine, a new allylamine agent. *Jpn J Med Mycol* 32:323–332, 1991.

Hofmann H, Brautigam M, Weidinger G, Zaun H, Lagos II. Treatment of toenail onychomycosis. *Arch Dermatol* 131:919–922, 1995.

Hull P R, Vismer H F. Treatment of cutaneous sporotrichosis with terbinafine. *Br J Dermatol* 126:51–55, 1992.

Hull P R, Vismer H F. Potential use of terbinafine in the treatment of cutaneous sporotrichosis. *Rev Contemp Pharmacother* 8:343–347, 1997.

Humbert H, Cabiac M D, Denouel J, Kirkesseli S. Pharmacokinetics of terbinafine and its five main metabolites in plasma and urine, following a single oral dose in healthy subjects. *Biopharm Drug Dispos* 16:685–694, 1995.

Jensen J C. Clinical pharmacokinetics of terbinafine. *Clin Exp Dermatol* 14:110–114, 1989.

Jessup C J, Ryder N S, Ghannoum M A. An evaluation of the in vitro activity of terbinafine. *Mycol* 38:155–159, 2000.

Katz H I. Drug interactions of the newer oral antifungal agents. *Br J Dermatol* 141(Suppl. 56):26–32, 1999.

Kovacs M J, Alshammari S, Guenther L, Bourcier M. Neutropenia and pancytopenia associated with oral terbinafine. *J Am Acad Dermatol* 31:806, 1994.

Kudoh K, Kamei E, Terunama A, Nakagawa S, Tagami H. Successful treatment of cutaneous sporotrichosis with terbinafine. *J Dermatol Treat* 7:33–35, 1996.

Nejjam F, Zagula M, Cabiac M D, Guessous N, Humbert H, Lakhdar H. Pilot study of terbinafine in children suffering from tinea capitis: evaluation of efficacy, safety and pharmacokinetics. *Br J Dermatol* 132:98–105, 1995.

Pappas P G, Bustamante B, Nolasco D, Restrepo A, Toban A, Tiraboschi Foss N, Dietze R, Fothergill A, Perez A, Felser J. Treatment of lymphocutaneous sporotrichosis with terbinafine: results of randomized double-blind trial. 39th Annual Infectious Diseases Society of America Meeting, San Francisco, CA, Abstract #648, 2001.

Petranyi G, Ryder N S, Stutz A. Allylamine derivatives: new class of synthetic antifungal agents inhibiting fungal squalene epoxidase. *Science* 224:1239–1241, 1984.

Petranyi G, Meingassner J G, Mieth H. Antifungal activity of the allylamine derivative terbinafine in vitro. *Antimicrob Agents Chemother* 31:1365–1368, 1987.

Restrepo A, Robledo J, Gomez I, Tabares A M, Gutierrez R. Itraconazole therapy in lymphangitic and cutaneous sporotrichosis. *Arch Dermatol* 122:413–417, 1986.

Rinaldi M G. In vitro susceptibility of dermatophytes to antifungal drugs. *Int J Dermatol* 32:502–503, 1993.

Roberts D T. The clinical efficacy of terbinafine in the treatment of fungal infections of nails. *Rev Contemp Pharmacother* 8:299–312, 1997.

Ryder N S, Dupont M C. Inhibition of squalene epoxidase by allylamine antimycotic compounds: a comparative study of fungal and mammalian enzymes. *Biochem J* 230:765–770, 1985.

Ryder N S. Terbinafine: mode of action and properties of the squalene epoxidase inhibition. *Br J Dermatol* 126(suppl 39):2–7, 1992.

Ryder N S, Leitner L. Activity of terbinafine against *Aspergillus* in vitro, in combination with amphotericin B or triazoles. 36th Interscience Conference on Antimicrobial Agents and Chemotherapy. New Orleans, LA. American Society for Microbiology, Abstract E54, 1996.

Ryder N S, Favre B. Antifungal activity and mechanism of action of terbinafine. *Rev Contemp Pharmacother* 8:275–287, 1997.

Ryder N S, Wagner S, Leitner I. In vitro activities of terbinafine against cutaneous isolates of *Candida albicans* and other pathogenic yeasts. *Antimicrob Agents Chemother* 42:1057–1061, 1998.

Schiraldi G F, Lo Cicero S, Colombo M D, Rossato D, Ferrarese M, Soresi E. Refractory pulmonary aspergillosis: compassionate trial with terbinafine. *Br J Dermatol* 134(Suppl 46):25–29, 1996.

Schiraldi G F, Colombo M D. Potential use of terbinafine in the treatment of aspergillosis. *Rev Contemp Pharmacother* 8:349–356, 1997.

Schmitt H J, Bernard E M, Andrade J, Edwards F, Schmitt B, Armstrong D. MIC and fungicidal activity of terbinafine against clinical isolates of *Aspergillus* spp. *Antimicrob Agents Chemother* 32:1619–1623, 1987.

Schuster I. The interaction of representative members from two classes of antimycotics–the azoles and the allylamines–with cytochromes P450 in steroidogenic tissues and liver. *Xenobiotica* 15:29–46, 1985.

Shadomy S, Espinel-Ingroff A, Gebhart R J. In vitro studies with SF 86–327, a new orally active allylamine derivative. *Sabouraudia* 23:125–132, 1985.

Shapiro M, Li L, Miller J. Terbinafine-induced neutropenia. *Br J Dermatol* 140:1169–1199, 1999.

Venugopal P V, Venugopal T V, Ramakrishna E S, Illavarasin S. Antifungal activity of allylamines against agents of eumycetoma. *Indian J Dermatol Venereol Leprol* 59:239–242, 1993.

Weitzman I, Summerbell R C. The dermatophytes. *Clin Microbiol Rev* 8:240–259, 1995.

Wong P K, Ching W T, Gwon-Chung K J, Meyer R D. Disseminated *Phialophora parasitica* infection in humans: case report and review. *Rev Infect Dis* 11:770–775, 1989.

Zaias N, Serrano L. The successful treatment of finger *Trichophyton rubrum* onychomycosis with oral terbinafine. *Clin Exp Dermatol* 14:120–123, 1989.

Zehender H, Cabiac M D, Denouel J, Faergemann J, Donatsch P, Kutz K. Elimination kinetics of terbinafine from human plasma and tissue following multiple-dose administration, and comparison with 3 main metabolites. *Drug Invest* 8:203–210, 1994.

9

Resistance to antifungal drugs

DOMINIQUE SANGLARD

Fungal infections caused by fungal pathogens remain quite common in immunocompromised hosts, especially in HIV-infected individuals, and in patients given immunosuppressive drugs or broad-spectrum antibiotics. *Candida* spp. represent the major group of yeast species recovered from these infected individuals; however, other yeasts such as *Cryptococcus neoformans* are also pathogens (Fridkin and Jarvis, 1996). Among filamentous fungi causing infections in humans, *Aspergillus fumigatus* is a common pathogen and is associated with a high mortality (Latge, 1999). Not only are a restricted number of antifungal agents available to treat these infections, but also resistance to antifungal drugs can occur. Table 9–1 summarizes the activity of known antifungal agents against *Candida* spp., *C. neoformans*, and *A. fumigatus* and also includes drugs in the late stages of development. The data given in Table 9–1 indicate that most of the agents show some activity against these pathogens. However, weak antifungal activity can be seen for the pyrimidine analogue, flucytosine, and azole agent, fluconazole, against *A. fumigatus*, for fluconazole against *C. glabrata* and *C. krusei*, and for the echinocandins against *C. neoformans*.

Resistance to antifungal treatment can develop on the basis of clinical and microbiological factors. A persistent infection despite treatment with an antifungal drug at maximal dosage may be described as clinically resistant to the therapeutic agent. However, the infecting organism may show normal susceptibility to the agent in vitro (Rex et al, 1997). Clinical resistance to treatment may result from microbial resistance to an agent, but may also be the result of complex interactions between an antimicrobial agent and the infecting microbe in a human host. Microbiological resistance can be defined as a shift (i.e., a decrease) in antifungal drug susceptibility that can be measured in vitro by appropriate laboratory methods. Resistance to specific antifungal drugs can be intrinsic (primary resistance) in some fungal pathogens as indicated above, and resistance can be also acquired (secondary resistance) either in a transient or permanent manner. The distinction between a susceptible and a resistant yeast or mould iso-

late can be made when a threshold drug susceptibility value, i.e., the breakpoint minimal inhibitory concentration (MIC) is reached. In medical practice, breakpoint values should predict ideally the success or the failure of an antifungal drug. However, experiences accumulated with different antifungal agents showed that this association cannot always be applied (Rex et al, 1997). Table 9–2 gives interpretative MIC breakpoint values for fluconazole, itraconazole, and flucytosine against *Candida albicans*. An intermediate breakpoint is given, the so-called dose-dependent susceptible (DDS) MIC, indicating that the drug dosage is important when a fungal pathogen possessing a DDS MIC value is identified. The breakpoint MIC values of a given fungal pathogen for a specific drug are less relevant for the microbiologist or the molecular biologist, since only a modest shift of antifungal drug susceptibility measured by increase in MIC values can be the consequence of one or several cellular alterations linked to modifications of the genetic material. This chapter reviews the present knowledge about resistance of fungal pathogens to the major antifungal agents and details the current understanding of the mechanisms of resistance. Recent published reviews on this topic provide complementary information (Kontoyiannis and Lewis, 2002; Lupetti et al, 2002; Masia Canuto and Gutierrez Rodero, 2002; Perea and Patterson, 2002a; Sanglard, 2002a; Sanglard and Odds, 2002b).

ANTIFUNGAL DRUGS IN CURRENT USE: MODE OF ACTION AND RESISTANCE

Polyenes

Polyenes belong to a class of natural antifungal compounds discovered in the early 1950s. One of the most successful polyene derivatives, AmB, is produced by *Streptomyces nodosus*. Amphotericin B can form soluble salts in both basic and acidic environments, is not orally or intramuscularly absorbed, and is virtually insoluble in water. The primary mode of action of AmB is to bind ergosterol in the membrane bilayer of sus-

TABLE 9–1. *Activities of Antifungal Agents Against* Candida Species, Cryptococcus neoformans *and* Aspergillus fumigatus

Antifungal Agent	MIC$_{90}$* (μg/ml)							Reference
	C. albicans	C. glabrata	C. krusei	C. parapsilosis	C. tropicalis	C. neoformans	A. fumigatus	
Amphotericin B	0.5	1	0.5	0.5	0.5	1	4	Brandt et al, 2001; Coleman et al, 1998 Coleman et al, 1998; Gehrt et al, 1995)
Flucytosine	4	0.5	16–32	1	4	16	> 64	
Azoles								
Fluconazole	1	64	64	2	2	16	> 128	Brandt et al, 2001; Mosquera and Denning, 2002; Pfaller et al, 1998; Pfaller et al, 1999; Uchida et al, 2001; Yamazumi et al, 2000; Yildiran et al, 2000
Itraconazole	0.25	4.0	2.0	0.5	0.5	1	0.125	
Voriconazole	0.06	2.0	1.0	0.12	0.25	0.25	0.5	
Posaconazole	0.06	4.0	0.5	0.12	0.25	< 0.015	0.031	
Ravuconazole	0.03	4.0	0.5	0.12	0.25	0.25	1	
Lipopeptides								
Caspofungin	0.5	0.5	1	0.5	1	32	N.A.**	Bartizal et al, 1997; Chavez et al, 1999; Espinel-Ingroff, 1998; Mikamo et al, 2000; Pfaller et al, 1997; Tawara et al, 2000
Micafungin	0.0156	0.156	0.125	1	0.0313	> 64	N.A.	
Anidulafungin	0.125	0.5	0.25	4	0.125	> 16	N.A.	

*MIC$_{90}$ is defined as the minimum inhibitory concentration value to which 90% of a study population belongs.
**N.A., not available by means of standard MIC tests.

TABLE 9–2. *National Committee for Clinical Laboratory Standards Interpretive Breakpoints Against* Candida albicans*

Antifungal Agent	Susceptible	Dose-Dependent Susceptible	Resistant
Fluconazole	≤ 8	16–32	≥ 64
Itraconazole	≤ 0.125	0.25–0.5	≥ 1
Flucytosine	≤ 4		≤ 32

*Data in μg/ml.

ceptible organisms, presumably resulting in the production of aqueous pores consisting of polyene molecules linked to the membrane sterols. This configuration gives rise to a pore-like structure, leakage of vital cytoplasmic components (mono- or divalent cations), and death of the organism. Amphotericin B has a strong fungicidal effect on most important yeast pathogens. Time-kill curves in several studies showed that AmB induces a 3 to 4 log decrease in viable colony counts in a time span of 2 to 4 hours at supra-MIC concentrations. The MICs of AmB are dependent on several factors and among them is the composition of the testing medium. Rex and coworkers recommended the use of a special broth medium (AM3) to determine AmB MICs against *Candida* species (Rex et al, 1995). Presently, a standard protocol, M-27A using AM3 medium, has been recommended by the NCCLS. Recently, other investigators evaluated an agar diffusion method using E-test with RPMI or AM3 as media in order to discriminate AmB-resistant from AmB-susceptible *Candida* isolates (Peyron et al, 2001). The MIC_{90} values for AmB against various *Candida* species including *C. albicans*, *C. glabrata*, *C. parapsilosis*, or *C. tropicalis* range from 0.25 to 1 μg/ml (Table 9–1). Microbiological resistance to AmB can be intrinsic or acquired. Intrinsic resistance to AmB is common for some *C. lusitaniae* isolates (Pfaller et al, 1994) and for *Trichosporon* species (Walsh et al, 1990), while acquired resistance during antifungal treatment with AmB is still rarely reported among yeast isolates. Some *C. lusitaniae* isolates are also able to undergo rapid in vitro switches to AmB resistance when exposed to the drug (Yoon et al, 1999).

Acquired resistance to AmB is often associated with alteration of membrane lipids and especially sterols. *Candida albicans* clinical isolates resistant to AmB have been shown to lack ergosterol and to accumulate other sterols (3β-ergosta-7,22-dienol and 3β-ergosta-8-enol) typical for a defect in the sterol $\Delta^{5,6}$ desaturase system (Nolte et al, 1997). Such a defect is known in *S. cerevisiae* harboring a defect of the $\Delta^{5,6}$ desaturase gene *ERG3* (Arthington et al, 1991; Watson et al, 1988). Curiously, the disruption of the *ERG3* gene in *C. albicans* is not linked to AmB resistance (Sanglard, unpublished). This contrasts with the results obtained in clinical strains, which probably possess other compen-

satory mutations resulting in AmB resistance. A defect in Δ^{8-7} isomerase in a clinical *C. neoformans* isolate from an AIDS patient also was linked with AmB resistance (Kelly et al, 1994). A decrease in the content of cell membrane-associated ergosterol also can cause AmB resistance, since AmB requires the presence of ergosterol to damage fungal cells. Different investigations supported this possibility by demonstrating that (1) development of inducible resistance (induced by an adaptation mechanism) in a strain of *C. albicans* was accompanied by a decrease in the ergosterol content of the cells; and (2) polyene-resistant *C. albicans* clinical isolates obtained from neutropenic patients had a 74% to 85% decrease in their ergosterol content (Dick et al, 1980). Another mechanism accounting for the resistance of yeasts to AmB is thought to be mediated by increased catalase activity, which can contribute to diminished oxidative damage caused by AmB (Sokol-Anderson et al, 1986).

Flucytosine

Flucytosine (5-FC), which belongs to the class of pyrimidine analogues, was developed in the 1950s as a potential antineoplastic agent. Abandoned as an anticancer drug due to its lack of activity against tumors, 5-FC showed good in vitro and in vivo antifungal activity. Because 5-FC is highly water-soluble, it can be administered by oral and intravenous routes (Polak, 1990). Flucytosine is taken up by fungal cells by a cytosine permease and deaminated by a cytosine deaminase to 5-fluorouracil (5-FU), a potent antimetabolite, which is converted to a nucleoside triphosphate and, when incorporated into RNA, causes miscoding. In addition, 5-FU can be converted to a deoxynucleoside, which inhibits thymidylate synthase and thereby DNA synthesis. Flucytosine shows little toxicity in mammalian cells, since cytosine deaminase is absent or poorly active in these cells. However, while 5-FU is a potent anticancer agent, it is impermeable to fungal cells. The conversion of 5-FC to 5-FU is facilitated by intestinal bacteria; consequently, oral 5-FC is associated with toxicity. Flucytosine is fungicidal against susceptible yeasts and fungi. A high variability in 5-FC MICs is observed against *Candida* species and *C. neoformans* because of the occurrence of intrinsic resistance. MIC_{90} values for 5-FC range from 0.5 to 4 μg/ml for *Candida* species including *C. albicans*, *C. parapsilosis*, *C. tropicalis*, and *C. glabrata* and for *C. neoformans* (Coleman et al, 1998) (Table 9–1).

Flucytosine is not usually administered as a single agent because of rapid development of resistance; therefore, it is used mainly in combination with other agents, particularly with AmB. In vitro data regarding the combination of both drugs against *Candida* species and *C. neoformans* are numerous and somewhat contradictory, showing antagonistic, indifferent, or synergistic effects (Groll et al, 1998). Flucytosine is also an antifungal agent against which fungal resistance can be either intrinsic or acquired. Resistance may occur due to the deficiency or lack of enzymes implicated in the metabolism of 5-FC or may be due to the deregulation of the pyrimidine biosynthetic pathway, in which products can compete with the fluorinated metabolites of 5-FC. Detailed investigations on the molecular mechanisms of resistance to 5-FC have shown that intrinsic resistance to 5-FC by fungi can be due to a defect in the cytosine permease (as observed in *C. glabrata* but not in *C. albicans* and *C. neoformans*). By contrast, acquired resistance results from a failure to metabolize 5-FC to 5-fluorouridine triphosphate (5-FUTP) and 5-fluorodeoxyuridine monophosphate (5-FdUMP) or from the loss of feedback control of pyrimidine biosynthesis (Whelan, 1988).

Azoles

Azole antifungal agents, discovered in the late 1960s, are synthetic compounds that constitute the largest group of available antifungal agents. Azole drugs used in medicine are categorized into N-1 substituted imidazoles (ketoconazole, miconazole, clotrimazole) and triazoles (fluconazole, itraconazole). The new generation of broader spectrum azoles are also triazoles (voriconazole, posaconazole, and ravuconazole).

Azoles have a cytochrome P450 as a common cellular target in yeasts or moulds (Fig. 9–1). This cytochrome P450, now referred to as Erg11p, is the product of the *ERG11* gene. The unhindered nitrogen of the imidazole or triazole ring of azole antifungal agents binds to the heme iron of Erg11p as a sixth ligand, thus inhibiting the enzymatic reaction. The affinity of imidazole and triazole derivatives is not only dependent on this interaction, but is also determined by the N-1 substituent, which is actually responsible for the high affinity of azole antifungal agents to their target. Each of these agents has distinct pharmacokinetics and their antifungal efficacy is different against yeast and mould species of medical relevance. Azole antifungals have a broad spectrum of activity as indicated in Table 9–1. For an inclusive discussion about the azoles (pharmacology, spectrum of activity, toxicity and clinical indications), see Chapter 6.

Reports on resistance to azole antifungal agents were rare until the late 1980s. The first cases of resistance were reported in *C. albicans* after prolonged therapy with miconazole and ketoconazole. Following the widespread use of fluconazole in a variety of clinical settings in the 1990s, antifungal resistance to this azole has been reported more frequently (White et al, 1998). There are several mechanisms by which yeasts or filamentous fungi can become resistant to azole antifungal agents. These mechanisms are illustrated in Figure 9–1.

Resistance by Altered Drug Transport

Failure to accumulate azole antifungal drugs has been identified as a cause of azole resistance in several posttreatment clinical fungal isolates, including yeast species such as *C. albicans*, *C. glabrata*, *C. krusei*, *C. dubliniensis*, and *C. neoformans* (Sanglard and Bille, 2002c). In azole-resistant yeasts, genes encoding ATP binding cassette (ABC)-transporters were upregulated as compared to most azole-susceptible species (Fig. 9–1). So far, only *Candida* drug resistance 1 (*CDR1*) and *Candida* drug resistance 2 (*CDR2*) genes in C. albicans (Sanglard et al, 1997; Sanglard et al, 1995; White, 1997a), *CdCDR1* gene in *C. dubliniensis* (Moran et al, 1998; Perea et al, 2002b), a *CDR1* homologue in *C. tropicalis* (Barchiesi et al, 2000), *CgCDR1* and *CgCDR2* genes in *C. glabrata* (Sanglard et al, 1999; Sanglard et al, 2001) and *CnDR* gene in *C. neoformans* (Posteraro et al, 2003), have been identified as ABC-transporter genes upregulated in azole-resistant isolates. In *A. fumigatus*, itraconazole is able to induce an ABC-transporter gene, *atrF*; however, the role of this gene in the resistance of clinical isolates to itraconazole is still not clearly established (Slaven et al, 2002). Heterologous expression of ABC-transporter genes such as *CDR1* and *CDR2*, *CdCDR1*, *CgCDR1*, and *CgCDR2* in *S. cerevisiae* conferred resistance not only to several azole derivatives (fluconazole, itraconazole, ketoconazole) but also to a wide range of other compounds including antifungal drugs and metabolic inhibitors (Sanglard et al, 1997; Sanglard et al, 1999; Nakamura et al, 2001). With the sequence data available from the genomes of yeast pathogens (*C. albicans*, *C. glabrata*, *C. tropicalis*, *C. neoformans*), it is possible that additional multidrug transporter genes involved in antifungal resistance will be characterized in the future.

Besides upregulation of ABC-transporter genes, several laboratories have also observed that a multidrug transporter gene named *CaMDR1* (Multidrug Resistance 1, previously known as *BEN^r* for Benomyl resistance) and belonging to the family of Major Facilitators, was upregulated in some *C. albicans* azole-resistant clinical isolates (Sanglard et al, 1995; White, 1997a) (Fig. 9–1). Deletion of *CaMDR1* in C. albicans isolates with acquired azole resistance by *CaMDR1* upregulation resulted in a sharp increase in azole susceptibility, thus supporting by a genetic approach, the involvement of this specific gene in azole resistance (Wirsching et al, 2000b). Deletion of *CaMDR1* in an azole-susceptible laboratory strain of *C. albicans* did not result in a significant increase in azole susceptibil-

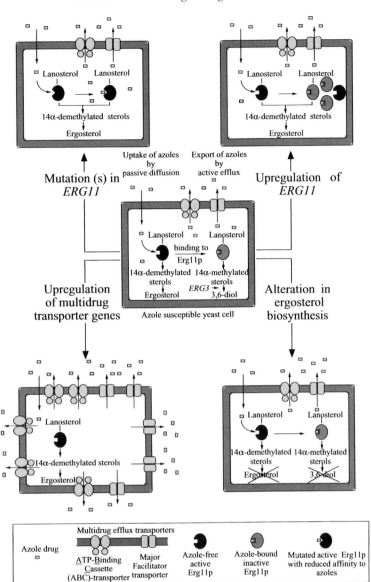

FIGURE 9–1. Schematic view of the four main resistance mechanisms to azole antifungals in yeast pathogens. Erg11p, the cellular target of azole antifungals, is responsible for the demethylation of lanosterol. 14α-demethylated sterols serve as further substrates in the formation of ergosterol. When azole drugs bind Erg11p, lanosterol demethylation is blocked and sterol metabolites remain methylated at the position 14α. The toxic metabolite 3,6-diol (14α-methylergosta-8,24(28)-dien-3β,6α-diol) is formed from the action of ERG3 on 14α-methylfecosterol. Details on specific resistance mechanisms are given in the text.

ity, providing further evidence that *CaMDR1* is almost not expressed in this type of strain and more generally, in azole-susceptible clinical isolates (Sanglard et al, 1996). Upregulation of a *CaMDR1*-like gene has also been observed in a fluconazole-exposed *C. tropicalis* isolate, which acquired cross-resistance to fluconazole and itraconazole (Barchiesi et al, 2000). Upregulation of another *CaMDR1*-like gene (*CdMDR1*) has been reported in fluconazole-resistant *C. dubliniensis* isolates (Wirsching et al, 2001; Perea et al, 2002b). In addition, *CdMDR1* has been deleted in this yeast species, al-

lowing a genetic correlation between the presence of this gene and acquired azole-resistance (Wirsching et al, 2001).

In most cases, azole resistance acquired in clinical situations by multidrug transporters in yeast pathogens is maintained over a high number of generations in vitro without drug selection. Azole resistance can be, however, a reversible phenomenon. Marr and collaborators obtained *C. albicans* isolates developing azole resistance from bone marrow transplant patients receiving fluconazole treatment (Marr et al, 1998). Increase in fluconazole MIC was coupled with upregulation of *CDR1* but the MIC decreased with a parallel decrease in *CDR1* expression in drug-free subculture. Azole-susceptible isolates from these type of patients, when exposed in vitro to fluconazole, developed reversible azole resistance by the same *CDR1* upregulation mechanism. Interestingly, only a portion of individually exposed colonies were rendered less susceptible to fluconazole, thus indicating that heteroresistance, which had already been described in azole-exposed *C. neoformans* isolates, could also occur in specific *C. albicans* isolates (Marr et al, 2001). Another interesting acquisition of azole resistance in a clinical context by multidrug transporter upregulation has been provided by *C. glabrata*. This yeast can convert to azole resistance by loss of mitochondrial DNA. The phenomenon, also called high frequency azole resistance (HFAR) because it occurs in vitro at high frequencies, was coupled with upregulation of both *CgCDR1* and the novel ABC-transporter gene *CgCDR2* (Sanglard et al, 2001).

The molecular basis for the upregulation of multidrug transporters belonging to the ABC and Major Facilitator families is being actively pursued in yeast pathogens. Investigators believe that the mutation(s) leading to gene upregulation might rather be caused by alterations in trans (i.e., those involving transcription factors). Using the *Renilla* luciferase reporter system fused to *CDR1* and *CDR2* promoters cloned from azole-susceptible isolates, de Micheli and colleagues showed that the expression of these genes was enhanced in an azole-resistant strain, in which these genes are constitutively upregulated (de Micheli et al, 2002). With another reporter system (i.e., gene-encoding green fluorescent protein fused to the *CaMDR1* promoter from an azole-susceptible strain), investigators showed that high fluorescence could be obtained when the chimeric construct was introduced into azole-resistant strains upregulating *CaMDR1* (Wirsching et al, 2000a). Until now, only the *CDR1* and *CDR2* promoters have been dissected systematically for the presence of regulatory elements. A common drug responsive element (DRE) in both promoters could be experimentally delimited with the consensus 5'-CGGA(A/T)ATCG-GATATTTTTTT-3', which has no equivalent in eukaryotic promoter databases (de Micheli et al, 2002). This DRE is necessary for *CDR1* and *CDR2* transient upregulation by drugs and for constitutive upregulation in an azole-resistant isolate. However, the detailed pathway resulting in *CDR* gene upregulation and the identity of proteins binding to the DRE remain to be determined.

No published data are yet available on the dissection of the *CaMDR1* promoter. In this promoter however, a AP1–like binding site (TTAGTAA) is present at −470 from the ATG start codon, suggesting that an AP1-like

transcription factor might interact with the regulation of *CaMDR1* (Sanglard, unpublished). *Saccharomyces cerevisiae* possesses an AP1-like transcription factor, *YAP1*, which mediates the expression of fluconazole resistance 1 (*FLR1*), a gene similar to *CaMDR1* in *S. cerevisiae* (Alarco et al, 1997a). This transcription factor shuffles from the cytoplasm to the nucleus under oxidative stress conditions and thus activates the transcription of target genes (Kuge et al, 2001). A *C. albicans* homologue of *YAP1*, *CAP1*, has been isolated and its disruption affects survival under oxidative stress stimulated by exposure to H_2O_2 (Alarco and Raymond, 1997b). Deletion of *CAP1* also affects, but not abolishes, responsiveness of *CaMDR1* in the presence of benomyl, thus suggesting that *CAP1* and yet unknown factors have the ability to interact with *CaMDR1* (Sanglard, unpublished). In an azole-resistant isolate in which *CaMDR1* upregulation was detected, *CAP1* deletion has been performed. In this case, however, no decrease of *CaMDR1* expression could be measured, thus suggesting that *CaMDR1* upregulation can be caused by *CAP1*-independent upregulation pathway(s) (Sanglard, unpublished).

Multidrug transporter genes can be upregulated in *C. glabrata* by the HFAR phenomenon as mentioned above. High frequency azole resistance strains show high constitutive expression of the ABC-transporters *CgCDR1* and *CgCDR2*, thus explaining the high level fluconazole resistance measured in these strains of *C. glabrata* (Sanglard et al, 2001). *CgCDR1* and *CgCDR2* promoters contain DNA regulatory elements, so-called pleotropic drug responsive elements (PDRE), first described in the promoter of the *S. cerevisiae PDR5* gene, the product of which is an important ABC transporter having similar functions as the *C. albicans CDR1* and the *C. glabrata CgCDR1* genes (Katzmann et al, 1996). The regulatory circuit of *PDR5* involves two transcription factors (*PDR1* and *PDR3*). Thus, it is likely that similar factors could function for the upregulation of *CgCDR1* and *CgCDR2* in *C. glabrata*. Multidrug transporter upregulation in *C. glabrata* can be considered as basically different from transporter upregulation in *C. albicans*, given that *CDR* genes do not possess PDRE-like sequences, but rather unrelated DRE sequences in their promoters, making it likely that different transcription factors will bind to these sequences. Surprisingly, *C. albicans* genes related to *PDR1* and *PDR3* have been isolated by functional complementation in *S. cerevisiae* and can activate the transcription of *PDR5* via the PDRE sequences (Yang et al, 2001).

One of the implications of the involvement of multidrug efflux transporters in resistance to azole antifungal drugs is that these transporters have the ability to mediate cross-resistance to unrelated antifungals or metabolic inhibitors. In order to determine whether or not a given substance is a potential substrate for multidrug efflux transporters, different approaches have been taken. One approach consists of functional expression of the *C. albicans* multidrug efflux transporters in baker's yeast, *S. cerevisiae*, carrying a deletion of the *PDR5* gene (Sanglard et al, 1996; Sanglard et al, 1997). Depending on the acquisition of resistance of *S. cerevisiae* mutants expressing these specific transporters against a given compound, the substance can be considered as a potential substrate for the expressed multidrug transporter. Potential substrates for the multidrug efflux transporters encoded by *CDR1* and *CDR2* include almost all antifungal azoles of medical importance (fluconazole, itraconazole, posaconazole, voriconazole, ravuconazole) as well as other antifungal agents such as terbinafine and amorolfine. For the multidrug transporter encoded by *CaMDR1*, fluconazole was the only relevant substrate among azole antifungals. Data suggest that the upregulation of *CaMDR1* is responsible for the specific resistance to fluconazole among *Candida* isolates, consistent with the observation that *CaMDR1* overexpression in *S. cerevisiae* was only conferring resistance to fluconazole (Sanglard et al, 1997). Since not only azole antifungal drugs but other antifungal agents can be taken simultaneously as substrates by several multidrug efflux transporters, these genes, when upregulated in yeast clinical isolates, have the potential of mediating cross-resistance to different antifungal agents.

Resistance Involving Alterations of the Cellular Target

Alterations in the affinity of azole derivatives to Erg11p is another important mechanism of resistance and has been described in different posttreatment yeast species, namely *C. albicans* (Vanden Bossche et al, 1990) and *C. neoformans* (Lamb et al, 1995). Affinity alterations are thought to be due to mutations in the gene encoding Erg11p (*ERG11*), which, by conformational changes, can affect the binding of azole derivatives (Fig. 9–1). When comparing *ERG11* sequences from matched pairs of azole-susceptible and azole-resistant *C. albicans* isolates, several laboratories have described nucleotide substitutions in *ERG11* alleles from azole-resistant *C. albicans* isolates, resulting in amino acid changes. A total of 83 amino acids substitutions have been reported by these studies (Sanglard and Bille, 2002c), illustrating the high allelic variability for *ERG11*, which still has few equivalents in other genes in lower eukaryotes. Functional expression of PCR-amplified *ERG11* alleles in *S. cerevisiae* as described by azole susceptibility assays is a convenient alternative to reveal mutations coupled with the development of azole resistance (Sanglard et al, 1998). In vitro methods consisting of binding assays of azoles with mutant

Erg11p protein variants have been carried out for the substitutions found in *ERG11* alleles of azole-resistant isolates. The introduction of the following substitutions, Arg467 to Lys, Gly464 to Ser, and Tyr132 to His, into *C. albicans* Erg11p resulted in decreased azole binding capacity (Kelly et al, 1999a; Kelly et al, 1999b; Lamb et al, 2000). While some *ERG11* alleles of azole-resistant isolates contained a single mutation responsible for azole resistance, other *ERG11* alleles were found to contain several mutations with potential additive effects. Alteration of the cellular target appears to be an important resistance mechanism in *A. fumigatus* clinical isolates that acquire resistance to itraconazole. Recently, investigators reported that a mutation in one of the *ERG11* alleles (Cyp51A) at amino acid position 54 could be responsible for resistance to itraconazole and posaconazole (Mann et al, 2002; Mellado et al, 2002). Interestingly however, this mutation is not associated with changes in voriconazole susceptibility. *Aspergillus fumigatus* isolates resistant to voriconazole remain rare (Mosquera and Denning, 2002).

Upregulation of *ERG11* has been mentioned as a possible cause of azole resistance among a few *C. albicans* and *C. glabrata* clinical isolates (Fig. 9–1). Upregulation of *ERG11* does not exceed a factor of 3–5 in azole-resistant isolates when compared to *ERG11* expression in related azole-susceptible strains (Sanglard et al, 1995). Upregulation of *ERG11* can be achieved in principle by deregulating gene transcription or by gene amplification. This latter possibility has been demonstrated in a *C. glabrata* isolate resistant to azole derivatives (Marichal et al, 1997). Upregulation of *ERG11* can also be obtained by exposure of *C. albicans* to ergosterol biosynthesis inhibitors, especially azole agents. Exposure of *C. albicans* to these type of drugs affects the expression of other *ERG* genes, as recently confirmed by genomewide expression studies performed in *C. albicans* (De Backer et al, 2001).

Resistance Involving Alterations in the Ergosterol Biosynthetic Pathway

Analysis of the sterol composition of azole-resistant yeasts has provided several hypotheses about specific alterations of enzymes involved in the complex ergosterol biosynthetic pathway. Accumulation of ergosta-7,22-dienol-3β-ol was observed in two separate azole-resistant *C. albicans* clinical isolates, which is a feature consistent with an absence of sterol $\Delta^{5,6}$ desaturase activity encoded by *ERG3* (Nolte et al, 1997). Interestingly, azole resistance in these two cases was coupled with resistance to AmB, which was expected because of the absence of ergosterol in these cells. An *ERG3* defect and cross-resistance between azoles and AmB were also reported in other *C. albicans* isolates from

AIDS patients (Kelly et al, 1996; Kelly et al, 1997). *ERG3* deletion by targeted mutagenesis in laboratory strains of *C. albicans* (Sanglard, unpublished) and *C. glabrata* (Geber et al, 1995) is not linked to AmB resistance, in contrast to the analysis of *C. albicans* clinical strains. In addition, the role of *ERG3* in azole resistance originates from the observation that treatment with azoles of a normal yeast cell inhibits Erg11p, resulting in accumulation of 14α-methylated sterols and 14α-methylergosta-8,24(28)-dien-3β,6α-diol. Formation of this latter sterol metabolite is thought to be catalyzed by the *ERG3* gene product (the sterol $\Delta^{5,6}$ desaturase). Thus, inactivation of this gene suppresses toxicity and causes azole resistance (Kelly et al, 1995; Lupetti et al, 2002) (Fig. 9–1). This specific mechanism of resistance to azole derivatives among *C. albicans* seems to mimic azole resistance obtained in laboratory conditions among *S. cerevisiae* by mutations of the *ERG3* gene (Watson et al, 1988). Loss of functional mutations in *ERG3* alleles from the known *C. albicans* azole-resistant Darlington strain were characterized recently (Miyazaki et al, 1999). Unfortunately, the effect of these mutations on azole resistance were masked by other azole resistance mechanisms in this strain, making it difficult to assess the contribution of *ERG3* in these conditions (Miyazaki et al, 1999).

Multiple Azole Resistance Mechanisms in Clinical Isolates

In some studies investigating resistance mechanisms to azoles among clinical isolates, sequential isolates from patients treated with these compounds may show a stepwise increase in azole resistance, as measured by susceptibility testing. This stepwise increase in azole resistance indicates that different resistance mechanisms could operate and, through their sequential addition, explain the increase in azole MIC values. Several examples have documented the multifactorial basis of azole resistance in clinical isolates (Sanglard et al, 1995; White, 1997a; White, 1997b; Sanglard et al, 1998; Perea et al, 2001). The combination of resistance mechanisms seems to be associated with a high level of azole resistance, e.g., MIC values for fluconazole exceeding 64 μg/ml (Perea et al, 2001). Alterations of the target enzymes by several distinct single or multiple mutations and upregulation of multidrug transporters from two different families provide a large flexibility for the potential combinations of resistance mechanisms. Molecular epidemiologic studies of azole resistance performed mainly with *C. albicans* isolates demonstrated that the diversity of resistance mechanism combinations was high enough to indicate that only a very few azole resistant isolates have identical patterns of *ERG11* mutations and profiles of multidrug transporter genes expression. The

relative frequency of resistance mechanisms in large populations of azole-resistant isolates has been investigated in a few studies. Perea and coworkers showed that 85% of azole-resistant isolates were upregulating multidrug transporter genes and that 65% contained *ERG11* mutations linked to azole resistance (Perea et al, 2001). Overall, 75% of the azole-resistant isolates combined resistance mechanisms. These results matched our own data obtained on azole-resistant isolates from 18 HIV-positive patients; 82% of these isolates showed upregulation of multidrug transporter genes; 63% contained *ERG11* mutations linked to azole resistance; and 50% showed combinations of resistance mechanisms (Sanglard, unpublished). The relative distribution of the type of multidrug transporter genes upregulated in these populations favors the ABC-transporters *CDR1* and *CDR2*; these transporters are upregulated in approximately twice as many azole-resistant isolates than in isolates with *CaMDR1* upregulation.

Combination of resistance mechanisms is not always linked to high levels of resistance. In *C. glabrata* azole-resistant isolates, a single resistance mechanism (i.e., upregulation of the *CgCDR1* ABC-transporter gene) is responsible for acquisition of high level azole resistance. Genetic evidence has also been provided for the occurrence of this single resistance mechanism by deletion of *CgCDR1* in an azole-resistant strain, which results in a decrease of fluconazole MIC values near to those obtained in the parental azole-susceptible isolate (Sanglard et al, 1999).

Alternative Mechanisms of Resistance

Besides the resistance mechanisms described above, alternative pathways for the acquisition of azole resistance can be used by yeasts and moulds. One interesting alternative for development of azole resistance is the ability of fungal pathogens to form biofilms on synthetic or natural surfaces. Biofilms are organized as a dense network of differentiated cells onto which a layer of extracellular matrix can form. Biofilms can constitute a physical barrier for the efficient penetration of antifungal drugs, which could explain why fungal cells embedded in the biofilm become recalcitrant to the antifungal action of the drugs. Measurement of drug susceptibilities of *C. albicans* or *C. dubliniensis* obtained from biofilms yielded high MIC values for azoles and AmB as compared to planktonic cells (Ramage et al, 2002). As reported for *C. albicans*, the expression of genes involved in azole resistance (i.e., multidrug transporter genes) can also be altered in biofilms and may contribute to the relatively high azole resistance measured in the fungal cell population of these dense structures (Ramage et al, 2002). The clinical relevance of biofilm formation and the potential contribution of biofilm to resistance to the action of antifungal agents is still under debate. There are at least two situations where biofilms can form in vivo: when fungal cells grow as multilayers on mucosal surfaces (as in oropharyngeal candidiasis) or grow on synthetic surfaces of catheters. Resistance to antifungal agents by fungal-associated biofilm formation is therefore limited to specific clinical presentations.

Genome Approaches to the Study of Azole Resistance

Azole resistance among fungal pathogens until now has been correlated with the upregulation of a limited number of genes belonging mainly to two distinct multidrug transporter families or to the ergosterol biosynthesis pathway. Microarray experiments, with their ability to deliver collections of genes differentially expressed in a genome, represent an attractive tool to identify clusters of genes coregulated between azole-susceptible and azole-resistant isolates. The expression of coregulated genes might be controlled by common regulatory circuits converging to similar regulatory sequences in the promoters of these genes. In one study of microarrays representing almost the entire C. albicans genome, gene expression profiles of individual C. albicans isolates with reduced azole susceptibility were investigated; these isolates were upregulating either CDR1/CDR2 or CaMDR1 (Cowen et al, 2002). Interestingly, in an isolate upregulating CDR2, other upregulated genes were found and, under them, three genes (YPL88 [LPG20], YOR49 [RTA3], and YLR63) contained in their promoter a consensus for a DRE, which is necessary for CDR1 and CDR2 upregulation. In other isolates upregulating CaMDR1, several genes involved in oxidative stress response were also upregulated, suggesting that the oxidative stress pathway, to which CAP1 also belongs, is contributing to CaMDR1 upregulation. With another microarray study, other sets of C. albicans azole-resistant and azole-susceptible isolates were compared for differential gene expression (Rogers and Barker, 2002). These investigators confirmed some of the earlier results by Cowen et al related to the coordinate upregulation of CDR1/CDR2 and YOR49 (RTA3) LPG20 (IFD5), and also enlarged the analysis to other upregulated genes such as the ergosterol biosynthesis gene ERG2, and the cell stress genes, CRD2 and GPX1. Microarray experiments also represent a valuable tool to investigate the mode of action of current or investigational antifungal drugs. This technique was used with S. cerevisiae cells exposed to fluconazole (Bammert and Fostel, 2000) and to AmB (Zhang et al, 2002) or with C. albicans cells exposed to itraconazole (De Backer et al, 2001). Beside confirming the mode of action of these drugs, these microarray studies can also

reveal other side effects (so-called off-targets) of the drugs on the metabolism of the entire cell.

Future microarray experiments will likely evaluate other azole-resistant isolates as tester strains for expression profile analyses. These analyses will be helpful not only because they may cluster genes under the control of specific regulatory pathways, but also they may reveal still unmasked azole resistance mechanisms.

Cyclic Lipopeptides: The Echinocandins

The fungal cell wall is an essential component for the maintenance of turgor pressure of the cell and is absent from mammalian cells. The fundamental components of the cell wall of most fungi are chitin, α- and β-linked glucans, mannoproteins, and glycosylphosphatidylinositol (GPI)-anchored proteins. Cyclic lipopeptide antifungal agents target the biosynthesis of individual cell wall components, which are attractive novel targets. The echinocandins are noncompetitive inhibitors of β-1,3 glucan synthase, which is part of an enzyme complex that forms the major glucan polymers of most pathogenic fungi. β-1,3 glucan synthases in S. cerevisiae are encoded by 2 separate genes, FKS1 and FKS2 (Kurtz and Douglas, 1997), whose simultaneous deletion results in nonviable cells. FKS-like genes have been cloned from other fungal pathogens, including C. albicans, C. neoformans, and Paracoccidioides brasiliensis (Douglas et al, 1997; Mio et al, 1997; Thompson et al, 1999; Pereira et al, 2000). Synthetic variations on the echinocandin moiety have produced several molecules with improved water solubility, antifungal potency and efficacy in animal models. Caspofungin (MK-0991) is the only currently approved echinocandin; two other drugs in this class are in various stages of development, micafungin (FK 463) and anidulafungin (VER 002). Caspofungin, a semisynthetic analogue of pneumocandin Bo (Onishi et al, 2000), is water-soluble, only available in parenteral form, and has very good fungicidal activity against a large number of Candida spp. and Aspergillus spp. The MIC values for these pathogens range between 0.12 and 2 μg/ml (Table 9–1).

The MICs for caspofungin against A. fumigatus are however atypical. Since the drug is active against experimental in vivo models of aspergillosis (Bowman et al, 2002), other criteria for measuring its activity have been developed (Arikan et al, 2001), such as the minimal effective concentration (MEC), which estimates microscopic cell damage rather than decrease in growth as classically measured by standard MIC tests. Pneumocandin resistance was first demonstrated in the model yeast S. cerevisiae; a mutant R560-1C was shown to be resistant to the semisynthetic pneumocandin derivative L-733,560. Glucan synthesis catalyzed by a crude membrane fraction prepared from the *S. cerevisiae* was resistant to inhibition by L-733,560; a nearly 50-fold increase in the inhibitory concentration 50% (IC_{50}) against glucan synthase was paralleled by an increase in whole-cell resistance (Douglas et al, 1994).

Pneumocandin resistance has been established in *C. albicans* either by mutagenesis or by spontaneous selection at low frequency of resistant mutants on pneumocandin-containing medium. Resistant mutants increased their MIC values to pneumocandin derivatives by 50- to 100-fold. The IC_{50} of glucan synthase activity was affected to variable degrees, from 4- to over 5000-fold, in these mutants, suggesting that alterations in this enzyme were responsible for resistance. With the cloning of the *CaFKS1* gene encoding a subunit of β-1,3 glucan synthase, genetic evidence was provided for this possibility since disruption of *CaFKS1* echinocandin-resistant alleles in a *C. albicans* resistant mutant resulted in loss of resistance (Douglas et al, 1997; Mio et al, 1997). These experiments also provided the evidence that echinocandin derivatives were targeting the product of the *CaFKS1* gene in *C. albicans*. Not only was the development of echinocandin resistance a rare event in *C. albicans*, but also it was coupled with reduced virulence in animal models (Frost et al, 1997). Other echinocandin-resistant mutants have been produced without significant loss of virulence. These mutants were more refractory but still susceptible to treatment with the echinocandin L-733,560 than fully susceptible wild types (Kurtz et al, 1996). Since the introduction of caspofungin for the treatment of fungal diseases is a very recent event, it is too early to speculate on the impact of the clinical use of this drug on the potential emergence of resistance.

SURVIVING IN THE PRESENCE OF ANTIFUNGAL DRUGS

Some important antifungal agents in use (fluconazole, itraconazole) have a fungistatic activity in *C. albicans*, while other compounds have strong (e.g., AmB) or moderate (e.g., caspofungin) fungicidal activities in *C. albicans*. The fungistatic nature of azoles limits the efficacy of these substances especially in patients with serious immunosuppression, since the immune system participates actively with azoles in the elimination of *C. albicans* from infected sites. Recently, a screening of different types of drugs encountered in medical practice and capable of potentiating the activity of azoles was done. Among these different drugs, cyclosporin A was found to act in synergism with fluconazole and converted the in vitro fungistatic antifungal effect of fluconazole into a potent fungicidal effect (Marchetti et al, 2000b). This conversion into a fungicidal effect is due to a loss of tolerance, which is generally defined

as the capacity of an organism to survive in the presence of a drug at growth-inhibiting concentrations. The impact of the loss of fluconazole tolerance on drug efficacy was tested in a rat model of endocarditis due to *C. albicans* infection (Marchetti et al, 2000a). The results of animal experiments confirmed those results observed in vitro: the combination of fluconazole with cyclosporin A greatly increased the efficacy of fluconazole treatment and reduced fungal load to undetectable levels in infected organs. The molecular mechanism of cyclosporin A on fluconazole tolerance in *C. albicans* infection is thought to be exerted at the level of the cyclophilin–cyclosporin A complex, which inhibits calcineurin functions. Calcineurin, a protein phosphatase conserved among eukaryotic organisms, is activated by a calcium-dependent pathway (Rusnak and Mertz, 2000). Recent studies indicate that calcineurin is essential for survival of *C. albicans* exposed to different environmental stresses; among these, exposure to antifungal agents is of special relevance (Cruz et al, 2002) (Sanglard, unpublished). Calcineurin seems to be involved in the survival of other fungal pathogens (i.e., *C. krusei* and *C. glabrata*) in the presence of antifungal drugs (Bonilla et al, 2002; Cruz et al, 2002). Inhibition of calcineurin could therefore be utilized in the future for increasing the efficacy of specific antifungal drugs. The exact mechanisms by which calcineurin protects *C. albicans* from cell death in the presence of antifungal drugs remain to be elucidated.

CURRENT SITUATION OF RESISTANCE TO ANTIFUNGAL DRUGS

Antifungal resistance over the last 10 to 15 years has been seen with triazole antifungals (fluconazole, itraconazole) in relation to oropharyngeal candidiasis associated with HIV infection. However, with the introduction of highly active antiretroviral therapy (HAART) for AIDS, oral candidiasis has decreased in frequency (Martins et al, 1998) and azole-resistant isolates from AIDS patients are now rarely isolated. The extensive use of azole antifungals during this period, either for treatment or prophylaxis of fungal diseases, could have been a predisposing factor for the emergence of yeast species intrinsically resistant, such as *C. krusei* or *C. glabrata*. However, available prospective data from oral and vaginal samples from more than 1220 HIV positive women between 1993 and 1995 showed little shift in the spectrum of *Candida* species, with *C. albicans* accounting for 87% of isolates at the start of the study, 84% after 1 year and 83% after 2 years (Sobel et al, 2000). The data for HIV-negative patients showed a similar (82%–87%) prevalence of *C. albicans*. Accordingly, azole usage appears to have little effect on the prevalence of *Candida* species originating from mucosal surfaces and has not predisposed to the predominance of non-*C. albicans* species associated with intrinsic resistance. Large surveillance studies performed in North America and in Europe have also looked at the problem of antifungal resistance in disseminated infections. A recent study of *Candida* bloodstream isolates in North America and Latin America indicated that less than 2% and 9% of *Candida* spp. were resistant to fluconazole and itraconazole, respectively (Pfaller et al, 2000). An overview of available data from population-based surveillance programs of *Candida* bloodstream infections indicate little, if any, resistance to fluconazole emerged among bloodstream isolates of *Candida* spp. between 1992 and 2000 (Pfaller and Diekema, 2002). In a recent review of this issue, the main conclusion was that *C. albicans*, which is the principal species to cause candidemia, has undergone no significant shift in fluconazole or itraconazole MICs (Sanglard and Odds, 2002b).

Some population shift toward intrinsically resistant non-*C. albicans* species has been reported in specific institutions. Compilation of data by Sanglard and Odds supports a correlation of *C. glabrata* and *C. krusei* prevalence with the introduction of fluconazole therapy (Sanglard and Odds, 2002b). Other less common fungi, many of which are intrinsically resistant to the currently available antifungal agents, are being increasingly reported as causes of fungal infections and therefore deserve more attention. These fungi include Zygomycetes (*Rhizopus arrhizus*, *Mucor* spp., *Rhizomucor pusillus*), *Fusarium* spp., *Trichosporon asahii*, *Scedosporium* spp., *Acremonium* spp. and dematiaceous fungi (Fridkin and Jarvis, 1996; Groll and Walsh, 2001; Perea and Patterson, 2002a).

CONCLUSIONS AND PERSPECTIVES

Studies on mechanisms of resistance of fungal organisms to antifungal agents have documented the many different resources utilized by simple microorganisms to circumvent the effect of growth inhibitory substances. Expectations are that other mechanisms will soon be revealed, either by use of novel technologies (i.e., genomewide analysis with DNA microarrays) or by continued isolation of resistant isolates in hospital environments. Clinicians faced with the treatment of fungal diseases have to take into account that fungal pathogens have versatile tools for evolving resistance mechanisms. This phenomenon was seen with azole resistance in AIDS patients before the introduction of HAART. Even if the incidence of antifungal drug resistance among fungal pathogens is now low, studies on surveillance of antifungal resistance are still necessary. New antifungal agents with improved properties (voriconazole) or with a new mode of action (echinocandins) are now available and offer attractive alternatives for the treatment of fungal diseases. In addition, combinations of these newer antifungal agents with older agents can be better rationalized since each of the individual drugs has a different mode of action. These antifungal drug combinations will likely offer novel alternative therapeutic approaches for refractory fungal infections.

ACKNOWLEDGMENTS

D.S. is supported by a grant No 3100-055901 from the Swiss National Foundation and from the Howard Hughes Medical Institute.

REFERENCES

Alarco A M, Balan I, Talibi D, Mainville N, Raymond M. AP1-mediated multi-drug resistance in *Saccharomyces cerevisiae* requires FLR1 encoding a transporter of the major facilitator superfamily. *J Biol Chem* 272:19304–19313, 1997a.

Alarco, A M, Raymond M. The bZip transcription factor Cap1p is involved in multi-drug resistance and oxidative stress response in *Candida albicans*. *J Bacteriol* 181:700–708, 1997b.

Arikan S, Lozano-Chiu M, Paetznick V, Rex J H. In vitro susceptibility testing methods for caspofungin against *Aspergillus* and *Fusarium* isolates. *Antimicrob Agents Chemother* 45:327–330, 2001.

Arthington B A, Bennett L G, Skatrud P L, Guynn C J, Barbuch R J, Ulbright C E, Bard M. Cloning, disruption and sequence of the gene encoding yeast C-5 sterol desaturase. *Gene* 102: 39–44, 1991.

Bammert G F, Fostel J M. Genome-wide expression patterns in *Saccharomyces cerevisiae*: comparison of drug treatments and genetic alterations affecting biosynthesis of ergosterol. *Antimicrob Agents Chemother* 44:1255–1265, 2000.

Barchiesi F, Calabrese D, Sanglard D, Falconi Di Francesco L, Caselli F, Giannini D, Giacometti A, Gavaudan S, Scalise G. Experimental induction of fluconazole resistance in *Candida tropicalis* ATCC 750. *Antimicrob Agents Chemother* 44:1578–1584, 2000.

Bartizal K, Gill C J, Abruzzo G K, Flattery A M, Kong L, Scott P M, Smith J G, Leighton C E, Bouffard A, Dropinski J F, Balkovec J. In vitro preclinical evaluation studies with the echinocandin antifungal MK-0991 (L-743,872). *Antimicrob Agents Chemother* 41:2326–2332, 1997.

Bonilla M, Nastase K K, Cunningham K W. Essential role of calcineurin in response to endoplasmic reticulum stress. *EMBO J* 21:2343–2353, 2002.

Bowman J C, Hicks P S, Kurtz M B, Rosen H, Schmatz, D M, Liberator P A, Douglas C M. The antifungal echinocandin caspofungin acetate kills growing cells of *Aspergillus fumigatus* in vitro. *Antimicrob Agents Chemother* 46:3001–3012, 2002.

Brandt M E, Pfaller M A, Hajjeh R A, Hamill R J, Pappas, P G., Reingold, A.L., Rimland, D. and Warnock, D.W. Trends in antifungal drug susceptibility of *Cryptococcus neoformans* isolates in the United States: 1992 to 1994 and 1996 to 1998. *Antimicrob Agents Chemother* 45:3065–3069, 2001.

Chavez M, Bernal S, Valverde A, Gutierrez M J, Quindos G, Mazuelos E M. In-vitro activity of voriconazole (UK-109,496), LY303366 and other antifungal agents against oral *Candida* spp. isolates from HIV-infected patients. *J Antimicrob Chemother* 44:697–700, 1999.

Coleman D C, Rinaldi M G, Haynes K A, Rex J H, Summerbell R C, Anaissie E J, Li A, Sullivan D J. Importance of *Candida* species other than *Candida albicans* as opportunistic pathogens. *Med Mycol* 36:156–165, 1998.

Cowen L E, Nantel A, Whiteway M S, Thomas D Y, Tessier D C, Kohn L M, Anderson J B. Population genomics of drug resistance in *Candida albicans*. *Proc Natl Acad Sci U S A* 99: 9284–9289, 200_.

Cruz M C, Goldstein A L, Blankenship J R, Del Poeta M, Davis D, Cardenas M E, Perfect J R, McCusker J H, Heitman J. Calcineurin is essential for survival during membrane stress in *Candida albicans*. *EMBO J* 21:546–559, 2002.

De Backer M D, Ilyina T, Ma X J, Vandoninck S, Luyten W H, Vanden Bossche H. Genomic profiling of the response of *Candida albicans* to itraconazole treatment using a DNA microarray. *Antimicrob Agents Chemother* 45:1660–1670, 2001.

de Micheli M, Bille J, Schueller C, Sanglard D. A common drug-responsive element mediates the upregulation of the *Candida albicans* ABC transporters CDR1 and CDR2, two genes involved in antifungal drug resistance. *Mol Microbiol* 43:1197–1214, 2002.

Dick J D, Merz W G, Saral R. Incidence of polyene-resistant yeasts recovered from clinical specimens. *Antimicrob Agents Chemother* 18:158–163, 1980.

Douglas C M, Marrinan J A, Li W, Kurtz M B. A *Saccharomyces cerevisiae* mutant with echinocandin-resistant 1,3-beta-D-glucan synthase. *J Bacteriol* 176:5686–5696, 1994.

Douglas C M, D'Ippolito J A, Shei G J, Meinz M, Onishi J, Marrinan J A, Li W, Abruzzo G K, Flattery A, Bartizal K, Mitchell A, Kurtz M B. Identification of the *FKS1* gene of *Candida albicans* as the essential target of 1,3-beta-D-glucan synthase inhibitors. *Antimicrob Agents Chemother* 41:2471–2479, 1997.

Espinel-Ingroff A. Comparison of in vitro activities of the new triazole SCH56592 and the echinocandins MK-0991 (L-743,872) and LY303366 against opportunistic filamentous and dimorphic fungi and yeasts. *J Clin Microbiol* 36:2950–2956, 1998.

Fridkin S K, Jarvis W R. Epidemiology of nosocomial fungal infections. *Clin Microbiol Rev* 9:499–511, 1996.

Frost D J, Knapp M, Brandt K, Shadron A, Goldman R C. Characterization of a lipopeptide-resistant strain of *Candida albicans*. *Can J Microbiol* 43:122–128, 1997.

Geber A, Hitchcock C A, Swartz J E, Pullen F S, Marsden K E, Kwon-Chung K J, Bennett J E. Deletion of the *Candida glabrata ERG3* and *ERG11* genes: effect on cell viability, cell growth, sterol composition, and antifungal susceptibility. *Antimicrob Agents Chemother* 39:2708–2717, 1995.

Gehrt A, Peter J, Pizzo P A, Walsh T J. Effect of increasing inoculum sizes of pathogenic filamentous fungi on MICs of antifungal agents by broth microdilution method. *J Clin Microbiol* 33:1302–1307, 1995.

Groll A H, Piscitelli S C, Walsh T J. Clinical pharmacology of systemic antifungal agents: a comprehensive review of agents in clinical use, current investigational compounds, and putative targets for antifungal drug development. *Adv Pharmacol* 44:343–500, 1998.

Groll A H, Walsh T J. Uncommon opportunistic fungi: new nosocomial threats. *Clin Microbiol Infect* 7(Suppl 2):8–24, 2001.

Katzmann D J, Hallstrom T C, Mahe Y, Moye-Rowley W S. Multiple Pdr1p/Pdr3p binding sites are essential for normal expression of the ATP binding cassette transporter protein-encoding gene *PDR5*. *J Biol Chem* 271:23049–23054, 1996.

Kelly S L, Lamb D C, Taylor M, Corran A J, Baldwin B C, Powderly W G. Resistance to amphotericin B associated with defective sterol delta 8–7 isomerase in a *Cryptococcus neoformans* strain from an AIDS patient. *FEMS Microbiol Lett* 122:39–42, 1994.

Kelly S L, Lamb D C, Corran A J, Baldwin B C, Kelly D E. Mode of action and resistance to azole antifungals associated with the formation of 14a-methylergosta-8,24(28)-dien-3β,6a-diol. *Biochem Biophys Res Commun* 207:910–915, 1995.

Kelly S L, Lamb D C, Kelly D E, Loeffler J, Einsele H. Resistance to fluconazole and amphotericin in *Candida albicans* from AIDS patients. *Lancet* 348:1523–1524, 1996.

Kelly S L, Lamb D C, Kelly D E, Manning N J, Loeffler J, Hebart H, Schumacher U, Einsele H. Resistance to fluconazole and cross-resistance to amphotericin B in *Candida albicans* from AIDS patients caused by defective sterol delta 5,6-desaturation. *FEBS Lett* 400:80–82, 1997.

Kelly S L, Lamb D C, Kelly D E. Y132H substitution in *Candida albicans* sterol 14alpha-demethylase confers fluconazole resistance by preventing binding to haem. *FEMS Microbiol Lett* 180:171–175, 1999a.

Kelly S L, Lamb D C, Loeffler J., Einsele H, Kelly D E. The G464S amino acid substitution in *Candida albicans* sterol 14alpha-demethylase causes fluconazole resistance in the clinic through reduced affinity. *Biochem Biophys Res Commun* 262:174–179, 1999b.

Kontoyiannis D P, Lewis R E. Antifungal drug resistance of pathogenic fungi. *Lancet* 359:1135–1144, 2002.

Kuge S, Arita M, Murayama A, Maeta K, Izawa S, Inoue Y, Nomoto A. Regulation of the yeast Yap1p nuclear export signal is mediated by redox signal-induced reversible disulfide bond formation. *Mol Cell Biol* 21:6139–6150, 2001.

Kurtz M B, Abruzzo G., Flattery A, Bartizal K, Marrinan J A, Li W, Milligan J, Nollstadt K, Douglas C M. Characterization of echinocandin-resistant mutants of *Candida albicans*: genetic, biochemical, and virulence studies. *Infect Immun* 64:3244–3251, 1996.

Kurtz M B, Douglas C M. Lipopeptide inhibitors of fungal glucan synthase. *J Med Vet Mycol* 35:79–86, 1997.

Lamb D C, Corran A, Baldwin B C, Kwon-Chung J, Kelly S L. Resistant P450A1 activity in azole antifungal tolerant *Cryptococcus neoformans* from AIDS patients. *FEBS Lett* 368:326–330, 1995.

Lamb D C, Kelly D E, White T C, Kelly S L. The R467K amino acid substitution in *Candida albicans* sterol 14alpha-demethylase causes drug resistance through reduced affinity. *Antimicrob Agents Chemother* 44:63–67, 2000.

Latge J P. *Aspergillus fumigatus* and *aspergillosis*. *Clin Microbiol Rev* 12:310–350, 1999.

Lupetti A, Danesi R, Campa M, Del Tacca M, Kelly S. Molecular basis of resistance to azole antifungals. *Trends Mol Med* 8:76–81, 2002.

Mann P A, Wei S, Walker S S, Mendrick C A, Cramer C, Loebenberg D, Li X, Didomenico B, Parmegiani R, Hare R S and McNicholas P M. Mutations that result in reduced susceptibility to posaconazole in *Aspergillus fumigatus* appear to be restricted to a single amino acid in cyp51a. Interscience Conference on Antimicrobial Agents and Chemotherapy. San Diego, CA. American Society of Microbiology, Abstract M-219, 2002.

Marchetti O, Entenza J M, Sanglard D, Bille J, Glauser M P, Moreillon P. Fluconazole plus cyclosporine: a fungicidal combination effective against experimental endocarditis due to *Candida albicans*. *Antimicrob Agents Chemother* 44:2932–2938, 2000a.

Marchetti O, Moreillon P, Glauser M P, Bille J, Sanglard D. Potent synergism of the combination of fluconazole and cyclosporine in *Candida albicans*. *Antimicrob Agents Chemother* 44:2373–2381, 2000b.

Marichal P, Vanden Bossche H, Odds F C, Nobels G, Warnock D W, Timmerman V, Van Broeckhoven C, Fay S and Mose-Larsen P. Molecular biological characterization of an azole-resistant *Candida glabrata* isolate. *Antimicrob Agents Chemother* 41:2229–2237, 1997.

Marr K A, Lyons C N, Rustad T R, Bowden R A, White T C, Rustad T. Rapid, transient fluconazole resistance in *Candida albicans* is associated with increased mRNA levels of CDR. *Antimicrob Agents Chemother* 42:2584–2589, 1998.

Marr K A, Lyons C N, Ha K, Rustad T R, White T C. Inducible

azole resistance associated with a heterogeneous phenotype in *Candida albicans*. *Antimicrob Agents Chemother* 45:52–59, 2001.

Martins M D, Lozano-Chiu M, Rex J H. Declining rates of oropharyngeal candidiasis and carriage of *Candida albicans* associated with trends toward reduced rates of carriage of fluconazole-resistant *C. albicans* in human immunodeficiency virus-infected patients. *Clin Infect Dis* 27: 1291–1294, 1998.

Masia Canuto M, Gutierrez Rodero F. Antifungal drug resistance to azoles and polyenes. *Lancet Infect Dis* 2:550–563, 2002.

Mellado E, Cuenca-Estrella M, Diaz-Guerra T M, Rodriguez-Tudela J L. Clinical isolates of *Aspergillus fumigatus* with a 14-a sterol demethylase (cyp51A) point mutation showed in vitro cross-resistance to itraconazole and posaconazole. Interscience Conference on Antimicrobial Agents and Chemotherapy. San Diego, CA, American Society of Microbiology, Abstract M-218, 2002.

Mikamo H, Sato Y, Tamaya T. In vitro antifungal activity of FK463, a new water-soluble echinocandin-like lipopeptide. *J Antimicrob Chemother* 46:485–487, 2000.

Mio T, Adachi-Shimizu M, Tachibana Y, Tabuchi H, Inoue S B, Yabe T, Yamada-Okabe T, Arisawa M, Watanabe T, Yamada-Okabe H. Cloning of the *Candida albicans* homolog of *Saccharomyces cerevisiae GSC1/FKS1* and its involvement in beta-1,3-glucan synthesis. *J Bacteriol* 179:4096–4105, 1997.

Miyazaki Y, Geber A, Miyazaki H, Falconer D, Parkinson T, Hitchcock C, Grimberg B, Nyswaner K, Bennett J E. Cloning, sequencing, expression and allelic sequence diversity of *ERG3* (C-5 sterol desaturase gene) in *Candida albicans*. *Gene* 236:43–51, 1999.

Moran G P, Sanglard D, Donnelly S, Shanley D B, Sullivan D J, Coleman D C. Identification and expression of multi-drug transporters responsible for fluconazole resistance in *Candida dubliniensis*. *Antimicrob Agents Chemother* 42:1819–1830, 1998.

Mosquera J, Denning D W. Azole cross-resistance in *Aspergillus fumigatus*. *Antimicrob Agents Chemother* 46:556–557, 2002.

Nakamura K, Niimi M, Niimi K, Holmes A R, Yates J E, Decottignies A, Monk B C, Goffeau A, Cannon R D.Functional expression of *Candida albicans* drug efflux pump Cdr1p in a *Saccharomyces cerevisiae* strain deficient in membrane transporters. *Antimicrob Agents Chemother* 45:3366–3374, 2001.

Nolte F S, Parkinson T, Falconer D J, Dix S, Williams J, Gilmore C, Geller R, Wingard J R. Isolation and characterization of fluconazole- and amphotericin B-resistant *Candida albicans* from blood of two patients with leukemia. *Antimicrob Agents Chemother* 44:196–199, 1997.

Onishi J, Meinz M, Thompson J, Curotto J, Dreikorn S, Rosenbach M, Douglas C, Abruzzo G, Flattery A, Kong L, Cabello A, Vicente F, Pelaez F, Diez M T, Martin I, Bills G, Giacobbe R, Dombrowski A, Schwartz R, Morris S, Harris G, Tsipouras A, Wilson K, Kurtz M B. Discovery of novel antifungal (1,3)-beta-D-glucan synthase inhibitors. *Antimicrob Agents Chemother* 44:368–377, 2000.

Perea S, Lopez-Ribot J L, Kirkpatrick W R, McAtee R K, Santillan R A, Martinez M, Calabrese D, Sanglard D, Patterson T F. Prevalence of molecular mechanisms of resistance to azole antifungal agents in *Candida albicans* strains displaying high-level fluconazole resistance isolated from human immunodeficiency virus-infected patients. *Antimicrob Agents Chemother* 45: 2676–2684, 2001.

Perea S, Patterson T F. Antifungal resistance in pathogenic fungi. *Clin Infect Dis* 35:1073–1080, 2002a.

Perea S, Lopez-Ribot J L, Wickes B L, Kirkpatrick W R, Dib O P, Bachmann S P, Keller S M, Martinez M, Patterson T F. Molecular mechanisms of fluconazole resistance in *Candida dubliniensis* isolates from human immunodeficiency virus-infected patients with oropharyngeal candidiasis. *Antimicrob Agents Chemother* 46:1695–1703, 2002b.

Pereira M, Felipe M S, Brigido M M, Soares C M, Azevedo M O.

Molecular cloning and characterization of a glucan synthase gene from the human pathogenic fungus *Paracoccidioides brasiliensis*. *Yeast* 16:451–462, 2000.

Peyron F, Favel A, Michel-Nguyen A, Gilly M, Regli P, Bolmstrom A. Improved detection of amphotericin B-resistant isolates of *Candida lusitaniae* by Etest. *J Clin Microbiol* 39:339–342, 2001.

Pfaller M A, Messer S A, Hollis R J. Strain delineation an antifungal susceptibilities of epidemiologically releated and unrelated isolates of *Candida lusitaniae*. *Diagn Microbiol Infect Dis* 20: 127–133, 1994.

Pfaller M A, Messer S A, Coffman S. In vitro susceptibilities of clinical yeast isolates to a new echinocandin derivative, LY303366, and other antifungal agents. *Antimicrob Agents Chemother* 41: 763–766, 1997.

Pfaller M A, Messer S A, Hollis R J, Jones R N, Doern G V, Brandt M E, Hajjeh R A. In vitro susceptibilities of *Candida* bloodstream isolates to the new triazole antifungal agents BMS-207147, SCH 56592, and voriconazole. *Antimicrob Agents Chemother* 42: 3242–3244, 1998.

Pfaller M A, Messer S A, Hollis R J, Jones R N, Doern G V, Brandt M E, Hajjeh R A. Trends in species distribution and susceptibility to fluconazole among bloodstream isolates of *Candida* species in the United States. *Diagn Microbiol Infect Dis* 33:217–222, 1999.

Pfaller M A, Jones R N, Doern G V, Sader HS, Messer S A, Houston A, Coffman S, Hollis R J. Bloodstream infections due to *Candida* species: SENTRY antimicrobial surveillance program in North America and Latin America, 1997–1998. *Antimicrob Agents Chemother* 44:747–751, 2000.

Pfaller M A, Diekema D J. Role of sentinel surveillance of candidemia: trends in species distribution and antifungal susceptibility. *J Clin Microbiol* 40:3551–3557, 2002.

Polak A, Mode of action studies. In Ryley J F, (ed.), *Chemotheray of Fungal Diseases*. Springer-Verlag, Berlin, pp. 153–182, 1990.

Posteraro B, Sanguinetti M, Sanglard D, La Sorda M, Boccia S, Romano L, Morace G, Giovanni F. Identification and characterization of a *Cryptococcus neoformans* ATP Binding Cassette (ABC) Transporter-encoding gene, *CnDR1*, involved in the resistance to fluconazole. *Mol Microbiol* 47:357–371, 2003.

Ramage G, Bachmann S, Patterson T F, Wickes B L, Lopez-Ribot J L. Investigation of multi-drug efflux pumps in relation to fluconazole resistance in *Candida albicans* biofilms. *J Antimicrob Chemother* 49:973–980, 2002.

Rex J H, Cooper C R, Jr, Merz W G., Galgiani J N, Anaissie E J. Detection of amphotericin B-resistant *Candida* isolates in a broth-based system. *Antimicrob Agents Chemother* 39: 906–909, 1995.

Rex J H, Pfaller M A, Galgiani J N, Bartlett M S, Espinel-Ingroff A, Ghannoum M A, Lancaster M, Odds F C, Rinaldi M G, Walsh T J, Barry A L. Development of interpretive breakpoints for antifungal susceptibility testing: conceptual framework and analysis of in vitro-in vivo correlation data for fluconazole, itraconazole, and *Candida* infections. Subcommittee on Antifungal Susceptibility Testing of the National Committee for Clinical Laboratory Standards. *Clin Infect Dis* 24:235–247, 1997.

Rogers P D, Barker K S. Evaluation of differential gene expression in fluconazole-susceptible and -resistant isolates of *Candida albicans* by cDNA microarray analysis. *Antimicrob Agents Chemother* 46:3412–3417, 2002.

Rusnak F, Mertz P. Calcineurin: form and function. *Physiol Rev* 80:1483–1521, 2000.

Sanglard D, Kuchler K, Ischer F, Pagani J L, Monod M, Bille J. Mechanisms of resistance to azole antifungal agents in *Candida albicans* isolates from AIDS patients involve specific multi-drug transporters. *Antimicrob Agents Chemother* 39:2378–2386, 1995.

Sanglard D, Ischer F, Monod M, Bille J. Susceptibilities of *Candida albicans* multi-drug transporter mutants to various antifungal agents and other metabolic inhibitors. *Antimicrob Agents Chemother* 40:2300–2305, 1996.

Sanglard D, Ischer F, Monod M, Bille J. Cloning of *Candida albicans* genes conferring resistance to azole antifungal agents: characterization of CDR2, a new multi-drug ABC-transporter gene. *Microbiol* 143:405–416, 1997.

Sanglard D, Ischer F, Koymans L, Bille J. Amino acid substitutions in the cytochrome P450 lanosterol 14a-demethylase (CYP51A1) from azole-resistant *Candida albicans* clinical isolates contributing to the resistance to azole antifungal agents. *Antimicrob Agents Chemother* 42:241–253, 1998.

Sanglard D, Ischer F, Calabrese D, Majcherczyk P A, Bille J. The ATP binding cassette transporter gene *CgCDR1* from *Candida glabrata* is involved in the resistance of clinical isolates to azole antifungal agents. *Antimicrob Agents Chemother* 43:2753–2765, 1999.

Sanglard D, Ischer, F, Bille J, Role of ATP-binding-cassette transporter genes in high-frequency acquisition of resistance to azole antifungals in *Candida glabrata*. *Antimicrob Agents Chemother* 45:1174–1183, 2001.

Sanglard D. Resistance of human fungal pathogens to antifungal drugs. *Curr Opin Microbiol* 5:379–385, 2002a.

Sanglard D, Odds F C. Resistance of *Candida* species to antifungal agents: molecular mechanisms and clinical consequences. *Lancet Infect Dis* 2:73–85, 2002b.

Sanglard D, Bille J. Current understanding of the mode of action and of resistance mechanisms to conventional and emerging antifungal agents for treatment of *Candida* infections. In Calderone R, (ed.), *Candida and Candidiasis*. ASM press, Washington, DC, pp. 349–383, 2002c.

Slaven J W, Anderson M J, Sanglard D, Dixon G K, Bille J, Roberts I S, Denning D W. Induced expression of a novel *Aspergillus fumigatus* ABC transporter gene, atrF, in response to itraconazole. *Fungal Genet Biol* 36:199–206, 2002.

Sobel J D, Ohmit S E, Schuman P, Klein R S, Mayer K, Duerr A, Vazquez J A, Rompalo A. The evolution of *Candida* species and fluconazole susceptibility among oral and vaginal isolates recovered from human immunodeficiency virus (HIV)-seropositive and at-risk HIV-seronegative women. *J Infect Dis* 183:286–293, 2000.

Sokol-Anderson M L, Brajtburg J, Medoff G. Amphotericin B-induced oxidative damage and killing of *Candida albicans*. *J Infect Dis* 154:76–83, 1986.

Tawara S, Ikeda F, Maki K, Morishita Y, Otomo K, Teratani N, Goto T, Tomishima M, Ohki H, Yamada A, Kawabata K, Takasugi H, Sakane K, Tanaka H, Matsumoto F, Kuwahara S. In vitro activities of a new lipopeptide antifungal agent, FK463, against a variety of clinically important fungi. *Antimicrob Agents Chemother* 44:57–62, 2000.

Thompson J R, Douglas C M, Li W, Jue C K, Pramanik B, Yuan X, Rude T H, Toffaletti D L, Perfect J R, Kurtz M. A glucan synthase FKS1 homolog in *Cryptococcus neoformans* is single copy and encodes an essential function. *J Bacteriol* 181:444–453, 1999.

Uchida K, Yokota N, Yamaguchi H. In vitro antifungal activity of posaconazole against various pathogenic fungi. *Int J Antimicrob Agents* 18:167–172, 2001.

Vanden Bossche H, Marichal P, Gorrens J, Bellens D, Moereels H,

Janssen P A J. Mutation in cytochrome P450-dependent 14a-demethylase results in decreased affinity for azole antifungals. *Biochem Soc Trans* 28:56–59, 1990.

Walsh T J, Melcher G P, Rinaldi M G, Lecciones J, McGough D A, Kelly P, Lee J, Callender D, Rubin M, Pizzo P A. *Trichosporon beigelii*, an emerging pathogen resistant to amphotericin *Br J Clin Microb* 28:1616–1622, 1990.

Watson P F, Rose M E, Kelly S L. Isolation and analysis of ketoconazole resistant mutants of *Saccharomyces cerevisiae*. *J Med Vet Mycol* 26:153–162, 1988.

Whelan W L. The genetic basis of resistance to 5-fluorocytosine in *Candida* species and *Cryptococcus neoformans*. *Crit Rev Microb* 15:45–56, 1988.

White T C. Increased mRNA levels of *ERG16*, *CDR*, and *MDR1* correlate with increases in azole resistance in *Candida albicans* isolates from a patient infected with human immunodeficiency virus. *Antimicrob Agents Chemother* 41:1482–1487, 1997a.

White T C. The presence of an R467K amino acid substitution and loss of allelic variation correlate with an azole-resistant lanosterol 14-alpha-demethylase in *Candida albicans*. *Antimicrob Agents Chemother* 41:1488–1494, 1997b.

White T C, Marr K A, Bowden R A. Clinical, cellular, and molecular factors that contribute to antifungal drug resistance. *Clin Microbiol Rev* 11:382–402, 1998.

Wirsching S, Michel S, Kohler G, Morschhauser J. Activation of the multiple drug resistance gene *MDR1* in fluconazole-resistant, clinical *Candida albicans* strains is caused by mutations in a trans-regulatory factor. *J Bacteriol* 182:400–404, 2000a.

Wirsching S, Michel S, Morschhauser J. Targeted gene disruption in *Candida albicans* wild-type strains: the role of the *MDR1* gene in fluconazole resistance of clinical *Candida albicans* isolates. *Mol Microbiol* 36:856–865, 2000b.

Wirsching S, Moran G P, Sullivan D J, Coleman D C, Morschhauser J. *MDR1*-mediated drug resistance in *Candida dubliniensis*. *Antimicrob Agents Chemother* 45:3416–3421, 2001.

Yamazumi T, Pfaller M A, Messer S A, Houston A, Hollis R J, Jones R N. In vitro activities of ravuconazole (BMS-207147) against 541 clinical isolates of *Cryptococcus neoformans*. *Antimicrob Agents Chemother* 44:2883–2886, 2000.

Yang X, Talibi D, Weber S, Poisson G, Raymond M. Functional isolation of the *Candida albicans* FCR3 gene encoding a bZip transcription factor homologous to *Saccharomyces cerevisiae* Yap3p. *Yeast* 18:1217–1225, 2001.

Yildiran S T, Saracli M A, Fothergill A W, Rinaldi M G. In vitro susceptibility of environmental *Cryptococcus neoformans* variety neoformans isolates from Turkey to six antifungal agents, including SCH56592 and voriconazole. *Eur J Clin Microbiol Infect Dis* 19: 317–319, 2000.

Yoon S A, Vazquez J A, Steffan P E, Sobel J D, Akins R A. High-frequency, in vitro reversible switching of *Candida lusitaniae* clinical isolates from amphotericin B susceptibility to resistance. *Antimicrob Agents Chemother* 43:836–845, 1999.

Zhang L, Zhang Y, Zhou Y, An S, Cheng J. Response of gene expression in *Saccharomyces cerevisiae* to amphotericin B and nystatin measured by microarrays. *J Antimicrob Chemother* 49:905–915, 2002.

10

Adjunctive antifungal therapy

EMMANUEL ROILIDES, JOHN DOTIS, JOANNA FILIOTI, AND ELIAS ANAISSIE

Invasive fungal infections (IFIs) have become an important problem in recent years, particularly among immunocompromised patients, such as those with cancer and those undergoing transplantation or chemotherapy. Corticosteroid treatment and phagocytic dysfunction occurring in patients with chronic granulomatous disease (CGD), human immunodeficiency virus (HIV), graft vs. host disease (GVHD) and birth prematurity are some other conditions that are associated with high frequency of IFIs. Invasive candidiasis and aspergillosis are the most frequent opportunistic IFIs. Despite recent progress in antifungal therapy with the development of new potent antifungal drugs and establishment of novel antifungal strategies of prevention and early treatment, their outcome remains dismal and mortality can be up to 90% (Denning, 1998). Reconstitution of immune host defense is a critical factor for recovery from IFIs (Roilides et al, 1998a).

Host defense against fungi is through both innate and acquired immunity. Innate immunity is based on the antifungal action of mononuclear and polymorphonuclear phagocytes. Both the number and the function of these cells can be up-regulated by hematopoietic growth factors (HGFs) and proinflammatory cytokines. By contrast, antiinflammatory cytokines exert an overall suppressive effect on antifungal function of phagocytes. Table 10–1 provides the names with abbreviations of clinically relevant HGFs and cytokines. Acquired immunity is based on T lymphocytes and antibody production by B lymphocytes and has been studied best in the cases of the fungal pathogens, *Candida albicans* and *Cryptococcus neoformans* (Aguirre and Johnson, 1997).

The immune system responds to challenges by fungi with secretion of a number of cytokines. For example in the case of *Aspergillus fumigatus*, one of the commonest pathogenic fungi, inhalation of conidia results in the production of interleukin (IL)-18, IL-12, and interferon (IFN)-γ, which play a protective role in pulmonary aspergillosis (Brieland et al, 2001). On the other hand, conidia, hyphae, and even fungal cell wall components result in secretion of high levels of IFN-γ, granulocyte-macrophage colony-stimulating factor (GM-CSF), tumor necrosis factor (TNF)-α, IL-2, and IL-6, especially by macrophages and monocytes (Grazziutti et al, 1997; Schelenz et al, 1999) orchestrating the host response to the invading fungus (Fig. 10–1). The immune responses to medically relevant fungi are summarized in Table 10–2.

HEMATOPOIETIC GROWTH FACTORS AND OTHER CYTOKINES

The most important biologic properties of HGFs and cytokines related to antifungal host defense are reviewed here. Granulocyte colony-stimulating factor (G-CSF) acts upon polymorphonuclear neutrophils (PMNs), promoting their maturation and increasing their number in peripheral blood (Lieschke and Burgess, 1992; Nemunaitis, 1997). In vitro studies have demonstrated that G-CSF also regulates the function of intact PMNs against fungi, such as *C. albicans* and *A. fumigatus* hyphae, mainly by enhancement of PMN superoxide anion (O_2^-) production (Roilides et al, 1995a; Roilides et al, 1993a; Liles et al, 1997). This enhancement occurs even when PMNs have been previously suppressed by corticosteroids (Roilides et al, 1993b).

Polymorphonuclear neutrophils from patients treated with G-CSF have been found to possess enhanced in vitro activity not only against *A. fumigatus* but also against *Rhizopus arrhizus*, *C. albicans* (Liles et al, 1997), and *C. neoformans* (Vecchiarelli et al, 1995). The latter two fungal organisms were killed even by PMNs from HIV-infected patients who had received G-CSF (5 μg/kg), a finding suggesting that this cytokine restores the suppressed function (Vecchiarelli et al, 1995). The effect of G-CSF has been also tested in combination with fluconazole and voriconazole in vitro and an additive effect has been found against *C. albicans* and *A. fumigatus* (Natarajan et al, 1997; Vora et al, 1998). Similar effect has been demonstrated in a neutropenic murine model of invasive aspergillosis given G-CSF and posaconazole (Graybill et al, 1998).

Granulocyte-macrophage colony-stimulating factor acts on both granulocytic and monocytic lineages, reg-

TABLE 10–1. *Clinically Relevant Hematopoietic Growth Factors and Cytokines with Potential Utility as Adjunctive Antifungal Therapy*

Hematopoietic Growth Factors	Cytokines	
G-CSF	IFN-γ	IL-4
GM-CSF	TNF-α	IL-10
M-CSF	IL-12	IL-15

G-CSF, granulocyte colony-stimulating factor; GM-CSF, granulocyte-macrophage colony-stimulating factor; M-CSF, macrophage colony-stimulating factor; IFN-γ, interferon-γ; TNF-α, tumor necrosis factor-α; IL, interleukin.

ulating the number not only of PMNs but also of eosinophils and monocytes. Granulocyte-macrophage colony-stimulating factor enhances antifungal activities of intact PMNs and mononuclear cells (MNCs) against *C. albicans* (Smith et al, 1990), *A. fumigatus* (Roilides et al, 1994), and other less common fungi. The effect of GM-CSF has been tested in vitro in combination with voriconazole and an additive effect, similar to that with G-CSF, has been found against *A. fumigatus* (Vora et al, 1998). Granulocyte-macrophage colony-stimulating factor also primes macrophages to release mediators of inflammation such as IL-1 and TNF-α (Rodriguez-Adrian et al, 1998) that can overcome dexamethasone-mediated suppression of antifungal monocytic activity against *Aspergillus* (Roilides et al, 1996a). On the other hand, these mediators may be responsible for the toxicity associated with GM-CSF therapy.

Macrophage colony-stimulating factor (M-CSF), which promotes the differentiation, proliferation, and activation of MNCs and macrophages, enhances the antifungal in vitro activity of MNCs and macrophages against *Candida* spp. (Karbassi et al, 1987), *A. fumigatus* (Roilides et al, 1995b) and other fungi. This enhancement also has been shown in vivo (Cenci et al, 1991; Roilides et al, 1996b).

Interferon-γ is a potent activator of both PMN and macrophage function (Murray, 1994) that can enhance phagocytic activity against a number of fungal pathogens both in vitro and in vivo (Kullberg and Anaissie, 1998a). An up-regulatory role of IFN-γ on both PMNs and MNCs against *Aspergillus* hyphae has been shown as well as an additive effect of the combination of IFN-γ and G-CSF at high concentrations (Roilides et al, 1994; Roilides et al, 1993a). Compared to G-CSF and GM-CSF, IFN-γ has been shown to be a very potent activator of phagocytes against opportunistic fungal pathogens (Gaviria et al, 1999). Synergy between IFN-γ and antifungal agents against *Candida* species, *A. fumigatus*, *C. neoformans*, *Paracoccidioides brasiliensis*, and *Blastomyces dermatiditis* has been demonstrated in vitro by use of macrophages (Rodriguez-Adrian et al, 1998) and in vivo for experimental cryptococcosis (Lutz et al, 2000).

Interleukin-12 can enhance fluconazole efficacy against *Candida* infections in mice with neutropenia (Mencacci et al, 2000) and has activity alone in experimental murine cryptococcosis (Clemons et al, 1994), histoplasmosis (Zhou et al, 1995), coccid-

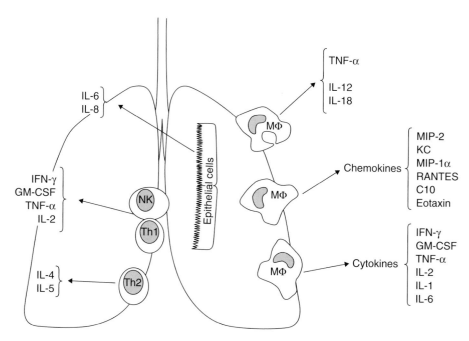

FIGURE 10–1. Cytokine response of host pulmonary immune cells after challenge with conidia of *A. fumigatus*, a typical airborne fungus.

TABLE 10–2. *Immune Response to Specific Groups of Fungi*

Fungi	Immune Response
Candida albicans and other *Candida* spp.	Macrophages (liver, spleen, etc.) phagocytose and kill blastoconidia intracellularly by nonoxidative mechanisms, produce monokines (i.e., TNF-α) Neutrophils (circulating in blood stream and in tissues) phagocytose and kill blastoconidia intracellularly, damage pseudohyphae and hyphae extracellularly by oxidative burst and nonoxidative mechanisms T lymphocytes produce lymphokines (i.e., IL-18, IFN-γ)
Airborne fungi (i.e., *Aspergillus* spp., Zygomycetes, *Fusarium* spp., *Scedosporium* spp.)	Pulmonary alveolar macrophages phagocytose and kill conidia intracellularly by nonoxidative mechanisms, produce monokines (i.e., TNF-α) Neutrophils damage escaping hyphae extracellularly by oxidative burst and nonoxidative mechanisms T lymphocytes produce lymphokines (i.e., IL-18, IFN-γ)
Cryptococcus neoformans (and *Trichosporon* spp.)	Polysaccharide-specific antibody mediated response, phagocytosis by macrophages and neutrophils, inhibition of immune functions

TNF-α, tumor necrosis factor-α; IL, interleukin; IFN, interferon.

ioidomycosis (Magee and Cox, 1996), and early in the course of aspergillosis. Thus, IL-12 may be useful adjunctive therapy against various IFIs in the setting of neutropenia. However, IL-12 can be detrimental in hosts that are not neutropenic because IL-12 can induce an excessive inflammatory response (Romani et al, 1997).

Interleukin-15 shares biological activities with IL-2, and appears to be important in up-regulation of host defenses against opportunistic fungal infections. Interleukin-15 has been shown to enhance O_2^- production and antifungal activities of PMNs and MNCs, including their abilities to phagocytose and inhibit growth of *C. albicans* (Musso et al, 1998; Vazquez et al, 1998b). Similarly, IL-15 enhances PMN-induced hyphal damage in a variety of fungi including *A. fumigatus*, *Scedosporium prolificans*, and *Fusarium* spp., but not *Aspergillus flavus* or *Scedosporium apiospermum* (*Pseudallescheria bodyii*) (Roilides et al, 2001a).

Tumor necrosis factor-α is another potent immunoenhancing cytokine that can augment the production of other cytokines, such as GM-CSF as well as enhance several PMN functions, mainly by increasing O_2^- and H_2O_2 release (Roilides et al, 1998b). In vitro studies have demonstrated that TNF-α enhances the antifungal activities of all the phagocytes against *A. fumigatus*. For example, TNF-α stimulates PMNs to damage hyphae, enhances pulmonary alveolar macrophage

(PAM) phagocytosis of conidia, and also increases O_2^- production by MNCs, although the effects on MNC functions are moderate (Roilides et al, 1998b). Fungicidal activity of PMNs against blastoconidia of *C. albicans* and *Candida glabrata* also have been enhanced by TNF-α (Djeu et al, 1986; Ferrante, 1989), whereas the results against pseudohyphae of *C. albicans* have been equivocal (Diamond et al, 1991).

Interleukin-4, a cytokine with antiinflammatory properties, has been shown to suppress the oxidative burst of MNCs and the killing of *C. albicans* blastoconidia (Roilides et al, 1997b). In the case of *A. fumigatus*, IL-4 significantly suppresses MNC-induced damage of hyphae, but did not alter phagocytic activity or inhibition of conidial germination. These findings suggest a lack of pathogenic role of IL-4 on the host response in the early phase of invasive aspergillosis and a suppressive role in the late phase. In murine models of candidiasis and aspergillosis, IL-4 had detrimental effects (Cenci et al, 1999; Cenci et al, 1993) and inhibition of IL-4 improves outcome.

Interleukin-10 is a similarly potent cytokine that affects MNCs by suppressing O_2^- production and antifungal activity of MNCs against *A. fumigatus* hyphae, a late host response event. IFN-γ and GM-CSF appear to counteract the suppressive effects of IL-10 (Roilides et al, 1997a). Interleukin-10 also affects PMN function against *C. albicans* by suppressing phagocytosis of blastoconidia and by reducing PMN-induced damage of *C. albicans* pseudohyphae (Roilides et al, 2000).

ADJUNCTIVE ANTIFUNGAL THERAPY WITH HEMATOPOIETIC GROWTH FACTORS AND OTHER CYTOKINES

Two patient population groups are at high risk for IFIs: those with neutropenia and those without neutropenia but with a variety of functional deficiencies of lymphocytes and phagocytes. Hematopoietic growth factors and other cytokines have a role in prophylaxis in both patient groups and in treatment of IFIs in combination with antifungal drugs.

Neutropenia

Patients with malignancies and disease or therapy-related neutropenia constitute the largest group of persons with acquired defects in host defenses and the group with greatest need for immune reconstitution. Thus, most of the preclinical and clinical studies have focused on this patient population. Although various cytokines have been evaluated extensively in preclinical studies, to date no randomized studies have been performed to specifically examine their roles against IFIs. The fact is that the number of IFIs as infectious sequelae of immune compromise is relatively small, and no study has had the statistical power to demonstrate significant differences in the two treatment groups (cytokine vs. placebo). Thus, conclusive clinical data are still missing, making the issue of cytokine use in the management of IFIs controversial.

The clinical use of G-CSF and GM-CSF has been based on the ability of either factor to abbreviate the depth and duration of neutropenia (American Society of Clinical Oncology, 1994; Boogaerts and Demuynck, 1996). In particular, G-CSF has been used to promote bone marrow recovery in patients with neutropenia and for the treatment of chronic neutropenia, myelodysplastic syndrome, and aplastic anemia (Nemunaitis, 1997). Both GM-CSF and G-CSF are used clinically in patients with neutropenia associated with chemotherapy and/or hematopoietic stem cell transplantation (HSCT), myelodysplastic syndromes, and aplastic anemia in order to promote bone marrow recovery. Both HGFs have assumed a central role in the supportive care of neutropenic patients associated with cancer, transplantation, aplastic anemia, and congenital defi-

ciencies. Since susceptibility to IFIs is proportional to the duration and degree of neutropenia (Nemunaitis, 1998a), the outcome of neutropenic patients with IFIs who receive a HGF may be better.

Hematopoietic growth factors have been administered in different settings of immunosuppression for the management of IFIs (Fig. 10–2). For prophylaxis against infections, HGFs have been given at the beginning of neutropenia (Antman et al, 1988; Crawford et al, 1991; Rowe et al, 1995; Seipelt, 2000). Although beneficial effects were noted in some of these studies, the number of IFIs that developed was too small to evaluate any potential effect. As shown in Table 10–3, in a retrospective study of prophylactic administration of GM-CSF to patients with autologous bone marrow transplantation (BMT) for lymphoid cancer (Nemunaitis et al, 1998b), GM-CSF resulted in a trend toward fewer IFIs and decreased use of amphotericin B. In this study, the 28-day post-BMT incidence of overall infections occurring in those who had taken GM-CSF was compared with those who had no GM-CSF.

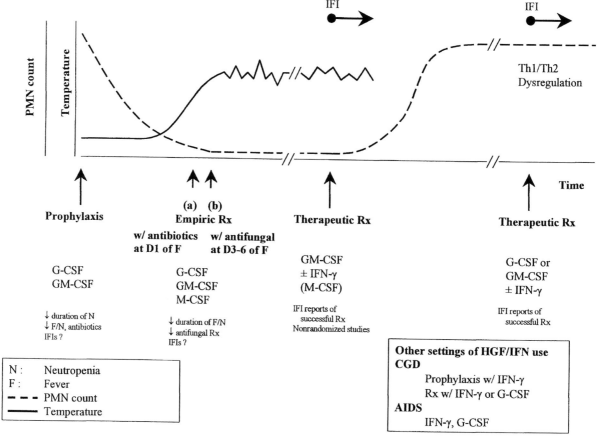

FIGURE 10–2. Settings where hematopoietic growth factors (HGFs) and interferon-γ (IFN-γ) have been used and may have potential clinical efficacy. Typical course of a hematopoietic stem cell transplant (HSCT) patient consisting of neutropenic and nonneutropenic periods and settings when invasive fungal infections (IFIs) may occur. Cytokine administration has been suggested at times indicated by arrows; the few clinical data published are summarized below. (Modified from Roilides et al, in press, 2003).

TABLE 10–3. *Clinical Studies on Use of Cytokines for Prophylaxis Against Invasive Fungal Infections in Cancer Patients*

Reference	Cytokine	Outcome
Nemunaitis et al, 1998b	GM-CSF	Overall ↓ infections, a trend of ↓ IFIs, ↓ intravenous antibiotics and ↓ days of amphotericin B usage
Rowe et al, 1995	GM-CSF	More complete responses, ↑ survival, ↓ IFI-related mortality
Peters et al, 1996	GM-CSF*	Overall ↓ infections, more complete responses, prevention of IFIs in patients receiving high-dose chemotherapy

*Retrospective analysis of GM-CSF vs. nonmacrophage enhancing cytokines
GM-CSF, granulocyte-macrophage colony-stimulating factor; IFI, invasive fungal infection.

Overall, fewer infections were observed with GM-CSF treatment as well as a trend of fewer IFIs and fewer days of amphotericin B usage.

Granulocyte-macrophage colony-stimulating factor has been used in patients with malignancies undergoing chemotherapy or BMT, and has been found to improve survival and decrease the rate of bacterial and fungal infections (Giles, 1998). A retrospective study (Peters et al, 1996) suggested that GM-CSF has some advantages compared to G-CSF as preventive therapy of IFIs in patients receiving high-dose chemotherapy, with or without stem cell transplantation (Table 10–3).

The only prospective, randomized study that had enough IFIs to show significant differences has been the Eastern Cooperative Oncology Group study (Rowe et al, 1995) (Table 10–3). In this placebo-controlled study, GM-CSF administration to 124 elderly patients with myelogenous leukemia resulted in a reduction in the IFI-related mortality (2% in the GM-CSF group as compared to 19% in the placebo group), and a higher rate of complete remission of neutropenia. Among the patients with IFIs, there were 11 patients with aspergillosis, 7 with candidiasis and 2 with other IFIs. Only 1 of 8 patients who had been randomized to receive GM-CSF and developed IFI died (13%) as compared to 9 among 12 patients on placebo (75%). No significant differences between aspergillosis and candidiasis were noted.

Similar lack of consistent beneficial effects to support routine use of HGFs exists in the case of preemptive administration of G-CSF or GM-CSF to patients at the onset of febrile neutropenia (Maher et al, 1994; Aviles et al, 1996; Anaissie et al, 1996; Ohno et al, 1997) (Table 10–4). In this setting, however, significantly less usage of antifungal drugs was observed probably due to the effect of the cytokines on the incidence and duration of febrile neutropenia. Again, the

numbers of IFIs diagnosed in the treated or the control arms were too small for any meaningful comparisons. Granulocyte colony-stimulating factor also was studied in a randomized trial in which patients with hematological malignancies and febrile neutropenia received either G-CSF with antibiotics or antibiotics alone (Aviles et al, 1996). Although only four IFIs occurred, all were encountered in the group receiving antibiotics alone. The patients receiving G-CSF plus antibiotics fared better by every outcome parameter.

In a double–blind controlled study, the administration of M-CSF to patients with myelogenous leukemia and febrile neutropenia decreased incidence and duration of febrile neutropenia and significantly decreased the use of systemic antifungal drugs (Ohno et al, 1997). However, no impact on disease-free survival was found, an outcome heavily dependent on many confounding factors in these high-risk patients.

Based on the data cited above, strong evidence for success with prophylactic or preemptive therapy with HGFs does not currently exist. On the other hand, when a febrile neutropenic episode is complicated and IFI is suspected, adjunctive use of a HGF with empirical antifungal therapy may be justified according to the American Society of Clinical Oncology (ASCO) updated recommendations regarding the use of HGFs (Ozer et al, 2000). In this document, ASCO does not recommend the use of HGFs for routine purposes in patients with afebrile neutropenia.

REFRACTORY INVASIVE FUNGAL INFECTIONS

Both in vitro and experimental animal models have suggested the utility of cytokine treatment as adjunc-

TABLE 10–4. *Clinical Use of Cytokines as Adjunctive Management of Febrile Neutropenia**

Reference	Cytokine	Outcome
Maher et al., 1994	G-CSF	↓ Number of days of neutropenia, ↓ time to resolution of febrile neutropenia, ↓ risk for prolonged hospitalization, accelerated neutrophil recovery
Aviles et al, 1996	G-CSF	More clinical responses, ↓ superinfections, ↓ hospitalization, ↓ antibiotic use, ↓ mortality IFIs in the group treated with antibiotics plus G-CSF
Anaissie et al, 1996	GM-CSF	No effect on clinical response and survival
Ohno et al, 1997	M-CSF	↓ Incidence and duration of febrile neutropenia, ↓ ↓ use of systemic antifungal drugs

Early or preemptive treatment of a possible invasive fungal infection in cancer patients
G-CSF, granulocyte colony-stimulating factor; GM-CSF, granulocyte-macrophage colony-stimulating factor; M-CSF, macrophage colony-stimulating factor.

tive therapy in combination with conventional anti-fungal chemotherapy against refractory IFIs (Kullberg and Anaissie, 1998a; Roilides et al, 1998a; Stevens, 1998; Stevens et al, 2000; Farmaki and Roilides, 2001). There are several small series and case reports suggesting the use of G-CSF as adjunctive therapy for certain IFIs with very poor prognosis in combination with amphotericin B or fluconazole and in some cases in addition to surgical debridement (Grauer et al, 1994; Fukushima et al, 1995; Dornbusch et al, 1995; Niitsu and Umeda, 1996; Sahin et al, 1996; Gonzalez et al, 1997; Hennequin et al, 1994; Boutati and Anaissie, 1997). Similarly, other reports have suggested a potential beneficial effect of the combination of GM-CSF and antifungal drugs (Spielberger et al, 1993; Pagano et al, 1996; Vazquez et al, 1998a; Abu Jawdeh et al, 2000) and GM-CSF and IFN-γ plus antifungal therapy (Poynton et al, 1998). Other clinical case reports of combination therapy with IFN-γ and conventional antifungal therapy have had mixed results.

In addition to the anecdotal reports cited above, three somewhat larger trials have addressed this issue. In the first clinical trial examining combination immunotherapy, M-CSF was administered to patients at escalating dosages (50–2000 mg/m^2, IV) in combination with the appropriate antifungal agent (amphotericin B, fluconazole, or flucytosine) at maximally tolerated doses (Nemunaitis et al, 1991). Among the 45 patients with IFIs, 30 had candidiasis, 15 had aspergillosis, and 1 had another. There was a trend toward better survival in the patients receiving M-CSF (Nemunaitis et al, 1993; Nemunaitis, 1998b). Moreover, this increase in survival was significant in patients with candidiasis and a Karnofsky score > 20% when compared with historical controls.

In another pilot study in which GM-CSF and amphotericin B were administered to 8 patients with IFIs and severe neutropenia, 6 had a PMN response, 4 were completely cured, and 2 were improved. Unfortunately, 3 patients developed a capillary leak syndrome, suggesting that the dosage of GM-CSF was excessive (Bodey et al, 1993). However, a subsequent open study of GM-CSF plus amphotericin B in 17 neutropenic cancer patients with proven IFIs did not show similar favorable outcomes; 6 of 17 died. Eight of the patients had candidemia, 8 had pulmonary aspergillosis, and 1 had fusariosis (Maertens et al, 1997). Clearly, statistically powered randomized clinical trials examining the utility of cytokine therapy in combination with conventional antifungal agents remain to be done.

The issue of cost effective use of cytokines as adjunctive therapy in combination with antifungal agents has not been thoroughly studied and does not allow specific recommendations. In 29 neutropenic patients with IFIs following chemotherapy or BMT, combined

therapy of amphotericin B and G-CSF (3–5 μg/kg per day) was associated with an improved response rate (62% vs. 33% controls) (Hazel et al, 1999). This study showed a greater cost-effectiveness of combination regimen, based on drug acquisition, hospital stay, and treatment duration (Flynn et al, 1999).

In immunocompetent patients, G-CSF is the only HGF that has been investigated. In a multicenter clinical trial addressing the utility of G-CSF as adjunctive therapy of invasive candidiasis, 51 nonneutropenic patients were randomized to receive either fluconazole alone or fluconazole with G-CSF. There was a trend (not statistically significant) toward an earlier resolution of infection as well as reduced mortality in the patients receiving combination therapy (Kullberg et al, 1998b). Results of this study support in vitro and in vivo results that have shown that not only number, but also function, of host immune cells is important to recovery from IFIs (Rodriguez-Adrian et al, 1998; Mencacci et al, 2000).

Phagocytic Dysfunction

Certain nonneutropenic patients have phagocytic dysfunction and are also at high risk for IFIs. Among them, patients with HSCT after recovery from neutropenia and especially during corticosteroid treatment of post-engraftment GVHD are the most susceptible hosts (Rodriguez-Adrian et al, 1998). Apart from a decrease in the function of circulating phagocytes, these patients present abnormal cell-mediated immunity related to defective function of MNCs, T, and NK cells. Indeed, IFIs, particularly aspergillosis, occur frequently in HSCT patients after the resolution of neutropenia (Wald et al, 1997), presumably related to an existing cytokine network dysregulation (Roilides et al, 2001b). These high-risk HSCT patients may benefit from cytokines administered during IFIs developed in the nonneutropenic phase after transplantation (Fig. 10–2).

Patients with qualitative phagocytic defects (most importantly CGD) are also at increased risk of IFIs, especially invasive aspergillosis, a main cause of mortality in these patients (Winkelstein et al, 2000). In one large prospective, randomized, placebo-controlled clinical trial, long-term administration of IFN-γ has been shown to reduce significantly the incidence of serious infections in CGD patients (The International Chronic Granulomatous Disease Cooperative Study Group, 1991). Patients in this study tended to have a reduced incidence of *Aspergillus* pneumonia compared with controls.

In addition, there is anecdotal evidence suggesting that IFN-γ can be an effective adjunctive therapy for the treatment of certain unusual IFIs (Phillips et al, 1991; Williamson et al, 1992; Tsumura et al, 1999; Roilides et al, 1999; Touza Rey et al, 2000). Adjunctive therapy with IFN-γ has proven to be most useful in patients with defects in their cellular immune function. For example, this cytokine has been used successfully for therapy of invasive aspergillosis in CGD patients in combination with antifungal agents (Cohen-Abbo and Edwards, 1995; Pasic et al, 1996).

Other nonneutropenic patients at high risk for IFIs who might benefit from immunotherapy, such as those with AIDS, lymphoma, solid organ transplant recipients, and patients receiving corticosteroids or other immunosuppressants, have dysfunctional phagocytes along with cytokine dysregulation and lymphocytic defects. In patients with AIDS, administration of recombinant IFN-γ showed a trend of decreased incidence of oral/esophageal candidiasis compared to control subjects (Riddell et al, 2001).

Recommendations of Cytokine Administration

As sufficient clinical data do not exist on the use of cytokines in the management of IFIs, no definite guidelines for their routine use can be established. Nevertheless, reconstitution of the immune response by exogenous administration of HGFs and proinflammatory cytokines or inhibition of immunoregulatory cytokines appears to be a promising adjunct to our armamentarium against life-threatening IFIs. In its 1994 guidelines, followed by its 1996 and 2000 updates (American Society of Clinical Oncology, 1994, 1996; Ozer et al, 2000), ASCO recommends that only high-risk patients (more than 40% risk of febrile neutropenia) receive G-CSF or GM-CSF prophylactically. Similarly, during the onset of febrile neutropenia in patients not receiving a HGF, G-CSF, or GM-CSF is suggested only when the duration of neutropenia is predicted to be long. Although no data exist, patients who have had an episode of IFI in the past and become neutropenic again should be treated with a HGF.

With regard to the management of documented IFIs in neutropenic patients, the 1997 Guidelines of the Infectious Diseases Society of America state that these HGFs "may be indicated" (Hughes et al, 1997). Up to now, potential direct applications of cytokines and HGFs against IFIs are limited to the following indications:

1. Use of G-CSF, GM-CSF, or M-CSF in the prevention and treatment of IFIs in neutropenic patients, especially those with myelogenous leukemia or HSCT. Granulocyte-colony stimulating factor may not be as effective as the macrophage-stimulating HGFs. In addition, patients with other types of neoplastic diseases including AIDS-related malignancies, which are associated with high probability of development of IFIs, may benefit from HGF therapy. Macrophage-colony stimulating factor is used in Japan. Since M-CSF has not been licensed in the United States and Europe, it cannot be used clinically in these countries.
2. Prophylactic use of IFN-γ in patients with CGD.
3. Under certain conditions of defective host defenses even without neutropenia (i.e., GVHD), a HGF with or without IFN-γ may be justified as adjunctive therapy for IFIs.

With completion of more clinical studies, indications also might include surgical and other nonneutropenic immunodeficient patients with IFIs, i.e., those with solid organ transplants, AIDS, neonates, and others. The role of administration of neutralizing antibodies or inhibitors of immunoregulatory cytokines on prevention and outcome of IFIs needs further clinical study.

Pharmacology of Hematopoietic Growth Factors and Interferon-γ

Two forms of G-CSF are commercially available. One is a recombinant nonglycosylated protein expressed in *Escherichia coli* (filgrastim). The other is a glycosylated form expressed in Chinese hamster ovarian cells in vitro (lenograstim). Both products have the same net effect, acceleration of myelopoiesis and enhancement of functional responses. Granulocyte colony-stimulating factor causes an immediate actual decrease of PMN count, which is followed by a sustained dose-dependent rise in the PMN count.

Granulocyte colony-stimulating factor has been recommended at a dose of 5 μg/kg/day subcutaneously or intravenously for high-risk patients after cytotoxic cancer chemotherapy. Administration of G-CSF begins the day after the last chemotherapy dose and continues with subsequent individualized adjustment of dosage depending on the PMN count until PMN count increases to 1000 per μl for 3 consecutive days. A higher dosage of 10 μg/kg/day can be used in early phases of HSCT followed by a standard dose of 5 μg/kg/day or when G-CSF is administered as adjunctive therapy for a documented IFI.

Granulocyte-macrophage colony-stimulating factor exists as a recombinant nonglycosylated protein expressed in *E. coli* (molgramostim) and a glycosylated protein expressed in *Saccharomyces cerevisiae* (sargramostim) or in mammalian cells (regramostim). Granulocyte-macrophage colony-stimulating factor transiently decreases leukocyte counts immediately after administration and afterwards causes sustained rises of PMN, eosinophil, and MNC counts.

Various dosing regimens of GM-CSF have been used in different studies. The recommended dosage is 250 μg per m² daily during the period of profound neutropenia or when a documented IFI is treated. The dosage is individualized depending on response and development of adverse effects. Interferon-γ has been administered at a dose of 50 μg per m² 3 times a week subcutaneously as prophylaxis in CGD patients (The International Chronic Granulomatous Disease Cooperative Study Group, 1991). Doses up to 100 μg per m² 3 times a week have been subsequently suggested. Similar doses have been used as adjunctive therapy.

Toxicity

Granulocyte-macrophage colony-stimulating factor has been described in some cases as inducing pleuritic pain, pulmonary edema, and a capillary leak syndrome. Another potential complication of its use stems from its activity in stimulating recovery of leukocyte function. Massive fatal hemoptysis has been reported to follow (Groll et al, 1992). Although bone pain is described in 20% of patients receiving G-CSF, the other adverse effects associated with GM-CSF are not commonly observed in G-CSF treated patients. The toxicity of GM-CSF appears to be related to the nonglycosylated preparations expressed in *E. coli*. By comparison, the glycosylated form of GM-CSF is not associated with these adverse effects. The toxicity profile of recombinant GM-CSF is consistent with priming of macrophages for increased formation and release of inflammatory cytokines, whereas G-CSF induces production of antiinflammatory factors, such as IL-1 receptor antagonist and soluble TNF receptor. Granulocyte colony-stimulating factor is protective against endotoxin- and sepsis- induced organ injury.

Although administration of G-CSF to patients with acute myeloid leukemia (AML) carries the theoretical risk of accelerating the leukemic blast cells, this has not been observed. Indeed, G-CSF has been used safely in patients with AML and myelodysplasia (Giralt et al, 1993). The adverse effect of GM-CSF accelerating HIV replication in MNCs may be offset by simultaneous administration of antiretroviral agents.

With regard to the IFN-γ therapy, the most common adverse effects are minor and consist of flu-like or constitutional symptoms such as fever, headache, chills, myalgia, or fatigue. These symptoms may decrease in severity as treatment continues.

WHITE BLOOD CELL TRANSFUSIONS

Based on the observation linking therapy-induced neutropenia with an increased risk for serious bacterial and fungal infection in cancer patients (Bodey et al, 1966), infusion of donor PMNs was attempted initially in an effort to combat progressive life-threatening infections in persistently neutropenic patients (Freireich et al 1964; Strauss, 1978; DiNubile, 1985; Schiffer, 1990). The findings supported the use of white blood cell transfusions (WBCTx) in persistently neutropenic patients with progressive bacterial infection, but were less com-

pelling for IFIs. This approach to immunotherapy was not used widely because of toxicity, cost, efficacy, alloimmunization, lack of readily available donors, and the development of potent alternative antibacterial strategies.

In the 1990s, use of WBCTx was reconsidered due to the increased incidence of neutropenia-related IFIs in combination with the limited efficacy of antifungal agents. At the same time, there were new developments, namely, the commercial availability of recombinant HGFs and modern transfusion practices. Studies supported the use of WBCTx in neutropenic patients with a progressive bacterial infection. In a review of 32 studies, the overall efficacy was 62% in 206 patients with bacterial infection (Strauss, 1994). For IFIs, the data were less encouraging. A positive clinical outcome was observed in only 29% of recipients. Investigators reported data on 50 patients; there was no significant improvement in outcome of IFIs, despite showing the feasibility of administering WBCTx (Bhatia et al, 1994). However, recent reports have provided encouraging data with G–CSF elicited WBCTx as compared to studies that used conventional WBCTx stimulated with corticosteroids (Catalano et al, 1997; Di Mario et al, 1997; Dignani et al, 1997; Ozsahin et al, 1998; Peters et al, 1999; Price et al, 2000) (Table 10–5).

A pilot study evaluated the safety and efficacy of G–CSF-elicited WBCTx in patients with neutropenia-related IFIs that were refractory to therapy with amphotericin B alone (Dignani et al, 1997). A favorable response was reported in 11 of 15 patients at the end of therapy. However, only 3 of the 11 patients were alive 3 months after starting WBCTx, and the IFI contributed to the cause of death in 6 of 8 patients in the setting of persistent or progressive immunosuppression (relapsed or refractory leukemia, or allogeneic BMT). The beneficial effect of WBCTx seemed to be enhanced by their administration to patients with good performance status, as well as administration early during neutropenia and soon after the onset of the IFI.

A separate small prospective multicenter phase I/II clinical trial evaluated the feasibility and tolerability of WBCTx in neutropenic patients with infection, 13 of whom had IFIs (Peters et al, 1999). A favorable outcome was observed in 5 of 9 patients with aspergillosis, and 2 of 4 patients with *Candida* infections. In addition to WBCTx, treatment consisted of antifungal agents, as well as surgical resection of the lesions in 5 patients following stabilization of the septic condition. In addition, as shown in Table 10–5, a number of successful cases using G-CSF-mobilized WBCTx have recently been reported. For example, a CGD patient with invasive aspergillosis due to *A. nidulans*, who failed 5 months of treatment with liposomal amphotericin B and IFN-γ, was treated successfully with BMT, G-CSF-mo-

TABLE 10–5. *Treatment of Neutropenia-Related Invasive Fungal Infections with G–CSF Stimulated White Blood Cell Transfusions*

Reference	Underlying Condition	No of Patients	Fungus	Outcome
Catalano et al, 1997	Aplastic anemia/BMT	1	*Aspergillus*	CR
Di Mario et al, 1997	Neutropenia	2	*C. tropicalis*	2/2 CR
Dignani et al, 1997	Neutropenia	15	11 moulds 4 yeasts	11/15 PR; (only 3/11 survived > 3 months post WBCTx)
Ozsahin et al, 1998	CGD	1	*Aspergillus*	CR
Peters et al, 1999	Neutropenia	13	9 *Aspergillus* 4 *Candida*	5/9 CR 2/4 CR
Price et al, 2000	Stem cell transplantation	15	8 moulds 7 yeasts	0/8 R 4/7 CR
Total		47	30 moulds 17 yeasts	7/19 CR (37%) 8/13 CR (62%)

CR, complete response; R, response; PR, partial response; BMT, bone marrow transplantation; CGD, chronic granulomatous disease; WBCTx, white blood cell transfusions.

bilized PMNs, and liposomal amphotericin B (Ozsahin et al, 1998). Overall in these two small trials and several case studies, yeast infections tended to respond to WBCTx better than did mould infections (62% vs. 37%) (Table 10–5). The rapid increase in PMNs coupled with the relatively low side effects suggest that WBCTx in combination with cytokines may be a useful approach and deserves further study in the setting of refractory IFIs.

Patients with evidence of alloimmunization (platelet refractoriness, antileukocyte antibodies, repeated febrile transfusion reactions, or posttransfusion pulmonary infiltrates) may not benefit from WBCTx (Strauss, 1994). This questionable benefit may result because such patients usually have a low posttransfusion increment, more pulmonary reactions, and transfused PMNs, which are unable to migrate to the sites of infection.

The higher the number of cells transfused per m^2 of body surface area, the better the clinical response to WBCTx (Freireich et al, 1964; Higby et al, 1976; Aisner et al, 1978; Appelbaum et al, 1978). For mobilization of PMNs in healthy donors, most experts have favored G-CSF, which is indeed, the standard of blood processing centers (Hubel et al, 2001). Both forms of G-CSF commercially available have the same net effect: acceleration of myelopoiesis and enhancement of functional PMN responses (including bactericidal activity, chemotaxis, phagocytosis, respiratory burst, and surface expression of low affinity Fc receptors) (Nathan, 1989; Roilides et al, 1991; Allen et al, 1997). Granulocyte colony-stimulating factor also delays apoptosis in PMNs, which is particularly important for harvested PMNs. It appears that G-CSF-stimulated PMNs have a longer shelf life and perhaps, once transfused, persist longer in vivo (Colotta et al, 1992; Kasahara et al, 1997).

Granulocyte colony-stimulating factor increases the yield of PMNs by roughly fivefold, which is greater than the 2–3-fold increase accomplished with corticosteroids (Liles et al, 1997; Peters et al, 1999; Price et al, 2000). The recommended optimal safe dose required to mobilize PMNs in adults is 450 μg (Liles et al, 1997). Only one dose is needed 12–24 hours prior to collection. Several recent studies have evaluated the role of the combination of G-CSF and corticosteroids, suggesting that the higher dose of G-CSF along with corticosteroids results in the highest yield (12-fold above premobilization) (Dale et al, 1998). With this approach, the functional properties of G-CSF-mobilized PMNs are essentially unchanged. Specifically, the respiratory burst activity is normal or elevated due to priming of PMNs. The half-life of transfused PMNs previously mobilized with G-CSF is at least twice as long (Dale et al, 1998). Single dose exposure to corticosteroids probably does not represent a major suppressant of PMN function in mobilized products. No G-CSF-related long-term effects have been observed in donors, even 1 year later, when all hematological measurements were comparable to pre-G-CSF levels (Bensinger et al, 1993; MacHida et al, 2000). Preliminary data suggest that storage at 10°C might lengthen the shelf-life of mobilized PMNs and may preserve antifungal and PMN function better (Hubel et al, 2000).

The leukapheresis technique used today is continuous flow centrifugation with the addition of a rouleauxing agent such as hydroxyethyl, which produces a better quality PMN (Bensinger et al, 1993). This technique, very advantageous over previous techniques, allows processing of larger volumes of blood, which has been translated into increased yields. Traditionally, related donors have been preferred to avoid toxicity related to incompatibility. More recently, community donors have been used effectively to safely and rapidly mobilize PMNs, thus increasing the availability of WBCTx to a larger number of potential recipients (Price et al, 2000).

White blood cell transfusions have been associated with a low incidence of complications. Mild reactions to the transfusion product are common, including fever and chills, which can be reduced if the infusion rate is reduced. Severe side effects, namely hypotension or respiratory distress, are estimated to occur in ~1% of recipients.

In two reports, respiratory complications have been temporally linked to coadministration of deoxycholate amphotericin B (Wright et al, 1981; Bow et al, 1984). Transfusion-related acute lung injury is rare and probably not associated with G-CSF mobilization (Dry et al, 1999). Graft vs. host disease is prevented by irradiation of the product preinfusion with 15–30 Gy, which does not appear to adversely affect the function of the transfused PMNs (Anderson and Weinstein, 1990). Alloimmunization can be a formidable problem in CGD patients, but interestingly does not occur in cancer or transplant recipients who have received immunosuppressive therapy. A recent study in HSCT recipients reported that those who received G-CSF-mobilized PMNs from an incompatible donor had a delayed engraftment (Adkins et al, 2000).

The major indication for WBCTx continues to be restricted to progressive, documented infection in the profoundly and persistently neutropenic host (Strauss, 1994). Antifungal drug-refractory IFIs in patients with an underlying phagocytic defect, namely CGD, are a particularly important indication for WBCTx adjunctive therapy. Prophylactic use of WBCTx therapy has not yet been incorporated into clinical practice, primarily because of cost and toxicity. It is still unclear that WBCTx should be widely embraced until further studies are completed and better define the niche of WBCTx in supportive care.

INTRAVENOUS IMMUNOGLOBULIN AND MONOCLONAL ANTIBODIES

Antibody-mediated host defense contributes to fighting against some IFIs. Mice with experimental *Candida* infection treated with human intravenous immunoglobulin (IVIG) combined with amphotericin B had modest prolongation of survival, suggesting the potential efficacy of serum antibodies against fungi (Neely and Holder, 1992). In humans, IVIG has been used in liver transplant recipients receiving anticytomegalovirus prophylaxis and in patients who had undergone BMT. In the first group, IVIG therapy was associated with a significant reduction in the incidence of IFIs (Stratta et al, 1992), whereas in the second group, IVIG therapy was not associated with a significant reduction (Klaesson et al, 1995). This latter finding was in disagreement with a previous finding that oral administration of bovine anti-*C. albicans* antibodies to BMT recipi-

ents reduced *Candida* colonization in 7 of 10 patients (Tollemar et al, 1999), suggesting that pathogen-specific antibodies can be effective in patients with immune defects.

For both *C. albicans* and *C. neoformans*, several protective monoclonal antibodies have been described, but the benefits of these are unclear (Casadevall, 1995). Studies have demonstrated that human serum antibodies and a mouse monoclonal antibody to hsp90 were protective against candidiasis in mice and a human recombinant antibody to an hsp90 linear epitope mediated protection against invasive murine candidiasis (Matthews et al, 1995). Antibodies to *C. albicans* polysaccharides have also been shown to be protective in murine models of infection (Han and Cutler, 1995).

Antibody efficacy against *C. neoformans* is a function of antibody isotype, idiotype, specificity, inoculum, and antibody dose. Another approach to antibody therapy has been to engineer antibodies with dual functions, or bispecific antibodies. A bispecific antibody that binds both the Fcα receptor (CD89) and *C. albicans* has been shown to enhance PMN-mediated antifungal activity in G–CSF-primed cells (van Spriel et al, 1999).

Although serum antibodies may promote natural resistance to infection, they may not necessarily ameliorate established or chronic infections. Hence, their efficacy against some fungi may be dependent on intact cellular immunity (Vecchiarelli and Casadevall, 1998). To date, the clinical use of antibodies has not been recommended in the management of IFIs.

CONCLUSION

In parallel with using antifungal agents to destroy fungi, helping immune response by either exogenous modulation of enhancing/regulatory cytokines or transfusion of cytokine-elicited allogeneic phagocytes appears to be a promising adjunct to antifungal chemotherapy. Potential application of these adjunctive therapies could be:

1. use of GM-CSF or M-CSF in prevention and therapy of IFIs in neutropenic patients with myelogenous leukemia or hematopoietic stem cell transplantation; and
2. use of IFN-γ in patients with CGD as prevention and therapy; and
3. infusion of G-CSF-elicited WBCTx to profoundly neutropenic patients with refractory IFIs.

The management of IFIs, which is still a great challenge for clinicians, may be greatly facilitated by various means to enhance host defense mechanisms. This approach has been experimentally achieved by reconstitution of effector cells numerically and/or functionally with cytokines and/or WBCTx, or by manipulation of cytokine dysbalance. Undoubtedly, immunotherapy opens new avenues and the interest in use of immune therapies as an adjunct to antifungal agents has greatly increased. Continued investigation of the safety and efficacy of these modalities as well as the most likely patients to benefit from adjunctive therapy are urgent priorities for research.

REFERENCES

Abu Jawdeh L, Haidar R, Bitar F, Mroueh S, Akel S, Nuwayri-Salti N, Dbaibo G S. *Aspergillus* vertebral osteomyelitis in a child with a primary monocyte killing defect: response to GM-CSF therapy. *J Infect* 41:97–100, 2000.

Adkins D R, Goodnough L T, Shenoy S, Brown R, Moellering J, Khoury H, Vij R, DiPersio J. Effect of leukocyte compatibility on neutrophil increment after transfusion of granulocyte colony-stimulating factor-mobilized prophylactic granulocyte transfusions and on clinical outcomes after stem cell transplantation. *Blood* 95:3605–3612, 2000.

Aguirre K M, Johnson L L. A role for B cells in resistance to *Cryptococcus neoformans* in mice. *Infect Immun* 65:525–530, 1997.

Aisner J, Schiffer C, Wiernik P. Granulocyte transfusions: Evaluation of factors influencing results and a comparison of filtration and intermittent centrifugation leukapheresis. *Br J Haematol* 38:121–129, 1978.

Allen R C, Stevens P R, Price T H, Chatta G S, Dale D C. In vivo effects of recombinant human granulocyte colony-stimulating factor on neutrophil oxidative functions in normal human volunteers. *J Infect Dis* 175:1184–1192, 1997.

American Society of Clinical Oncology. Recommendations for the use of hematopoietic colony stimulating factors: evidence-based, clinical practice guidelines. *J Clin Oncol* 12:2471–2508, 1994.

American Society of Clinical Oncology. Update of recommendations for the use of hematopoietic colony stimulating factors: evidence-based clinical practice guidelines. *J Clin Oncol* 14:1957–1960, 1996.

Anaissie E J, Vartivarian S, Bodey G P, Legrand C, Kantarjian H, Abi-Said D, Karl C, Vadhan-Raj S. Randomized comparison between antibiotics alone and antibiotics plus granulocyte-macrophage colony-stimulating factor (*Escherichia coli*-derived) in cancer patients with fever and neutropenia. *Am J Med* 100:17–23, 1996.

Anderson K C, Weinstein H J. Transfusion-associated graft-versus-host disease. *N Engl J Med* 323:315–321, 1990.

Antman K S, Griffin J D, Elias A, Socinski M, Ryan L, Cannista S A, Oette D, Whittey M, Frei E, Schnipper L. Effect of recombinant human granulocyte-macrophage colony stimulating factor on chemotherapy-induced myelosuppression. *N Engl J Med* 319:593–598, 1988.

Appelbaum F, Bowles C, Makuch R, Deisseroth A. Granulocyte transfusion therapy of experimental *Pseudomonas* septicemia: Study of cell dose and collection technique. *Blood* 52:323–331, 1978.

Aviles A, Guzman R, Garcia E L, Talavera A, Diaz-Maqueo J C. Results of a randomized trial of granulocyte colony-stimulating factor in patients with infection and severe granulocytopenia. *Anti-Cancer Drugs* 7:392–397, 1996.

Bensinger W I, Price T H, Dale D C, Appelbaum F R, Clift R, Lilleby K, Williams B, Storb R, Thomas E D, Buckner C D. The effects of daily recombinant human granulocyte colony-stimulating factor adminstration on normal granulocyte donors undergoing leukapheresis. *Blood* 81:1883–1888, 1993.

Bhatia S, McCullough J, Perry E H, Clay M, Ramsay N K, Neglia J P. Granulocyte transfusions: efficacy in treating fungal infections in neutropenic patients following bone marrow transplantation. *Transfusion* 34:226–232, 1994.

Bodey G P, Anaissie E, Gutterman J, Vadhan Raj S. Role of granulocyte-macrophage colony-stimulating factor as adjuvant therapy for fungal infection in patients with cancer. *Clin Infect Dis* 17:705–707, 1993.

Bodey G P, Buckley M, Sathe Y S, Freireich E J. Quantitative relationships between circulating leukocytes and infections in patients with acute leukemia. *Ann Intern Med* 64:328–340, 1966.

Boogaerts M A, Demuynck H M. Consensus on the clinical use of myeloid growth factors. *Curr Opin Hematol* 3:241–246, 1996.

Boutati E I, Anaissie E J. *Fusarium*, a significant emerging pathogen in patients with hematologic malignancy: ten years' experience at a cancer center and implications for management. *Blood* 90:999–1008, 1997.

Bow E J, Schroeder M L, Louie T J. Pulmonary complications in patients receiving granulocyte transfusions and amphotericin B. *Can Med Assoc J* 130:593–597, 1984.

Brieland J K, Jackson C, Menzel F, Loebenberg D, Cacciapuoti A, Halpern J, Hurst S, Muchamuel T, Debets R, Kastelein R, Churakova T, Abrams J, Hare R, O'Garra A. Cytokine networking in lungs of immunocompetent mice in response to inhaled *Aspergillus fumigatus*. *Infect Immun* 69:1554–1560, 2001.

Casadevall A. Antibody immunity and invasive fungal infections. *Infect Immun* 63:4211–4218, 1995.

Catalano L, Fontana R, Scarpato N, Picardi M, Rocco S, Rotoli B. Combined treatment with amphotericin-B and granulocyte transfusion from G-CSF-stimulated donors in an aplastic patient with invasive aspergillosis undergoing bone marrow transplantation. *Haematologica* 82:71–72, 1997.

Cenci E, Bartocci A, Puccetti P, Mocci S, Stanely E R, Bistoni F. Macrophage colony-stimulating factor in murine candidiasis: Serum and tissue levels during infection and protective effect of exogenous administration. *Infect Immun* 59:868–872, 1991.

Cenci E, Romani L, Mencacci A, Spaccapelo R, Schiaffella E, Puccetti P, Bistoni F. Interleukin-4 and interleukin-10 inhibit nitric oxide-dependent macrophage killing of *Candida albicans*. *Eur J Immunol* 23:1034–1038, 1993.

Cenci E, Mencacci A, Del Sero G, Bacci A, Montagnoli C, Fe d'Ostiani C, Mosci P, Bachmann M, Bistoni F, Kopf M, Romani L. Interleukin-4 causes susceptibility to invasive aspergillosis through suppression of protective type 1 responses. *J Infect Dis* 180:1957–1968, 1999.

Clemons K V, Brummer E, Stevens D A. Cytokine treatment of central nervous system infection: efficacy of interleukin-12 alone and synergy with conventional antifungal therapy in experimental cryptococcosis. *Antimicrob Agents Chemother* 38:460–464, 1994.

Cohen-Abbo A, Edwards K M. Multifocal osteomyelitis caused by *Paecilomyces varioti* in a patient with chronic granulomatous disease. *Infection* 23:55–57, 1995.

Colotta F, Re F, Polentarutti N, Sozzani S, Mantovani A. Modulation of granulocyte survival and programmed cell death by cytokines and bacterial products. *Blood* 80:2012–2020, 1992.

Crawford J, Ozer H, Stoller R, Johnson D, Lyman G, Tabbara I, Kris M, Grous J, Picozzi V, Rausch G, Smith R, Gradishar W, Yahanda A, Vincent M, Stewart M, Glaspy J. Reduction by granulocyte colony-stimulating factor of fever and neutropenia induced by chemotherapy in patients with small-cell lung cancer. *N Engl J Med* 325:164–170, 1991.

Dale D C, Liles W C, Llewellyn C, Rodger E, Price T H. Neutrophil transfusions: kinetics and functions of neutrophils mobilized with granulocyte colony-stimulating factor and dexamethasone. *Transfusion* 38:713–721, 1998.

Denning D W. Invasive aspergillosis. *Clin Infect Dis* 26:781–803, 1998.

Di Mario A, Sica S, Salutari P, Ortu La Barbera E, Marra R, Leone G. Granulocyte colony-stimulating factor-primed leukocyte transfusions in *Candida tropicalis* fungemia in neutropenic patients. *Haematologica* 82:362–363, 1997.

Diamond R D, Lyman C A, Wysong D R. Disparate effects of interferon-gamma and tumor necrosis factor-alpha on early neutrophil respiratory burst and fungicidal responses to *Candida albicans* hyphae in vitro. *J Clin Invest* 87:711–720, 1991.

Dignani M C, Freireich E J, Andersson B S, Lichtiger B, Jendiroba D B, Kantarjian H, Rex J H, Vartivarian S E, O'Brien S, Hester J P, Anaissie E J. Treatment of neutropenia-related fungal infections with granulocyte colony-stimulating factor-elicited white blood cell transfusions: a pilot study. *Leukemia* 11:1621–1630, 1997.

DiNubile, M J. Therapeutic role of granulocyte transfusions. *Rev Infect Dis* 7:232–242, 1985

Djeu J Y, Blanchard D K, Halkias D, Friedman H. Growth inhibition of *Candida albicans* by human polymorphonuclear neutrophils: activation by interferon-gamma and tumor necrosis factor. *J Immunol* 137:2980–2984, 1986.

Dornbusch H J, Urban C E, Pinter H, Ginter G, Fotter R, Becker H, Miorini T, Berghold C. Treatment of invasive pulmonary aspergillosis in severely neutropenic children with malignant disorders using liposomal amphotericin B, granulocyte colony-stimulating factor and surgery: report of 5 cases. *Pediatr Hematol Oncol* 12:577–586, 1995.

Dry S M, Bechard K M, Milford E L, Churchill W H, Benjamin R J. The pathology of transfusion-related acute lung injury. *Am J Clin Pathol* 112:216–221, 1999.

Farmaki E, Roilides E. Immunotherapy in patients with systemic mycoses: a promising adjunct. *Bio Drugs* 15:207–214, 2001.

Ferrante A. Tumor necrosis factor alpha potentiates neutrophil antimicrobial activity: Increased fungicidal activity against *Torulopsis glabrata* and *Candida albicans* and associated increases in oxygen radical production and lysosomal enzyme release. *Infect Immun* 57:2115–2122, 1989.

Flynn T N, Kelsey S M, Hazel D L, Guest J F. Cost effectiveness of amphotericin B plus G-CSF compared with amphotericin B monotherapy. Treatment of presumed deep-seated fungal infection in neutropenic patients in the UK. *Pharmacoeconomics* 16:543–550, 1999.

Freireich E J, Levin R H, Whang J, Carbone P P, Bronson W, Morse E E. The function and fate of transfused leukocytes from donors with chronic myelocytic leukemia in leukopenic recipients. *Ann NY Acad Sci* 113:1081–1089, 1964.

Fukushima T, Sumazaki R, Shibasaki M, Saitoh H, Fujigaki Y, Kaneko M, Akaogi E, Mitsui K, Ogata T, Takita H. Successful treatment of invasive thoracopulmonary mucormycisis in a patient with acute lymphoblastic leukemia. *Cancer* 76:895–899, 1995.

Gaviria J M, van Burik J A, Dale D C, Root R K, Liles W C. Comparison of interferon-gamma, granulocyte colony-stimulating factor, and granulocyte-macrophage colony-stimulating factor for priming leukocyte-mediated hyphal damage of opportunistic fungal pathogens. *J Infect Dis* 179:1038–1041, 1999.

Giles F J. Monocyte-macrophages, granulocyte-macrophage colony stimulating factor, and prolonged survival among patients with acute myeloid leukemia and stem cell transplants. *Clin Infect Dis* 26:1282–1289, 1998.

Giralt S, Escudier S, Kantarjian H, Deisseroth A, Freireich E J, Andersson B S, O'Brien S, Andreeff M, Fisher H, Cork A, et al. Preliminary results of treatment with filgrastim for relapse of leukemia and myelodysplasia after allogeneic bone marrow transplantation. *N Engl J Med* 329:757–761, 1993.

Gonzalez C E, Couriel D R, Walsh T J. Successful treatment of disseminated zygomycosis in a neutropenic patient with amphotericin B lipid complex and granulocyte colony-stimulating factor. *Clin Infect Dis* 24:192–196, 1997.

Grauer M E, Bokemeyer C, Bautsch W, Freund M, Link H. Successful treatment of a *Trichosporon beigelii* septicemia in a granulocytopenic patient with amphotericin B and granulocyte colony-stimulating factor. *Infection* 22:283–286, 1994.

Graybill J R, Bocanegra R, Najvar L K, Loebenberg D, Luther M F. Granulocyte colony-stimulating factor and azole antifungal therapy in murine aspergillosis: role of immune suppression. *Antimicrob Agents Chemother* 42:2467–2473, 1998.

Grazziutti M L, Savary C A, Ford A, Anaissie E J, Cowart R E, Rex J H. *Aspergillus fumigatus* conidia induce a Th1–type cytokine response. *J Infect Dis* 176:1579–1583, 1997.

Groll A, Renz S, Gerein V, Schwabe D, Katschan G, Schneider M, Hubner K, Kornhuber B. Fatal haemoptysis associated with invasive pulmonary aspergillosis treated with high-dose amphotericin B and granulocyte-macrophage colony-stimulating factor (GM-CSF). *Mycoses* 35:67–75, 1992.

Han Y, Cutler J E. Antibody response that protects against disseminated candidiasis. *Infect Immun* 63:2714–2719, 1995.

Hazel D L, Newland A C, Kelsey S M. Malignancy: Granulocyte colony-stimulating factor increases the efficacy of conventional amphotericin in the treatment of presumed deep-seated fungal infection in neutropenic patients following intensive chemotherapy or bone marrow transplantation for haematological malignancies. *Hematol* 4:305–311, 1999.

Hennequin C, Benkerrou M, Gaillard J L, Blanche S, Fraitag S. Role of granulocyte colony-stimulating factor in the management of infection with *Fusarium oxysporum* in a neutropenic child. *Clin Infect Dis* 18:490–491, 1994.

Higby D J, Freeman A, Henderson E S, Sinks L, Cohen E. Granulocyte transfusions in children using filter-collected cells. *Cancer* 38:1407–1413, 1976.

Hubel K, Dale D C, Rodgers E, Gaviria J M, Price T, Liles W C. Preservation of function in granulocyte concetrates collected from donors stimulated with G-CSF /dexamethasone during storage at reduced temperature [abstract]. *Blood* 96:820a, 2000.

Hubel K, Dale D C, Engert A, Liles W C. Current status of granulocyte (neutrophil) transfusion therapy for infectious diseases. *J Infect Dis* 183:321–328, 2001.

Hughes W T, Armstrong D, Bodey G P, Brown A E, Edwards J E, Feld R, Pizzo P, Rolston K V, Shenep J L, Young L S. 1997 guidelines for the use of antimicrobial agents in neutropenic patients with unexplained fever. Infectious Diseases Society of America. *Clin Infect Dis* 25:551–573, 1997.

Karbassi A, Becker J M, Foster J S, Moore R N. Enhanced killing of *Candida albicans* by murine macrophages treated with macrophage colony-stimulating factor: Evidence for augmented expression of mannose receptors. *J Immunol* 139:417–421, 1987.

Kasahara Y, Iwai K, Yachie A, Ohta K, Konno A, Seki H, Miyawaki T, Taniguchi N. Involvement of reactive oxygen intermediates in spontaneous and CD95 (Fas/APO-1)-mediated apoptosis of neutrophils. *Blood* 89:1748–1753, 1997.

Klaesson S, Ringden O, Markling L, Tammik L. Intravenous immunoglobulin: immune modulatory effects in vitro and clinical effects in allogeneic bone marrow transplant recipients. *Transplant Proc* 27:3536–3537, 1995.

Kullberg B J, Anaissie E J. Cytokines as therapy for opportunistic fungal infections. *Res Immunol* 149:478–488, 1998a.

Kullberg B J, van de Woude K, Aoun M, Jacobs F, Herbrecht R, Kujath P, for the European Filgrastim Candidiasis Study Group. A double-blind, randomized, placebo-controlled phase II study of filgrastim (recombinant granulocyte colony-stimluating factor) in combination with fluconazole for treatment of invasive candidiasis and candidemia in nonneutropenic patients. In: Program and

Abstracts of the 38th Interscience Conference on Antimicrobial Agents and Chemotherapy; San Diego CA. Abstract J-100, 1998b.

Lieschke G J, Burgess A W. Granulocyte colony-stimulating factor and granulocyte-macrophage colony-stimulating factor. N Engl J Med 327:28–35, 1992.

Liles W C, Huang J E, van Burik J A, Bowden R A, Dale D C. Granulocyte colony-stimulating factor administered in vivo augments neutrophil-mediated activity against opportunistic fungal pathogens. J Infect Dis 175:1012–1015, 1997.

Lutz J E, Clemons K V, Stevens D A. Enhancement of antifungal chemotherapy by interferon-gamma in experimental systemic cryptococcosis. J Antimicrob Chemother 46:437–442, 2000.

MacHida U, Tojo A, Takahashi S, Iseki T, Ooi J, Nagayama H, Shirafuji N, Mori S, Wada Y, Ogami K, Yamada Y, Sakamaki H, Maekawa T, Tani K, Asano S. The effect of granulocyte colony-stimulating factor administration in healthy donors before bone marrow harvesting. Br J Haematol 108:747–753, 2000.

Maertens J, Demuynck H, Verhoef G, Vandenberhe P, Zachee P, Boogaerts M. GM-CSF fails to improve outcome in invasive fungal infections in neutropenic cancer patients. In: 13th Congress of the Intern Soc Hum Animal Mycol; Parma Italy; Abstr. 560, 1997.

Magee D M, Cox R A. Interleukin-12 regulation of host defenses against Coccidioides immitis. Infect Immun 64:3609–3613, 1996.

Maher D W, Lieschke G J, Green M, Bishop J, Stuart-Harris R, Wolf M, Sheridan W P, Kefford R F, Cebon J, Olver I, McKendrick J, Toner G, Bradstock K, Lieschke M, Bruickshank S, Tomita D K, Hoffman E W, Fox R M, Morstyn G. Filgrastim in patients with chemotherapy-induced febrile neutropenia. A double-blind, placebo-controlled trial. Ann Intern Med 121:492–501, 1994.

Matthews R, Hodgetts S, Burnie J. Preliminary assessment of a human recombinant antibody fragment to hsp90 in murine invasive candidiasis. J Infect Dis 171:1668–1671, 1995.

Mencacci A, Cenci E, Bacci A, Bistoni F, Romani L. Host immune reactivity determines the efficacy of combination immunotherapy and antifungal chemotherapy in candidiasis. J Infect Dis 181:686–694, 2000.

Murray H W. Interferon-gamma and host antimicrobial defense: current and future clinical applications. Am J Med 97:459–467, 1994.

Musso T, Calosso L, Zucca M, Millesimo M, Puliti M, Bulfone-Paus S, Merlino C, Savoia D, Cavallo R, Ponzi A N, Badolato R. Interleukin-15 activates proinflammatory and antimicrobial functions in polymorphonuclear cells. Infect Immun 66:2640–2647, 1998.

Natarajan U, Brummer E, Stevens D A. Effect of granulocyte colony-stimulating factor on the candidacidal activity of polymorphonuclear neutrophils and their collaboration with fluconazole. Antimicrob Agents Chemother 41:1575–1578, 1997.

Nathan C F. Respiratory burst in adherent human neutrophils: triggering by colony-stimulating factors CSF-GM and CSF-G. Blood 73:301–306, 1989.

Neely A N, Holder I A. Effects of immunoglobulin G and low-dose amphotericin B on Candida albicans infections in burned mice. Antimicrob Agents Chemother 36:643–646, 1992.

Nemunaitis J, Meyers J D, Buckner D, Shannon-Dorcy K, Mori M, Shulman H, Bianco J A, Higano C S, Groves E, Storb R, Hansen J, Appelbaum F R, Singer J W. Phase I trial of recombinant human macrophage colony-stimulating factor in patients with invasive fungal infections. Blood 78:907–913, 1991.

Nemunaitis J, Shannon-Dorcy K, Appelbaum F R, Meyers J D, Owens A, Day R, Ando D, O'Neill C, Buckner D, Singer J W. Long-term follow-up of patients with invasive fungal disease who received adjunctive therapy with recombinant human macrophage colony-stimulating factor. Blood 82:1422–1427, 1993.

Nemunaitis J. A comparative review of colony-stimulating factors. Drugs 54:709–729, 1997.

Nemunaitis J. Use of macrophage colony-stimulating factor in the treatment of fungal infections. Clin Infect Dis 26:1279–1281, 1998a.

Nemunaitis J, Buckner C D, Dorsey K S, Willis D, Meyer W, Appelbaum F. Retrospective analysis of infectious diseases in patients who received recombinant human granulocyte-macrophage colony-stimulating factor versus patients not receiving a cytokine who underwent autologous bone marrow transplantation for treatment of lymphoid cancer. Am J Clin Oncol 21:341–346, 1998b.

Niitsu N, Umeda M. Fungemia in patients with hematologic malignancies: therapeutic effects of concomitant administration of fluconazole and granulocyte colony-stimulating factor. Chemotherapy 42:215–219, 1996.

Ohno R, Miyawaki S, Hatake K, Kuriyama K, Saito K, Kanamaru A, Kobayashi T, Kodera Y, Nishikawa K, Matsuda S, Yamada O, Omoto E, Takeyama H, Tsukuda K, Asou N, Tanimoto M, Shiozaki H, Tomonaga M, Masaoka T, Miura Y, Takaku F, Ohashi Y, Motoyoshi K. Human urinary macrophage colony-stimulating factor reduces the incidence and duration of febrile neutropenia and shortens the period required to finish three courses of intensive consolidation therapy in acute myeloid leukemia: a double-blind controlled study. J Clin Oncol 15:2954–2965, 1997.

Ozer H, Armitage J O, Bennett C L, Crawford J, Demetri G D, Pizzo P A, Schiffer C A, Smith T J, Somlo G, Wade J C, Wade J L, 3rd, Winn R J, Wozniak A J, Somerfield M R. 2000 update of recommendations for the use of hematopoietic colony-stimulating factors: evidence-based, clinical practice guidelines. American Society of Clinical Oncology Growth Factors Expert Panel. J Clin Oncol 18:3558–3585, 2000.

Ozsahin H, von Planta M, Muller I, Steinert H C, Nadal D, Lauener R, Tuchschmid P, Willi U V, Ozsahin M, Crompton N E, Seger R A. Successful treatment of invasive aspergillosis in chronic granulomatous disease by bone marrow transplantation, granulocyte colony-stimulating factor-mobilized granulocytes, and liposomal amphotericin-B. Blood 92:2719–2724, 1998.

Pagano L, Morace G, Ortu-La Barbera E, Sanguinetti M, Leone G. Adjuvant therapy with rhGM-CSF for the treatment of Blastoschizomyces capitatus systemic infection in a patient with acute myeloid leukemia. Ann Hematol 73:33–34, 1996.

Pasic S, Abinun M, Pistignjat B, Vlajic B, Rakic J, Sarjanovic L, Ostojic N. Aspergillus osteomyelitis in chronic granulomatous disease: treatment with recombinant gamma-interferon and itraconazole. Pediatr Infect Dis J 15:833–834, 1996.

Peters B G, Adkins D R, Harrison B, Velasquez W S, Dunphy F R, Petruska P J, Bowers C E, Niemeyer R, McIntyre W, Vrahnos D, Auberry S E, Spitzer G. Antifungal effects of yeast-derived rhu-GM-CSF in patients receiving high-dose chemotherapy given with or without autologous stem cell transplantation: a retrospective analysis. Bone Marrow Transplant 18:93–102, 1996.

Peters C, Minkov M, Matthes-Martin S, Potschger U, Witt V, Mann G, Hocker P, Worel N, Stary J, Klingebiel T, Gadner H. Leucocyte transfusions from rhG-CSF or prednisolone stimulated donors for treatment of severe infections in immunocompromised neutropenic patients. Br J Haematol 106:689–696, 1999.

Phillips P, Forbes J C, Speert D P. Disseminated infection with Pseudallescheria boydii in a patient with chronic granulomatous disease: response to gamma-interferon plus antifungal chemotherapy. Pediatr Infect Dis J 10:536–539, 1991.

Poynton C H, Barnes R A, Rees J. Interferon gamma and granulocyte-macrophage colony-stimulating factor for the treatment of hepatosplenic candidosis in patients with acute leukemia. Clin Infect Dis 26:239–240, 1998.

Price T H, Bowden R A, Boeckh M, Bux J, Nelson K, Liles W C, Dale D C. Phase I/II trial of neutrophil transfusions from donors stimulated with G-CSF and dexamethasone for treatment of patients with infections in hematopoietic stem cell transplantation. *Blood* 95:3302–3309, 2000.

Riddell L A, Pinching A J, Hill S, Ng T T, Arbe E, Lapham G P, Ash S, Hillman R, Tchamouroff S, Denning D W, Parkin J M. A phase III study of recombinant human interferon gamma to prevent opportunistic infections in advanced HIV disease. *AIDS Res Hum Retroviruses* 17:789–797, 2001.

Rodriguez-Adrian L J, Grazziutti M L, Rex J H, Anaissie E J. The potential role of cytokine therapy for fungal infections in patients with cancer: is recovery from neutropenia all that is needed? *Clin Infect Dis* 26:1270–1278, 1998.

Roilides E, Walsh T J, Pizzo P A, Rubin M. Granulocyte colony-stimulating factor enhances the phagocytic and bactericidal activity of normal and defective human neutrophils. *J Infect Dis* 163:579–583, 1991.

Roilides E, Uhlig K, Venzon D, Pizzo P A, Walsh T J. Enhancement of oxidative response and damage caused by human neutrophils to *Aspergillus fumigatus* hyphae by granulocyte colony-stimulating factor and gamma interferon. *Infect Immun* 61:1185–1193, 1993a.

Roilides E, Uhlig K, Venzon D, Pizzo P A, Walsh T J. Prevention of corticosteroid-induced suppression of human polymorphonuclear leukocyte-induced damage of *Aspergillus fumigatus* hyphae by granulocyte colony-stimulating factor and interferon-gamma. *Infect Immun* 61:4870–4877, 1993b.

Roilides E, Holmes A, Blake C, Venzon D, Pizzo P A, Walsh T J. Antifungal activity of elutriated human monocytes against *Aspergillus fumigatus* hyphae: Enhancement by granulocyte-macrophage colony-stimulating factor and interferon-gamma. *J Infect Dis* 170:894–899, 1994.

Roilides E, Holmes A, Blake C, Pizzo P A, Walsh T J. Effects of granulocyte colony-stimulating factor and interferon-gamma on antifungal activity of human polymorphonuclear neutrophils against pseudohyphae of different medically important *Candida* species. *J Leukoc Biol* 57:651–656, 1995a.

Roilides E, Sein T, Holmes A, Blake C, Pizzo P A, Walsh T J. Effects of macrophage colony-stimulating factor on antifungal activity of mononuclear phagocytes against *Aspergillus fumigatus*. *J Infect Dis* 172:1028–1034, 1995b.

Roilides E, Blake C, Holmes A, Pizzo P A, Walsh T J. Granulocyte-macrophage colony-stimulating factor and interferon-gamma prevent dexamethasone-induced imunosuppression of antifungal monocyte activity against *Aspergillus fumigatus* hyphae. *J Med Vet Mycol* 34:63–69, 1996a.

Roilides E, Lyman C A, Mertins S D, Cole D J, Venzon D, Pizzo P A, Chanock S J, Walsh T J. Ex vivo effects of macrophage colony-stimulating factor on human monocyte activity against fungal and bacterial pathogens. *Cytokine* 8:42–48, 1996b.

Roilides E, Dimitriadou A, Kadiltsoglou I, Sein T, Karpouzas J, Pizzo P A, Walsh T J. IL-10 exerts suppressive and enhancing effects on antifungal activity of mononuclear phagocytes against *Aspergillus fumigatus*. *J Immunol* 158:322–329, 1997a.

Roilides E, Kadiltsoglou I, Dimitriadou A, Hatzistilianou M, Manitsa A, Karpouzas J, Pizzo P A, Walsh T J. Interleukin-4 suppresses antifungal activity of human mononuclear phagocytes against *Candida albicans* in association with decreased uptake of blastoconidia. *FEMS Immunol Med Microbiol* 19:169–180, 1997b.

Roilides E, Dignani M C, Anaissie E J, Rex J H. The role of immunoreconstitution in the management of refractory opportunistic fungal infections. *Med Mycol* 36:12–25, 1998a.

Roilides E, Dimitriadou-Georgiadou A, Sein T, Kadiltzoglou I, Walsh T J. Tumor necrosis factor alpha enhances antifungal activities of polymorphonuclear and mononuclear phagocytes against *Aspergillus fumigatus*. *Infect Immun* 66:5999–6003, 1998b.

Roilides E, Sigler L, Bibashi E, Katsifa H, Flaris N, Panteliadis C. Disseminated infection due to *Chrysosporium zonatum* in a patient with chronic granulomatous disease and review of non-*Aspergillus* infections in these patients. *J Clin Microbiol* 37:18–25, 1999.

Roilides E, Katsifa H, Tsaparidou S, Stergiopoulou T, Panteliadis C, Walsh T J. Interleukin-10 suppresses phagocytic and antihyphal activities of human neutrophils. *Cytokine* 12:379–387, 2000.

Roilides E, Maloukou A, Gil-Lamaignere C, Winn R M, Panteliadis C, Walsh T J. Differential effects of interleukin 15 on hyphal damage of filamentous fungi induced by human neutrophils. In: 41st Interscience Conference on Antimicrobial Agents and Chemotherapy, Chicago IL. Abstract J-468, 2001a.

Roilides E, Sein T, Roden M, Schaufele R L, Walsh T J. Elevated serum concentrations of interleukin-10 in nonneutropenic patients with invasive aspergillosis. *J Infect Dis* 183:518–520, 2001b.

Roilides, E, Lyman C A, Panagopoulou P, Chanock S. Immunomodulation of invasive fungal infections. *Infect Dis Clin N Am*, In Press, 2003.

Romani L, Mencacci A, Cenci E, Spaccapelo R, Del Sero G, Nicoletti I, Trinchieri G, Bistoni F, Puccetti P. Neutrophil production of IL-12 and IL-10 in candidiasis and efficacy of IL-12 therapy in neutropenic mice. *J Immunol* 158:5349–5356, 1997.

Rowe J M, Anderson J W, Mazza J J, Bennett J M, Paietta E, Hayes F A, Oette R, Cassileth P A, Stadtmauer E A, Wiernik P H. A randomized placebo-controlled phase III study of granulocyte-macrophage colony-stimulating factor in adult patients (> 55 to 70 years) with acute myelogenous leukemia: a study by the Eastern Co-operative Oncology Group (E1490). *Blood* 86:457–462, 1995.

Rowe J M. Treatment of acute myeloid leukemia with cytokines: effect on duration of neutropenia and response to infections. *Clin Infect Dis* 26:1290–1294, 1998.

Sahin B, Paydas S, Cosar E, Bicacki K, Hazar B. Role of granulocyte colony-stimulating factor in the treatment of mucormycosis. *Eur J Clin Microbiol Infect Dis* 15:866–869, 1996.

Schelenz S, Smith D A, Bancroft G J. Cytokine and chemokine responses following pulmonarry challenge with *Aspergillus fumigatus*: obligatory role of TNF-a and GM-CSF in neutrophil recruitment. *Med Mycol* 37:183–194, 1999.

Schiffer, C. A. Granulocyte transfusions: An overlooked therapeutic modality. *Transfusion Med Rev* IV:2–7, 1990.

Seipelt G. Clinical use of hematopoietic growth factors. *Antibiot Chemother* 50:94–105, 2000.

Smith P D, Lamerson C L, Banks S M, Saini S S, Wahl L M, Calderone R A, Wahl S M. Granulocyte-macrophage colony-stimulating factor augments human monocyte fungicidal activity for *Candida albicans*. *J Infect Dis* 161:999–1005, 1990.

Spielberger R T, Falleroni M J, Coene A J, Larson R A. Concomitant amphotericin B therapy, granulocyte transfusions, and GM-CSF administration for disseminated infection with *Fusarium* in a granulocytopenic patient. *Clin Infect Dis* 16:528–530, 1993.

Stevens D A. Combination immunotherapy and antifungal chemotherapy. *Clin Infect Dis* 26:1266–1269, 1998.

Stevens D A, Kullberg B J, Brummer E, Casadevall A, Netea M G, Sugar A M. Combined treatment: antifungal drugs with antibodies, cytokines or drugs. *Med Mycol* 38:305–315, 2000.

Stratta R J, Shaefer M S, Cushing K A, Markin R S, Reed E C, Langnas A N, Pillen T J, Shaw B W. A randomized prospective trial of acyclovir and immune globulin prophylaxis in liver transplant recipients receiving OKT3 therapy. *Arch Surg* 127:55–63, 1992.

Strauss, R G. Therapeutic neutrophil transfusions: are controlled studies no longer appropriate? *Am J Med* 65:1001–1006, 1978.

Strauss R G. Granulocyte transfusion therapy for hematology/oncology patients. *Hem Onc Ann* 2:304–309, 1994.

The International Chronic Granulomatous Disease Cooperative

Study Group. A controlled trial of interferon gamma to prevent infection in chronic granulomatous disease. *N Engl J Med* 324: 509–516, 1991.

Tollemar J, Gross N, Dolgiras N, Jarstrand C, Ringden O, Hammarstrom L. Fungal prophylaxis by reduction of fungal colonization by oral administration of bovine anti-Candida antibodies in bone marrow transplant recipients. *Bone Marrow Transplant* 23:283–290, 1999.

Touza Rey F, Martinez Vazquez C, Alonso Alonso J, Mendez Pineiro M J, Rubianes Gonzalez M, Crespo Casal M. The clinical response to interferon-gamma in a patient with chronic granulomatous disease and brain abcesses due to *Aspergillus fumigatus*. *Anales de Medicina* 17:86–87, 2000.

Tsumura N, Akasu Y, Yamane H, Ikezawa S, Hirata T, Oda K, Sakata Y, Shirahama M, Inoue A, Kato H. *Aspergillus* osteomyelitis in a child who has p67-phox-deficient chronic granulomatous disease. *Kurume Med J* 46:87–90, 1999.

van Spriel A B, van den Herik-Oudijk I E, van Sorge N M, Vile H A, van Strijp J A, van de Winkel J G. Effective phagocytosis and killing of *Candida albicans* via targeting FcgammaRI (CD64) or FcalphaRI (CD89) on neutrophils. *J Infect Dis* 179:661–669, 1999.

Vazquez J A, Gupta S, Villanueva A. Potential utility of recombinant human GM-CSF as adjunctive treatment of refractory oropharyngeal candidiasis in AIDS patients. *Eur J Clin Microbiol Infect Dis* 17:781–783, 1998a.

Vazquez N, Walsh T J, Friedman D, Chanock S J, Lyman C A. Interleukin-15 augments superoxide production and microbicidal activity of human monocytes against *Candida albicans*. *Infect Immun* 66:145–150, 1998b.

Vecchiarelli A, Morani C, Baldelli F, Pietrella D, Retini C, Tascini C, Francisci D, Bistoni F. Beneficial effect of recombinant human granulocyte colony-forming factor on fungicidal activity of polymorphonuclear leukocytes from patients with AIDS. *J Infect Dis* 171:1448–1454, 1995.

Vecchiarelli A, Casadevall A. Antibody-mediated effects against *Cryptococcus neoformans*: evidence for interdependency and collaboration between humoral and cellular immunity. *Res Immunol* 149:321–333, 1998.

Vora S, Chauhan S, Brummer E, Stevens D A. Activity of voriconazole combined with neutrophils or monocytes against *Aspergillus fumigatus*: effects of granulocyte colony-stimulating factor and granulocyte-macrophage colony-stimulating factor. *Antimicrob Agents Chemother* 42:2299–2303, 1998.

Wald A, Leisenring W, van Burik J A, Bowden R A. Epidemiology of *Aspergillus* infections in a large cohort of patients undergoing bone marrow transplantation. *J Infect Dis* 175:1459–1466, 1997.

Williamson P R, Kwon-Chung K J, Gallin J I. Successful treatment of *Paecilomyces varioti* infection in a patient with chronic granulomatous disease and a review of *Paecilomyces* species infections. *Clin Infect Dis* 14:1023–1026, 1992.

Winkelstein J A, Marino M C, Johnston R B, Boyle J, Curnutte J, Gallin J I, Malech H L, Holland S M, Ochs H, Quie P, Buckley R H, Foster C B, Chanock S J, Dickler H. Chronic granulomatous disease. Report on a national registry of 368 patients. *Medicine (Baltimore)* 79:155–169, 2000.

Wright D G, Robichaud K J, Pizzo P A, Deisseroth A B. Lethal pulmonary reactions associated with the combined use of amphotericin B and leukocyte transfusions. *New Engl J Med* 304:1185–1189, 1981.

Zhou P, Sieve M C, Bennett J, Kwon-Chung K J, Tewari R P, Gazzinelli R T, Sher A, Seder R A. IL-12 prevents mortality in mice infected with *Histoplasma capsulatum* through induction of IFN-gamma. *J Immunol* 155:785–795, 1995.

III

MYCOSES CAUSED BY YEASTS

11

Candidiasis

JOSE A. VAZQUEZ AND JACK D. SOBEL

Within a few decades, *Candida* species have progressed from infrequent pathogens that were largely considered nuisance contaminants to important and common human pathogens causing a wide spectrum of superficial and deep disease. Superficial infections are frequently community acquired and responsible for considerable morbidity. In contrast, deep seated, invasive, and systemic *Candida* infections are usually nosocomial in origin. Pathogenic and risk factors for superficial and deep candidiasis, although overlapping, are markedly different; hence superficial infection uncommonly results in systemic disease. Matching the increased incidence of *Candida* infections has been the availability in the last 2 decades of successive generations of antifungal agents.

ORGANISM

Candida are small (4–6 μm), oval, thin-walled yeast-like fungi that reproduce by budding or fission. The genus *Candida* is comprised of over 200 species and constitutes an extremely diverse yeast species whose common bond is the absence of a sexual cycle (Berkhout, 1923). Only a few species cause disease in humans (Odds, 1988). The medically significant *Candida* species include: *Candida albicans, Candida (Torulopsis) glabrata, Candida parapsilosis, Candida tropicalis, Candida krusei, Candida kefyr, Candida guilliermondii, Candida lusitaniae, C. stellatoidea,* and *Candida dubliniensis.*

Candida organisms grow readily in blood culture bottles and on agar plates. In most situations, they do not require special conditions for growth. On culture media, *Candida* species form smooth, creamy white, glistening colonies (Rippon, 1988; Kwon-Chung and Bennett, 1992). The numerous species of *Candida* are easily identified on the basis of growth characteristics and commercial kits that evaluate carbohydrate assimilation and fermentation reactions and provide species identification of *Candida* isolates within 2–4 days. A rapid, but nonspecific identification of *C. albicans* can be made by testing for germ tube production. This test is performed by growing the yeast in serum at 37°C and observing for the growth of small projections from the cell wall that develop after 60–90 minutes of incubation (Odds, 1988). *Candida stellatoidea* and *C. dubliniensis* also generate germ tubes, thus eliciting false-positive results (Sullivan,1995). CHROMagar, a culture media utilized to rapidly identify many common *Candida* species (Pfaller et al, 1996), employs a chemical colorimetric reaction on agar that allows distinction between *C. albicans, C. glabrata, C. krusei, C. tropicalis,* and other non-*albicans Candida* species.

Candida albicans (Robin) (synonyms: *Oidium albicans,* Robin, 1853; *Monilia albicans,* Zopf, 1890; *Endomyces albicans,* Vuillemin, 1898) remains the major fungal pathogen of man and the most common cause of mucosal and systemic fungal infection (Pfaller, 2001), and is the best characterized of the *Candida* species (Odds, 1994).

Candida glabrata (Anderson) Meyer and Yarrow, 1978 (synonym: *Torulopsis glabrata (Anderson) Lodder et De Vries, 1938)* has become important because of its increasing incidence worldwide and decreased susceptibility to antifungals. Its emergence is largely due to an increased immunocompromised patient population and widespread use of antifungal drugs (Fidel et al, 1999; Gumbo et al, 1999). In the most recent SENTRY Trial data, *C. glabrata* emerged as the second most common cause of candidemia following *C. albicans* (Pfaller, 2001).

Candida parapsilosis (Ashford) Camargo, 1934 (synonyms: *Monilia parapsilosis,* Ashford, 1928; *M. parakrusei,* Castellani and Chalmers, 1934; *C. brumpti,* Langeron and Guerra, 1935) in most parts of the world is the third most common cause of candidemia (Pfaller et al, 2001), especially in patients with intravenous catheters, prosthetic devices, and intravenous drug use (Girmenia et al, 1996; Levy et al,1998). *Candida parapsilosis* is one of the most common causes of candidemia in neonatal intensive care units (Levy et al, 1998). This species produces slime as a virulence factor enabling it to adhere to environmental surfaces and skin of hospital personnel (Sanchez et al, 1993; Girmenia et al, 1996).

Candida tropicalis (Castellani) (synonyms: *Monilia candida*, Hansen, 1888; *Oidium tropicalis*, Castellani, 1910; *Mycotorula dimorpha*, Redaelli and Ciferri, 1935; *M. trimorpha*, Redaelli and Ciferri,1935) is the third or fourth most commonly recovered *Candida* species from blood cultures (Pfaller et al, 2001). Leukemia, prolonged neutropenia, and prolonged intensive care unit (ICU) days are major risk factors for *C. tropicalis* candidemia (Kontoyiannis et al, 2001).

Candida krusei (Castellani) (synonyms: *Saccharomyces krusei*, Castellani, 1910; *Monilia krusei*, Castellani and Chambers, 1913; perfect state *Pichia kudriavezii*) is the fifth most common bloodstream isolate. Although less common (1%–2%), *C. krusei* is of clinical significance because of its intrinsic resistance to fluconazole, and reduced susceptibility to most other antifungal drugs (Pfaller et al, 2001). *Candida krusei* is frequently recovered from patients with hematological malignancies complicated by neutropenia (Merz et al, 1986; Wingard et al, 1991; Abbas et al, 2000), and tends to be associated with higher mortality rates (49% vs. 28% with *C. albicans*), and lower response rates (51% vs. 69% with *C. albicans*).

Candida kefyr (Beijerinck) van Uden et Buckley, 1970 (synonyms: *C. pseudotropicalis* [Castellani] Basgal, 1931; *Endomyces pseudotropicalis*, Castellani, 1911; *Monilia pseudotropicalis*, Castellani and Chambers, 1913; perfect state *Kluveromyces fragilis*) is a rare species that occasionally causes disease in immunocompromised host (Hazen, 1995).

Candida guilliermondii (Castellani) Langeron et Guerra, 1938 (synonym: *Endomyces guilliermondii*, Castellani, 1912; perfect state *Pichia guilliermondii*), is another rare species. While infections due to *C. guilliermondii* are uncommon, candidemia and invasive disease in the neutropenic host (Vazquez et al, 1995) are reported occasionally as is endocarditis in intravenous drug addicts.

Candida lusitaniae van Uden et do Carmo-Sousa, 1959 (synonyms: *C. parapsilosis* [Ashford] Langeron et Talice var *obtusa* [Dietrichson] 1954; *Candida obtusa* (Dietrichson) van Uden et do Carmo-Sousa ex van Udeen et Buckley, 1970), perfect state: *Clavispora lusitaniae*. Although uncommon (< 1%–2%), *C. lusitaniae* is of clinical importance because of intrinsic or secondary resistance acquisition to amphotericin B (Hazen, 1995; Yoon et al, 1999) and is typically found in patients with hematological malignancies and patients in intensive care units (Sanchez et al, 1992; Hazen, 1995).

Candida stellatoidea (Jones and Martin, 1938) (synonym: *C. albicans*) is closely related to *C. albicans* (Bodey et al, 1993), by producing germ tubes in vitro, a morphologic characteristic seen only in *C. albicans* and some *C. dubliniensis* strains (Sullivan et al, 1995).

C. stellatoidea is a heterogeneous species with at least two confirmed subtypes, subtype I and II (Kwon-Chung et al, 1989). Type I differs from *C. albicans* in several genetic characteristics and is not considered a mutant of *C. albicans*. Type II *C. stellatoidea* is a sucrose-negative mutant of *C. albicans* serotype A (Kwon-Chung et al, 1990). Additionally, type II isolates appear to have lower virulence and are slower growers than either type I *C. stellatoidea* or *C. albicans* (Kwon-Chung et al, 1988; Kwon-Chung et al, 1989; Rikkerink et al, 1990).

Candida dubliniensis is a recently identified species of *Candida*, previously hidden among the germ tube positive strains of *C. albicans*. Identified initially from the oral cavity of HIV-positive patients (Sullivan and Coleman, 1998), *C. dubliniensis* has been recovered from HIV-positive patients throughout the world at rates ranging from 19% to 32% (Sullivan and Coleman, 1998), has also been recovered from 3% to 14% of oral cavities of HIV-negative individuals, and rarely is associated with candidemia or invasive disease (Hidalgo et al, 2000). However, recently *Candida dubliniensis* was recovered from 14 patients with either solid organ or hematological malignancies (Sebti et al, 2001). *C. dubliniensis* is identified by germ tube and chlamydospore production, by an inability to grow at 45°C, and occasionally by a specific colony color on CHROM-agar *Candida* medium (Pfaller et al,1996). This species can also be identified easily using commercially available yeast identification kits (Jabra-Rizk et al, 1999).

Less common non-*albicans Candida* species are listed in Table 11–1, and their unique features and diseases are described briefly.

Virulence Factors

Biologic features that contribute to *Candida's* ability to cause disease were previously defined phenotypically. Total genome sequencing of *C. albicans* has allowed measurement of the effects of gene knockouts on the virulence of *Candida* in animal models. Genes required for virulence are regulated in response to environmental signals indigenous to the host environment (Mekalanos, 1992). These signals include temperature, pH, osmotic pressure, and iron and calcium ion concentrations. Adaptation to a changing environment facilitates the ability of *Candida* to survive within the host niche (De Bernardis et al, 1998).

Candida albicans undergoes reversible morphological transition between budding pseudohyphal and hyphal growth forms (Brown and Gow, 1999). All forms are present in clinical disease tissue specimens. Yeast cells may be disseminated more effectively, whereas hyphae are thought to promote invasion of epithelial and endothelial tissue and help evade macrophage engulf-

TABLE 11–1. *Characteristics and Disease States Associated with the Uncommon Non-Albicans Candida Species*

Candida Species	Characteristics/Disease States	In vitro Susceptibilities					
		AmB	5-FC	Flz	Itz	Clz	Ktz
C. catenulata	A natural contaminant of dairy products, especially camembert cheeses; causes cutaneous, and mucosal infection; candidemia (1 case report in a patient with gastric carcinoma who frequently ate cheese)	S	S	DD-S	S		
C. ciferii	Cutaneous, onychomycosis	S	R	R	R	S	S
C. famata (*Torulopsis candida*)	Candidemia, endophthalmitis, peritonitis due to CAPD	S	S	S	S	S	S
C. haemulonii	Candidemia, cutaneous						
C. inconspicua	Candidemia in neutropenics, oropharyngeal, esophageal, and vaginal candidiasis in diabetics and HIV-positive patients	S		R	R		
C. lipolytica	Low virulence, catheter-related candidemia, commonly colonizes the stool, sputum, and mouth, although not associated with mucosal infections	S	S	S	S	S	S
C. norvegensis	Recovered from the GI and respiratory tract, rarely causes candidemia and peritonitis	S	S	DD-S or or R	S		S
C. pelliculosa Telomorph: *Hansenula anomola* the sexual state of *Pichia anomola*	The most frequent of the uncommon causes of invasive candidiasis; > 20 cases of invasive candidiasis including: candidemia, endocarditis, intraabdominal abscess, pyelonephritis, cerebral ventriculitis	Broad range MICs (0.04–1.56 µg/ml)	S	S	S	S	
C. pulcherrima	Recovered from skin and nails of normal host						
C. rugosa (*Mycoderma rugosa*)	Associated with nosocomial candidemia and invasive candidiasis in burn patients, neutropenics, and catheter-associated infections	S	S	Broad range MICs (2–32 µg/ml)	S		S
C. utilis Telomorph: *Hansenula jadinii, Pichia jadinii*	Utilized primarily in industry; a rare cause with only 2 cases of invasive candidiasis	S		S			
C. viswanathii	Recovered from respiratory tract and rare cause of meningitis						
C. zeylanoides	Low virulence, associated with catheter-related infections and septic arthritis	S		S	S		

S, susceptible; R, resistant; DD-S, dose dependent susceptible; MIC, minimum inhibitory concentration; AmB, amphotericin B; 5-FC, flucytosine; Flz, fluconazole; Itz, itraconazole; Clz, clotrimazole; Ktz, ketoconazole; CAPD, continuous ambulatory peritoneal dialysis.
References: Bodey et al, 1993; D'Antonio et al, 1998; Dube et al, 1994; Hazen, 1995.

ment (Sherwood et al, 1992). *Candida* double mutants (chp1/chp1, efg1/efg1) that are locked in the yeast form are avirulent in a mouse model (Lo et al, 1997). The ability to switch from one form to another appears to have a direct influence on the organism's capacity to cause disease. Drugs that inhibit yeast-hyphal transformation without fungicidal activity have a role in suppressing clinical disease. At least 15 genes are recognized as playing a role in morphogenesis, including TUP1 regulated genes (Brown and Gow, 1999).

The first step in a *Candida* infection is epithelial colonization, in turn dependent upon microorganism adherence to epithelial cells and proteins, allowing them to withstand fluid forces that serve to expel particulates (Sundstrom, 1999). Adhesive ability of *C. albicans* has been correlated with pathogenesis of infection. A hierarchy exists among *Candida* species, with more frequently isolated pathogenic species exhibiting greater adhesive capacity. Several genes and their products have been identified to play a role in cell adhesion, including the adhesion like sequence (ALS) family of protein encoding cell-surface adhesion glycoproteins (x-agglutinins) and HWP-1, which encodes a protein (Hwp1), an adhesin attaching to buccal epithelial cells (Staab et al, 1999).

Invasion of host cells by *Candida* involves penetration and damage of the outer cell envelope. Transmigration is most likely mediated by physical and/or enzymatic processes. Phospholipids and proteins represent the major chemical constituents of the host cell membrane. Phospholipases, by cleaving phospholipids, induce cell lysis and thereby facilitate tissue invasion (Leidich et al, 1998). Phospholipase activity is concentrated at the hyphal growing tip and extracellular phospholipase is considered necessary for the invasion of tissue. Three genes have been cloned and encode candidal phospholipases. In 1969, Staib first reported that proteolytic activity in *C. albicans* was related to strain pathogenicity (Staib, 1969). A family of at least 9 genes makes up the secreted aspartyl proteinase isoenzymes (SAP) (Monod et al, 1994). SAP1 and SAP3 are regulated during phenotypic transformation. Several studies have confirmed the importance of secreted aspartyl proteinases in the pathogenesis of tissue invasion by *C. albicans*. SAP-gene knockout experiments demonstrate attenuated virulence in both guinea pig and murine models of disseminated candidiasis.

The ability of *Candida* species to overcome the suppressive effect of antifungal chemotherapy is considered a virulence attribute (See Chapter 9).

EPIDEMIOLOGY AND PATHOGENESIS

Candida species are important opportunistic pathogens because of their ability to infect seriously ill hospitalized patients (Pfaller et al, 2001). *Candida* accounts for approximately 15% of all hospital-acquired infections and over 72% of all nosocomial fungal infections (Jarvis, 1995).

During the 1980s, data from the National Center for Health Statistics (NCHS) reported bloodstream infections as the 13th leading cause of death in the United States, with an attributable mortality rate of approximately 35% (Edmond et al, 1999). During this period, fungal infections (particularly due to *Candida* spp.) increased dramatically, accounting for 8%–15% of all nosocomial bloodstream infections (BSIs) (Beck-Sague et al, 1993; Fisher-Hoch and Hutwagner, 1995; Fridkin and Jarvis, 1996). The National Hospital Discharge Survey reported rates of oropharyngeal and disseminated candidiasis to have increased more than 4-fold and 11-fold, respectively, between 1980 and 1989 (Fisher-Hoch and Hutwagner, 1995). In 1997, systemic mycoses ranked seventh as the underlying cause of death due to infections, compared with tenth in 1980

(Pinner et al, 1996; McNeil et al, 2001). The Surveillance and Control of Pathogens of Epidemiologic Importance (SCOPE) study reported that for the 3–year period ending 1998, *Candida* species remained the fourth (7.7%) most common cause of nosocomial BSI in the United States (Edmond et al, 1999; Wenzel and Edmond, 2001). Although this incidence is low when compared to bacteremias, candidemia had the highest (40%) crude mortality rate of all nosocomial BSIs (Edmond et al, 1999; Wenzel and Edmond, 2001). Autopsy studies have also confirmed the increase in the incidence of disseminated candidiasis, reflecting the parallel increase in candidemia (Singh, 2001; McNeil et al, 2001). Candidemia is also associated with a prolongation of hospital length of stay (70 days vs. 40 days) in comparable nonfungemic patients (Wey et al, 1988).

Disease usually originates from gastrointestinal tract or the skin. Most organisms that colonize endogenous reservoirs are acquired exogenously. *Candida* species are frequently recovered from the hospital environment, including food, counter tops, air-conditioning vents, floors, respirators, and from medical personnel (Mahayni et al, 1995). *Candida* species are also commensals of diseased skin and mucosal surfaces of the gastrointestinal, genitourinary, and respiratory tracts (Odds, 1994). Serious candidal infections are more frequent in burn patients, low birth–weight infants, recipients of parenteral nutrition, patients with hematological or solid organ malignancies, patients with indwelling intravascular catheters or undergoing hemodialysis, and patients in the postoperative period (Jarvis, 1995), especially following transplantation (Singh, 2001).

Until recently, epidemiologic data of *Candida* colonization, transmission, and infection were incomplete because of a lack of a reliable strain delineation (genotyping) system (Soll, 2000). Molecular biology tools have improved the understanding of *Candida* epidemiology; isolates of a single strain type (genotype) have the same or very similar DNA patterns, while epidemiologically unrelated isolates have distinctly different patterns (Soll, 2000). Prospective molecular epidemiologic studies of *Candida* using longitudinal cultures have shown that individual patient tends to harbor the same genotype of *Candida* over long periods of time (Pfaller et al, 1990; Vazquez et al, 1993a; Soll, 2000). More than 60% of patients with candidemia have positive cultures for the same *Candida* genotype as the genotype isolated from various anatomic sites prior to developing fungemia (Pfaller et al, 1990).

DNA typing has also confirmed acquisition of nosocomial *Candida* species from environmental and human sources. *Candida* species have been recovered from 25% to 50% of inanimate surfaces sampled (Vazquez et al, 1993b), and *Candida* was cultured from patients' rooms prior to patient acquisition of the same strain (Vaudry et al, 1988; Vazquez et al, 1993b). Surfaces commonly harboring *Candida* spp. were those in contact with hands of personnel or patients. Identical strains of *Candida* have also been recovered from patient food prior to patient acquisition (Berger et al, 1988; Vazquez et al, 1993b). Considerable strain diversity in *Candida*, specifically among *C. albicans* is evident. In one study of nosocomial acquisition of *Candida*, approximately 70% of patients were colonized with multiple strains of *C. albicans*, including 40% of patients with multiple *Candida* species at different anatomical sites (Vazquez et al, 1993).

CLINICAL MANIFESTATIONS

Oropharyngeal Candidiasis

Hippocrates is credited with first describing oral thrush in debilitated individuals (Hippocrates and Adams, 1989). Nineteenth-century authorities recognized that thrush invariably arose as a consequence of preexisting illness (Trousseau, 1869; Parrot, 1877). The initial discovery of the organism causing thrush was not made until 1839, when Langenbeck described a fungus in buccal aphthae in a case of typhus (Langenbeck, 1939), but it was left to Berg in 1846 to establish a cause–effect relationship between the fungus and oral lesions (Berg, 1846). The taxonomic confusion continued until 1933 when Berkhout proposed the genus name *Candida*, separating this genus from the universal *Monilia* genus that affects fruit and vegetables (Berkhout, 1923).

Oropharyngeal candidiasis (OPC) is most prevalent in infants, the elderly, and compromised hosts and occurs in association with serious underlying conditions including diabetes, leukemia, neoplasia, steroid use, antimicrobial therapy, radiation therapy, and HIV-infection (Silverman et al, 1984; Sobel, 1995). Persistent OPC in infants may be the first manifestation of childhood AIDS or chronic mucocutaneous candidiasis. One group of investigators reported that 28% of cancer patients not receiving antifungal prophylaxis developed OPC (Samonis and Bodey, 1990) and another group observed OPC in 57% of immunocompromised patients (Yeo et al, 1985). Patients at greatest risk of developing OPC include those receiving corticosteroids and with prolonged neutropenia who are colonized with a *Candida* species (Yeo et al, 1985). Approximately 80%–90% of patients with HIV-infection will develop OPC at some stage of their disease (Feigal et al, 1991; Vazquez, 2000); 60% of untreated patients develop an AIDS-related infection or Kaposi's sarcoma within two years of the appearance of OPC (Klein et al, 1984).

Candida albicans remains the most common species responsible for OPC (80%–90%) (Coleman et al, 1993). The ability of *C. albicans* to adhere to buccal epithelial cells is critical in establishing oral colonization; *C. albicans* adheres better to epithelial cells than non-*albicans Candida* species. Low numbers of organisms are the result of effective antifungal host defense mechanisms in the oral cavity. Low salivary flow rates correlate with higher prevalence rate of *Candida*. Genotyping of *Candida* strains obtained from HIV-positive patients with OPC and esophageal candidiasis compared to isolates from healthy individuals indicate an identical distribution frequency, suggesting that HIV-associated candidiasis is not caused by unique or particularly virulent strains, but from defects in host defenses (Whelan et al, 1990).

Profound differences exist between HIV-positive and negative patients with regard to natural history, diagnosis and management of OPC (Vazquez et al, 1999; Vazquez, 2000) including an increase in non-*albicans Candida* species recovered from HIV-positive individuals (Barchiesi et al, 1993; van't Wout et al, 1996). HIV-positive patients experience recurrent episodes of OPC and esophageal candidiasis as immunodeficiency progresses; these patients may also receive multiple courses of antifungal drugs contributing to antifungal resistance. In these patients, antifungal agents are also less efficacious and take longer to achieve a clinical response (Darouiche, 1998).

Symptoms of oral thrush are variable, including a sore, painful mouth, burning tongue and dysphagia (Vazquez, 2000). Frequently, patients with severe objective intraoral lesions are aymptomatic. Signs include diffuse erythema with white patches that appear as discrete lesions on the surfaces of the mucosa, throat, tongue, and gums. With some difficulty, the plaques can be wiped off revealing a raw, erythematous and sometimes bleeding base. Constitutional signs of infection are absent. Oropharyngeal candidiasis can impair the quality of life by reduction in fluid or food intake.

Acute Pseudomembranous Candidiasis (Exudative). This most common form of OPC, especially in HIV-positive persons, presents with a whitish-yellow thick curd–like exudate on mucosal surfaces (See Color Fig. 11–1a in separate color insert). Plaques may be small and discrete or confluent lesions involving the entire oral mucosa, and consist of necrotic material and desquamated epithelial cells, penetrated by hyphae and yeast cells which continue their invasion into the stratum corneum (Letiner, 1964).

Chronic Atrophic Stomatitis (Denture Stomatitis). This common form of OPC is frequently asymptomatic, but may be associated with chronic soreness and burning of the mouth. Diffuse erythema and edema of the portion of the palate in contact with dentures is evident (see Color Fig. 11–1b in separate color insert). For unknown reasons, the lower denture is rarely involved. Chronic atrophic stomatitis was recorded in 24%–60% of denture wearers and is several-fold more frequent in females than in males (Budtz-Jorgensen et al, 1975). Candida is detected by culture or microscopy in over 90% of symptomatic subjects. Even in the absence of signs or symptoms, the prevalence of yeast is higher in denture wearers. Maximum concentrations of yeast are found on the denture fitting surface. Candida species readily adhere to plastic objects including orthodontic appliances. The pathogenesis of this form of OPC remains unclear (Odds, 1988).

Angular Cheilitis (Perleche).   Angular cheilitis or cheilosis is characterized by soreness, erythema, and fissuring at the corners of the mouth (see Color Fig. 11–1c in separate color insert). Cheilitis may accompany oral thrush or denture stomatitis, or may appear in the absence of oral disease (Cawson, 1965). Vitamin deficiency and iron-deficiency anemia are also associated with cheilitis, with Candida as a secondary colonizer (Russotto, 1980).

Chronic Hyperplastic Candidiasis (Candida Leukoplakia).   Oral white patches are discrete, transparent to whitish raised lesions of variable sizes found on the inner surface of the cheeks and, less frequently, on the tongue. These lesions are found predominantly in males and are highly associated with smoking. Most leukoplakia lesions are not related to Candida infection (Daftary et al, 1972; Russotto, 1980) and may be premalignant. Importantly, there is no known association between Candida and either dysplasia or malignancy. Biopsy of Candida-related leukoplakia lesions reveals parakeratosis and epithelial hyperplasia with Candida invasion.

Midline Glossitis (Median Rhomboid Glossitis, Acute Atrophic Stomatitis).   This form of OPC manifests as symmetrical lesions on the center dorsum of the tongue, characterized by erythema and loss of papillae (Cernea et al, 1965).

Candida species have also been incriminated in an oral "burning mouth" syndrome, characterized by a raw or sore tongue, especially following antibiotic administration (Lehner, 1966). This self-limiting entity, although common, has not been shown to be due to primary or secondary Candida infection in spite of positive smears or cultures. Since Candida can be expected to be cultured in 20%–50% of asymptomatic patients, the etiology of this syndrome is probably multifactorial (Lamey and Lamb, 1988a; Lamey et al, 1988b).

Physical signs of OPC are insufficient to allow reliable diagnosis. Oral lesions resembling candidiasis occur with severe mucositis accompanying chemotherapy (reflecting tissue necrosis), viral and bacterial infections (Smith and Meech, 1984). Oropharyngeal Candida infections can complicate Herpes simplex virus infection or leukoplakia. Diagnosis requires mycological confirmation, achieved by 10% potassium hydroxide or normal saline microscopic examination. Cultures are not essential for diagnosis and do not distinguish colonization and infection.

Esophageal Candidiasis
The prevalence of Candida esophagitis has increased because of AIDS, as well as the increased pool of transplant recipients, cancer and other severely immunocompromised patients. Candida microorganisms are frequently recovered from the esophageal surface and reach the esophagus in oral secretions. Little is known about host and yeast factors operative in the pathogenesis of esophageal candidiasis (EC) and experimental models have not been established. Predisposing factors include exposure to local irradiation, recent cytotoxic chemotherapy, antibiotics, corticosteroids, and neutropenia (Wheeler et al, 1987). The high prevalence of EC in patients with AIDS indicates the critical role of cell mediated immunity in normally protecting the esophagus from Candida invasion. Esophageal candidiasis in an HIV-positive patient may be the first manifestation of AIDS (Coleman et al, 1993), typically occurring at lower CD4 counts, < 100 cells/mm^3 (Wheeler et al, 1987; Coleman et al, 1993). Histological sections reveal yeast hyphae in the mucosal epithelium, accompanied by a neutrophilic response as seen in oral thrush.

Candida esophagitis presents with dysphagia, odynophagia, and retrosternal pain. Constitutional findings, including fever, only occasionally occur. Rarely, epigastric pain is the dominant symptom. Although EC may arise as an extension of OPC, in more than 66% of cases, the esophagus was the only site involved and more often in the distal 2/3 than in the proximal 1/3 of the esophagus. Candida esophagitis in patients with AIDS may be entirely asymptomatic in spite of extensive esophageal involvement (Clotet et al, 1986). Esophageal candidiasis is classified on the basis of endoscopic appearance: Type I, a few white or beige plaques, up to 2 mm in diameter; Type II, plaques are more numerous, larger than 2 mm in diameter; Type III, confluent, linear and nodular elevated plaques with hyperemia and frank ulceration (See Color Fig. 11–2 in separate color insert); and Type IV, similar to Type III but with increased mucosal friability and occasional narrowing of the lumen (Kodsi et al, 1976). Uncommon complications of esophagitis include perforation, aortic-esophageal fistula (Lefkowitz et al, 1964; Sehhat et al, 1976), and rarely, extensive necrosis destroying the entire esophageal mucosa. In neutropenic patients, bacteremia and candidemia may arise from EC.

A reliable diagnosis of EC can only be made by histological evidence of tissue invasion in biopsy material. Antifungal therapy is frequently initiated empirically in a high-risk patient. The finding of *Candida* within an esophageal lesion by smear or culture or in esophageal brushings does not allow distinction between *Candida* as a commensal or invasive pathogen. Positive esophageal brushings are highly sensitive but very nonspecific in the diagnosis of EC.

Radiologic features, which previously formed the basis for diagnosis of EC, are rarely used today. A barium contrast upper GI study may reveal shaggy mucosal irregularities and nodular filling defects (Athey et al, 1977; Pagani and Libshitz, 1981). The sensitivity of barium swallow is relatively low and radiologic abnormalities are often absent in mild to moderate esophagitis, especially in patients with AIDS (Athey et al, 1977; Wheeler et al, 1987). Radiology has been replaced by endoscopy, which not only provides a rapid and highly sensitive method of diagnosis, but is also the only reliable method of differentiating among the various other causes of esophagitis (Wheeler et al, 1987). The characteristic endoscopic appearance of EC is described as yellow-white plaques on an erythematous background, with varying degrees of ulceration.

Differential diagnosis of EC includes radiation esophagitis, reflux esophagitis, and esophagitis caused by *Cytomegalovirus* or *Herpes simplex virus* infection. In patients with AIDS, multiple etiologic agents causing esophagitis are not uncommon.

Gastric Candidiasis
Since normal gastric microbial flora is derived from oropharyngeal secretions, saliva and food, *Candida* organisms are normal components of gastric flora. Factors that enhance oral carriage of *Candida* similarly increase gastroduodenal colonization with *Candida* species. The role of acid in influencing gastric carriage rates of *Candida* remains controversial. However, *Candida* infections of the stomach are documented less frequently than in the esophagus, implying greater gastric mucosal resistance to *Candida* infection. Generally, *C. albicans* usually invades pre-existing gastric lesions, particularly gastric ulcers, both benign and malignant, as well as sites of gastric resection.

In patients with AIDS and *Candida* esophagitis, gastric thrush is not uncommon, and manifests with epigastric pain, nausea and vomiting. It is difficult to establish what role, if any, these symptoms can be attributed to candidiasis. Most patients are asymptomatic or only experience symptoms of the associated gastric abnormality (Sobel and Vazquez, 1995b;

Vazquez, 2000). There is scant information about the need for or efficacy of antifungal therapy.

Candida Enterocolitis and Diarrhea Syndromes
Autopsies of adults with hematological malignancy and other debilitating diseases, including AIDS, show that *Candida* invasion of enteric and colonic mucosa rarely occurs. In one study, infection of the small bowel was found at autopsy in 22 of 109 patients with GI candidiasis (Eras et al, 1972). The most common abnormality was ulceration of the mucosa, which led to fungal penetration into the submucosa in some patients. Symptoms included nausea, abdominal pain and diarrhea.

Candida-associated diarrhea has been reported to develop during hospitalization (Gupta and Ehrinpreis, 1990). Diarrhea developed in elderly, malnourished, critically or chronically ill patients. The diarrhea was secretory in nature, and characterized by frequent watery stools, without blood, mucus, tenesmus, or abdominal pain. All patients had received therapy with multiple antibiotics or chemotherapeutic agents. Colonoscopy failed to reveal evidence of colitis. Not all authorities agree with the evidence supporting the existence of this syndrome.

Cutaneous Candidiasis
Candida can invade any body surface and cause superficial infection of the skin, hair, and nails. Symptomatic mucocutaneous candidiasis will occur if dysfunction or local reduction in host resistance promotes an overgrowth of indigenous flora and there is a breach in the anatomical barriers (skin and mucosa). Dry intact skin is a potent barrier to fungal invasion, and hydration of the epidermis decreases resistance.

Candida albicans and *C. tropicalis* are the most common causes of superficial infections of the skin and the nails. These organisms favor growth in warm, moist areas such as the skin folds of obese individuals, between the fingers and toes, perineal areas, and genitocrural folds. Infections in these areas occur with much greater frequency in HIV-positive and diabetic patients, and are exacerbated by occlusion, moisture, epidermal barrier dysfunction, hormonal manipulation, antibiotic use, and immunosuppression.

Generalized Cutaneous Candidiasis. This syndrome is a rare form of candidiasis that manifests as a diffuse eruption over the trunk, thorax, and extremities. Patients have a history of generalized pruritus, with increased severity in the genitocrural folds, anal region, axillae, hands, and feet. Examination reveals a widespread rash that begins as individual vesicles that evolve into large confluent areas (Alteras et al, 1979).

Intertrigo. One of the most common skin infections due to *Candida*, intertrigo affects sites where skin surfaces are in close proximity providing a warm and moist environment. Infection begins with a vesiculopustular pruritic rash that enlarges and frequently progresses to maceration and erythema. The involved area has a scalloped border with a white rim consisting of necrotic epidermis that surrounds the erythematous macerated base. Satellite lesions are frequently found and may coalesce and extend into larger lesions.

Erosio Interdigitalis Blastomycetica. This form of intertrigo that occurs in the areas between the fingers and toes manifests as an erythematous painful rash. The affected skin reveals a tender, erythematous area of erosion, that may extend onto the sides of the digits and may be surrounded by maceration (Domonkos et al, 1982; Fitzpatrick et al, 1997).

Candida Folliculitis. This infection, which is predominantly found in the hair follicles and rarely becomes extensive (Kapdagli et al, 1997), should be differentiated from more common bacterial folliculitis.

Paronychia and Onychomycosis. Nail plate infection is generally not due to *Candida* species, unless it is associated with congenital candidiasis or chronic mucocutaneous candidiasis (Arbegast et al, 1990). *Candida* paronychia and onychomycosis are seen typically in patients with prolonged immersion of extremities in water and in patients with diabetes mellitus. *Candida* paronychia tends to be chronic, presenting as a painful and erythematous area around and underneath the nail and nailfold. Physical examination reveals an area of inflammation that is warm, glistening, tense, and erythematous and extends underneath the nail. Chronic manifestations of this infection include loss of seal of the proximal nail-fold, nail thickening, ridging, discoloration, and occasional nail loss.

Chronic Mucocutaneous Candidiasis. This syndrome involves multiple superficial sites, primarily the mouth, facial skin, hair and nails, which are simultaneously infected with *Candida* over a prolonged period of time. Chronic mucocutaneous candidiasis (CMC) is not a single disease entity, but is a consequence of multiple defects in anti-*Candida* host defenses. The final outcome is a chronic, superficial *Candida* infection at sites where *Candida* normally resides as a commensal organism (Wells, 1973; Kirkpatrick, 1993; Kirkpatrick, 1994). Chronic mucocutaneous candidiasis is a rare entity, and links between increased incidence of CMC and families of either Iranian, Jewish or Finnish descent are described (Ahonen et al, 1990; Bjorses et al, 1996).

Most CMC infections begin in infancy or the first 2 decades of life; onset after 30 years of age is rare. Chronic and recurrent infections frequently result in a disfiguring form of CMC called *Candida* granuloma (Wells, 1973). Most patients with CMC survive for prolonged periods of time and rarely experience visceral or disseminated fungal infections. The most common cause of death is bacterial sepsis. A wide spectrum of CMC clinical syndromes have been described. Newer classifications are based on inheritance as well as clinical factors (Hermans and Ritts, 1970; Wells, 1973; Kirkpatrick, 1993; Kirkpatrick, 1994). Group 1 is chronic oral candidiasis associated with HIV, inhaled steroids and denture-stomatitis. Group 2 comprises CMC associated with endocrinopathy (autosomal recessive) and has also been called "*Candida* endocrinopathy syndrome" or autoimmune polyendocrinopathy candidiasis syndrome. It is now known to be due to mutations in the autoimmune regulator (AIRE) gene. Group 3 is localized CMC that is characterized by hyperkeratosis and cutaneous horn formation that affects both hands. This group is not associated with endocrine dysfunction. Group 4 is diffuse CMC, and tends to include patients with widespread and the most severe infections and in whom familial factors are unknown or obscure. Group 5 includes CMC associated with thymoma, and usually manifests during the third decade of life. In addition, Group 5 CMC is also associated with myasthenia gravis, hypogammaglobulinemia, red cell aplasia, aplastic anemia, and neutropenia. Group 6 is CMC associated with interstitial keratitis (Okamoto et al, 1977). Group 7 is CMC associated with keratitis, icthyosis, and deafness (KID syndrome).

A variety of *Candida* antigen-specific defects have been described in CMC patients. The commonest abnormality is a negative delayed-type cutaneous (hyposensitive) reaction to *Candida* antigen and is evident in > 80% of patients tested (controls 16%–37%), regardless of clinical type of CMC. Approximately 70% of patients tested showed defective in vitro lymphocyte blastogenesis in response to *Candida* antigen (Holt et al, 1972). The nature of the T-cell defect has not been clarified. A subpopulation of T-suppressor cells has been described that respond to *Candida* mannoproteins by inhibiting T-helper cell function (Fischer, 1978; Durandy et al, 1988). These investigators reported a serum inhibitory factor in CMC patients that suppressed T-cell function. The majority of patients with CMC have normal or high serum antibodies to *Candida* and no consistent B-cell dysfunction has been reported.

Chronic mucocutaneous candidiasis is frequently associated with endocrinopathies such as: hypoparathyroidism (80%), hypoadrenalism (72%), chronic lymphocytic thyroiditis and hypothyroidism (5%), ovarian failure (60%), growth hormone deficiency, gonad insufficiency (15%), and diabetes mellitus (12%) (Hermans and Ritts, 1970; Wells, 1973). Autoimmune antibodies may be found to adrenal, thyroid, and gastric tissues, and melanin-producing cells (vitiligo). Other features include thymomas and dental dysplasias, polyglandular autoimmune diseases, and antibodies. T-cell dysfunction is often reversible, with improvement in immunological parameters following clinical remission achieved by antimycotic therapy.

The onset of CMC is usually within the first year of life in nonendocrinopathy cases, and within the first decade when associated with endocrinopathies. Approximately 90% of all cases of CMC have their onset before the age of 20 years, and about 33% of cases are associated with endocrinopathies.

The earliest lesion to appear is chronic pseudomembranous oral candidiasis (Shama and Kirkpatrick, 1980). Angular cheilitis and lip fissures may develop and infection may spread to involve the esophagus and larynx. In postmenarchal females, *Candida* vaginitis supervenes, but is not a common feature. These superficial infections tend to be severe, chronic and recurrent in nature. Persistent onychia and paronychia are nearly as common as oral lesions. Lesions of the fingers vary from discoloration and dystrophy of the nails to crusting and hyperkeratotic horns (See Color Fig. 11–3a in separate color insert). Skin lesions, when present, are found mainly on the face, neck, ears, and shoulders, and less often involve the scalp and groin. In severe forms of CMC, there are hyperkeratotic crusts or *Candida* granuloma producing severe disfigurement (See Color Fig. 11–3b in separate color insert). The latter findings are invariably found in the idiopathic, infant or juvenile-onset cases and rarely in association with endocrinopathy or mature-onset cases. A striking feature of CMC is the lack of invasive candidiasis.

Other associated disorders include autoimmune hepatitis, iron deficiency and malabsorption syndromes; aplastic anemia, hemolytic anemia, pernicious anemia, neutropenia, and thrombocytopenia; thymomas and oropharyngeal tumors; and ectodermal abnormalities such as alopecia and dental dysplasias. Patients with CMC are also prone to superinfections caused by *Herpes simplex*, *Herpes zoster*, pyogenic infections including bacteremia, disseminated *Mycobacterium avium* infections, dermatophytosis and occasionally, invasive fungal infections.

The evaluation of persons suspected of having any form of CMC should include a complete blood count with differential, lymphocyte phenotyping, T-lymphocyte response to *Candida* and tetanus, DTH testing with *Candida*, tetanus, and mumps, lymphokine production by antigen or mitogen-stimulated cells, T and B lymphocyte counts, and serum immunoglobulins. In adults, HIV antibody testing and a CT scan of the chest to rule out a thymus tumor should be done (Kirkpatrick, 1993).

Vulvovaginal Candidiasis

In the United States, *Candida* vaginitis is the second most common vaginal infection. During the childbearing years, 75% of women experience at least one episode of vulvovaginal candidiasis (VVC), and 40%–50% of these women experience a second attack (Hurley and De Louvois, 1979). *Candida* is isolated from the genital tract of approximately 10%–20% of asymptomatic, healthy women of childbearing age. *Candida* organisms gain access to the vagina from the adjacent perianal area and then adhere to vaginal epithelial cells. *Candida albicans* adheres to vaginal epithelial cells in significantly greater numbers than non-*albicans Candida* species (Sobel, 1985a).

Several factors are associated with increased rates of asymptomatic vaginal colonization with *Candida* as well as *Candida* vaginitis including pregnancy (30%–40%), oral contraceptives with a high estrogen content, and uncontrolled diabetes mellitus (Fig. 11–4). The hormonal dependence of VVC is illustrated by the fact that *Candida* is seldom isolated from premenarchial girls, and the prevalence of *Candida* vaginitis is lower after the menopause, except in women taking hormone replacement therapy. Other predisposing factors include corticosteroids, antimicrobial therapy, intrauterine devices, and high frequency of coitus (Reed, 1992).

Germination of *Candida* enhances colonization and tissue invasion. Factors that enhance or facilitate germination (e.g., estrogen therapy, pregnancy) tend to precipitate symptomatic vaginitis whereas measures that inhibit germination (e.g., bacterial flora) may prevent acute vaginitis in women who are asymptomatic carriers of *Candida*. A precipitating factor that explains the transformation from asymptomatic carriage to symptomatic vaginitis is identified in only a few patients (Fig. 11–4).

During pregnancy, the incidence of clinical episodes reaches a maximum in the third trimester, but symptomatic recurrences are common throughout pregnancy. The high levels of reproductive hormones are thought to increase the glycogen content of the vaginal environment and provide a carbon source for *Candida* growth and germination. Estrogens enhance vaginal epithelial cell avidity for *Candida* adherence, and a yeast cytosol receptor or binding system for female reproductive hormones has been documented. In addition, estrogens enhance yeast-mycelial transformation. Low-estrogen oral contraceptives may also cause an increase in *Candida* vaginitis. Hormone replacement therapy may contribute to vaginitis in postmenopausal women. Vaginal colonization with *Candida* is more common in diabetic patients, and poorly controlled diabetes pre-

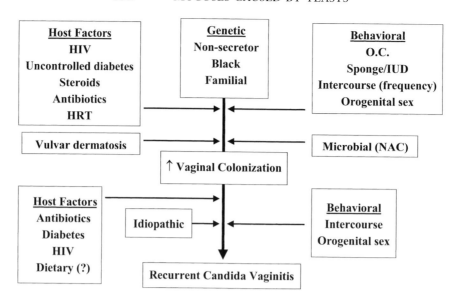

FIGURE 11–4. Pathogenesis of recurrent vulvovaginal candidiasis.

disposes to symptomatic vaginitis. Glucose tolerance tests have been recommended for women with recurrent vulvovaginal candidiasis (RVVC); however, the yield is low and testing is not justified in otherwise healthy premenopausal women. Diets high in refined sugar may precipitate symptomatic *Candida* vaginitis.

Symptomatic VVC is often observed during or after use of systemic or intravaginal antibiotics. Although no antimicrobial agent is free of this complication, the broad-spectrum antibiotics are mainly responsible; they act by eliminating the normal protective vaginal bacterial flora. *Lactobacillus spp.* in the natural flora provides a colonization-resistance mechanism and prevents germination of *Candida*. However, most women taking antibiotics do not develop *Candida* vaginitis. Environmental factors that predispose to *Candida* vaginitis may include tight, poorly ventilated clothing and nylon underclothing, which increase perineal moisture and temperature. Chemical contact, local allergy and hypersensitivity reactions may also predispose to symptomatic vaginitis. Iron deficiency is said to predispose to *Candida* infection, but there is no evidence to support this view. In patients who are debilitated or immunosuppressed, oral and vaginal candidiasis correlates well with reduced cell-mediated immunity, as evident in CMC and AIDS. Based on these observations, T-lymphocytes may contribute to normal vaginal defense mechanisms preventing mucosal invasion by *Candida*.

Several theories have been proposed to explain RVVC (Sobel et al, 1985a; Sobel, 1992). The intestinal reservoir theory is based on recovery of *Candida* on rectal culture in almost 100% of women with vulvovaginal candidiasis. DNA typing of vaginal and rectal cultures obtained simultaneously usually reveals identical strains. However, other studies have shown a lower concordance between rectal and vaginal cultures in patients with RVVC. In a maintenance study of women with RVVC who were receiving ketoconazole, recurrence of *Candida* vaginitis often occurred with no evidence of *Candida* in the rectum. Also, oral nystatin, which reduces intestinal yeast carriage, fails to prevent RVVC. Repeated reintroduction of yeast into the vagina from the gut is therefore no longer considered a likely cause of recurrent *Candida*.

The sexual transmission theory is based on (1) penile colonization with *Candida* organisms, which are present in approximately 20% of male partners of women with RVVC, and (2) infected partners often carry identical strains. Oral colonization of partners with an identical strain of *Candida* also occurs, and may be a source of orogenital transmission. However, in most studies involving treatment of partners, there was no reduction in the frequency of episodes of vaginitis.

The vaginal relapse theory to explain RVVC is also an alternative. Although antimycotic therapy may reduce the number of *Candida* and alleviate signs and symptoms of inflammation, the eradication or clearance of *Candida* from the vagina is incomplete because most of the antimycotic agents are fungistatic. The small number of organisms that persist in the vagina result in continued carriage of the organism; when host environmental conditions permit, the colonizing organisms increase in number and undergo mycelial transformation, resulting in a new clinical episode. Drug resistance is seldom responsible for RVVC in women infected with *C. albicans*. Current vaginal relapse theories regarding the pathogenesis of RVVC include qualitative and quantitative deficiency in the normal protective vaginal bacterial flora (unproven), and an acquired, often transient, antigen-specific deficiency in T lymphocyte function that permits unchecked yeast proliferation and germination. Reduced T lymphocyte reactivity to *Candida* antigen may result from the elaboration of prostaglandin E2 by the patient's macrophages which blocks *Candida* antigen-induced lymphocyte proliferation, possibly by inhibiting interleukin-2 production. Abnormal macrophage function could be the result of histamine produced as a consequence of local IgE *Candida* antibodies or a serum factor (Witkin, 1991).

Vulvar pruritus is the most common symptom of VVC. Vaginal discharge is often minimal and sometimes absent. Although described as being typically "cottage cheese-like" in character (See Color Fig. 11–5 in separate color insert), the discharge may vary from watery to homogeneously thick. Vaginal soreness, irritation, vulvar burning, dyspareunia, and external dysuria are other common symptoms. If there is an odor, it is minimal and unoffensive. Characteristically, the symptoms are exacerbated during the week before the onset of menses. The onset of menstrual flow brings some relief. Examination reveals erythema and swelling of the labia and vulva, often with discrete pustulopapular peripheral lesions. The cervix is normal with vaginal mucosal erythema with adherent whitish discharge.

In most symptomatic patients with VVC, diagnosis is readily made on the basis of microscopic examination of vaginal secretions. A wet mount with saline has a sensitivity of only 40%–60%. A preparation of 10% potassium hydroxide (KOH) is even more sensitive (50%–70%) in identifying the presence of yeast cells. Patients with *Candida* vaginitis have a normal vaginal pH, 4.0–4.5. A pH > 4.5 suggests the possibility of bacterial vaginosis, trichomoniasis, or mixed infection. Routine cultures are unnecessary, but vaginal culture should be performed in suspicious cases with negative microscopy. Although vaginal culture is the most sensitive method available for detecting *Candida*, a positive culture does not necessarily indicate that *Candida* is responsible for the vaginal symptoms. There is no reliable serological technique for the diagnosis of symptomatic VVC. Commercial tests (including latex agglutination slide tests) are less sensitive than culture and have no advantages over microscopy.

Candidemia and Disseminated Candidiasis

Candidemia or systemic candidiasis has been divided into four groups or syndromes, namely, catheter-related candidiasis, acute disseminated candidiasis, chronic disseminated candidiasis (hepatosplenic candidiasis), and deep organ candidiasis (Rex et al, 2000). Although hematogenous involvement occurs at some stage in the evolution of each, only the first two syndromes are associated strongly with documented candidemia. Hence use of the term candidemia only as a marker of invasive candidiasis results in the underestimation of the true incidence of invasive candidiasis (Rex et al, 2000).

The last 4 decades have witnessed a dramatic increase in the incidence of candidemia, originating in tertiary care centers and now observed in virtually all type hospitals (Fraser et al, 1992; Sandven, 2000). Approximately 20,000 cases of candidemia in adults occur annually in the United States. A published population-based survey reported that the incidence of nosocomial candidemia in the United States is 8 cases/ 100,000 population (Kao et al, 1999). If defined on the basis of candidemia, the incidence of invasive candidiasis has a bimodal age distribution with peaks at extremes of age, 75 cases/100,000 infants < 1 year old and 26 cases/ 100,000 individuals > 65 years (Kao et al, 1999).

Within the hospital setting, not all departments report high rates of candidemia. Patients in ICUs, especially surgical units (Voss et al, 1995; Vincent et al, 1998), trauma units, and neonatal ICUs, have the highest rates (Beck-Sague and Jarvis,1993; Fridkin and Jarvis, 1996). Twenty-five percent to fifty percent of nosocomial candidemia now occurs in critical care units (Rangel-Frausto et al, 1999). Neutropenic patients, previously the highest risk population, are no longer the most vulnerable subpopulation, due to the widespread use of fluconazole prophylaxis during neutropenia (Abi-Said et al, 1997). In some tertiary care centers, *C. albicans* is no longer the most frequent bloodstream isolate, being replaced by *C. glabrata*, which surpassed *C. tropicalis* as the most prevalent non-*albicans* species and currently cause 3%–35% of all candidemias (Valdivieso et al,1976; Wingard,1995; Abi-Said et al,1997; Pfaller et al, 2001; Bodey et al, 2002). Non-*albicans Candida* species have also become an increasing problem in ICUs, attributed to the more widespread use of fluconazole prophylaxis in this population (Nguyen et al, 1996a; Bodey et al, 2002). Antifungal prophylaxis, usually fluconazole, primarily in patients with acute leukemia and following BMT transplantation, has been associated with increased gut colonization and infection with *C. glabrata* (Abi-Said et al, 1997).

Risk factors for *Candida* bloodstream infections include systemic antibiotics, chemotherapy, corticosteroids, presence of intravascular catheters, total parenteral nutrition (TPN), recent abdominal surgery, hospitalization in ICU, malignancy, neutropenia, and fungal colonization (Bross et al, 1989; Beck-Sague et al, 1993; Pittet et al, 1994; Fridkin and Jarvis, 1996; Nguyen et al, 1996a; Nguyen et al, 1996b). In a recent prospective study conducted in six surgical ICUs, multivariate analysis revealed increased risk with prior abdominal surgery (R.R. 7.3) acute renal failure (R.R.

4.2), TPN (R.R. 3.6), and triple lumen catheter (R.R. 5.4) (Blumberg et al, 2001). In contrast to other studies, prior fungal colonization could not be demonstrated as a risk factor, whereas receipt of any systemic antifungal drug was associated with reduced risk (Blumberg et al, 2001). *Candida parapsilosis* is the most frequent cause of *Candida* bloodstream infection in neonates (Pappas et al, 1997; Rowen et al, 1999; Sandven, 2000). Neonatal candidemia (< 1 year of age) represents 12% of the cases of candidemia (Kao et al, 1999).

The source of candidemia remains poorly understood in spite of the aforementioned risk factors. In neutropenic individuals, gut colonization is likely responsible for most cases of candidemia. The gut is also likely to be the source of candidemia following abdominal surgery and in patients without intravascular central catheters. In contrast, in patients with skin colonization and contaminated intravascular catheters, the skin is thought to serve as the source. Other sources include intraabdominal abscesses, peritonitis, and rarely, urinary tract and contaminated IV solution. A recently published study estimated the attributable cost in 1997 U.S. dollars of each case of candidemia at $34,000 to $44,000, with a national annual total attributable cost for nosocomial candidemia of approximately $800 million in the United States (Rentz et al, 1998).

Clinical aspects of candidemia are extremely variable. Patients present with fever alone without organ-specific manifestations, or a wide spectrum of symptoms and signs, including fulminant sepsis. Accordingly, acute candidemia is indistinguishable from bacterial sepsis and septic shock. Clinical manifestations of fungemia are frequently superimposed on those due to the underlying pathology. Concomitant bacterial infections including bacteremia are not uncommon. In general, there are no specific clinical features of candidemia associated with individual *Candida* species.

At the time of documented candidemia, manifestations of systemic and invasive metastatic candidiasis may be present, although frequently when the latter is evident, blood cultures have become negative. Hence, candidemia is a marker, although an insensitive one of deeply invasive candidiasis (Berenguer et al, 1993). Only 50% of patients with disseminated candidiasis have positive blood cultures (Hockey et al, 1982) and antemortem diagnosis is relatively infrequent in the absence of candidemia (15%–40%). The likelihood of systemic invasion has been correlated with increasing numbers of positive blood cultures (Lecciones et al, 1992), although not all patients with candidemia have the same risk of dissemination. Patients with neutropenia have a significantly higher rate of visceral and cutaneous dissemination (Anaissie et al, 1998). Dissemination to multiple organs often involves skin, kidney, eye, brain, myocardium, and bone (See Color Fig. 11–6 in separate color insert). In leukemia patients, dissemination to liver and spleen is especially common, and may occasionally involve lungs, skin, and endocardium.

The possibility of asymptomatic disseminated infection drives the treatment principles of candidemia, even when candidemia is transient. Transient candidemia can occur from any source but most frequently follows intravascular catheter infection with prompt resolution following catheter removal. In general, in most prospective studies of nosocomial candidemia, approximately half the patients will have cleared candidemia within 72 hours without receiving systemic fungal therapy. Prolonged candidemia, especially when blood cultures remain persistently positive on appropriate antifungal therapy, suggests: *(1)* a persistent focus or source, e.g., intravascular catheter, abscess, suppurative thrombophlebitis; *(2)* endocarditis; *(3)* severe neutropenia; and *(4)* rarely, antifungal resistance especially with some non-*albicans Candida* species (Wingard, 1995; Pfaller et al, 2001). At the time of diagnosis of candidemia, general physical examination rarely reveals clinical signs of dissemination. However, a thorough examination, including a dilated funduscopic examination, is mandatory.

Occasionally, blood cultures obtained via central catheters may represent contamination; hence the importance of obtaining multiple blood cultures, especially cultures from peripheral vein sites. Nevertheless, febrile patients with a single positive blood culture for *Candida* species should always initially be considered to have a proven infection. In reviewing 155 episodes of catheter-related candidiasis, investigators observed a similar frequency of autopsy-proven candidiasis whether blood cultures were obtained from central catheter or peripheral site (Lecciones et al, 1992).

Improving blood culture yield can also be enhanced by increasing blood volume and utilizing newer techniques and media (Murray, 1991). Given the insensitivity of blood cultures, together with the lack of test for the diagnosis of invasive candidiasis, detection of hematogenous dissemination remains poor (Krick and Remington, 1976; Bennett, 1978; Edwards, 1991; Mitsutake et al, 1996).

The crude mortality rates reported in patients with candidemia represent a range of 40%–60% (Komshian et al, 1989; Wey et al, 1988; Fraser et al, 1992; Fridkin and Jarvis, 1996; Edmond et al, 1999; Blumberg et al, 2001) with an attributable mortality of 38%, exceeding that of most bacteremias. Since 1989, a 50% reduction in national mortality rates for invasive candidiasis has been reported, following a steady increase in mortality in the previous decades reaching 0.62 deaths/100,000 population (McNeil et al, 2001). A similar decline in rates of death from systemic candidiasis associated with HIV infection occurred (0.04/100,000). The explanation for decreased mortality in both HIV positive and negative patients in spite of increased *Candida* invasive disease may be related to increased awareness, earlier diagnosis and an enhanced therapeutic armamentarium. Non-*albicans Candida* infections in general tend to be associated with reduced lethality.

Ocular Candidiasis

Candida organisms gain access to the eye by one of two routes, either direct inoculation during eye surgery or trauma, or as the result of hematogenous spread (endogenous) (Edwards et al, 1974; Samiy and D'Amico, 1996). Any eye structure may be involved including conjunctiva, cornea, lens, ciliary body, vitreous humor, and uveal tract. Eye involvement may be unilateral or bilateral. Once endophthalmitis occurs, therapy, especially if delayed, is often insufficient to prevent blindness. Given the recent increased incidence of nosocomial candidemia, a parallel increase in endophthalmitis has occurred in all population groups (Donahue et al, 1994; Menezes et al, 1994; Coskuncan et al, 1994; Papanicolaou et al, 1997; Wolfensberger and Gonvers, 1998; Noyola et al, 2001), including neonates, and intravenous drug addicts (Hogeweg and de Jong, 1983). *Candida* endophthalmitis should raise the suspicion of concomitant widely disseminated candidiasis. Estimates of the incidence of eye involvement during candidemia have been as high as 28%–37% (Brooks et al, 1989; Penk and Pittrow, 1998); moreover in only half the cases of endophthalmitis is there a history of recent culture proven candidemia. In a prospective study of 50 patients with fungemia, incidence of ocular candidiasis was 26%, all manifested as chorioretinitis (Krishna et al, 2000). Some of the patients with an initially negative eye examination developed signs of ocular candidiasis within 2 weeks. *Candida albicans* is the commonest species responsible for ocular involvement, but other *Candida* species have been incriminated (Joshi and Hamory, 1991). In experimental animal models, a tropism of *C. albicans* for chorioretinal blood vessels has been demonstrated.

Symptoms of chorioretinitis are variable and often absent in patients too ill to complain. Symptoms include visual blurring, floaters, scotomata and blindness. Funduscopic examination usually reveals white, cotton ball-like lesions situated in the chorioretinal layer which may rapidly progress to extend into the posterior vitreous (See Color Fig. 11–7 in separate color insert). Indirect ophthalmoscopy with pupillary dilation is necessary to achieve complete visualization. Ocular lesions require the presence of leukocytes for development; presence of neutropenia inhibits the formation of ocular lesions in experimental rabbit models (Henderson et al, 1980).

Diagnosis of *Candida* endophthalmitis is usually made on the basis of clinical context and characteristic fundoscopic picture. Aspiration of the anterior chamber is rarely diagnostic whereas vitrectomy, often performed for therapeutic purposes, usually yields positive culture for *Candida* (McDonald et al, 1990).

Cardiac and Endovascular Candidiasis

Myocarditis and Pericarditis. *Candida* myocarditis is the result of hematogenous dissemination with development of one or more abscesses within the myocardium. Most frequently, abscesses are microabscesses usually diagnosed at autopsy. One group reported 62% of 50 patients with disseminated candidiasis had myocardial involvement at autopsy and other retrospective autopsy studies reported myocardial abscesses in 8%–93% (Franklin et al, 1976; Hofman et al, 1992).

Candida spp. may reach the pericardium from adjacent endocarditis or myocarditis but most frequently pericardial involvement is the result of hematogenous seeding or direct inoculation at the time of cardiac surgery (Rubin and Moellering, 1975; McNamee et al, 1998). Pericarditis is purulent in nature, resembles bacterial infection, and may be complicated by constrictive disease. Successful therapy requires pericardiectomy in addition to antifungal drugs. Medical therapy alone is associated with an extremely poor prognosis (Schrank and Dooley, 1995).

Endocarditis. Although previously rare, the advent of prosthetic cardiac valve surgery in the late 1960s together with the worldwide increase in intravenous drug abuse, especially heroin, resulted in a dramatic increase in incidence of *Candida* endocarditis (Rubinstein et al, 1975). In a large retrospective review of fungal endocarditis from 1965 to 1995, investigators determined that fungal endocarditis was responsible for fewer than 10% of all cases of infective endocarditis (Ellis et al, 2001). This review documented the changing epidemiology of fungal endocarditis. Although *Candida* spp. were previously responsible for > 66% of fungal endocarditis cases, the frequency of fungal endocarditis due to *Candida* species now accounts for less than half the cases (48%), and infection due to non-*albicans Candida* is as common as *C. albicans* (Ellis et al, 2001). The increase in non-*albicans Candida* endocarditis reflects the changing epidemiology of nosocomial candidemia, although it would appear that *C. parapsilosis* has a unique tropism for prosthetic endovascular surfaces. Another major factor determining the epidemiology of *Candida* endocarditis is the recent acceptance by clinicians that all candidemia episodes should be treated.

The pathogenesis of *Candida* endocarditis is complex, and several risk factors have been confirmed (Hallum and Williams, 1993; Ellis et al, 2001). *Candida* organisms rarely adhere to and colonize normal valvular endothelium. Predisposing factors include: *(1)* underlying valvular disease; *(2)* prosthetic cardiac valves, including homografts, which provide an abnormal surface once coated with platelets and fibronectin for *Candida* adherence; *(3)* prolonged presence of intravascular catheters, resulting in persistent high inoculum candidemia; *(4)* heroin addiction, still responsible for sporadic cases and occasional epidemics of *Candida* endocarditis (Rubinstein et al, 1975); and *(5)* other risk factors such as cancer chemotherapy, pre-existing bacterial endocarditis, immunocompromised hosts and temporally related noncardiac surgery, especially abdominal surgery (Ellis et al, 2001). *Candida* endocarditis is rare in the setting of granulocytopenia (Chim et al, 1998). Possible explanations include the short duration of undiagnosed candidemia together with universal aggressive therapy; however, it is also likely that the accompanying thrombocytopenia may prevent vegetation formation.

Postoperative endocarditis, especially following prosthetic valve surgery, so-called prosthetic valve endocarditis (PVE) remains the most common form of *Candida* endocarditis (> 50%). However, Ellis and colleagues in their review concluded that cardiac valve surgery showed the largest decrease in incidence as a risk factor. Most episodes of *Candida* PVE occur within 2 months of valve surgery, although endocarditis may occur much later (> 12 months) (Gilbert et al, 1996; Nasser et al, 1997). Specific risk factors for PVE include complicated surgery, perioperative antibiotics, prolonged postoperative use of catheters, and candidemia even if transient. Non-*albicans Candida* species are increasingly responsible for PVE, especially *C. parapsilosis*. Damaged endocardium, especially suture line and prosthetic material, serve as foci for *Candida* adherence (Calderone et al, 1978; Yeaman et al, 1996). Rarely, contamination of homografts and heterografts occurs before insertion. Pacemaker endocarditis due to *Candida* has also been described (Joly et al, 1997).

Clinical findings and complications in *Candida* endocarditis are similar to those seen in bacterial endocarditis with the exception of increased frequency of large emboli to major vessels in *Candida* endocarditis (Nguyen et al, 1996b). The higher incidence of embolization is manifested as either focal or global neurological deficits. Aortic and mitral valve involvement are most common. The classical findings of bacterial endocarditis are reported including Osler nodes, Janeway lesions, splinter hemorrhages, splenomegaly, hematuria and embolic manifestations. Some studies have found a reduced incidence of cardiac failure, changing heart murmurs and splenomegaly (Ellis et al,

2001). *Candida* endophthalmitis can complicate endocarditis but is usually seen in the absence of endocarditis. Rarely, polymicrobial *Candida* endocarditis occurs and may follow or accompany bacterial endocarditis. A patient with *Candida* PVE may relapse several years following a putative cure with medical therapy (Galgiani and Stevens, 1977; Nguyen et al, 1996b); hence long-term follow-up is necessary.

Most patients with *Candida* endocarditis have positive blood cultures. An analysis of 91 published cases of *Candida* endocarditis following cardiac surgery revealed that 26% of patients had negative blood cultures (Seelig et al, 1974). In the culture negative patients, frequently a history was obtained of recent documented but untreated candidemia that resolved without antifungal therapy. Improved diagnosis of *Candida* endocarditis has followed greater awareness of the significance of candidemia, newer blood culture techniques and more frequent use of echocardiography. Accordingly, increased preoperative diagnosis has been noted in the last decade (Ellis et al, 2001). Although not specific for microorganisms, both transthoracic and transesophogeal echocardiography have made an enormous contribution to facilitating diagnosis and avoiding the usual delayed diagnosis. Visualizing large vegetations via ECHO in patients with negative blood cultures is strong circumstantial evidence of *Candida* endocarditis. Mycological exam should be performed on all surgically removed emboli.

Mortality of *Candida* endocarditis remains high. Prior to availability of cardiac surgery, mortality was in excess of 90%. With combined treatment employing surgery and aggressive antifungal therapy, mortality rates of ~45% are now universal (see later under TREATMENT).

Noncardiac Endovascular *Candida* Infections. The increased incidence of nosocomial candidemia has resulted in an inevitable increase in *Candida* endovascular infections involving large and medium sized arteries and veins (Friedland, 1996; Khan et al, 1997). Phlebitis due to all *Candida* species is common and often is associated with tunneled subcutaneous catheters. Delay in treatment often results in extensive vascular thrombosis and suppuration, and persistent candidemia in spite of treatment with high doses of fungicidal agents. Venous thrombi, even after removal of responsible catheters, impair drug penetration and allow microabscesses to persist within the thrombi with resultant persistent candidemia (Walsh et al, 1986). For cure, surgical excision of thrombi is often required in addition to prolonged antifungal therapy. Complications include superior vena cava obstruction, tricuspid valve endocarditis, right-sided mural endocarditis, and pulmonary vein thrombosis. Small peripheral vein thrombophlebitis is not uncommon.

Arterial involvement may occur as a result of candidemia seeding prosthetic aortic valves and other large arterial grafts (Doscher et al, 1987). Uncontrolled diabetes in high-risk patients further facilitates the development of true mycotic aneurysms localized and originating at the graft suture line. In addition to pain, fever, and signs of systemic infection, the mycotic aneurysm may rupture resulting in catastrophic hemorrhage or in large vessel occlusion. *Candida* mycotic aneurysms have been reported in the cerebral circulation, pulmonary arteries (following use of Swan-Ganz catheter), and iliac vessels (of intravenous drug users). *Candida* mycotic aneurysms may also complicate dialysis shunts.

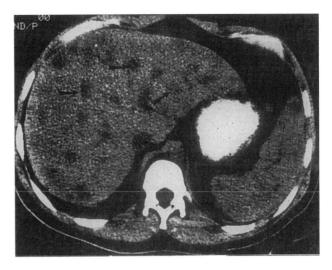

FIGURE 11–8. Hepatosplenic candidiasis. Note multiple "bull's-eye" lesions shown on CT scan.

Chronic Systemic Candidiasis

Hepatosplenic candidiasis (HSC) is a chronic form of disseminated candidiasis that develops as a complication of invasive candidiasis during granulocytopenia. Many authorities now prefer the term chronic systemic candidiasis since other organs (eyes, skin, and soft tissue) may be involved (Gorg et al, 1994; Bjerke et al, 1994; Anttila et al, 1994; Chanock and Pizzo, 1997). In the last 2 decades, there have been increasing reports of HSC, possibly due to improved diagnostic imaging, but also reflecting increased rates of candidemia. Candidemia, the cornerstone of this syndrome, frequently follows *Candida* colonization of the gut, complicated by gastrointestinal mucosa disruption and lamina propria invasion by *Candida*, which reach submucosal blood vessels that drain into the portal venous system and then into the liver where focal *Candida* abscesses are established. Many of the patients with chronic systemic candidiasis have no history of documented previous peripheral vein or catheter-associated candidemia. Following recovery from neutropenia, the *Candida* lesions established during neutropenia do not resolve, but become more prominent, especially in the liver, spleen, and kidneys. At the time of diagnosis of HSC, both acute and chronic inflammatory cells are found to surround the outer border of *Candida* pseudohyphae and an expanding zone of tissue necrosis between the inflammatory infiltrate and fungal cells. Occasionally calcification occurs at the center of lesions within nonviable fungal elements.

Clinically, patients with HSC usually have a history of hematologic malignancy (ALL > AML), cytotoxic chemotherapy and have recent recovery from neutropenia, during which time they were febrile and received antibacterial therapy. After recovery from neutropenia, symptoms of antibiotic resistant fever and gastrointestinal upset (nausea, vomiting, abdominal pain) increase as neutrophils infiltrate foci of *Candida* invasion in liver and spleen. Laboratory findings often include elevation in serum alkaline phosphatase and leukocytosis. Hepatic transaminases are not commonly elevated. In one study of leukemic subjects, 6.8% developed HSC (Anttila et al, 1994).

Lesions of HSC may be detected by several diagnostic imaging modalities, computed tomographies (CT), ultrasonography (U/S) and magnetic resonance imaging (Fig. 11–8). The characteristic "bulls-eye" lesions seen on U/S and CT are not detectable until neutrophil recovery. However, these lesions are not specific for HSC. As the lesions resolve during therapy, they may either disappear completely or undergo calcification. Ultrasonography appears to be less sensitive but possibly more specific than CT scanning in demonstrating characteristic target lesions (Helton et al, 1986; Semelka et al, 1992; Gorg et al, 1994). Diagnosis is confirmed by histopathological examination and culture of hepatic tissue obtained by percutaneous biopsy and occasionally laparoscopy. The appearance of hyphae in a granulomatous lesion is in itself not specific for *C. albicans* and may be caused by other *Candida* spp. as well as non-*Candida* fungi such as *Trichosporon* spp., *Fusarium* spp. and *Aspergillus* spp. Among *Candida* species, *C. albicans* is most common and *C. tropicalis* is next most common. Metastatic tumors may simulate the appearance of HSC.

Neonatal Candidiasis

Two distinct *Candida* syndromes are seen in neonates, and especially in preterm, low birth–weight neonates.

The most serious of these syndromes is neonatal systemic candidiasis. Developing either via ascending infection of the uterine contents prior to birth or from colonization acquired during passage through the birth canal, hematogenous dissemination of *Candida* presents in the first days or weeks of life with symptoms identical to those of neonatal bacterial sepsis (Faix, 1992a; Jin et al, 1995; van den Anker et al, 1995). Involvement of the lung, skin, and particularly the central nervous system (CNS) is common.

By contrast, neonates with congenital cutaneous candidiasis present within a few hours of birth with a diffuse maculopapular, erythematous rash involving almost any part of the skin (Johnson et al, 1981; Almeida-Santos et al, 1991; Glassman and Muglia, 1993). The initial rash can evolve to pustular or vesicular lesions with subsequent desquamation. Culture and microscopic examination of scrapings of the skin reveal *Candida* species, usually *C. albicans*. If the affected neonate is preterm (< 1500 g), systemic involvement is frequent and the neonate should be evaluated repeatedly with blood, urine and cerebrospinal fluid (CSF) cultures in order to rule out neonatal systemic candidiasis (Johnson et al, 1981; Faix, 1992a). In full-term neonates, infection is usually limited to the skin and gastrointestinal tract (Barone and Krilov, 1995).

Central Nervous System Candidiasis

Candida is the most prevalent cerebral mycosis at postmortem examination and was found in 48% of autopsied subjects with systemic candidiasis (Lipton et al, 1984). In the same study, in less than 25% of the subjects, the diagnosis of CNS involvement was made antemortem. Hence, diagnosis is often difficult and frequently delayed in all age groups but especially in preterm low birth–weight neonates, resulting in considerable morbidity and mortality.

Central nervous system candidiasis involves both brain tissue and/or meninges, and, except for occasional association with neurosurgery and head trauma, is invariably the result of hematogenous dissemination (Treseler and Sugar, 1992; Voice et al, 1994; Burgert et al, 1995; Chimelli and Mahler-Araujo, 1997). Autopsy studies observed a correlation between cardiac and cerebral involvement; 80% of patients with myocardial or valve infection also had CNS candidiasis (Lipton et al, 1984). Cerebral parenchymal infection occurs as a single or multiple micro- or macroabscesses scattered throughout the brain (Pendlebury et al, 1989; Lai et al, 1997). Rarely, larger abscesses are visualized on CT scan (Hagensee et al, 1994). Other *Candida* CNS presentations include thrombosis, vasculitis, hemorrhage, fungus balls of both white and gray matter, and mycotic aneurysms. *Candida parapsilosis* has a predilection

for cerebral vascular involvement (Lipton et al, 1984). As part of systemic candidiasis syndrome, *Candida* brain abscess presents with a variable picture, including fever, altered mental status (obtundation or coma), and/or focal manifestations depending on size and site of the abscess(es).

Acute *Candida* meningitis presents with meningismus and may be indistinguishable from bacterial infection. *Candida* meningitis has been reported with all species of *Candida*, although a higher representation of *C. tropicalis* has been noted in leukemic children with *Candida* meningitis (McCullers et al, 2000). In non-neutropenic patients, especially postsurgical patients, meningitis is most commonly caused by *C. albicans*. CSF findings in acute *Candida* meningitis include hypoglycorrhachia, increased protein and variable pleocytosis (mean 600/mm^3) with lymphocytic dominance. Yeasts are seen on Gram stain in only 40% of patients (Lipton et al, 1984). In premature neonates, acute *Candida* meningitis is indistinguishable from bacterial infection or systemic infection, and meningitis is especially severe in this population (Fernandez et al, 2000). Occasional cases that are diagnosed early may present with normal CSF findings. Because of the paucity of signs indicating acute meningitis in neonates, and severe morbidity associated with delay in diagnosis, lumbar puncture should be obligatory in this high-risk population in the presence of positive blood cultures for *Candida*. Complications include hydrocephalus.

A chronic form of *Candida* meningitis, which may mimic tuberculous or cryptococcal meningitis, has also been reported. Patients presented with chronic headache, fever, and nuchal rigidity (Voice et al, 1994). Analysis of CSF showed either mononuclear or neutrophilic pleocytosis, elevated protein and hypoglycorrhachia. Only 17% of CSF Gram stains were positive and only 44% of initial CSF cultures yielded *Candida* species. Overall mortality was 53% (Voice et al, 1994). *Candida* species are not uncommon isolates in postneurosurgical infections including meningitis and wound or deep surgical-site infections, especially following trauma and in patients with brain tumors (Nguyen and Yu, 1995a). An even more frequent scenario is the patient with fever and positive *Candida* CSF cultures in the presence of an indwelling CSF shunt or device (Gower et al, 1986). The clinical significance of a single positive CSF sample drawn through an indwelling device is problematic and a definitive diagnosis may require repeated positive cultures of CSF samples obtained by lumbar puncture (Geers and Gordon, 1999). Shunt-associated infections include ventriculitis and meningitis (Sugarman and Massanari, 1980). Anecdotal case reports of *Candida* meningitis following lumbar puncture are extremely rare (Chmel, 1973).

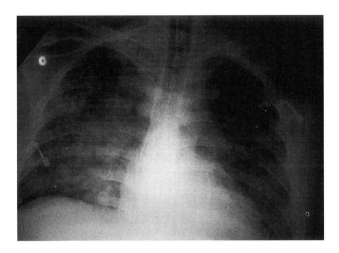

FIGURE 11–9. *Candida* bronchopneumonia associated with aspiration.

Pulmonary Candidiasis

Candida species are frequently found in sputum and aspirates of endotracheal tube secretions, and their role as a possible cause of pulmonary disease is a frequent clinical dilemma. Although invasive lung parenchymal disease, pneumonitis or pneumonia due to *Candida* undoubtedly occurs, these entities are rare. Two forms of *Candida* pneumonia are described (Masur et al, 1977). One form is local or diffuse bronchopneumonia as a consequence of bronchogenic spread (Haron et al, 1993; Heurlin et al, 1996) (Fig. 11–9). This infrequent event is rarely the consequence of aspiration even in heavily colonized high-risk patients (Kontoyiannis et al, 2001). The second form is pneumonia resulting from widespread seeding of the lung in a patient with candidemia. The second syndrome is characterized by diffuse, often nodular infiltrates, and usually misdiagnosed as *Pneumocystis carinii* pneumonia or congestive cardiac failure (Cairns and Durack, 1986; Zeluff, 1990). Other rare clinical manifestations include necrotizing pneumonia, *Candida* pulmonary mycetoma, and transient infiltrates attributed to allergic bronchopulmonary candidiasis (Cairns and Durack, 1986; Lee et al, 1987).

X-ray and CT scan studies are nonspecific and not useful in diagnosis. Diagnosis of pulmonary candidiasis is extremely difficult and requires biopsy with histopathology demonstrating fungal tissue invasion (McAdams et al, 1995; von Eiff et al, 1995). Diagnosis cannot be made on the basis of radiologic findings and/or recovery of yeast from sputum or aspirates of endotracheal tube secretions because of the frequency of both upper and lower respiratory tract colonization with *Candida* (el-Ebiary et al, 1997). Even quantitative cultures are of little help. Similarly cultures of BAL

specimens and recovery of *Candida* from lung biopsy specimens are of low sensitivity and specificity and have a poor positive predictive value (Kontoyiannis et al, 2001). Finally, even when *Candida* infection is confirmed histopathologically, pulmonary invasion is uncommonly of clinical significance and in the few instances of extensive pulmonary involvement, pneumonitis usually occurs in the setting of a terminally ill patient. *Candida* has rarely been reported to cause epiglottitis, laryngitis, and bronchitis (Wengrower et al, 1985; Walsh and Gray, 1987; Wang et al, 1997).

Urinary Tract Candidiasis

Candiduria is a relatively rare finding in otherwise healthy people; funguria was found in only 15 of 1500 patients (Guze and Harley, 1957). In another study, the results of urine cultures were positive for 10 of 440 healthy adults, but the positive cultures reverted to negative when clean-catch techniques were used (Schonebeck, 1972). The incidence of fungal urinary tract infections, and specifically candiduria, has dramatically increased among hospitalized patients, especially those patients with indwelling drainage devices (Michigan, 1976; Platt et al, 1986; Schaberg et al, 1991). A study by Platt and colleagues showed that 26.5% of all urinary infections related to indwelling catheters were caused by fungi. Another study found that 2% of all urine specimens submitted to a hospital microbiology laboratory tested positive for yeast vs. 11% of the urine samples obtained from patients in the leukemia and bone marrow transplantation unit in the same hospital (Rivett et al, 1986). *Candida* species are the microbial pathogens that are most frequently isolated from the urine samples of patients in surgical ICUs. Presently, 10%–15% of nosocomial urinary tract infections are caused by *Candida* species (Phillips and Karlowicz, 1997; Febre et al, 1999).

Diabetes mellitus may predispose patients to candiduria by predisposing them to *Candida* colonization of the vulvovestibular area (in women), enhancing urinary fungal growth in the presence of glycosuria, lowering host resistance to invasion by fungi as a consequence of impaired phagocytic activity, and promoting stasis of urine in a neurogenic bladder (Johnson, 1954). *Candida* species colonization of the gastrointestinal tract is present in ~30% of normal adults. However, among patients who are receiving antibiotics, colonization rates approach 100%. Because there is little evidence that systemic antibiotics directly influence *Candida* proliferation or virulence, it is likely that antibiotics contribute to colonization by *Candida* species by suppressing endogenous bacterial flora, primarily in the gut and lower genital tract, and possibly in superficial areas adjacent to the urethral meatus (Stamm et al, 1991). The same risk factors for nosocomial can-diduria also predispose to bacteriuria (Fisher et al, 1982; Kauffman et al, 2000). Candiduria per se is al-most invariably preceded by bacteriuria. Factors that predispose to candiduria, but not to bacteriuria, other than duration of hospitalization, have not been identi-fied, and more studies on the pathogenesis of can-diduria are needed.

Indwelling urinary catheters serve as a portal of en-try for microorganisms into the urinary drainage sys-tem. All catheters become colonized if left in place long enough (Stamm et al, 1991). Other risk factors for candiduria include extremes of age, female sex, use of immunosuppressive agents, intravenous catheters, in-terruption of urine flow, radiation therapy, and geni-tourinary tuberculosis (Fisher et al, 1982; Kauffman et al, 2000).

The overwhelming majority of fungal infections of the urinary tract involve *Candida* species. In a large multicenter study, *C. albicans* was found in 446 (51.8%) of 861 patients with funguria (Kauffman et al, 2000). The second most common pathogen (found in 134 of patients) was *Candida glabrata*. A second study reported a slightly higher proportion of isolates due to *C. glabrata* (Storfer et al, 1994). Risk factors for *C. glabrata* UTI are similar to those that predispose a patient to *C. albicans* infection (Kauffman et al, 1984; Frye et al, 1988). Although *C. albicans* is the most com-mon species encountered, virtually all epidemiologic studies have concluded that non-*albicans Candida* species are also extremely common and more prevalent than in other sites (i.e., oropharynx and vagina), pos-sibly as a function of urine composition and pH se-lecting for non-*albicans* species. In ~10% of patients, more than one species of *Candida* are found simulta-neously and candiduria frequently coexists with or fol-lows bacteriuria (Sobel et al, 2000).

Ascending infection is by far the most common route for *Candida* infection of the urinary tract and occurs more often in women due to a shorter urethra and frequent vulvovestibular colonization with *Candida* (10%–35%). Catheterization can cause infection by al-lowing migration of organisms into the bladder along the surface of the catheter from the external peri-urethral surfaces. Ascending infection that originates in the bladder can also lead to infection of the upper urinary tract, especially if vesicoureteral reflux or ob-struction of urinary flow occurs, and may result in acute pyelonephritis and, rarely, candidemia. A fungus ball consisting of yeast, hyphal elements, epithelial and inflammatory cells, and, sometimes, renal medullary tissue secondary to papillary necrosis, may complicate ascending or descending infections. The fungus ball tends to be found in dilated areas of the urinary tract, especially in the bladder in the presence of obstruction.

Renal candidiasis most commonly follows hematoge-nous dissemination of *Candida* to the kidneys. *Candida* species have a tropism for the kidneys; one study re-vealed that 90% of patients with fatal disseminated candidiasis had renal involvement at autopsy (Letiner, 1964). Rarely, isolated hematogenous renal infection after transient candidemia can occur, and often when renal candidiasis is suspected, blood cultures are no longer positive.

The finding of *Candida* organisms in the urine may represent contamination, colonization of the drainage device, or infection. Contamination of a urine speci-men is common, especially with suboptimal urine col-lection from a catheterized patient or a woman who has heavy yeast colonization of the vulvovestibular area. Given the capacity of yeast to grow in urine, small numbers of yeast that find their way into the collected urine sample may multiply quickly. Therefore, high colony counts could be the result of yeast contamina-tion or colonization. Colonization refers to the asymp-tomatic adherence and settlement of yeast, usually on drainage catheters or other foreign bodies in the uri-nary tract (i.e., stents and nephrostomy tubes), and may spuriously result in a high concentration of the organ-isms on urine culture. Simply finding or culturing the organism does not imply clinical significance, regard-less of the concentration of organisms in the urine. Accordingly, some clinicians require confirmation of *Candida* presence by means of a second urine sample examination before they initiate treatment or further investigation. Infection is caused by tissue invasion, both superficial and deep. Colony counts of $> 10^4$ cfu/ml of urine are associated with infection in patients without indwelling urinary catheters, although clini-cally significant renal candidiasis has been reported with colony counts of 10^3 cfu/ml of urine (Schonebeck, 1972; Kozinn et al, 1978). While pyuria supports the diagnosis of infection in the presence of a urinary catheter, pyuria can be explained by mechanical injury of the bladder mucosa by the catheter, and is frequently the result of coexistent bacteriuria. Absence of pyuria and low colony counts tend to rule out *Candida* infec-tion, but the low specificity of pyuria and counts $> 10^3$ cfu/ml require that results be interpreted in the clinical context (Schonebeck, 1972; Kozinn et al, 1978).

The number of yeasts in urine has little value in lo-calizing the anatomical level of infection. Rarely, a granular cast containing *Candida* hyphal elements is found in urine that localizes the infection to renal parenchyma. Declining renal function suggests urinary obstruction or renal invasion (Michigan, 1976). For candiduric patients with sepsis, not only is it necessary to obtain blood cultures, but given the frequency that obstruction and stasis coexist, radiographic imaging of the upper tract is essential. Any febrile patient for whom therapy for candiduria is considered necessary should be evaluated to find the anatomic source of candiduria. In contrast, a patient without sepsis requires performance of no additional studies unless candiduria persists after removal of the catheter.

Candiduria is most often asymptomatic and usually occurs in hospitalized patients with indwelling catheters. These patients usually show none of the signs or symptoms associated with urinary tract infection. Occasionally, patients may present with symptoms of bladder irritation including dysuria, hematuria, frequency, urgency, and suprapubic tenderness. Cystoscopy reveals soft, pearly white, elevated patches with underlying friable mucosa. Hyperemia of the bladder mucosa is common (See Color Fig. 11–10 in separate color insert). Symptomatic Candida cystitis is extremely rare in both catheterized and noncatheterized patients, implying that the bladder is relatively resistant to invasion by Candida species. Emphysematous cystitis is a rare complication of lower tract infection, whereas prostatic abscess caused by Candida species is occasionally seen, especially among patients with diabetes.

Upper urinary tract infection presents with fever, leukocytosis, and costovertebral angle tenderness. On clinical grounds, ascending pyelonephritis and urosepsis with Candida species are indistinguishable from bacterial pyelonephritis. Ascending infection almost invariably occurs in the presence of urinary obstruction and stasis, especially in patients with diabetes or nephrolithiasis. Candida pyelonephritis is often complicated by local suppurative disease, resulting in pyonephrosis or focal abscess formation. A major complication of upper urinary tract involvement is obstruction caused by fungal balls (bezoars), which can also be visualized by ultrasound (Fisher et al, 1979). Renal colic may occur with the passage of fungal "stones" which are actually portions of fungal balls.

Patients with hematogenous seeding of the kidneys from candidemia may present with high fever, hemodynamic instability, and variable renal insufficiency. Blood cultures are positive for Candida in half of these patients. Retinal or skin involvement may suggest dissemination, but candiduria and a decline in renal function are often the only clues to systemic candidiasis in a febrile, high-risk patient. A reliable means for diagnosing invasive candidiasis continues to be elusive.

Abdominal Candidiasis Including Peritonitis
Candida infection has been increasingly recognized as a cause of abdominal sepsis and is associated with a high mortality. Abdominal sepsis may occur as monomicrobial or polymicrobial peritonitis and result in single or multiple abscesses (McClean et al, 1994). Translocation of Candida across the intact intestinal mucosa has been shown experimentally in animals and human volunteers (Stone et al, 1974). Peritoneal contamination with Candida species usually follows spontaneous gastrointestinal perforation on surgical opening of gut (Calandra et al, 1989). After contamination of the peritoneal cavity, Candida organisms do not inevitably result in peritonitis and clinical infection. Peritonitis is more likely to follow proliferation of accompanying bacterial pathogens but can occur with Candida alone. Several risk factors have been recognized in the development of peritonitis including recent or concomitant antimicrobial therapy, inoculum size and surgery for acute pancreatitis (Calandra et al, 1989). Pancreatic transplantation, especially with enteric drainage, is associated with intraabdominal Candida abscess formation (Benedetti et al, 1996). Candida species appear to have unique affinity for the inflamed pancreas, resulting in intrapancreatic abscesses or infection of a pseudocyst. With Candida peritonitis, Candida usually remains localized to the peritoneal cavity; dissemination occurs in approximately 25% of patients. Candidemia complicating intraabdominal infection is associated with a high mortality.

The clinical significance of Candida isolated from the peritoneal cavity at the time of surgery or in the postoperative period is controversial. Several earlier studies concluded that the finding of a positive culture did not require antifungal therapy (Peoples, 1986). In a review of Candida isolates from the peritoneal cavity, investigators determined that Candida caused intraabdominal infection in 39% (19/49) of patients. In 61% of patients, Candida isolation occurred without signs of peritonitis (Calandra et al, 1989). Accordingly, in each individual patient, judgement based upon the presence of clinical signs of infection and other risk factors should be taken into consideration in deciding to initiate antifungal therapy (Eggimann et al, 1999).

Candida peritonitis complicating peritoneal dialysis (CAPD) is more common, but uncommonly results in positive blood cultures and hematogenous dissemination. In a series of patients on CAPD followed for 5 years, fungal peritonitis, most commonly caused by Candida species, accounted for 7% of episodes of peritonitis and eight associated deaths (Rubin et al, 1987). Others have reported that fungal infections account for between 1% and 15% of episodes of peritonitis in patients on CAPD (Kerr et al, 1983; Eisenberg et al, 1986; Goldie et al, 1996). Few risk factors for CAPD associated fungal peritonitis have emerged except for hospitalization and recent prior episodes of peritonitis and antibacterial therapy (Eisenberg et al, 1986). An extraperitoneal site of fungal infection is rarely identified. Clinically, fungal peritonitis cannot be differentiated from bacterial peritonitis except by Gram stain and dialysate culture.

Biliary Candidiasis

Yeast isolated from the bile is not uncommon, especially following biliary surgery, and has the same significance as asymptomatic bactobilia, that is, colonization without invasion is typical. While a potential source of future infection, the finding of yeast in the bile in itself is not a justification for antifungal therapy (Ehrenstein et al, 2002). *Candida* is an infrequent cause of cholecystitis and cholangitis usually following extrahepatic biliary tract obstruction (Irani and Truong, 1986). Other risk factors for biliary candidiasis include diabetes, immunosuppression and abdominal malignancy. A major contributory factor is use of biliary stents placed to relieve obstruction; *Candida* infection usually supervenes when stent drainage is compromised. In this setting, infection is usually polymicrobial and *Candida* is a pathogen that cannot be ignored. An uncommon complication of biliary candidiasis is development of fungus balls in the gall bladder and dilated bile ducts (Magnussen et al, 1979; Irani and Truong, 1986; Morris et al, 1990). Candidemia is an infrequent complication of biliary candidiasis. Cholecystitis due to *Candida* has been reported in AIDS patients with cholangiopathy. Morris and colleagues reviewed 31 cases of biliary candidiasis and classified disease as uncomplicated and complicated. Uncomplicated cholecystitis implied that *Candida* organisms were confined to bile and the gall bladder without extrabiliary spread. In contrast, complicated infections implied spread to adjacent structures, including liver and peritoneum. Uncomplicated disease has minimal mortality and cure is achieved by cholecystectomy alone.

Candida Osteomyelitis and Arthritis

Although previously rare, *Candida* osteomyelitis has become more common. Most cases result from hematogenous dissemination with seeding of long bones in children and the axial skeleton in adults. Sites of bone infection include spine (vertebral and intervertebral disks) wrist, femur, humerus, and costochondral junctions (Collette et al, 1989; Herzog et al, 1989). Osteomyelitis may present weeks or months following the causal candidemic episode; hence at the time of the presentation, blood cultures are usually negative and radiologic findings nonspecific. Diagnosis usually requires percutaneous biopsy or open biopsy.

Occasionally, postoperative wound infections may spread to contiguous bone such as sternum and vertebrae (Clancy et al, 1997). Regardless of source, manifestations resemble bacterial infection, but run a more insidious course, with a significant delay in diagnosis. Hematogenous vertebral osteomyelitis most commonly (95%) affects the lower thoracic or lumbar spine. In one series, 83% of patients had back pain lasting more

than 1 month, only 32% presented with fever and 19% had associated neurologic complications (Miller and Mejicano, 2001). Species identified were *C. albicans* (57%), *C. tropicalis* (17%), and *C. glabrata* (12%). A prior history of positive blood cultures was present in 51%–61% of cases (Hendrickx et al, 2001).

Candida arthritis also represents a complication of hematogenous candidiasis. It rarely follows local trauma, surgery, or intraarticular injections (Silveira et al, 1993; Hansen and Anderson, 1995; Murphy et al, 1997; Fukasawa and Shirakura, 1997). Patients with underlying joint disease are at increased risk, e.g., those with rheumatoid arthritis and prosthetic joints. Non-*albicans Candida* species account for a higher than expected frequency of cases of fungal arthritis. *Candida* arthritis can occur in any joint and involves multiple joints in up to 27% of cases. The knee is the most commonly involved joint. Infection resembles bacterial septic arthritis, but frequent delays in diagnosis and suboptimal therapy often lead to chronic infection with secondary bone involvement.

Rarely hematogenous candidiasis may involve single or multiple muscles resulting in *Candida* pyomyositis (Belzunegui et al, 1997). Abscesses may be large or small, and this complication is frequently seen in patients with AIDS.

Candida Infections in Burns

Fungal infection is a serious complication of major burns (Spebar and Pruitt, 1981; Prasad et al, 1987; Desai et al, 1987; Grube et al, 1988). Risk factors include the use of broad-spectrum antibiotics, TPN, and intravascular catheters. An additional risk is related to the surface area of the burn. Increased survival of patients with extensive burns has expanded the pool of at risk subjects. *Candida* species causing burn-associated infection are similar to those involved in other nosocomial *Candida* infections. Burn colonization rates are usually less than 20% (range 13%–65%), with rates of candidemia ranging from 1.8% to 5%. Candidemia and bacteremia frequently coexist in burn patients (Spebar and Pruitt, 1981; Prasad et al, 1987; Desai et al, 1987). Mortality attributable to invasive candidiasis in burn patients is low (< 1%) with concomitant bacterial pathogens playing a more important role. However, candidemia should be viewed as a prognostic indicator of high mortality. During the decade of the 1980s, many burn units utilized antifungal prophylaxis with oral nystatin or topical nystatin incorporated into silver sulfadiazine with considerable efficacy in reducing both burn wound colonization by *Candida* species and candidemia (Desai et al, 1987). Unfortunately, outbreaks have been reported of nystatin-resistant *Candida* species (Dube et al, 1994). Given the risk of antifungal resistance and the availability of less toxic antifungal agents, prophylaxis in burn patients is no longer widely practiced.

DIAGNOSIS

Candida species grow readily when cultures are obtained from body fluids or tissues, and results are usually available in 48–72 hours. Isolation of *Candida* species from nonsterile sites such as wounds, skin, urine, sputum, vaginal secretions, and stool is not diagnostic of *Candida* infection. A positive culture only indicates that *Candida* species are present in the tissues examined. On the other hand, positive *Candida* cultures from sterile sites (blood, CSF, pleural fluid, peritoneal fluid) are almost always indicative of infection.

Blood cultures are only positive in 50%–60% of autopsy-proven cases of disseminated candidiasis; thus, negative blood cultures do not rule out invasive disease. In one study, the highest sensitivity reported to date was achieved using the lysis centrifugation technique (Berenguer et al, 1993). Other methods with at least equal efficacy include the BACTEC high blood volume fungal media and the BacT/Alert system (Wilson et al, 1993; Rowen et al, 1999).

Deep-seated organ *Candida* infection may require tissue biopsy to establish a definitive diagnosis. Unfortunately, tissue samples may contain small numbers of organisms with resultant negative cultures. Fixed tissues can be stained with hematoxylin and eosin. In addition, yeasts and fungal hyphae may be demonstrated with Gomori silver-methenamine, methylene blue, or periodic acid-Schiff stains.

Species identification of *Candida* is required for all infections because of the variable susceptibility to antifungal drugs that is species specific. *C albicans, C dubliniensis,* and *C stellatoidea* can be identified morphologically by germ-tube formation (hyphae are produced from yeast cells after 2–3 hours of incubation) or biochemical assays. CHROMagar *Candida* media allows for the presumptive identification of several *Candida* species by using color reactions in specialized media that demonstrate different colony colors, depending on the species of *Candida* (Pfaller et al, 1996), but use of this method as an alternative to assimilation assays is controversial. Commercially available carbohydrate fermentation and assimilation assays such as the API 20C AUX, API 32C, Vitek 2 ID-YST, RapidID yeast Plus, and ID32C are several biochemical assays that allow the identification of the different *Candida* species with more precision (Ponton, 2002).

Serologic assays include testing for *Candida* antibodies, antigens and metabolites. The *Candida* antibody assays are nonstandardized and are generally detected late in the course of infection. Unfortunately, they are less sensitive in immunocompromised patients. The *Candida* mannan antigen assay has a reported sensitivity of 31%–90% (even less for non-*albicans Candida species*) and is difficult to perform (Kerkering et al, 1979; Gentry et al, 1983). *Candida* heat labile glycoprotein antigen (CAND-TEC *Candida* Detection System) is relatively easy to perform, with a sensitivity of 40%–70%. Unfortunately, colonization produces false-positive results and testing of sequential specimens is necessary to increase the sensitivity of the test (Escuro, 1989). The test for *Candida* enolase antigen has a low sensitivity (55%–70%) and specificity and requires serial assays to increase its sensitivity (Walsh et al, 1991; van Deventer et al, 1994). The Glucatell assay for $(1–3)\beta$-D-glucan or the amebocyte lysis assay detects the presence of glucan in blood. The assay appears to have excellent sensitivity (75%–95%) and a specificity of 88%–100%. Its drawback is cross-reaction with other fungi such as *Aspergillus, Cryptococcus, Fusarium, Acremonium,* and *Saccharomyces* (Obayashi et al, 1995). D-arabinatol is a metabolite of *Candida* and testing for D-arabinatol has a sensitivity of approximately 50% (not useful for infection with *C. krusei* or *C. glabrata*). This assay has higher sensitivity in patients with fungemia and lower sensitivity with tissue invasion (Walsh et al, 1994).

Polymerase chain reaction (PCR) and DNA probes have the advantage of being able to detect small amounts of *Candida* DNA in either blood or tissues (Sandhu et al, 1995; van Burik et al, 1998; Polanco et al, 1999). Despite the fact that PCR assays have been shown to be highly sensitive, they continue to have problems of false-positivity, are technically difficult to perform, and are not yet commercially available.

TREATMENT

In Vitro Susceptibility

Currently available systemic agents with anti-*Candida* activity are amphotericin B, ketoconazole, itraconazole, fluconazole, voriconazole, caspofungin, and flucytosine. In vitro susceptibility data for the most common *Candida* species are shown in Table 11–2 (NCCLS, 1997; Rex et al, 1993). The drug of choice depends on the infecting species and the clinical setting. *Candida albicans* is the most susceptible species. The pattern for *C. tropicalis* and *C. parapsilosis* is quite similar, with just slightly higher MICs for most antifungal drugs. *Candida parapsilosis* tends to have higher MICs and in vitro is less susceptible to all echinocandin agents (Kurtz and Rex, 2001; Pfaller et al, 2001). *Candida glabrata* tends to have fluconazole MICs that are 16–64-fold

TABLE 11–2. *In Vitro Susceptibility of* Candida *spp. to Antifungal Agents*

MIC$_{50}$	Amphotericin B	Fluconazole	Itraconazole	Flucytosine	Caspofungin
C. albicans	0.5	0.5	0.12	≤ 0.25	0.12
C. tropicalis	0.25	1	0.06	≤ 0.25	0.25
C. glabrata	0.5	16	0.25	≤ 0.25	0.12
C. parapsilosis	0.25	1	0.12	≤ 0.25	1.0
C. krusei	0.25	64	0.5	16	0.5
C. lusitaniae	≤ 1	2	0.25	≤ 0.25	1.0

MIC, minimum inhibitory concentration.
Sources: NCCLS, 1997; Rex et al, 1993.

higher than those for *C. albicans*. *Candida krusei* isolates have the highest fluconazole and flucytosine MICs of any of the species. In addition, *C. krusei* is also less susceptible to amphotericin B (Bhargava and Vazquez, 2000).

For three drugs, fluconazole, itraconazole, and flucytosine, interpretive breakpoints when tested by NCCLS-M27 have been proposed and are summarized in the footnotes of Table 11–3 (Rex et al, 1997). For fluconazole and itraconazole, the designation S-DD implies that susceptibility is dependent on obtaining the maximal possible drug level. For fluconazole, this designation implies use of doses of ≥ 400 mg/day in adults with normal renal function. Utilizing these breakpoints, *C. albicans*, *C. parapsilosis*, *C. tropicalis*, and *C. lusitaniae* are susceptible to fluconazole, whereas MICs of *C. glabrata* typically are in the S-DD category (Table 11–3). For itraconazole, *C. glabrata*, *C. krusei*, and *C. lusitaniae* often have MICs in the S-DD category, while the other common *Candida* species are generally susceptible. In general, virtually all azoles, including the latest generation triazoles, voriconazole and posaconazole, are 10–100 times less active against *C. glabrata* strains compared to *C. albicans*. Finally, most species, except for *C. krusei*, are susceptible to flucytosine.

Measurement of MICs of amphotericin B utilizing the NCCLS M27 method is unreliable in detecting amphotericin B-resistant isolates (Rex et al, 1997). Recent

modifications based on the use of Antibiotic Medium 3 may resolve this problem (Rex et al, 1997). Available data indicate that *Candida* isolates with NCCLS-M27 amphotericin B MICs > 1 μg/mL are likely resistant to amphotericin B (Rex et al, 1997).

Development of resistance to azole antifungal agents is not uncommon following prolonged therapy of recurrent mucocutaneous disease (See Chapter 9). Emergence of resistance during a course of therapy in other settings, e.g., candidemia, appears uncommon (Pfaller et al, 1995) but has been reported occasionally (Marr et al, 1997; Mori et al, 1997). Primary infection with a resistant strain of *C. albicans* has been described (Xu et al, 2000). Resistance to amphotericin B is uncommon (Law et al, 1997), but has been described for all *Candida* species, particularly *C. tropicalis*, *C. lusitaniae*, *C. parapsilosis*, and *C. glabrata* isolates from immunocompromised patients treated extensively with amphotericin B (Merz and Sanford, 1979; Pappagianis et al, 1979; Dick et al, 1980; Guinet et al, 1983; Sterling et al, 1996). Resistance to amphotericin B appears to be common with *C. lusitaniae* (Minari et al, 2001), implying that *C. lusitaniae* is also likely to be resistant to the newer lipid-based formulations of amphotericin B (Karyotakis et al, 1994). Testing for susceptibility to amphotericin B should use deoxycholate amphotericin B, rather than a lipid associated form of amphotericin

TABLE 11–3. *General Patterns of Susceptibility of* Candida *Species*

Candida Species	Fluconazole	Itraconazole	Flucytosine	Amphotericin B
C. albicans	S	S	S	S
C. tropicalis	S	S	S	S
C. parapsilosis	S	S	S	S
C. glabrata	S-DD to R	S-DD to R	S	S-I
C. krusei	R	S-DD to R	I-R	S-I
C. lusitaniae	S	S	S	S to R

Drug	Interpretive Breakpoints for Isolates of *Candida* (minimum inhibitory concentration, μg/mL)		
	Susceptible (S)	(S-DD or I)	Resistant (R)
Fluconazole	≤ 8	S-DD, 16–32	> 32
Itraconazole	≤ 0.125	S-DD, 0.25–0.5	> 0.5
Flucytosine	≤ 4	1, 8–16	>16

I-R, intermediate-resistant; R, resistant; S, susceptible; S-DD, susceptible-dose dependent; S-I, susceptible-intermediate.

B (Swenson et al, 1998). Intrinsic or primary resistance to flucytosine may be present in any species of *Candida* (Stiller et al, 1982). Acquisition of resistance by susceptible isolates is not uncommon during flucytosine monotherapy (Polak, 1987).

Routine susceptibility testing of all *Candida* isolates is not indicated although all invasive isolates should be identified to the species level. Susceptibility testing is justified in patients with refractory disease, e.g., refractory OPC in AIDS patients or persistent candidemia while on antifungal therapy. Likewise testing of selected isolates from invasive or deep sites might be useful in selecting alternatives to amphotericin B.

Combination of flucytosine with either amphotericin B or an azole has been used, and these combinations often appear at least additive in vitro (Bennett et al, 1979; Polak, 1987). The combination of flucytosine and amphotericin B is used less for synergy and more to exploit the superior penetrating ability of flucytosine (e.g., CSF). The use of amphotericin B and azoles in combination for treatment of candidiasis is controversial (Sugar, 1995a). The overlapping mechanisms of action of these agents raise the possibility of antagonism. Antagonism has been seen under some circumstances, especially when ketoconazole or itraconazole are combined with amphotericin B (Schaffner and Bohler, 1993; Scheven and Schwegler, 1995). In particular, preincubation of the fungus with the azole in vitro often raises the MIC to amphotericin B. Interactions ranging from antagonism to synergy have been reported depending on dose, experimental model, design and microorganism (Sugar et al, 1995b). A recently completed trial evaluated the observation that antagonism is not seen with simultaneous exposure to therapeutic concentrations of both fluconazole and amphotericin B (Rex et al, in press 2003) (for results, see section on TREATMENT).

Choice of an antifungal agent is based on consideration of relative drug toxicity, patient status, and microbiological information. Amphotericin B is generally fungicidal in vitro for *Candida* isolates (Witt et al, 1993). Both the deoxycholate and lipid-based derivatives of amphotericin B are active against *Candida* species (Anaissie et al, 1991; Karyotakis and Anaissie, 1994; Ng and Denning, 1995; Beovic et al, 1997), although higher doses of the lipid-based formulations are required. The azoles are fungistatic against *Candida* species (Hughes and Beggs, 1987) and the echinocandins are fungicidal and exhibit a broad spectrum of activity against all *Candida* species.

Pediatric Dosing for Candida Infections

Dosing regimens in pediatric and neonatal patients are incompletely defined (van den Anker et al, 1995). The kinetics of amphotericin B in neonates appear similar to those in adults, and therapy with daily dosing of 0.5–1.0 mg/kg/day is usually well tolerated (van den Anker et al, 1995). The half-life of flucytosine is variable, but tends to be prolonged in neonates. While doses of 50–200 mg/kg/day have been used, careful monitoring of serum levels (< 100 μg/ml) is important. Marked variation occurs between patients (including patients with very slow elimination); accordingly, the recommendation is to administer flucytosine at q 24-hour intervals in newborns and dose adjust after checking serum levels (Baley et al, 1990). The pharmacokinetics of fluconazole have been studied in several groups of pediatric patients (Saxen et al, 1993; Brammer and Coates, 1994; Seay et al, 1995). In neonates the volume of distribution is 2–3 fold higher than adults and falls to adult levels by 3 months of age. Clearance rates in children are highly variable compared with adults: neonates have a $T^{1}/_{2}$ of 55–90 hours, children above the age of 3 months have a $T^{1}/_{2}$ of 21–22 hours, and adults have a $T^{1}/_{2}$ of approximately 30 hours (Grant and Clissold, 1990). Accordingly, daily doses approximately double those used in adults are advised in children older than 1 month of age. Neonates should be given this doubled dose every 72 hours during the first 1–2 weeks of life and every 48 hours during the remainder of the first month of life (Saxen et al, 1993; Brammer and Coates, 1994).

Oropharyngeal Candidiasis

Oropharyngeal candidiasis (OPC) may be treated with either topical antifungal agents (nystatin, clotrimazole, amphotericin B oral suspension) or systemic oral azole drugs (fluconazole, itraconazole). In patients who are HIV-positive, oropharyngeal candidiasis infections tend to respond more slowly, and about 60% of patients experience a recurrence within 6 months of the initial episode (Vazquez, 2000).

Numerous antifungal agents are available for the treatment of OPC (Table 11–4). Gentian violet was introduced as a topical treatment for OPC in 1925, and is less effective than newer antifungals (Kozinn et al, 1957). Topical gentian violet and nystatin have been replaced by more active and rapidly acting topical azoles, especially clotrimazole and miconazole (Kozinn et al, 1957). Clotrimazole 10 mg troches administered five times a day have been successful in treating mild to moderate OPC (Yap and Badey, 1979; Schectman et al, 1984). Ketoconazole 200 mg daily was the first oral systemic azole used and is highly effective even in debilitated patients including those with malignancy, AIDS and CMC with cure rates $> 80\%$ (Hughes et al, 1983; Horsburgh and Kirkpatrick, 1983). However, ketoconazole use has been limited by hepatotoxicity and concerns about the reliability of gastric absorption, especially in patients receiving H2-blockers.

TABLE 11–4. *Oropharyngeal and Esophageal Candidiasis Treatment Option*

Treatment Options	Dosing Guidelines	Patient/Prescribing Issues
Nystatin		
Pastilles or lozenge	200,000 U qid × 7–14 days	Unpleasant taste; may cause nausea and GI disturbances.
Suspension	500,000 U by swish & swallow qid × 7–14 days	
Vaginal tablets	100,000 U dissolve 1 tab tid	Vaginal tablets in combination with unsweetened mints or chewing gum better tolerated. Not recommended for esophagitis.
Clotrimazole	Suck on 1 troche 5 × d × 7–14 days	More palatable than nystatin but contains dextrose, which may promote dental caries. Not recommended for esophagitis.
Fluconazole	100 mg/day × 7–14 days (up to 21 days for esophagitis). Loading dose of 200 mg for severe OPC and esophagitis.	Superior to nystatin, clotrimazole, ketoconazole. High doses (up to 800 mg/day) can be used in difficult cases. Success has been obtained even in cases of in vitro resistance.
Itraconazole		
Solution	200 mg (20 mL) qd by swish & swallow without food × 7–14 days (up to 21 days for esophagitis)	Limited bioavailability; absorption improved if taken with fatty meal. Efficacy of capsules is thought equal to ketoconazole. Solution has been tested only among HIV patients, but is much better absorbed and has shown efficacy equivalent to fluconazole.
Capsules	200 mg/day (with food) × 2–4 weeks	
Ketoconazole	200–400 mg/day × 7–14 days (up to 21 days for esophagitis)	Limited bioavailability; requires acidic environment for best absorption; liver toxicity. Less efficacious than fluconazole and itraconazole and less frequently used.
Amphotericin B		
Suspension	1 mg/ml, 1 mL swish & swallow qid	Agent considered second-line option; reserved for severe cases and documented failures to azoles. Parenteral dosing necessary for esophagitis.
Lozenge	100 mg qid	
Tablet	10 mg qid	
Parenteral	0.4–0.6 mg/kg/day	

qid, four times daily; tid, three times daily; bid, twice daily; qd, once daily.

Itraconazole and fluconazole have markedly improved safety profiles and have become the standard of care, especially for patients with moderate to severe OPC (Hay, 1990; Darouiche, 1998; Vazquez, 2000). These drugs are considered equivalent in efficacy. Although most studies on fluconazole efficacy for OPC utilized an initial loading dose of 200 mg followed by 100 mg daily, success has been achieved with 50 mg daily (Hay, 1990). Fluconazole treatment is characterized by rapid response. Slower response rates have been described with both ketoconazole and clotrimazole troches in OPC patients with solid tumors (Yap and Bodey, 1979; Meunier-Carpentier et al, 1983). In all published studies, fluconazole 100 mg/day, was at least equal in efficacy and in some studies superior to clotrimazole or ketoconazole (Darouiche, 1998; Vazquez, 2000). The goal of antimycotic therapy in OPC is rapid relief of symptoms, prevention of complications and prevention of early relapse following cessation of therapy. The goal is not to achieve sterilization of the oral cavity, since treatment uncommonly achieves negative cultures (Vazquez, 2000).

Esophageal Candidiasis

Candida esophagitis requires systemic therapy; topical drugs are of little value (Ginsburg et al, 1981). Parenteral therapy may be required initially if the patient is unable to take oral medication. Ketoconazole 200 mg bid was shown to be effective in esophageal candidiasis (EC) (Fazio et al, 1983). However, ketoconazole has now been replaced by the triazoles, fluconazole, and itraconazole, because of greater efficacy of the latter and the adverse side effect profile of ketoconazole. Fluconazole has become the standard of care in the management of *Candida* esophagitis. Oral fluconazole at a dose of 200 mg/day for 14–21 days enjoys a superior safety profile with bioavailability of > 92%. In several clinical trials, EC patients treated with itraconazole oral solution 100–200 mg/day had a high clinical response rate, 94%, comparable to 91% for patients treated with fluconazole tablets 100–200 mg/day (Barbaro et al, 1995; Barbaro, et al, 1996; Wilcox et al, 1997).

Given the high success rate achieved with fluconazole and itraconazole, iv amphotericin B is generally reserved for endoscopically proven cases of EC that fail azole therapy. Low-dose amphotericin B (0.3–0.5 mg/kg or 10–20 mg/day for 10 days) is often sufficient for moderate disease, but higher doses may be necessary for some patients with AIDS and refractory EC (Medoff et al, 1972; Vazquez, 2000).

Patients with AIDS are at high risk of developing symptomatic recurrences of EC (Tavitian et al, 1986; Glatt, 1993; Maenza et al, 1996; Maenza et al, 1997).

Accordingly, many clinicians, following a single episode of EC, begin secondary prophylaxis with either fluconazole or itraconazole. Daily suppressive antifungal therapy with fluconazole 100–200 mg/day is effective in preventing recurrent episodes, but should only be used if the recurrences are frequent or are associated with malnutrition due to poor oral intake and wasting syndrome.

New antifungal agents have also been evaluated in patients with EC. In a randomized, multicenter trial comparing voriconazole to fluconazole for the treatment of EC in 391 immunocompromised patients, voriconazole 200 mg bid was as effective as fluconazole 200 mg daily, 98.3% and 95.1%, respectively, and well tolerated (Ally et al, 2001). Similarly, IV caspofungin regimens were equivalent to amphotericin B 0.5 mg/kg/day in 123 immunocompromised patients with EC. Clinical success was achieved in 74% and 89% of patients receiving caspofungin at 50 mg and 70 mg/day, respectively, and in 63% of patients receiving amphotericin B (Villanueva et al, 2001).

Management of Antifungal Refractory Oropharyngeal and Esophageal Candidiasis

Management of fluconazole-resistant OPC and EC is frequently unsatisfactory and any response is short lived, with periodic and rapid recurrences. The clinical impact of antifungal resistance in patients with AIDS has been reviewed (Koletar et al, 1994). After the onset of fluconazole-resistant thrush, AIDS patients had a median survival of 184 days. Moreover, after the onset of clinical resistance to amphotericin B, the patients had a median survival of only 83 days. Although mucosal candidiasis does not produce death directly, clinical failure acts as a comorbid factor in the rapid demise of these patients. Clinical failure is also a marker of severe immunosuppression and a nonfunctional immune system.

Several studies reveal a good correlation between in vitro susceptibility (MIC) and response of OPC to antifungal treatment in HIV-infected patients (Cameron et al, 1993; Quereda et al, 1996). On the other hand, therapeutic antifungal successes and failures were noted in patients with OPC and *Candida* isolates with both low and high MIC values (Revankar et al, 1998). Risk factors for the development of fluconazole-resistant mucosal candidiasis in patients with AIDS include: greater number of episodes of OPC (6.1 vs. 1.8); lower median CD4 cell count (11 vs. 71 cells/mm^3); longer median duration of antifungal therapy (419 vs. 118 days); and longer duration of systemic azole exposure (272 vs. 14 days) (Maenza et al, 1996). When the investigators studied two control groups matched by CD4 cell count, resistant cases also had a greater median exposure time to azoles (272 vs. 88 days; $p = 0.005$) as

the most significant risk factor (Maenza et al, 1996; Maenza et al, 1997).

Fluconazole refractory candidiasis may respond to doses of fluconazole from 200 mg/day to ≥ 400 mg/day but with a short-term clinical response only. Occasionally, fluconazole suspension may be beneficial as a swish and swallow approach (Martins and Rex, 1997; Parving, 1997). Several studies have demonstrated good response rates with itraconazole oral solution 200mg bid (Eichel et al, 1996; Phillipps et al, 1996; Cartledge et al, 1997). Clinical cure or improvement occurred in 55%–70% of patients; however, mycological cure rates were low (< 30%) and almost inevitably, relapses following treatment cessation were rapid, usually within 14 days. In vitro ketoconazole and itraconazole cross-resistance is common. Amphotericin B oral suspension is another therapeutic option in patients with azole-refractory mucosal candidiasis (Dewsnup and Stevens, 1994; Nguyen et al, 1996c) but this formulation is no longer available in all countries. In several small studies, clinical improvement rates varied from 50%–75%, but the relapse rate was high, usually within 4 weeks of discontinuing therapy.

In patients with severe refractory OPC or EC, parenteral amphotericin B at dosages of 0.4–0.6 mg/kg/day may be used. After clinical improvment, it is essential to continue suppressive therapy in an attempt to achieve disease-free intervals. In occasional patients, parenteral amphotericin B may not ameliorate OPC and EC. These patients generally have advanced-HIV disease. Lipid-based preparations may prove useful in patients unable to tolerate deoxycholate amphotericin B (Brajtburg et al, 1990). The newer triazoles, voriconazole, and posaconazole, have excellent in vitro activity against fluconazole-resistant *C. albicans* isolates (Ruhnke et al, 1997; Vazquez, 2000; Ernst, 2001). Caspofungin and micafungin are also being evaluated in clinical trials.

Highly active antiretroviral therapy is an essential component of therapy of refractory disease. Treatment with HAART alone without antifungal drugs has been shown to eradicate refractory OPC in patients with advanced HIV-infection (Zingman, 1996). In addition, several cytokines produced by recombinant technology show promise in assisting the host response to fungal infections (Vecchiarelli et al, 1995). Human recombinant granulocyte-macrophage colony-stimulating factor (rhuGM-CSF) has demonstrated encouraging results in patients with refractory OPC and EC (Swindells et al, 1997; Vazquez et al, 1998).

Vulvovaginal Candidiasis

Treatment of VVC predominantly involves use of the imidazole and triazole agents available as topical or oral formulations (Table 11–5). Azoles achieve higher success rates even over shorter duration of therapy than

TABLE 11–5. *Azole Therapy for Vaginal Candidiasis*

Drug	Formulation	Dosage
Butoconazole	2% cream (5 g)	5 g × 3 days
	2% vaginal suppository	1 suppository once
Clotrimazole	1% cream (5 g)	5 g × 7–14 days
	10% cream	5 g single application
	100 mg vaginal tablet	1 tablet × 7 days
	100 mg vaginal tablet	2 tablets × 3 days
	500 mg vaginal tablet	1 tablet once
Miconazole	2% cream (5 g)	5 g × 7 days
	100 mg vaginal suppository	1 suppository × 7 days
	200 mg vaginal suppository	1 suppository × 3 days
	1200 mg vaginal suppository	1 suppository once
Econazole	150 mg vaginal tablet	1 tablet × 3 days
Fenticonazole	2% cream (5 g)	5 g × 7 days
Tioconazole	2% cream (5 g)	5 g × 3 days
	6.5% cream (5 g)	5 g single dose
Terconazole	0.4% cream (5 g)	5 g × 7 days
	0.8% cream (5 g)	5 g × 3 days
	80 mg vaginal suppository	80 mg × 3 days
Fluconazole	150 mg tablet oral	150 mg single dose
Ketoconazole	200 mg tablet oral	400 mg × 5 days
Itraconazole	100 mg tablet oral	200 mg × 3 days

nystatin vaginal suppositories or creams. Little evidence exists that the choice of formulation of the topical azoles influences cure rates. Topical agents previously prescribed for 7–14 days are now available as single dose or short course (3–5 day) regimens. Topical azoles when appropriately prescribed are remarkably free of systemic side effects and toxicity.

The oral azoles used for systemic therapy are ketoconazole, itraconazole, and fluconazole, but only fluconazole (150 mg given as a single dose) is approved by the FDA for this indication in the United States. Oral azoles have been shown to be at least as effective as topical agents and are more convenient, more popular among users and free of local side effects (Silva-Cruz et al, 1991; Sobel et al, 1995a).

In selecting an antifungal agent, it is useful to define VVC as uncomplicated or complicated disease (Sobel et al, 1998). The majority of episodes of VVC are uncomplicated (90%). These are sporadic, mild-to-moderate infections caused by *C. albicans* that occur in normal hosts who lack predisposing factors. Uncomplicated infections can be successfully treated with any of the available topical or oral antifungal agents including short course and single dose regimens. Complicated infections are defined as those that *(1)* have a moderate to severe clinical presentation, *(2)* are recurrent in nature (≥ 4 episodes per year), *(3)* are caused by non-*albicans Candida* species, or *(4)* occur in abnormal hosts, e.g., diabetic patients with poor glucose control. Complicated infections are far less likely to respond to abbreviated courses of therapy (Sobel et al, 1998) and should be treated more intensively for 7 to 14 days in order to achieve a clinical response. In a recent study of almost 500 women with complicated

VVC, prolonging fluconazole therapy by adding a second dose of 150 mg fluconazole 72 hours after the initial dose resulted in significantly higher clinical and mycological cure rates in women with severe VVC (Sobel et al, 2001a). Non-*albicans Candida* species, especially *C. glabrata*, are less susceptible in vitro to azoles and VVC caused by these species is less likely to respond clinically, especially to short course azole therapy. Encouraging results have been obtained with boric acid 600 mg capsules given vaginally qd for 14 days (Sobel and Chaim, 1997) or topical 17% flucytosine (Horowitz, 1986).

Vulvovaginal candidiasis in HIV-infected women is incompletely understood. One large study found it to behave in a fashion similar to that in seronegative women (Schuman et al, 1998). Vaginal carriage of *Candida* is more common in HIV seropositive women, but symptomatic VVC was not more frequent or modestly increased only and did not increase with progressive immunosuppression. Others have, however, noted increased rates of VVC with increasing immunosuppression (Rhoads et al, 1987; Carpenter et al, 1989; Imam et al, 1990; Duerr et al, 1997; Sobel et al, 2001b) The differences in results may be due to differences in study design and diagnostic criteria (White, 1996; Schuman et al, 1998). Longitudinal cohort studies of vaginal candidiasis in HIV-positive women show a progressive increase in colonization with *C. glabrata* and diminished fluconazole susceptibility (Sobel et al, 2001a). Therapy of VVC in HIV-infected women remains the same as that for seronegative women. Vulvovaginal candidiasis, even if recurrent, is not considered a sentinel of HIV infection and its presence does not justify HIV testing.

Recurrent VVC is usually caused by susceptible strains of *C. albicans*. Although more intensive prolonged induction therapy lasting up to 14 days invariably induces remission, the fungistatic nature of the available agents combined with persistence of the underlying defect makes relapse within 3 months almost inevitable unless a maintenance antifungal regimen is employed. Successful regimens include ketoconazole 100 mg daily or fluconazole 150 mg weekly (Sobel, 1992).

Male genital candidiasis presents in two forms, and most commonly as a transient pruritic and erythematous penile cutaneous reaction that may follow unprotected intercourse with exposure to *Candida* antigens present in the partner's vagina and represents a hypersensitivity reaction. Successful treatment entails eradication of yeast in the vagina. True superficial penile *Candida* infection, the second form, occurs infrequently and usually in diabetic and uncircumcised males who develop balanoposthitis that responds promptly to topical or systemic azole therapy.

Cutaneous Candidiasis
Localized, cutaneous candidiasis infections may be treated with any number of topical antifungal agents (e.g., clotrimazole, econazole, miconazole, ketoconazole, ciclopirox). *Candida* paronychia requires drainage of the abscess, followed by oral therapy with either fluconazole or itraconazole. However, *Candida* folliculitis, onychomycosis, and extensive cutaneous infections in patients who are immunocompromised require systemic antifungal therapy. For Candida onychomycosis, oral itraconazole appears to be the most efficacious, either daily 100 mg itraconazole for 3–6 months or as a pulse-dose regimen that requires a higher dose, 200 mg bid for 7 days, followed by 3 weeks off therapy. The cycle is repeated every month for 3–6 months (Rex et al, 2000).

Chronic Mucocutaneous Candidiasis
Oral azoles have revolutionized the prognosis and treatment of CMC. Ketoconazole, fluconazole, and itraconazole induce long, treatment-free remission of CMC and can be used continuously or intermittently in cases requiring chronic maintenance therapy (Hay and Clayton, 1982; Hay and Clayton, 1988; Burke, 1989). Over the last decade, a variety of therapeutic approaches aimed at improving cell mediated immunity have been attempted, with inconsistent results and only moderate success as compared to oral azole therapy. Thymus transplantation has been reported to provide improvement in CMC patients suffering from DiGeorge syndrome (Cleveland et al, 1968; Aiuti et al, 1990). White blood cell transfusions produced transient improvement in CMC symptoms only (Kirkpatrick et al, 1971); however, bone marrow transplantation has been successful (Buckley et al, 1968; Deeg et al, 1986; Hoh et al, 1996).

Candidemia and Acute Disseminated Candidiasis
In the nonneutropenic patient, candidemia is related to the presence of an intravascular catheter in up to 80% of patients (Rex et al, 1994). Removal of all intravascular catheters appears to shorten duration of candidemia (Komshian et al, 1989) and has been associated with reduced mortality (Nguyen et al, 1995b; Luzzatti et al, 2000; Rex et al, 2000). Some patients have even been cured by catheter removal alone (Klein and Watanakunakorn, 1979; Berkowitz et al, 1987). However, even the most transient episodes of candidemia can be associated with hematogenous dissemination causing endophthalmitis or osteomyelitis. Thus, all episodes of candidemia merit antifungal therapy (Edwards et al, 1997; Luzzati et al, 2000). A dilated fundoscopic examination is important in all candidemic patients (Rex et al, 2000).

While amphotericin B has been the standard therapy of candidemia (Meunier, 1994), two prospective randomized trials (Rex et al, 1994; Phillips et al, 1997), and two retrospective reviews (Nguyen et al,1995b; Anaissie et al, 1996), compared amphotericin B with fluconazole. These studies have demonstrated that amphotericin B at 0.5–0.6 mg/kg/d and fluconazole at 400 mg/day are highly effective and not significantly different as therapy of candidemia in non-neutropenic patients. In all four studies, the majority of isolates were *C. albicans* and the strength of the data is less for non-*albicans* species, but similar trends hold (Rex et al, 2000). Non-*albicans* species especially *C. glabrata* have higher fluconazole MICs and higher antifungal doses may be required for optimal outcome. Many clinicians treat *C. glabrata* fungemia with iv fluconazole 800 mg/day (12 mg/kg) in adults with normal renal function. The results of one small noncomparative study suggest that fluconazole 800 mg/day may produce a better response rate than 400 mg/day for *C. albicans* fungemia (Graninger et al, 1993).

Accordingly, iv amphotericin B at 0.6–0.7 mg/kg/day or fluconazole at 400–800 mg/day is recommended as initial therapy for candidemia (Rex et al, 2000). If the isolate is found to be *C. albicans*, then fluconazole at 400 mg/day may be continued since fluconazole resistance in bloodstream *Candida* isolates is uncommon. Choosing between initial amphotericin B and fluconazole is somewhat arbitrary since amphotericin B has not been shown to be superior in eradicating candidemia or reducing mortality in any comparative study. However, in unstable, critically ill patients with little margin for error or in patients previously exposed to fluconazole, initiating treatment with amphotericin

B is recommended (Rex et al, 2000). Moreover, a recent large, randomized and blinded study suggests an advantage in initiating treatment with a combination of fluconazole and amphotericin B versus fluconazole alone (Rex et al, 2003). Nonneutropenic adults with candidemia were randomized to receive either fluconazole alone (800 mg/day) or fluconazole plus amphotericin B (0.7 mg/kg/day). No evidence of antagonism was noted and the combination arm produced more rapid clearance of the fungemia. The combination was, however, more nephrotoxic. Many clinicians who currently treat candidemia with amphotericin B initially, and then switch to fluconazole when the patient is more stable and the *Candida* species is known, may consider initiating therapy with both amphotericin B and fluconazole and then discontinuing one of the two drugs. The combination of either fluconazole or amphotericin B with flucytosine at 100–150 mg/kg/day may be useful in selected patients, but the precise role of this combination is unclear.

The required duration of antifungal therapy is undetermined, but therapy is usually continued for approximately 2 weeks after the last positive blood culture. With this approach, the rate of subsequent recurrent infection at hematogenously seeded sites is about 1% (Rex et al, 1994). Although use of itraconazole for invasive forms of candidiasis would seem logical, clinical data are limited and there appears to be no advantage of itraconazole over fluconazole. Recent data support the efficacy of caspofungin, a recently licensed ecchinocandin drug, as therapy of candidemia and other forms of invasive candidasis (Mora-Duarte et al, 2002).

In the neutropenic patient with candidemia, less data are available to guide management. Although the gut has been implicated as an occasional source of candidemia in nonneutropenic patients (Berkowitz et al, 1987), it appears likely that the gastrointestinal tract is the most common source of candidemia in neutropenic patients (Nucci and Colombo, 2002). One notable exception is that *C. parapsilosis* fungemia is highly associated with intravascular catheters in cancer patients (Girmenia et al, 1996). Moreover, in neutropenic patients, removal of intravascular catheters, if possible, is still recommended (Lecciones et al, 1992). Recovery of bone marrow function is critical, and no therapeutic approach is consistently successful in the face of persistent leukopenia. Most experience is with amphotericin B at 0.6–1.0 mg/kg/day until recovery of marrow function. The optimal dose of amphotericin B is not certain, but non-*albicans Candida* species require higher doses (0.8–1.0 mg/kg/day) of amphotericin B, especially *C. krusei* and *C. glabrata*, the two species that also are the least susceptible to fluconazole (Goldman et al, 1993). Data comparing this approach with

fluconazole are limited, but one recent retrospective matched cohort study found that median daily doses of 400 mg for fluconazole and 0.6 mg/kg for amphotericin B were associated with similar outcomes in a mixed group of neutropenic and nonneutropenic cancer patients (Anaissie et al, 1996). Because of flucytosine's potential for marrow suppression and the lack of a readily available intravenous formulation, flucytosine is infrequently used.

Patients may develop candidemia while on antifungal therapy including prophylactic antifungal drugs. Such breakthrough candidemia may be due to infection of an intravascular catheter, in which case the infecting isolate is usually susceptible to the apparently failing drug (Blumberg and Reboli, 1996). In cancer patients, breakthrough candidemia was associated with a higher mortality and occurred more often in the setting of an intensive care unit stay, prolonged neutropenia, and use of corticosteroids (Uzun et al, 2001). In this setting, immunosuppression should be reduced and factors that might alter antifungal drug delivery or clearance excluded. Intravenous catheters should be changed. Since non-*albicans Candida* species are frequently responsible, the possibility of drug resistance should be considered. If resistance is likely or MIC data document resistance, therapy should be changed to an antifungal drug of a different class.

Nonsubcutaneous tunneled central intravascular catheters should be removed in nonneutropenic patients with candidemia, and suspect catheters should not be replaced over a guide wire. In contrast, central tunneled catheters in febrile neutropenic patients do not require mandatory removal since in this setting alternate vascular access sites are less available and removal is more difficult. Most importantly, such catheters are less likely to be the source of candidemia although they may become infected secondary to bloodstream infection. Occasionally, these valuable access sites may be salvaged using the controversial antibiotic lock method utilizing amphotericin B (Arnow and Kushner, 1991; Mermel et al, 1993; Viale et al, 2001). However, results are unpredictable. The importance of a positive catheter tip is similarly controversial. In afebrile patients at low risk of candidemia, antifungal treatment does not appear to be indicated. On the other hand, in a high-risk patient with unexplained antibiotic-resistant fever, the finding of a positive catheter tip culture for *Candida* often results in initiation of empirical antifungal therapy.

Presumptive Therapy of Febrile Neutropenia
Invasive *Candida* infections are an important cause of antibiotic resistant fever in neutropenic patients. The likelihood of *Candida* as the cause is diminished in the presence of azole prophylaxis. Nevertheless, antifungal

therapy should include coverage of *Candida* species. For more detailed information, see Chapter 29.

Chronic Disseminated Candidiasis

Therapy has usually consisted of prolonged amphotericin B alone; however, this approach has not been uniformly successful (Haron et al, 1987). Amphotericin B, total dose 0.5–1.0 g, followed by a protracted course of fluconazole (200–400 mg/day for 2–14 months) is associated with cure rates of > 90% (Anaissie et al, 1991b; Kauffman et al, 1991). This regimen is preferred by many experts. Use of fluconazole is sometimes successful when amphotericin B was not. Lipid-based amphotericin B has also been used successfully (Walsh et al, 1997). Provided that the *Candida* hepatic and splenic lesions have stabilized, the patient is clinically improved, and antifungal therapy is continued, antineoplastic therapies (including those that will induce neutropenia) may be continued (Walsh et al, 1995). Duration of antifungal therapy is determined by results of imaging studies of liver and spleen.

Neonatal Candidiasis

Amphotericin B at 0.5–1.0 mg/kg/day for a total dose of 10–25 mg/kg, with or without flucytosine, is the therapy of choice for neonated candidiasis. The excellent penetration of amphotericin B into the CSF in neonates is presumably part of the reason that amphotericin B alone is often successful (Baley et al, 1990). The utility of the lipid-formulations of amphotericin B for this condition is still unknown. Fluconazole is also attractive in this setting, and has been used successfully at doses of 6–12 mg/kg/day (Viscoli et al, 1991; Driessen et al, 1996; Wainer et al, 1997; Huang et al, 2000). Comparative data between amphotericin B and fluconazole for neonatal candidiasis are lacking. Topical and oral therapy with agents such as nystatin or an antifungal azole often are adequate therapy for full-term infants with candidiasis limited to skin and the GI tract (Barone and Krilov, 1995).

Urinary Candidiasis

Treatment of candiduria requires differentiating between colonization and superficial and deep tissue infection as well as the anatomical level of infection. Candiduria in catheterized subjects usually represents catheter or superficial bladder colonization only, is extremely common, almost invariably asymptomatic, and of little clinical significance. Asymptomatic candiduria in this context should not be treated since the sequelae of ascending or invasive *Candida* infections are rare (Ang et al, 1993) and any effects of treatment are short lived (Sobel et al, 2000). Asymptomatic candiduria should be treated in neutropenic patients, those undergoing elective urinary instrumentation, and following renal transplantation.

Symptomatic lower urinary tract infections due to *Candida* are rare and should be treated, especially in noncatheterized patients. Therapeutic options include oral fluconazole 200 mg/day for 7–14 days, iv amphotericin B as 0.3 mg/kg single dose (Fisher et al, 1982), or iv amphotericin B 0.3 mg/kg for 5–7 days (Fan-Havard et al, 1995). Amphotericin B bladder irrigation with 1 L/day of a solution of 50 mg amphotericin B/L of sterile water or D5W through a triple lumen catheter for 7 days is an effective but inconvenient option (Sanford, 1993). Shorter courses may prove to be an alternative (Leu and Huang, 1995). Ketoconazole and itraconazole achieve low urine drug concentrations and yield unreliable results (Wong-Beringer et al, 1992). Oral flucytosine is rarely indicated because of emergence of resistance during therapy, but has been useful in eradicating non-*albicans Candida* infections.

Ascending pyelonephritis, although uncommon, represents a serious infection that may be complicated by candidemia and disseminated infection (Ang et al, 1993). Therapy for this form of *Candida* pyelonephritis consists of relieving any urinary obstruction plus fluconazole or systemic amphotericin B in doses similar to those used for disseminated candidiasis. Finally, candiduria may be the result of renal candidiasis secondary to previous or ongoing candidemia (hematogenous pyelonephritis). Therapy is identical to that of disseminated candidiasis.

Candida Endophthalmitis

Penetration of amphotericin B into the eye is variable but generally poor (Fisher et al, 1983; O'Day et al, 1985). Even so, courses of at least 1 gram of amphotericin B have been curative in > 90% of infected eyes (Edwards et al, 1974). However, intravenous therapy alone is not uniformly successful and intravitreal amphotericin B following vitrectomy has been helpful either as monotherapy or in conjunction with systemic therapy. Vitrectomy may be especially valuable in endophthalmitis associated with intravenous drug abuse (Martinez-Vazquez et al, 1998). Vitrectomy in therapy of *Candida* endophthalmitis is in part based upon benefits reported in bacterial endophthalmitis (Endophthalmitis Vitrectomy Study Group, 1995). Intravitreal doses of amphotericin B of 5–10 μg are indicated for vision threatening disease (Stern et al, 1977; Cantrill et al, 1980; Perraut et al, 1981; Brod et al, 1990).

Fluconazole diffuses well into all parts of the eye (Savani et al, 1987; O'Day et al, 1990; Urbak and Degn, 1992). Fluconazole, given as sole therapy at ~200 mg/day for approximately 2 months, cured 15 of 16 patients with *Candida* endophthalmitis (Akler et al, 1995). Fluconazole was also effective following short

(~200 mg total dose) courses of amphotericin B. Patients requiring vitrectomy generally have more severe disease, and fluconazole monotherapy was curative when given at ~200 mg/day for 3 months after vitrectomy. If an ocular implant is present in the infected eye, implant removal appears critical to resolution of the infection (Kauffman et al, 1993). Ketoconazole and itraconazole penetrate the eye less readily than fluconazole in animal models (Savani et al, 1987) and clinical experience is limited.

Candida Endocarditis, Pericarditis, and Suppurative Thrombophlebitis

Medical therapy alone has rarely been curative for these cardiac or vascular infections (Zenker et al, 1991; Faix, 1992b; Hallum and Williams, 1993; Melamed et al, 2000). The inability of prolonged courses of high dose amphotericin B to cure either native or prosthetic valve endocarditis (Utley et al, 1975; Nguyen et al, 1996d) has led to the recommendation that patients be treated with a combination of mandatory valve replacement and prolonged antifungal therapy (Johnston et al, 1991; Muehrcke, 1995a; Muehrcke et al, 1995b; Ellis et al, 2001). Preoperative therapy usually consists of high dose amphotericin B often in combination with flucytosine, followed by one of the azole drugs. Fluconazole has been the most frequently employed long-term oral agent, given its superior safety profile (Cancelas et al, 1994; Muehrcke, 1995a; Nguyen et al, 1996d). A similar strategy is applicable in children. Medical therapy alone is often pursued in neonates due to their complicated, overlapping medical problems (Zenker et al, 1991; Faix, 1992b; Mayayo et al, 1996). Late recurrence, especially following medical treatment only, has been described even several years after the initial episode (Johnston et al, 1991), emphasizing the need for prolonged follow-up. Chronic suppressive therapy with fluconazole is recommended for patients in whom cardiac surgery is contraindicated (Roupie et al, 1991; Hernandez et al, 1992; Castiglia et al, 1994).

Candida infections of transvenous pacemakers require both surgical removal of the infected device and prolonged systemic antifungal therapy (4–6 weeks) (Joly et al, 1997). Purulent *Candida* pericarditis is treated with a combination of surgical drainage (pericardiocentesis or pericardiectomy) together with prolonged antifungal therapy (Schrank and Dooley, 1995; Rabinovici et al, 1997).

Persistent candidemia is sometimes due to *Candida* suppurative phlebitis of either central or peripheral veins. In the case of peripheral phlebitis, the involved vein is not always tender, although usually thrombosed. Treatment consists of catheter removal, aspiration, resection, or incision and drainage of the vein, followed by a 14-day course of amphotericin B or fluconazole

(Torres-Rojas, 1982; Walsh et al, 1986; Berkowitz et al, 1987; Friedland, 1996). When a central vein is involved, surgery is not an option, and systemic therapy for 10–14 days is generally successful (Jarrett et al, 1978; Strinden et al, 1985; Berg and Stein, 1989). Systemic anticoagulation has been used in some patients. *Candida* infections of arteriovenous dialysis fistulas (Nguyen et al, 1996b) are rare, and effective therapy generally requires both antifungal therapy and removal of the fistula.

Abdominal Candida Infections

Removal of the dialysis catheter is usually required for successful therapy of CAPD-related fungal peritonitis (Eisenberg, 1988; Michel et al, 1994; Montenegro et al, 1995; Goldie et al, 1996). Occasionally, some patients are cured via this maneuver alone (Bayer et al, 1976; Eisenberg et al, 1986; Sugar, 1991). However, short courses of either parenteral or intraperitoneal amphotericin B have been used successfully. Intraperitoneal therapy with the infusate containing 0.5–5 g/mL of amphotericin B is often associated with significant abdominal pain and the development of adhesions (Arfania et al, 1981; Eisenberg et al, 1986). Several reports have documented the utility of fluconazole in combination with flucytosine as therapy for dialysis catheter-related peritonitis (Levine et al, 1989; Thomas and Ellis-Pegler, 1989; Corbella et al, 1991; Michel et al, 1994). Dosages of fluconazole are 100–200 mg/day and dosages of flucytosine range from 15 mg/kg after hemodialysis to 50–100 mg/L in the peritoneal dialysate (Eisenberg, 1988; Michel et al, 1994).

The potential for untreated *Candida* peritoneal isolates to cause peritonitis has now been clearly demonstrated (Solomkin et al, 1980a; Solomkin and Simmons, 1980b; Alden et al, 1989; Calandra et al, 1989). While no specific criteria identify the patients in whom *Candida* is significant, factors such as presence of sepsis, multiple operations, pancreatic involvement, and heavy growth of *Candida* from peritoneal culture strongly suggest that antifungal therapy is indicated (Alden et al, 1989; Calandra et al, 1989; Rantala et al, 1991). Thus, isolation of *Candida* from an intra-abdominal specimen should not be ignored. Therapy with amphotericin B (0.5–1 g total) (Solomkin et al, 1980; Alden et al, 1989; Calandra et al, 1989) or fluconazole 200–400 mg/day (Thomas and Ellis-Pegler, 1989; Kujath et al, 1990; Aguado et al, 1994) has been used successfully.

While *Candida* is isolated from the bile in up to 2% of cholecystectomies (Gupta and Jain, 1985), the mere isolation of the organism does not mandate therapy. However, if the patient has biliary obstruction or gangrenous cholecystitis, then isolation of *Candida* merits systemic therapy. Amphotericin B achieves bile concentrations that are two- to sevenfold higher than serum concentrations (Adamson et al, 1989). *Candida* fungus balls can cause biliary obstruction of the collecting system and may require surgical removal (Magnussen et al, 1979; Gupta and Jain, 1985).

The association between increased mortality and *Candida* superinfections in patients with acute necrotizing pancreatitis (Hoerauf et al, 1998; Grewe et al, 1999) provides strong support for the use of an antifungal agent if *Candida* is isolated from pancreatic tissue. After suitable debridement and/or drainage, amphotericin B at standard doses (0.5–1.0 mg/kg/day to a total of 1–2 grams) or parenteral fluconazole is indicated.

Candida Osteomyelitis, Arthritis, and Mediastinitis
Surgical debridement of infected bone is extremely useful (Gathe et al, 1987) whereas medical therapy alone for vertebral osteomyelitis has a failure rate approaching 33% (Hendrickx et al, 2001). Most investigators recommend amphotericin B as the primary agent for *Candida* osteomyelitis. Courses of 1–1.5 g total dose are usually given (Edwards et al, 1975; Fogarty, 1983; Gathe et al, 1987; Almekinders and Greene, 1991; Ferra et al, 1994). There is no consensus regarding duration of therapy, but treatment is usually continued for at least 2–4 weeks after resolution of clinical signs and symptoms of infection or microbiologic evidence of eradication of infection (Rex et al, 2000). In general, total duration of therapy is usually 6–10 weeks. A recent report suggested that amphotericin B might safely be added to bone cement in complicated cases (Marra et al, 2001). Several investigators have used a course of amphotericin B, followed by 6–12 months with either ketoconazole (200–600 mg/day) (Gathe et al, 1987; Almekinders and Greene, 1991) or fluconazole (400 mg/day) (Sugar et al, 1990). There is also some experience with azole drugs as sole therapy. Ketoconazole has been used successfully at 50 mg/day for 3 months in a 3-year-old boy with phalangeal osteomyelitis (Bannatyne and Clarke, 1989) and at 400–1600 mg/day for 3–7 months in adults (Dijkmans et al, 1982). While fluconazole has been successful therapy at 200–400 mg/day for 6–12 months (Hennequin et al, 1996), occasional failures have been reported (Dan and Priel, 1994; Arranz-Caso et al, 1996). There is little published experience with itraconazole for *Candida* osteomyelitis.

Systemic antifungal therapy and joint drainage or joint lavage may be necessary to achieve cure of septic *Candida* arthritis. Open drainage is particularly important in *Candida* infection of the native hip (Rex et al, 2000). For infection involving a prosthetic joint, resection arthroplasty is virtually always required (Tunkel et al, 1993). Successful medical treatment with

fluconazole for 17 months of a hip prosthesis that was infected with *C. albicans* has been described, but post-therapy follow-up was only 11 months and this type of response appears to be the exception rather than the rule (Merrer et al, 2001). Most treatment experience for *Candida* arthritis has been with iv amphotericin B (Bayer and Guze, 1978). Substantial synovial fluid levels (20%–100% of serum levels) are achieved with amphotericin B. Intraarticular amphotericin B, typically 5–10 mg, is given at intervals in association with joint aspiration, but may be associated with joint surface irritation (Bayer and Guze, 1978). Experience with azole therapy is limited, but a few reports indicate success (Katzenstein, 1985; Tunkel et al, 1993; Weers-Pothoff et al, 1997). Good drug penetration with fluconazole has been documented.

Candida mediastinitis, a rare entity, has recently been reviewed (Clancy et al, 1997). Based on a small number of cases, surgical debridement followed by either amphotericin B or fluconazole appears appropriate.

Candida Meningitis
Most experience with the therapy of *Candida* meningitis has been with amphotericin B, often in combination with flucytosine because of the latter agent's ability to penetrate the blood-brain barrier (Buchs and Pfister, 1982; Smego et al, 1984). Amphotericin B is usually given intravenously, although occasional patients have required intrathecal therapy. Fluconazole with flucytosine was successful in one case (Marr et al, 1994), and fluconazole monotherapy has been used (Gurses and Kalayci, 1996). For *Candida* meningitis following neurosurgical procedures, especially in association with CSF devices such as shunts or drains, device removal plus antifungal therapy is required (Chiou et al, 1994; Sanchez-Portocarrero et al, 1994; Geers and Gordon, 1999). Distinguishing between specimen contamination and true infection can be difficult, as neither increased CSF cellularity nor hypoglycorrhachia are consistently present (Geers and Gordon, 1999). Most patients with true infections more often have repeatedly positive cultures. For *Candida* meningitis associated with neurosurgery or devices, intravenous amphotericin B is usually effective, but some patients may require the addition of flucytosine or intrathecal amphotericin B. A regimen of 0.5 mg/kg/day of amphotericin B and ≥ 75 mg/kg/day flucytosine for three or more weeks has been recommended (Nguyen and Yu, 1995a). The excellent penetration of fluconazole into the CSF suggests that it might be a useful agent in this setting, although some fluconazole failures have been reported (Cruciani et al, 1992; Nguyen and Yu, 1995a). Treatment of *Candida* brain abscess (Black, 1970; Burgert et al, 1995), epidural abscess (Bonomo et al, 1996), and intramedullary abscess (Lindner et al, 1995)

has been with amphotericin B and flucytosine, occasionally followed by oral azole therapy.

PREVENTION

Primary and secondary prophylaxis is directed at preventing symptomatic superficial or deep disease, and not colonization.

Oropharyngeal Candidiasis and Esophageal Candidiasis

Chronic suppressive therapy with fluconazole is effective in prevention of OPC in both AIDS (Powderly et al, 1995; Schuman et al, 1997; Revankar et al, 1998) and cancer patients (Philpott-Howard et al, 1993). Maintenance fluconazole has been prescribed daily (100 mg/day), two or three times weekly or even once weekly at 200 mg/week. All regimens reduce relapse frequency, but have the potential to select for resistant C. albicans strains and may be associated with appearance of C. glabrata. Given costs of long-term therapy and concern for resistance development, chronic suppressive therapy is only recommended in patients with frequent and disabling recurrences, especially EC, as an alternative to early treatment of each recurrent episode. In spite of numerous reports of refractory mucosal candidiasis due to resistant C. albicans during the 1990s, risk of refractory disease in patients receiving maintenance fluconazole and adhering to HAART therapy appears small (Goldman et al, 2002).

Recurrent Vulvovaginal Candidiasis

Every effort should be made to identify causal factors in women with recurrent infection. Controlled studies have not shown any benefit of treating male partners with antifungal drugs. In the majority of women no identifiable or treatable causes are found and repeated episodes usually occur with susceptible strains of C. albicans. Recommended prophylaxis is fluconazole 150 mg/week for 6 months (MMWR, 2002).

Patients with Neutropenia

Given the high frequency of superficial and systemic fungal infections, especially candidiasis in neutropenic patients, antifungal prophylaxis has been widely utilized (Anaissie et al, 1998). Early studies of prophylactic use of oral antifungals, e.g., amphotericin B, nystatin, clotrimazole, miconazole, and ketoconazole, yielded unsatisfactory results because of poor absorption and tolerance. However, prophylaxis with fluconazole is frequently used and well tolerated. The best results have been obtained with fluconazole 400 mg/day in neutropenic BMT recipients, in whom reduction in superficial and deep fungal infections is achieved, but with variable effects on mortality. Results

of two large studies gave conflicting results; one study showed that fluconazole improved survival (Slavin et al, 1995) and a second study showed no survival benefit (Goodman et al, 1992). Even more controversial is the use of fluconazole as prophylaxis in non-BMT neutropenic patients. Fluconazole prophylaxis reduced systemic fungal infection twofold compared with placebo (Winston et al, 1993) and was similarly protective in a large Canadian study (Rotstein et al, 1999). However, a meta-analysis of 16 randomized controlled trials concluded that fluconazole prophylaxis in neutropenic non-BMT patients did not decrease fungus-related mortality or systemic fungal infections (Kanda et al, 2000). This disparity in outcomes appears to be the consequence of patient selection. Not all neutropenic patients are at high risk, e.g., patients with acute myeloid leukemia receiving cytarabine are particularly vulnerable. Oral itraconazole solution appears equivalent in efficacy to fluconazole in neutropenic patients, and has the added potential of preventing Aspergillus infection. However, use of itraconazole in non-BMT patients is also controversial (Nucci and Columbo, 2000; Harousseau et al, 2000).

The risk of invasive candidiasis is largest during the neutropenic period following BMT. Fluconazole 400 mg/day administered for 75 days following BMT was associated with improved survival, attributed to reduced invasive candidiasis and decreased graft versus host disease involving the GI tract (Marr et al, 2000).

Patients in Intensive Care Units

Twenty five percent to 50% of nosocomial Candida infections occur in patients in ICUs (Rangel-Frausto et al, 1999), particularly in surgical patients (Beck-Sague and Jarvis, 1993). Fluconazole use has increased dramatically in the ICU both as prophylaxis and as empiric therapy in the febrile antibiotic-resistant patient (Gleason et al, 1997; Rocco and Simms, 2000). Until recently, no data supporting this practice was available with multiple studies failing to show any benefit, due in part to inclusion of low-risk patients in SICU trials and studies lacking adequate power (Savino et al, 1994; Garbino et al, 1997; Ables et al, 2000; Rocco and Simms, 2000).

At least two recent studies have shown the benefit of fluconazole prophylaxis by either using highly selective entry criteria (Eggimann et al, 1999) or high-risk surgical patients (Pelz et al, 2001). The majority of patients in a surgical ICU are at low risk of invasive Candida infection with an overall 1% incidence of candidemia. Patients at highest risk are those who undergo liver transplantation (Kung et al, 1995; Tollemar et al, 1995), pancreas transplantation (Benedetti et al, 1996), and those with persistent or refractory gastrointestinal leakage (Eggimann et al, 1999). The NEMIS study observed that exposure to antifungal drugs in the SICU was associated with reduced risk of *Candida* bloodstream infection (Blumberg et al, 2001). While liver and pancreas transplant recipients are easy to identify, as are surgical patients with persistent GI leakage, the largest group of ICU patients who may benefit from fluconazole prophylaxis remains difficult to select. Recently, investigators have identified critically ill postsurgery patients likely to remain in SICU for at least 72 hours, especially but not exclusively following abdominal surgery, and in association with acute renal failure, use of intravascular catheters, TPN, and broad-spectrum antibiotics, as a high-risk group (Pelz et al, 2001). Specific laboratory tests to identify the patients at highest risk that may benefit from antifungal prophylaxis are not yet available. *Candida* surveillance cultures are currently not recommended.

Neonatal Candidiasis

Prophylactic administration of fluconazole during the first 6 weeks of life is effective in preventing fungal colonization and invasive candidiasis in infants with birth weights of less than 1000 g (Kaufman et al, 2001). Similar studies in older infants and children are needed.

REFERENCES

Abbas J, Bodey G P, Hanna H A, Mardani M, Girgawy E, Abi-Said D, Whimbey E, Hachem R, Raad I. *Candida krusei* fungemia. An escalating serious infection in immunocompromised patients. *Arch Intern Med* 160:2659–2664, 2000.

Abi-Said D, Anaissie E, Uzun O, Raad I, Pinzcowski, Vartivarian O. The epidemiology of hematogenous candidiasis caused by different *Candida* species. *Clin Infect Dis* 24:1122–1128, 1997.

Ables A Z, Blumer N A, Valainis G T. Fluconazole prophylaxis of severe *Candida* infection in trauma and postsurgical patients: a prospective, double blind, randomized, placebo-controlled trial. *Infect Dis Clin Pract* 9:169–173, 2000.

Adamson P C, Rinaldi M G, Pizzo P A, Walsh T J. Amphotericin B in the treatment of *Candida* cholecystitis. *Pediatr Infect Dis J* 8:408–411,1989.

Aguado J M, Hidalgo M, Ridriguez-Tudela J L. Successful treatment of *Candida* peritonitis with fluconazole. *J Antimicrob Chemother* 34:847, 1994.

Ahonen P, Myllarniemi S, Sipila I, Perheentupa J. Clinical variation of autoimmune polyendocrinopathy-candidiasis-ectodermal dystrophy (APECED) in a series of 68 patients. *N Engl J Med* 322:1829–1836, 1990.

Aiuti F, Businco L, Gatti R A. Reconstitution of T-cell disorders following thymus transplantation. *Birth Defects Orig Artic Ser* 11:370–376, 1975.

Akler M E, Vellend H, McNeely D M, Walmsley S L, Gold W L. Use of fluconazole in the treatment of candidal endophthalmitis. *Clin Infect Dis* 20:657–664, 1995.

Alden S M, Frank E, Flancbaum L. Abdominal candidiasis in surgical patients. *Am Surg* 55:45–49, 1989.

Ally R, Schurmann D, Kreisel W, Carosi G, Aguirrebengoa K, Dupont B, Hodges M, Troke P, Romero A J. A randomized, double-blind, double-dummy, multicenter trial of voriconazole and fluconazole in the treatment of esophageal candidiasis in im-

munocompromised patients. *Clin Infect Dis* 33:1447–1454, 2001.

Almeida-Santos L, Beceiro J, Hernandez R, Salas S, Escriba R, Garcia-Frias E, Perez-Rodriguez J, Quero J. Congenital cutaneous candidiasis: report of four cases and review of the literature. *Eur J Pediatr* 150:336–338, 1991.

Almekinders L C, Greene W B. Vertebral *Candida* infections. A case report and review of the literature. *Clin Orthop* 267:174–178, 1991.

Alteras I, Feuerman E J, David M, Shohat B, Livni E. Widely disseminated cutaneous candidosis in adults. *Sabouraudia* 17:383–388, 1979.

Anaissie E, Paetznick V, Bodey G P. Fluconazole susceptibility testing of *Candida albicans*: microtiter method that is independent of inoculum size, temperature, and time of reading (published erratum appears in *Antimicrob Agents Chemother* 36:1170, 1992). *Antimicrob Agents Chemother* 35:1641–1646, 1991a.

Anaissie E, Bodey G P, Kantarjian H, David C, Barnett K, Bow E, Defelice R, Downs N, File T, Karam G, Potts D, Shelton M, Sugar A. Fluconazole therapy for chronic disseminated candidiasis in patients with leukemia and prior amphotericin B therapy. *Am J Med* 91:142–150, 1991b.

Anaissie E J, Vartivarian S E, Abi-Said D, Uzon O, Pinczowski H, Kontoyiannis D P, Khoury P, Papadakis K, Gardner A, Raad II, Gilbreath J, Bodey G P. Fluconazole versus amphotericin B in the treatment of hematogenous candidiasis: a matched cohort study. *Am J Med* 101:170–176, 1996.

Anaissie E J, Rex J H, Uzun O, Vartivarian S. Predictors of adverse outcome in cancer patients with candidemia. *Am J Med* 104:238–245, 1998.

Ang B S, Telenti A, King B, Steckelberg J M, Wilson W R. Candidemia from a urinary tract source: microbiological aspects and clinical significance. *Clin Infect Dis* 17:662–666, 1993.

Anttila V J, Ruutu P, Bondestam S, Jansson S E, Nordling S, Farkkila M, Sivonen A, Castren M, Ruutu T. Hepatosplenic yeast infection in patients with acute leukemia: a diagnostic problem. *Clin Infect Dis* 18:979–981, 1994.

Arbegast K D, Lamberty L F, Koh J K, Pergram J M, Braddock J W. Congenital candidiasis limited to the nail plates. *Pediat Dermatol* 7:310–312, 1990.

Arfania D, Everett E D, Nolph K D, Rubin J. Uncommon causes of peritonitis in patients undergoing peritoneal dialysis. *Arch Intern Med* 141:61–64, 1981.

Arnow P M, and Kushner R. *Malassezia furfur* catheter infection cured with antibiotic lock therapy. *Am J Med* 90:128–130, 1991.

Arranz-Caso J A, Lopez-Pizarro V M, Gomez-Herruz P, Garcia-Altozano J, Martinez-Martinez. *Candida albicans* osteomyelitis of the zygomatic bone. A distinctive case with a possible peculiar mechanism of infection and therapeutic failure with fluconazole. *Diagn Microbiol Infect Dis* 24:161–164, 1996.

Athey P A, Goldstein H M, Dodd G D. Radiologic spectrum of opportunistic infections of the upper gastrointestinal tract. *Am J Roentgenol* 129:419–424, 1977.

Baley J E, Meyers C, Kliegman R M, Jacobs MR, Blumer J L. Pharmacokinetics, outcome of treatment, and toxic effects of amphotericin B and 5-fluorocytosine in neonates. *J Pediatr* 116:791–797, 1990.

Bannatyne R M, Clarke H M. Ketoconazole in the treatment of osteomyelitis due to *Candida albicans*. *Can J Surg* 32:201–202, 1989.

Barbaro G, Barbarini G, DiLorenzo G. Fluconazole compared with itraconazole in the treatment of esophageal candidiasis in AIDS patients: a double-blind, randomized, controlled clinical study. *Scand J Infect Dis* 27:613–617, 1995.

Barbaro G, Barbarini G, Calderon W, Grisorio B, Alcini P, DiLorenzo G. Fluconazole versus itraconazole for *Candida* esophagitis in acquired immunodeficiency syndrome. *Gastroenterol* 111:1169–1177, 1996.

Barchiesi F, Morbiducci V, Ancarani F, Scalise G. Emergence of oropharyngeal candidiasis caused by non-*albicans* species of *Candida* in HIV-infected patients (letter). *Eur J Epidemiol* 9:455–456, 1993.

Barone S R, Krilov L R. Neonatal candidal meningitis in a full-term infant with congenital cutaneous candidiasis. *Clin Ped* 34:217–219, 1995.

Bayer A S, Blumenkrantz M J, Montgomerie J Z, Galpin J E, Coburn J W, Guze L B. *Candida* peritonitis. Report of 22 cases and review of the English literature. *Am J Med* 61:832–840, 1976.

Bayer A S, Guze L B. Fungal arthritis. I. *Candida* arthritis: diagnostic and prognostic implications and therapeutic considerations. *Semin Arthritis Rheum* 8:142–150, 1978.

Beck-Sague C M, Jarvis T R, the National Nosocomial Infections Surveillance System. Secular trends in the epidemiology of nosocomial fungal infections in the United States. *J Infect Dis* 167:1247–1251, 1993.

Belzunegui J, Gonzalez C, Lopez L, Plazaola I, Maiz O, Figueroa M. Osteoarticular and muscle infectious lesions in patients with the human immunodeficiency virus. *Clin Rheumatol* 16:450–453, 1997.

Benedetti E, Gruessner A C, Troppmann C, Papalois B E, Sutherland D E, Dunn D L, Gruessner R W. Intra-abdominal fungal infections after pancreatic transplantation: incidence, treatment, and outcome. *J Am Coll Surg* 183:307–316, 1996.

Bennett J E, Dismukes W E, Duma R J, Medoff G, Sande M A, Gallis H, Leonard J, Fields B T, Bradshaw M, Haywood H, McGee Z A, Cate T R, Cobbs C G, Warner J F, Alling D W. A comparison of amphotericin B alone and combined with flucytosine in the treatment of cryptococcal meningitis. *New Engl J Med* 301:126–131, 1979.

Bennett J E. Diagnosis and management of candidiasis in the immunosuppressed host. *Scand J Infect Dis.* 16(Suppl):83–86, 1978.

Beovic B, Lejko-Zupanc T, Pretnar J. Sequential treatment of deep fungal infections with amphotericin B deoxycholate and amphotericin B colloidal dispersion. *Appl Microbiol Biotechnol* 48:23–26, 1997.

Berenguer J, Buck M, Witebsky F, Stock F, Pizzo P A, and Walsh T J. Lysis-centrifugation blood cultures in the detection of tissue-proven invasive candidiasis. Disseminated versus single-organ infection. *Diagn Microbiol Infect Dis* 17:103–109, 1993.

Berg F T. *GM Torsk hos Barn. L.J. Hjerta, Stockholm,* 1846.

Berg R A, Stein J M. Medical management of fungal suppurative thrombosis of great central veins in a child. *Pediatr Infect Dis J* 8:469–470, 1989.

Berger C, Frei R, Gratwohl A, Scheidegger C. Bottled lemon juice—a cryptic source of invasive *Candida* infections in the immunocompromised host. *J Infect Dis* 158:654–655, 1988.

Berkhout C M. De Schimmelgeschlachter Monilia, Oidium, Vospora, en Torula. *Dissertation: University of Utrecht,* 1923.

Berkowitz F E, Argent A C, Baise T. Suppurative thrombophlebitis: a serious nosocomial infection. *Pediatr Infect Dis J* 6:64–67, 1987.

Bhargava P, Vazquez J A. Amphotericin B-resistant *Candida krusei?* A comparison of standardized testing and time kill studies. 40th Interscience Conference on Antimicrobial Agents and Chemotherapy, Toronto, Ontario, Canada. American Society for Microbiology, Abstract 924, 2000.

Bjerke J W, Meyers J D, Bowden R A. Hepatosplenic candidiasis—a contraindication to marrow transplantation? *Blood* 84:2811–2814, 1994.

Bjorses P, Aaltonen J, Vikman A, Perheentupa J, Ben-Zion G, Chiumello G, Dahl N, Heideman P, Hoorweg-Nijman J J, Mathivon L, Mullis P E, Pohl M, Ritzen M, Romeo G, Shapiro M S, Smith C S, Solyom J, Zlotogora J, Peltonen L. Genetic homogeneity of autoimmune polyglandular disease type I. *Am J Hum Genet* 59:879–886, 1996.

Black J T. Cerebral candidiasis: case report of brain abscess secondary to *Candida albicans*, and review of literature. *J Neurol Neurosurg Psychiatry* 33:864–870, 1970.

Blumberg E A, Reboli A C. Failure of systemic empirical treatment with amphotericin B to prevent candidemia in neutropenic patients with cancer. *Clin Infect Dis* 22:462–466, 1996.

Blumberg H M, Jarvis W R, Soucie J M, Edwards J E, Patterson J E, Pfaller M A, Rangel-Frausto M S, Rinaldi M G, Saiman L, Wiblin R T, Wenzel R P. Risk factors for candidal bloodstream infections in surgical intensive care unit patients: the NEMIS prospective multicenter study. The National Epidemiology of Mycosis Survey. *Clin Infect Dis* 33:177–186, 2001.

Bodey G P, Anaissie E J, Edwards J E. Candidiasis: pathogenesis, diagnosis, and treatment. In: Bodey G P ed. *Definitions of Candida Infections.* New York: Raven Press Ltd, 407–409, 1993.

Bodey, G P, Mardani M, Hanna H A, Boktour M, Abbas J, Girgawy E, Hachem R Y, Kontoyiannis D P, Raad, I I. The epidemiology of *Candida glabrata* and *Candida albicans* fungemia in immunocompromised patients with cancer. *Am J Med* 112:380–385, 2002.

Bonomo R A, Strauss M, Blinkhorn R, Salata R A. *Torulopsis (Candida) glabrata*: a new pathogen found in spinal epidural abscess. *Clini Infect Dis* 22:588–589, 1996.

Brajtburg J, Powderly W G, Kobayashi G S, Medoff G. Amphotericin B: delivery systems. *Antimicrob Agents Chemother* 34:381–384, 1990.

Brammer K W, Coates P E. Pharmacokinetics of fluconazole in pediatric patients. *Eur J Clin Microbiol Infect Dis* 13:325–329, 1994.

Brod R D, Flynn Jr. H W, Clarkson J G, Pflugfelder S C, Culbertson W W, and Miller D. Endogenous *Candida* endophthalmitis. Management without intravenous amphotericin B. *Ophthalmol* 97:666–672, 1990.

Brooks R G. Prospective study of *Candida* endophthalmitis in hospitalized patients with candidemia. *Arch Intern Med* 149:2226–2228, 1989.

Bross J, Talbot G H, Maislin G, Hurwitz S, Strom B L. Risk factors for nosocomial candidemia: a case control study in adults without leukemia. *Am J Med* 87:614–620, 1989.

Brown A J, Gow N A. Regulatory networks controlling *Candida albicans* morphogenesis. *Trends Microbiol* 7:333–338, 1999.

Buchs S, Pfister P. *Candida* meningitis. Course, prognosis and mortality before and after introduction of the new antimycotics. *Mykosen* 26:73–81, 1982.

Buckley R H, Lucas Z J, Hattler Jr. B G, Zmijewski C M, Amos D B. Defective cellular immunity associated with chronic mucocutaneous moniliasis and recurrent staphylococcal botryomycosis: immunological reconstitution by allogeneic bone marrow. *Clin Exp Immunol* 3:153–169, 1968.

Budtz-Jorgensen E, Stenderup A, Grabowski M. An epidemiological study of yeasts in elderly denture wearers. *Community Dent Oral Epidemiol* 3:115–119, 1975.

Burgert S J, Classen D C, Burke J P, Blatter D D. Candidal brain abscess associated with vascular invasion: a devastating complication of vascular catheter-related candidemia. *Clin Infect Dis* 21:202–205, 1995.

Burke W A. Use of itraconazole in a patient with chronic mucocutaneous candidiasis. *J Am Acad Dermatol* 21:1309–1310, 1989.

Cairns M R, Durack D T. Fungal pneumonia in the immunocompromised host. *Semin Respir Infect* 1:166–185, 1986.

Calandra T, Bille J, Schneider R, Mosimann F, Francioli P. Clinical significance of *Candida* isolated from peritoneum in surgical patients. *Lancet* 2:1437–1440, 1989.

Calderone R A, Rotondo M F, Sande M A. *Candida albicans* endocarditis: ultrastructural studies of vegetation formation. *Infect Immun* 20:279–289, 1978.

Cameron M L, Schell W A, Bruch S, Bartlett J A, Waskin H A, Perfect J R. Correlation of in vitro fluconazole resistance of *Candida* isolates in relation to therapy and symptoms of individuals seropositive for human immunodeficiency virus type 1. *Antimicrob Agents Chemother* 37:2449–2453, 1993.

Cancelas J A, Lopez J, Cabezudo E, Navas E, Garcia-Larana J, Jimenez-Mena M, Diz P, Perez de Oteyza J, Villalon L, Sanchez-Sousa A. Native valve endocarditis due to *Candida parapsilosis*: a late complication after bone marrow transplantation-related fungemia. *Bone Marrow Transplant* 13:333–334, 1994.

Cantrill H L, Rodman W P, Ramsay R C, Knobloch W H. Postpartum *Candida* endophthalmitis. *JAMA* 243:1163–1165, 1980.

Carpenter C C, Mayer K H, Fisher A, Desai M B, Durand L. Natural history of acquired immunodeficiency syndrome in women in Rhode Island. *Am J Med* 86: 771–775, 1989.

Castiglia, M, Smego R A, Sames E L. *Candida* endocarditis and amphotericin B intolerance: Potential role for fluconazole. *Infect Dis Clin Pract* 3:248–253, 1994.

Cartledge J D, Midgley J, Gazzard B G. Itraconazole cyclodextrin solution: the role of in vitro susceptibility testing in predicting successful treatment of HIV-related fluconazole-resistant and fluconazole-susceptible oral candidosis. *AIDS* 11:163–168, 1997.

Cawson R A. Symposium on denture sore mouth. II. The role of *Candida*. *Dent Pract Dent Rec* 16:138–142, 1965.

Cernea P, Crepy C, Kuffer R. Aspects peu connus des candidoses buccales. *Rev Stomat Chir Maxillofac* 66:103–138, 1965.

Chanock SJ, Pizzo PA. Infectious complications of patients undergoing therapy for acute leukemia: current status and future prospects. *Semin Oncol* 24:132–140, 1997.

Chim C S, Ho P L, Yuen P T, Yuen K Y. Fungal endocarditis in bone marrow transplantation: case report and review of literature. *J Infect* 37:287–291, 1998.

Chimelli L, Mahler-Araujo M B. Fungal infections. *Brain Pathol* 7:613–627, 1997.

Chiou C C, Wong T T, Lin H H, Hwang B, Tang R B, Wu K G, Lee B H. Fungal infection of ventriculoperitoneal shunts in children. *Clin Infect Dis* 19:1049–1053, 1994.

Chmel H. *Candida albicans* meningitis following lumbar puncture. *Am J Med Sci* 266: 465–467, 1993.

Clancy C J, Nguyen M H, Morris A J. Candidal mediastinitis: an emerging clinical entity. *Clin Infect Dis* 25:608–613, 1997.

Cleveland W W, Fogel B J, Brown W T, Kay H E. Foetal thymic transplant in a case of Digeorge's syndrome. *Lancet* 2:1211–1214, 1968.

Clotet B, Grifol M, Parra O, Boix J, Junca J, Tor J, Foz M. Asymptomatic esophageal candidiasis in the acquired-immunodeficiency-syndrome-related complex. *Ann Intern Med* 105:145, 1986.

Coleman D C, Bennett D E, Sullivan D J, Gallagher P J, Henman M C, Shanley D B, Russell R J. Oral *Candida* in HIV infection and AIDS: new perspectives/new approaches. *Crit Rev Microbiol* 19:61–82, 1993.

Collette N, van der Auwera P, Lopez A P, Heymans C, and Meunier F. Tissue concentrations and bioactivity of amphotericin B in cancer patients treated with amphotericin B-deoxycholate. *Antimicrob Agents Chemother* 33:362–368, 1989.

Corbella X, Sirvent J M, Carratala J. Fluconazole treatment without catheter removal in *Candida albicans* peritonitis complicating peritoneal dialysis. *Am J Med* 90: 277, 1991.

Coskuncan N M, Jabs D A, Dunn J P, Haller J A, Green W R, Vogelsang G B, SantosG W. The eye in bone marrow transplantation. VI. Retinal complications. *Arch Ophthalmol* 112:372–379, 1994.

Cruciani M, Di Perri G, Molesini M, Vento S, Concia E, Bassetti D.

Use of fluconazole in the treatment of *Candida albicans* hydrocephalus shunt infection. *Eur J Clin Microbiol Infect Dis* 11:957, 1992.

Dan M, Priel I. Failure of fluconazole therapy for sternal osteomyelitis due to *Candida albicans*. *Clin Infect Dis* 18:126–127, 1994.

Daftary D K, Mehta F S, Gupta P C, Pindborg J J. The presence of *Candida* in 723 oral leukoplakias among Indian villagers. *Scand J Dent Res* 80:75–79, 1972.

D'Antonio D, Violante B, Mazzoni A, Bonfini T, Capuani M A, D'Aloia F, Iacone A, Schioppa F, Romano F. A nosocomial cluster of *Candida inconspicua* infections in patients with hematological malignancies. *J Clin Microbiol* 36:792–795, 1998.

Darouiche R O. Oropharyngeal and esophageal candidiasis in immunocompromised patients: treatment issues. *Clin Infect Dis* 26:259–272, 1998.

De Bernardis F, Muhlschlegel F A, Cassone A, Fonzi W A. The pH of the host niche controls gene expression in and virulence of *Candida albicans*. *Infect Immun* 66:3317–3325, 1998.

Deeg H J, Lum L G, Sanders J, Levy G J, Sullivan K M, Beatty P, Thomas E D, Storb R.Severe aplastic anemia associated with chronic mucocutaneous candidiasis. Immunologic and hematologic reconstitution after allogeneic bone marrow transplantation. *Transplant* 41:583–586, 1986.

Desai M H, Herndon D N, Abston S. *Candida* infection in massively burned patients. *J Trauma* 27:1186–1188, 1987.

Dewsnup D H, Stevens D A. Efficacy of oral amphotericin B in AIDS patients with thrush clinically resistant to fluconazole. *J Med Vet Mycol* 32: 389–393, 1994.

Dick J D, Rosengard B R, Merz W G, Stuart R K, Hutchins G M, Saral R. Fatal disseminated candidiasis due to amphotericin-B-resistant *Candida guilliermondii*. *Ann Intern Med* 102:67–68, 1985.

Dijkmans B A, Koolen M I, Mouton R P, Falke T H, van den Broek PJ, van der Meer J W. Hematogenous *Candida* vertebral osteomyelitis treated with ketoconazole. *Infect* 10:290–292, 1982.

Domonkos A N, Arnold Jr H L, Odom R B. Disease due to fungi. In: Domonkos A N, Arnold H L, Jr, Odom R B, ed. *Andrew's Diseases of the Skin. Clinical Dermatology.* Philadelphia: WB Saunders, 341–403, 1982.

Donahue S P, Greven C M, Zuravleff J J, Eller A W, Nguyen M H, Peacock J E, Wagener Jr MW, Yu VL. Intraocular candidiasis in patients with candidemia. Clinical implications derived from a prospective multicenter study. *Ophthalmol* 101:1302–1309, 1994.

Doscher W, Krishnasastry K V, Deckoff S L. Fungal graft infections: case report and review of the literature. *J Vasc Surg* 6:398–402, 1987.

Driessen M, Ellis J B, Cooper P A, Wainer S, Muwazi F, Hahn D, Gous H, De Villiers F P. Fluconazole vs. amphotericin B for the treatment of neonatal fungal septicemia: a prospective randomized trial. *Pediatr Infect Dis J* 15:1107–1112, 1996.

Dube M P, Heseltine P N, Rinaldi M G, Evans S, Zawacki B. Fungemia and colonization with nystatin-resistant *Candida rugosa* in a burn unit. *Clin Infect Dis* 1:77–82, 1994.

Duerr A, Sierra M F, Feldman J, Clarke L M, Ehrlich I, DeHovitz J. Immune compromise and prevalence of *Candida* vulvovaginitis in human immunodeficiency virus-infected women. *J Bacteriol* 179:4654–4663, 1997.

Durandy A, Fischer A, LeDeist F, Drouhet E, Griscelli C. Mannan-specific and mannan-induced T-cell suppressive activity in patients with chronic mucocutaneous candidiasis. *J Clin Immunol* 7:400–419, 1987.

Edmond M B, Wallace S E, McClish D K, Pfaller M A, Jones R N, Wenzel R P. Nosocomial bloodstream infections in United States hospitals: a three-year analysis. *Clin Infect Dis* 29:239–244, 1999.

Edwards J E Jr, Foos R Y, Montgomerie J Z, Guze L B. Ocular manifestations of *Candida* septicemia: review of seventy-six cases of hematogenous *Candida* endophthalmitis. *Medicine (Baltimore)* 53:47–75, 1974.

Edwards J E Jr, Turkel S B, Elder H A, Rand R W, Guze L B. Hematogenous *Candida* osteomyelitis. Report of three cases and review of the literature. *Am J Med* 59:89–94, 1975.

Edwards J E Jr. Invasive *Candida* infections—evolution of a fungal pathogen (editorial; comment). *N Engl J Med* 324:1060–1062, 1991.

Edwards J E Jr, Bodey G P, Bowden R A, Buchner T, de Pauw B E, Filler S G, Ghannoum M A, Glauser M, Herbrecht R, Kauffman C A, Kohno S, Martino P, Meunier F, Mori T, Pfaller M A, Rex J H, Rogers T R, Rubin R H, Solomkin J, Viscoli C, WalshT J, and White M. International Conference for the Development of a Consensus on the Management and Prevention of Severe Candidal Infections. *Clin Infect Dis* 25:43–59, 1997.

Eggimann P, Francioli P, Bille J, Schneider R, Wu M M, Chapuis G, Chiolero R, Pannatier A, Schilling J, Geroulanos S, Glauser M P, Calandra T. Fluconazole prophylaxis prevents intra-abdominal candidiasis in high-risk surgical patients. *Crit Care Med* 27:1066–1072, 1999.

Ehrenstein B P, Salamon L, Linde H J, Messmann H, Scholmerich J, Gluck T. Clinical determinants for the recovery of fungal and mezlocillin-resistant pathogens from bile specimens. *Clin Infect Dis* 34:902–908, 2002.

Eichel M, Just-Nubling G, Helm E B, Stille W. Itraconazole suspension in the treatment of HIV-infected patients with fluconazole-resistant oropharyngeal candidiasis and esophagitis. *Mycoses* 39(Suppl 1):102–106, 1996.

Eisenberg E S, Leviton I, Soeiro R. Fungal peritonitis in patients receiving peritoneal dialysis: experience with 11 patients and review of the literature. *Rev Infect Dis* 8:309–321, 1986.

Eisenberg E S. Intraperitoneal flucytosine in the management of fungal peritonitis in patients on continuous ambulatory peritoneal dialysis. *Am J Kidney Dis* 11: 465–467, 1988.

el-Ebiary M, Torres A, Fabregas N, de la Bellacasa J P, Gonzalez J, Ramirez J, del Bano D, Hernandez C, Jimenez de Anta M T. Significance of the isolation of *Candida* species from respiratory samples in critically ill, non-neutropenic patients. An immediate postmortem histologic study. *Am J Neuroradiol* 18:1303–1306, 1997.

Ellis M E, Al-Abdely H, Sandridge A, Greer W, Ventura W. Fungal endocarditis: evidence in the world literature, 1965–1995. *Clin Infect Dis* 32:50–62, 2001.

Endophthalmitis Vitrectomy Study Group. Results of the Endophthalmitis Vitrectomy Study. A randomized trial of immediate vitrectomy and of intravenous antibiotics for the treatment of postoperative bacterial endophthalmitis. *Arch Ophthalmol* 113: 1479–1496, 1995.

Eras P, Goldstein M J, Sherlock P. *Candida* infection of the gastrointestinal tract. *Medicine (Baltimore)* 51:367–379, 1972.

Ernst EJ. Investigational antifungal agents. *Pharmacotherapy* 21: 165S–174S, 2001.

Escuro R S, Jacobs S M, Gerson S L, Machicao A R, Lazarus H M. Prospective evaluation of a *Candida* antigen detection test for invasive candidiasis in immunocompromised adult patients with cancer. *Am J Med* 87:621–627, 1989.

Faix R G. Invasive neonatal candidiasis: comparison of *albicans* and *parapsilosis* infection. *Pediatr Infect Dis J* 11:88–93, 1992a.

Faix R G. Nonsurgical treatment of *Candida* endocarditis. *J Pediatr* 120:665–666, 1992b.

Fan-Havard P, O'Donovan C, Smith S M, Oh J, Bamberger M, Eng R H. Oral fluconazole versus amphotericin B bladder irrigation for treatment of candidal funguria. *Clin Infect Dis* 21:960–965, 1995.

Fazio R A, Wickremesinghe P C, Arsura E L. Ketoconazole treatment of *Candida* esophagitis—a prospective study of 12 cases. *Am J Gastroenterol* 78:261–264, 1983.

Febre N, Silva V, Medeiros E A, Wey S B, Colombo A L, Fischman O. Microbiological characteristics of yeasts isolated from urinary tracts of intensive care unit patients undergoing urinary catheterization. *J Clin Microbiol* 37:1584–1586, 1999.

Feigal DW, Katz MH, Greenspan D, Westenhouse J, Winkelstein Jr. W, Lang W, Samuel M, Buchbinder SP, Hessol NA, Lifson AR, and et al. The prevalence of oral lesions in HIV-infected homosexual and bisexual men: three San Francisco epidemiological cohorts. *AIDS* 5:519–525, 1991.

Fernandez M, Moylett E H, Noyola D E, and Baker C J. Candidal meningitis in neonates: a 10-year review. *Clin Infect Dis* 31:458–463, 2000.

Ferra C, Doebbeling B N, Hollis R J, Pfaller M A, Lee C K, Gingrich R D. *Candida tropicalis* vertebral osteomyelitis: a late sequela of fungemia. *Clin Infect Dis* 19:697–703, 1994.

Fidel P L, Jr., Lynch M E, Conaway D H, Tait L, Sobel J D. Mice immunized by primary vaginal *Candida albicans* infection develop acquired vaginal mucosal immunity. *Infect Immun* 63:547–553, 1995.

Fidel P L, Jr., Vazquez J A, Sobel, J D. Candida glabrata: Review of epidemiology, pathogenesis, and clinical disease with comparison to *C. albicans*. *Clin Microbiol Rev* 12:80–96, 1999.

Fischer A, Ballet J J, Griscelli C. Specific inhibition of in vitro *Candida*-induced lymphocyte proliferation by polysaccharidic antigens present in the serum of patients with chronic mucocutaneous candidiasis. *J Clin Invest* 62:1005–1013, 1978.

Fisher J, Mayhall G, Duma R, Shadomy S, Shadomy J, Watlington C. Fungus balls of the urinary tract. *South Med J* 72:1281–1284, 1979.

Fisher J F, Chew W H, Shadomy S, Duma R J, Mayhall C G, House W C. Urinary tract infections due to *Candida albicans*. *Rev Infect Dis* 4:1107–1118, 1982.

Fisher J F, Taylor A T, Clark J, Rao R, Espinel-Ingroff A. Penetration of amphotericin B into the human eye. *J Infect Dis* 147:164, 1983.

Fisher-Hoch S P, Hutwagner L. Opportunistic candidiasis: an epidemic of the 1980s. *Clin Infect Dis* 21:897–904, 1995.

Fitzpatrick T B, Johnson R A, Wolff K, Polano M K, Suurmond D. *Color Atlas and Synopsis of Clinical Dermatology: Common and Serious Diseases*, 3rd ed. New York: McGraw Hill, 1997.

Fogarty M. Candidial osteomyelitis: a case report. *Aust N Z J Surg* 53:141–143, 1983.

Franklin W G, Simon A B, Sodeman T M. *Candida* myocarditis without valvulitis. *Am J Cardiol* 38:924–928, 1976.

Fraser V J, Dunkel J, Jones M, Storfer S, Medoff G, Dunagan W C. Candidemia in a tertiary care hospital; epidemiology, risk factors, and predictors of mortality. *Clin Infect Dis* 15:414–421, 1992.

Fridkin S K, Jarvis W R. Epidemiology of nosocomial fungal infections. *Clin Microbiol Rev* 9:499–511, 1996.

Friedland I R. Peripheral thrombophlebitis caused by *Candida*. *Pediatr Infect Dis J* 15:375–377, 1996.

Frye K R, Donovan J M, Drach G W. *Torulopsis glabrata* urinary infections: a review. *J Urol* 139:1245–1249, 1988.

Fukasawa N, Shirakura K. *Candida* arthritis after total knee arthroplasty—a case of successful treatment without prosthesis removal. *J Ind Microbiol Biotechnol* 18:360–363, 1997.

Galgiani J N, Stevens D A. Fungal endocarditis: need for guidelines in evaluating therapy. Experience with two patients previously reported. *J Thorac Cardiovasc Surg* 73:293–296, 1977.

Garbino T, Lew D, Romand J A. Fluconazole prevents severe *Candida* spp. infections in high risk critically ill patients. Paper presented at the American Society Microbiology, Washington, D.C., 1997.

Gathe Jr. J C, Harris R L, Garland B, Bradshaw M W, Williams Jr. T W. *Candida* osteomyelitis. Report of five cases and review of the literature. *Am J Med* 82:927–937, 1987.

Geers T A, Gordon S M. Clinical significance of *Candida* species isolated from cerebrospinal fluid following neurosurgery. *Clin Infect Dis* 28:1139–1147, 1999.

Gentry L O, Wilkinson I D, Lea A S, Price M F. Latex agglutination test for detection of *Candida* antigen in patients with disseminated disease. *Eur J Clin Microbiol Infect Dis* 2:122–128, 1983.

Gilbert H M, Peters E D, Lang S J, Hartman B J. Successful treatment of fungal prosthetic valve endocarditis: case report and review. *Clin Infect Dis* 22:348–354, 1996.

Ginsburg C H, Braden G L, Tauber A I, Trier J S. Oral clotrimazole in the treatment of esophageal candidiasis. *Am J Med Sci* 71: 891–895, 1981.

Girmenia C, Martino P, De Bernardis F, Gentile G, Boccanera M, Monaco M, Antonucci G, Cassone A. Rising incidence of *Candida parapsilosis* fungemia in patients with hematologic malignancies: clinical aspects, predisposing factors, and differential pathogenicity of the causative strains. *Clin Infect Dis* 23:506–514, 1996.

Glassman B D, Muglia J J. Widespread erythroderma and desquamation in a neonate. Congenital cutaneous candidiasis (CCC). *Arch Dermatol* 129:899–902, 1993.

Glatt A E. Therapy for oropharyngeal candidiasis in HIV-infected patients. *J AIDS* 6:1317–1318, 1993.

Gleason T G, May A K, Caparelli D, Farr B M, Sawyer R G. Emerging evidence of selection of fluconazole-tolerant fungi in surgical intensive care units. *Arch Surg* 132:1197–1201; discussion p.1202, 1997.

Goldie S J, Kiernan-Tridle L, Torres C, Gorban-Brennan N, Dunne D, Kliger A S, and Finkelstein F O. Fungal peritonitis in a large chronic peritoneal dialysis population: a report of 55 episodes. *Am J Kidney Dis* 28:86–91, 1996.

Goodman J L, Winston D, Greenfield R A, Chandrasekar P H, Fox B, Kaizer H, Shadduck R K, Shea T C, Stiff P, Friedman D J. A controlled trial of fluconazole to prevent fungal infections in patients undergoing bone marrow transplantation. *N Engl J Med* 326:845–851, 1992.

Goldman M, Pottage Jr. J C, Weaver D C. *Candida krusei* fungemia. Report of 4 cases and review of the literature. *Medicine (Baltimore)* 72:143–150, 1993.

Goldman M, Filler S G, Cloud G A, ACTG 323, Mycoses Study Group 40. Randomized study of long-term chronic suppressive fluconazole vs. episodic fluconazole for patients with advanced HIV infection and history of oropharyngeal candidiasis. 42nd Interscience Conference on Antimicrobial Agents and Chemotherapy, San Diego, CA. American Society for Microbiology. Abstract M-1241, 2002.

Gorg C, Weide R, Schwerk W B, Koppler H, Havemann K. Ultrasound evaluation of hepatic and splenic microabscesses in the immunocompromised patient: sonographic patterns, differential diagnosis, and follow-up. *J Clin Ultrasound* 22:525–529, 1994.

Gower D J, Crone K, Alexander Jr. E, Kelly Jr. D L. *Candida albicans* shunt infection: report of two cases. *Neurosurgery* 19:111–113, 1986.

Graninger W, Presteril E, Schneeweiss B, Teleky B, Georgopoulos A. Treatment of *Candida albicans* fungaemia with fluconazole. *J Infect* 26:133–146, 1993.

Grant S M, Clissold S P. Fluconazole. A review of its pharmacodynamic and pharmacokinetic properties, and therapeutic potential in superficial and systemic mycoses. *Drugs* 39:877–916, 1990.

Grewe M, Tsiotos G G, Luque de-Leon E, Sarr M G. Fungal infection in acute necrotizing pancreatitis. *J Am Coll Surg* 188:408–414, 1999.

Grube B J, Marvin J A, Heimbach D M. Candida. A decreasing problem for the burned patient? *Arch Surg* 123:194–196, 1988.

Guinet R, Chanas J, Goullier A, Bonnefoy G, Ambroise-Thomas P. Fatal septicemia due to amphotericin B-resistant *Candida lusitaniae*. *J Clin Microbiol* 18:443–444, 1983.

Gumbo T, Isada C M, Hall G, Karafa M T, Gordon S M. *Candida glabrata* fungemia: Clinical features of 139 patients. *Medicine (Baltimore)* 78:220–227, 1999.

Gupta S, Jain P K. Low-dose heparin in experimental peritonitis. *Eur Surg Res* 17:167–172, 1985.

Gupta T P, Ehrinpreis MN. *Candida*-associated diarrhea in hospitalized patients. *Gastroenterol* 98:780–785, 1990.

Gurses N, Kalayci A G. Fluconazole monotherapy for candidal meningitis in a premature infant. *Clin Infect Dis* 23:645–646, 1996.

Guze L B, Harley L D. Fungus infections of the urinary tract. *Yale J Biol Med* 30:292–305, 1957.

Hagensee M E, Bauwens J E, Kjos B, Bowden R A. Brain abscess following marrow transplantation: experience at the Fred Hutchinson Cancer Research Center, 1984–1992. *Clin Infect Dis* 19:402–408, 1994.

Hallum J L, Williams T W, Jr. Candida endocarditis. In: Bodey GP, ed. *Candidiasis: Pathogenesis, Diagnosis and Treatment*, 2nd ed. New York: Raven, 357–370, 1993.

Hansen B L, Anderson K. Fungal arthritis. A review. *Scand J Rheumatol* 24:248–250, 1995.

Haron E, Feld R, Tuffnell P, Patterson B, Hasselback R, Matlow A. Hepatic candidiasis: an increasing problem in immunocompromised patients. *Am J Med* 83:17–26, 1987.

Haron E, Vartivarian S, Anaissie E, Dekmezian R, Bodey G P. Primary *Candida* pneumonia. Experience at a large cancer center and review of the literature. *Medicine (Baltimore)* 72:137–142, 1993.

Harousseau J L, Dekker A W, Stamatoullas-Bastard A, Fassas A, Linkesch W, Gouveia J, De Bock R, Rovira M, Seifert W F, Joosen H, Peeters M, De Beule K. Itraconazole oral solution for primary prophylaxis of fungal infections in patients with hematological malignancy and profound neutropenia: a randomized, double-blind, double-placebo, multicenter trial comparing itraconazole and amphotericin B. *Antimicrob Agents Chemother* 44:1887–1893, 2000.

Hay R J, Clayton Y M. The treatment of patients with chronic mucocutaneous candidosis and candida onychomycosis with ketoconazole. *Clin Exp Dermatol* 7:155–162, 1982.

Hay R J, Clayton Y M. Fluconazole in the management of patients with chronic mucocutaneous candidosis. *Br J Dermatol* 119:683–684, 1988.

Hay R J. Overview of studies of fluconazole in oropharyngeal candidiasis. *Rev Infect Dis.* 3(Suppl 3):334–337, 1990.

Hazen K C. New and emerging yeast pathogens. *Clin Microbiol Rev* 8:462–478, 1995.

Helton W S, Carrico C J, Zaveruha P A, Schaller R. Diagnosis and treatment of splenic fungal abscesses in the immune-suppressed patient. *Arch Surg* 121: 580–586, 1986.

Henderson D K, Hockey L J, Vukalcic L J, Edwards J E, Jr. Effect of immunosuppression on the development of experimental hematogenous *Candida* endophthalmitis. *Infect Immun* 27:628–631, 1980.

Hendrickx L, Van Wijngaerden E, Samson I, Peetermans W E. Candidal vertebral osteomyelitis: report of 6 patients, and a review. *Clin Infect Dis* 32:527–533, 2001.

Hennequin C, Bouree P, Hiesse C, Dupont B, Charpentier B. Spondylodiskitis due to *Candida albicans*: report of two patients who were successfully treated with fluconazole and review of the literature. *Clin Infect Dis* 23:176–178, 1996.

Hermans P E, Ritts R E, Jr. Chronic mucocutaneous candidiasis. Its association with immunologic and endocrine abnormalities. *Minn Med* 53:75–80, 1970.

Hernandez J A, Gonzalez-Moreno M, Llibre J M, Aloy A, Casan C M. Candidal mitral endocarditis and long-term treatment with fluconazole in a patient with human immunodeficiency virus infection. *Clin Infect Dis* 15:1062–1063, 1992.

Herzog W, Perfect J, Roberts L. Intervertebral diskitis due to *Candida tropicalis*. *South Med J* 82:270–273, 1989.

Heurlin N, Bergstrom SE, Winiarski J, Ringden O, Ljungman P, Lonnqvist B, Andersson J. Fungal pneumonia: the predominant lung infection causing death in children undergoing bone marrow transplantation. *Acta Paediatrica* 85: 168–172, 1996.

HidalgoJ A, Brown W, Vazquez J A. Invasive *Candida dubliniensis* in an HIV-negative patient: A new opportunistic fungal pathogen. *Infect Dis Clin Pract* 9:176–179, 2000.

Hipocrates C A, Adams F. *Epidemics 460–377 BC, Book 3.* Baltimore, MD: Williams and Wilkins, 1939.

Hockey L J, Fujita N K, Gibson T R, Rotrosen D, Montgomerie J Z, Edwards J E, Jr. Detection of fungemia obscured by concomitant bacteremia: in vitro and in vivo studies. *J Clin Microbiol* 16:1080–1085, 1982.

Hoerauf A, Hammer S, Muller-Myhsok B, and Rupprecht H. Intra-abdominal *Candida* infection during acute necrotizing pancreatitis has a high prevalence and is associated with increased mortality. *Crit Care Med* 26:2010–2015, 1998.

Hofman P, Gari-Toussaint M, Bernard E, Michiels J F, Gibelin P, Le Fichoux Y, Morand P, Loubiere R. Fungal myocarditis in acquired immunodeficiency syndrome. *Arch Mal Coeur Vaiss* 85: 203–208, 1992.

Hogeweg M, de Jong P T. *Candida* endophthalmitis in heroin addicts. *Doc Ophthalmol* 55:63–71, 1983.

Hoh M C, Lin H P, Chan L L, Lam S K. Successful allogeneic bone marrow transplantation in severe chronic mucocutaneous candidiasis syndrome. *Bone Marrow Transplant* 18:797–800, 1996.

Holt PJ, Higgs JM, Munro J, Valdimarsson H. Chronic mucocutaneous candidiasis: a model for the investigation of cell mediated immunity. *Br J Clin Pract* 26:331–336, 1972.

Horowitz B J. Topical flucytosine therapy for chronic recurrent *Candida tropicalis* infections. *J Reprod Med* 31:821–824, 1986.

Horsburgh C R, Kirkpatrick C H. Long term therapy of chronic mucocutaneous candidiasis with ketoconazole; experience with 21 patients. *Am J Med* 74(Suppl 1B):23–29, 1983.

Huang Y C, Lin T Y, Lien R I, Chou Y H, Kuo CY, Yang P H, Hsieh W S. Candidaemia in special care nurseries: comparison of albicans and parapsilosis infection. *J Infect* 40:171–175, 2000.

Hughes W T, Bartley D L, Patterson G G, Tufenkeji H. Ketoconazole and candidiasis: a controlled study. *J Infect Dis* 147:1060–1063, 1983.

Hughes C E, Beggs W H. Action of fluconazole (UK-49,858) in relation to other systemic antifungal azoles. *J Antimicrob Chemother* 19:171–174, 1987.

Hurley R, De Louvois J. *Candida* vaginitis. *Postgrad Med J* 55:645–647, 1979.

Imam N, Carpenter C C, Mayer K H, Fisher A, Stein M, Danforth SB. Hierarchical pattern of mucosal *Candida* infections in HIV-seropositive women. *Am J Med* 89: 142–146, 1990.

Irani M, Truong L D. Candidiasis of the extrahepatic biliary tract. *Arch Pathol Lab Med* 110:1087–1090, 1986.

Jabra-Rizk M A, Baqui A A, Kelley J I, Falkler W A, Merz W G, Jr., Meiller T F. Identification of *Candida dubliniensis* in a prospective study of patients in the United States. *J Clin Microbiol* 37: 321–326, 1999.

Jarrett F, Maki D G, Chan CK. Management of septic thrombosis of the inferior vena cava caused by *Candida*. *Arch Surg* 113:637–639, 1978.

Jarvis W R. Epidemiology of nosocomial fungal infections, with emphasis on *Candida* species. *Clin Infect Dis* 20:1526–1530, 1995.

Jin Y, Endo A, Shimada M, Minato M, Takada M, Takahashi S, Harada K. Congenital systemic candidiasis. *Pediatr Infect Dis J* 14:818–820, 1995.

Johnson D E, Thompson T R, Ferrieri P. Congenital candidiasis. *Am J Dis Child* 135:273–275, 1981.

Johnston P G, Lee J, Domanski M, Dressler F, Tucker E, Rothenberg M, Cunnion R E, Pizzo P A, Walsh T J. Late recurrent *Candida* endocarditis. *Chest* 99:1531–1533, 1991.

Joly V, Belmatoug N, Leperre A, Robert J, Jault F, Carbon C, Yeni P. Pacemaker endocarditis due to *Candida albicans*: case report and review. *Clin Infect Dis* 25:1359–1362, 1997.

Joshi N, Hamory B H. Endophthalmitis caused by non-*albicans* species of *Candida*. *Rev Infect Dis* 13:281–287, 1991.

Kanda Y, Yamamoto R, Chizuka A, Hamaki T, Suguro M, Arai C, Matsuyama T, Takezako N, Miwa A, Kern W, Kami M, Akiyama H, Hirai H, Togawa A. Prophylactic action of oral fluconazole against fungal infection in neutropenic patients. A meta-analysis of 16 randomized, controlled trials. *Cancer* 89:1611–1625, 2000.

Kao A S, Brandt M E, Pruitt W R, Conn L A, Perkins B A, Stephens D S, Baughman W S, Reingold A L, Rothrock G A, Pfaller M A, Pinner R W, Hajjeh R A. The epidemiology of candidemia in two United States cities: results of a population-based active surveillance. *Clin Infect Dis* 29:1164–1170, 1999.

Kapdagli H, Ozturk G, Dereli T. *Candida folliculitis* mimicking tinea barbae. *Int J Dermatol* 36:295–297, 1997.

Katzenstein D. Isolated *Candida* arthritis: report of a case and definition of a distinct clinical syndrome. *Arthritis Rheum* 28:1421–1424, 1985.

Karyotakis N C, Anaissie E J. Efficacy of escalating doses of liposomal amphotericin B (AmBisome) against hematogenous *Candida lusitaniae* and *Candida krusei* infection in neutropenic mice. *Antimicrob Agents Chemother* 38:2660–2662, 1994.

Kauffman C A, Jones P G, Bergman A G, McAuliffe L S, Liepman M K. Effect of prophylactic ketoconazole and nystatin on fungal flora. *Mykosen* 27:165–172, 1984.

Kauffman C A, Bradley S F, Ross S C, Weber D R. Hepatosplenic candidiasis: successful treatment with fluconazole. *Am J Med* 91:137–141, 1991.

Kauffman C A, Bradley S F, Vine A K. *Candida* endophthalmitis associated with intraocular lens implantation: efficacy of fluconazole therapy. *Mycoses* 36:13–17, 1993.

Kauffman C A, Vazquez J A, Sobel J D, Gallis H A, McKinsey D S, Karchmer A W, Sugar A M, Sharkey P K, Wise G J, Mangi R, Mosher A, Lee J Y, Dismukes W E. Prospective multicenter surveillance study of funguria in hospitalized patients. The National Institute for Allergy and Infectious Diseases (NIAID) Mycoses Study Group. *Clin Infect Dis* 30:14–18, 2000.

Kaufman D, Boyle R, Hazen K C, Patrie J T, Robinson M, Donowitz L G. Fluconazole prophylaxis against fungal colonization and infection in preterm infants. *N Engl J Med* 345:1660–1666, 2001.

Kerkering T M, Espinel-Ingroff A, Shadomy S. Detection of *Candida* antigenemia by counterimmunoelectrophoresis in patients with invasive candidiasis. *J Infect Dis* 140:659–664, 1979.

Kerr C M, Perfect J R, Craven P C, Jorgensen J H, Drutz D J, Shelburne J D, Gallis H A, Gutman R A. Fungal peritonitis in patients on continuous ambulatory peritoneal dialysis. *Ann Intern Med* 99:334–336, 1983.

Khan,EA, Correa AG, Baker CJ. Suppurative thrombophlebitis in children: a ten-year experience. *Pediatr Infect Dis J* 16:63–67, 1997.

Kirkpatrick C H, Rich R R, Graw R G, Jr., Smith K, Mickenberg I, Rogentine G N. Treatment of chronic mucocutaneous moniliasis by immunologic reconstitution. *Clin Exp Immunol* 9:733–748, 1971.

Kirkpatrick C H. Chronic mucocutaneous candidiasis. In: Bodey G P, ed. *Candidiasis: Pathogenesis, Diagnosis and Treatment*, New York: Raven Press Ltd., 167–184, 1993.

Kirkpatrick C H. Chronic mucocutaneous candidiasis. *J Am Acad Dermatol* 31:S14–S17, 1994.

Klein J J, Watanakunakorn C. Hospital-acquired fungemia. Its natural course and clinical significance. *Am J Med* 67:51–58, 1979.

Klein RS, Harris CA, Small CB, Moll B, Lesser M, and Friedland GH. Oral candidiasis in high-risk patients as the initial manifestation of the acquired immunodeficiency syndrome. *N Engl J Med* 311:354–358, 1984.

Kodsi B E, Wickremesinghe C, Kozinn P J, Iswara K, Goldberg P K.

Candida esophagitis: a prospective study of 27 cases. *Gastroenterol* 71:715–719, 1976.

Koletar S L, Weed H G, Raimundo M B. Thrush unresponsive to treatment with fluconazole in HIV-infected patients. 1st National Conference on Human Retroviruses, Washington DC, 1994.

Komshian S V, Uwaydah A K, Sobel J D, Crane L R. Fungemia caused by *Candida* species and *Torulopsis glabrata* in the hospitalized patient: frequency, characteristics, and evaluation of factors influencing outcome. *Rev Infect Dis* 11:379–390, 1989.

Kontoyiannis D P, Vaziri I, Hanna H A, Boktour M, Thornby J, Hachem R, Bodey G P, and Raad, I I. Risk Factors for *Candida tropicalis* fungemia in patients with cancer. *Clin Infect Dis* 33:1676–1681, 2001.

Kozinn P J, Taschdjian C L, Dragutsky D. Therapy of oral thrush; a comparative evaluation of gentian violet, mycostatin, and amphotericin B. *Monogr Ther.* 2:16–24, 1957.

Kozinn P J, Taschdjian C L, Goldberg P K, Wise G J, Toni E F, Seelig M S. Advances in the diagnosis of renal candidiasis. *J Urol* 119:184–187, 1978.

Krick J A, Remington J S. Opportunistic invasive fungal infections in patients with leukaemia lymphoma. *Clin Haematol* 5:249–310, 1976.

Krishna R, Amuh D, Lowder C Y, Gordon S M, Adal K A, Hall G. Should all patients with candidaemia have an ophthalmic examination to rule out ocular candidiasis? *Eye* 14:30–34, 2000.

Kujath P, Kochendorfer P, Kreiskother E, Dammrich J. Fungal peritonitis. *Chirurg* 61:900–905, 1990.

Kung N, Fisher N, Gunson B, Hastings M, Mutimer D. Fluconazole prophylaxis for high-risk liver transplant recipients. *Lancet* 345: 1234–1235, 1995.

Kurtz M B, Rex J H. Glucan synthase inhibitors as antifungal agents. *Adv Protein Chem* 56:423–475, 2001.

Kwon-Chung K J, Wickes B L, Merz W G. Association of electrophoretic karyotype of *Candida stellatoidea* with virulence for mice. *Infect Immun* 56:1814–1819, 1988.

Kwon-Chung K J, Riggsby W S, Uphoff R A, Hicks J B, Whelan W L, Reiss E, Magee B B, Wickes B L. Genetic differences between type I and type II *Candida stellatoidea*. *Infect Immun* 57:527–532, 1989.

Kwon-Chung K J, Wickes B L, Salkin I F, Kotz H L, Sobel J D. Is *Candida stellatoidea* disappearing from the vaginal mucosa? *J Clini Microbiol* 28:600–601, 1990.

Kwon-Chung K J, Bennett J E. *Medical Mycology*. Lea & Febiger, Philadelphia, 1992.

Lai P H, Lin SM, Pan H B, Yang C F. Disseminated miliary cerebral candidiasis. *J Periodontol* 68:729–733, 1997.

Lamey P J, Lamb A B. Prospective study of aetiological factors in burning mouth syndrome. *Br Med J Clin Res Ed* 296:1243–1246, 1988a.

Lamey P J, Darwaza A, Fisher B M, Samaranayake L P, Macfarlane T W, Frier B M. Secretor status, candidal carriage and candidal infection in patients with diabetes mellitus. *J Oral Path* 17:354–357, 1988b.

Langenbeck B. Auffingung von Pilzer aus der Schleimhaut der Speiserohre einer Typhus-Leiche. *Neue Not Geb. Natur-u-Heilk (Froorief)* 12:145–147, 1939.

Law D, Moore C B, Denning D W. Amphotericin B resistance testing of *Candida* spp.: a comparison of methods. *J Antimicrob Chemother* 40:117–119, 1997.

Lecciones J A, Lee J W, Navarro E E, Witebsky F G, Marshall D, Steinberg S M, Pizzo P A, Walsh T J. Vascular catheter-associated fungemia in patients with cancer: analysis of 155 episodes. *Clin Infect Dis* 14:875–883, 1992.

Lee T M, Greenberger P A, Oh S, Patterson R, Roberts M, Liotta J L. Allergic bronchopulmonary candidiasis: case report and suggested diagnostic criteria. *J Allergy Clin Immunol* 80:816–820, 1987.

Lefkowitz M, Elsas L J, Levine R J. *Candida* infection complicating peptic esophageal ulcer. Infection in an aortic-esophageal fistula. *Arch Intern Med* 113:672–675, 1964.

Lehner T. Symposium on *Candida* Infections. Hurley R, Winner H, eds. *Classification and clinico-pathological features of Candida infections in the mouth*. Livingstone, Edinburgh, 1966.

Leidich S D, Ibrahim A S, Fu Y, Koul A, Jessup C, Vitullo J, Fonzi W, Mirbod F, Nakashima S, Nozawa Y, Ghannoum M A. Cloning and disruption of caPLB1, a phospholipase B gene involved in the pathogenicity of *Candida albicans*. *J Biol Chem* 273:2678–2686, 1998.

Letiner T. Oral thrush or acute pseudomembranous candidiasis; a clinical-pathologic study of 44 cases. *Oral Surg* 18:27–37, 1964.

Leu HS, and Huang CT. Clearance of funguria with short-course antifungal regimens: a prospective, randomized, controlled study. *Clin Infect Dis* 20:1152–1157, 1995.

Levine J, Bernard D B, Idelson B A, Farnham H, Saunders C, Sugar A M. Fungal peritonitis complicating continuous ambulatory peritoneal dialysis: successful treatment with fluconazole, a new orally active antifungal agent. *Am J Med* 86: 825–827, 1989.

Levy I, Rubin L G, Vasishtha S, Tucci V, Sood S K. Emergence of *Candida parapsilosis* as the predominant species causing candidemia in children. *Clin Infect Dis* 26:1086–1088, 1998.

Lindner A, Becker G, Warmuth-Metz M, Schalke B C, Bogdahn U, Toyka K V. Magnetic resonance image findings of spinal intramedullary abscess caused by *Candida albicans*: case report. *Neurosurgery* 36:411–412, 1995.

Lipton S A, Hickey W F, Morris J H, Loscalzo J. Candidal infection in the central nervous system. *Am J Med* 76:101–108, 1984.

Lo H J, Kohler J R, DiDomenico B, Loebenberg D, Cacciapuoti A, Fink G R. Nonfilamentous *Candida albicans* mutants are avirulent. *Cell* 90:939–949, 1997.

Luzzati R, Amalfitano G, Lazzarini L, Soldani F, Bellino S, Solbiati M, Danzi M C, Vento S, Todeschini G, Vivenza C, Concia E. Nosocomial candidemia in non-neutropenic patients at an Italian tertiary care hospital. *Eur J Clin Microbiol Infect Dis* 19:602–607, 2000.

Maenza J R, Keruly J C, Moore R D, Chaisson R E, Merz W G, Gallant J E. Risk factors for fluconazole-resistant candidiasis in human immunodeficiency virus-infected patients. *J Infect Dis* 173:219–225, 1996.

Maenza J R, Merz W G, Romagnoli M J, Keruly J C, Moore R D, Gallant J E. Infection due to fluconazole-resistant *Candida* in patients with AIDS: prevalence and microbiology. *Clin Infect Dis* 24:28–34, 1997.

Magnussen C R, Olson J P, Ona F V, and Graziani A J. *Candida* fungus balls in the common bile duct. Unusual manifestation of disseminated candidiasis. *Arch Intern Med* 139:821–822, 1979.

Mahayni R, Vazquez J A, Zervos M J. Nosocomial candidiasis: epidemiology and drug resistance. *Infect Agents Dis* 4:248–253, 1995.

Marr B, Gross S, Cunningham C, Weiner L. Candidal sepsis and meningitis in a very-low-birth-weight infant successfully treated with fluconazole and flucytosine. *Clin Infect Dis* 19:795–796, 1994.

Marr K A, White T C, Van Burik J A, Bowden R A. Development of fluconazole resistance in *Candida albicans* causing disseminated infection in a patient undergoing marrow transplantation. *Clin Infect Dis* 25:908–910, 1997.

Marr K A, Seidel K, Slavin M A, Bowden R A, Schoch H G, Flowers M E, Corey L, Boeckh M. Prolonged fluconazole prophylaxis is associated with persistent protection against candidiasis-related death in allogeneic marrow transplant recipients: long-term follow-up of a randomized, placebo-controlled trial. *Blood* 96:2055–2061, 2000.

Marra F, Robbins G M, Masri B A, Duncan C, Wasan K M, Kwong E H, Jewesson P J. Amphotericin B-loaded bone cement to treat osteomyelitis caused by *Candida albicans*. *Can J Surg* 44:383–386, 2000.

Martinez-Vazquez C, Fernandez-Ulloa J, Bordon J, Sopena B, de la Fuente J, Ocampo A. *Candida albicans* endophthalmitis in brown heroin addicts: response to early vitrectomy preceded and followed by antifungal therapy. *Clin Infect Dis* 27:1130–3, 1998.

Martins, M D, Rex J H. Fluconazole suspension for oropharyngeal candidiasis unresponsive to tablets. *Ann Intern Med* 126:332–333, 1997.

Masur H, Rosen P P, Armstrong D. Pulmonary disease caused by *Candida* species. *Am J Med* 63:914–925, 1977.

Mayayo E, Moralejo J, Camps J, Guarro J. Fungal endocarditis in premature infants: case report and review. *Clin Infect Dis* 22:366–368, 1996.

McAdams H P, Rosado-de-Christenson M L, Templeton P A, Lesar M, Moran C A. Thoracic mycoses from opportunistic fungi: radiologic-pathologic correlation. *Radiographics* 15:271–286, 1995.

McClean K L, Sheehan G J, Harding G K. Intraabdominal infection: a review. *Clin Infect Dis* 19:100–116, 1994.

McCullers J A, Vargas S L, Flynn P M, Razzouk B I, Shenep J L. Candidal meningitis in children with cancer. *Clin Infect Dis* 31:451–457, 2000.

McDonald H E, De Bustros S, Sipperley J O. Vitrectomy for epiretinal membrane with *Candida* chorioretinitis. *Ophthalmol* 97:466–469, 1990.

McNamee C J, Wang S, Modry D. Purulent pericarditis secondary to *Candida parapsilosis* and *Peptostreptococcus* species. *Can J Cardiol* 14:85–86, 1998.

McNeil M M, Nash SL, Hajjeh RA, Phelan MA, Conn LA, Plikaytis BD, and Warnock DW. Trends in mortality due to invasive mycotic diseases in the United States, 1980–1997. *Clin Infect Dis* 33:641–647, 2001.

Medoff G, Dismukes W E, Meade RH, III, Moses J M. A new therapeutic approach to *Candida* infections, a preliminary report. *Arch Intern Med.* 130:241–245, 1972.

Mekalanos J J. Environmental signals controlling expression of virulence determinants in bacteria. *J Bacteriol* 174:1–7, 1992.

Melamed R, Leibovitz E, Abramson O, Levitas A, Zucker N, Gorodisher R. Successful non-surgical treatment of *Candida tropicalis* endocarditis with liposomal amphotericin-B (AmBisome). *Scand J Infect Dis* 32:86–89, 2000.

Menezes A V, Sigesmund D A, Demajo W A, Devenyi R G. Mortality of hospitalized patients with *Candida* endophthalmitis. *Arch Intern Med* 154:2093–2097, 1994.

Mermel L A, Stolz S M, Maki D G. Surface antimicrobial activity of heparin-bonded and antiseptic-impregnated vascular catheters (published erratum appears in *J Infect Dis* 168:1342,1993). *J Infect Dis* 167:920–924, 1993.

Merrer J, Dupont B, Nieszkowska A, De Jonghe B, Outin H. *Candida albicans* prosthetic arthritis treated with fluconazole alone. *J Infect* 42:208–209, 2001.

Merz W G, Sandford G R. Isolation and characterization of a polyene-resistant variant of *Candida tropicalis*. *J Clin Microbiol* 9:677–680, 1979.

Merz W G, Karp J E, Schron D, Saral R. Increased incidence of fungemia caused by *Candida krusei*. *J Clin Microbiol* 24:581–584, 1986.

Meunier-Carpentier F, Cruciani M, and Klastersky J. Oral prophylaxis with miconazole or ketoconazole of invasive fungal disease in neutropenic cancer patients. *Eur J Cancer Clin Oncol* 19:43–48, 1983.

Meunier F. Management of candidemia. *N Engl J Med* 331:1371–372, 1994.

Michel C, Courdavault L, al Khayat R, Viron B, Roux P, and Mignon F. Fungal peritonitis in patients on peritoneal dialysis. *Am J Nephrol* 14:113–120, 1994.

Michigan S. Genitourinary fungal infections. *J Urol* 116:390–397, 1976.

Miller L G, Hajjeh R A, Edwards J E Jr. Estimating the cost of nosocomial candidemia in the United States. *Clin Infect Dis* 32:1110, 2001.

Miller D J, Mejicano G C. Vertebral osteomyelitis due to *Candida* species: case report and literature review. *Clin Infect Dis* 33:523–530, 2001.

Minari A, Hachem R, Raad I. *Candida lusitaniae*: a cause of breakthrough fungemia in cancer patients. *Clin Infect Dis* 32:186–190, 2001.

Mitsutake K, Miyazaki T, Tashiro T, Yamamoto Y, Kakeya H. Enolase antigen, mannan antigen, Cand-Tec antigen, and beta-glucan in patients with candidemia. *J Clin Microbiol* 34:1918–1921, 1996.

Monod M, Togni G, Hube B, Sanglard D. Multiplicity of genes encoding secreted aspartic proteinases in *Candida* species. *Molec Microbiol* 13:357–368, 1994.

Montenegro J, Aguirre R, Gonzalez O, Martinez I, Saracho R. Fluconazole treatment of *Candida* peritonitis with delayed removal of the peritoneal dialysis catheter. *Clin Nephrol* 44:60–63, 1995.

Mora-Duarte J, Betts R, Rotstein C, Columbo AL, Thompson-Moya L, Smietana J, Lupinacci R, Sable C, Kartsonis N, Perfect J for the Caspofungin Invasive Candidiasis Study Group. Comparison of caspofungin and amphotericin B for invasive candidiasis. *N Engl J Med* 347;2020–2029, 2002.

Morbidity and Mortality Weekly Report. CDC. Sexually transmitted diseases: Treatment Guidelines 2002. *MMWR* 51:45–48, 2002.

Mori T, Matsumura M, Kanamaru Y, Miyano S, Hishikawa T, Irie S, Oshimi K, Saikawa T, Oguri T. Myelofibrosis complicated by infection due to *Candida albicans*: emergence of resistance to antifungal agents during therapy. *Clin Infect Dis* 25: 1470–1471, 1997.

Morris A B, Sands M L, Shiraki M, Brown R B, Ryczak M. Gallbladder and biliary tract candidiasis: nine cases and review. *Rev Infect Dis* 12:483–489, 1998.

Muehrcke D D. Fungal prosthetic valve endocarditis. *Semin Thorac Cardiovasc Surg* 7:20–24, 1995a.

Muehrcke D D, Lytle B W, Cosgrove D M, III. Surgical and long-term antifungal therapy for fungal prosthetic valve endocarditis. *Ann Thorac Surg* 60:538–543, 1995b.

Murphy O, Gray J, Wagget J, Pedler SJ. *Candida* arthritis complicating long term total parenteral nutrition. *Pediatr Infect Dis J* 16:329, 1997.

Murray P R. Comparison of the lysis-centrifugation and agitated biphasic blood culture systems for detection of fungemia. *J Clin Microbiol* 29:96–98, 1991.

National Committee for Clinical Laboratory Standards (NCCLS). Reference method for broth dilution antifungal susceptibility testing of yeasts. Approved standard M27-A. National Committee for Clinical Laboratory Standards, Wayne, PA, 1997.

Nasser R M, Melgar G R, Longworth D L, Gordon S M. Incidence and risk of developing fungal prosthetic valve endocarditis after nosocomial candidemia. *Dermatol Surg* 23:527–535; discussion 535–536, 1997.

Ng T T, Denning D W. Liposomal amphotericin B (AmBisome) therapy in invasive fungal infections. Evaluation of United Kingdom compassionate use data. *Arch Intern Med* 155:1093–1098, 1995.

Nguyen MH, and Yu VL. Meningitis caused by *Candida* species: an emerging problem in neurosurgical patients. *Clin Infect Dis* 21:323–327, 1995a.

Nguyen MH, Peacock Jr, JE, Tanner DC, Morris AJ, Nguyen ML, Snydman DR, Wagener MM, and Yu VL. Therapeutic approaches in patients with candidemia. Evaluation in a multicenter, prospective, observational study. *Arch Intern Med* 24:29–35, 1995b.

Nguyen MH, Morris AJ, Peacock JE, Tanner DC, Nguyen ML, Snydman DR, Wagener MM, Rinaldi MG, Yu VL. The changing face of candidemia; emergence of non-*albicans Candida* species and antifungal resistance. *Am J Med* 100:617–623, 1996a.

Nguyen M T, Yu V L, Morris A J. *Candida* infection of the arteriovenous fistula used for hemodialysis. *Am J Kidney Dis* 27:596–598, 1996b.

Nguyen M T, Weiss P J, LaBarre R C, Wallace M R. Orally administered amphotericin B in the treatment of oral candidiaisis in HIV-infected patients caused by azole-resistant *Candida albicans*. *J AIDS* 10:1745–1747, 1996c.

Nguyen M H, Nguyen M L, Yu V L, McMahon D, Keys T F, Amidi M. *Candida* prosthetic valve endocarditis: prospective study of six cases and review of the literature. *Clin Infect Dis* 22:262–267, 1996d.

Noyola DE, Fernandez M, Moylett EH, and Baker CJ. Ophthalmologic, visceral, and cardiac involvement in neonates with candidemia. *Clin Infect Dis* 32:1018–1023, 2001.

Nucci M, Colombo A L. Risk factors for breakthrough candidemia. *Eur J Clin Microbiol Infect Dis* 21:209–211, 2002.

Obayashi T, Yoshida M, Mori T, Goto H, Yasuoka A, Iwasaki H, Teshima H, Kohno S, Horiuchi A, Ito A. Plasma (1, 3)-beta-D-glucan measurement in diagnosis of invasive deep mycosis and fungal febrile episodes. *Lancet* 345:17–20, 1995.

O'Day DM, Head WS, Robinson RD, Stern WH, and Freeman JM. Intraocular penetration of systemically administered antifungal agents. *Curr Eye Res* 4:131–134, 1985.

O'Day D M, Foulds G, Williams T E, Robinson R D, Allen R H, Head W S. Ocular uptake of fluconazole following oral administration. *Arch Ophthalmol* 108:1006–1008, 1990.

Odds F C. Ecology of *Candida* and Epidemiology of Candidosis. Odds FC, ed. *Candida and Candidosis*, 2nd ed. London: Bailliere Tindall, 1988.

Odds F C. *Candida albicans*, the life and times of a pathogenic yeast. *J Med Veterin Mycol* 32(Suppl 1):1–8, 1994.

Okamoto G A, Hall J G, Ochs H, Jackson C, Rodaway K, Chandler J. New syndrome of chronic mucocutaneous candidiasis. *Birth Defects Orig Artic Ser* 13:117–125, 1977.

Pagani J J, Libshitz H I. Radiology of *Candida* infections. In: *Candidiasis*, Bodey G P, Fainstein V, eds. New York: Raven Press, 71–84, 1981.

Pappagianis D, Collins M S, Hector R, Remington J. Development of resistance to amphotericin B in *Candida lusitaniae* infecting a human. *Antimicrob Agents Chemother* 16:123–126, 1979.

Papanicolaou G A, Meyers B R, Fuchs W S, Guillory S L, Mendelson M H, Sheiner P, Emre S, Miller C. Infectious ocular complications in orthotopic liver transplant patients. *Clin Infect Dis* 24:1204–1207, 1997.

Pappas,P G, Rex J H, Hamil R J, Larsen R A, Powderly W G, Horowitz H, Kauffman C A, Chapman S W, Lee J, the NIAID-Mycoses Study Group Candidiasis Subproject. Current trends in nosocomial candidemia: Results of a large multicenter study. 35th Annual Meeting of Infectious Diseases Society of America, San Francisco, CA. Abstract 13, 1997.

Parving H. Fluconazole suspension for oropharyngeal candidiasis unresponsive to tablets. *Ann Intern Med* 126:332–333, 1997.

Parrot J. *Cliniques des Noruvea-n s L'athrepsie.*, Leçons Recuellies par Dr. Troisier. G. Masson, Paris, 1877.

Pelz R K, Hendrix C W, Swoboda S M, Diener-West M, Merz W G, Hammond J, Lipsett P A. Double-blind placebo controlled trial of prophylactic fluconazole to prevent *Candida* infections in critically ill surgical patients. *Ann Surg* 233:542–548, 2001.

Pendlebury W W, Perl D P, Munoz D G. Multiple microabscesses in the central nervous system: a clinicopathologic study. *J Neuropathol Exp Neurol* 48:290–300, 1989.

Penk A, Pittrow L. Status of fluconazole in the therapy of endogenous *Candida* endophthalmitis. *Mycoses* 41(Suppl 2):41–44, 1998.

Peoples J B. *Candida* and perforated peptic ulcers. *Surgery* 100:758–764, 1986.

Perraut L E, Jr, Perraut L E, Bleiman B, Lyons J. Successful treatment of *Candida albicans* endophthalmitis with intravitreal amphotericin B. *Arch Ophthalmol* 99:1565–1567, 1991.

Pfaller M A, Cabezudo I, Hollis R, Huston B, Wenzel RP. The use of biotyping and DNA fingerprinting in typing *Candida albicans* from hospitalized patients. *Diagn Microbiol Infect Dis* 13:481–489, 1990.

Pfaller M A, Messer S A, Hollis R J. Variations in DNA subtype, antifungal susceptibility, and slime production among clinical isolates of *Candida parapsilosis*. *Diagn Microbiol Infect Dis* 21:9–14, 1995.

Pfaller MA, Houston A, and Coffmann S. Application of CHRO-Magar *Candida* for rapid screening of clinical specimens for *Candida albicans, Candida tropicalis, Candida krusei,* and *Candida (Torulopsis) glabrata J Clin Microbiol* 34:58–61, 1996.

Pfaller M A, Diekema D J, Jones R N, Sader H S, Fluit A C, Hollis R J, Messer S A, SENTRY Participant Group. International surveillance of bloodstream infections due to *Candida* species: frequency of occurrence and in vitro susceptibilities to fluconazole, ravuconazole, and voriconazole of isolates collected from 1997 through 1999 in the SENTRY Antimicrobial Surveillance Program. *J Clin Microbiol* 39:3254–3259, 2001.

Phillips P, Zemcov J, Mahmood W, Montaner J S, Craib K, Clarke A M. Itraconazole cyclodextrin solution for fluconazole-refractory oropharyngeal candidiasis in AIDS: correlation of clinical response with in vitro susceptibility. *AIDS* 10:1369–1376, 1996.

Phillips P, Shafran S, Garber G, Rotstein C, Smaill F, Fong I, Salit I, Miller M, Williams K, Conly J M, Singer J, Ioannou S. Multicenter randomized trial of fluconazole versus amphotericin B for treatment of candidemia in non-neutropenic patients. Canadian Candidemia Study Group. *Eur J Clin Microbiol Infect Dis* 16:337–345, 1997.

Phillips J R, Karlowicz M G. Prevalence of *Candida* species in hospital-acquired urinary tract infections in a neonatal intensive care unit. *Pediatr Infect Dis J* 16:190–194, 1997.

Philpott-Howard J N, Wade J J, Mufti G J, Brammer K W, Ehninger G. Randomized comparison of oral fluconazole versus oral polyenes for the prevention of fungal infection in patients at risk of neutropenia. Multicentre Study Group. *J Antimicrob Chemother* 31:973–984, 1993.

Pinner R W, Teutsch S M, Simonsen L, Klug L A, Graber J M, Clarke M J, Berkelman R L. Trends in infectious diseases mortality in the United States. *JAMA* 275: 189–193, 1996.

Pittet D, Monod M, Suter PM, Frenk E, and Auckenthaler R. *Candida* colonization and subsequent infections in critically ill surgical patients. *Ann Surg* 220: 751–758, 1994.

Platt R, Polk B F, Murdock B, Rosner B. Risk factors for nosocomial urinary tract infection. *Am J Epidemiol* 124:977–985, 1986.

Polanco A, Mellado E, Castilla C, Rodriguez-Tudela J L. Detection of *Candida albicans* in blood by PCR in a rabbit animal model of disseminated candidiasis. *Diagn Microbiol Infect Dis* 34:177–183, 1999.

Polak A. Multicenter study of the standardization of sensitivity testing of fungi to 5-fluorocytosine and amphotericin B. *Mykosen* 30:306–308, 311–314, 1987.

Ponton J. Diagnostico microbiologico de las micosis. *Rev Iberoam Micol* 19:25–29, 2002.

Powderly W G, Finkelstein D M, Feinberg J, Frame P, He W, van der Horst C, Koletar S L, Eyster M E, Carey J, Waskin H. A randomized trial comparing fluconazole with clotrimazole troches for the prevention of fungal infections in patients with advanced human immunodeficiency virus infection. *N Engl J Med* 332:700–705, 1995.

Prasad J K, Feller I, Thomson P D. A ten-year review of *Candida* sepsis and mortality in burn patients. *Surgery* 101:213–216, 1987.

Quereda C, Polanco A M, Giner C, Sanchez-Sousa A, Pereira E, Navas E, Fortun J, Guerrero A, Baquero F. Correlation between in vitro resistance to fluconazole and clinical outcome of oropharyngeal candidiasis in HIV-infected patients. *Eur J Clin Microbiol Infect Dis*15: 30–37, 1996.

Rabinovici R, Szewczyk D, Ovadia P, Greenspan J R, Sivalingam J J. *Candida* pericarditis: clinical profile and treatment. *Ann Thorac Surg* 63: 1200–1204, 1997.

Rangel-Frausto M S, Wiblin T, Blumberg H M, Saiman L, Patterson J, Rinaldi M, Pfaller M, Edwards JE, Jr, Jarvis W, Dawson J, Wenzel R P. National Epidemiology of Mycoses Survey (NEMIS): variations in rates of bloodstream infections due to *Candida* species in seven surgical intensive care units and six neonatal intensive care units. *Clin Infect Dis* 29:253–258, 1999.

Rantala A, Lehtonen O P, Kuttila K, Havia T, Niinikoski J. Diagnostic factors for postoperative candidosis in abdominal surgery. *Ann Chirurg Gynaecol* 80:323–328, 1991.

Reed B D. Risk factors for *Candida* vulvovaginitis. *Obstet Gynecol Surv* 47:551–559, 1992.

Rentz A M, Halpern M T, Bowden R. The impact of candidemia on length of hospital stay, outcome, and overall cost of illness. *Clin Infect Dis* 27:781–788, 1998.

Revankar S G, Dib O, Kirkpatrick W R, McAtee R K, Fothergill A W, Rinaldi M G, Redding S W, Patterson T F. Clinical evaluation and microbiology of oropharyngeal infection due to fluconazole-resistant *Candida* in human immunodeficiency virus-infected patients. *Clin Infect Dis* 26:960–963, 1998.

Rex J H, Pfaller M A, Rinaldi M G, Polak A, Galgiani J N. Antifungal susceptibility testing. *Clin Microbiol Rev* 6:367–381, 1993.

Rex J H, Bennett J E, Sugar A M, Pappas P G, van der Horst C M, Edwards J E, Washburn R G, Scheld W M, Karchmer A W, Dine A P. A randomized trial comparing fluconazole with amphotericin B for the treatment of candidemia in patients without neutropenia. Candidemia Study Group and the National Institute of Allergy and Infectious Diseases Mycoses Study Group. *N Engl J Med* 331: 325–330, 1994.

Rex J H, Pfaller M A, Galgiani J N, Bartlett M S, Espinel-Ingroff A, Ghannoum M A, Lancaster M, Odds F C, Rinaldi M G, Walsh T J, Barry A L. Development of interpretive breakpoints for antifungal susceptibility testing: conceptual framework and analysis of in vitro-in vivo correlation data for fluconazole, itraconazole, and *Candida* infections. Subcommittee on Antifungal Susceptibility Testing of the National Committee for Clinical Laboratory Standards. *Clin Infect Dis* 24:235–247, 1997.

Rex J H, Walsh T J, Sobel J D, Filler S G, Pappas P G, Dismukes W E, Edwards J E. Practice guidelines for the treatment of candidiasis. Infectious Diseases Society of America. *Clin Infect Dis* 30: 662–678, 2000.

Rex J H, Pappas P G, Karchmer A W, Sobel J D, Edwards J E, Hadley S, Brass C, Vazquez J A, Chapman S W, Horowitz H, Zervos M, Lee J, for the National Institute of Allergy and Infectious Diseases Mycoses Study Group. A randomized and blinded multicenter trial of high-dose fluconazole plus placebo vs. fluconazole plus amphotericin B as therapy of candidemia and its consequences in non-neutropenic patients. In Press, *Clin Infect Dis*, 2003.

Rhoads J L, Wright D C, Redfield R R, Burke D S. Chronic vaginal candidiasis in women with human immunodeficiency virus infection. *JAMA* 257:3105–3107, 1987.

Rikkerink E H, Magee B B, Magee P T. Genomic structure of *Candida stellatoidea*: extra chromosomes and gene duplication. *Infect Immun* 58:949–954, 1990.

Rippon J W. *The Pathogenic Fungi and Pathogenic Actinomycetes*, 3rd ed. Philadelphia, PA: W B Saunders Co., 1988.

Rivett A G, Perry J A, Cohen J. Urinary candidiasis: a prospective study in hospital patients. *Urol Res* 14:183–186, 1986.

Rocco T R, Simms H H. Inadequate proof of adverse outcome due to the use of fluconazole in critically ill patients. *Arch Surg* 135:1114, 2000.

Rotstein C, Bow E J, Laverdiere M, Ioannou S, Carr D, Moghaddam N. Randomized placebo-controlled trial of fluconazole prophylaxis for neutropenic cancer patients: benefit based on purpose and intensity of cytotoxic therapy. The Canadian Fluconazole Prophylaxis Study Group. *Clin Infect Dis* 28:331–340, 1999.

Roupie E, Darmon J Y, Brochard L, Saada M, Rekik N, Brun-Buisson C. Fluconazole therapy of candidal native valve endocarditis. *Eur J Clin Microbiol Infect Dis* 10:458–459, 1991.

Rowen J L, Tate J M, Nordoff N, Passarell L, McGinnis M R. *Candida* isolates from neonates: frequency of misidentification and reduced fluconazole susceptibility. *J Clin Microbiol* 37:3735–3737, 1999.

Rubin R H, Moellering RC, Jr. Clinical, microbiologic and therapeutic aspects of purulent pericarditis. *Am J Med* 59:68–78, 1975.

Rubin J, Kirchner K, Walsh D, Green M, Bower J. Fungal peritonitis during continuous ambulatory peritoneal dialysis: a report of 17 cases. *Am J Kidney Dis* 10:361–368, 1987.

Rubinstein E, Noriega E R, Simberkoff M S, Holzman R, Rahal J J, Jr. Fungal endocarditis: analysis of 24 cases and review of the literature. *Medicine (Baltimore)* 54:331–344, 1975.

Ruhnke M, Schmidt-Westhausen A, Trautmann M. In vitro activities of voriconazole (UK-109,496) against fluconazole-susceptible and -resistant *Candida albicans* isolates from oral cavities of patients with human immunodeficiency virus infection. *Antimicrob Agents Chemother* 41:575–577, 1997.

Russotto S B. The role of *Candida albicans* in the pathogenesis of angular cheilosis. *J Prosthet Dent* 44:243–246, 1980.

Samiy N, D'Amico D J. Endogenous fungal endophthalmitis. *Int Ophthalmol Clin* 36:147–162, 1996.

Samonis G, Anaissie EJ, Rosenbaum B, Bodey G P. A model of sustained gastrointestinal colonization by *Candida albicans* in healthy adult mice. *Infect Immun* 58:1514–1517, 1990.

Sanchez V, Vazquez J A, Barth-Jones D, Dembry L, Sobel J D, Zervos M J. Epidemiology of nosocomial acquisition of *Candida lusitaniae*. *J Clin Microbiol* 30:3005–3008, 1992.

Sanchez V, Vazquez J A, Barth-Jones D, Dembry L, Sobel J D, Zervos M J. Nosocomial acquisition of *Candida parapsilosis*: an epidemiologic study. *Am J Med* 94:577–582, 1993.

Sanchez-Portocarrero J, Martin-Rabadan P, Saldana C J, Perez-Cecilia E. *Candida* cerebrospinal fluid shunt infection. Report of two new cases and review of the literature. *Diagn Microbiol Infect Dis* 20:33–40, 1994.

Sandhu G S, Kline B C, Stockman L, Roberts G D. Molecular probes for diagnosis of fungal infections (published erratum appears in *J Clin Microbiol* 34:1350, 1996.) *J Clin Microbiol* 33:2913–2919, 1995.

Sandven P. Epidemiology of candidemia. *Rev Iberoam Micol* 17:73–81, 2000.

Sanford J P. The enigma of candiduria: evolution of bladder irrigation with amphotericin B for management—from Anecdote to Dogma and a lesson from Machiavelli. *Clin Infect Dis* 16:145–147, 1993.

Savani D V, Perfect J R, Cobo L M, Durack D T. Penetration of new azole compounds into the eye and efficacy in experimental *Candida* endophthalmitis. *Antimicrob Agents Chemother* 31:6–10, 1987.

Savino J A, Agarwal N, Wry P, Policastro A, Cerabona T, Austria L. Routine prophylactic antifungal agents (clotrimazole, ketoconazole, and nystatin) in nontransplant/nonburned critically ill surgical and trauma patients. *J Trauma* 36:20–25; discussion 25–26, 1994.

Saxen H, Hoppu K, Pohjavuori M. Pharmacokinetics of fluconazole in very low birth weight infants during the first two weeks of life. *Clin Pharmacol Ther* 54:269–277, 1993.

Schaberg D R, Culver D H, Gaynes R P. Major trends in the microbial etiology of nosocomial infection. *Am J Med* 91:72S-75S, 1991.

Schaffner A, Bohler A. Amphotericin B refractory aspergillosis after itraconazole: evidence for significant antagonism. *Mycoses* 36:421–424, 1993.

Schectman L B, Funaro L, Robin T, Bottone E J, Cuttner J. Clotrimazole treatment of oral candidiasis in patients with neoplastic disease. *Am J Med* 76:91–94, 1984.

Scheven M, Schwegler F. Antagonistic interactions between azoles and amphotericin B with yeasts depend on azole lipophilia for special test conditions in vitro. *Antimicrob Agents Chemother* 39:1779–1783, 1995.

Schonebeck J. Asymptomatic candiduria. Prognosis, complications and some other clinical considerations. *Scand J Urol Nephrol* 6:136–146, 1972.

Schrank J H, Jr., Dooley D P. Purulent pericarditis caused by *Candida* species: case report and review. *Clin Infect Dis* 21:182–187, 1995.

Schuman P, Capps L, Peng G, Vazquez J, el-Sadr W, Goldman AI, Alston B, Besch C L, Vaughn A, Thompson M A, Cobb M N, Kerkering T, Sobel J D. Weekly fluconazole for the prevention of mucosal candidiasis in women with HIV infection. A randomized, double-blind, placebo-controlled trial. Terry Beirn Community Programs for Clinical Research on AIDS. *Ann Intern Med* 126:689–696, 1997.

Schuman P, Sobel J D, Ohmit S E, Mayer K H, Carpenter CC, Rompalo A, Duerr A, Smith D K, Warren D, Klein R S. Mucosal candidal colonization and candidiasis in women with or at risk for human immunodeficiency virus infection. HIV Epidemiology Research Study (HERS) Group. *Clin Infect Dis* 27:1161–1167, 1998.

Seay R E, Larson T A, Toscano J P, Bostrom B C, O'Leary M C, Uden D L. Pharmacokinetics of fluconazole in immune-compromised children with leukemia or other hematologic diseases. *Pharmacother* 15:52–58, 1995.

Sebti A, Kiehn T E, Perlin D, Chaturvedi V, Wong M, Doney A, Park S, Sepkowitz K A. *Candida dubliniensis* at a cancer center. *Clin Infect Dis* 32:1034–1038, 2001.

Seelig M S, Speth C P, Kozinn P J, Taschdjian C L, Toni E F, Goldberg P. Patterns of *Candida* endocarditis following cardiac surgery: Importance of early diagnosis and therapy (an analysis of 91 cases). *Prog Cardiovasc Dis* 17:125–160, 1974.

Sehhat S, Hazeghi K, Bajoghli M, Touri S. Oesophageal moniliasis causing fistula formation and lung abscess. *Thorax* 31:361–364, 1976.

Semelka R C, Shoenut J P, Greenberg H M, Bow E J. Detection of acute and treated lesions of hepatosplenic candidiasis: comparison of dynamic contrast-enhanced CT and MR imaging. *J Magn Reson Imaging* 2:341–345, 1992.

Shama SK, and Kirkpatrick CH. Dermatophytosis in patients with chronic mucocutaneous candidiasis. *J Am Acad Dermatol* 2:285–294, 1980.

Sherwood J, Gow N A, Gooday G W, Gregory D W, Marshall D. Contact sensing in *Candida albicans*: a possible aid to epithelial penetration. *J Med Veterin Mycol* 30:461–469, 1992.

Silva-Cruz A, Andrade L, Sobral L, Francisca A. Itraconazole versus placebo in the management of vaginal candidiasis. *Int J Gynaecol Obstet* 36:229–232, 1991.

Silveira L H, Cuellar M L, Citera G, Cabrera G E, Scopelitis E, Espinoza LR. *Candida* arthritis. *Rheum Dis Clin North Am* 19:427–437, 1993.

Silverman S, Jr., Luangjarmekorn I, Greenspan D. Occurrence of oral *Candida* in irradiated head and neck cancer patients. *J Oral Med* 39:194–196, 1984.

Singh N. Trends in the epidemiology of opportunistic fungal infections: predisposing factors and the impact of antimicrobial use practices. *Clin Infect Dis* 33:1692–1696, 2001.

Slavin M A, Osborne B, Adams R, Levenstein M J, Schoch H G, Feldman A R, Meyers J D, Bowden R A. Efficacy and safety of fluconazole prophylaxis for fungal infections after marrow transplantation—a prospective, randomized, double-blind study. *J Infect Dis* 171:1545–552, 1995.

Smego R A, Jr., Perfect J R, Durack D T. Combined therapy with amphotericin B and 5-fluorocytosine for *Candida* meningitis. *Rev Infect Dis* 6:791–801, 1984.

Smith J M, Meech R J. The polymicrobial nature of oropharyngeal thrush. *N Z Med J* 97:335–336, 1984.

Sobel J D. Epidemiology and pathogenesis of recurrent vulvovaginal candidiasis. *Am J Obstet Gynecol* 152:924–935, 1985a.

Sobel J D, Muller G, McCormick J F. Experimental chronic vaginal candidosis in rats. *Sabouraudia* 23:199–206, 1985b.

Sobel J D. Pathogenesis and treatment of recurrent vulvovaginal candidiasis. *Clin Infect Dis* 14(Suppl 1):S148–S153, 1992.

Sobel J D, Brooker D, Stein G E, Thomason J L, Wermeling D P, Bradley B, Weinstein L. Single oral dose fluconazole compared with conventional clotrimazole topical therapy of *Candida* vaginitis. Fluconazole Vaginitis Study Group. *Am J Obstet Gynecol* 172:1263–1268, 1995a.

Sobel J D, Vazquez J A. Gastrointestinal and hepatic infections. In: Surawicz CM, Owen RL, eds. *Fungal Infections of the Gastrointestinal Tract*. Philadelphia: W B Saunders, 219–246, 1995b.

Sobel J D, Chaim W. Treatment of *Torulopsis glabrata* vaginitis: retrospective review of boric acid therapy. *Clin Infect Dis* 24:649–652, 1997.

Sobel J D, Faro S, Force R W, Foxman B, Ledger W J, Nyirjesy P R, Reed BD, Summers P R. Vulvovaginal candidiasis: epidemiologic, diagnostic, and therapeutic considerations. *Am J Obstet Gynecol* 178:203–121, 1998.

Sobel J D, Kauffman C A, McKinsey D, Zervos M, Vazquez J A, Karchmer A W, Lee J, Thomas C, Panzer H, Dismukes W E. Candiduria: a randomized, double-blind study of treatment with fluconazole and placebo. The National Institute of Allergy and Infectious Diseases (NIAID) Mycoses Study Group. *Clin Infect Dis* 30:19–24, 2000.

Sobel J D, Kapernick P S, Zervos M, Reed B D, Hooton T, Soper D, Nyirjesy P, Heine M W, Willems J, Panzer H, Wittes H. Treatment of complicated *Candida* vaginitis: comparison of single and sequential doses of fluconazole. *Am J Obstet Gynecol* 185:363–369, 2001a.

Sobel J D, Ohmit S E, Schuman P, Klein R S, Mayer K, Duerr A, Vazquez J A, Rampalo A. The evolution of *Candida* species and fluconazole susceptibility among oral and vaginal isolates recovered from human immunodeficiency virus (HIV)-seropositive and at-risk HIV-seronegative women. *J Infect Dis* 183:286–293, 2001b.

Soll D R. The ins and outs of DNA fingerprinting the infectious fungi. *Clin Microbiol Rev* 13:332–370, 2000.

Solomkin J S, Flohr A B, Quie P G, Simmons R L. The role of *Candida* in intraperitoneal infections. *Surgery* 88:524–530, 1980a.

Solomkin J S, Simmons R L. *Candida* infection in surgical patients. *World J Surg* 4:381–394, 1980b.

Spebar M J, Pruitt BA, Jr. Candidiasis in the burned patient. *J Trauma* 21:237–239, 1981.

Staab J F, Bradway S D, Fidel P L, Sundstrom P. Adhesive and mammalian transglutaminase substrate properties of *Candida albicans* Hwp1. *Science* 283:1535–1538, 1999.

Staib F. Proteolysis and pathogenicity of *Candida albicans* strains. *Mycopathol Mycol Appl* 37:345–348, 1969.

Stamm W E, McKevitt M, Roberts P L, White N J. Natural history of recurrent urinary tract infections in women. *Rev Infect Dis* 13:77–84, 1991.

Sterling T R, Gasser RA, Jr. Ziegler A. Emergence of resistance to amphotericin B during therapy for *Candida glabrata* infection in an immunocompetent host. *Clin Infect Dis* 23:187–188, 1996.

Stern G A, Fetkenhour C L, O'Grady R B. Intravitreal amphotericin B treatment of *Candida* endophthamitis. *Arch Ophthalmol* 95:89–93, 1977.

Stiller R L, Bennett J E, Scholer H J, Wall M, Polak A, Stevens D A. Susceptibility to 5-fluorocytosine and prevalence of serotype in 402 *Candida albicans* isolates from the United States. *Antimicrob Agents Chemother* 22:482–487, 1982.

Strinden W D, Helgerson R B, Maki D G. *Candida* septic thrombosis of the great central veins associated with central catheters. Clinical features and management. *Ann Surg* 202:653–658, 1985.

Stone H H, Kolb L D, Currie C A, Geheber C E, Cuzzell J Z. *Candida* sepsis: pathogenesis and principles of treatments. *Ann Surg* 179:697–711, 1974.

Storfer S P, Medoff G, Fraser V J. Candiduria: Retrospective review in hospitalized patients. *Inf Dis Clin Pract* 3:23–29, 1994.

Sugar A M, Saunders C, Diamond R D. Successful treatment of *Candida* osteomyelitis with fluconazole. A noncomparative study of two patients. *Diagn Microbiol Infect Dis* 13:517–520, 1990.

Sugar A M. Antifungal therapy in CAPD peritonitis-do we have a choice? *Sem in Dialysis* 4:145–146, 1991.

Sugar A M. Use of amphotericin B with azole antifungal drugs: what are we doing? *Antimicrob Agents Chemother* 39:1907–1912, 1995a.

Sugar A M, Hitchcock C A, Troke P F, Picard M. Combination therapy of murine invasive candidiasis with fluconazole and amphotericin B. *Antimicrob Agents Chemother* 39:598–601, 1995b.

Sugarman B, Massanari R M. *Candida* meningitis in patients with CSF shunts. *Arch Neurol* 37:180–181, 1980.

Sullivan D, Coleman D. *Candida dubliniensis*: Characteristics and identification. *J Clin Microbiol* 36:329–334, 1998.

Sullivan D J, Westerneng T J, Haynes K A, Bennett D E, Coleman D C. *Candida dubliniensis* sp. nov.: phenotypic and molecular characterization of a novel species associated with oral candidosis in HIV-infected individuals. *Microbiol* 141:1507–1521, 1995.

Sundstrom P. Adhesins in *Candida albicans*. *Curr Opin Microbiol* 2:353–357, 1999.

Swenson C E, Perkins W R, Roberts P, Ahmad I, Stevens R, Stevens D A, Janoff S. In vitro and in vivo antifungal activity of amphotericin B lipid complex: are phospholipases important? *Antimicrob Agents Chemother* 42:767–771, 1998.

Swindells S, Kleinschmidt D R, Hayes F A. Pilot Study of adjunctive GM-CSF (yeast derived) for fluconazole-resistant oral candidiasis in HIV-infection. *Infect Dis Clin Pract* 6:278–279, 1997.

Tavitian A, Raufman J P, Rosenthal L E, Weber J, Webber C A, Dincsoy H P. Ketoconazole resistant *Candida* esophagitis in patients with acquired immunodefieiency syndrome. *Gastroenterol* 90:443–445, 1986.

Thomas M G, and Ellis-Pegler R B. Fluconazole treatment of *Candida glabrata* peritonitis (letter). *J Antimicrob Chemother* 24:94–96, 1989.

Tollemar J, Hockerstedt K, Ericzon B G, Jalanko H, Ringden O. Liposomal amphotericin B prevents invasive fungal infections in liver transplant recipients. A randomized, placebo-controlled study. *Transplant* 59:45–50, 1995.

Torres-Rojas J R, Stratton C W, Sanders C V, Horsman T A, Hawley H B, Dascomb H E, and Vial L J, Jr. Candidal suppurative peripheral thrombophlebitis. *Ann Intern Med* 96:431–435, 1982.

Treseler C B, Sugar A M. Fungal meningitis. *Infect Dis Clin N Am* 4:789–808, 1990.

Trousseau A. Lectures on Clinical Medicine, delivered on the Hôtel-Dieu, Paris. Trans by Cormack Jr., ed. from 1865 ed., Vol.2., New Sydenham Society, London, 1869.

Tunkel A R, Thomas C Y, Wispelwey B. *Candida* prosthetic arthritis: report of a case treated with fluconazole and review of the literature. *Am J Med* 94:100–103, 1993.

Urbak S F, Degn T. Fluconazole in the treatment of *Candida albicans* endophthalmitis. *Acta Ophthalmol (Copenh)* 70:528–529, 1992.

Utley J R, Mills J, Roe B B. The role of valve replacement in the treatment of fungal endocarditis. *J Thorac Cardiovasc Surg* 69:255–258, 1975.

Uzun O, Ascioglu S, Anaissie E J, Rex J H. Risk factors and predictors of outcome in patients with cancer and breakthrough candidemia. *Clin Infect Dis* 32: 1713–1717, 2001.

Valdivieso M, Luna M, Bodey G P, Rodriguez V, Groschel D. Fungemia due to *Torulopsis glabrata* in the compromised host. *Cancer* 8:1750–1756, 1976.

van Burik J A, Myerson D, Schreckhise R W, Bowden R A. Panfungal PCR assay for detection of fungal infection in human blood specimens. *J Clin Microbiol* 36: 1169–1175, 1998.

van den Anker J N, van Popele N M, Sauer P J. Antifungal agents in neonatal systemic candidiasis. *Antimicrob Agents Chemother* 39:1391–1397, 1995.

van Deventer A J, van Vliet H J, Hop W C, Goessens W H. Diagnostic value of anti-*Candida* enolase antibodies. *J Clin Microbiol* 32:17–23, 1994.

van't Wout J W, Meynaar I, Linde I, Poell R, Mattie H, Van Furth R. Effect of amphotericin B, fluconazole and itraconazole on intracellular *Candida albicans* and germ tube development in macrophages. *J Antimicrob Chemother* 25:803–811, 1990.

Vaudry W L, Tierney A J, Wenman W M. Investigation of a cluster of systemic *Candida albicans* infections in a neonatal intensive care unit. *J Infect Dis* 158:1375–1379, 1988.

Vazquez J A, Beckley A, Donabedian S, Sobel J D, Zervos M J. Comparison of restriction enzyme analysis versus pulsed-field gradient gel electrophoresis as a typing system for *Torulopsis glabrata* and *Candida* species other than *C. albicans*. *J Clin Microbiol* 31: 2021–2030, 1993a.

Vazquez J A, Sanchez V, Dmuchowski C, Dembry L M, Sobel J D, Zervos M J. Nosocomial acquisition of *Candida albicans*: an epidemiologic study. *J Infect Dis* 168:195–201, 1993b.

Vazquez J A, Lundstrom T, Dembry L, Chandrasekar P, Boikov D, Parri M B, Zervos M J. Invasive *Candida guilliermondii* infection: in vitro susceptibility studies and molecular analysis. *Bone Marrow Transplant* 16:849–853, 1995.

Vazquez J A, Gupta S, Villanueva A. Potential utility of recombinant human GM-CSF as adjunctive treatment of refractory oropharyngeal candidiasis in AIDS patients. *Eur J Clin Microbiol Infect Dis* 17:781–783, 1998.

Vazquez J A, Sobel J D, Peng G, Steele-Moore L, Schuman P, Holloway W, Neaton J D. Evolution of vaginal *Candida* species recovered from human immunodeficiency virus-infected women receiving fluconazole prophylaxis: the emergence of *Candida glabrata*? Terry Beirn Community Programs for Clinical Research in AIDS (CPCRA). *Clin Infect Dis* 28:1025–1031, 1999.

Vazquez J A. Therapeutic options for the management of oropharyngeal and esophageal candidiasis in HIV/AIDS patients. *HIV Clin Trials* 1:47–59, 2000.

Vecchiarelli A, Monari C, Baldelli F, Pietrella D, Retini C, Tascini C, Francisci D, Bistoni F. Beneficial effect of recombinant human granulocyte colony-stimulating factor on fungicidal activity of polymorphonuclear leukocytes from patients with AIDS. *J Infect Dis* 171:1448–1454, 1995.

Viale P, Petrosillo N, Signorini L, Puoti M, Carosi G. Should lock therapy always be avoided for central venous catheter-associated fungal bloodstream infections? *Clin Infect Dis* 33:1947–1948; discussion 1949–1951, 2001.

Villanueva A, Arathoon E G, Gotuzzo E, Berman R S, DiNubile M J, Sable C A. A randomized double-blind study of caspofungin versus amphotericin for the treatment of candidal esophagitis. *Clin Infect Dis* 33:1529–1535, 2001.

Vincent J L, Anaissie E, Bruining H, Demajo W, el-Ebiary M, Haber

J. Epidemiology, diagnosis and treatment of systemic *Candida* infection in surgical patients under intensive care. *Intensive Care Med* 24:206–216, 1998.

Viscoli C, Castagnola E, Fioredda F, Ciravegna B, Barigione G, and Terragna A. Fluconazole in the treatment of candidiasis in immunocompromised children. *Antimicrob Agents Chemother* 35: 365–367, 1991.

Voice R A, Bradley S F, Sangeorzan J A, Kauffman C A. Chronic candidal meningitis: an uncommon manifestation of candidiasis. *Clin Infect Dis* 19: 60–66, 1994.

von Eiff M, Zuhlsdorf M, Roos N, Hesse M, Schulten R, van de Loo J. Pulmonary fungal infections in patients with hematological malignancies—diagnostic approaches. *Ann Hematol* 70:135–141, 1995.

Voss A, Pfaller M A, Hollis R J, Rhine-Chalberg J, Doebbeling B N. Investigation of *Candida albicans* transmission in a surgical intensive care unit cluster by using genomic DNA typing methods. *J Clin Microbiol* 33:576–580, 1995.

Wainer S, Cooper P A, Gouws H, Akierman A. Prospective study of fluconazole therapy in systemic neonatal fungal infection. *Pediatr Infect Dis J* 16:763–767, 1997.

Walsh TJ, Bustamente C I, Vlahov D, Standiford H C. Candidal suppurative peripheral thrombophlebitis: recognition, prevention, and management. *Infect Control* 7:16–22, 1986.

Walsh T J, Gray W C. *Candida* epiglottitis in immunocompromised patients. *Chest* 91:482–485, 1987.

Walsh T J, Hathorn J W, Sobel J D, Merz W G, Sanchez V, Maret S M, Buckley H R, Pfaller M A, Schaufele R, Sliva C. Detection of circulating *Candida* enolase by immunoassay in patients with cancer and invasive candidiasis (see comments). *N Engl J Med* 324:1026–1031, 1991.

Walsh T J, Lee J W, Sien T, Schaufele R, Bacher J, Switchenko A C, Goodman T C, Pizzo PA. Serum D-arabinitol measured by automated quantitative enzymatic assay for detection and therapeutic monitoring of experimental disseminated candidiasis: correlation with tissue concentrations of *Candida albicans*. *J Med Veterin Mycol* 32:205–215, 1994.

Walsh T J, Whitcomb P O, Revankar S G, Pizzo P A. Successful treatment of hepatosplenic candidiasis through repeated cycles of chemotherapy and neutropenia. *Cancer* 76:2357–2362, 1995.

Walsh T J, Whitcomb P, Piscitelli S, Figg W D, Hill S, Chanock S J, Jarosinski P, Gupta R, PA. Safety, tolerance, and pharmacokinetics of amphotericin B lipid complex in children with hepatosplenic candidiasis. *Antimicrob Agents Chemother* 41:1944–1948, 1997.

Wang J N, Liu C C, Huang T Z, Huang S S, and Wu J M. Laryngeal candidiasis in children. *Scand J Infect Dis* 29:427–429, 1997.

Weers-Pothoff G, Havermans J F, Kamphuis J F, Sinnige H A, Meis J F. *Candida tropicalis* arthritis in a patient with acute myeloid leukemia successfully treated with fluconazole: case report and review of the literature. *Infection* 25:109–111, 1997.

Wells R S. Chronic mucocutaneous candidiasis: a clinical classification. *Proc R Soc Med* 66:801–802, 1973.

Wengrower D, Or R, Segal E, Kleinman Y. Bronchopulmonary candidiasis exacerbating asthma. Case report and review of the literature. *Respiration* 47: 209–213, 1985.

Wenzel R P, Edmond M B. Severe sepsis-national estimates. *Crit Care Med* 29:1472–1474, 2001.

Wey S B, Mori M, Pfaller M A, Woolson R F, Wenzel R P. Hospital-acquired candidemia. The attributable mortality and excess length of stay. *Arch Intern Med* 148:2642–2645, 1988.

Wheeler R R, Peacock J E, Jr., Cruz J M, Richter J E. Esophagitis in the immunocompromised host: role of esophagoscopy in diagnosis. *Rev Infect Dis* 9:88–96, 1987.

Whelan W L, Kirsch D R, Kwon-Chung K J, Wahl S M, Smith P D. *Candida albicans* in patients with the acquired immunodeficiency

syndrome: absence of a novel of hypervirulent strain. *J Infect Dis* 162:513–518, 1990.

Whelan W L, Delga J M, Wadsworth E, Walsh T J, Kwon-Chung K J, Calderone R, Lipke P N. Isolation and characterization of cell surface mutants of *Candida albicans*. *Infect Immun* 58:1552–1557, 1990.

White M H. Is vulvovaginal candidiasis an AIDS-related illness? *Clin Infect Dis* 22 (Suppl 2):S124–S127, 1996.

Wilcox C M, Darouiche R O, Laine L, Moskovitz B L, Mallegol I, Wu J A. randomized, double-blinded comparison of itraconazole oral solution and fluconazole tablets in the treatment of esophageal candidiasis. *J Infect Dis.* 176:227–232, 1997.

Wilson M L, Davis T E, Mirrett S, Reynolds J, Fuller D, Allen S D, Flint K K, Koontz F, Reller L B. Controlled comparison of the BACTEC high-blood-volume fungal medium, BACTEC Plus 26 aerobic blood culture bottle, and 10-milliliter isolator blood culture system for detection of fungemia and bacteremia. *J Clin Microbiol* 31:865–871, 1993.

Wingard J R, Merz W G, Rinaldi M G, Johnson T R, Karp J E, Saral R. Increase in *Candida krusei* infection among patients with bone marrow transplantation and neutropenia treated prophylactically with fluconazole. *Antimicrob Agents Chemother.* 37:1847–1849, 1991.

Wingard J R. Importance of *Candida* species other than *C. albicans* as pathogens in oncology patients. *Clin Infect Dis* 20:115–125, 1995.

Winston D J, Chandrasekar P H, Lazarus H M, Goodman J L, Silber J L, Horowitz H, Shadduck R K, Rosenfeld C S, Ho W G, Islam, M Z. Fluconazole prophylaxis of fungal infections in patients with acute leukemia. Results of a randomized placebo-controlled, double-blind, multicenter trial. *Ann Intern Med* 118, 7: 495–503, 1993.

Witkin S S. Immunologic factors influencing susceptibility to recurrent candidal vaginitis. *Clin Obstet Gynecol* 34:662–668, 1991.

Witt M D, Imhoff T, Li C, Bayer A S. Comparison of fluconazole and amphotericin B for treatment of experimental *Candida* endocarditis caused by non-*C. albicans* strains. *Antimicrob Agents Chemother* 37:2030–2032, 1993.

Wolfensberger T J, Gonvers M. Bilateral endogenous *Candida* endophthalmitis. *Retina* 18:280–281, 1998.

Wong-Beringer A, Jacobs R A, Guglielmo B J. Treatment of funguria. *JAMA* 267:2780–2785, 1992.

Xu J, Ramos A R, Vilgalys R, Mitchell T G. Clonal and spontaneous origins of fluconazole resistance in *Candida albicans*. *J Clin Microbiol* 38:1214–1220, 2000.

Yap B S, Bodey G P. Oropharyngeal candidiasis treated with a troche form of clotrimazole. *Arch Int Med* 139:656–657, 1979.

Yeaman M R, Soldan S S, Ghannoum M A, Edwards J E Jr., Filler S G, Bayer A S. Resistance to platelet microbicidal protein results in increased severity of experimental *Candida albicans* endocarditis. *Infect Immun* 64:1379–1384, 1996.

Yeo E, Alvarado T, Fainstein V, Bodey G P. Prophylaxis of oropharyngeal candidiasis with clotrimazole. *J Clin Oncol* 3:1668–1671, 1985.

Yoon S A, Vazquez J A, Steffan P E, Sobel J D, Akins R A. High-frequency, in vitro reversible switching of *Candida lusitaniae* clinical isolates from amphotericin B susceptibility to resistance. *Antimicrob Agents Chemother* 43:836–845, 1999.

Zeluff B J. Fungal pneumonia in transplant recipients. *Semin Respir Infect* 5:80–89, 1990.

Zenker P N, Rosenberg E M, Van Dyke R B, Rabalais G P, Daum R S. Successful medical treatment of presumed *Candida* endocarditis in critically ill infants. *J Pediatr* 119:472–477, 1991.

Zingman B S. Resolution of refractory AIDS-related mucosal candidiasis after initiation of didanosine plus saquinavir. *N Eng J Med* 334:1674–1675, 1996.

12

Cryptococcosis

JOHN W. BADDLEY AND WILLIAM E. DISMUKES

Cryptococcosis is a systemic mycosis caused by the encapsulated yeast *Cryptococcus neoformans*, an organism found in soil, often associated with pigeon droppings. Infection most often involves the lungs or central nervous system, and less frequently the blood, skin, skeletal system, and prostate. Since the incidence of cryptococcosis is greatly increased in immunocompromised patients, especially among patients with AIDS and organ transplant recipients, cryptococcosis is considered an opportunistic fungal disease. Treatment of cryptococcosis is based on anatomic site of disease and immune status of the patient. Cryptococcal meningitis is typically treated with induction therapy of amphotericin B with or without flucytosine, followed by a prolonged course of fluconazole. For pulmonary disease, fluconazole is effective therapy in most patients. Chronic maintenance therapy with fluconazole may be required in HIV-infected patients who remain immunosuppressed.

ORGANISM

Microbiology

At least 19 species of the genus *Cryptococcus* have been described (Rippon, 1988), but few are recognized as causing infection in humans. The predominant pathogen is *C. neoformans*, but two other species, *C. albidus*, and *C. laurentii*, have been reported to rarely cause disease in humans (Gluck et al, 1987; Johnson et al, 1998; Kordossis et al, 1998). *Cryptococcus neoformans* is a round or oval encapsulated yeast, measuring approximately 4–6 μm in diameter in clinical specimens, and having a capsule ranging in size from 1 to > 30 μm. In specimens isolated from nature, organisms tend to be smaller and poorly encapsulated (Neilson et al, 1977). Four serotypes, A, B, C, and D, of *C. neoformans* are recognized based on antigenic determinates on the polysaccharide capsule, with serotype A most common. *Cryptococcus neoformans* is further classified into pathogenic varieties: *C. neoformans* var. *neoformans* traditionally included serotypes A and D; and *C. neoformans* var. *gattii* includes serotypes B and C.

Serotype A has been recently identified as a new variety, *C. neoformans* var. *grubii* (Franzot et al, 1999). The *C. neoformans* varieties differ in epidemiology, ecology, and certain biochemical properties. In contrast to var. *neoformans*, variety *gattii* uncommonly infects AIDS patients, is found in tropical areas, and is able to assimilate malate. For a more detailed description of differences between *C. neoformans* varieties, see these two comprehensive references (Kwon-Chung and Bennett, 1984; Mitchell and Perfect, 1995).

The sexual, or perfect state of *C. neoformans*, *Filobasidella neoformans*, a basidiomycete, can be demonstrated by mating the fungus under certain defined conditions (Kwon-Chung, 1976). In this perfect state, mycelia are produced that bear basidiospores 1–3 μm in size. The perfect state has not yet been demonstrated in patients or in nature, so the importance of inhalation of basidiospores in disease acquisition is unknown.

Identification

Cryptococcus neoformans produces white to cream-colored, smooth, mucoid colonies when grown on solid culture media such as blood agar or Sabouraud's dextrose agar. The amount of mucoidness of the colonies is related to the thickness of the capsule. Growth of *Cryptococcus* usually occurs in 36 to 72 hours, and is typically slower than that of *Candida* and *Saccharomyces* species under the same conditions. *Cryptococcus neoformans* grows at 37°C, whereas nonpathogenic species of *Cryptococcus* do not. A distinguishing feature of *C. neoformans* is the ability to produce melanin. On selective media supplemented with niger seed (birdseed agar), smooth brown colonies are formed after several days of incubation. Color reactions on solid media are also useful to distinguish between *C. neoformans* var. *neoformans* (serotypes A, D, and AD), and *C. neoformans* var. *gattii* (serotypes B and C). For example, colonies of serotypes B and C on canavanine-glycine-bromthymol blue (CGB) agar turn the agar blue, while colonies of serotypes A, D, and AD do not illicit a color change (Min and Kwon-Chung, 1986).

Ecology

Cryptococcus neoformans is ubiquitous in the environment. The organism was isolated initially in nature from peach juice in 1894 by Francisco Sanefelice, and was first isolated from soil by Emmons in 1951 (Levitz, 1991). *Cryptococcus neoformans* was isolated from pigeon excrement in 1955, and has since been isolated from multiple geographic sites worldwide, many of which are contaminated by pigeon or other bird excrement. Pigeon droppings are commonly colonized with *C. neoformans*, and may contain greater than 10^6 organisms per gram of fecal material. Pigeons do not appear to develop cryptococcal disease, perhaps due to the pigeon's high body temperature (Emmons, 1955). Although *C. neoformans* is most frequently isolated from pigeon excreta and soil, it has been isolated less commonly from other sources, including fruits and vegetables, dairy products, and excrement from a wide variety of avian species (Staib and Heissenkuber, 1989a).

In contrast to the numerous geographic sites of isolation of *C. neoformans* var. *neoformans*, the isolation of *C. neoformans* var. *gattii* has been more restricted (Levitz, 1991). Variety *gattii* has been isolated from leaves, wood, bark, and air associated with *Eucalyptus camaldulensis* (red river gum) trees, but has not been isolated from bird droppings. The distribution of *E. camaldulensis*, in tropical and subtropical regions such as Southern California, Australia, Southeast Asia, Central Africa, and Brazil, corresponds to areas where cases of cryptococcosis due to *C. neoformans* var. *gattii* are recognized as endemic (Ellis and Pfeiffer, 1990b; Levitz, 1991). However, infections caused by *C. neoformans* var. *gattii* occur in areas without eucalyptus trees, suggesting an additional unidentified environmental source (Chen et al, 1997; Fyfe et al, 2002).

EPIDEMIOLOGY

Because *C. neoformans* is isolated primarily from pigeon droppings and soil, the assumption has been made that infection arises via aerosolized particles from pigeon excrement. This hypothesis has been difficult to confirm, as most patients who develop cryptococcosis do not recall a history of recent exposure to pigeons or their excreta. Exposure to *C. neoformans*, on the basis of serum antibody levels or skin testing, is common among pigeon handlers; however, the incidence of active cryptococcal infections among this population does not appear to be increased (Newberry et al, 1967; Fink et al, 1968). No particular occupational predisposition to cryptococcosis is currently recognized, although data from recent population-based surveillance suggest that outdoor occupations may be associated with an increased risk of cryptococcosis (Hajjeh et al, 1999). Association with pigeons, pigeon excrement, soil, or dust does not increase the likelihood of proven cryptococcosis (Hajjeh et al, 1999).

In the majority of cases, infection with *C. neoformans* is thought to be caused by inhalation of the organism, either in yeast form or perhaps as basidiospores, from an environmental source such as bird droppings or soil. Evidence for this mechanism of acquisition is supported by isolation of cryptococci measuring less than 4 μm, ideal for alveolar deposition, from aerosols associated with soil and pigeon excreta (Powell et al, 1972; Neilson et al, 1977). Unlike other mycoses transmitted by aerosolized particles, outbreaks of cryptococcosis from a particular environmental source rarely occur (Swinne et al, 1989; Levitz, 1991; Fyfe et al, 2002).

While *C. neoformans* has been frequently isolated from pulmonary and skin cultures of healthy, asymptomatic individuals, this fungal organism is not regarded as normal microbial flora in animals or humans (Duperval et al, 1977). Rarely, skin infection can occur after local inoculation, but in most cases, skin disease results from blood-borne dissemination after an initial lung focus of infection. Person-to-person transmission via inhalation of aerosols has not yet been documented, but in several cases, other sources of presumed human-to-human transmission have been described (Beyt and Waltman, 1978; Glaser and Garden, 1985; Kanj et al, 1996). In one report, a recipient of a corneal transplant from a donor with cryptococcosis developed cryptococcal endophthalmitis greater than 2 months after transplantation (Beyt and Waltman, 1978). In a second case, a health-care worker developed cryptococcal skin lesions at the site of an inoculation of blood from a patient with cryptococcemia (Glaser and Garden, 1985). A more recent case was described in which the recipient of a lung transplant developed cryptococcal left lower lobe pneumonia 2 days after transplantation (Kanj et al, 1996). Endotracheal cultures from postoperative day two were positive for *C. neoformans*, although donor lung cultures were positive only for *Rhodotorula* species. However, development of pulmonary cryptococcosis this early in the posttransplant period suggests transmission by the donor organ. Evidence supporting zoonotic transmission of *Cryptococcus* has been recently reported (Nosanchuk et al, 2000). In their description, a clinical isolate from a renal transplant recipient with cryptococcal meningitis was indistinguishable on the basis of molecular genotyping from an isolate present in the feces of the patient's pet cockatoo.

Cryptococcosis occurs in many patients without a recognized immunologic defect, but the large majority of patients have a predisposing factor or underlying disease (Fig. 12–1; Pappas et al, 2001). Evidence is convincing that patients with defects in T-cell-mediated immunity are at increased risk of developing cryptococcal

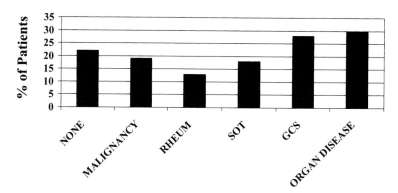

FIGURE 12–1. Underlying conditions in HIV-negative patients with cryptococcosis. RHEUM, rheumatologic disease; SOT, solid organ transplant; GCS, glucocorticosteroid use; ORGAN DISEASE, chronic liver, renal, or lung disease. Adapted from Pappas et al, 2001.

infection. Predisposing conditions include AIDS, systemic corticosteroids, organ transplantation, lymphoreticular malignancies, and sarcoidosis independent of steroid use (Fig. 12–1; Lewis and Rabinovich, 1972; Perfect et al, 1989; Mitchell and Perfect, 1995; Kontoyiannis et al, 2001; Pappas et al, 2001). While diabetes mellitus has been alleged to be a predisposition for cryptococcosis, this association is less clear. Prior to the AIDS epidemic, up to 50% of patients with cryptococcosis had no recognized T-cell immune defect or dysfunction (Lewis and Rabinovich, 1972; Dismukes et al, 1987). In a recent observational study of 306 HIV-negative patients with cryptococcosis, 21% had no significant immune dysfunction or other predisposing condition to cryptococcosis (Fig. 12–1; Pappas et al, 2001). In contrast, among patients with a predisposing condition, chronic organ disease and glucocorticosteroid use were most common (Pappas et al, 2001). Recently, idiopathic CD4 lymphocytopenia has been associated with cryptococcosis in patients with no other predisposing conditions for cryptococcosis (Smith et al, 1993; Kumlin et al, 1997). It is unclear if immune cytopenias predate the onset of disease or result from it.

Before the era of highly active antiretroviral therapy (HAART), the prevalence of cryptococcosis among patients with AIDS was estimated to be between 5% and 10% (Dismukes, 1993; Currie and Casadevall, 1994). With the widespread use of HAART in the United States, the prevalence of cryptococcosis may be decreasing, but is currently unknown. Recent data from four United States geographic areas, prior to use of HAART, showed the annual incidence of cryptococcosis among patients with AIDS to range from 17 to 66 cases per 1000 persons (Hajjeh et al, 1999). By contrast, in non-HIV-infected persons, the annual incidence ranged from 0.2 to 0.9 per 100,000 persons. In Europe, the prevalence of cryptococcosis among AIDS patients is lower than that in the United States (Ellis and Pfeiffer, 1990a; Dromer et al, 1996b). In Africa

and other developing areas, the prevalence of cryptococcosis in patients with AIDS approaches 30%, and is often an AIDS-defining illness (Heyderman et al, 1998).

PATHOGENESIS

Virulence

Among several factors of virulence and pathogenicity for *C. neoformans*, the best characterized include the polysaccharide capsule, thermotolerance (ability to grow at 37°), melanin production, mannitol production, and soluble extracellular constituents. Two in-depth reviews are recommended for more detailed information about factors of virulence and pathogenicity (Mitchell and Perfect, 1995; Buchanan and Murphy, 1998). Here, only two of these factors are discussed. For a particular *C. neoformans* isolate, virulence is attributed to these different factors plus the interaction of the host's immune responses.

The polysaccharide capsule of *C. neoformans* is composed of a backbone of α-1,3-D mannopyranose units with single residues of β-D-xylopyranosyl and β-D-glucuronopyranosyl, and referred to as glucuronoxylomannan (GXM). The capsule is probably the key virulence factor for *C. neoformans*; acapsular mutants are typically avirulent, whereas encapsulated isolates have varying degrees of virulence (Chang and Kwon-Chung, 1994). However, capsule size does not correlate with virulence (Dykstra et al, 1977). The capsule may sometimes protect the organism from host defenses. For example, encapsulated *C. neoformans* cells are not phagocytized or killed by neutrophils, monocytes, or macrophages to the same degree as acapsular mutants (Bulmer and Sans, 1968). In addition, highly encapsulated strains are less able to stimulate T-cell proliferation, and do not enhance the production of cytokines as well as poorly encapsulated or acapsular strains (Collins and Bancroft, 1991; Levitz et al, 1994). Paradoxically, the capsule may also benefit the host response by activation of the alternative complement pathway, therefore enhancing the ability of leukocytes to kill cryptococci (Kozel and Pfrommer, 1986).

Melanin production also appears to be an important virulence factor of *C. neoformans*, based on in vitro and animal in vivo systems. For example, the role of melanin was first demonstrated when naturally occurring *C. neoformans* mutants lacking melanin were found to be less virulent in mice than melanin-producing strains (Kwon-Chung et al, 1982). Melanin is deposited in the inner cell wall of *C. neoformans*, and may resist oxidation, or reactive nitrogen intermediates produced by phagocytes (Wang et al, 1995).

Host Response

Once *C. neoformans* is inhaled, transient colonization of the airways occurs before subsequent spread and establishment of respiratory infection. Given the widespread presence of *Cryptococcus* in the environment, exposure is likely common. However, the incidence of infection is very low, suggesting that most people mount an appropriate host response when exposed to the organism. Development of disease appears to depend on inoculum of inhaled organisms, virulence of the organism, and interaction with the host's cellular immune response. As noted earlier, host defense, especially cell-mediated immunity, is fundamental to protection from cryptococcal infections. After inhalation of the organism, the first line of defense is the alveolar macrophage. In addition, complement-mediated phagocytosis appears to have an important role in initial defense (Kwon-Chung et al, 1992). In vitro, alveolar macrophages are able to bind and phagocytize *C. neoformans* in the presence of human serum containing opsonins such as C3 (Bolanos and Mitchell, 1989). Macrophages from patients with HIV infection tend to be impaired, or defective in both oxidative-dependent and oxidative-independent killing of *C. neoformans* (Harrison and Levitz, 1997). Furthermore, the presence of HIV envelope protein gp 120 inhibits killing of cryptococci by normal macrophages (Pietrella et al, 1998). If initial defense mechanisms in alveoli are ineffective, cryptococci reach the bloodstream and disseminate to other organs, such as the central nervous system (CNS) or prostate. In such sites, additional defense mechanisms are needed to thwart progressive infection. In vitro and in animal models, other cells, including neutrophils, natural-killer cells, macrophage-like microglial cells, and T-cell lymphocytes can kill or inhibit growth of cryptococci (Levitz et al, 1995). Cytokines, especially interleukin-2 and γ-interferon, released by phagocytic cells and lymphocytes, also appear to play an important role in enhancing the killing of *C. neoformans* (Mitchell and Perfect, 1995).

The role of humoral immunity in protection against cryptococcal infections is controversial, but increasing data indicate that this facet of the immune response may play an important role. Antibodies to capsular constituents facilitate clearance of cryptococcal antigen, enhancing antibody-dependent cell-mediated killing, and increasing antifungal activity of leukocytes and natural killer cells (Cassadeval et al, 1995; Lendvai et al, 1998). Preliminary studies with murine monoclonal antibodies directed at cryptococcal capsular polysaccharide are being conducted in humans to assess the potential to decrease circulating cryptococcal antigen (Larsen et al, 2002).

CLINICAL MANIFESTATIONS

Pulmonary Infection

Pulmonary cryptococcal involvement can manifest in a variety of ways, ranging from asymptomatic airway colonization to fulminant respiratory failure with acute respiratory distress syndrome (ARDS)(Murray et al, 1988; Visnegarwala et al, 1998). Most patients are asymptomatic, or will have only mild to moderate respiratory symptoms such as dyspnea, cough, pleuritic chest pain, or rarely, hemoptysis (Campbell, 1966). Constitutional symptoms, such as fever, night sweats, malaise, and weight loss are uncommon in HIV-negative patients unless extrapulmonary disease is also present.

In the immunologically normal host, a diagnosis of respiratory colonization with *Cryptococcus* can be made on the basis of a positive respiratory tract culture without evidence of pulmonary symptoms or abnormalities on chest radiography. Limited data suggest that patients with colonization often may have underlying pulmonary pathology, such as chronic obstructive pulmonary disease (Tynes et al, 1968). The diagnosis of colonization, particularly in the immunocompromised patient, must be interpreted with caution. Because of the propensity of *Cryptococcus* for dissemination to the CNS, a thorough evaluation for extrapulmonary sites of cryptococcal involvement in the immunocompromised host is recommended.

Chest radiography of pulmonary cryptococcal infection may reveal lobar or patchy infiltrates (Fig. 12–2); single or multiple nodular lesions (Fig. 12–3); interstitial infiltrates; mediastinal or hilar adenopathy (Fig. 12–4); circumscribed mass lesions (0.5–7 cm) (Fig. 12–5); or less commonly, pleural effusions or cavitary lesions (Fig. 12–6). In HIV-negative patients, solitary or multiple pulmonary nodules and lobar infiltrates are frequently seen on chest radiography (Feigin, 1983; Khoury et al, 1984; Baddley et al, 2000). By contrast, in patients with AIDS, the most common radiographic

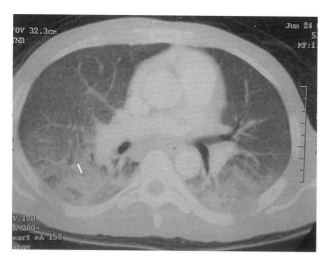

FIGURE 12–2. CT scan showing severe bilateral cryptococcal lobar pneumonia and prominent adenopathy in AIDS patient with fatal disseminated cryptococcosis.

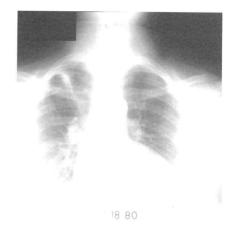

FIGURE 12–4. Cryptococcal lung disease manifest as prominent bilateral hilar adenopathy plus nodule in right upper lobe and patchy pneumonitis in right lower lobe in immunocompetent host.

abnormalities are diffuse, interstitial infiltrates, and lobar, often mass-like, infiltrates (Cameron et al, 1991; Woodring et al, 1996). Pulmonary nodules are less common, but are more likely to cavitate than nodules in patients without immune compromise.

Comparison of pulmonary cryptococcal infection in AIDS patients versus HIV-negative patients reveals important distinctions. In AIDS patients, pulmonary disease plus other sites of involvement are more common. These patients may have a more rapid clinical course, often associated with high mortality (Cameron et al, 1991; Meyohas et al, 1995). The majority of AIDS patients with cryptococcal pneumonia have constitutional symptoms (Cameron et al, 1991), in part explained by increased frequency of concomitant extrapulmonary sites of cryptococcal infection, for example, dissemination to the CNS. The finding of pulmonary cryptococ-

cosis in an AIDS patient warrants thorough evaluation for CNS disease, even in the asymptomatic patient.

Central Nervous System Infection

The most common clinical manifestation of cryptococcosis is central nervous system infection, typically manifested as meningitis, which can be subacute, or chronic in nature. The clinical presentation and course of cryptococcal meningitis vary greatly, and often are related to the immune status or underlying condition of the patient. In general, the signs and symptoms of cryptococcal meningitis among AIDS patients and HIV-negative patients are similar. However, in AIDS pa-

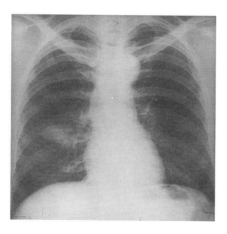

FIGURE 12–3. Well-circumscribed small mass/nodule in patient with underlying systemic lupus erythematosus treated with corticosteroids.

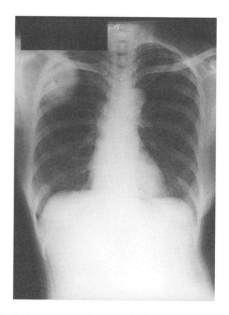

FIGURE 12–5. Large, well circumscribed cryptococcal mass lesion in right upper lobe of immunocompetent host. Mass was excised surgically.

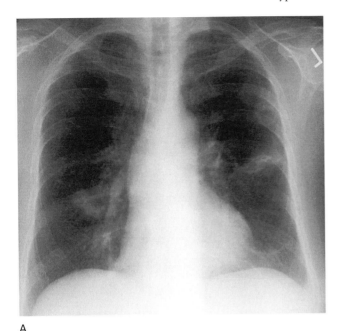

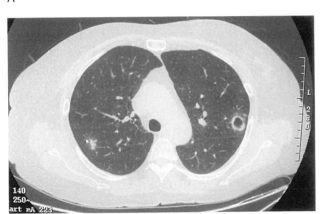

FIGURE 12–6. (*a*) Cryptococcal lung disease manifest as several irregular nodules. (*b*) Note the cavitation of left lung nodule shown on CT scan.

creased intracranial pressure, cryptococcal invasion of cranial nerves, or brain parenchymal lesions (cryptococcomas). The most common symptoms and signs of cranial nerve involvement include decreased visual acuity, blindness (Rex et al, 1993), diplopia, hearing loss, and facial weakness. Seizures, often a reflection of increased intracranial pressure or focal mass lesions, tend to occur later in the course of disease.

Increased intracranial pressure associated with cryptococcal meningitis, especially among patients with AIDS, is a prominent finding. An opening CSF pressure of > 200 mmHg is found in 70% of patients with AIDS (Denning et al, 1991; Graybill et al, 2000). In AIDS patients, high fungal burden is felt to be a contributing factor to increased intracranial pressures. Cryptococci may cause outflow obstruction by blocking passage of CSF across arachnoid villi. In addition, soluble cryptococcal capsular polysaccharide may accumulate in arachnoid villi, leading to alterations in CSF drainage (Graybill et al, 2000). Consequently, routine assessment of suspected cryptococcal meningitis should always include manometry. Imaging of the brain is also important to evaluate for hydrocephalus and potential mass lesions (Fujita et al, 1981). In AIDS patients, other causes of brain lesions, such as *Toxoplasma gondii*, and lymphoma, should be considered. Among AIDS patients with cryptococcal meningitis and increased intracranial pressure, hydrocephalus is an uncommon finding on brain imaging (Poprich et al, 1990). By contrast, in HIV-negative patients with subacute or chronic cryptococcal meningitis, the course is more likely complicated by hydrocephalus caused by obstruction of flow due to inflammation of the basilar meninges (Park et al, 1999), but normal ventricular size in the setting of increased intracranial pressure is not uncommon (Liliang et al, 2002).

Prognostic factors for cryptococcal meningitis have been well characterized in both HIV-negative and HIV-infected patients (Diamond and Bennett, 1974; Dismukes et al, 1987; Saag et al, 1992; van der Horst et al, 1997). Important prognostic factors include the patient's underlying disease or predisposing condition, the burden of organisms, titer(s) of CSF cryptococcal antigen, mental status at baseline, and the ability to amount an inflammatory response in CSF (Saag et al, 1992). For example, in AIDS patients, fewer cells on initial lumbar puncture may signify poor prognosis (Saag et al, 1992). Cryptococcal antigen detection in the CSF may be of prognostic value in certain patient populations. In HIV-negative patients with meningitis, a CSF cryptococcal antigen titer of ≥ 1:8 at the conclusion of ≥ 1 month of therapy correlated with likelihood of relapse (Dismukes et al, 1987). Likewise, in AIDS patients, higher titers of CSF cryptococcal antigen (> 1:1024) at baseline are predictive of poorer out-

tients, onset tends to be more acute, and the course more rapidly progressive, perhaps explained by poor inflammatory response and high burden of organisms in these patients. A wide range of symptoms and signs can be seen with CNS cryptococcosis, but complaints are often mild or nonspecific, and include headache, nausea and vomiting, and malaise. In some instances, patients are even asymptomatic. Altered mental status, somnolence and obtundation may signify advanced disease and a poor prognosis (Saag et al, 1992). Fever is typically low grade, and is more likely to be present in HIV-infected patients (Saag et al, 1992; van der Horst et al, 1997). Unlike in bacterial meningitis, meningismus is uncommon. Cranial nerve dysfunction may occur in up to 30% of patients, and may result from incomes (Saag et al, 1992). However, in AIDS patients with meningitis, serial measurement of cryptococcal antigen titers obtained during acute therapy or prolonged suppression has little role in management (Powderly et al, 1992; Powderly et al, 1994).

Among patients with cryptococcal meningitis, mortality varies from 5% to 25% and most deaths occur within the first few weeks of illness (Saag et al, 1992; van der Horst et al, 1997; Graybill et al, 2000). Recent data suggest that mortality in AIDS patients due to cryptococcosis appears to be decreasing (McNeil et al, 2001).

Skin Infection

Cryptococcal skin lesions are seen in up to 15% of patients with disseminated cryptococcosis, and are most common in HIV patients (Mitchell and Perfect, 1995). Skin disease may manifest as a variety of cutaneous lesions, including pustules, papules, purpura, ulcers, cellulitis, superficial granulomas or plaques, abscesses, and sinus tracts (Mitchell and Perfect, 1995). In AIDS patients, umbilicated papules resembling molluscum contagiosum are frequently present (See Color Fig. 12–7 in separate color insert; Pema et al, 1994; Concus et al, 1998). Cellulitis, characterized by prominent erythema and induration, is often present in patients receiving systemic corticosteroids or other immunosuppressive therapy (See Color Fig. 12–8 in separate color insert; Anderson et al, 1992). Although the majority of cryptococcal skin lesions result from disseminated infection, primary cryptococcal skin infection either by laboratory accidents or other inoculations is well-described (Glaser and Garden, 1995; Casadeval et al, 1994; Neuville et al, 2003).

Skeletal

Cryptococcal lesions of the skeletal system are present in less than 10% of patients with disseminated cryptococcosis (Nottebart et al, 1974; Behrman et al, 1990). Lesions often manifest with soft tissue swelling and tenderness, but lack of symptoms is not uncommon. A single skeletal site is involved most often, with vertebral infection occurring most frequently (Behrman et al, 1990). On radiography, well-circumscribed, osteolytic lesions, which may resemble malignancy, are seen. Cryptococcal septic arthritis is rare, and most often involves the knee joint (Stead et al, 1988).

Other Sites of Infection

Cryptococcal infection can involve many other sites and organ systems. Because of the frequency of positive blood cultures and disseminated disease, particularly in AIDS patients, infection may involve virtually any organ. Not infrequently, cryptococcemia in the absence of a proven site is discovered (Perfect et al, 1983). Additional nonmeningeal, extrapulmonary sites of involvement include the prostate, kidneys, muscle, liver, peritoneum, adrenals, esophagus, heart and aorta, and eyes (Randall et al, 1968; Braman, 1981; Shah et al, 1986; Poblete and Kirby, 1987; Leavitt and Kauffman, 1988; Hurd et al, 1989; Crump et al, 1992). The prostate gland may also serve as a "sanctuary" for *Cryptococcus* pre- and posttreatment (Larsen et al, 1989; Staib et al, 1989b). In one series of HIV-infected patients successfully treated for cryptococcal meningitis, cultures of urine were positive in 9 (22%) of 41 patients at the end of therapy (Larsen et al, 1989).

LABORATORY FINDINGS

A definitive diagnosis of cryptococcosis is made by culture and identification of the organism. Clinical specimens can be examined with an India Ink preparation, a rapid test performed by mixing an equal amount of fluid, CSF, or blood, and nigrosin or Pelikan India ink on a slide. After adding a coverslip and upon viewing, the polysaccharide capsule of *Cryptococcus* will exclude the ink particles and appear as a halo around the organism (See Color Fig. 12–9 in separate color insert). In patients with cryptococcal meningitis, a positive India ink preparation showing budding yeasts surrounded by a capsule is a useful presumptive test for diagnosis. In AIDS patients with cryptococcal meningitis, India ink preparation of CSF will be positive in 60% to 80% of cases (Saag et al, 1992; van der Horst et al, 1997); whereas, in HIV-negative patients the positivity rate is lower (Bennett et al, 1979; Pappas et al, 2001). Presumptive diagnosis of cryptococcosis can also be made by wet preparations of fresh clinical samples, or with the use of Gram stain. However, with these methods, the appearance of cryptococci may be highly variable; therefore, culture should be used for confirmation. Although not specific for the cryptococcal cell wall, Calcofluor white staining may be useful, particularly if few yeast cells are present.

The presumptive diagnosis of cryptococcosis is frequently made on examination of tissue sections. On routine hematoxylin and eosin staining, C. neoformans is difficult to identify. However, Gomori-methenamine silver or periodic acid-Schiff staining does allow identification; the organism can be recognized by its oval shape, and narrow-based budding. With the use of mucicarmine staining (See Color Fig. 12–10 in separate color insert), the cryptococcal capsule will stain rose to burgundy in color and help differentiate C. neoformans from yeast organisms, especially *Blastomyces dermatiditis*, and *Histoplasma capsulatum*.

The diagnosis of cryptococcal meningitis is easier to establish than the diagnosis of pulmonary cryptococcosis. If cryptococcal meningitis is suspected, a lumbar puncture should be performed. Abnormalities in CSF commonly include elevated opening pressure, hypoglycorrhachia, elevated protein, and a lymphocytic pleocytosis. In AIDS patients with cryptococcal meningitis, the CSF formula may be normal, or show only minimal abnormalities (Saag et al, 1992). However, elevated opening pressure is common, and may be seen in 50%–70% of AIDS patients (Graybill et al, 2000). In AIDS patients, lack of white blood cells in the CSF is not unusual and may reflect decreased or absent inflammatory response; furthermore, few white blood cells in CSF is a poor prognostic sign (Saag et al, 1992).

The detection of cryptococcal polysaccharide antigen in CSF or serum is useful in patients with suspected cryptococcosis. After infection is established, cryptococcal polysaccharide becomes solubilized in fluids and can be detected by latex agglutination and quantified. Any positive cryptococcal antigen titer in CSF, or a positive antigen in undiluted CSF should be correlated with clinical findings. A titer of $\geq 1:4$ strongly suggests cryptococcal infection, particularly in the immunocompromised patient. In cryptococcal meningitis, antigen testing is highly sensitive and specific, and may be particularly useful if CSF cultures are negative. Cryptococcal antigen is found in CSF in $> 90\%$ and in serum in $> 70\%$ of patients with cryptococcal meningitis. In AIDS patients with cryptococcal meningitis, sensitivity of the CSF antigen test is even greater (approaching 95%–99%), and titers are often higher, up to $1:10^6$ (Saag et al, 1992; van der Horst et al, 1997). In HIV-negative patients with pulmonary cryptococcosis, serum cryptococcal antigen will be positive in 25%–56% of patients (Aberg et al, 1999; Pappas et al, 2001).

With cryptococcal antigen testing, it is important to use proper controls to eliminate errors in testing. The presence of rheumatoid factor may cause a false-positive result, as will the presence of polysaccharide from *Trichosporon asahii* (*beigelii*) (Campbell et al, 1985). In addition, false-negative cryptococcal antigen results, although rare, may be due to low numbers of organisms invading the CSF, infection by poorly or nonencapsulated strains, high titers of antigen (prozone phenomenon), low titers of antigen, and immune complexes (Mitchell and Perfect, 1995).

Either routine bacteriologic or mycologic media will facilitate culture of *C. neoformans*. In patients with AIDS and cryptococcal meningitis, blood and CSF cultures will be positive in 55% and 95%, respectively (Saag et al, 1992; van der Horst et al, 1997). In a recent study of HIV-negative patients with cryptococcal meningitis, CSF cultures were positive in 89% of patients tested (Pappas et al, 2001). For blood cultures, the lysis-centrifugation (isolator) technique appears to be the most sensitive method to identify *C. neoformans* (Tarrand et al, 1991).

The methods of in vitro antifungal susceptibility testing for *C. neoformans* against a variety of antifungal agents have been standardized (National Committee for Clinical Laboratory Standards, 1997), although interpretive breakpoints for the antifungal agents against *C. neoformans* have yet to be defined. Most *C. neoformans* isolates appear susceptible to common antifungal agents, including amphotericin B, flucytosine, fluconazole, and itraconazole (Brandt et al, 2001). The newer triazoles voriconazole, ravuconazole, and posaconazole, also appear active in vitro against *C. neoformans* (Pfaller et al, 1999), while the echinocandin class of antifungals has poor activity (Bartizal et al, 1998). Several recent reports indicate the potential for microbiological resistance to fluconazole and clinical failure among patients with cryptococcosis (Witt et al, 1996; Armengou et al, 1997; Aller et al, 2000). Susceptibility testing, although not routinely recommended, may be useful to evaluate relapse or recurrence of disease among AIDS patients receiving maintenance fluconazole therapy.

TREATMENT

Treatment of cryptococcosis is based on the sites of involvement and the underlying immunologic status of the patient. For patients with pulmonary disease, the aims of therapy are to eradicate disease, and to prevent dissemination to the CNS. For patients with CNS disease, the aims of therapy are to eradicate or control the infection, adequately manage elevated intracranial pressure, and prevent long-term neurologic sequelae. Prior to 1950, before the availability of amphotericin B, surgical intervention for pulmonary disease was the only therapeutic option available, and cryptococcosis was associated with high mortality. With the availability of amphotericin B in the 1950s and its use as a single agent for cryptococcosis, outcomes were significantly improved, but adverse reactions to amphotericin B were frequently encountered. Flucytosine was found to be an effective drug in vitro for cryptococcosis, and became available for clinical use in 1972. It was used with moderate success for cryptococcal meningitis and pneumonia; however, single-drug therapy with flucytosine led to rapid emergence of resistance, and flucytosine use as a single agent has, for the most part, been abandoned (Hospenthal and Bennett, 1998). Combination therapy with amphotericin B and flucytosine, first employed in a large clinical trial in 1979, was successful in 60%–85% of patients (Bennett et al, 1979; Dismukes et al, 1987). In addition, the availability of the triazoles in the early 1990s led to simplification of the primary regimen for cryptococcal meningitis, utilizing, for example, shorter courses of combination amphotericin B and flucytosine followed by prolonged oral

TABLE 12–1. *Treatment of Cryptococcal Infection in the HIV-Negative Patient*

Pulmonary Disease

A. Colonization*
   1) Observation in the immunocompetent patient
   2) Fluconazole 200–400 mg daily for 6–12 months

B. Asymptomatic or minimally symptomatic disease
   1) Fluconazole 200–400 mg/day for 6–12 months (Dromer et al, 1996a; Pappas et al, 2001)
   Alternative: Close observation without therapy is a consideration

C. Mild to moderate disease
   1) Fluconazole 200–400 mg/day for 6–12 months (Yamaguchi et al, 1996; Dromer et al, 1996a; Saag et al, 2000)
   Alternative: Itraconazole 200–400 mg/day for 6–12 months (Denning et al, 1989)

D. Severe or progressive disease, or azole drug not an option
   Amphotericin B 0.5–1.0 mg/kg/day for a total dose of 1–2 g. This may be followed by oral fluconazole in selected patients (Kerkering et al, 1981; Dromer et al, 1996a; Saag et al, 2000)
   Alternative: 1) regimens similar to those used for CNS disease, as described below
                2) Surgical resection in selected cases refractory to chemotherapy

CNS Disease

Amphotericin B 0.5–1.0 mg/kg/day plus flucytosine 100 mg/kg/day for 2 weeks followed by fluconazole 400 mg/day for 8–12 weeks[†] (White et al, 1992; van der Horst et al, 1997)
Alternative: Amphotericin B 0.5–1.0 mg/kg/day plus flucytosine 100 mg/kg/day for 4–6 weeks (Bennett et al, 1979; Dismukes et al, 1987)
Adjunctive therapy: see text

*Colonization is defined as a positive respiratory tract culture without signs or symptoms of pulmonary disease or radiographic abnormalities.
[†]Chronic suppressive fluconazole for 3–6 months should be considered for patients with persistent immunosuppression, i.e., transplant recipients.

therapy with azoles, primarily fluconazole, and good efficacy (Saag et al, 1992; Dismukes, 1993; van der Horst et al, 1997). Recently, concensus guidelines for the treatment of cryptococcosis have been developed (Saag et al, 2000).

Treatment in the HIV-Negative Patient

Pulmonary Disease. The presentation of pulmonary cryptococcosis in the HIV-negative patient can vary widely, ranging from colonization, to asymptomatic disease, to fulminant pneumonia or ARDS (Table 12–1; Kerkering et al, 1981). Treatment data from clinical trials among HIV-negative patients with pulmonary infection are limited (Yamaguchi et al, 1996; Dromer et al, 1996a; Pappas et al, 2001), and questions remain about which populations require therapy, and the optimal dosage and duration of therapy. Although few clinical trials, particularly in the era of effective azole therapy, have addressed risk factors for CNS dissemination among patients with pulmonary cryptococcal infection (Kerkering et al, 1981; Baddley et al, 2000), most authorities recommend lumbar puncture in immunocompromised patients and those with systemic symptoms.

In patients with normal immunologic function and colonization (defined as positive respiratory tract cultures with negative CXR and absence of symptoms), observation is recommended. Prior to the availability of potent oral azole antifungal agents, immunocompetent patients with an abnormal CXR and asymptomatic disease or mild disease were frequently observed, as many such patients did well without therapy (Hammerman et al, 1973; Kerkering et al, 1981). However, with the availability of oral azole therapy, currently most immunocompetent patients with pulmonary disease are treated (Pappas et al, 2001). In contrast, all patients with immune compromise and colonization (i.e., asymptomatic with negative CXR and positive respiratory tract cultures) should receive therapy. If a decision to treat is made, oral fluconazole at a dose of 200–400 mg/day for 6–12 months is recommended (Saag et al, 2000; Dromer et al, 1996a; Yamaguchi et al, 1996). In HIV-negative patients with immunocompromising conditions and asymptomatic or mild-to-moderate disease, treatment should be initiated both to prevent CNS dissemination as well as eradicate symptoms (Kerkering et al, 1981; Aberg et al, 1999; Saag et al, 2000). Fluconazole at a dose of 200–400 mg daily is a suitable regimen and is associated with improvement in > 80% of cases (Dromer et al, 1996a; Yamaguchi et al, 1996; Pappas et al, 2001). Therapy should continue beyond resolution of symptoms and CXR abnormalities. Most experts recommend therapy for 6–12 months duration (Dromer et al, 1996a; Yamaguchi et al, 1996; Saag et al, 2000). The optimal length of therapy has not yet been determined from clinical trials, but factors to be considered include resolution of symptoms and radiographic findings, persistent immunosuppression, underlying disease, and a persistently elevated serum cryptococcal antigen titer. Itraconazole 200–400 mg daily, although not FDA approved for the treatment of cryptococcosis, is an alternative oral drug to fluconazole (Denning et al, 1989).

For HIV-negative patients with severe pulmonary disease or progressive disease, or for whom azole therapy is not an option, amphotericin B should be given at a dose of 0.5–1.0 mg/kg/day for a total dose of 1 to 2 grams (Saag et al, 2000). In HIV-negative patients with renal insufficiency, lipid preparations of amphotericin B should be substituted (Coker et al, 1993; Sharkey et al, 1996; Leenders et al, 1997; Hamill et al, 2002). Other drug regimens for severe cryptococcal disease are similar to those of patients with CNS disease and are described below, and in Table 12–1.

Surgical intervention for pulmonary cryptococcosis may be required for removal of large mass lesions or areas of severe consolidation that are refractory to antifungal therapy (Temeck et al, 1994).

CNS Infection. Early studies among HIV-negative patients with CNS cryptococcosis were important in defining the efficacy of combination therapy with amphotericin B and flucytosine, and duration of therapy among immunocompromised patients (Bennett et al, 1979; Dismukes et al, 1987). In the first prospective study of cryptococcal meningitis in 50 HIV-negative patients (Bennett et al, 1979), combination therapy with low-dose amphotericin B (0.3 mg/kg/day) plus high-dose flucytosine (150 mg/kg/day) given for 6 weeks was compared to amphotericin B therapy alone (0.4 mg/kg/day) given for 10 weeks. Combination therapy resulted in higher rates of cure and improvement, fewer relapses, and more rapid sterilization of CSF (P < 0.001). Adverse reactions to flucytosine were seen in 11 (32%) of 34 patients, necessitating discontinuation of flucytosine in 6. While the authors concluded that combination therapy was superior to amphotericin B alone, concerns were expressed about the low dosage of amphotericin B and high dosage of flucytosine used in the two arms of the study.

The next prospective study attempted to better address duration of therapy among patients with cryptococcal meningitis by comparing combination therapy with amphotericin B (0.3 mg/kg/day) and flucytosine (150 mg/kg/day) for 4 vs. 6 weeks (Dismukes et al, 1987). Note that the treatment regimens employed here were similar to those used in the initial trial (Bennett et al, 1979). In the second study, 91 patients were randomized to receive either 4 (45 patients) or 6 (46 patients) weeks of therapy. Among randomized patients treated for 4 weeks, cure or improvement was noted in 75%, compared with 85% cure or improvement among patients treated for 6 weeks. Patients who received 4 weeks of therapy had a higher relapse rate (27%) when compared with patients who received 6 weeks of therapy (16%). Toxicities of the regimens in both groups were similar, and were most often azotemia, leukopenia, and diarrhea (Stamm et al, 1987). Among 23 non-

randomized transplant recipients who were protocol-adherent, 16 (70%) of 23 were cured or improved, but 7 (30%) relapsed. From this study, significant baseline predictors of a favorable response included headache, normal mental status, and a CSF white cell count above 20/mm³. The authors concluded that important considerations in determining duration of therapy should include the patient's underlying disease and immune status, and severity of meningitis.

Few other studies are available that address treatment of cryptococcal CNS disease in HIV-negative patients (Dromer et al, 1996a; Pappas et al, 2001). Dromer and colleagues reviewed retrospectively 83 cases of meningeal and extrameningeal cryptococcosis in HIV-negative French patients, with emphasis on the comparison of efficacy of amphotericin B and fluconazole (Dromer et al, 1996a). Patients with more severe infections, such as meningitis, or those with higher CSF cryptococcal antigen titers, were more likely to receive amphotericin B. However, a subgroup of 25 patients received fluconazole alone for cryptococcal meningitis; 68% were cured with this regimen. A more recent retrospective study by Pappas and colleagues reported findings in 306 patients from 15 U.S. medical centers, comprising the largest series to date of HIV-negative patients with cryptococcosis (Pappas et al, 2001). As in the Dromer study, patients with CNS disease were more likely to receive amphotericin B, alone, or in combination. The most common regimen employed was induction therapy with amphotericin B and flucytosine, followed by consolidation therapy with fluconazole as described for HIV-infected patients. Of 107 patients who received induction therapy with amphotericin B and flucytosine, 90 (84%) were cured or improved. In the Pappas study, only 8 of 154 patients with meningitis were treated with fluconazole alone; 7 were cured or improved.

Rarely, intrathecal or intraventricular therapy with amphotericin B is required for refractory cases in addition to systemic therapy, and may be administered directly, or via a subcutaneous Ommaya reservoir. (Diamond and Bennett, 1973; Polsky et al, 1986). Amphotericin B at a maximum dose of 0.5 mg is given daily for intraventricular therapy, and two to three times weekly for intrathecal therapy; the maximum daily dose should be achieved after gradually increasing from an initial dose of 0.025 mg. Difficulties in administration and complications of therapy are frequently encountered (Polsky et al, 1986).

Much of the recent treatment recommendations for HIV-negative patients with CNS cryptococcal disease have been extrapolated from results of more recent studies in HIV-infected patients (Coker et al, 1993; Leenders et al, 1997; Sharkey et al, 1996; Saag et al, 1992; van der Horst et al, 1997; Hamill et al, 2002).

Specific issues addressed by these studies include use of higher doses of amphotericin B (0.5–1.0 mg/kg/day) (Saag et al, 1992; van der Horst et al, 1997); substitution of lipid amphotericin B formulations in patients with renal insufficiency (Coker et al, 1993; Sharkey et al, 1996; Leenders et al, 1997; Hamill et al, 2002); and treatment with an induction regimen of amphotericin B plus flucytosine for 2 weeks followed by a consolidation regimen with fluconazole for an additional 8–12 weeks (van der Horst et al, 1997). For details, see the section on treatment of CNS disease in HIV-infected patients. The authors favor the induction/consolidation approach for the treatment of cryptococcal meningitis in HIV-negative patients.

Although no prospective studies have addressed the use of maintenance or suppressive therapy for HIV-negative patients who have been successfully treated for cryptococcal disease, many experts recommend several months of additional maintenance therapy with oral fluconazole, 200 mg/day, for selected patients who remain persistently immunocompromised after initial treatment. A recent observation noted that cryptococcal CNS parenchymal lesions may persist radiographically for months or years after completion of therapy, and do not necessarily signify relapse or recurrence of disease (Hospenthal and Bennett, 2000).

Other Sites of Disease. HIV-negative patients infrequently present with cryptococcal disease at other sites in the absence of pulmonary or CNS infection. Other infections may include skin lesions, abscesses, cryptococcemia, or positive urine cultures. In HIV-negative patients, few studies address treatment for these entities (Pappas et al, 2001). For the majority of patients, treatment is recommended; however, no preferred regimen has been identified. In a retrospective review of 40 HIV-negative patients with cryptococcal disease at non-CNS and nonpulmonary sites, 36 (90%) received antifungal therapy, and 25 (63%) were successfully treated (Pappas et al, 2001). Multiple regimens were used: 20 evaluable patients received amphotericin B alone or in combination with flucytosine or fluconazole, and 12 (60%) of these 20 were cured or improved; 12 other patients received fluconazole alone and all were cured or improved.

Treatment in the HIV-Infected Patient

Pulmonary Disease. The diagnosis of cryptococcal pneumonia in HIV-infected patients is difficult, as the clinical signs and symptoms and radiographic findings can often be nonspecific and mimic disease by other pathogens (Table 12–2). Since there have been no controlled trials that evaluate the treatment of pulmonary

cryptococcal infection in HIV-infected patients, the treatment of choice and duration of therapy have yet to be defined. Because of the advanced immunosuppressed state of the HIV-infected patient and the propensity of Cryptococcus to cause CNS disease, all patients with pulmonary disease should be treated (Saag et al, 2000).

Patients who are asymptomatic, or have mild-to-moderate symptoms with positive respiratory tract cultures appear to be good candidates for therapy with oral fluconazole 200–400 mg daily (Jones et al, 1991; Saag et al, 2000). Itraconazole 200–400 mg daily may be used as a second-line oral therapy (Denning et al, 1991). While fluconazole plus flucytosine for 10 weeks has been used for HIV-infected patients with cryptococcal meningitis, there is minimal evidence to suggest it as an alternative therapy for patients with pulmonary disease (Larsen et al, 1994). For patients with severe or progressive pulmonary disease, or for patients who cannot tolerate azole therapy, treatment should be similar to recommendations for CNS disease, as described below, and in Table 12–2.

Length of therapy should be lifelong, unless immune reconstitution occurs as a consequence of HAART (Masur et al, 2002). For a detailed discussion of this topic, see section on maintenance therapy under treatment of the HIV-infected patient with CNS infection.

CNS Infection. Given the increased number of cases of cryptococcal meningitis in AIDS patients, many important trials focusing on treatment have been conducted in this population during the last 2 decades. These studies have demonstrated the efficacy of higher doses of amphotericin B, the safety and efficacy of oral azole antifungal drugs in the treatment of CNS disease, and the importance of adequate management of elevated intracranial pressure associated with cryptococcal meningitis.

Based on success rates of 75% to 85% in earlier studies of combination therapy with amphotericin B and flucytosine among HIV-negative patients with cryptococcal meningitis (Bennett et al, 1979; Dismukes et al, 1987), AIDS patients with CNS disease were initially treated with combination therapy for prolonged periods. However, early reports during the late 1980s suggested that use of flucytosine in HIV-infected patients was frequently associated with cytopenias, and offered no survival benefit or improvement in relapse rate when compared to single therapy with amphotericin B (Chuck and Sande, 1989). Moreover, success rates with amphotericin B (0.3–0.5 mg/kg/day) with or without flucytosine were only 40%–50% among patients with AIDS (Kovacs et al, 1985; Zuger et al, 1986). Because of concerns for toxicity of flucytosine, decreased success rates, and the evolving availability of potent oral

TABLE 12–2. *Treatment of Cryptococcal Infection in the HIV-infected Patient*

Pulmonary Disease

A. Asymptomatic or mild to moderate disease

Fluconazole 200–400 mg/day as lifelong therapy* (Jones et al, 1991)
  Alternatives: Itraconazole 400 mg/day as lifelong therapy* (Denning et al, 1989)
  Fluconazole 400 mg/day plus flucytosine 100–150 mg/kg/day for 10 weeks (Larsen et al, 1994)

B. Severe, progressive disease

Regimens similar to those for CNS disease

CNS Disease

Amphotericin B 0.7–1.0 mg/kg/day plus flucytosine 100 mg/kg/day for 2 weeks followed by fluconazole 400 mg/day for 8–12 weeks (Saag et al, 1992; van der Horst et al, 1997).
  Alternative: Itraconazole 400 mg/day may be substituted for fluconazole
Amphotericin B 0.7–1.0 mg/kg/day plus flucytosine 100 mg/kg/day for 6–10 weeks (Larsen et al, 1990; Saag et al, 1992; White et al, 1992)
Amphotericin B 0.7–1.0 mg/kg/day for 6–10 weeks (Saag et al, 1992)
Fluconazole 400 mg/day plus flucytosine 150 mg/kg/day for 10 weeks (Larsen et al, 1994; Mayanja-Kizza et al, 1998)
Fluconazole 400–1000 mg/day for 10–12 weeks (Berry et al, 1992; Saag et al, 1992; Haubrich et al, 1994; Menichetti et al, 1996)
Itraconazole 200 mg/day for 10–12 weeks (Denning et al, 1989; de Gans et al, 1992)

Maintenance Therapy*

Fluconazole 200 mg/day (Bozzette et al, 1991; Powderly et al, 1992; Saag et al, 1999)
  Alternatives: Amphotericin B 1 mg/kg/week (Powderly et al, 1992)
       Itraconazole 200–400 mg/day (Saag et al, 1999)

*Lifelong maintenance therapy may be discontinued in selected patients who achieve immune reconstitution with highly active antiretroviral therapy (Aberg et al, 2002; Masur et al, 2002)
  Note: Lipid formulations of amphotericin B should be substituted for amphotericin B in patients with renal insufficiency (Coker et al, 1993; Sharkey et al, 1996; Leenders et al, 1997; Hamill et al, 2002).
  Note: Patients receiving flucytosine should have renal function routinely monitored, as plasma concentrations of flucytosine may increase to toxic levels in patients with renal impairment. Dose adjustment should be made as necessary with use of a nomogram, or monitoring of flucytosine levels. Serum flucytosine levels should be measured 2 hours after the dose, with optimal levels between 50 and 100 μg/ml.
  Adapted from Saag et al, 2000.

azoles, fluconazole and itraconazole, subsequent studies evaluated novel regimens for primary therapy of CNS cryptococcal disease (Larsen et al, 1990; de Gans et al, 1992; Saag et al, 1992).

In a small study of 21 patients with AIDS and cryptococcal meningitis, Larsen and colleagues (1990) compared combination therapy with amphotericin B (0.7–1.0 mg/kg/day) plus flucytosine (150 mg/kg/day) to fluconazole (400 mg/day) alone. Clinical and mycologic failure was more common in patients who received fluconazole, particularly in patients with severe disease. In fact, the study was discontinued prematurely because of the higher mortality rate in fluconazole-treated patients. Perhaps the most important finding in this study, reported in 1990, was the successful treatment in all 6 patients who received higher doses of amphotericin B as part of the combination regimen. In a second small study of 28 patients with presumed cryptococcal meningitis by De Gans and colleagues, reported in 1992, itraconazole 200 mg twice daily was compared to combination therapy with amphotericin B (0.3 mg/kg/day) plus flucytosine (150 mg/kg/day), both administered for 6 weeks (de Gans et al, 1992). Among patients who received itraconazole, 5 (42%) of 12 achieved a complete response, compared with all 10 patients who received amphotericin B plus flucytosine.

In contrast to these two small trials, two large sequential trials were jointly conducted by the National Institute of Allergy and Infectious Diseases (NIAID) Mycoses Study Group (MSG) and the NIAID AIDS Clinical Trials Group (ACTG) in the 1990s. The initial trial compared amphotericin B (0.3 mg/kg/day) with fluconazole (200 mg/d) in the treatment of AIDS-associated cryptococcal meningitis (Saag et al, 1992). Flucytosine as combination therapy with amphotericin B was optional, and was utilized in only 9 patients. Treatment was successful in 34% of 131 fluconazole recipients, compared with 40% of 63 amphotericin B recipients. Overall mortality was similar in both groups, 18% in patients who received fluconazole, vs. 14% in patients who received amphotericin B (p = 0.48). However, mortality during the first 2 weeks was higher among patients receiving fluconazole, and conversion of CSF cultures to negative was less rapid in fluconazole-treated patients. While this study showed no significant difference between the 2 arms, the results emphasized the need for a more effective primary regimen for the treatment of cryptococcal meningitis. In addition, this study also demonstrated the potential role of fluconazole as part of a new treatment regimen.

The second joint study was conducted to evaluate higher doses of amphotericin B, lower doses of flucytosine, and the safety and efficacy of oral azoles in the treatment of AIDS-associated CNS cryptococcosis (van der Horst et al, 1997). Patients were randomized to receive 2 weeks of induction therapy with combination amphotericin B (0.7 mg/kg/day) plus flucytosine (100 mg/kg/day) (202 patients) or amphotericin B alone (0.7 mg/kg/day) (179 patients). At the end of 2 weeks of therapy, if entry criteria were met, patients were again randomized to receive 8 weeks of consolidation treatment with oral fluconazole 400 mg per day or oral itraconazole 400 mg per day. At the end of 2 weeks, CSF cultures for *C. neoformans* were negative in 60% of patients who received combination amphotericin B and flucytosine, compared with 51% of amphotericin B alone treated patients ($p = 0.06$). However, clinical outcomes at 2 weeks did not differ significantly between the 2 groups. At the end of the 10-week induction and consolidation treatment period, clinical responses were also similar between the two groups, with 68% of fluconazole-treated patients responding, compared with 70% response among itraconazole-treated patients. Negative CSF cultures were observed in 72% of patients who received fluconazole, compared with 60% of patients who received itraconazole. The addition of flucytosine in the first 2 weeks and treatment with fluconazole over the next 8 weeks were independently associated with CSF sterilization. The use of higher dose amphotericin B plus lower-dose flucytosine was associated with more effective CSF sterilization and decreased mortality at 2 weeks when compared with previous studies of combination therapy. Fluconazole and itraconazole were both effective as consolidation therapy, although fluconazole appeared to be more rapid in terms of CSF sterilization. This trial established the concept of induction and consolidation therapy as an attractive treatment regimen for CNS cryptococcosis.

For HIV-infected patients with cryptococcal meningitis and renal insufficiency, use of lipid formulations of amphotericin B should be considered based on the results of 4 trials (Coker et al, 1993; Sharkey et al, 1996; Leenders et al, 1997; Hamill et al, 2002). Response rates of 86% were seen in patients receiving amphotericin B lipid complex at a dose of 5mg/kg/day (Sharkey et al, 1996), and in 65% to 80% of patients receiving liposomal amphotericin B at a dose of 3–6 mg/kg/day (Coker et al, 1993; Leenders et al, 1997; Hamill et al, 2002). The optimal doses of lipid preparations for cryptococcosis have not yet been established.

Although less well studied, other therapeutic options for CNS cryptococcal disease in AIDS patients have been employed, but are considered second-line options. These include fluconazole alone at higher doses (800–1000 mg daily) (Berry et al, 1992; Haubrich et al, 1994; Menichetti et al, 1996), itraconazole alone (Denning et al, 1989; de Gans et al, 1992), and com-

bination therapy with fluconazole and flucytosine (Larsen et al, 1994; Mayanja-Kizza et al, 1998). Combination therapy with fluconazole and flucytosine appears more effective than fluconazole alone, but is also more toxic (Larsen et al, 1994; Mayanja-Kizza et al, 1998). Itraconazole at a dose of 400 mg daily has been used to treat a small number of HIV-infected patients with CNS disease, with varying results (Denning et al, 1989; de Gans et al, 1992).

Maintenance Therapy

After initial successful treatment of cryptococcal meningitis in AIDS patients, high relapse rates have been demonstrated in patients who did not receive lifelong suppressive or chronic maintenance therapy (Bozette et al, 1991). A placebo-controlled trial evaluated the effectiveness of fluconazole as maintenance therapy for AIDS patients who received successful therapy for cryptococccal meningitis with amphotericin B with or without flucytosine (Bozette et al, 1991). Relapse occurred in 15% of patients in the placebo group, compared with 0% in fluconazole-treated patients, thereby establishing the need for maintenance therapy in this population.

Subsequently, a randomized comparative trial conducted by the NIAID-MSG demonstrated the superior efficacy of oral fluconazole 200 mg daily to intravenous amphotericin B 1 mg/kg weekly for maintenance therapy (Powderly et al, 1992). Relapses of symptomatic cryptococcal disease were seen in 18% and 2% of patients receiving amphotericin B and fluconazole, respectively ($p < 0.001$). In addition, patients receiving amphotericin B had more frequent adverse events and associated bacterial infections.

The NIAID-MSG and NIAID-ACTG conducted another trial comparing oral fluconazole 200 mg daily to oral itraconazole 200 mg daily for 12 months as maintenance therapy for CNS cryptococcal disease (Saag et al, 1999). Fluconazole proved to be superior; the trial was terminated prematurely after interim analysis revealed that 23% of itraconazole-treated patients relapsed, compared with only 4% of fluconazole-treated patients ($p = 0.006$). Furthermore, the trial showed that risk of relapse was increased if the patient had not received flucytosine during the initial 2 weeks of primary therapy for cryptococcal meningitis ($p = 0.04$). These 2 large NIAID-MSG/ACTG trials established fluconazole as the drug of choice for maintenance therapy for cryptococcosis in AIDS patients.

Until recently, maintenance or lifelong suppressive therapy has been recommended for all AIDS patients after successful completion of therapy for acute cryptococcosis (Table 12–2; Saag et al, 2000; Masur et al, 2002). Preliminary studies suggest that risk of recurrence of cryptococcosis in AIDS patients is low, provided patients have successfully completed primary therapy for cryptococcosis, are free of symptoms of cryptococcosis, and have achieved immune reconstitution with HAART therapy (Mussini et al, 2001; Aberg et al, 2002). Data to support discontinuation of chronic maintenance or lifelong therapy have come from small series of patients with cryptococcosis; therefore, caution and close observation of the patient are important until additional long-term data emerge. Some authorities recommend a lumbar puncture to confirm CSF sterility prior to discontinuation of maintenance therapy.

Adjunctive Therapy

As mentioned previously, elevated intracranial pressure is a common finding, especially among AIDS patients with cryptococcal meningitis. Furthermore, a very high opening pressure at baseline may be associated with more frequent headaches and meningismus, pathologic reflexes, early death, and overall increased mortality (Graybill et al, 2000). The treatment of elevated intracranial pressure is aimed at reduction of CSF volume, either by repeated lumbar puncture, or ventricular or lumbar drainage. If intracranial pressures cannot be adequately reduced with frequent lumbar punctures, a lumbar drain placement or ventriculostomy may be necessary for CSF removal. Ventricular fluid shunting, via ventriculo-peritoneal shunt, is often reserved for patients with hydrocephalus. In addition, in patients with increased intracranial pressure and no evidence of hydrocephalus on imaging studies, placement of a ventriculo-peritoneal shunt may be extremely useful and help to reverse neurologic sequelae (Liliang et al, 2002). Moreover, shunting is not typically associated with dissemination of cryptococcal infection into the peritoneum or bloodstream (Park et al, 1999). Medical therapy, including the use of acetazolamide, mannitol, or corticosteroids, is less helpful than mechanical intervention in lowering intracranial pressure. A recent trial comparing acetazolamide vs. placebo for treatment of elevated intracranial pressure in patients with cryptococcal meningitis was terminated prematurely because patients who received acetazolamide developed significantly lower venous bicarbonate levels, increased chloride levels, and increased serious adverse events when compared to patients who received placebo (Newton et al, 2002).

The addition of cytokines and other immunomodulatory approaches to antifungal therapy of cryptococcosis are actively being explored (Casadevall and Pirofski, 2001; Lutz et al, 2000; Clemons et al, 2001). Studies currently are ongoing in animal models and phase I/II human trials with recombinant human gene product interferon-γ, and monoclonal antibodies directed against cryptococcal capsular polysaccharide (Lutz et al, 2000; Clemons et al, 2001; Pappas et al,

2001; Larsen et al, 2002). Given the increased number of immunosuppressed patients over the past 2 decades at risk for opportunistic fungal infections such as cryptococcosis, results of studies involving immunomodulatory approaches are eagerly awaited.

PREVENTION

Prevention of cryptococcal disease is difficult, because *C. neoformans* is ubiquitous in the environment and only causes sporadic disease. Because of the morbidity and mortality associated with CNS cryptococcal disease, and the increased incidence of cryptococcosis in patients with advanced HIV infection, primary prophylaxis has been studied in AIDS patients in several prospective trials (Nightingale et al, 1992; Powderly et al, 1995; McKinsey et al, 1999). Although data suggest that prophylaxis with antifungal agents such as fluconazole and itraconazole may be effective in reducing the incidence of cryptococcosis, a survival advantage has not yet been established. Moreover, concern exists for the development of azole-resistant fungi, especially *Candida* species, if widespread antifungal prophylaxis is employed. Currently, primary prophylaxis in HIV-infected patients is not routinely recommended.

REFERENCES

Aberg J A, Mundy L M, Powderly W G. Pulmonary cryptococcosis in patients without HIV infection. *Chest* 115:734–40, 1999.
Aberg J A, Price R W, Heeren D M, Bredt B. A pilot study of the discontinuation of antifungal therapy for disseminated cryptococcal disease in patients with acquired immunodeficiency syndrome, following immunologic response to antiretroviral therapy. *J Infect Dis* 185:1179–1182, 2002.
Aller A I, Martin-Mazuelos E, Lozano F, Gomez-Mateos J, Steele-Moore I, Holloway W J, Gutierrez M J, Recio F J, Espinel-Ingroff A. Correlation of fluconazole MICs with clinical outcome in cryptococcal infection. *Antimicrob Agents Chemother* 44: 1544–1548, 2000.
Anderson D J, Schmidt C, Goodman J, Pomeroy C. Cryptococcal disease presenting as cellulitis. *Clin Infect Dis* 14:666–672, 1992.
Armengou A, Porcar C, Mascaro J, Garcia-Bragado F. Possible development of resistance to fluconazole during suppressive therapy for AIDS-associated cryptococcal meningitis. *Clin Infect Dis* 23:1337–1338, 1996.
Baddley J W, Perfect J, Warren R, Pankey G, Larsen R, Henderson H, Pappas P G. Pulmonary cryptococcosis in patients without HIV infection: when is a lumbar puncture needed? 40th Interscience Conference on Antimicrobial Agents and Chemotherapy, Toronto, Canada, Abstract #707, 2000.
Bartizal K, Gill CJ, Abruzzo G K, Flattery A M, Kong L, Scott P M, Smith J G, Leighton C E, Bouffard A, Dropinski J F, Balkovec J. In vitro preclinical evaluation studies with the echinocandin antifungal MK-0991 (L-743,872). *Antimicrob Agents Chemother* 41:2326–2332, 1998.
Behrman R E, Masci J R, Nicholas P. Cryptococcal skeletal infections: case report and review. *Rev Infect Dis* 12:181–190, 1990.
Bennett J E, Dismukes W E, Duma R J, Medoff G, Sande M A, Gallis H A, Leonard J, Fields B T, Bradshaw M, Haywood H B,

McGee Z A, Cate T R, Cobbs C G, Warner J F, Alling D A. A comparison of amphotericin B alone and combined with flucytosine in the treatment of cryptococcal meningitis. *N Engl J Med* 301:126–131, 1979.

Berry A J, Rinaldi M G, Graybill J R. Use of high-dose fluconazole as salvage therapy for cryptococcal meningitis in patients with AIDS. *Antimicrob Agents Chemother* 36:690–692, 1992.

Beyt B E Jr, Waltman S R. Cryptococcal endophthalmitis after corneal transplantation. *N Engl J Med* 298:825–826, 1978.

Bolaños B, Mitchell T G. Phagocytosis of *Cryptococcus neoformans* by rat alveolar macrophages. *J Med Vet Mycol* 27:219–228, 1989.

Bozzette S A, Larsen R A, Chiu J, Leal M A E, Jacobsen J, Rothman P, Robinson P, Gilbert G, McCutchan J A, Tilles J, Leedom J M, Richman D D, The California Collaborative Treatment Group. A placebo-controlled trial of maintenance therapy with fluconazole after treatment of cryptococcal meningitis in the acquired immunodeficiency syndrome. *N Engl J Med* 324:580–584, 1991.

Braman R T. Cryptococcosis (torulosis) of the prostate. *Urology* 17:284–286, 1981.

Brandt M E, Pfaller M A, Hajjeh R A, Hamill R J, Pappas P G, Reingold A L, Rimland D, Warnock D W, Cryptococcal Disease Active Surveillance Group. Trends in antifungal drug susceptibility of *Cryptococcus neoformans* isolates in the United States 1992 to 1994 and 1996 to 1998. *Antimicrob Agents Chemother* 45:3065–3069, 2001.

Buchanan K L, Murphy J W. What makes *Cryptococcus neoformans* a pathogen? *Emerg Infect Dis* 4:71–83, 1998.

Bulmer G S, Sans M D. *Cryptococcus neoformans*. III. Inhibition of phagocytosis. *J Bacteriol* 95:5–8, 1968.

Cameron M L, Bartlett J A, Gallis H A, Waskin H A. Manifestations of pulmonary cryptococcosis in patients with acquired immunodeficiency syndrome. *Rev Infect Dis* 13:64–67, 1991.

Campbell C K, Payne A I, Teall A J, Brownell A, Mackenzie D W R. Cryptococcal latex antigen test positive in patient with *Trichosporon beigelii* infection. *Lancet* ii:43–44, 1985.

Campbell G D. Primary pulmonary cryptococcosis. *Am Rev Respir Dis* 94:236–243, 1966.

Casadevall A, Mukherjee J, Yuan R R, Perfect J R. Management of injuries caused by *Cryptococcus neoformans*-contaminated needles. *Clin Infect Dis* 19:951–953, 1994.

Casadevall A. Antibody immunity and invasive fungal infections. *Infect Immun* 63:4211, 1995.

Casadevall A, Pirofski L A. Adjunctive immune therapy for fungal infections. *Clin Infect Dis* 33:1048–1056, 2001.

Chang Y C, Kwon-Chung K J. Complementation of a capsule-deficient mutation of *Cryptococcus neoformans* restores its virulence. *Mol Cell Biol* 14:4912–4919, 1994.

Chen S C, Currie B J, Campbell H M, Fisher D A, Pfeiffer T J, Ellis D H, Sorrell T C. *Cryptococcus neoformans* var. *gattii* infection in northern Australia: existence of an environmental source other than known host eucalyptus. *Trans R Soc Trop Med Hyg* 91:547–550, 1997.

Chuck S L, Sande M A. Infections with *Cryptococcus neoformans* in the acquired immunodeficiency syndrome. *N Engl J Med* 321:794–799, 1989.

Clemons K V, Lutz J E, Stevens D A. Efficacy of recombinant gamma interferon for treatment of systemic cryptococcosis in SCID mice. *Antimicrob Agents Chemother* 45:686–689, 2001.

Coker R J, Viviani M, Gazzard B G, DuPont B, Pohle H D, Murphy S M, Atouguia J, Champalimaud J L, Harris J R. Treatment of cryptococcosis with liposomal amphotericin B (AmBisome) in 23 patients with AIDS. *AIDS* 7:829–835, 1993.

Collins H L, Bancroft G J. Encapsulation of *Cryptococcus neoformans* impairs antigen-specific T-cell responses. *Infect Immun* 59:3883–3888, 1991.

Concus A P, Helfand R F, Imber M J, Lerner S A, Sharpe R J. Cu-

taneous cryptococcosis mimicking molluscum contagiosum in a patient with AIDS. *J Infect Dis* 158:897–898, 1988.

Crump J R C, Elner S G, Elner V M, Kauffman C A. Cryptococcal endophthalmitis: case report and review. *Clin Infect Dis* 14:1069–1073, 1992.

Currie B P, Casadevall A. Estimation of the prevalence of cryptococcal infection among patients infected with the human immunodeficiency virus in New York City. *Clin Infect Dis* 19:1029–1033, 1994.

De Gans J, Portegies P, Tiessens G, Schattenkerk J K M E, Van Boxtel C J, Van Ketel, R J, Stam J. Itraconazole compared with amphotericin B plus flucytosine in AIDS patients with cryptococcal meningitis. *AIDS* 6:185–190, 1992.

Denning D W, Tucker R M, Hanson L H, Hamilton J R, Stevens D A. Itraconazole therapy for cryptococcal meningitis and cryptococcosis. *Arch Intern Med* 149:2301–2308, 1989.

Denning D W, Armstrong R W, Lewis B H, Stevens D A. Elevated cerebrospinal fluid pressures in patients with cryptococcal meningitis and acquired immunodeficiency syndrome. *Am J Med* 91:267–272, 1991.

Diamond R D, Bennett J E. A subcutaneous reservoir for intrathecal therapy of fungal meningitis. *N Engl J Med* 288:186–188, 1973.

Diamond R D, Bennett J E. Prognostic factors in cryptococcal meningitis: a study in 111 cases. *Ann Intern Med* 80:176–181, 1974.

Dismukes W E, Cloud G, Gallis H A, Kerkering T M, Medoff G, Craven P C, Kaplowitz L G, Fisher J F, Gregg C R, Bowles C A, Shadomy S, Stamm A M, Diasio R B, Kaufman L, Soon S-J, Blackwelder W C, National Institute of Allergy and Infectious Diseases Mycoses Study Group. Treatment of cryptococcal meningitis with combination amphotericin B and flucytosine for four as compared with six weeks. *N Engl J Med* 317:334–341, 1987.

Dismukes W E. Management of cryptococcosis. *Clin Infect Dis* 17(Suppl 2):S507–S512, 1993.

Dromer F, Mathoulin S, Dupont B, Brugiere O, Letenneur L, the French Cryptococcosis Study Group. Comparison of the efficacy of amphotericin B and fluconazole in the treatment of cryptococcosis in human immunodeficiency virus-negative patients: retrospective analysis of 83 cases. *Clin Infect Dis* 22(Suppl 2):S154–S160, 1996a.

Dromer F, Mathoulin S, Dupont B, Laporte A, the French Cryptococcosis Study Group. Epidemiology of cryptococcosis in France: a 9-year survey (1985–1993). *Clin Infect Dis* 23:82–90, 1996b.

Duperval R, Hermans P E, Brewer N S, Roberts G D. Cryptococcosis with emphasis on the significance of isolation of *Cryptococcus neoformans* from the respiratory tract. *Chest* 72:13–19, 1977.

Dykstra M A, Friedman L, Murphy J W. Capsule size of *Cryptococcus neoformans*: control and relationship to virulence. *Infect Immun* 16:239–135,1977.

Ellis D H, Pfeiffer T J. Ecology, life cycle, and infectious propagule of *Cryptococcus neoformans*. *Lancet* 336:923–925, 1990a.

Ellis D H, Pfeiffer T J. Natural habitat of *Cryptococcus neoformans* var. *gattii*. *J Clin Microbiol* 28:1642–1644, 1990b.

Emmons C W. Saprophytic sources of *Cryptococcus neoformans* associated with the pigeon (*Columbia livia*). *Am J Hyg* 62:227–232, 1955.

Feigin D S. Pulmonary cryptococcosis; radiologic-pathologic correlates of its three forms. *Am J Roentgenol* 141:1262–1272, 1983.

Fink J N, Barboriak J J, Kaufman L. Cryptococcal antibodies in pigeon breeders' disease. *J Allergy Clin Immunol* 41:297–301, 1968.

Franzot S P, Salkin I F, Casadevall A. *Cryptococcus neoformans* var. *grubii*: separate varietal status for cryptococcus neoformans serotype A isolates. *J Clin Micro* 37:838–40, 1999.

Fujita N K, Reynard M, Sapico F L, Guze L B, Edwards J E. Cryptococcal intracerebral mass lesions. The role of computed tomography and nonsurgical management. *Ann Int Med* 94:382–388, 1981.

Fyfe, M W, MacDougall L, Barlett K, Romney M, Kibsey P, Pearce M, Starr M, Stephen C, Stein L, Kidd S, Patrick D, Black W. Emergence of *Cryptococcus neoformans* var. *gattii* infections in British Columbia, Canada. 42nd Interscience Conference on Antimicrobial Agents and Chemotherapy, San Diego, CA. Abstract #1242, 2002.

Glaser J B, Garden A. Inoculation of cryptococcosis without transmission of the acquired immunodeficiency syndrome. *N Engl J Med* 313:264, 1985.

Gluck J L, Myers J P, Pass L M. Cryptococcemia due to *Cryptococcus albidus*. *South Med J* 80:511–513, 1987.

Graybill J R, Sobel J, Saag M, Van der Horst C, Powderly W, Cloud G, Riser L, Hamill R, Dismukes W, the NIAID Mycoses Study Group and AIDS Cooperative Treatment Group. Diagnosis and management of increased intracranial pressure in patients with AIDS and cryptococcal meningitis. *Clin Infect Dis* 30:47–54, 2000.

Hajjeh R A, Conn L A, Stephens D S, Baughman W, Hamill R, Graviss E, Pappas P G, Thomas C, Reingold A, Rothrock G, Hutwagner L C, Schuchat A, Brandt M E, Pinner R W. Cryptococcosis: population-based multistate active surveillance and risk factors in human immunodeficiency virus-infected persons. Cryptococcal Active Surveillance Group. *J Infect Dis* 179:449–454, 1999.

Hamill R J, Sobel J, El-Sadr W, Johnson P, Graybill J R, Javaly K, Bardker D. Randomized double-blind trial of Ambisome (Liposomal Amphotericin B) and amphotericin B in acute cryptococcal meningitis in AIDS paients. 39th Interscience Conference on Antimicrobial Agents and Chemotherapy, San Francisco, CA. Abstract #1161, 1999.

Hammerman K J, Powell K E, Christianson C S, Huggin P M, Larsh H W, Vivas J R, Tosh F E. Pulmonary cryptococcosis: clinical forms and treatment (a Center for Disease Control cooperative mycoses study). *Am Rev Respir Dis* 108:1116–1123, 1973.

Harrison T S, Levitz S M. Mechanisms of impaired anticryptococcal activity of monocytes from donors infected with human immunodeficiency virus. *J Infect Dis* 176:537–540, 1997.

Haubrich R H, Haghighat D, Bozzette S A, Tilles J, McCutchan J A, the California Collaborative Treatment Group. High-dose fluconazole for treatment of cryptococcal disease in patients with human immunodeficiency virus infection. *J Infect Dis* 170:2380–242, 1994.

Heyderman R S, Gangaidzo I T, Hakim J G, Mielke J, Taziwa A, Musvaire P, Robertson V J, Mason P R. Cryptococcal meningitis in human immunodeficiency virus-infected patients in Harare Zimbabwe. *Clin Infect Dis* 26:284–289, 1998.

Hospenthal D, Bennett J. Flucytosine monotherapy for cryptococcosis. *Clin Infect Dis* 27:260–264, 1998.

Hospenthal D, Bennett J E. Persistence of cryptococcomas on neuroimaging. *Clin Infect Dis* 31:1303–1306, 2000.

Hurd D D, Staub D B, Roelofs R I, Dehner L P. Profound muscle weakness as the presenting feature of disseminated cryptococcal infection. *Rev Infect Dis* 11:970974, 1989.

Johnson L B, Bradley S F, Kauffman C A. Fungaemia due to *Cryptococcus laurentii* and a review of non-neoformans cryptococcaemia. *Mycoses* 41:277–280, 1998.

Jones B, Larsen R A, Forthal D, Haghighat D, Bozzette S. Treatment of nonmeningeal cryptococcal disease in HIV-infected persons. Proceedings of the 91st Annual Meeting of the American Society for Microbiology, Dallas, TX. abstract F4, 1991.

Kanj S S, Welty-Wolf K, Madden J, Tapson V, Baz M, Davis D, Perfect J R. Fungal infections in lung and heart-lung transplant recipients: Report of 9 cases and review of the literature. *Medicine* 75:142–156, 1996.

Kerkering T M, Duma R J, Shadomy S. The evolution of pulmonary cryptococcosis: clinical implications from a study of 41 patients with and without compromising host factors. *Ann Intern Med* 94:611–616, 1981.

Khoury M B, Godwin J D, Ravin C E, Gallis H A, Halvorsen R A, Putnam C E. Thoracic cryptococcosis: immunologic competence and radiologic appearance. *Am J Roentgenol* 142:893–896, 1984.

Kontoyiannis D P, Peitsch W K, Reddy B T, Whimbey E E, Han X Y, Bodey G P, Rolston K V. Cryptococcosis in patients with cancer. *Clin Infect Dis* 32:e145–e150, 2001.

Kordossis T, Avlami A, Velegraki A, Stefanou I, Georgakopoulos G, Papalambrou C, Legakis N J. First report of *Cryptococcus laurentii* meningitis and a fatal case of *Cryptococcus albidus* cryptococcaemia in AIDS patients. *Med Mycology* 36:335–339, 1998.

Kovacs J A, Kovacs A A, Polis M, Wright W C, Gill V J, Tuazon C U, Gelmann E P, Lane H C, Longfield R, Overturf G. Cryptococcosis in the acquired immunodeficiency syndrome. *Ann Intern Med* 103:533–538, 1985.

Kozel T R, Pfrommer G S. Activation of the complement system by *Cryptococcus neoformans* leads to binding of iC3b to the yeast. *Infect Immun* 52:1–5, 1986.

Kumlin U, Elmqvist L G, Granlund M, Olsen B, Tarnvik A. CD4 lymphopenia in a patient with cryptococcal osteomyelitis. *Scandinavian J Infect Dis* 29:205–206, 1997.

Kwon-Chung K J. A new species of *Filobasidiella neoformans*, the sexual state of *Cryptococcus neoformans* B and C serotypes. *Mycologia* 68:942–946, 1976.

Kwon-Chung K J, Polacheck I, Popkin T J. Melanin-lacking mutants of *Cryptococcus neoformans* and their virulence for mice. *J Bacteriol* 150:1414–1421, 1982.

Kwon-Chung K J, Bennett J E. Epidemiologic differences between the two varieties of *Cryptococcus neoformans*. *Am J Epidemiol* 120:123–130, 1984.

Kwon-Chung K J, Kozel T R, Edman J C, Polacheck I, Ellis D, Shinoda T, Dromer F. Recent advances in biology and immunology of *Cryptococcus neoformans*. *J Med Vet Mycol* 30(Suppl 1):133–142, 1992.

Larsen R A, Bozzette S A, McCutchan A, Chiu J, Leal M A E, Richman D D. Persistent *Cryptococcus neoformans* infection of the prostate after successful treatment of meningitis. *Ann Intern Med* 111:125–128, 1989.

Larsen R A, Leal M A E, Chan L S. Fluconazole compared with amphotericin B plus flucytosine for cryptococcal meningitis in AIDS. A randomized trial. *Ann Intern Med* 113:183–187, 1990.

Larsen R A, Bozzette S A, Jones B E, Haghighat D, Leal M A, Forthal D, Bauer M, Tilles J G, McCutchan J A, Leedom J M. Fluconazole combined with flucytosine for the treatment of cryptococcal meningitis in patients with AIDS. *Clin Infect Dis* 19:741–745, 1994.

Larsen R A, Pappas P, Perfect J, Aberg J A, Casadevall A, Dismukes W E, The National Institute of Allergy and Infectious Diseases (NIAID) and the Mycoses Study Group. Passive immunization for therapy: the MSG 43 study. Fifth International Conference on *Cryptococcus* and Cryptococcosis, Adelaide, Australia. Abstract #S3.3. March, 2002.

Leavitt A D, Kauffman C A. Cryptococcal aortitis. *Am J Med* 85:108–110, 1988.

Leenders A C, Reiss P, Portegies P, Clezy K, Hop W C J, Hoy J, Borleffs J C C, Allworth T, Kauffmann R H, Jones P, Kroon F P, Verbrugh H A, de Marie S. Liposomal amphotericin B (AmBisome) compared with amphotericin B followed by oral fluconazole in the treatment of AIDS-associated cryptococcal meningitis. *AIDS* 11:1463–1471, 1997.

Lendvai N, Casadevall A, Liang Z, Goldman D L, Mukherjee J, Zuckier L. Effect of immune mechanisms on the pharmacokinetics and organ distribution of cryptococcal polysaccharide. *J Infect Dis* 177:1647–1659, 1998.

Levitz S M. The ecology of *Cryptococcus neoformans* and the epidemiology of cryptococcosis. *Rev Infect Dis* 13: 1163–1169, 1991.

Levitz S M, Tabuni A, Kornfield H, Reardon C C, Golenbock D T. Production of tumor necrosis factor alpha in human leukocytes stimulated by *Cryptococcus neoformans*. *Infect Immun* 62:1975–1981, 1994.

Levitz S M, Matthews H L, Murphy J W. Direct antimicrobial activity of T cells. *Immunol Today* 16:387–391, 1995.

Lewis J L, Rabinovich S. The wide spectrum of cryptococcal infections. *Am J Med* 53:315–322, 1972.

Liliang P, Liang C, Chang W, Lu K, Lu C. Use of ventriculoperitoneal shunts to treat uncontrollable intracranial hypertension in patients who have cryptococcal meningitis without hydrocephalus. *Clin Infect Dis* 34:e64–68, 2002.

Lutz J E, Clemons K V, Stevens D A. Enhancement of antifungal chemotherapy by interferon-gamma in experimental systemic cryptococcosis. *J Antimicrob Chemother* 46:437–442, 2000.

Masur H, Kaplan J E, Holmes K K. Recommendations of the U.S. Public Health Service and the Infectious Diseases Society of America. Guidelines for preventing opportunistic infections among HIV-infected persons—2002. *Ann Intern Med* 137:435–477, 2002.

Mayanja-Kizza H, Kazunori O, Mitarai S, Yamashita H, Nalongo K, Watanabe K, Izumi T, Ococi-Jungala, Augustine K, Mugerwa R, Nagatake T, Matsumoto K. Combination therapy with fluconazole and flucytosine for cryptococcal meningitis in Ugandan patients with AIDS. *Clin Infect Dis* 26:1362–1366, 1998.

McKinsey D S, Wheat L J, Cloud G A, Pierce M, Black J R, Bamberger D M, Goldman M, Thomas C J, Gutsch H M, Moskovitz B, Dismukes W E, Kauffman C A, the National Institute of Allergy and Infectious Diseases Mycoses Study Group. Itraconazole prophylaxis for fungal infections in patients with advanced human immunodeficiency virus infection: randomized, placebo-controlled, double-blind study. *Clin Infect Dis* 28:1049–1056, 1999.

McNeil M M, Nash S L, Hajjeh R A, Phelan M A, Conn L A, Plikaytis B D, Warnock D W. Trends in mortality due to invasive mycotic diseases in the United States, 1980–1997. *Clin Infect Dis* 33:641–647, 2001.

Menichetti F, Fiorio M, Tosti A, Gatti G, Pasticci M B, Miletich F, Marroni M, Bassetti D, Pauluzzi S. High-dose fluconazole therapy for cryptococcal meningitis in patients with AIDS. *Clin Infect Dis* 22:838–840, 1996.

Meyohas M, Roux P, Bollens D, Chouaid C, Rozenbaum W, Meynard J, Poirot J, Frottier J, Mayaud C. Pulmonary cryptococcosis: localized and disseminated infection in 27 patients with AIDS. *Clin Infect Dis* 21:628–633, 1995.

Min K H, Kwon-Chung K J. The biochemical basis for the distinction between the two *Cryptococcus neoformans* varieties with CGB medium. *Zentralbl Bakteriol Mikrobiol Hyg [A]* 26:471–480, 1986.

Mitchell T G, Perfect J R. Cryptococcosis in the era of AIDS—100 years after the discovery of *Cryptococcus neoformans*. *Clin Microbiol Rev* 8:515–548, 1995.

Murray R J, Becker P, Furth P, Criner G J. Recovery from cryptococcemia and the adult respiratory distress syndrome in the acquired immunodeficiency syndrome. *Chest* 93:1304–1306, 1988.

Mussini C, Cossarizza A, Pezzotti P, Antinori A, De Luca A, Ortolani P, Rizzardini G, Mongiardo N, Esposito R. Discontinuation or continuation of maintenance therapy for cryptococcal meningitis in patients with AIDS treated with HAART. Program and Abstracts of the 8th Conference on Retroviruses and Opportunistic Infections, Chicago, IL. Abstract # 546, 2001.

National Committee for Clinical Laboratory Standards. Reference method for broth dilution antifungal susceptibility testing of yeasts. Approved standard NCCLS document M27–A. *National Committee for Clinical Laboratory Standards*, Wayne, PA, 1997.

Neilson J B, Fromtling R A, Bulmer G S. *Cryptococcus neoformans*: size range of infectious particles from aerosolized soil. *Infect Immun* 17:634–638, 1977.

Neuville S, Dromer F, Morin O, Dupont B, Ronin O, Lortholary O, and the French Cryptococcus Study Group. Primary cutaneous cryptococcosis: a distinct clinical entity. *Clin Infect Dis* 36:337–347, 2003.

Newberry W M Jr., Walter J E, Chandler J W Jr, Tosh F E. Epidemiologic study of *Cryptococcus neoformans*. *Ann Intern Med* 67:724–732, 1967.

Newton P N, Thai L H, Tip N Q, Short J M, Chierakul W, Rajanuwong A, Pitisuttithum P, Chasombat S, Phonrat B, Maek-A-Nantawat W, Teaunadi R, Lalloo D G, White N J. A randomized, double-blind, placebo-controlled trial of acetazolamide for the treatment of elevated intracranial pressure in cryptococcal meningitis. *Clin Infect Dis* 35:769–772, 2002.

Nightingale S D, Cal S X, Peterson D M, Loss S D, Gamble B A, Watson D A, Manzone C P, Baker J E, Jockusch J D. Primary prophylaxis with fluconazole against systemic fungal infections in HIV-positive patients. *AIDS* 6:191–194, 1992.

Nosanchuk J D, Shoham S, Fries B C, Shapiro D S, Levitz S M, Casadevall A. Evidence of zoonotic transmission of *Cryptococcus neoformans* from a pet cockatoo to an immunocompromised patient. *Ann Intern Med* 132:205–208, 2000.

Nottebart H C, McGehee R F, Utz J P. *Cryptococcus neoformans* osteomyelitis: case report of two patients. *Sabouraudia* 12:127–132, 1974.

Pappas P G, Bustamante B, Ticona E, Hamill R, Johnson P, Reboli A, Ellner J, Hsu H. Adjunctive interferon gamma (IFNγ) for treatment of cryptococcal meningitis (Crypto): a randomized, double-blind pilot trial. 41st Interscience Conference on Antimicrobial Agents and Chemotherapy, Chicago, IL. Abstract LB-10, 2001.

Pappas P G, Perfect J R, Cloud G A, Larsen R A, Pankey G A, Lancaster D J, Henderson H, Kauffman C A, Haas D W, Saccente M, Hamill R J, Holloway M S, Warren R M, Dismukes W E. Cryptococcosis in human immunodeficiency virus-negative patients in the era of effective azole therapy. *Clin Infect Dis* 33:690–699, 2001.

Park M K, Hospenthal D R, Bennett J E. Treatment of hydrocephalus secondary to cryptococcal meningitis by use of shunting. *Clin Infect Dis* 28:629–633, 1999.

Pema K, Diaz J, Guerra L G, Nabhan D, Verghese A. Disseminated cutaneous cryptococcosis: comparison of clinical manifestations in the pre-AIDS and AIDS eras. *Arch Intern Med* 154:1032–1034, 1994.

Perfect J R. Cryptococcosis. *Infect Dis Clin N Am* 3:77–102, 1989.

Perfect J R, Durack D T, Gallis H A. Cryptococcemia. *Medicine* (Baltimore) 62:98–109, 1983.

Pfaller M A, Zhang J, Messer S A, Brandt M E, Hajjeh R A, Jessup C J, Tumberland M, Mbidde E K, Ghannoum M A. In vitro activities of voriconazole, fluconazole, and itraconazole against 566 clinical isolates of *Cryptococcus neoformans* from the United States and Africa. *Antimicrob Agents Chemother* 43:169–171, 1999.

Pietrella D, Monari C, Retini C, Palazzetti B, Bistoni F, Vecchiarelli A. Human immunodeficiency virus type 1 envelope protein gp120 impairs intracellular antifungal mechanisms in human monocytes. *J Infect Dis* 177:347–354, 1998.

Poblete R B, Kirby B D. Cryptococcal peritonitis. Report of a case and review of the literature. *Am J Med* 82:665–667, 1987.

Polsky B, Depman M R, Gold J W M, Galicich J H, Armstrong D. Intraventricular therapy of cryptococcal meningitis via a subcutaneous reservoir. *Am J Med* 81:24–28, 1986.

Poprich M J, Arthur R H, Helmer E. CT of intracranial cryptococcosis. *Am J Roentgenol* 54:603–606, 1990.

Powderly W G, Saag M S, Cloud G A, Robinson P, Meyer R D, Jacobson J M, Graybill J R, Sugar A M, McAuliffe V J, Follansbee S E, Tuazon C U, Stern J J, Feinberg J, Hafner R, Dismukes W E, NIAID AIDS Clinical Trials Group, NIAID Mycoses Study Group. A controlled trial of fluconazole or amphotericin B to prevent relapse of cryptococcal meningitis in patients with the acquired immunodeficiency syndrome. *N Engl J Med* 326:793–798, 1992.

Powderly W G, Cloud G A, Dismukes W E, Saag M S. Measurement of cryptococcal antigen in serum and cerebrospinal fluid: value in the management of AIDS-associated cryptococcal meningitis. *Clin Infect Dis* 18:789–792, 1994.

Powderly W G, Finkelstein D, Feinberg J, Frame P, He W, van der Horst C, Kolestar S L, Eyster M E, Carey J, Waskin H. A randomized trial comparing fluconazole with clotrimazole troches for the prevention of fungal infections in patients with advanced human immunodeficiency virus infection. *N Engl J Med* 332:700–705, 1995.

Powell K E, Dahl B A, Weeks R J, Tosh F E. Airborne *Cryptococcus neoformans*: particles from pigeon excreta compatible with alveolar deposition. *J Infect Dis* 125:412–415, 1972.

Randall R E Jr., Stacy W K, Toone E C, Prout G R Jr., Madge G E, Shadomy H J, Shadomy S, Utz J P. Cryptococcal pyelonephritis. *N Engl J Med* 279:60–65, 1968.

Rex J H, Larsen R A, Dismukes W E, Cloud G A, Bennett J E. Catastrophic visual loss due to *Cryptococcus neoformans* meningitis. *Medicine* 72:207–224, 1993.

Rippon J W. *Medical mycology. The pathogenic fungi and the pathogenic actinomycetes.* 3rd ed. Philadelphia: W B Saunders, 1988: 582–609.

Saag M S, Powderly W G, Cloud G A, Robinson P, Grieco M H, Sharkey P K, Thompson S E, Sugar A M, Tuazon C U, Fisher J F, Hyslop N, Jacobson J M, Hafner R, Dismukes W E, The NIAID Mycoses Study Group and The AIDS Clinical Trials Group. Comparison of amphotericin B with fluconazole in the treatment of acute AIDS-associated cryptococcal meningitis. *N Engl J Med* 326:83–89, 1992.

Saag M S, Cloud G A, Graybill J R, Sobel J D, Tuazon C U, Johnson P C, Fessel W J, Moskovitz B L, Weisinger B, Cosmatos D, Riser L, Thomas C, Hafner R, Dismukes W E, the National Institute of Allergy and Infectious Diseases Mycoses Study Group. A comparison of itraconazole vs. fluconazole as maintenance therapy for AIDS-associated cryptococcal meningitis. *Clin Infect Dis* 28:291–296, 1999.

Saag M S, Graybill R J, Larsen R A, Pappas P G, Perfect J R, Powderly W G, Sobel J D, Dismukes W E. Practice guidelines for the management of cryptococcal disease. *Clin Infect Dis* 30:710–718, 2000.

Shah B, Taylor H C, Pillay I, Chung-Park M, Dobrinich R. Adrenal insufficiency due to cryptococcosis. *JAMA* 256:3247–3249, 1986.

Sharkey P K, Graybill J R, Johnson E S, Hausrath S G, Pollard R B, Kolokathis A, Mildvan D, Fan-Havard P, Eng R H K, Patterson T F, Pottage J C, Jr, Simberkoff M S, Wolf J, Meyer R D, Gupta R, Lee L W, Gordon D S. Amphotericin B lipid complex compared with amphotericin B in the treatment of cryptococcal meningitis in patients with AIDS. *Clin Infect Dis* 22:315–321, 1996.

Smith D K, Neal J J, Holmberg S D. Unexplained opportunistic infections and CD4+ T-lymphocytopenia without HIV infection.

An investigation of cases in the United States. *N Engl J Med* 328:373–379, 1993.

Staib F, Heissenkuber M. *Cryptococcus neoformans* in bird droppings: a hygienic-epidemiological challenge. *AIDS-Forschung* 12:649–655, 1989a.

Staib F, Seibold M, L'age M, Heise W, Skorde J, Grosse G, Nurnberger F, Bauer G. *Cryptococcus neoformans* in the seminal fluid of an AIDS patient: a contribution in the clinical course of cryptococcosis. *Mycoses* 32:171–180, 1989b.

Stamm A M, Diasio R B, Dismukes W E, Shadomy S, Cloud G A, Bowles C A, Karam G H, Espinel-Ingroff A, National Institute of Allergy and Infectious Diseases Mycoses Study Group. Toxicity of amphotericin B plus flucytosine in 194 patients with cryptococcal meningitis. *Am J Med* 83:236–242, 1987.

Stead K J, Klugman K P, Painter M L, Koornhof H J. Septic arthritis due to *Cryptococcus neoformans*. *J Infect* 17:139–145, 1988.

Swinne D, Deppner M, Laroche R, Floch J-J, Kadende P. Isolation of *Cryptococcus neoformans* from houses of AIDS-associated cryptococcosis patients in Bujumbura (Burundi). *AIDS* 3:389–390, 1989.

Tarrand J J, Guillot C, Wengler M, Jackson J, Lajeunesse J D, Rolston K V. Clinical comparison of the resin-containing BACTEC 26 Plus and the Isolater 10 blood culturing system. *J Clin Microbiol* 29:2245–2249, 1991.

Temeck B K, Venzon D J, Moskaluk C A, Pass H I. Thoracotomy for pulmonary mycoses in non-HIV-immunosuppressed patients. *Ann Thorac Surg* 58:333–338, 1994.

Tynes B, Mason K N, Jennings A E, Bennett J E. Variant forms of pulmonary cryptococcosis. *Ann Intern Med* 69:1117–1125, 1968.

van der Horst C, Saag M S, Cloud G A, Hamill R J, Graybill J R, Sobel J D, Johnson P C, Tuazon C U, Kerkering T, Moskovitz B L, Powderly W G, Dismukes W E, The National Institute of Allergy and Infectious Diseases Mycoses Study Group and AIDS Clinical Trials Group. Treatment of cryptococcal meningitis associated with the acquired immunodeficiency syndrome. *N Engl J Med* 337:15–21, 1997.

Visnegarwala F. Graviss E A, Lacke C E, Dural A T, Johnson P C, Atmar A L, Hamill R J. Acute respiratory failure associated with cryptococcosis in patients with AIDS: analysis of predictive factors. *Clin Infect Dis* 27:1231–1237, 1998.

Wang Y, Aisen P, Casadevall A. *Cryptococcus neoformans* melanin and virulence: mechanism of action. *Infect Immun* 63:3131–3136, 1995.

White M, Cirrincione C, Blevins A, Armstrong D. Cryptococcal meningitis: outcome in patients with AIDS and patients with neoplastic disease. *J Infect Dis* 165:960–963, 1992.

Witt M D, Lewis R J, Larsen R A, Milefchik E N, Leal M A E, Haubrich R H, Richie J A, Edwards J E Jr, Ghannoum M A. Identification of patients with acute AIDS-associated cryptococcal meningitis who can be effectively treated with fluconazole: the role of antifungal susceptibility testing. *Clin Infect Dis* 22:322–328, 1996.

Woodring J H, Ciporkin G, Lee C, Worm B, Woolley S. Pulmonary cryptococcosis. *Sem Roentgenol* 31:67–75, 1996.

Yamaguchi H, Ikemoto H, Watanabe K, Ito A, Hara K, Kohno S. Fluconazole monotherapy for cryptococcosis in non-AIDS patients. *Eur J Clin Microbiol Infect Dis* 15:787–792, 1996.

Zuger A, Louie E, Holzman R S, Simberkoff M S, Rahal J J. Cryptococcal disease in patients with the acquired immunodeficiency syndrome: diagnostic features and outcome of treatment. *Ann Intern Med* 104:234–240, 1986.

13

Rhodotorula, malassezia, trichosporon, and other yeast-like fungi

JOSE A. VAZQUEZ

Yeasts are found ubiquitously in nature, in association with plants, mammals, and insects. Accordingly, humans are continually exposed to multiple genera of yeasts via various routes. Depending on the interaction between host mucosal defense mechanisms and fungal virulence factors, yeast colonization may be transient or persistent, with either systemic or local disease.

Yeast organisms are usually of low virulence, and frequently require a significant alteration or reduction in host defenses prior to tissue invasion. Recently, because of the increased population of immunocompromised patients, the frequency of yeast infections as well as the organisms causing disease continues to grow.

RHODOTORULOSIS

Rhodotorulosis results from infection with the genus *Rhodotorula*. Although the yeast is recovered worldwide from a variety of sources, infection is generally only seen in the immunocompromised host.

Pathogen

The fungi from the genus *Rhodotorula* are imperfect basidiomycetous yeast belonging to the family Cryptococcaceae.

There are 8 species in the genus *Rhodotorula* (Fell, 1984a; Kreger-van Rij, 1984). *Rhodotorula rubra (R. mucilaginosa)* is the species most frequently associated with human infection. The other less commonly isolated species include *R. glutinis, R. pilimanae, R. pallida, R. aurantiaca, R. minuta* (syn, *R. marina*). The majority of *Rhodotorula* species produce red-to-orange colonies due to the presence of carotenoid pigments (Rippon, 1988; Kwon-Chung and Bennett, 1992). The yeast is mucoid, encapsulated, rarely forms mycelia, and readily grows on almost all types of culture media. *Rhodotorula* is very similar to the *Cryptococcus* in rate of growth, cell size and shape, presence of capsule, and the ability to split urea. The difference includes *Rhodotorula's* inability to assimilate inositol and ferment sugars (Kwon-Chung and Bennett, 1992). *Rhodotorula* can be differentiated from other red-pigmented yeast, such as *Sporobolomyces*, by the lack of ballistospore formation.

In vitro susceptibility studies (Table 13–1) reveal that *Rhodotorula* is susceptible to amphotericin B (MIC range 0.8–1.6 μg/ml) (Hazen, 1995). *Rhodotorula* are less susceptible to azoles, with MIC to fluconazole (range 0.5–> 64 μg/ml), itraconazole (range 0.5–12.8 μg/ml), ketoconazole (range 0.4–0.8 μg/ml), posaconazole (0.5–4.0 μg/ml), and voriconazole (0.25–4.0 μg/ml) (Espinel-Ingroff, 1998a). In addition, *Rhodotorula* species are susceptible to flucytosine (MIC < 0.1 μg/ml) (Kiehn et al, 1992).

Epidemiology

Rhodotorula species are commonly recovered from seawater, plants, air, food (cheese and milk products, fruit juices) (Volz et al, 1974; Rippon, 1988; Kwon-Chung and Bennett, 1992), and occasionally from humans. They are frequently recovered as an airborne laboratory contaminant (Rippon, 1988; Kwon-Chung and Bennett, 1992). Additionally, *Rhodotorula* are commonly recovered from shower curtains, bathtub–wall junctions, and toothbrushes. In humans, *Rhodotorula* spp. have been recovered from the skin (Mackenzie, 1961), nails, respiratory tract, urinary tract (Ahearn et al, 1966; Kiehn et al, 1992), gastrointestinal tract (Saez, 1979), and bloodstream (Kares and Biava, 1979; Anaissie et al, 1989; Kiehn et al, 1992).

R. rubra and *R. glutinis* account for approximately 0.5% of yeast isolated from the oral cavity and more than 12% of yeast isolates from stool and rectal swabs (Rose and Kurup, 1989). It is important to note that the recovery of *Rhodotorula* species from human sources, especially mucosal sites has frequently been of questionable clinical significance, although isolation from numerous sterile body sites has now been described (Gyaurgieva et al, 1996).

TABLE 13–1. In vitro Antifungal Activity Against Emerging Yeast Isolates

Organism	MIC (μg/ml)							
	FLU	ITRA	VORI	POSA	RAVU	AMB	5-FC	References
Rhodotorula rubra	0.5–>64	0.25–>16	0.25–4.0	2.0–4.0	0.25–2.0	0.25–1.0	<0.1	Hazen, 1995
Saccharomyces cerevisiae	0.5–16	0.25–1.0	0.06–0.25	0.12–1.0	na	0.5–2.0	0.06–0.12	Hazen, 1995 Tawara et al, 2000 Espinel, 1998a Pfaller et al, 1997
Malassezia furfur	1.0–16	0.06–0.25	0.03–0.125	na	0.015–0.03	0.25–2.0	na	Marcon et al, 1987 Gupta et al, 2000
Trichosporon asahii	0.5–>64	0.125–1.56	0.03–1.24	0.12–1.0	0.008–0.78	0.39–>12.5	16–>32	Hazen, 1995 Tawara et al, 2000 Espinel, 1998a McGinnis et al, 1997
Blastoschizomyces capitatus	8–32	0.25–0.50	0.06–0.25	0.12–0.25	na	0.15–0.62	0.4–>64	Espinel, 1998a Hazen, 1995
Sporobolomyces	1.25–>64	1.0–2.0	0.25–4.0	na	na	0.14–1.0	na	Espinel, 1998a Hazen, 1995

FLU, fluconazole; ITRA, itraconazole; VORI, voriconazole; POSA, posaconazole; RAVU, ravuconazole; AMB, amphotericin B; 5-FC, flucytosine; na, not available.

Clinical Manifestations

Clinical signs and symptoms of *Rhodotorula* infection are nonspecific, and vary from subtle and mild, to severe, including septic shock. *Rhodotorula* have been incriminated in a wide spectrum of infections including fungemia (Louria et al, 1960; Shelbourne and Carey, 1962; Leeber and Scher, 1969; Young et al, 1974; Anaissie et al, 1989; Kiehn et al, 1992), endocarditis (Naveh et al, 1975), peritonitis (Eisenberg et al, 1983), meningitis (Gyaurgieva et al, 1996), and disseminated disease (Rusthoven et al, 1984).

Rhodotorula fungemia is the most common form of infection. In most cases, it is associated with intravascular catheters in patients receiving either chemotherapy or long-term antimicrobials (Louria et al, 1960; Louria et al, 1967; Anaissie et al, 1989; Braun and Kauffman, 1992; Kiehn et al, 1992). Fever is the most clinical frequent manifestation associated with fungemia.

Endocarditis. A fatal case of aortic valve endocarditis in a patient with underlying rheumatic heart disease has been described (Louria et al, 1960). In addition, a second case of endocarditis in a 7-year-old boy has also been reported. This case however, was treated successfully with 5-flucytosine (Naveh et al, 1975).

Central Nervous System Infections. Several cases of meningitis have been described. *Rhodotorula rubra* was reported in a fatal case of meningitis in a patient with acute leukemia (Pore and Chen, 1976). The patient presented with epistaxis, frontal headaches, right tympanic membrane perforation, followed by fever and chills. The organism was recovered from the cerebrospinal

fluid (CSF) on culture, and seen on an India ink stain. The patient was treated with amphotericin B, but did not respond. In a second case of meningitis, *R. rubra* was recovered from the CSF of an HIV-positive patient (Gyaurgieva et al, 1996). The diagnosis was made with a positive CSF culture for *R. rubra.* The patient responded clinically to 15 days of 5-flucytosine, but relapsed 8 months later. *R. rubra* has also been implicated in a case of postoperative ventriculitis in a woman with benign meningioma. The patient was treated successfully with 5-flucytosine and amphotericin B (Donald and Sharp, 1988).

Peritonitis. Three case of *R. rubra* peritonitis have been described in patients undergoing continuous ambulatory peritoneal dialysis (Eisenberg et al, 1983). Environmental cultures revealed a possible common source outbreak. In all patients, the symptoms were subtle and intermittent at first, and consisted of abdominal pain, anorexia, nausea, and occasional diarrhea.

Diagnosis

In the majority of proven infections, *Rhodotorula* is recovered from a sterile site of infection. In these cases, the decision to attribute a causal role to *Rhodotorula* is relatively simple, and the patient should be treated appropriately for an invasive fungal infection. More difficult is when the organism is recovered from body sites that may normally harbor *Rhodotorula* species, especially in the absence of signs or symptoms of infection. In this setting, it is necessary to establish true infection instead of colonization.

Rhodotorula species grow readily in blood cultures and any media suitable for yeast, such as Sabouraud dextrose agar. There are no serological diagnostic tests available.

Treatment

It is difficult to assess the role of antifungal therapy in patients with infection due to the genus *Rhodotorula*. Optimal management of patients with indwelling catheters infected with *Rhodotorula* has not been well defined. There are several reports that document clearance of fungemia and resolution of infection by removing the intravascular catheter in the absence of antifungal therapy (Braun and Kauffman, 1992; Kiehn et al, 1992). On the other hand, several reports suggest antifungal treatment alone may suffice (Kiehn et al, 1992; Hazen, 1995). Given that infections due to *Rhodotorula* can be severe and life threatening, it is probably best to manage these infections aggressively by discontinuing the indwelling venous catheter if possible and the use of systemic antifungal therapy.

SACCHAROMYCES

Saccharomyces is an ascomycetous yeast, and is widespread in nature. The species includes *S. cerevisiae*, *S. fragilis* and *S. carlsbergensis*, and are occasionally part of the normal flora of the human gastrointestinal and genitourinary tracts (Mackenzie, 1961; Sobel et al, 1993). *Saccharomyces cerevisiae*, also known as brewer's yeast or baker's yeast, has been reported to cause infection in humans. *Saccharomyces cerevisiae* is better known for its commercial uses, i.e., beer and wine production, health food supplementation, and recently by its use in DNA recombinant technology, rather than as a human pathogen (Kwon-Chung and Bennett, 1992). Recently, however, *S. cerevisiae* has been found to be a cause of mucosal and disseminated infection in humans, primarily in immunocompromised hosts (Cimolai et al, 1987; Tawfik et al, 1989; Nielsen et al, 1990; Sobel et al, 1993; Nyirjesy et al, 1995).

Pathogen

Cells are oval to spherical, measure 3 to 9 μm by 5 to 20 μm and exist as multilateral budding cells as either haploids or diploids. Cells may form short chains and elongate as rudimentary pseudohyphae or no pseudohyphae. Ascospores, one to four in number, are in either tetrahedral or linear arrangement and are gram negative (vegetative cells are gram positive). Colonies are smooth, moist, and either white or cream-colored.

Saccharomyces are almost invariably nonpathogenic. Kiehn and coworkers reviewed more than 3300 yeast cultures from cancer patients and found only 19 isolates of *S. cerevisiae* (Kiehn et al, 1992). In a more recent review from the University of Minnesota bone marrow transplant program, only two *S. cerevisiae* infections were found out of 138 documented fungal infections over a 15-year period (Morrison et al, 1993).

In the majority of situations the organism is nonpathogenic due to innate low virulence. In early experimental studies, subcutaneous inoculation with *S. cerevisiae* was neither lethal nor invasive for normal and cortisone-treated mice (Holzschu et al, 1979). More recent studies have demonstrated that some clinical isolates of *S. cerevisiae* in CD-1 mice can proliferate and resist clearance in vivo and thus, supports *S. cerevisiae* as a cause of clinical infection (Clemons et al, 1994).

Epidemiology

Recovery of *Saccharomyces* from human mucosal surfaces rarely is of clinical significance. On the other hand, isolation from sterile body sites has now been described (Eng et al, 1984; Morrison et al, 1993). *Saccharomyces* has been recovered from the bloodstream, lungs, peritoneal cavity, esophagus, urinary tract, and vagina (Eng et al, 1984; Morrison et al, 1993; Sobel et al, 1993).

Recent DNA typing studies evaluating the relatedness between clinical strains and commercial strains of *S. cerevisiae* have demonstrated that commercial products may be a contributing factor in human colonization and infection (McCullough et al, 1998). Four women suffering from recurrent *S. cerevisiae* vaginitis also had exposure to bread dough that contained *S. cerevisiae* genotypes that were identical to those found in the vagina. Furthermore, in one of the women, her husband, who worked at a pizza shop was also colonized subungually by the same strain of *S. cerevisiae* recovered from her vagina (Nyirjesy et al, 1995).

The risk factors associated with *Saccharomyces* infections are similar to the risk factors associated with candidemia and systemic candidiasis, including central venous catheters, neutropenia, antimicrobials, and gastrointestinal tract surgery (Eschete and West, 1980; Cimolai et al, 1987; Nielsen et al, 1990; Aucott et al, 1990). There have also been several reports of *S. cerevisiae* fungemia in HIV-positive individuals (Sethi and Mandell, 1988). Possible portals of entry for invasive disease include the oropharynx, gastrointestinal tract and skin (Aucott et al, 1990).

Clinical Manifestations

Clinical signs and symptoms of infection are nonspecific and vary from subtle and mild to severe. *Saccharomyces* species have been incriminated in bloodstream infections (Eschete and West, 1980; Cimolai et al, 1987; Sethi and Mandell, 1988; Kwon-Chung and Bennett, 1992), endocarditis (Stein et al, 1970; Rubenstein et al, 1975), peritonitis (Canafax et al, 1982; Dougherty and Simmons, 1982), disseminated disease (Eng et al,

1984; Aucott et al, 1990), pneumonia (Cimolai et al, 1987) and vaginitis (Sobel et al, 1993; Nyirjesy et al, 1995).

Fungemia, the most common form of infection, is seen in the immunocompromised host and is associated with intravascular catheters and either chemotherapy or antimicrobials (Aucott et al, 1990; Nielsen et al, 1990). Manifestations are similar to those of systemic candidiasis and candidemia. Fever of unknown etiology is the most frequent symptom associated with fungemia, and in the majority of cases, the patients have survived.

Respiratory Tract Infections. Four suspected cases of pneumonia due to *S. cerevisiae* have been reported. In three out of the four, the patients had underlying hematologic malignancies, and the diagnosis was made on biopsy of lung tissue (Cimolai et al, 1987; Aucott et al, 1990). There have also been two cases of empyema. In one patient, the empyema resulted from a complication during sclerotherapy for esophageal varices (Chertow et al, 1991).

Peritonitis. There have been two surgical cases in which *S. cerevisiae* was recovered from the peritoneal fluid of symptomatic patients (Cimolai et al, 1987; Aucott et al, 1990). In both patients, the organism was recovered after surgery for a malignant neoplasm. Both were cured with surgical drainage and antifungal therapy. There has been one reported case of cholecystitis in a patient with diabetes mellitus (Katras et al, 1992). *Saccharomyces cerevisiae* was recovered from the gallbladder and from the stone inside the gallbladder. The patient did well postcholecystectomy and required no antifungal therapy.

Endocarditis. Three documented cases of endocarditis have been reported (Stein et al, 1970; Aucott et al, 1990). All were associated with prosthetic valves, and two were intravenous heroin users. All three patients were apparently cured with antifungal therapy; in only one patient was the valve replaced.

Genitourinary Tract Infections. There have been three reported cases of urinary tract infections due to *S. cerevisiae* (Eng et al, 1984; Aucott et al, 1990). One patient had a bilateral ureteral obstruction, and developed fungus balls due to *S. cerevisiae*. Two renal abscesses associated with fungemia have also been documented (Aucott et al, 1990).

Vaginitis due to *S. cerevisiae* has been reported in 17 women (Sobel et al, 1993; Nyirjesy et al, 1995), including 9 women with symptomatic vaginitis indistinguishable from that caused by *C. albicans* (Sobel et al, 1993). All patients had a history of chronic vaginitis

unresponsive to standard antifungal drugs, and all but two had systemic or local predisposing factors. Additionally, eight other women were reported with refractory vaginitis due to *S. cerevisiae* (Nyirjesy et al, 1995).

Diagnosis

The decision to attribute a causal role to *S. cerevisiae* is simple, and the patient should be treated for an invasive fungal infection. Diagnostic difficulty occurs when the organism is recovered from body sites that may be colonized by *Saccharomyces*, especially in the absence of symptoms of infection. In this setting, it is necessary to establish true infection instead of colonization with this organism.

Saccharomyces cerevisiae readily grows in blood cultures and on Sabouraud dextrose media. No serologic diagnostic tests are available to assist in the diagnosis.

Treatment

As with many nonpathogenic yeast infections, it is difficult to assess the role of antifungal therapy in patients with infection due to the genus *Saccharomyces*. Optimal management of patients with prosthetic valve infections and infected indwelling catheters has not been established. There are several reports that document clearance of fungemia and resolution of infection by removing the intravascular catheter without providing antifungal therapy (Cimolai et al, 1987; Aucott et al, 1990). Most experts advocate the removal of the indwelling catheter and the use of antifungal agents (Aucott et al, 1990). Although in vitro susceptibility tests have not been standardized, *Saccharomyces* are susceptible to most antifungal drugs including amphotericin B, 5-flucytosine, ketoconazole, clotrimazole, miconazole, and terconazole (Table 13–1). However, *Saccharomyces* have higher MICs to most antifungal drugs than do *Candida albicans* (Sobel et al, 1993).

MALASSEZIA INFECTIONS

Malassezia furfur (*Pityrosporum orbiculare, Pityrosporum ovale*) and other *Malassezia* are common yeasts frequently found on normal human skin. *Malassezia* are well known to cause superficial skin infections such as tinea (pityriasis) versicolor, dermatophytosis, and folliculitis; occasionally in the immunocompromised host it may also cause fungemia and disseminated infection.

Pathogen

Malassezia furfur is a dimorphic lipophilic yeast that cannot synthesize medium or long chain fatty acids and has strict in vitro requirements for exogenous fatty acids of the C_{12} and C_{14} series (Nazzaro-Porro et al, 1976). The genus *Malassezia* consists of several species, including *M. furfur* and *M. pachydermatis*. *M. furfur* and other *Malassezia* exist primarily in the yeast form, but may form filamentous structures on the skin when the organism is associated with superficial infections (Marcon and Powell, 1992). Because of its nutritional requirements, *M. furfur* is not frequently isolated from clinical specimens in the microbiology laboratory unless its presence is suspected and special preparations are made. *M. pachydermatis* is generally associated with infections in dogs, where it produces otitis externa (Nazzaro-Porro et al, 1976). This species, however, has occasionally been implicated in human infections (Redline and Dahms, 1981; Gueho et al, 1987). Both organisms, when grown under favorable conditions, produce clusters of oval to round, thick-walled yeast cells, with unipolar buds that form repeatedly from the same pole of the parent cell, giving rise to the characteristic "collarette" at the bud site. The cells measure ~6 µm in their largest dimension (Marcon and Powell, 1992). Optimal growth for *M. furfur* occurs between 35°C to 37°C. Media such as Sabouraud dextrose agar, chocolate agar, trypticase soy agar with 5% sheep blood all require the addition of supplements such as olive oil, in order to permit growth of this organism (Ingham and Cunningham, 1993). *M. pachydermatis*, does not require exogenous lipids for growth and can be recovered on standard fungal media. In addition, *M. pachydermatis* does not have known filamentous forms (Marcon and Powell, 1992). Colonies are dry and white to creamy in color.

In vitro susceptibility studies (Table 13–1) of *M. furfur* strains report that the majority of the isolates are susceptible to amphotericin B (MIC range 0.3–2.5 µg/ml), ketoconazole (MIC range ≤ 0.05–0.4 µg/ml), miconazole (MIC range 0.4–> 50 µg/ml), and fluconazole (MIC range 1–16 µg/ml). However, most isolates are intrinsically resistant to flucytosine (MIC > 100 µg/ml) (Faergeman, 1984; Marcon et al, 1987a; Klotz, 1989; Gupta et al, 2000).

Epidemiology

Malassezia frequently colonizes the skin of normal hosts over the scalp, shoulders, chest, and back (Ingham and Cunningham, 1993). The distribution of colonization correlates with oily areas of the skin, due to the organisms' requirement of exogenous fatty acids which it obtains from sebum. The highest incidence of colonization has been found in young teenagers, with rates greater than 90% (Marcon and Powell, 1987b). The low incidence of colonization in preadolescent children has been postulated to be due to immature sebum production.

Isolation of *M. furfur* from newborns is reported to be less than 10%, in nonintensive care settings. However, isolation of *M. furfur* has been reported to be greater than 80% in neonatal intensive care units (Powell et al, 1987; Marcon and Powell, 1992; Ingham and Cunningham, 1993). The reason for this increased colonization rate may be because sick infants are handled frequently by adult personnel (Klotz, 1989).

Risk factors that correlate with increased colonization rates in neonates include prematurity, duration of hospitalization in the intensive care unit, use of occlusive dressings, and prolonged use of antimicrobials (Roberts, 1969; Marcon and Powell, 1992). Although the epidemiology of disseminated infection has not been well studied, there are several risk factors frequently associated with deep-seated infection due to *M. furfur*. These include: prematurity, central venous catheters (Garcia et al, 1987; Weiss et al, 1991; Marcon and Powell, 1992; Barber et al, 1993), total parenteral nutrition, parenteral lipid preparations (Garcia et al, 1987; Weiss et al, 1991; Barber et al, 1993), and immunocompromised state (Marcon and Powell, 1992).

Molecular epidemiologic studies using PCR-mediated DNA fingerprinting have concluded that within the neonatal intensive care unit there is longitudinal persistence of both *M. furfur* and *M. pachydermatis* strains (van Belkum et al, 1994).

Clinical Manifestations

Malassezia produces superficial skin infections, such as tinea (pityriasis) versicolor or a distinctive folliculitis, and on occasion a deep-seated or hematogenous infection (Klotz, 1989). Cutaneous infections are discussed in Chapter 24.

The first reported case of systemic infection was described in 1981, in a premature neonate who developed vasculitis while on lipid therapy (Redline and Dahms, 1981). Since then, numerous reports describing disseminated infection due to *M. furfur* have been reported (Klotz, 1989; Marcon and Powell, 1992).

The manifestations of disseminated or deep-seated infection vary from subclinical and mild symptomatology such as fever, to sepsis with multiorgan dysfunction (Klotz, 1989; Marcon and Powell, 1992). Although the majority of these infections are seen in premature infants, they may occur occasionally in the immunocompromised adult. The most commonly reported signs and symptoms of systemic infection include fever, bradycardia and respiratory distress (> 50%), apnea (37%), hepatosplenomegaly (25%), and lethargy (12%) (Powell et al, 1987). Laboratory findings include leukocytosis, thrombocytopenia, and bilateral pulmonary infiltrates (> 50%) (Powell et al, 1987). Deep-seated organ dissemination is rare.

Diagnosis

The diagnosis of disseminated infection can be made by gram stain of the buffy coat of blood. The budding yeast cells may be observed using specific fungal stains such as Giemsa, PAS, or Calcofluor. Blood cultures will usually be negative, unless the infection is suspected previously and the laboratory adds sterile olive oil to the media. Recovery of the organism may be enhanced by using lysis centrifugation blood culture tubes to support the growth of the yeast (Nelson et al, 1995). In addition, palmitic acid (3%) supplementation may improve the recovery of *Malassezia* (Nelson et al, 1995).

Treatment

Management principles of *M. furfur* fungemia and disseminated infection are controversial. Most authorities recommend prompt removal of the central venous catheter and discontinuation of intravenous lipids (Klotz, 1989; Marcon and Powell, 1992). In most cases without deep-seated infection, removal of the central venous catheter and discontinuation of lipids is all that is needed to clear the infection. This treatment approach accomplishes two objectives: eradication of the nidus of infection, and removal of the nutritional requirements of the organism. If fungemia persists or there is evidence of deep-seated infection, antifungal therapy should be initiated. Fortunately, *Malassezia* species are susceptible to azoles and polyenes (Klotz, 1989; Marcon and Powell, 1992). Although randomized clinical trials have not been undertaken, in most situations, either fluconazole 400 mg per day or amphotericin B 0.7 mg/kg/day intravenously should be sufficient to eradicate the infection.

TRICHOSPORONOSIS

Infections due to the genus *Trichosporon* may be classified as superficial or deep. Superficial infection of the hair shafts, generally due to *Trichosporon asahii* (*T. beigelii*), is commonly known as white piedra because of the soft white nodules characteristic of this infection. Deep seated or disseminated *Trichosporon* infections have been recognized in the compromised host with increasing frequency over the past decade and are life threatening.

The organism now known as *Trichosporon asahii* was first described in 1865 by Beigel, who identified it as the causative agent of the hair shaft infection (Beigel, 1936). The first reported case of disseminated infection appears to be a 39 year-old female with adenocarcinoma of the lung who developed a brain abscess (Watson and Kallichurum, 1970).

Pathogen

The genus *Trichosporon*, initially described by Behrend, currently contains two main species: *(1)* T. *asahii* (formerly, *T. beigelii*, *T. cutaneum*) (Behrend, 1890), and *(2) Blastoschizomyces capitatus,* previously called *Tri-*

chosporon capitatum or *Geotrichum capitatum* (Salkin et al, 1985; Kwon-Chung and Bennett, 1992; Gueho et al, 1997). For a discussion of *Blastoschizomyces,* see the following section. Gueho and colleagues have also suggested that the species known as *T. asahii* may include several different *Trichosporon* species with epidemiological and pathogenic differences (Gueho et al, 1997). In 1991, investigators using isoenzyme delineation and PCR DNA fingerprinting techniques suggested that the strains that generally produce superficial infections are distinctly different from those strains that produce invasive disease (Kemeker et al, 1991).

Trichosporon species are characterized by true hyphae, pseudohyphae, arthroconidia, and blastoconidia (Kwon-Chung and Bennett, 1992), and are commonly found in soil, animals, and on human skin (Rippon, 1988). *T. asahii* grows readily on Sabouraud dextrose agar as rapidly growing smooth, shiny gray to cream colored yeast-like colonies with cerebriform radiating furrows that become dry and membranous with age (Kwon-Chung and Bennett, 1992). *T. asahii* is readily identified using commercially available carbohydrate assimilation assays.

In 1963, investigators described the presence of common antigens between *T. asahii* and *Cryptococcus neoformans* (Seeliger and Schroter, 1963). Immunodiagnosis of trichosporonosis using the anticryptococcal latex-agglutination test of the serum has also been reported (Campbell et al, 1985; McManus et al, 1985).

Epidemiology

While *Trichosporon asahii* is generally found in the soil, it may also be recovered from air, rivers and lakes, sewage, and bird droppings (Walsh, 1989). It rarely colonizes the inanimate environment, but may occasionally colonize the mucosal surfaces of the oropharynx, the lower gastrointestinal tract, and the skin in approximately 4% of humans (Rose and Kurup, 1977; Haupt et al, 1983).

There have been more than 100 documented cases of disseminated infection due to *T. asahii* (Rippon, 1988; Walsh, 1989; Kwon-Chung and Bennett, 1992; Krcmery et al, 1999; Ebright et al, 2001). In most cases the major risk factors include underlying neoplastic disease (acute leukemia, chronic leukemia, multiple myeloma, solid tumors) and neutropenia (Keay et al, 1991; Fisher et al, 1993; Mirza, 1993; Hajjeh and Blumberg, 1995; Lussier et al, 2000; Chan et al, 2000; Ebright et al, 2001). In nonneoplastic, nonneutropenic patients, the major risk factors include corticosteroids, prosthetic valve surgery, solid organ transplant recipients (kidney, heart, liver), chronic active hepatitis, and intravenous drug use. In the majority of cases, the proposed portal of entry appears to be the respiratory or gastrointestinal tract, and occasionally central venous catheters and percutaneous vascular devices (Walsh et al, 1993; Ebright et al, 2001).

Clinical Manifestations

Trichosporonosis can be classified into superficial infections such as white piedra (hair shaft), onychomycosis and otomycosis, and invasive infection. Invasive infection can be further divided into localized deep tissue infection and disseminated (hematogenous) infection.

Deep tissue infection results from the invasion of *Trichosporon* into deep nonmucosal tissues. The infection may involve a single organ infection or multiple organs. The most frequently affected organ is the lungs, representing approximately 33% of localized deep tissue infections (Marin et al, 1989). Other sites of deep organ infection include the peritoneum (Cheng et al, 1989; Parsonnet, 1989), heart valves (natural and prosthetic) (Keay et al, 1991), eyes (Sheikh et al, 1986), brain, liver, and spleen (Bhansali et al, 1986), stomach (Szili and Domjan, 1982), kidneys (Lussier et al, 2000), uterine tissue, gallbladder (Patel et al, 1990; Chan et al, 2000), and central nervous system (chronic fungal meningitis) (Surmont et al, 1990; Walsh et al, 1993).

The clinical spectrum of disseminated infection resembles systemic candidiasis and includes fungemia associated with organ infection. In addition, disseminated infections may be either acute or chronic. Acute disseminated trichosporonosis frequently has a sudden onset and progresses rapidly, primarily in patients who are persistently neutropenic with fungemia characterized by persistent fever despite broad-spectrum antibacterial agents. Patients frequently develop cutaneous lesions (~ 33%), pulmonary infiltrates (~30%–60%), and hypotension, with renal and ocular involvement.

The metastatic cutaneous lesions begin as an erythematous rash with raised papules on the trunk and the extremities. As the infection progresses, the rash evolves into macronodular lesions, followed by central necrosis of the nodules and rarely, the formation of hemorrhagic bullae (Yung et al, 1981). Pulmonary infiltrates frequently accompany the disseminated infection (Walsh et al, 1993), and may manifest as either a lobar consolidation, bronchopneumonia, or a reticulonodular pattern.

Renal involvement in disseminated infection is quite common and occurs in > 75% of the cases. Renal disease may manifest as proteinuria, hematuria, red blood cell casts, acute renal failure, and glomerulonephritis (Haupt et al, 1983; Walsh et al, 1993). Urine cultures are frequently positive for *Trichosporon* and should suggest disseminated disease in a neutropenic patient.

Chorioretinitis is frequently seen in disseminated disease (Walsh et al, 1982), and may cause decreased or complete loss of vision due to retinal vein occlusion and retinal detachment. In experimental studies, *Trichosporon* has been found to have tropism for the choroid and retina (Walsh, 1989). However, unlike candidal endophthalmitis, *Trichosporon* infects uveal tissues including the iris, but spares the vitreous (Walsh et al, 1982; Walsh et al, 1993).

During disseminated infection, virtually any tissue in the body may be infected with *Trichosporon*. The organs that have been documented to be involved include the liver, spleen, gastrointestinal tract, lymph nodes, myocardium, bone marrow, pleura, brain, adrenal gland, thyroid gland, and skeletal muscle (Walsh et al, 1986; Ito et al, 1988; Mochizuki et al, 1988; Liu et al, 1990; Ebright et al, 2001).

In chronic disseminated trichosporonosis, symptoms may be present for several weeks to months and include persistent fever despite broad-spectrum antimicrobial therapy (Walsh, 1989). This infection is similar to the entity known as chronic disseminated (hepatosplenic) candidiasis (Thaler et al, 1988; Meyer et al, 2002), and tends to be a chronic infection of the liver, spleen, and other tissues after recovery from neutropenia. Laboratory studies frequently reveal an elevated alkaline phosphatase. Imaging the abdomen with either a CT scan or MR reveals hepatic or splenic lesions compatible with abscesses. If lesions are demonstrated, a biopsy is needed to confirm the diagnosis.

Diagnosis

The diagnosis is made with a biopsy for histopathology and culture of the skin or involved organs. Blood cultures may also be useful in diagnosing disseminated infection, and on occasion in deep-tissue infection. *Trichosporon* will grow readily in blood culture and on fungal specific media such as Sabouraud dextrose agar (Kwon-Chung and Bennett, 1992). The presence of *Trichosporon* in the urine of a high-risk patient should increase the suspicion of disseminated infection.

Although there are no standardized serologic assays for *Trichosporon*, the serum latex agglutination test for *Cryptococcus neoformans* may be positive in patients (Seeliger and Schroter, 1963). The initial clinical observations suggesting the usefulness of this test was reported by McManus and coworkers who demonstrated a positive serum latex agglutination test for *C. neoformans* in several patients with disseminated *Trichosporon* infection (McManus et al, 1985).

Management

Trichosporonosis has a mortality rate of 60%–70%. The underlying disease, persistent neutropenia and concurrent infections also contribute to overall mortality. The initial step in the management of disseminated *Trichosporon* infection should be to decrease or reverse immunosuppression. Optimal therapy has not been established. Until recently, however, most patients received amphotericin B, occasionally in combination with flucytosine (Walsh, 1989). Several investigators, however, have reported amphotericin B tolerant or resistant isolates of *T. asahii* (Walsh et al, 1990, 1992).

Several antifungal options are now available. In vitro susceptibility studies and animal models suggest that azoles and not polyenes are more effective in the eradication of *Trichosporon* species in neutropenic and nonneutropenic models (Keay et al, 1991; Walsh et al, 1992). In vitro susceptibility studies of *T. asahii* (Table 13–1) reveal fluconazole MIC$_{50}$ of 8.0 μg/ml (MIC range 4–> 64 μg/ml) and itraconazole MIC$_{50}$ of 0.25 μg/ml (range 0.12–> 16 μg/ml) at 48 hours (Paphitou et al, 2002). In the same study, amphotericin B MIC$_{50}$ for *T. asahii* was 4.0 μg/ml (range 1.0–8.0 μg/ml) in AM3 media. Although there are no established breakpoints to define susceptibility, the majority of the strains evaluated thus far demonstrate relatively high MIC for polyenes and relatively low MIC for azoles. Accordingly, one therapeutic approach is to use fluconazole 400–800 mg/day, or itraconazole 400–600 mg/day, for the treatment of disseminated trichosporonosis (Anaissie et al, 1992).

A second approach, especially in the nonneutropenic patient, is to utilize amphotericin B at 1.0–1.5 mg/kg/day (Walsh et al, 1993). Bearing in mind, that at these dosages, amphotericin B is fungistatic, not fungicidal (Walsh et al, 1990). If a patient remains fungemic despite therapy with amphotericin B, it may prove useful to add either flucytosine or fluconazole, since these combinations in vitro have demonstrated some synergy. In a recent study in a murine model of disseminated trichosporonosis, combination therapy was superior to single agent therapy using either fluconazole or amphotericin B alone (Louie et al, 2001). The combination of fluconazole, amphotericin B and levofloxacin was the most effective regimen in reducing fungal burden in kidneys and improving survival in the experimental murine model. The other combinations, such as fluconazole and levofloxacin and fluconazole and amphotericin B, were also more effective than monotherapy (Louie et al, 2001). A recent case illustrates this point. A bone marrow transplant recipient developed breakthrough trichosporonosis while receiving prophylaxis against invasive fungal infection with caspofungin. Subsequent treatment of the trichosporonosis with the combination regimen of fluconazole and amphotericin B lipid complex resulted in complete cure (Goodman et al, 2002).

Among the newer triazoles, voriconazole, posaconazole, and ravuconazole have demonstrated broader in vitro activity against more yeast and moulds than prior triazoles. All three triazoles have excellent in vitro activity against most isolates of *T. asahii*. Voriconazole MIC$_{50}$ at 48 hours was 0.25 μg/ml (range 0.06–> 16 μg/ml), posaconazole MIC$_{50}$ at 48 hours was 1 μg/ml (range 0.25–> 16 μg/ml), and ravuconazole MIC$_{50}$ at 48 hours was 4 μg/ml (range 0.25–> 16 μg/ml) (Paphitou et al, 2002). In a patient with disseminated trichosporonosis, it may be clinically useful to determine in vitro susceptibilities, as a helpful adjunct in the management of this serious infection, especially in light of recent case reports describing multidrug resistant *T. asahii* infections (Wolf et al, 2001).

BLASTOSCHIZOMYCES CAPITATUS

Infections due to *Blastoschizomyces capitatus,* although not as common as *T. asahii,* have been recognized in the immunocompromised host over the past 20–35 years (Gemeinhardt, 1965). Most cases appear to be very similar to either disseminated candidiasis or disseminated *T. asahii* infection.

Pathogen

Trichosporon capitatum (syn. *Geotrichum capitatum*) (Behrend, 1890; Kwon-Chung and Bennett, 1992) is now known as *Blastoschizomyces capitatus* (Salkin et al, 1985; Gueho et al, 1997). This organism is difficult to differentiate from *Geotrichum candidum* and *T. asahii. Blastoschizomyces capitatus* produces smooth to wrinkled, raised hyaline colonies with short and finely funiculose aerial mycelium. Hyphae are septate and branching and often form anelloconidia, instead of arthroconidia (Martino et al, 1990).

Epidemiology

Blastoschizomyces capitatus is found in wood and poultry, but has also been recovered from sputum and normal intact skin (Kwon-Chung and Bennett, 1992). Geographically, *B. capitatus* appears to be the opposite of *T. asahii,* with *B. capitatus* infections found more commonly in Europe, and *T. asahii* infections found in North America (Martino et al, 1990). In most cases, the major risk factors include neutropenia and underlying hematologic malignancies (Martino et al, 1990).

The portal of entry is unknown, but is suspected to be the respiratory tract, gastrointestinal tract, and possibly infected central venous catheters (Martino et al, 1990; Kwon-Chung and Bennett, 1992).

In vitro susceptibility studies (Table 13–1) indicate that *B. capitatus* is susceptible to amphotericin B (MIC$_{90}$ 0.62 μg/ml, MIC range 0.15–0.78 μg/ml); less susceptible to azoles such as fluconazole (MICs > 32 μg/ml) and ketoconazole (MIC$_{90}$ 3.12 μg/ml, MIC range 0.04–50 μg/ml); and susceptible to itraconazole (MIC 0.2 μg/ml). Most isolates are resistant to flucytosine (MIC range 0.04–100 μg/ml) (D'Antonio et al, 1994; Hazen, 1995). The newer triazoles, voriconazole and posaconazole, demonstrate good in vitro activity (Espinel-Ingroff, 1998a; Espinel-Ingroff, 1998b).

Clinical Manifestations

Blastoschizomyces capitatus infection may involve a single organ or multiple organs and may be associated with fungemia. The most frequently affected organs are the lungs, liver, skin, and central nervous system. In addition, other involved organs include the spleen, epididymis, kidney, gastrointestinal tract, vertebral body and disk, and prosthetic heart valves (Hazen, 1995).

The clinical spectrum of disseminated infection is similar to that of systemic candidiasis and includes fungemia with or without organ infection (Martino et al, 1990; Hazen, 1995). Generally, the manifestations begin with fever unresponsive to antibacterial therapy, in a neutropenic patient. In addition, in the largest series from Italy, many patients presented with pulmonary disease characterized by cavitary lung lesions and focal hepatosplenic lesions (Martino et al, 1990). Skin lesions similar to those found in systemic candidiasis were also seen. Less commonly described infections include endocarditis, especially involving prosthetic valves, urinary tract infection, vertebral osteomyelitis with discitis of the lumbar spine, cerebritis, and brain abscess (Walsh, 1989; Martino, 1990; Polacheck et al, 1992; D'Antonio et al, 1996).

Diagnosis

Diagnosis is made by positive blood cultures or by biopsy with histopathology and culture of the skin or affected organs. In a series from Italy, blood cultures were positive in 20 of 22 cases (Martino et al, 1990). Blastoschizomyces capitatus will grow easily in blood culture bottles and on fungal specific media such as Sabouraud dextrose agar (Kwon-Chung and Bennett, 1992). Although skin lesions are common, fungal stains and cultures of these lesions are usually negative (Martino et al, 1990; Kwon-Chung and Bennett, 1992).

Management

Infections with B. capitatus have mortality rates between 60% and 70% (Martino et al, 1990). However, underlying disease, persistent neutropenia, and concurrent infections are also significant contributing factors to overall mortality. Optimal therapy has not been established. Until recently, however, most patients received amphotericin B (Walsh, 1989).

The initial step in the management of disseminated infection should be to decrease or reverse the immunocompromised state. Since most isolates are susceptible to amphotericin B, the recommended therapy is amphotericin B at a dose of 1.0–1.5 mg/kg/day (Hazen, 1995). Based on their promising in vitro activity, voriconazole and posaconazole may be suitable alternatives for therapy (Espinel-Ingroff, 1998a; Espinel-Ingroff, 1998b).

SPOROBOLOMYCES

Sporobolomyces are yeast-like organisms that belong to the family Sporobolomycetaceae. These yeasts, which are found throughout the world in soil, bark, and decaying organic material, rarely have been associated with infections in humans. There are seven known species of Sporobolomyces, but only three have been reported to cause human disease, S. salmonicolor, S. holsaticus, and S. roseus. To date, there have been six cases of documented Sporobolomyces infections: a nasal polyp (Plazas et al, 1994), one case of dermatitis (Bergman and Kauffman, 1984), one case of infected skin blisters, one case of Madura foot, and two cases of disseminated infection (lymph node and bone marrow) in patients with AIDS (Morris et al, 1991; Plazas et al, 1994). Despite the fact that Sporobolomyces are saprophytic, these case reports indicate the potential ability of these organisms to produce invasive infection in humans, especially, in a compromised host.

Sporobolomyces produces pink–orange colonies due to the production of carotenoid pigments, and should be differentiated from R. rubra, which also produces a similar color. The genus Sporobolomyces is differentiated from yeast by their reproductive ballistoconidia (Fell and Tallman, 1984). In vitro susceptibility studies (Table 13–1) show that S. salmonicolor is susceptible to amphotericin B, fluconazole, and ketoconazole (Morris et al, 1991). All patients reported thus far have responded to therapy with either amphotericin B or ketoconazole (Hazen, 1995).

REFERENCES

Ahearn D G, Jannach J R, Roth F J. Speciation and densities of yeasts in human urine specimens. Sabouraudia 5:110–119, 1966.

Anaissie E, Bodey G P, Kantarjiani H, Ro J, Vartivarian S E, Hopfer R, Hoy J, Rolston K. New spectrum of fungal infections in patients with cancer. Rev Infect Dis 11:369–378, 1989.

Anaissie E, Gokaslan A, Hachem R, Rubin R, Griffin G, Robinson R, Sobel J, Bodey G. Azole therapy for trichosporonosis: clinical evaluation of eight patients, experimental therapy for murine infection, and review. Clin Infect Dis 15:781–787, 1992.

Aucott J N, Fayen J, Grossnicklas H, Morrissey A, Lederman M M, Salata R A. Invasive infection with Saccharomyces cerivisiae: report of three cases and review. Rev Infect Dis 12:406–411, 1990.

Barber G R, Brown A E, Kiehn T E, Edwards F F, Armstrong D. Catheter-related Malassezia furfur fungemia in immunocompromised patients. Am J Med 95:365–370, 1993.

Behrend G. Ubertrichomycosis nodosa. Berlin Lin Wochenschr 27:464, 1890.

Beigel H. The human hair: Its growth and structure (1865), as cited by Langenon M. In: Darier S et al *Nouvelle Praqt Dermatol* (Paris, Masson, Cie) 2:377, 1936.

Bergman A G, Kauffman C A. Dermatitis due to *Sporobolomyces* infection. *Arch Dermatol* 120:1059–1060, 1984.

Bhansali S, Karanes K, Palutke W, Crane L, Kiel R, Ratanatharathorn V. Successful treatment of disseminated *Trichosporon beigelii* (cutaneum) infection with associated splenic involvement. *Cancer* 58:1630–1632, 1986.

Braun D K, Kauffman C A. *Rhodotorula* fungaemia: a life-threatening complication of indwelling central venous catheters. *Mycoses* 35:305–308, 1992.

Campbell C K, Payne A L, Teall A J, Brownell A, Mackenzie D W. Cryptococcal latex antigen test positive in a patient with *Trichosporon beigelii. Lancet* 2:43–44, 1985.

Canafax D M, Mann H J, Dougherty S H. Postoperative peritonitis due to *Saccharomyces cerevisiae* treated with ketoconazole. *Drug Intell Clin Pharm* 16:698–699, 1982.

Chan R M, Lee P, Wroblewski J. Deep-seated trichosporonosis in an immunocompetent patient: A case report of uterine trichosporonosis. *Clin Infect Dis* 31:621, 2000.

Cheng I K P, Fang G, Chan T, Chan P C, Chan M K. Fungal peritonitis complicating peritoneal dialysis: Report of 27 cases and review of the literature. *Quart J Med* 71:407–416, 1989.

Chertow G M, Marcantonio E R, Wells R G. *Saccharomyces cerevisiae* empyema in a patient with esophago-pleural fistula complicating variceal sclerotherapy. *Chest* 99:1518–1519, 1991.

Cimolai N, Gill M J, Church D. *Saccharomyces cerevisiae* fungemia: case report and review of the literature. *Diagn Microbiol Infect Dis* 8:113–117, 1987.

Clemons K V, McCusker J H, Davis R W, Stevens DA. Comparative pathogenesis of clinical and non-clinical isolates of *Saccharomyces cerevisiae. J Infect Dis* 169:859–867, 1994.

D'Antonio D, Piccolomini R, Fioritoni G, Iacone A, Betti S, Fazii P, Mazzoni A. Osteomyelitis and intervertebral discitis caused by *Blastoschizomyces capitatus* in a patient with acute leukemia. *J Clin Microbiol* 32:224–227, 1994.

D'Antonio D, Mazzoni A, Iacone A, Violante B, Assunta Capuani M, Schioppa F, Romano, F. Emergence of fluconazole-resistant strains of *Blastoschizomyces capitatus* causing nosocomial infections in cancer patients. *J Clin Microbiol* 34:753–755, 1996.

Donald F E, Sharp J F. *Rhodotorula rubra* ventriculitis. *J Infect* 16:187–191, 1988.

Dougherty S H, Simmons R L. Postoperative peritonitis caused by *Saccharomyces cerevisiae. Arch Surg* 117:248–249, 1982.

Ebright J R, Fairfax M R, Vazquez J A. *Trichosporon asahii*, a non-*Candida* yeast that caused fatal septic shock in a patient without cancer or neutropenia. *Clin Infect Dis* 33:28–30, 2001.

Eisenberg E S, Alpert B E, Weiss R A, Mittman N, Soeiro R. *Rhodotorula rubra* peritonitis in patients undergoing continuous ambulatory peritoneal dialysis. *Am J Med* 75:349–352, 1983.

Eng R H, Drehmel R, Smith S M, Goldstein E J C. *Saccharomyces cerevisiae* infections in man. *Sabouraudia* 22:403–407, 1984.

Eschete M L, West B C. *Saccharomyces cerevisiae* septicemia. *Arch Intern Med* 140:1539, 1980.

Espinel-Ingroff A. In vitro activity of the new triazole voriconazole (UK-109,496) against opportunistic filamentous and dimorphic fungi and common and emerging yeast pathogens. *J Clin Microbiol* 36:198–202, 1998a.

Espinel-Ingroff A. Comparison of in vitro activities of the new triazole SCH56592 and the echinocandins MK-0991 (L-743,872) and LY303366 against opportunistic filamentous and dimorphic fungi and yeast. *J Clin Microbiol* 36:2950–2956, 1998b.

Faergemann J. In vitro and in vivo activities of ketoconazole and itraconazole against *Pityrosporum orbiculare. Antimicrob Agents Chemother* 26:773–774, 1984.

Fell J W, Tallman A S. Genus 13. *Sporobolomyces* Kluyver et van Niel. In: Kreiger-van Rij N J W, ed. *The Yeasts: a Taxomonic Study*, 3rd Ed. Amsterdam: Elsevier Science Publishers, 911–920, 1984a.

Fell J W, Tallman A S, Ahearn D G. *Rhodotorula* Harrison. In: Kreiger-van Rij N J W, ed. *The Yeasts: A Taxonomic Study*, 3rd Ed. Amsterdam: Elsevier Science Publishers, 893–905, 1984b.

Fisher D J, Christy C, Spafford P, Maniscalo W M, Hardy D J, Graman P S. Neonatal *Trichosporon beigelii* infection. Report of a cluster of cases in a neonatal intensive care unit. *Pediatr Infect Dis J* 12:149–155, 1993.

Garcia C R, Johnston B L, Corvi G, Walker L J, George W L. Intravenous catheter-associated *Malassezia furfur* fungemia. *Am J Med* 83:790–792, 1987.

Gemeinhardt H. Lungenpathogenitat von *Trichosporon capitatum* beim menschen. *Zentrablatt fur Bakteriolgie* (Series A) 196:121–133, 1965.

Goodman D, Pamer E, Jakubowski A, Morris C, Sepkowitz. Breakthrough trichosporonosis in a bone marrow transplant recipient receiving caspofungin acetate. *Clin Infect Dis* 35: e35–e36, 2002.

Gueho E, Simmons R B, Pruitt W R, Meyer S A, Ahearn D G. Association of *Malassezia pachydermatis* with systemic infections of humans. *J Clin Microbiol* 25:1789–1790, 1987.

Gueho E, de Hoog G S, Smith M T, Meyer S A. DNA relatedness, taxonomy, and medical significance of *Geotrichum capitatum. J Clin Microbiol* 25:1191–1194, 1997.

Gupta A K, Kohli Y, Li A, Faergemann J, Summerbell R C. In vitro susceptibility of the seven *Malassezia* species to ketoconazole, voriconazole, itraconazole and terbinafine. *Br J Dermatol* 142(4): 758–765, 2000.

Gyaurgieva O H Bogomolova T S, Gorshkova G I. Meningitis caused by *Rhodotorula rubra* in an HIV-infected patient. *J Med Vet Mycol* 34:357–359, 1996.

Hajjeh R A, Blumberg H M. Bloodstream infection due to *Trichosporon beigelii* in a burn patient: Case report and review of therapy. *Clin Infect Dis* 20:913–916, 1995.

Haupt H M, Merz W G, Beschorner W E, Vaughan W P, Saral R. Colonization and infection with *Trichosporon* species in the immunosuppressed host. *J Infect Dis* 147:199–203, 1983.

Hazen K C. New and emerging yeast pathogens. *Clin Microbiol Rev* 8:462–478, 1995.

Holzschu D L, Chandler F W, Ajello L, Ahearn D G. Evaluation of industrial yeast for pathogenicity. *Sabouradia* 17:71–78, 1979.

Ingham E, Cunningham A C. *Malassezia furfur. J Med Vet Mycol* 31:265–288, 1993.

Ito T, Ishikawa Y, Fujii R, Hattori T, Konno M, Kawakami S, Kosakai M. Disseminated *Trichosporon capitatum* infection in a patient with acute leukemia. *Cancer* 61:585–588, 1988.

Kares L, Biava M F. Levures isolees dans les hemocultures de 1962 a Mar 1979 in laboratoire de mycologie du CHU de Nancy. *Bull Soc Fr Mycol Med* 8:153–155, 1979.

Katras T, Hollier P P, Stanton P E. Calculous cholecystitis associated with *Saccharomyces cerevisiae. Infect Med* 9(2):38–39, 1992.

Keay S, Denning D, Stevens D A. Endocarditis due to *Trichosporon beigelii*: In-vitro susceptibility of isolates and review. *Rev Infect Dis* 13:383–386, 1991.

Kemeker B J, Lehman P F, Lee J W, Walsh T J. Distinction of deep vs. superficial clinical and non-clinical environmental isolates of *Trichosporon beigelii* by isoenzymes and restriction fragment length polymorphisms of rDNA generated by the polymerase chain reaction. *J Clin Microbiol* 29:1677–1683, 1991.

Kiehn T E, Gorey E, Brown A E, Edwards F F, Armstrong D. Sepsis due to *Rhodotorula* related to use of indwelling central venous catheters. *Clin Infect Dis* 14:841–846, 1992.

Klotz SA. *Malassezia furfur. Infect Dis Clin Am* 3:53–63, 1989.

Kreger-van Rij N J W. *Trichosporon* Behrend. In: Kreiger-van Rij N J W, ed. *The Yeasts: A Taxonomic Study*, 3rd Ed. Amsterdam, Elsevier Science Publishers, 933–962, 1984.

Krcmery V, Mateicka F, Kunova A, Spanik S, Gyarfas J, Sycova Z, Trupl J. Hematogenous trichosporonosis in cancer patients: report of 12 cases including 5 during prophylaxis with itraconazole. *Support Care Cancer* 7:39–43, 1999.

Kwon-Chung K J, Bennett J E. Infections due to *Trichosporon* and other miscellaneous yeast-like fungi. In: Kwon-Chung, KJ, Bennett, JE, eds. *Medical Mycology*, 1st Ed. Philadelphia: Lea & Febiger, 768–782, 1992.

Leeber D A, Scher I. *Rhodotorula* fungemia presenting as "endotoxic" shock. *Arch Intern Med* 123:78–81, 1969.

Liu K L, Herbrecht R, Bergerat J P, Koenig H, Waller J, Oberling F. Disseminated *Trichosporon capitatum* infection in a patient with acute leukemia undergoing bone marrow transplantation. *Bone Marrow Transplant* 6:219–221, 1990.

Louie A, Banerjee P, Liu Q F, Drusano G. Efficacies of fluconazole (Flu), Amphotericin B lipid complex (AmB), and the quinolone Levofloxacin (Levo) as single, double, and triple drug regimens in murine disseminated trichosporonosis. In: Programs and Abstracts of the 41st Interscience Conference on Antimicrobial Agents and Chemotherapy, Chicago, IL, Abstract #J-1619, page 392, 2001.

Louria D B, Greenberg S M, Molander D W. Fungemia caused by certain nonpathogenic strains of the family Cryptococcaceae. *N Engl J Med* 263:1281–1284, 1960.

Louria D B, Blevins A, Armstrong D, Burdick R, Lieberman P. Fungemia caused by non-pathogenic yeasts. *Arch Intern Med* 119:247–252, 1967.

Lussier N, Laverdiere M, Delorme J, Weiss K, Dandavino R. *Trichosporon beigelii* funguria in renal transplant recipients. *Clin Infect Dis* 31:1299–1301, 2000.

Mackenzie D W H. Yeasts from human sources. *Sabouraudia* 1:8–14, 1961.

Marcon M J, Durrell D E, Powell D A, Buesching W J. In vitro activity of systemic antifungal agents against *Malassezia furfur*. *Antimicrob Agents Chemother* 31:951–953, 1987a.

Marcon M J, Powell D A. Epidemiology, diagnosis and management of *M. furfur* systemic infection. *Diagn Microbiol Infect Dis* 10:161–175, 1987b.

Marcon M J, Powell D A. Human infections due to *Malassezia* spp. *Clin Microbiol Rev* 5:101–119, 1992.

Marin J, Chiner E, Franco J, Borras R. *Trichosporon beigelii* pneumonia in a neutropenic patient. *Eur J Clin Microbiol Infect Dis* 8:631–633, 1989.

Martino P, Venditti M, Micozzi A, Morace G, Polonelli L, Mantovani M P, Petti M C, Burgio V L, Santini C, Serra P. *Blastoschizomyces capitatus*: an emerging cause of invasive fungal disease in leukemia patients. *Rev Infect Dis* 12:570–582, 1990.

McCullough M J, Clemens K V, Farina C, McCusker J H, Stevens D A. Epidemiological investigation of vaginal *Saccharomyces cerevisiae* isolates by a genotypic method. *J Clin Microbiol* 36:557–562, 1998.

McGinnis M R, Pasarell L, Sutton D A, Fothergill A W, Cooper C R, Rinaldi M G. In vitro evaluation of voriconazole against some clinically important fungi. *Antimicrob Agents Chemother* 41:1832–1834, 1997.

McManus E J, Bozdech M J, Jones J M. Role of the latex agglutination test for cryptococcal antigen in diagnosing disseminated infection with *Trichosporon beigelii*. *J Infect Dis* 151:1167–1169, 1985.

Meyer M H, Letscher-Bru V, Waller J, Lutz P, Marcellin L, Herbrecht R. Chronic disseminated *Trichosporon asahii* infection in a leukemic child. *Clin Infect Dis* 35: e22–e25, 2002.

Mirza S H. Disseminated *Trichosporon beigelii* infection causing skin lesions in a renal transplant patient. *J Infect* 27:67–70, 1993.

Mochizuki T, Sugiura H, Watanabe S, Takada M, Hodohara K, Kushima R. A case of disseminated trichosporonosis: A case report and immunohistochemical identification of fungal elements. *J Med Vet Mycol* 26:343–349, 1988.

Morris J T, Beckius M, McAllister C K. *Sporobolomyces* infection in an AIDS patient. *J Infect Dis* 164:623–624, 1991.

Morrison V A, Haake R J, Weisdorf D J. The spectrum of non-*Candida* fungal infections following bone marrow transplantation. *Medicine* 72:78–89, 1993.

Naveh Y A, Friedman A, Merzbach D, Hashman N. Endocarditis caused by *Rhodotorula* successfully treated with 5-flucytosine. *Br Heart J* 37:101–104, 1975.

Nazzaro-Porro M N, Passi S, Caprilli F, Morpurgo G. Growth requirements and lipid metabolism of *Pityrosporum orbiculare*. *J Invest Dermatol* 66:178–182, 1976.

Nelson S C, Yau Y C W, Richardson S E, Matlow A G. Improved detection of *Malassezia* species in lipid-supplemented peds plus blood culture bottles. *J Clin Microbiol* 33:1005–1007, 1995.

Nielsen H, Stenderup J, and Bruun B. Fungemia with Saccharomycetaceae. Report of four cases and review of the literature. *Scand J Infect Dis* 22:581–584, 1990.

Nyirjesy P, Vazquez J A, Ufberg D D, Sobel J D, Boikov D A, Buckley H R. *Saccharomyces cerevisiae* vaginitis: transmission from yeast used in baking. *Obstet Gynecol* 86:326–329, 1995.

Paphitou N I, Ostrosky-Zeichner L, Paetznick V L, Rodriguez J R, Chen E, Rex J H. In vitro antifungal susceptibilities of *Trichosporon* species. *Antimicrob Agents Chemother* 46:1144–1146, 2002.

Patel S A, Borges M C, Batt M D, Rosenblate H J. *Trichosporon* cholangitis associated with hyperbilirubinemia, and findings suggesting primary sclerosing cholangitis on endoscopic retrograde cholangiopancreatography. *Gastroenterol* 85:84–87, 1990.

Pfaller M A, Messer S, Jones R N. Activity of a new triazole, Sch 56592, compared with those of four other antifungal agents tested against clinical isolates of *Candida* spp. and *Saccharomyces cerevisiae*. *Antimicrob Agents Chemother* 41:233–235, 1997.

Plazas J, Portilla J, Boix V, Perez-Mateo M. *Sporobolomyces salmonicolor* lymphadenitis in an AIDS patient: pathogen or passenger? *AIDS* 8:387–398, 1994.

Polacheck I, Salkin I F, Kitzes-Cohen, Raz R. Endocarditis caused by *Blastoschizomyces capitatus* and taxonomic review of the genus. *J Clin Microbiol* 30:2318–2322, 1992.

Pore R S, Chen J. Meningitis caused by *Rhodotorula*. *Sabouraudia* 14:331–335, 1976.

Powell D A, Hayes J, Durrell D E, Miller M, Marcon M J. *Malassezia furfur* skin colonization of infants hospitalized in intensive care units. *J Pediatr* 111:217–220, 1987.

Redline R W, Dahms B B. *Malassezia* pulmonary vasculitis in an infant on long-term intralipid therapy. *N Engl J Med* 305:1395, 1981.

Rippon J W. *Medical Mycology*. The pathogenic fungi and Pathogenic actinomycetes, 3rd Ed. Philadelphia: W. B. Saunders, 148–152, 1988.

Roberts W. *Pityrosporum orbiculare*: incidence and distribution on clinically normal skin. *Br J Dermatol* 81:264, 1969.

Rose H D, Kurup V P. Colonization of hospitalized patients with yeast-like organisms. *Sabouraudia* 15:251–256, 1977.

Rubinstein E, Noriega E R, Simberkoff M S, Holzman R, Rahal J J. Fungal endocarditis: analysis of 24 cases and review of the literature. *Medicine* 54:331–344, 1975.

Rusthoven J J, Feld R, Tuffnell P G. Systemic infection by *Rhodotorula* spp. in the immunocompromised host. *J Infect* 8:241–246, 1984.

Saez H. Etude ecologique sur les *Rhodotorula* des homotherms. *Rev Med Vet* 130:903–908, 1979.

Salkin I F, Gordon M A, Samsonoff W A, Rieder C L. *Blastoschizomyces capitatus*, a new combination. *Mycotaxon* 22:375–380, 1985.

Seeliger H P R, Schroter R. A serologic study on the antigenic relationship of the form genus *Trichosporon. Sabouraudia* 2:248, 1963.

Sethi N, Mandell W. *Saccharomyces* fungemia in a patient with AIDS. *NY State J Med* 88:278–279, 1988.

Sheikh H A, Mahgoub S, Badi K. Postoperative endophthalmitis due to *Trichosporon cutaneum. Brit J Ophthalmol* 58:591–594, 1986.

Shelbourne P F, Carey R J. *Rhodotorula* fungemia complicating staphylococcal endocarditis. *JAMA* 180:38–42, 1962.

Sobel J D, Vazquez J, Lynch M, Meriwether C, Zervos M J. Vaginitis due to *Saccharomyces cerevisiae*: epidemiology, clinical aspects, and therapy. *Clin Infect Dis* 16:93–99, 1993.

Stein P D, Folkens A T, Hruska K A. *Saccharomyces* fungemia. *Chest* 58:173–175, 1970.

Surmont I, Vergauwen B, Marcelis L, Verbist L, Verhoef G, Boogaerts M. First report of chronic meningitis caused by *Trichosporon beigelii. Eur J Clin Microbiol Infect Dis* 9:226–229, 1990.

Szili M, Domjan L. Primary gastric mycosis caused by *Trichosporon cutaneum. Mykosen* 25:189–193, 1982.

Tawara S, Ikeda F, Maki K, Morishita Y, Otomo K, Teratani N, Goto T, Tomishima M, Ohki H, Yamada A, Kawabata K, Takasugi H, Sakane K, Tanaka H, Matsumoto F, Kuwahara S. In vitro activities of a new lipopeptide antifungal agent, FK463, against a variety of clinically important fungi. *Antimicrob Agents Chemother* 44:57–62, 2000.

Tawfik O W, Papasian C, Dixon A Y, Potter L M. *Saccharomyces cerevisiae* pneumonia in a patient with acquired immune deficiency syndrome. *J Clin Microbiol* 27:1689–1691, 1989.

Thaler M, Pastakia B, Shawker T H, O'Leary T O, Pizzo P A. Hepatic candidiasis in cancer patients: The evolving picture of the syndrome. *Ann Intern Med* 108:88–100, 1988.

van Belkum A, Boekhout T, Bosboom R. Monitoring spread of *Malassezia* infections in a neonatal intensive care unit by PCR-medicated genetic typing. *J Clin Microbiol* 32:2528–2532, 1994.

Volz P A, Jerger D E, Wurzburger A J, Hiser J L. A preliminary study of yeasts isolated from marine habitats at Abaco Island, The Bahamas. *Mycopathologia et Mycologia Applicata* 54:313–316, 1974.

Walsh T J, Orth D H, Shapiro C M, Levine R A. Metastatic fungal chorioretinitis developing during *Trichosporon* sepsis. *Ophthalmol* 89:152–156, 1982.

Walsh T J, Newman K R, Moody M, Wharton R, Wade J C. Trichosporonosis in patients with neoplastic disease. *Medicine* 65:268–279, 1986.

Walsh T J. Trichosporonosis. *Infect Dis Clin North Am* 3:43–52, 1989.

Walsh T J, Melcher G P, Rinaldi M G, Lecciones J, McGough D A, Kelly P, Lee J, Callender D, Rubin M, Pizzo P A. *Trichosporon beigelii*, an emerging pathogen resistant to amphotericin B. *J Clin Microbiol* 28:1616–1622, 1990.

Walsh T J, Lee J W, Melcher G P, Navarro E, Bacher J, Callender D, Reed K D, Wu T, Lopez-Berestein V, Pizzo P A. Experimental *Trichosporon* infection in persistently granulocytopenia rabbits: Implications for pathogenesis, diagnosis, and treatment of an emerging opportunistic mycosis. *J Infect Dis* 166:121–133, 1992.

Walsh T J, Melcher G P, Lee J W, Pizzo P A. Infections due to *Trichosporon* species: new concepts in mycology, pathogenesis, diagnosis and treatment. *Curr Top Med Mycol* 5:79–113, 1993.

Watson K C, Kallichurum S. Brain abscess due to *Trichosporon cutaneum. J Med Microbiol* 3:191, 1970.

Weiss S J, Schoch P E, Cunha B A. *Malassezia furfur* fungemia associated with central venous catheter lipid emulsion infusion. *Heart and Lung* 20:87–90, 1991.

Wolf D G, Falk R, Hacham M, Theelen B, Boekhout T, Scorzetti G, Shapiro M, Block C, Salkin I F, Polacheck I. Multidrug-resistant *Trichosporon asahii* infection of nongranulocytopenic patients in three intensive care units. *J Clin Microbiol* 39:4420–4425, 2001.

Young R C, Bennett J E, Geelhoed G W, Levine A S. Fungemia with compromised host resistance: a study of 70 cases. *Ann Intern Med* 80:605–612, 1974.

Yung C W, Hanauer S B, Fretzin D, Rippon J W, Shapiro C, Gonzalez M. Disseminated *Trichosporon beigelii (cutaneum). Cancer* 48:2107–2111, 1981.

IV

MYCOSES CAUSED BY MOULDS

14

Aspergillosis

THOMAS F. PATTERSON

The opportunistic mould *Aspergillus* is the etiologic agent responsible for a variety of infections and conditions referred to as aspergillosis. These manifestations include allergic responses following exposure to the organisms (allergic bronchopulmonary aspergillosis), colonization with *Aspergillus* spp. (aspergilloma or fungus ball due to *Aspergillus* and other conditions such as external ear colonization) and invasive infection (invasive pulmonary aspergillosis and other clinical syndromes of tissue invasion).

The importance of *Aspergillus* as a clinically important pathogen has increased dramatically in recent decades. Invasive aspergillosis is a significant cause of morbidity and mortality in high risk patients (Denning, 1998). A major factor associated with the increased number of cases of invasive aspergillosis is the increase in patients at risk for this disease, such as patients undergoing bone marrow or organ transplantation and patients with other immunodeficiencies. Unfortunately, definitive diagnosis of invasive aspergillosis remains difficult and is compounded by the fact that antifungal agents must be begun promptly if therapy is likely to be successful (von Eiff et al, 1995; Stevens et al, 2000a). However, as rapid diagnostic tools are not widely available to effectively establish a definite diagnosis of invasive aspergillosis, consideration of risk factors in specific epidemiological settings may be useful in suggesting a clinical diagnosis. In high-risk patients, clinical presentation as well as the use of alternative diagnostic procedures such as radiology may be useful in establishing a presumptive diagnosis of infection (Caillot et al, 1997; Patterson, 1998; Stevens et al, 2000a). Cultures may not always be positive in patients with invasive aspergillosis, but it is important to recognize that a positive culture result in high-risk patients may suggest the presence of infection (Patterson, 1999b). However, even when therapy is begun promptly, therapeutic outcomes with current agents remain poor, particularly in patients with disseminated disease (Denning, 1998; Patterson et al, 2000b; Stevens et al, 2000a). Recently, significant advances in the therapy of aspergillosis have been reported and therapeutic guidelines using currently available drugs have been published.

HISTORICAL REVIEW

Micheli in Florence first recognized *Aspergillus* in 1729 (Micheli, 1729). In his historic monograph *Nova Geneva Plantarum*, Micheli, a priest, noted the resemblance between the sporing head of the organism he described as *Aspergillus* and an aspergillum used to sprinkle holy water (with the name derived from the Latin *aspergo*, to sprinkle) (Micheli, 1729; Mackenzie, 1987). Later, Rayer and Montagne identified *Aspergillus candidus* from a bird air sac in 1842, but the first detailed microscopic descriptions of *Aspergillus* were provided by Virchow in 1856 who also published the first detailed descriptions of human infection (Virchow, 1856; Kwon-Chung, 1987). Virchow examined tissues described in earlier reports of animal disease by Bennett in 1844 and Sluyter in 1847 and concluded the organisms were closely related to those that he observed in human infection (Kwon-Chung and Bennett, 1992). Fresenius introduced the term aspergillosis in 1863 in his work describing avian infection (Fresenius, 1863).

Initial descriptions of clinical cases (some of which were likely colonization) were first detailed in workers that had been occupationally exposed to the organism and the association was made with infection and certain occupations—such as pigeon feeders, wig combers, farmers, feed-mill workers, and others exposed to dust or grains (Denning, 1998). Others noted the potential for *Aspergillus* to colonize or invade cavities that formed following other diseases such as tuberculosis. Deve described fungus balls due to *Aspergillus* (aspergilloma) in 1938 (Deve, 1938). The potential for allergic reactions to the organisms in the form of allergic bronchopulmonary aspergillosis was described in 1952 (Hinson et al, 1952). It was not until the mid-1950s with the introduction of immunosuppressive agents such as corticosteroids and cytotoxic chemotherapy that the first occurrences of invasive aspergillosis in immunocompromised hosts were recognized (Rankin, 1953). In recent decades the use of immunosuppressive therapies in increasing numbers of patients has resulted in a dramatic global increase in cases of invasive infections due to *Aspergillus* (Groll et al, 1996).

MYCOLOGY

After the initial early descriptions of the organism, *Aspergillus flavus* was formally named in 1809 (Link, 1809). Thom and Church first classified the genus in 1926 with 69 *Aspergillus* species in 11 groups—which has gradually increased to over 200 species (although some are not universally accepted) in 18 groups (Thom and Church, 1926; Raper and Fennel, 1965; Pitt, 1994; Denning, 2000). Most species of *Aspergillus* reproduce asexually but a teleomorph (or sexual form) has been identified for some species, including at least two pathogenic species *A. nidulans*—now correctly identified as *A. nidulellus*—(teleomorph, *Emericella nidulans*) and *A. amstelodami* (*Eurotium amstelodami*) (Klich and Pitt, 1988). The generic name *Aspergillus* is generally applied to all species regardless of their teleomorphs, rather than separating the organisms into a limited number of new (and unfamiliar) species based on discovery of a sexual state along with the majority of isolates without an identified teleomorph (Kwon-Chung, 1987).

The genus *Aspergillus* is classified in the family Moniliaceae of the form class Hyphomycetes in the phylum Deuteromycota. The teleomorphs of *Aspergillus* species are classified in 10 genera in the phylum Ascomycota. Specific species identification of the organism may be difficult and taxonomy of the species is undergoing revision with the use of molecular tools of identification. *Aspergillus* is distinct but is closely related to the genus *Penicillium* (Klich and Pitt, 1988). The most common species causing invasive infection include: *Aspergillus fumigatus* (historically causes approximately 90% of invasive aspergillosis), *A. flavus*, *A. niger*, and *A. terreus*. Recent studies have shown continued emergence of less common species, including *A. terreus* and unusual less pathogenic species as the etiologic agents of invasive infection (Table 14–1). With more prolonged and profound immunosuppression, the list of rare species causing invasive infection

continues to increase and includes: *A. amstelodami*, *A. avenaceus*, *A. caesiellus*, *A. candidus*, *A. carneus*, *A. chevalieri*, *A. clavatus*, *A. flavipes*, *A. glaucus*, *A. granulosus*, *A. nidulans* (*A. nidulellus*), *A. oryzae*, *A. quadrilineatus*, *A. restrictus*, *A. sydowii*, *A. ustus*, *A. versicolor*, *A. wentii*, *Neosartorya pseudofisheri* (previously *Aspergillus fischeri*), and others (Denning, 2000; Klich and Pitt, 1988; Kwon-Chung and Bennett, 1992; Denning, 1998, 2000; Stevens et al, 2000; Sutton et al, 1998; Sutton et al, 2000).

Pathogenic *Aspergillus* species grow easily and rapidly at a broad range of culture temperatures and on a wide variety of media, although blood cultures are uncommonly positive. Growth of pathogenic species at 37°C is a feature that differentiates the pathogenic from non-pathogenic isolates. *Aspergillus fumigatus* is able to grow at temperatures up to 50°C, which can be used in identification of that species (Sutton et al, 1998). Most species will initially appear as small, fluffy white colonies within 48 hours of culture. Presumptive identification at the genus level is usually performed based on morphological characteristics without difficulty, although species level identification of unusual species may be significantly more difficult.

Microscopic features and colony morphology for *A. fumigatus*, *A. flavus*, *A. terreus* and *A. niger* are shown in Color Figures 14–1 A–D and 14–2 A–D (see separate color insert), respectively. Specific identification of *Aspergillus* has become important, as differences in pathogenicity as well as susceptibility have been recognized. Key features of these four species most frequently associated with clinical manifestations of disease are outlined below.

Aspergillus fumigatus (See Color Figures 14–1A and 14–2A in separate color insert) is the most common species to cause invasive infection, comprising more than 90% of the isolates identified in some series. The organism is found widespread in nature—in soil, on decaying vegetation, in the air, and in water supplies (Anaissie et al, 2002). Its thermotolerance permits a wide range of suitable host conditions, which can also be used to identify the species. Colonies are a gray–green color with a wooly to cottony texture (Sutton et al, 1998). Hyphae are septate and hyaline with columnar conidial heads. Conidiophores are smooth-walled, uncolored and uniseriate with closely compacted phialides only on the upper portion of the vesicle. Conidia are smooth to finely roughened and are 2–3.5 μm in diameter. Hyphae, which are strongly angioinvasive, may not always branch at 45°C. Fruiting heads may occur rarely in clinical specimens in sites exposed to air (Sutton et al, 1998).

Aspergillus flavus (See Color Figs. 14–1B and 14–2B in separate color insert) is found in soil and decaying vegetation. Colonies are olive to lime green and grow

TABLE 14–1. *Identification of* Aspergillus *Species in 261 Cases of Invasive Infection*

Species	Number (%)
A. fumigatus	173 (66)
A. flavus	36 (14)
A. niger	17 (7)
A. terreus	11 (4)
Others	5 (2)
A. versicolor	2
A. nidulans	1
A. oryzae	1
A. glaucus	1
Not specified or not identified	19 (7)

Source: Patterson et al, 2000b.

at a rapid rate. This species is typically biseriate with rough conidiophores and smooth conidia 3–6 μm that serve to distinguish the species. Some isolates are uniseriate. The organism is a common cause of sinusitis as well as invasive infection in immunosuppressed hosts. *Aspergillus flavus* is also responsible for a mycotoxicosis as the species produces a potent aflatoxin (Denning, 1987).

Aspergillus terreus (See Color Figures 14–1C and 14–2C in separate color insert) is common in tropical and subtropical habitats and has been increasingly reported as a cause of invasive infection in immunocompromised hosts (Iwen et al, 1998). Colonies are buff to beige to cinnamon (Sutton et al, 1998). Conidial heads are biseriate and columnar. Conidiophores are smooth walled and hyaline. Globose, sessile aleurioconidia are frequently produced on submerged hyphae. Conidia are small (2–2.5 μm). The colony color and fruiting structures are characteristic for this species, notable for its decreased susceptibility to some antifungal agents including amphotericin B (Iwen et al, 1998; Sutton et al, 1999).

Aspergillus niger (See Color Figures 14–1D and 14–2D in separate color insert) is widespread in soil and on plants and is common in food (such as pepper). Colonies are initially white but quickly become black with the production of the fruiting structures. This species grows rapidly with a pale yellow reverse. Like other *Aspergillus* species, hyphae are hyaline and septate. Conidial heads are biseriate and cover the entire vesicle. Conidia are brown to black and are very rough (4–5 μm) (Sutton et al, 1998). This species, which is commonly associated with colonization and otic infections, produces oxalate crystals in clinical specimens (Geyer and Surampudi, 2002).

PATHOGENESIS AND HOST DEFENSES

Aspergillus infection is typically acquired through inhalation of conidia into the lungs although other routes of exposure may also occur, such as oral or aerosol exposure to contaminated water (Anaissie and Costa, 2001) or though local exposure, including surgical wounds, contaminated intravenous catheters or arm boards leading to cutaneous infection (Allo et al, 1987; Walsh, 1998; Gettleman et al, 1999).

Invasive aspergillosis is uncommon in immunocompetent patients, although infection in apparently normal hosts does occur (Clancy and Nguyen, 1998; Patterson et al, 2000b). Hence, despite the ubiquitous nature of the organism and frequent exposure to it, normal host defenses do not readily permit invasive pulmonary aspergillosis to occur.

Aspergillus species commonly produce toxins that may contribute to clinical manifestations of exposure to the organisms although they are unlikely to be major virulence determinants for systemic infection (Denning, 1987). These mycotoxins include aflatoxins, ochratoxin A, fumagillin, and gliotoxin. The latter particularly may reduce macrophage and neutrophil function (Denning, 2000). Aflatoxin, produced by *A. flavus*, is important as a carcinogenic and immunosuppressive agent but is not an important determinate of virulence of the organism (Denning, 1987). Other pathogenic features of the organisms include a variety of proteases and phospholipases (Latge, 1999), which contribute to pathogenicity of the organism. However, strains without these features are still capable of causing experimental infection (Monod et al, 1993; Tang et al, 1993; Smith et al, 1994; Birch et al, 1996).

The first lines of host defense against inhalation of *Aspergillus* conidia are ciliary clearance of the organism from the airways and the limited access to deep lung structures for larger, less pathogenic conidia. In the pulmonary tissues, the alveolar macrophage is a potent defense, capable of ingesting and killing inhaled *Aspergillus* conidia (Schaffner et al, 1982; Kan and Bennett, 1988). After germination, the major line of defense against both swollen conidia and hyphae is the polymorphonuclear leukocyte. However, hyphae are too large to be effectively ingested and hyphae damage occurs extracellularly (Levitz et al, 1986). Swollen conidia and hyphae are both able to fix complement, which is important in phagocytic killing of the organism. Notably, *Aspergillus fumigatus* produces a complement inhibitor, which may play a role in its pathogenicity (Washburn et al, 1986; Washburn et al, 1987). Antibody responses due to prior exposures to *Aspergillus* are common but antibodies are not protective against invasive infection nor are they useful for diagnosis of infection, due to the fact few immunosuppressed patients are able to mount an antibody response even in the setting of invasive disease (Young and Bennett, 1971).

The ability of phagocytes to oxidatively kill *Aspergillus* is a critical component of host defenses against the organism (Kan and Bennett, 1988). The use of corticosteroids substantially impairs neutrophil killing of hyphae and resistance to conidia by neutrophils, which may be reversed to some degree with the use of interferon-γ or with administration of granulocyte or granulocyte-macrophage growth factors (Schaffner, 1985; Roilides et al, 1993). Recent studies have also suggested a role for cellular immunity. In a murine model of invasive aspergillosis, a Th1 response induced by administration of soluble interleukin-4 was associated with a favorable response (Cenci et al, 1997).

In the clinical setting, prolonged neutropenia is a major risk factor for invasive aspergillosis (Gerson et al, 1984). Notably, without recovery from absolute neutropenia, response to even aggressive antifungal therapy is unlikely (Denning, 1998; Patterson et al, 2000b). Nevertheless, with changing patterns of immunosuppressive therapy, patients are less likely to remain neutropenic for extended periods of time and the use of growth factors has further limited the duration of neutropenia. In recent surveys, other immunosuppressive conditions have emerged as important risk factors for invasive aspergillosis, and the time period for risk of invasive aspergillosis is now greatly extended. In patients receiving hematopoietic stem cell or marrow transplants, the period at risk now extends for more than 100 days after immunosuppression (Wald et al, 1997; Baddley et al, 2001), and reflects long-term complications of high-dose steroid therapy and other immunosuppressive agents for chronic graft-vs.-host disease that occurs following nonmyeloablative transplant procedures.

In noninvasive or allergic forms of aspergillosis, the pathogenesis is not well defined but appears to relate to chronic allergic responses to the organism (Stevens et al, 2000; Denning, 2001). The most frequent organism associated with allergic bronchopulmonary aspergillosis is *A. fumigatus*, with usual manifestations including central bronchiectasis, with typical allergic features of bronchiolitis and chronic eosinophilic pneumonia (Rosenberg et al, 1977). Similarly, the pathogenesis of aspergilloma due to *Aspergillus* is not well defined but also seems to be associated with allergic reactions to chronic colonization. In aspergilloma, the organism does not usually invade the tissues but colonizes a pulmonary cavity. Although tissue invasion resulting in a chronic necrotizing form of aspergillosis can occur, the pathogenic features leading from colonization to invasive disease are not clearly understood (Tomlinson and Sahn, 1987).

EPIDEMIOLOGY

Aspergillus is a ubiquitous saprophytic mould that is found worldwide in a variety of habitats. *Aspergillus* is found in soil, water, food, and is particularly common in decaying vegetation. The inoculum for establishing infection is not known, but persons with normal pulmonary defense mechanisms can withstand even extensive exposure without any manifestation of disease, while severely immunocompromised hosts are susceptible to presumably lower inocula for establishing disease. Notably, patients may manifest infection due to prior asymptomatic colonization that leads to invasive infection with the occurrence of immunosuppressive conditions (such as neutropenia, corticosteroid use, or AIDS) (Walsh and Dixon, 1989).

Consideration of the epidemiology and host risk factors for aspergillosis may be useful in suggesting a clin-

ical diagnosis of invasive infection. Neutropenia remains a major risk factor for invasive aspergillosis, but increasing numbers of patients with other risk factors, including solid organ and bone marrow transplantation, develop infection (Patterson et al, 2000a; Patterson et al, 2000b; Stevens et al, 2000). In patients undergoing hematopoetic stem cell or marrow transplant, increased incidence of invasive aspergillosis has been reported (Marr et al, 2002). The epidemiology of invasive aspergillosis in those patients has shifted to the development of infection late in the course of transplant with cases occurring more than 100 days after transplant due to risk factors of chronic graft-vs.-host disease, steroid use and other factors leading to prolonged immunosuppression (Wald et al, 1997; Marr et al, 2002). Recent series have shown that patients undergoing bone marrow transplantation or receiving chemotherapy for hematological malignancies still constitute the majority of those patients diagnosed with invasive aspergillosis (Patterson et al, 2000a; Patterson et al, 2000b). Among patients with solid organ transplants, those undergoing lung transplantation are at particular risk for *Aspergillus* infection with a clinical presentation ranging from an ulcerative tracheobronchitis to disseminated infection (Paterson and Singh, 1999; Patterson et al, 2000a). Data from recent (1998–2001) liver transplant recipients indicate that invasive aspergillosis is more likely to involve the lung, occurs later in the post-transplantation period, and is associated with a lower mortality rate, compared to earlier liver transplant recipients (1990–1995) (Singh et al, 2003). In summary, specific risk factors include not only neutropenia and graft-vs.-host disease, but also high dose corticosteroids and other immunosuppressive therapies. In addition, invasive aspergillosis has been observed among patients with advanced AIDS, especially in those with CD4 cell counts below $50/mm^3$ (Denning et al, 1991). For further discussion of aspergillosis in AIDS patients, see Chapter 32.

Standards for air quality in bone marrow transplant units, particularly spore filtration with high-efficiency particulate air (HEPA) filtration, have been recommended during the period of most severe neutropenia in order to reduce the rates of nosocomial infection (Patterson et al, 2000a). Outbreaks of invasive aspergillosis have occurred in patients exposed to *Aspergillosis* in association with construction and other environmental risks. Air filtration and infection control measures such as construction barriers that reduce risks by limiting exposure to aerosols have been shown to reduce the incidence of infection. However, in the most severely immunosuppressed patients, aspergillosis may still occur either as a result of endogenous reactivation of latent tissue infection or due to other exposures, perhaps even related to aerosols of contaminated water

(Iwen et al, 1993; Patterson et al, 1997; Patterson et al, 2000a; Anaissie and Costa, 2001). In addition, because bone marrow transplant and other organ transplant patients frequently receive substantial portions of their care in the outpatient setting, control of air quality in those settings is not possible and may result in exposure to *Aspergillus* conidia.

CLINICAL SYNDROMES

Saprophytic and Superficial Aspergillosis
Pulmonary aspergilloma. A pulmonary fungus ball due to *Aspergillus* (aspergilloma) is characterized by chronic, extensive colonization of *Aspergillus* species in a pulmonary cavity or ectatic bronchus. Fungus balls may also develop in other sites such as the maxillary or ethmoid sinus or even in the upper jaw following endodontic treatment (de Carpentier et al, 1994; Ferguson, 2000; Gillespie and O'Malley, 2000). Typically *Aspergillus* fungus balls in the lung develop in cavities resulting from pre-existing diseases or infections such as tuberculosis, histoplasmosis, sarcoidosis, bullous emphysema, fibrotic lung disease, or *Pneumocystis carinii* pneumonia in AIDS. *Aspergillus* is more common as the etiologic agent although other organisms such as *Scedosporium apiospermum* (*Pseudallescheria boydii*) or agents of zygomycosis can also cause similar syndromes. The diagnosis of a pulmonary fungus ball is usually made radiographically; aspergilloma appears as a solid round mass inside a cavity. The detection of *Aspergillus* antibodies are further evidence that the radiographic findings are consistent with a diagnosis of fungus ball due to *Aspergillus* and a biopsy is not usually undertaken (Rafferty et al, 1983).

Although the presence of a fungus ball due to *Aspergillus* may be relatively asymptomatic, in some patients tissue invasion may occur, leading to invasive pulmonary aspergillosis or a subacute chronic necrotizing form of the disease (Tomlinson and Sahn, 1987). Hemoptysis is a common clinical symptom and can lead to a fatal complication (Aslam et al, 1971; Kauffman, 1996). Hemoptysis has been reported as the cause of death in up to 26% of patients with aspergilloma (Aslam et al, 1971; Kauffman, 1996). Management of aspergilloma is determined by the frequency and severity of hemoptysis as well as evaluation for risk factors that are associated with a poor prognosis. Complications are more likely in patients with severe underlying lung disease, immunosuppression or extensive disease, suggested by high titers of *Aspergillus* antibody. In these settings, specific therapies may be needed earlier in the course of management in order to attempt to avoid potential life-threatening hemoptysis (Kauffman, 1996).

Other Superficial or Colonizing Conditions of Aspergillosis. *Aspergillus* can also be associated with fungal balls of the sinuses without tissue invasion (Vennewald et al, 1999; Ferguson, 2000). The maxillary sinus is the most common site for a sinus aspergilloma (Ferguson, 2000). Clinical presentation is similar to that for any chronic sinusitis with chronic nasal discharge, sinus congestion and pain. The diagnosis of a fungal ball may be suggested on computed tomography of the sinuses along with positive cultures for the organism, which is usually *A. fumigatus* or *A. flavus*. Management is usually directed at surgical removal of the lesion with confirmation that the fungal ball has not caused bony erosion.

Otomycosis is a condition of superficial colonization by *Aspergillus*, most typically *A. niger* (Kaur et al, 2000). The usual clinical presentation is that of an external otitis media, with ear pain and drainage. Examination of the ear canal may reveal the black conidiophores of *A. niger*. Treatment involves cleaning of the external ear canal and the topical administration of a variety of agents including cleansing solutions and topical antifungal agents.

Other superficial or colonizing conditions due to *Aspergillus* include onychomycosis, which can be a chronic condition not responsive to antifungal agents directed at yeasts. Consequently, culture confirmation of *Aspergillus* as the etiologic agent will be useful in this setting.

In addition, *Aspergillus* species may colonize the airways in patients with a variety of lung conditions that do not have apparent disease. A recent report by the Mycoses Study Group showed that a large number of clinical isolates of *Aspergillus* are not associated with infection (Perfect et al, 2001). Many of those isolates come from sputum samples of patients without apparent invasive disease, although the role of *Aspergillus* in causing symptoms of occasional hemoptysis and bronchitis in those patients is unclear.

Allergic Manifestations of Disease
Allergic Bronchopulmonary Aspergillosis. Allergic bronchopulmonary aspergillosis (ABPA) is a chronic allergic response to colonization with *Aspergillus*. Specific criteria for establishing a diagnosis include: *(1)* episodic bronchial obstruction (asthma); *(2)* peripheral eosinophilia; *(3)* immediate skin test reactivity to *Aspergillus* antigen; *(4)* precipitating *Aspergillus* antibodies; *(5)* elevated serum immunoglobulin E (IgE); *(6)* history of or presence of pulmonary infiltrates; and *(7)* central bronchiectasis (Rosenberg et al, 1977). The detection of the first six criteria establishes a likely diagnosis, while the presence of all seven confirm the condition. Other secondary features that may be present include positive sputum cultures for *Aspergillus*, brown mucus plugs in sputa, elevated specific IgE antibodies against

Aspergillus, late skin reactivity to *Aspergillus*, and reactions following intrabronchial challenge with *Aspergillus* (Patterson et al, 1982).

In ABPA, typically the initiating event is for an asthmatic patient to develop an allergic reaction to inhaled *Aspergillus*. Following that reaction, mucus plugs develop in the bronchi and can be detected by the presence of hyphae in sputa. The impacted mucus causes atelectasis, which in turn causes transient pulmonary infiltrates; repeated bronchial reactions ultimately lead to bronchiectasis in the proximal bronchi. Characteristic "ring signs" (circular or oblong densities) or "tram lines" (parallel shadows) are seen on radiographs. These findings result from chronic peribronchial inflammation around dilated bronchi (Malo et al, 1977).

Allergic bronchopulmonary aspergillosis is reported to occur in up to 14% of patients with steroid-dependent asthma (Basich et al, 1981; Kumar and Gaur, 2000), and is also particularly common in patients colonized with *Aspergillus* such as those with cystic fibrosis who have a 7% prevalence of ABPA (Mroueh and Spock, 1994). In cystic fibrosis patients undergoing lung transplantation, the presence of *Aspergillus* colonization is an important risk for developing invasive pulmonary aspergillosis (Stevens et al, 2000).

Allergic bronchopulmonary aspergillosis typically progresses through a series of stages which can be useful in approaching management of the condition: *(1)* acute; *(2)* remission; *(3)* exacerbation; *(4)* steroid-dependent asthma; and *(5)* fibrosis (Patterson et al, 1982). The initial acute stage is usually responsive to corticosteroid therapy which may lead to a period of asymptomatic remission. Most patients will experience exacerbations and may eventually become steroid dependent. Late stage manifestations include pulmonary fibrosis that may be associated with substantially reduced pulmonary function and is associated with a poor long-term prognosis. Management of ABPA is directed at reducing acute asthmatic symptoms and avoiding end-stage fibrotic complications. Corticosteroid therapy is commonly used for treating exacerbations although few randomized trials have been conducted to evaluate its use (Stevens et al, 2000a). However, increasing serum IgE levels, worsening or new infiltrates, or worsening findings on spirometry suggest that steroids may be helpful (Stevens et al, 2000a). The role of antifungal agents is limited although itraconazole may be beneficial in reducing symptoms and reducing the use of steroids. A recent, randomized double-blind, placebo-controlled trial showed that itraconazole at 200 mg per day for 16 weeks significantly reduced daily corticosteroid use, reduced levels of serum IgE and improved exercise tolerance and pulmonary function (Stevens et al, 2000b).

Other Allergic Manifestations. Allergic responses can also contribute to symptoms of sinusitis (Katzenstein et al, 1983; Corey et al, 1995; DeShazo et al, 1997). Allergic sinusitis is similar in its presentation to sinusitis complicated with fungal balls due to *Aspergillus* (Houser and Corey, 2000). Frequently, in patients with allergic fungal sinusitis, polyposis or eosinophil-rich mucin containing Charcot-Leyden crystals may be seen (Washburn, 1998). Management is largely directed at confirming lack of invasive infection and in aerating the sinus (Kuhn and Javer, 2000b). The use of steroids or antifungal agents has not been conclusively demonstrated to be of benefit (Kuhn and Javer, 2000a; Kuhn and Javer, 2000b).

Invasive Syndromes Caused by Aspergillus
Infection with *Aspergillus* is usually acquired through inhalation of airborne conidia, which invade the lung tissue in the absence of an effective monocytic or neutrophilic immune response (Latge, 2001). The major infection is invasive pulmonary aspergillosis (IPA) which arises from spread of the organisms from a primary pulmonary inoculum or from the paranasal sinuses. Hyphal invasion into blood vessels is common, occurring in approximately a third of patients with IPA. Nonpulmonary sites become infected by contiguous spread or via hematogenous spread to the central nervous system (occurring in 10 to 40% of severely immunosuppressed patients such as those undergoing allogeneic stem cell or bone marrow transplant) or to other organs including the liver, spleen, kidney, skin, bone, and heart (Denning, 1998; Latge, 1999; Ribaud et al, 1999).

Response to antifungal therapy depends on several factors including the immune status of the host and extent of the infection at time of diagnosis. As shown in Table 14–2, favorable responses, defined as those with complete resolution of signs and symptoms attributed to invasive aspergillosis, and those with partial re-

TABLE 14–2. *Favorable Responses in Invasive Aspergillosis: Role of Immunosuppression and Extent of Disease*

Underlying Disease (n)	Complete/Partial Responses (%)
Overall (595)	37
Severe Immunosuppression (363)	28
Allogeneic BMT (151)	13
Hematological Malignancy (212)	39
Less Severe Immunosuppression (232)	51

Site of Infection (n)	Complete/Partial Responses (%)
Pulmonary (330)	40
Disseminated (without CNS) (114)	18
Central Nervous System (34)	9

Source: Patterson et al, 2000b.

TABLE 14–3. *Case Fatality Rates in Invasive Aspergillosis*

Underlying Disease/Site of Infection (n)	Case Fatality Rate (%)
Overall (1941)	57.6
Bone marrow transplantation (285)	86.1
Leukemia/lymphoma (288)	49.3
Pulmonary infection (1153)	59.4
CNS/disseminated infection (175)	88.1

Source: Lin et al, 2001.

sponses (substantial improvement), are seen in less than 40% of treated patients (Patterson et al, 2000b). Even more striking are the extremely poor responses seen in the most highly immunosuppressed patients. For example, in a survey of 595 patients with invasive aspergillosis, favorable responses were seen in only 13% of patients undergoing allogeneic bone marrow transplantation (Patterson et al, 2000b). Similarly poor responses have been reported in other recent series as well, although newer therapeutic modalities may improve the outcome even in patients with more severe immunosuppression (Maertens et al, 2000; Bowden et al, 2002; Herbrecht et al, 2002a). Extent of infection also correlates with likelihood of a favorable outcome: in patients with disseminated aspergillosis favorable responses decrease to less than 20% and to less than 10% in patients with central nervous system disease.

As might be predicted, the mortality rate of patients with invasive aspergillosis also correlates with immune status of the host and extent of disease. Lin and colleagues reviewed 1941 patients from 50 recent series of invasive aspergillosis and found an overall mortality rate of 60%, which rose to more than 80% in patients with severe immunosuppression and almost 90% in those with central nervous system involvement (Table 14–3) (Lin et al, 2001).

Invasive Pulmonary Aspergillosis. Invasive pulmonary aspergillosis is the most common manifestation of invasive aspergillosis. The temporal pattern of IPA is closely linked to changes in circulating neutrophils including both the degree and the duration of severe neutrophil depression. The incubation period of IPA is currently unknown and a significant number of patients are colonized at the time of admission or develop sinus/airway colonization with *Aspergillus* shortly after hospitalization suggesting prior community-acquired colonization or infection (Patterson et al, 2000a; Patterson et al, 1997). The disease rarely manifests before 10–12 days of profound neutropenia. The most frequent symptoms include progressive dry cough, fever despite coverage with broad-spectrum antibiotics (although fever may not be present in patients receiving corticosteroids), dyspnea, and pleuritic chest pain. Notably, extensive infection can develop before symptoms are prominent, which emphasizes the importance of clinical suspicion in establishing the diagnosis early. Other manifestations include hemoptysis and pneumothorax. Invasive pulmonary aspergillosis may resemble a pulmonary embolism with infarction with sudden onset chest pain and difficulty breathing. The physical exam is unfortunately nonspecific. Laboratory studies usually reflect neutropenia and thrombocytopenia secondary to chemotherapy. Occasional nonspecific findings include elevation in bilirubin and lactate dehydrogenase, coagulation abnormalities, and elevation in C-reactive protein and fibrinogen. Patients with more widespread pulmonary involvement may develop respiratory failure characterized by hypoxemia with compensatory hyperventilation, hypocapnea and respiratory alkalosis. The prognosis of patients with focal IPA is more favorable as the disease tends to progress more slowly and may be amenable to surgical intervention (Yeghen et al, 2000). The major problem for patients with focal disease is hemoptysis that may be explosive and life threatening.

Initially plain chest radiographs may be nonspecific or show few abnormalities. In extensive infection, diffuse nodular pulmonary infiltrates typically occur and are readily seen on chest radiograph (Fig. 14–3). Other pulmonary lesions include pleural-based, wedge-shaped densities and cavities. Pleural effusions have been considered rare (Denning, 1998), but recent studies suggest that pleural effusions are more common than has been recognized, although their association with infection has not been established (Herbrecht et al, 2002a). Chest CT scans are more sensitive for detecting early infection and in establishing extent of infection (Caillot et al, 1997). The presence of a "halo" of low attenuation surrounding a nodular lesion is an early find-

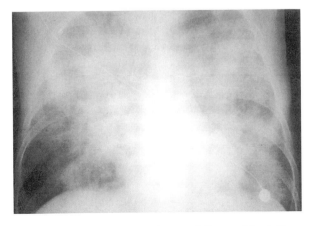

FIGURE 14–3. Chest radiograph showing diffuse nodular infiltrates in patient with invasive pulmonary aspergillosis.

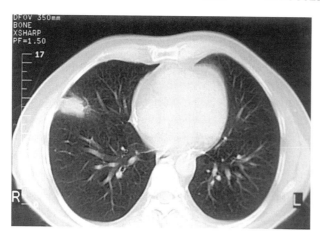

FIGURE 14–4. Computed tomography of chest showing "halo" sign of low attenuation surrounding a nodular lung lesion in patient with early invasive pulmonary aspergillosis.

ing in IPA and has been used as a marker for initiating early antifungal therapy (Caillot et al, 1997; Herbrecht et al, 2002a) (Fig. 14–4). Later in the course of infection, nodular lesions may cavitate (usually in temporal association with recovery of neutrophils), producing an "air-crescent" sign (Fig. 14–5). Despite the utility of these radiographic findings in establishing an early diagnosis, it should be recognized that their validity has been established in high risk, neutropenic and bone marrow transplant patients. In other groups, including solid organ transplant patients, other opportunistic etiologic agents can clearly cause similar findings; consequently, CT findings should be interpreted with caution.

Chronic IPA, less common than acute IPA, occurs most frequently in patients with AIDS, chronic granulomatous disease, alcoholism, and diabetes mellitus, but

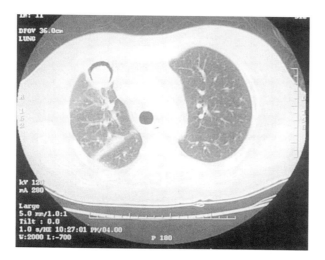

FIGURE 14–5. Computed tomography of chest showing classic "air crescent" sign in patient with invasive aspergillosis.

also has been observed in a significant number of immunocompetent persons (Binder et al, 1982; Karam and Griffin, 1986; Denning, 2001). The major manifestations of this indolent pulmonary process, characterized by symptoms over weeks to months, include low-grade fever, malaise, and chronic productive cough, with or without hemoptysis.

Tracheobronchitis. *Aspergillus* infection of the airways is more common in patients with advanced AIDS and in patients undergoing lung transplantation (Denning et al, 1991; Paterson and Singh, 1999). The syndromes in these patients range from colonization (which is particularly common in lung transplantation) to an extensive pseudomembranous tracheobronchitis and ulcerative tracheobronchitis that occur at the suture line of lung transplant patients (Kramer et al, 1991; Kanj et al, 1996). Symptoms of tracheobronchitis may be mild and may be confused with other causes including rejection in lung transplantation. Typically these patients have cough, fever, and dyspnea along with chest plan and hemoptysis. In more severe disease, unilateral wheezing or stridor may develop due to local obstruction (Denning, 1998). Plain radiographs are not sensitive for the diagnosis and clinical suspicion combined with change in pulmonary function capacity may be early clues for the diagnosis. Bronchoscopy with biopsy to document tissue invasion is needed to establish the diagnosis of invasive *Aspergillus* tracheobronchitis. Therapy with systemic antifungal agents is usually given for a prolonged period of time. While aerosols of amphotericin B are poorly tolerated, aerosols of lipid formulations of amphotericin B have been successfully used for localized disease (Palmer et al, 1998).

Sinusitis. Involvement of the nasal passages or sinuses are also relatively classic manifestations of invasive aspergillosis that may occur either as isolated syndromes or, more commonly, in the setting of IPA. *Aspergillus* infections of the sinuses and nasal cavities in immunocompromised patients usually present as acute invasive rhinosinusitis. The clinical manifestations are initially nonspecific and consist of fever, cough, epistaxis, sinus discharge, and headaches. Clinical examination is usually nondiagnostic. Identification of anesthetic areas and ulcers is particularly important. Frequently, the disease spreads to adjacent areas such as palate, orbit, or brain. The mortality in invasive cases is high, ranging from 20% in patients with leukemia in remission who are undergoing maintenance therapy, up to 100% in patients with relapsed leukemia or those undergoing bone marrow transplantation (Iwen et al, 1997). Plain radiographs are not sensitive for the diagnosis and do not distinguish fungal etiologies from other causes of sinusitis. Sinus CT scans are useful for establishing extent of infection and determining local invasion of bone and soft tissues. Diagnosis is established presumptively from culture of sinus or nasal material but requires tissue to document invasive disease.

Disseminated Infection. Widely disseminated invasive aspergillosis is a common end-stage complication of refractory IPA. In patients with severe immunosuppression including patients with profound granulocytopenia, grade III–IV graft-vs.-host disease, and progressive underlying malignancy, infection can disseminate rapidly and involve virtually every organ system as seen in autopsy series. In patients with extensive disseminated disease, favorable responses to therapy are uncommon and mortality rates approach 90% (Lin et al, 2001).

Cerebral Aspergillosis. Cerebral aspergillosis is one of the most dreaded complications of disseminated aspergillosis due to the extremely high mortality rates of more than 90% that have been reported in most series (Lin et al, 2001). Cerebral aspergillosis occurs in 10%–20% of all cases of invasive aspergillosis, usually associated with disseminated disease (Denning, 1998). In severely immunosuppressed patients such as those undergoing allogeneic transplantation, *Aspergillus* is a major cause of brain abscess and was found in 58% of biopsied lesions in one series (Hagensee et al, 1994). Importantly, cerebral aspergillosis was associated with pulmonary disease in 87% of the cases, with an overall mortality of 97% (Hagensee et al, 1994). Isolated cerebral aspergillosis can occur even in immunocompetent patients and may be associated with a slightly better prognosis provided the diagnosis is made early and surgical drainage or extirpation is performed. *Aspergillus* meningitis is rare. The clinical presentation of cerebral aspergillosis is in general nonspecific, characterized by focal neurological signs, alteration in mental status and headaches. Fever may occur but is usually related to other concomitant infections. On CT of the brain, *Aspergillus* lesions will appear similar to other infectious causes of brain abscess and manifest ring enhancement of the abscess along with surrounding edema (Fig. 14–6). Magnetic resonance scans may reveal additional lesions but the findings are also nonspecific. Although the diagnosis of cerebral aspergillosis is confirmed by biopsy, the etiology can be inferred in patients with widely disseminated infection. However, in highly immunosuppressed patients including those with organ or bone marrow transplants or advanced AIDS, the differential diagnosis is very broad and includes bacterial brain abscess, toxoplasmosis, other fungi, tuberculosis, and lymphoma; consequently a presumptive diagnosis should be entertained with caution. Formerly, the outcome of cerebral aspergillosis had been almost universally fatal; recent limited tri-

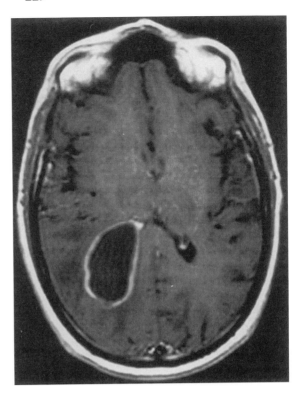

FIGURE 14–6. Brain abscess with ring enhancement and extensive edema in patient with cerebral aspergillosis.

als with the new triazole, voriconazole, have demonstrated responses in approximately 25% of patients with well-documented cerebral infection (Denning et al, 2002; Herbrecht et al, 2002a).

Cutaneous Disease. Skin involvement by *Aspergillus* can either represent disseminated hematogenous spread or local infection associated with an intravenous-catheter insertion site or the skin areas covered by adhesive dressings (Allo et al, 1987). While most cutaneous lesions occur in patients with neutropenia or in other immunocompromised patients such as neonates, *Aspergillus* can also invade burns or surgical wounds (Denning and Stevens, 1990). Clinically, the lesions appear as areas of rapidly increasing erythema with a necrotic, often ulcerated center, resembling pyoderma gangrenosum. Pathologically, there is invasion of blood vessels and cutaneous ulceration. In patients with cutaneous disease as a manifestation of widespread disseminated aspergillosis, a skin biopsy can be a relatively easy method to obtain tissue to establish the diagnosis.

Osteomyelitis. *Aspergillus* osteomyelitis is an uncommon manifestation of invasive aspergillosis. Bony involvement can occur in the setting of local extension (pulmonary, sinus, or brain lesion) resulting in extensive infection that requires long-term therapy, but is often refractory to therapy. *Aspergillus* osteomyelitis can also be seen as a complication of disseminated infection or as a primary infection in certain risk groups such as patients with chronic granulomatous disease (CGD) or intravenous drug use (Van't Wout et al, 1990). As a primary infection, the spine is often affected, usually the lumbar area (Vinas et al, 1999). The lesions can be seen on plain radiographs as well as CT or MR which can be useful to stage the infection and guide needle biopsy of the lesion. Favorable responses (≥ 60%) in *Aspergillus* osteomyelitis of the spine were reported in one review, although the need for long-term therapy and surgical intervention in medically nonresponsive patients was noted (Vinas et al, 1999).

Other Invasive Infections.   Invasive aspergillosis in a variety of other sites has been reported in case reports or small series (Denning, 1998). Endocarditis due to *Aspergillus* can occur on either native or prosthetic heart valves. The diagnosis of endocarditis is particularly difficult as blood cultures for *Aspergillus* usually remain negative despite extensive disease (Duthie and Denning, 1995). The prognosis of *Aspergillus* endocarditis is poor even with surgical intervention (Denning and Stevens, 1990). Pericarditis can also occur, usually secondary to local extension from IPA or in the setting of disseminated disease, and can be complicated by cardiac tamponade (Denning, 1998). Other unusual sites of *Aspergillus* infection include eye (keratitis, endophthalmitis), gastrointestinal tract, and kidneys, although invasive infection has been observed in virtually all body sites (Denning, 1998). Some of these infections appear more common in certain settings, e.g., renal infection appears more likely to occur in patients with AIDS (Halpern et al, 1992).

DIAGNOSIS

The diagnosis of invasive aspergillosis continues to be made largely on clinical grounds and histopathological findings, although extensive efforts are ongoing to establish a panel of tests and procedures to facilitate more rapid diagnosis. An important clue for the diagnosis of IPA, for example, is the presence of signs and symptoms that result from angioinvasion of pulmonary veins and arteries by the fungus. This process produces clinical features that may include acute dyspnea, pleuritic chest pain, or hemoptysis.

The diagnosis of invasive aspergillosis is proven with hyphal invasion of tissue specimens together with a positive culture for *Aspergillus* species (Ascioglu et al, 2002). However, tissue samples are often reluctantly undertaken because of the severe thrombocytopenia that is frequently present in patients at high risk for the

disease. Hyphal elements and morphology are usually easily demonstrated using fungal stains, such as Gomori methenamine silver or periodic acid-Schiff (See Color Fig. 14–7 in separate color insert). In acute invasive aspergillosis, the hyphae are typically hyaline, septate and 3–6 μm in width with parallel cross-walls and are dichotomously branched at acute angles (Sutton et al, 1998). These features usually allow distinction from Zygomycetes, which are much broader, exhibit right angle branching, and are rarely septate. In addition, agents of phaeohyphomycosis can be distinguished due to their black or darkly pigmented hyphae with specific melanin staining with the Fontana-Masson stain (Dixon and Polak-Wyss, 1991). However, it is important to note that a number of pathogenic moulds, including *Scedosporium*, *Fusarium*, *Geotrichium*, *Scopulariopsis* and others will have virtually identical appearances on histopathology regardless of the stains used. Although specific immunohistochemical stains using fluorescent antibodies to *Aspergillus* can distinguish the organism, they are not specific nor are they widely available for clinical use (de Repentigny et al, 1994; Kaufman et al, 1997).

Genus specific identification and susceptibility testing are becoming more important as antifungal therapies are increasingly directed at specific pathogens. For example, the newer triazoles, such as voriconazole, are extremely active against *Aspergillus* but variably active against Zygomycetes (Espinel-Ingroff et al, 2001; Pfaller et al, 2002). Similarly, the echinocandins are not active against Zygomycetes and have limited activity against moulds other than *Aspergillus*. Additionally, identification of the organism will also allow susceptibility testing to be performed.

Recently, susceptibility testing for moulds including *Aspergillus* has been validated (Espinel-Ingroff et al, 1997; Espinel-Ingroff et al, 2000), but correlation with clinical results has not yet been established. Antifungal resistance to itraconazole has been reported for a limited number of isolates, which correlates with lack of efficacy in an animal model. In addition, these isolates may not be cross-resistant to other azoles in vitro (Denning et al, 1997; Mosquera and Denning, 2002). In addition, *A. terreus* may be resistant to amphotericin B and susceptible to azoles so that testing of that species could also be of potential clinical utility (Sutton et al, 1998). Nevertheless, the need for routine susceptibility testing of *Aspergillus* species is limited at the present time.

A number of approaches can be utilized to obtain tissue samples for invasive aspergillosis. For pulmonary lesions and other sites, such as deep organs or bone, a fine needle biopsy can be attempted and guided by CT or fluoroscopy to increase the diagnostic yield and avoid a more invasive procedure. Bronchoscopy with bronchoalveolar lavage and transbronchial biopsies are useful in establishing a specific diagnosis and in evaluating for multiple pathogens in these high-risk patients (Albelda et al, 1984; Kahn et al, 1986). Brain lesions that are not accessible can be presumptively identified with the presence of invasive pulmonary aspergillosis and/or disseminated infection diagnosed elsewhere (Perea and Patterson, 2002).

Cultures for *Aspergillus* in respiratory samples may be associated with infection. Recent studies have demonstrated in high-risk patients with increased rates of infection, such as patients with neutropenia or those undergoing bone marrow transplantation, the presence of *Aspergillus* in a respiratory sample, particularly if obtained via bronchoalveolar lavage, is highly suggestive of the diagnosis of invasive aspergillosis (Yu et al, 1986; Horvath and Dummer, 1996). By contrast, blood cultures are rarely positive for *Aspergillus*. These features have led to standardized criteria developed by a joint Mycoses Study Group/European Organization for Research and Treatment of Cancer (MSG/EORTC) panel that has proposed that positive respiratory cultures in conjunction with clinical illness and pulmonary infiltrates in neutropenic or bone marrow transplant patients meet criteria for a probable diagnosis of invasive pulmonary aspergillosis (Ascioglu et al, 2002).

Radiographic findings can also be helpful in establishing a diagnosis of *Aspergillus* infection. Plain chest radiographs are insensitive as extensive pulmonary disease may be present with few findings on chest films. In neutropenic and bone marrow transplant patients with invasive aspergillosis and other angioinvasive moulds, chest computed tomography (CT) scans may demonstrate lesions that are not visible on plain radiographs. A "halo" of low attenuation surrounding a nodular lung lesion in a high risk patient has been associated with an early diagnosis of infection (Caillot et al, 1997) (Fig. 14–4). A nodular lesion may undergo cavitation and subsequently be associated with an "air crescent" sign that is associated with aspergillosis; this radiographic sign occurs later in the course of illness, usually after recovery of neutrophils (Fig. 14–5) (Caillot et al, 1997). Recent studies have demonstrated that the presence of a CT "halo" sign as a trigger to begin presumptive therapy for IPA in high-risk patients resulted in very favorable response rates particularly when combined with surgical resection of isolated lesions (Yeghen et al, 2000).

The utility of non-culture methods to establish a rapid diagnosis of invasive aspergillosis remains limited (Verweij et al, 1998). Antibody detection was initially evaluated, but a large proportion of patients have antibodies due to prior asymptomatic exposure to ubiq-

uitous *Aspergillus* conidia. Even more problematic for utilizing antibody for diagnosis of invasive disease is the fact that highly immunosuppressed patients will not develop a prompt antibody response to infection. A number of investigators have evaluated various methods to establish a diagnosis of invasive infection by detecting *Aspergillus* antigens or metabolites in serum, but the clinical utility of these methods remain limited, due in part to the lack of widespread availability of these tests (Patterson et al, 1997; Patterson et al, 1995; Verweij et al, 1998).

Recently, a sandwich ELISA technique that utilizes a monoclonal antibody to galactomannan antigen has been developed. The ELISA assay (Platelia *Aspergillus*, Sonofi Diagnostics Pasteur, Marnes-la-Coquette, France; BioRad, Redmond, WA) has been used most extensively in Europe where it is approved for clinical use (Verweij et al, 1995). This system uses the monoclonal antibody EB-A2 that is also used in the Pastorex *Aspergillus* latex agglutination test (Sonofi Diagnostics Pasteur), which has limited sensitivity for the detection of circulating antigen. However, in contrast to the latex agglutination test, the sandwich ELISA lowers the detection limit for antigen 10-fold, to 0.5–1.0 ng/ml of galactomannan in serum by using the antibody both as a captor and as a detector (Verweij et al, 1995). With this ELISA assay, sensitivity for detecting invasive aspergillosis is more than 90% with a positive predictive value of more than 80% (Maertens et al, 2001). False positive results have been reported, leading to recommendations from the manufacturer to consider the test a true positive at higher OD values or perhaps with more than one positive sample. Unfortunately, the higher cut-off value has resulted in low sensitivity, particularly in patients receiving empirical or prophylactic antifungal therapies (Herbrecht et al, 2002b). Recent studies have evaluated lower thresholds for positivity in an attempt to increase the sensitivity of this test (Herbrecht et al, 2002b). False positive results have been seen in some pediatric patients, which may be due to dietary intake (Verweij et al, 1995; Maertens et al, 2001). Although the ELISA method has been used to test other body fluids such as cerebrospinal fluid and bronchoalveolar lavage fluid, these fluids have been less extensively studied compared to serum (Verweij et al, 1998). Ongoing clinical trials are in progress to establish the clinical utility of the sandwich ELISA to detect galactomannan antigen as well as to establish guidelines regarding frequency of testing and interpretation of results.

The use of PCR to detect invasive fungal pathogens, including *Aspergillus*, has been reported, but false positive results for this very sensitive method have thus far limited its clinical utility (Hebart et al, 2000; Loeffler et al, 2001). Specifically, the ubiquitous nature of fungal conidia in patient samples as well as in air has resulted in patients or even in controls with false positive results. Preliminary studies have suggested that this method can be very sensitive but still specific for the diagnosis of invasive aspergillosis.

THERAPY

Over the past 40 years, amphotericin B deoxycholate has been the standard therapy for critically ill patients with invasive aspergillosis (Stevens et al, 2000a), but recent studies have demonstrated the significant dose-limiting toxicities of amphotericin B when given in high doses for opportunistic moulds like *Aspergillus*. In addition, the efficacy of amphotericin B deoxycholate in high-risk patients is also extremely limited (Wingard et al, 1999; Bates et al, 2001b; Herbrecht et al, 2002a). Fortunately, an extensive effort has resulted in development of new drugs to meet unmet medical needs (Patterson, 2002). New antifungal therapies with activity directed against *Aspergillus* have been developed including lipid formulations of amphotericin B, the newer triazoles (voriconazole, posaconazole, and ravuconazole), and the echinocandins (caspofungin, micafungin,

and anidulafungin) (Table 14–4). Recent studies have documented the high overall failure rates of current antifungal agents in invasive aspergillosis, with complete responses (cures) occurring in only 27% of patients (Patterson et al, 2000b). The response rate of amphotericin B, which has been used in the most severely immunosuppressed patients, is only about 25%. Thus, the mortality associated with invasive aspergillosis in high-risk patients remains high, even with the "gold standard therapy" of amphotericin B (Patterson, 1998).

Lipid formulations of amphotericin B offer the advantage of less toxicity and allow higher doses of drug, but the optimal dosage and/or use of these compounds is not known (Ellis et al, 1998; Leenders et al, 1998; Walsh et al, 1998; Walsh et al, 2001). The utility of liposomal amphotericin B at 5 mg/kg/day was compared to standard amphotericin B at 1.0 mg/kg/day for proven or suspected invasive mycoses (Leenders et al, 1998). Overall outcomes of both groups in this small study were equivalent; however, analysis of outcomes in those patients with proven invasive aspergillosis favored therapy with the liposomal preparation. Investigators have recently documented the increased morbidity associated with standard amphotericin B, primarily renal insufficiency, in patients receiving bone marrow trans-

TABLE 14–4. *Currently Available Antifungal Agents for Therapy of Invasive Aspergillosis*

Class/Agent	Route of Administration	Dose	Comment
Polyenes			
Amphotericin B	IV	1.0–1.5 mg/kg/day	Previous "gold standard" therapy; significant toxicity; limited efficacy in high risk patients (Wingard et al, 1999; Bates et al, 2001a)
Liposomal amphotericin	IV	3–5 mg/kg/day	Well tolerated; minimal infusion reactions or nephrotoxicity; higher doses (> 5 mg/kg/day) anecdotally more effective; expensive (Leenders et al, 1998)
Amphotericin B lipid complex	IV	5 mg/kg/day	Indicated for invasive mycoses intolerant or refractory to standard therapy (Walsh et al, 1998)
Amphotericin B colloidal dispersion	IV	3–6 mg/kg/day	More infusion-related toxicity than other lipid formulations; limited efficacy in single trial of primary treatment (Bowden et al, 2002)
Azoles			
Itraconazole	IV/oral	200 mg/day (IV) 200 mg bid (PO)	Oral solution improved bioavailability; limited efficacy data for intravenous preparation. Effective for "sequential" polyene to azole therapy (Patterson et al, 2000b; Caillot et al, 2001)
Voriconazole	IV/oral	4 mg/kg/day (IV) (6 mg/kg q12 h × 2 loading dose)	Effective in acute invasive aspergillosis; improved survival as compared with amphotericin B (Herbrecht et al, 2002a)
Echninocandins			
Caspofungin	IV	50–70 mg/day	Approved for use in patients with invasive aspergillosis refractory to or intolerant of standard therapy; well tolerated in clinical trials; possible interaction with cyclosporine (Maertens et al, 2000)

plantation and those receiving concomitant nephro-toxic agents (Wingard et al, 1999). These and other results suggest that while lipid formulations of amphotericin B are dramatically more expensive than standard amphotericin B deoxycholate, hidden costs of standard amphotericin B in terms of morbidity and mortality as well as resource utilization may justify the use of a lipid formulation of amphotericin B in certain high-risk patients (Rex and Walsh, 1999; Bates et al, 2001a).

Other investigators have evaluated the potential for lower doses of lipid formulations (1 mg/kg/day as compared with 4 mg/kg/day liposomal amphotericin B)(Ellis et al, 1998). While overall results were similar in the two arms of the study, the patients with suspected or proven invasive aspergillosis responded better to the higher dose of liposomal amphotericin B, which is consistent with preclinical studies in experimental aspergillosis documenting a dose response to the lipid drugs (Patterson et al, 1989; Walsh et al, 2000). On the basis of results of several studies with the lipid formulations, these agents are approved for salvage therapy of invasive aspergillosis. However, a recent study compared amphotericin B deoxycholate versus amphotericin B colloidal dispersion as primary therapy for invasive aspergillosis (Bowden et al, 2002). Results of this study were disappointing, in that the colloidal dispersion formulation had equal but no better efficacy than amphotericin B deoxycholate. Toxicity of the lipid formuatlion was minimally decreased, compared to that of the parent drug. Liposomal nystatin, an investigational polyene drug, has some promise against Aspergillus (Offner et al, 2000).

Itraconazole is approved for use in aspergillosis, but the utility of itraconazole has been limited. Until recently it had been available only in an oral formulation which is erratically or poorly absorbed and associated with potentially serious drug interactions. An intravenous itraconazole preparation has only recently been approved for clinical use (Caillot et al, 2001). Thus, itraconazole has not been frequently used as a single antifungal agent for severely immunosuppressed patients. In less immunosuppressed patients who are able to take oral therapy, itraconazole has been shown to be an effective agent (Patterson et al, 2000b). Moreover, the use of oral itraconazole, following an initial "induction" course of amphotericin B, has been shown to be effective (Patterson et al, 2000b).

The second generation triazoles have an expanded spectrum of activity that includes Aspergillus spp. (Sheehan et al, 1999; Denning et al, 2002). Recently, voriconazole, a potent, broad-spectrum triazole, was approved for the primary therapy of invasive aspergillosis based on a randomized trial comparing voriconazole to amphotericin B deoxycholate followed by other licensed antifungal therapy when necessary (Herbrecht et al, 2002a). Notably, this trial documented success in 52% of voriconazole treated patients compared to only 31% success in amphotericin B treated patients. Importantly, benefit was demonstrated in patients at high risk for mortality including those undergoing bone marrow transplantation and those with extrapulmonary disease including central nervous system involvement (Denning et al, 2002; Herbrecht et al, 2002a). In addition, a survival benefit of voriconazole was shown as compared with standard therapy (Herbrecht et al, 2002a). Thus, it seems likely that voriconazole will become a preferred therapy for invasive aspergillosis. Voriconazole, available in both oral and parenteral forms, has been evaluated in an extensive Phase III clinical evaluation for efficacy against a wide range of fungal pathogens (Ally et al, 2001; Herbrecht et al, 2002a). In vitro, voriconazole demonstrates fungicidal activity against clinically relevant Aspergillus species, including A. terreus, which may be resistant to amphotericin B (Espinel-Ingroff et al, 2001; Pfaller et al, 2002).

In clinical trials, voriconazole exhibits a favorable pharmacokinetic profile and has been reasonably tolerated. The most common adverse event has been a transient and reversible visual disturbance which has been reported in approximately one-third of patients receiving the drug (Ally et al, 2001; Herbrecht et al, 2002a; Walsh et al, 2002). This effect, which is dose related, is described as an altered or increased light perception that is temporary and not associated with pathologic sequelae. Other adverse events have been less common, including liver abnormalities in 10% of patients, skin rash in 6%, nausea and vomiting in 2%, and anorexia in 1%.

Investigational triazoles in clinical development include posaconazole (SCH 56592) and ravuconazole (BMS 207,147) (Patterson, 1999a; Kirkpatrick et al, 2000; Kirkpatrick et al, 2002b). Posaconazole, currently available in only an oral formulation, has been shown to have activity against Aspergillus in vitro as well as in preclinical animal in vivo studies (Kirkpatrick et al, 2000; Pfaller et al, 2002). In an open-label trial, posaconazole was also reported to have activity in patients with invasive aspergillosis (Hachem et al, 2000). Although human trials with ravuconazole are just beginning, this drug has shown activity in animal models of invasive aspergillosis, similar to that of voriconazole and posaconazole (Roberts et al, 2000; Kirkpatrick et al, 2002b).

The echinocandins are a new class of antifungal drugs that also have activity against Aspergillus (Petraitis et al, 2002; Kirkpatrick et al, 2002a; Petraitiene et al, 2002). These agents, which are administered intravenously, target glucan synthase, which is needed for synthesis of β-1,3-glucan in fungal cell walls (Bowman et al, 2002). Included in this class are caspofungin, micafungin (FK463) and anidulafungin (VER-002). The latter two drugs are investigational. Capsofungin has recently been approved for clinical use for treatment of patients refractory to or intolerant of standard therapies for invasive aspergillosis. In an open-label trial for such patients, caspofungin was demonstrated to produce satisfactory clinical responses in 41% (22/54) of patients studied (Maertens et al, 2000). This class of compounds has been extremely well tolerated in clinical trials; for example, drug discontinuations attributed to caspofungin intolerance or toxicity in the aspergillosis trial occurred in only 5% of patients. Nephrotoxicity appears to be minimal (Maertens et al, 2000).

The clinical availability of several new antifungal drugs and new drug classes with activity against *Aspergillus* has increased interest in combination antifungal therapy for this potentially lethal mould disease. As none of these potential combinations have been evaluated in clinical trials, caution for these approaches has arisen largely from previous studies showing in vivo (murine aspergillosis) and in vitro antagonism between amphotericin B and ketoconazole, an early imidazole with limited *Aspergillus* activity (Schaffner and Frick, 1985). This antagonism occurred with pre-treatment of *Aspergillus* with the azole, thereby reducing cell wall ergosterol and eliminating the site of action of amphotericin B. Other studies with the newer azoles have not shown this effect and clinical demonstrations of this antagonism are limited (George et al, 1993; Schaffner and Böhler, 1993).

In the past, other drug combinations as therapy of aspergillosis have been evaluated, including amphotericin B and rifampin, amphotericin B and flucytosine, and others (Denning and Stevens, 1990; Denning et al, 1992). Problems with rifampin combined with azoles include increased metabolism of the azole drugs, which obviates their use and makes that combination unattractive. Similarly, flucytosine has limited activity against *Aspergillus* and can cause pancytopenia that worsens immunosuppression. Recent animal model studies have demonstrated the potential efficacy in reducing burden of infection of echinocandins used in combination with amphotericin B or the new triazoles (Kohno et al, 2000; Nakajima et al, 2000; Kirkpatrick et al, 2002a). For example, voriconazole combined with the echinocandin, caspofungin, improved sterilization of tissues in a neutropenic animal model of infection (Kirkpatrick et al, 2002a). Clinical studies using combination antifungal therapy are ongoing.

The role of adjuvant therapies for invasive aspergillosis may be important in management although they have not been well studied. Surgical approaches of removing isolated pulmonary nodules prior to ad-

ditional immunosuppressive therapies have been shown to improve outcome of infection (Caillot et al, 1997; Yeghen et al, 2000). Other adjuvant therapies such as granulocyte transfusions (Bhatia et al, 1994), granulocyte and granulocyte-macrophage colony-stimulating factors (Vose et al, 1991; Pui et al, 1997; Rowe, 1998), and interferon-γ (Bernhisel-Broadbent et al, 1991) have been shown in anecdotal reports to improve outcome in individual patients but are not generally recommended for routine use as improved responses and survival have not been conclusively demonstrated (Stevens, 1998). Adjunctive immunotherapy is usually reserved for patients who have progressive infection despite aggressive antifungal chemotherapy (Stevens et al, 2000a).

Approach to Management

Guidelines for treating invasive aspergillosis have been published recently by the Infectious Diseases Society of America (Stevens et al, 2000). Notable in these guidelines are a striking absence of recommendations derived from large, placebo-controlled antifungal treatment trials, due to the difficulty of studying this relatively uncommon and difficult to diagnose infection. Nevertheless, these guidelines suggest that in high-risk patients a prompt diagnosis and aggressive antifungal therapy may be a means to improve the outcome of this disease (Stevens et al, 2000a). Unfortunately, even aggressive antifungal therapy is unlikely to be successful unless the underlying state of immunosuppression of the patient improves. Typically, the diagnosis of invasive aspergillosis is proven or probable in high risk patients in whom suggestive clinical findings develop. Adjunctive diagnostic measures such as CT scans, culture results, and non-culture-based methods can be used to facilitate earlier and more precise diagnosis. Although high doses of standard amphotericin B deoxycholate are often used as initial therapy, this therapy is toxic and often ineffective. Lipid formulations of amphotericin B, which are used in patients with renal insufficiency, progressive infection despite standard amphotericin B, or perhaps as initial therapy in patients at high risk for nephrotoxicity, may reduce toxicity and may be associated with an improved outcome of infection. Newer triazoles, such as voriconazole, posaconazole, and ravuconazole, and a new class of drugs, namely, the echinocandins, offer the potential for improved therapy of invasive aspergillosis. In patients treated with initial induction courses of amphotericin B, sequential therapy with oral azoles with *Aspergillus* activity such as itraconazole or one of the newer triazoles such as voriconazole, may prove be a useful option. The availability of these new compounds also offers the potential for combination antifungal therapy for invasive aspergillosis, but drug combinations have not yet been evaluated in clinical trials.

Improvement in underlying host defenses is crucial to successful therapy of invasive aspergillosis. While substantial advances have recently been made in the management of this disease, newer approaches to therapy, including drug–drug combinations or drug–immunotherapy combinations, as well as highly sensitive and specific methods of diagnosis are still needed to improve the outcome of this aggressive mould disease.

PREVENTION AND PROPHYLAXIS

Prevention of invasive aspergillosis in high-risk patients remains a difficult challenge. Outbreaks of *Aspergillus* infections have been linked to hospital construction, contaminated ventilation systems and operating rooms, and more recently to contaminated water (Sherertz et al, 1987; Walsh and Dixon, 1989; Anaissie and Costa, 2001; Dykewicz, 2001;). Nevertheless, it is important to recognize that high-risk immunosuppressed patients now spend much of their treatment course in the outpatient setting; consequently, community-acquired infection is also common (Patterson et al, 1997). Prevention of nosocomial aspergillosis in the highest risk populations is difficult even using state of the art air control systems including point of use HEPA filters, frequent air exchanges and positive pressure ventilation. Unfortunately, these high-risk patients have exposures in the hospital setting outside of their protective environment (Iwen et al, 1993).

Antifungal prophylaxis using agents with activity against moulds has been attempted, usually in the setting of an outbreak of *Aspergillus* infection that involves multiple other interventions to control the outbreak. Efficacy in that setting is usually compared to the incidence of infection during a prior historical setting. Agents evaluated in this setting include low dose amphotericin B, low doses of lipid formulations of amphotericin B, and nasal and aerosolized forms of amphotericin B. None of these have been conclusively demonstrated to have benefit in large, randomized clinical trials (Dykewicz et al, 2000; Palmer et al, 2001). Itraconazole has been suggested to have benefit in preventing mould infections but poor tolerance of itraconazole by high-risk patients has limited its use (Morgenstern et al, 1999). Thus, no agents are currently recommended for prevention of mould infections (Dykewicz et al, 2000), although studies are ongoing to evaluate the efficacy of the echinocandins and the newer triazoles in this setting.

REFERENCES

Albelda S M, Talbot G H, Gerson S L, Miller W T, Cassileth P A. Role of fiberoptic bronchoscopy in the diagnosis of invasive pulmonary aspergillosis in patients with acute leukemia. *Am J Med* 76:1027–1034, 1984.

Allo M D, Miller J, Townsend T, Tan C. Primary cutaneous aspergillosis associated with Hickman intravenous catheters. *N Engl J Med* 317:1105–1108, 1987.

Ally R, Schurmann D, Kreisel W, Carosi G, Aguirrebengoa K, Dupont B, Hodges M, Troke P, Romero A J. A randomized, double-blind, double-dummy, multicenter trial of voriconazole and fluconazole in the treatment of esophageal candidiasis in immunocompromised patients. *Clin Infect Dis* 33:1447–1454, 2001.

Anaissie E J, Costa SF. Nosocomial aspergillosis is waterborne. *Clin Infect Dis* 33:1546–1548, 2001.

Anaissie E J, Stratton S L, Dignani M C, Summerbell R C, Rex J H, Monson T P, Spencer T, Kasai M, Francesconi A, Walsh T J. Pathogenic *Aspergillus* species recovered from a hospital water system: A 3-year prospective study. *Clin Infect Dis* 34:780–789, 2002.

Ascioglu S, Rex J H, de Pauw B, Bennett J E, Bille J, Crokaert F, Denning D W, Donnelly J P, Edwards J E, Erjavec Z, Fiere D, Lortholary O, Maertens J, Meis J F, Patterson T F, Ritter J, Selleslag D, Shah P M, Stevens D A, Walsh T J. Defining opportunistic invasive fungal infections in immunocompromised patients with cancer and hematopoietic stem cell transplants: An international consensus. *Clin Infect Dis* 34:7–14, 2002.

Aslam P, Eastridge C, Hughes F. Aspergillosis of the lung—an 18 year experience. *Chest* 59:28–32, 1971.

Baddley J W, Stroud T P, Salzman D, Pappas P G. Invasive mold infections in allogeneic bone marrow transplant recipients. *Clin Infect Dis* 32:1319–1324, 2001.

Basich J, Graves T, Baz M N, Scanlon G, Hoffman R G, Patterson R, Fink J N. Allergic bronchopulmonary aspergillosis in corticosteroid-dependent asthmatics. *J Allergy Clin Immunol* 68:98–102, 1981.

Bates D W, Su L, Yu D T, Chertow G M, Seger D L, Gomes D R J, Dasbach E J, Platt R. Mortality and costs of acute renal failure associated with amphotericin B therapy. *Clin Infect Dis* 32:686–693, 2001a.

Bates D W, Su L, Yu D T, Chertow G M, Seger D L, Gomes D R, Platt R. Correlates of acute renal failure in patients receiving parenteral amphotericin B. *Kidney Int* 60:1452–1459, 2001b.

Bernhisel-Broadbent J, Camargo E E, Jaffe H S, Lederman H M. Recombinant human interferon-gamma as adjunct therapy for *Aspergillus* infection in a patient with chronic granulomatous disease. *J Infect Dis* 163:908–911, 1991.

Bhatia S, McCullough J, Perry E H, Clay M, Ramsey N K, Neglia J P. Granulocyte transfusion: efficacy in treating fungal infections in neutropenic patients following bone marrow transplantation. *Transfusion* 34:226–232, 1994.

Binder R E, Faling L J, Pugatch R D, Mahasen C, Snider G L. Chronic necrotizing pulmonary aspergillosis: a discrete clinical entity. *Medicine* (Baltimore) 61:109–124, 1982.

Birch M, Robson G, Law D, Denning D W. Evidence of multiple extracellular phospholipase activities of *Aspergillus fumigatus*. *Infect Immun* 64:751–755, 1996.

Bowden R, Chandrasekar P, White M H, Li X, Pietrelli L, Gurwith M, van Burik J, Laverdiere M, Safrin S, Wingard J R. A double-blind, randomized, controlled trial of amphotericin B colloidal dispersion versus amphotericin B for treatment of invasive aspergillosis in immunocompromised patients. *Clin Infect Dis* 35:359–366, 2002.

Bowman J C, Hicks P S, Kurtz M B, Rosen H, Schmatz D M, Liberator P A, Douglas C M. The antifungal echinocandin caspofungin acetate kills growing cells of *Aspergillus fumigatus* in vitro. *Antimicrob Agents Chemother* 46:3001–3012, 2002.

Caillot D, Casasnovas O, Bernard A, Couaillier J F, Durand C, Cuisenier B, Solary E, Piard F, Petrella T, Bonnin A, Couillault G, Dumas M, Guy H. Improved management of invasive pulmonary aspergillosis in neutropenic patients using early thoracic computed tomographic scan and surgery. *J Clin Oncol* 15:139–147, 1997.

Caillot D, Bassaris H, McGeer A, Arthur C, Prentice H G, Siefert W, DeBeule K. Intravenous itraconazole followed by oral itraconazole in the treatment of invasive pulmonary aspergillosis in patients with hematologic malignancies, chronic granulomatous disease, or AIDS. *Clin Infect Dis* 33:E83–E90, 2001.

Cenci E, Perito S, Enssle K H, Mosce P, Latge J P, Romani L, Bistoni F. Th1 and Th2 cytokines in mice with invasive aspergillosis. *Infect Immun* 65:564–570, 1997.

Clancy C J, Nguyen M H. Acute community-acquired pneumonia due to *Aspergillus* in presumably immunocompetent hosts—Clues for recognition of a rare but fatal disease. *Chest* 114:629–634, 1998.

Corey J, Delsupehe K, Ferguson B. Allergic fungal sinusitis: allergic, infectious, or both? *Otolaryngol Head Neck Surg* 1995:110–119, 1995.

de Carpentier J P, Ramamurthy L, Denning D W, Taylor P H. An algorithmic approach to *Aspergillus* sinusitis. *J Laryngol Otol* 108:314–318, 1994.

de Repentigny L, Kaufman L, Cole GT, Kruse D, Latge J P, Matthews R C. Immunodiagnosis of invasive fungal infections. *J Med Vet Mycol* 32 (Suppl. 1):239–252, 1994.

Denning DW. Aflatoxin and human disease. A review. *Adverse Drug Reactions and Acute Poisoning Reviews* 4:175–209, 1987.

Denning DW, Stevens DA. Antifungal and surgical treatment of invasive aspergillosis: Review of 2,121 published cases. *Rev Infect Dis* 12:1147–1201, 1990.

Denning D W, Follansbee S E, Scolaro M, Norris S, Edelstein H, Stevens D A. Pulmonary aspergillosis in the acquired immunodeficiency syndrome. *N Engl J Med* 324:654–662, 1991.

Denning D W, Hanson L H, Perlman A M, Stevens D A. In vitro susceptibility and synergy studies of *Aspergillus* species to conventional and new agents. *Diagn Microbiol Infect Dis* 15:21–34, 1992.

Denning D W, Radford S A, Oakley K L, Hall L, Johnson E M, Warnock D W. Correlation between in-vitro susceptibility testing to itraconazole and in-vivo outcome of *Aspergillus fumigatus* infection. *J Antimicrob Chemother* 40:401–414, 1997.

Denning D W. Invasive aspergillosis. *Clin Infect Dis* 26:781–803, 1998.

Denning D W. *Aspergillus* species. In: Mandell G L, Bennett J E, Dolin R, eds. *Principles and Practice of Infectious Diseases*, 5th Edition. Philadelphia: Churchill Livingstone. 2674–2685, 2000.

Denning D W. Chronic forms of pulmonary aspergillosis. *Clin Microbiol Infect* 7:25–31, 2001.

Denning D W, Ribaud P, Milpied N, Caillot D, Herbrecht R, Thiel E, Haas A, Ruhnke M, Lode H. Efficacy and safety of voriconazole in the treatment of acute invasive aspergillosis. *Clin Infect Dis* 34:563–571, 2002.

DeShazo R D, Chapin K, Swain R E. Fungal sinusitis. *N Engl J Med* 337:254–259, 1997.

Deve F. Une nouvelle forme anatomoradiologique de mycose pulmonaire primitive: le megamycetome intrabronchetasique. *Arch Med Chir Appl Respir* 13:337–361, 1938.

Dixon D M, Polak-Wyss A. The medically important dematiaceous fungi and their identification. *Mycoses* 34:1–18, 1991.

Duthie R, Denning D W. *Aspergillus* fungemia: Report of two cases and review. *Clin Infect Dis* 20:598–605, 1995.

Dykewicz C A, Jaffe H W, Kaplan J E. Guidelines for preventing opportunistic infections among hematopoietic stem cell transplant recipients—Recommendations of CDC, the Infectious Diseases Society of America, and the American Society of Blood and Mar-

row Transplantation. *Biol Blood Marrow Transplant* 6:659–713, 715, 717–727, 2000.

Dykewicz C A. Hospital infection control in hematopoietic stem cell transplant recipients. *Emerg Infect Dis* 7:263–267, 2001.

Ellis M, Spence D, de Pauw B, Meunier F, Marinus A, Collette L, Sylvester R, Meis J, Boogaerts M, Selleslag D, Kremery V, von Sinner W, MacDonald P, Doyen C, Vanderveam B. An EORTC international multicenter randomized trial (EORTC number 19923) comparing two dosages of liposomal amphotericin B for treatment of invasive aspergillosis. *Clin Infect Dis* 27:1406–1412, 1998.

Espinel-Ingroff A, Bartlett M, Bowden R, Chin N X, Cooper C, Fothergill A, McGinnis M R, Menezes P, Messer S A, Nelson P W, Odds F C, Pasarell L, Peter J, Pfaller M A, Rex J H, Rinaldi M G, Shankland G S, Walsh T J, Weitzman I. Multicenter evaluation of proposed standardized procedure for antifungal susceptibility testing of filamentous fungi. *J Clin Microbiol* 35:139–143, 1997.

Espinel-Ingroff A, Warnock D W, Vazquez J A, Arthington-Skaggs B A. In vitro antifungal susceptibility methods and clinical implications of antifungal resistance. *Med Mycol* 38 (Suppl. 1):293–304, 2000.

Espinel-Ingroff A, Boyle K, Sheehan D J. In vitro antifungal activities of voriconazole and reference agents as determined by NCCLS methods: Review of the literature. *Mycopathologia* 150:101–115, 2001.

Ferguson B J. Fungus balls of the paranasal sinuses. *Otolaryngol Clin N Amer* 33:389–398, 2000.

Fresenius G. *Beitrage zur Mykologie*. Frankfurt: H L Bronner, 1863.

George D, Kordick D, Miniter P, Patterson T F, Andriole V T. Combination therapy in experimental invasive aspergillosis. *J Infec Dis* 168:692–698, 1993.

Gerson S L, Talbot G H, Hurwitz S, Strom B L, Lusk E J, Cassileth P A. Prolonged granulocytopenia: the major risk factor for invasive pulmonary aspergillosis in patients with acute leukemia. *Ann Intern Med* 100:345–351, 1984.

Gettleman L K, Shetty A K, Prober C G. Posttraumatic invasive *Aspergillus fumigatus* wound infection. *Pediat Infect Dis J* 18:745–747, 1999.

Geyer S J, Surampudi R K. Photo quiz—Birefringent crystals in a pulmonary specimen. *Clin Infect Dis* 34:481, 551–552, 2002.

Gillespie M B, O'Malley B W. An algorithmic approach to the diagnosis and management of invasive fungal rhinosinusitis in the immunocompromised patient. *Otolaryngol Clin N Amer* 33:323–334, 2000.

Groll A H, Shah P M, Mentzel C, Schneider M, Just-Neubling G, Huebner K. Trends in the postmortem epidemiology of invasive fungal infections at a university hospital. *J Infect* 33:23–32, 1996.

Groll A H, Mickiene D, Petraitis V, Petraitiene R, Ibrahim K H, Piscitelli S C, Bekersky I, Walsh T J. Compartmental pharmacokinetics and tissue distribution of the antifungal echinocandin lipopeptide micafungin (FK463) in rabbits. *Antimicrob Agents Chemother* 45:3322–3327, 2001.

Hachem R Y, Raad I I, Afif C M, Negroni J, Graybill J, Hadley S, Kantarjian H, Adams S, Mukwaya G. An open, noncomparative multicenter study to evaluate efficacy and safety of posaconazole (SCH 56592) in the treatment of invasive fungal infections refractory to or intolerant of standard therapy. 40th Interscience Conference on Antimicrobial Agents and Chemotherapy, Toronto, CA, American Society for Microbiology, Abstract 1109, 2000.

Hagensee M E, Bauwens J E, Kjos B, Bowden R A. Brain abscess following marrow transplantation: experience at the Fred Hutchinson Cancer Research Center, 1984–1992. *Clin Infect Dis* 19:402–408, 1994.

Halpern M, Szabo S, Hochberg E, Hammer G S, Lin J, Gurtman

A C, Sacks H S, Shapiro R S, Hirschman S Z. Renal aspergilloma: an unusual cause of infection in a patient with the acquired immunodeficiency syndrome. *Am J Med* 92:437–440, 1992.

Hebart H, Loffler J, Meisner C, Seray F, Schmidt D, Böhme H, Martin H, Engel A, Bunjes D, Kern W V, Schumacher U, Kanz L, Einsele H. Early detection of *Aspergillus* infection after allogeneic stem cell transplantation by polymerase chain reaction screening. *J Infect Dis* 181:1713–1719, 2000.

Herbrecht R, Denning D W, Patterson T F, Bennett J E, Greene R E, Oestman J-W, Kern W V, Marr K A, Ribaud P, Lortholary O, Sylvester R, Rubin R H, Wingard J R, Stark P, Durand C, Caillot D, Thiel E, Chandrasekar P H, Hodges M R, Schlamm H T, Troke P F, de Pauw B. Voriconazole versus amphotericin B for primary therapy of invasive aspergillosis. *N Engl J Med* 347: 408–415, 2002a.

Herbrecht R, Letscher-Bru V, Oprea C, Lioure B, Waller J, Campos F, Villard O, Liu K L, Natarajan-Ame S, Lutz P, Dufour P, Bergerat J P, Candolfi E. *Aspergillus* galactomannan detection in the diagnosis of invasive aspergillosis in cancer patients. *J Clin Oncol* 20:1898–1906, 2002b.

Hinson K, Moon A, Plummer N. Broncho-pulmonary aspergillosis. A review and a report of eight new cases. *Thorax* 7:317–333, 1952.

Horvath J A, Dummer S. The use of respiratory-tract cultures in the diagnosis of invasive pulmonary aspergillosis. *Am J Med* 100: 171–178, 1996.

Houser S M, Corey J P. Allergic fungal rhinosinusitis—pathophysiology, epidemiology, and diagnosis. *Otolaryngol Clin N Amer* 33:399–408, 2000.

Iwen P C, Reed E C, Armitage J O, Bierman P J, Kessinger A, Vose J M, Arneson M A, Winfield B A, Woods G L. Nosocomial invasive aspergillosis in lymphoma patients treated with bone marrow or peripheral stem cell transplants. *Infect Control Hosp Epidemiol* 14:131–139, 1993.

Iwen P C, Rupp M E, Hinrichs S H. Invasive mold sinusitis: 17 cases in immunocompromised patients and review of the literature. *Clin Infect Dis* 24:1178–1184, 1997.

Iwen P C, Rupp M E, Langnas A N, Reed E C, Hinrichs S H. Invasive pulmonary aspergillosis due to *Aspergillus terreus*: 12-year experience and review of the literature. *Clin Infect Dis* 26:1092–1097, 1998.

Kahn F W, Jones J M, England D M. The role of bronchoalveolar lavage in the diagnosis of invasive pulmonary aspergillosis. *Am J Clin Pathol* 86:518–523, 1986.

Kan V L, Bennett J E. Lectin-like attachment sites on murine pulmonary alveolar macrophages bind *Aspergillus fumigatus* conidia. *J Infect Dis* 158:407–414, 1988.

Kanj S S, Welty-Wolf K, Madden J, Tapson V, Baz M A, Davis R D, Perfect J R. Fungal infections in lung and heart-lung transplant recipients. Report of 9 cases and review of the literature. *Medicine (Baltimore)* 75:142–156, 1996.

Karam G H, Griffin F M, Jr. Invasive pulmonary aspergillosis in nonimmunocompromised, nonneutropenic hosts. *Rev Infect Dis* 8:357–363, 1986.

Katzenstein A-L, Sale S, Greenberger P. Allergic *Aspergillus* sinusitis: a newly recognised form of sinusitis. *J Allergy Clin Immunol* 72:89–93, 1983.

Kauffman C A. Quandary about treatment of aspergillomas persists. *Lancet* 347:1640, 1996.

Kaufman L, Standard P G, Jalbert M, Kraft D E. Immunohistologic identification of *Aspergillus* spp. and other hyaline fungi by using polyclonal fluorescent antibodies. *J Clin Microbiol* 35:2206–2209, 1997.

Kaur R, Mittal N, Kakkar M, Aggarwal A K, Mathur M D. Otomycosis: a clinicomycologic study. *Ear Nose Throat J* 79:606–609, 2000.

Kirkpatrick W R, McAtee R K, Fothergill A W, Loebenberg D, Rinaldi M G, Patterson T F. Efficacy of SCH56592 in a rabbit model of invasive aspergillosis. *Antimicrob Agents Chemother* 44:780–782, 2000.

Kirkpatrick W R, Perea S, Coco B J, Patterson T F. Efficacy of caspofungin alone and in combination with voriconazole in a guinea pig model of invasive aspergillosis. *Antimicrob Agents Chemother* 46:2564–2568, 2002a.

Kirkpatrick W R, Perea S, Coco B J, Patterson T F. Efficacy of ravuconazole (BMS-207147) in a guinea pig model of disseminated aspergillosis. *J Antimicrob Chemother* 49:353–357, 2002b.

Klich M, Pitt J. A laboratory guide to common *Aspergillus* species and their teleomorphs. Commonwealth Scientific and Industrial Research Organization, North Ryde, New South Wales, Australia, 1988.

Kohno S, Maesaki S, Iwakawa J, Miyazaki Y, Nakamura K, Kakeya H, Yanagihara K, Ohno H, Higashiyama T. Synergistis effects of combination of FK463 with amphotericin B: Enhanced efficacy in murine model of invasive pulmonary aspergillosis. 40th Interscience Conference on Antimicrobial Agents and Chemotherapy, Toronto, CA, Abstract 1686, 2000.

Kramer M, Denning D, Marshall S, Ross D J, Berry G, Lewiston N J, Stevens D A, Theodore J. Ulcerative tracheobronchitis following lung transplantation: a new form of invasive aspergillosis. *Am Rev Resp Dis* 144:552–556, 1991.

Kuhn F A, Javer A R. Allergic fungal rhinosinusitis—Perioperative management, prevention of recurrence, and role of steroids and antifungal agents. *Otolaryngol Clin N Amer* 33:419–432, 2000a.

Kuhn F A, Javer A R. Allergic fungal sinusitis: a four-year followup. *Am J Rhinol* 2000:149–156, 2000b.

Kumar R, Gaur S N. Prevalence of allergic bronchopulmonary aspergillosis in patients with bronchial asthma. *Asian Pacific J Allergy Immunol* 18:181–185, 2000.

Kwon-Chung K J. *Aspergillus*: Diagnosis and description of the genus. Vanden Bossche H, Mackenzie D W R and Cauwenbergh G. *Proceedings of the Second International Symposium on Topics in Mycology*, Antwerp, Belguim, University of Antwerp, 1987.

Kwon-Chung K J, Bennett J E. *Medical Mycology*. Philadelphia, Lea & Febiger, 1992.

Latge J P. *Aspergillus fumigatus* and aspergillosis. *Clin Microbiol Rev* 12:310–350, 1999.

Latge J P. The pathobiology of *Aspergillus fumigatus*. *Trends Microbiol* 9:382–389, 2001.

Leenders A C, Daenen S, Jansen R L, Hop W C, Loebenberg B, Wijermans P W, Cornelissen J, Herbrecht R, van der Lelie H, Hoogsteden H C, Verbrugh H A, de Marie S. Liposomal amphotericin B compared with amphotericin B deoxycholate in the treatment of documented and suspected neutropenia-associated invasive fungal infections. *Brit J Haematol* 103:205–212, 1998.

Levitz S M, Selsted M E, Ganz T, Lehrer R I, Diamond R D. In vitro killing of spores and hyphae of *Aspergillus fumigatus* and *Rhizopus oryzae* by rabbit neutrophil cationic peptides and bronchoalveolar macrophages. *J Infect Dis* 154:483–489, 1986.

Lin S J, Schranz J, Teutsch S M. Aspergillosis case—fatality rate: systematic review of the literature. *Clin Infect Dis* 32:358–366, 2001.

Link H. Observations in ordines plantarum naturales. *Igesellschaft Naturforschender Freunde zu Berlin, Magazin* 3:1, 1809.

Loeffler J, Henke N, Hebart H, Schmidt D, Hagmeyer L, Schumacher U, Einsele H. Quantification of fungal DNA by using fluorescence resonance energy transfer and the Light Cycler system. *J Clin Microbiol* 38:586–590, 2000.

Loeffler J, Hebart H, Cox P, Flues N, Schumacher U, Einsele H. Nucleic acid sequence-based amplification of *Aspergillus* RNA in blood samples. *J Clin Microbiol* 39:1626–1629, 2001.

Mackenzie D W. *Aspergillus* in man. Vanden Bossche H, Mackenzie D W R, Cauwenbergh G. *Proceedings of the Second International Symposium on Topics in Mycology,* Antwerp, Belgium, University of Antwerp, 1987.

Maertens J, Raad I, Sable C A, Ngai A, Berman R, Patterson T F, Denning D, Walsh T. Multicenter, noncomparative study to evaluate safety and efficacy of caspofungin in adults with aspergillosis refractory or intolerant to amphotericin B, amphotericin B lipid formulations, or azoles. 40th Interscience Conference on Antimicrobial Agents and Chemotherapy, Toronto, CA, Abstract 1103, 2000.

Maertens J, Verhaegen J, Lagrou K, van Eldere J, Boogaerts M. Screening for circulating galactomannan as a noninvasive diagnostic tool for invasive aspergillosis in prolonged neutropenic patients and stem cell transplantation recipients: a prospective validation. *Blood* 97:1604–1610, 2001.

Malo J L, Pepys J, Simon G. Studies in chronic allergic bronchopulmonary aspergillosis. 2. Radiological findings. *Thorax* 32:262–268, 1977.

Marr K A, Carter R A, Crippa F, Wald A, Corey L. Epidemiology and outcome of mould infections in hematopoietic stem cell transplant recipients. *Clin Infect Dis* 34:909–917, 2002.

Micheli P. Nova plantarum genra juxta Tournefortii methodum disposita. *Bernardo Paperini,* 1729.

Monod M, Paris S, Sarfati J, Jaton-Ogay K, Ave P, Latge J P. Virulence of alkaline protease-deficient mutants of *Aspergillus fumigatus. FEMS Microbiol Lett* 80:39–46, 1993.

Morgenstern G R, Prentice A G, Prentice H G, Ropner J E, Schey S A, Warnock D W. A randomised controlled trial of itraconazole versus fluconazole for the prevention of fungal infections in patients with haematological malignancies. *Brit J Haematol* 105:901–911, 1999.

Mosquera J, Denning D W. Azole cross-resistance in *Aspergillus fumigatus. Antimicrob Agents Chemother* 46:556–557, 2002.

Mroueh S, Spock A. Allergic bronchopulmonary aspergillosis in patients with cystic fibrosis. *Chest* 105:32–36, 1994.

Nakajima M, Tamada S, Yoshida K, Wakai Y, Nakai T, Ikeda F, Goto T, Niki Y, Matsushima T. Pathological findings in a murine pulmonary aspergillosis model: Treatment with FK463, amphotericin B, and a combination of FK463 and amphotericin B. 40th Interscience Conference on Antimicrobial Agents and Chemotherapy, Toronto, CA, Abstract 1685, 2000.

Offner F C J, Herbrecht R, Engelhard D, Guiot H F L, Samonis G, Marinus A, Roberts R J, DePauw B E. EORTC-IFCT Phase II study on liposomal nystatin in patients with invasive aspergillosis infections, refractory to or intolerant of conventional/lipid amphotericin B. 40th Interscience Conference on Antimicrobial Agents and Chemotherapy, Toronto, CA, Abstract 1102, 2000.

Palmer S M, Perfect J R, Howell D N, Lawrence C M, Miralles A P, Davis R D, Tapson V F. Candidal anastomotic infection in lung transplant recipients: Successful treatment with a combination of systemic and inhaled antifungal agents. *J Heart Lung Transplant* 17:1029–1033, 1998.

Palmer S M, Drew R H, Whitehouse J D, Tapson V F, Davis R D, McDowell R R, Kanj S S, Perfect J R. Safety of aerosolized amphotericin B lipid complex in lung transplant recipients. *Transplantation* 72:545–548, 2001.

Paterson DL and Singh N. Invasive aspergillosis in transplant recipients. *Medicine (Baltimore)* 78:123–138, 1999.

Patterson J E, Zidouh A, Miniter P, Andriole V T, Patterson T F. Hospital epidemiologic surveillance for invasive aspergillosis: patient demographics and the utility of antigen detection. *Infect Control Hosp Epidemiol* 18:104–108, 1997.

Patterson J E, Peters J, Calhoon J H, Levine S, Anzueto A, Al-Abdely H, Sanchez R, Patterson T F, Rech M, Jorgensen J H, Rinaldi M G, Sako E, Johnson S, Speeg V, Halff G A, Trinkle J K. Investigation and control of aspergillosis and other filamentous

fungal infections in solid organ transplant recipients. *Transpl Infect Dis* 2:22–28, 2000a.

Patterson R, Greenberger P A, Radin R C, Roberts M. Allergic bronchopulmonary aspergillosis: Staging as an aid to management. *Ann Intern Med* 96:286–291, 1982.

Patterson T F, Miniter P, Dijkstra J, Szoka F C, Ryan J L, Andriole V T. Treatment of experimental invasive aspergillosis with novel amphotericin B/cholesterol-sulfate complexes. *J Infect Dis* 159:717–721, 1989.

Patterson T F, Miniter P, Patterson J E, Rappeport J M, Andriole V T. *Aspergillus* antigen detection in the diagnosis of invasive aspergilosis. *J Infect Dis* 171:1553–1558, 1995.

Patterson T F. Approaches to therapy for invasive mycoses—the role of amphotericin B. *Clin Infect Dis* 26:339–340, 1998.

Patterson T F. Role of newer azoles in surgical patients. *J Chemother* 11:504–512, 1999a.

Patterson T F. Approaches to fungal diagnosis in transplantation. *Transpl Infect Dis* 1:262–272, 1999b.

Patterson T F, Kirkpatrick W R, White M, Hiemenz J W, Wingard J R, Dupont B, Rinaldi M G, Stevens D A, Graybill J R. Invasive aspergillosis. Disease spectrum, treatment practices, and outcomes. I3 Aspergillus Study Group. *Medicine (Baltimore)* 79:250–260, 2000b.

Patterson T F. New agents for treatment of invasive aspergillosis. *Clin Infect Dis* 35:367–369, 2002.

Perea S, Patterson T F. Invasive *Aspergillus* infections in hematologic malignancy patients. *Semin Respir Infect* 17:99–105, 2002.

Perfect J R, Cox G M, Lee J Y, Kauffman C A, deRepentigny L, Chapman S W, Morrison V A, Pappas P, Hiemenz J W, Stevens D A, and the Mycoses Study Group. The impact of culture isolation of *Aspergillus* species: A hospital-based survey of aspergillosis. *Clin Infect Dis* 33:1824–1833, 2001.

Petraitiene R, Petraitis V, Groll A H, Sein T, Schaufele R L, Francesconi A, Bacher J, Avila N A, Walsh T J. Antifungal efficacy of caspofungin (MK-0991) in experimental pulmonary aspergillosis in persistently neutropenic rabbits: Pharmacokinetics, drug disposition, and relationship to galactomannan antigenemia. *Antimicrob Agents Chemother* 46:12–23, 2002.

Petraitis V, Petraitiene R, Groll A H, Rousillon K, Hemmings M, Lyman C A, Sein T, Bacher J, Bekersky I, Walsh T J. Comparative antifungal activities and plasma pharmacokinetics of micafungin (FK 463) against disseminated candidiasis and invasive pulmonary aspergillosis in persistently neutropenic rabbits. *Antimicrob Agents Chemother* 46:1857–1869, 2002.

Pfaller M A, Messer S A, Hollis R J, Jones R N, Sentry Participants Group. Antifungal activities of posaconazole, ravuconazole, and voriconazole compared to those of itraconazole and amphotericin B against 239 clinical isolates of *Aspergillus* spp. and other filamentous fungi: Report from SENTRY Antimicrobial Surveillance Program, 2000. *Antimicrob Agents Chemother* 46:1032–1037, 2002.

Pitt J. The current role of *Aspergillus* and *Penicillium* in human and animal health. *J Med Vet Mycol* 1:17–21, 1994.

Pui C H, Boyett J M, Hughes W T, Rivera G K, Hancock M L, Sandlund J T, Synold T, Relling M V, Ribeiro R C, Crist W M, Evans W E. Human granulocyte colony-stimulating factor after remission induction chemotherapy in children with acute lymphocytic leukemia. *N Engl J Med* 336:1822–1824, 1997.

Rafferty P, Biggs B, Crompton G, Grant I W. What happens to patients with pulmonary aspergilloma? Analysis of 23 cases. *Thorax* 38:579–583, 1983.

Rankin N. Disseminated aspergillosis and moniliasis associated with agranulocytosis and antibiotic therapy. *Br Med J* 183:918–919, 1953.

Raper B, Fennel J. *The Genus Aspergillus.* Baltimore: Williams & Wilkins, 1965.

Rex J H, Walsh T J. Editorial response: Estimating the true cost of amphotericin B. *Clin Infect Dis* 29:1408–1410, 1999.

Ribaud P, Chastang C, Latge J P, Baffroy-Lafitte L, Parquet N, Devergie A, Esperon H, Selimi F, Rocha V, Derouin F, Socie G, Gluckman E. Survival and prognostic factors of invasive aspergillosis after allogeneic bone marrow transplantation. *Clin Infect Dis* 28:322–330, 1999.

Roberts J, Schock K, Marino S, Andriole V T. Efficacies of two new antifungal agents, the triazole ravuconazole and the echinocandin LY-303366, in an experimental model of invasive aspergillosis. *Antimicrob Agents Chemother* 44:3381–3388, 2000.

Roilides E, Uhlig K, Venzon D, Pizzo P A, Walsh T J. Prevention of corticosteroid-induced suppression of human polymorphonuclear leukocyte-induced damage of *Aspergillus fumigatus* hyphae by granulocyte colony-stimulating factor and gamma interferon. *Infect Immun* 61:4870–4877, 1993.

Rosenberg M, Patterson R, Mintzer R, Cooper B J, Roberts M, Harris K E. Clinical and immunologic criteria for the diagnosis of allergic bronchopulmonary aspergillosis. *Ann Intern Med* 86:405–414, 1977.

Rowe J M. Treatment of acute myeloid leukemia with cytokines: Effect on duration of neutropenia and response to infections. *Clin Infect Dis* 26:1290–1294, 1998.

Schaffner A, Douglas H, Braude A. Selective protection against conidia by mononuclear and against mycelia by polymorphonuclear phagocytes in resistance to *Aspergillus*. Observations on these two lines of defense in vivo and in vitro with human and mouse phagocytes. *J Clin Invest* 69:617–631, 1982.

Schaffner A. Therapeutic concentrations of glucocorticoids suppress the antimicrobial activity of human macrophages without impairing their responsiveness to gamma interferon. *J Clin Invest* 76:1755–1764, 1985.

Schaffner A, Frick PG. The effect of ketoconazole on amphotericin B in a model of disseminated aspergillosis. *J Infect Dis* 151:902–910, 1985.

Schaffner A, Böhler A. Amphotericin B refractory aspergillosis after itraconazole: evidence for significant antagonism. *Mycoses* 36:421–424, 1993.

Sheehan D J, Hitchcock C A, Sibley C M. Current and emerging azole antifungal agents. *Clin Microbiol Rev* 12:40–79, 1999.

Sherertz R J, Belani A, Kramer B S, Elfenbein G J, Weiner R S, Sullivan M L, Thomas R G, Samsa G P. Impact of air filtration on nosocomial *Aspergillus* infections: unique risk of bone marrow transplant recipients. *Am J Med* 83:709–718, 1987.

Singh N, Avery R K, Munoz P, Pruett T L, Alexander B, Jacobs R, Tolleman J G, Dominguez E A, Yu C M, Paterson D L, Husain S, Kusne S, Linden P. Trends in risk profiles for and mortality associated with invasive aspergillosis among liver transplant recipients. *Clin Infect Dis* 36:46–52, 2003.

Smith J M, Tang C M, Van Noorden S, Holden D W. Virulence of *Aspergillus fumigatus* double mutants lacking restriction and an alkaline protease in a low-dose model of invasive pulmonary aspergillosis. *Infect Immun* 62:5247–5254, 1994.

Stevens D A. Combination immunotherapy and antifungal chemotherapy. *Clin Infect Dis* 26:1266–1269, 1998.

Stevens D A, Kan V L, Judson M A, Morrison V A, Dummer S, Denning D W, Bennett J E, Walsh T J, Patterson T F, Pankey G A. Practice guidelines for diseases caused by *Aspergillus*. *Clin Infect Dis* 30:696–709, 2000a.

Stevens D A, Schwartz H J, Lee J Y. A randomized trial of itraconazole in allergic bronchopulmonary aspergillosis. *N Engl J Med* 342:756–762, 2000b.

Sutton D A, Fothergill A W, Rinaldi M G. *Guide to Clinically Significant Fungi*. Baltimore, Williams & Wilkins, 1998.

Sutton D A, Sanche S E, Revankar S G, Fothergill A W, Rinaldi M G. In vitro amphotericin B resistance in clinical isolates of *Aspergillus terreus*, with a head-to-head comparison to voriconazole. *J Clin Microbiol* 37:2343–2345, 1999.

Tang C, Cohen J, Krausz T, Van Noorden S, Holden D W. The alkaline protease of *Aspergillus fumigatus* is not a virulence determinant in two murine models of the invasive pulmonary aspergillosis. *Infect Immun* 61:1650–1656, 1993.

Thom C, Church M. *The Aspergilli*. Baltimore: Williams & Wilkins, 1926.

Tomlinson J, Sahn S. Aspergilloma in sarcoid and tuberculosis. *Chest* 92:505–508, 1987.

Vanden Bossche H. Echinocandins—an update. *Expert Opin Ther Patents* 12:151–167, 2002.

Van't Wout J W, Raven E J, van der Meer J W. Treatment of invasive aspergillosis with itraconazole in a patient with chronic granulomatous disease. *J Infect* 20:147–150, 1990.

Vennewald I, Henker M, Klemm E, Seebacher C. Fungal colonization of the paranasal sinuses. *Mycoses* 42:33–36, 1999.

Verweij P E, Stynen D, Rijs A J, dePauw B E, Hoogkamp-Korstanje J A, Meis J F. Sandwich enzyme-linked immunosorbent assay compared with Pastorex latex agglutination test for diagnosing invasive aspergillosis in immunocompromised patients. *J Clin Microbiol* 33:1912–1914, 1995.

Verweij P E, Poulain D, Obayashi T, Patterson T F, Denning D W, Ponton J. Current trends in the detection of antigenaemia, metabolites and cell wall markers for the diagnosis and therapeutic monitoring of fungal infections. *Med Mycol* 36:146–155, 1998.

Vinas P C, King P K, Diaz F G. Spinal *Aspergillus* osteomyelitis. *Clin Infect Dis* 28:1223–1229, 1999.

Virchow V. Breitage zur lehre von den beim menschen vorkommenden pfanzlichen parasiten. *Virchows Archiv*:557, 1856.

von Eiff M, Roos N, Schulten R, Hesse M, Zuhlsdorf M, van de Loo J. Pulmonary aspergillosis: early diagnosis improves survival. *Respiration* 62:341–347, 1995.

Vose J M, Bierman P J, Kessinger A, Coccia P F, Anderson J, Oldham F B, Epstein C, Armitage J O. The use of recombinant human granulocyte-macrophage colony-stimulating factor for the treatment of delayed engraftment following high dose therapy and autologous hematopoietic stem cell transplantation for lymphoid malignancies. *Bone Marrow Transplant* 7:139–143, 1991.

Wald A, Leisenring W, van Burik J-A, Bowden R. Epidemiology of *Aspergillus* infections in a large cohort of patients undergoing bone marrow transplantation. *J Infect Dis* 175:1459–1466, 1997.

Walsh T J, Dixon D M. Nosocomial aspergillosis: environmental microbiology, hospital epidemiology, diagnosis and treatment. *Eur J Epidemiol* 5:131–142, 1989.

Walsh T J. Primary cutaneous aspergillosis—an emerging infection among immunocompromised patients. *Clin Infect Dis* 27:453–457, 1998.

Walsh T J, Hiemenz J W, Seibel N L, Perfect J R, Horwith G, Lee L, Silber J L, DiNubile M J, Reboli A, Bow E, Lister J, Anaissie E J. Amphotericin B lipid complex for invasive fungal infections: Analysis of safety and efficacy in 556 cases. *Clin Infect Dis* 26:1383–1396, 1998.

Walsh T J, Jackson A J, Lee J W, Amantea M, Sein T, Bacher J, Zech L. Dose-dependent pharmacokinetics of amphotericin B lipid complex in rabbits. *Antimicrob Agents Chemother* 44:2068–2070, 2000.

Walsh T J, Goodman J L, Pappas P, Bekersky I, Buell D N, Roden M, Barrett J, Anaissie E J. Safety, tolerance, and pharmacokinetics of high-dose liposomal amphotericin B (AmBisome) in patients infected with *Aspergillus* species and other filamentous fungi: Maximum tolerated dose study. *Antimicrob Agents Chemother* 45:3487–3496, 2001.

Walsh T J, Pappas P, Winston D J, Blumer J, Finn P, Raffali J, Yanovich S, Stiff P, Greenberg R, Donowitz G, Lee J, Schuster

M, Reboli A, Wingard J, Arndt C, Reinhart J, Hadley S, Finberg R, Laverdiere M, Perfect J, Garber G, Fioritini G, Anaissie E, for the NIAID Mycoses Study Group. Voriconazole compared with liposomal amphotericin B for empirical antifungal therapy in patients with neutropenia and persistent fever. *N Engl J Med* 346:225–234, 2002.

Washburn R G, Hammer C H, Bennett JE. Inhibition of complement by culture supernatants of *Aspergillus fumigatus*. *J Infect Dis* 154:944–951, 1986.

Washburn R G, Gallin J I, Bennett J E. Oxidative killing of *Aspergillus fumigatus* proceeds by parallel myeloperoxidase-dependent and -independent pathways. *Infect Immun* 55:2088–2092, 1987.

Washburn R G. Fungal sinusitis. *Curr Clin Topics Infect Dis* 18:60–74, 1998.

Wingard J R, Kubilis P, Lee L, Yee G, White M, Walshe L, Bowden R, Anaissie E, Hiemenz J, Lister J. Clinical significance of nephrotoxicity in patients treated with amphotericin B for suspected or proven aspergillosis. *Clin Infect Dis* 29:1402–1407, 1999.

Yeghen T, Kibbler C C, Prentice HG, Berger L A, Wallesby R K, McWhinney P H M, Lampe F C, Gillespie S. Management of invasive pulmonary aspergillosis in hematology patients: A review of 87 consecutive cases at a single institution. *Clin Infect Dis* 31:859–868, 2000.

Young R C, Bennett J E. Invasive aspergillosis. Absence of detectable antibody response. *Am Rev Resp Dis* 104:710–716, 1971.

Yu V L, Muder R R, Poorsattar A. Significance of isolation of *Aspergillus* from the respiratory tract in diagnosis of invasive pulmonary aspergillosis: results from a three-year prospective study. *Am J Med* 81:249–254, 1986.

15

Zygomycoses

ASHRAF S. IBRAHIM, JOHN E. EDWARDS JR, AND SCOTT G. FILLER

Zygomycosis is a group of fungal infections caused by a variety of mould organisms belonging to the class Zygomycetes. This class is further classified into two orders, Mucorales and Entomophthorales. Fungi belonging to the order Mucorales are distributed into six families all of which can cause cutaneous and deep infections in immunocompromised patients (Ribes et al, 2000) (Fig. 15–1). In contrast, the order Entomophthorales contains two families of organisms that cause subcutaneous and mucocutaneous infections primarily in immunocompetent children (Richardson and Shankland, 1999; Sugar, 2000) (Fig. 15–1).

For years, infections caused by the Zygomycetes class of fungi were described in the literature under the names phycomycosis or zygomycosis. The term phycomycosis is no longer used because the class Phycomycetes no longer exists. The use of the term zygomycosis is taxonomically correct to describe infections caused by organisms belonging to the order Mucorales or Entomophthorales. However, infections caused by organisms of the order Mucorales differ both clinically and pathologically from infections caused by organisms of the order Entomophthorales. Therefore, zygomycosis is too imprecise and vague to convey useful information to the clinician. We propose to use the term mucormycosis for infections caused by organisms belonging to the order Mucorales and entomophthoramycosis for infections caused by organisms of the order Entomophthorales. We discuss each of these types of infections separately.

MUCORMYCOSIS

Etiology

A variety of organisms has been implicated in mucormycosis. However, organisms belonging to the family Mucoraceae are isolated more frequently from patients with mucormycosis patients than any other family. *Rhizopus oryzae* (*Rhizopus arrhizus*) is the most common cause of infection followed by *Rhizopus microsporus* var. *rhizopodiformis* (Richardson and Shankland, 1999; Ribes et al, 2000). Other, less fre-

quently isolated species of the Mucoraceae family that cause a similar spectrum of infections include *Absidia corymbifera, Apophysomyces elegans, Mucor* species, and *Rhizomucor pusillus* (Kwon-Chung and Bennett, 1992; Ribes et al, 2000). Other organisms such as *Cunninghamella bertholletiae* (in Cunninghamellaceae family) have been increasingly isolated from patients with pulmonary and disseminated mucormycosis (Kwon-Chung et al, 1975; Ventura et al, 1986; Cohen-Abbo et al, 1993; Kontoyianis et al, 1994). Additionally, *Saksenaea vasiformis* (in Saksenaceae family) has been reported as a cause of cutaneous (Bearer et al, 1994), subcutaneous (Pritchard et al, 1986; Lye et al, 1996), rhinocerebral (Gonis and Starr, 1997), and disseminated infections (Torell et al, 1981; Hay et al, 1983). Rare cases of mucormycosis have been reported due to *Cokeromyces recurvatus* (Kemna et al, 1994) (in Thamnidiaceae family), *Mortierella* species (Ribes et al, 2000) (in Mortierellaceae family) and *Syncephalastrum* species (Kamalam and Thambiah, 1980) (in Syncephalastraceae family).

The agents of mucormycosis are classified into six different families (Fig. 15–1) based on morphologic analysis of the fungus, namely the presence and location of rhizoids, the presence of apophyses, and the morphology of the columellae (Sugar, 2000). Other taxonomically relevant features include carbohydrate assimilation and the maximal temperature compatible for growth. Because the diseases caused by the different families of Mucorales are clinically indistinguishable from each other, laboratory confirmation of the identity of the causative agent is the only way to differentiate among these fungi. The identification of organisms isolated from patients with mucormycosis to the species level will assist in clarifying the epidemiology of this infection, and may be helpful in determining the susceptibility of the different organisms to antifungal drugs.

Ecology and Epidemiology

Agents of mucormycosis are ubiquitous and thermotolerant organisms that usually grow in decaying matter, including bread, vegetables, fruits, and seeds. They

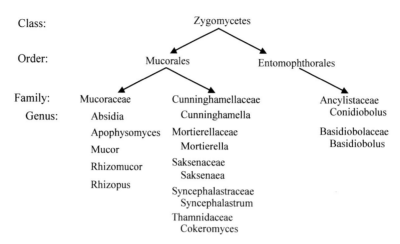

FIGURE 15–1. Taxonomy of Zygomycetes adapted from Ribes et al, 2000.

can also be recovered from soil, compost piles, and animal excreta. Most of the Mucorales can grow and sporulate abundantly on any carbohydrate-containing source. Abundant growth with sporulation is usually seen in culture media within 2–5 days. The spores are easily air-borne and Mucorales are readily recovered as contaminants in laboratory cultures. Indeed, the ability of *R. microsporus* var. *rhizopodiformis* to grow on nonsterile wooden sticks used for culturing stool samples from immunocompromised patients led to misdiagnosis of these patients with gastrointestinal mucormycosis (Verweij et al, 1997).

Members of Mucorales cause both localized and disseminated infections in immunocompromised patients. Only rare case reports of invasive mucormycosis in apparently normal hosts have been described (Al-Asiri et al, 1996; Del Valle et al, 1996). Allergic pulmonary disease does occur in immunocompetent hosts and reflects an acute hypersensitive immune response illness rather than invasive disease (Wimander and Belin, 1980; O'Connell et al, 1995).

Mucormycosis is relatively uncommon in neutropenic patients compared to other fungal infections. However, an increasing prevalence of mucormycosis cases in this population has been observed. Because the number of iatrogenically immunocompromised patients continues to rise, it is likely that the incidence of mucormycosis will also increase (Ribes et al, 2000). Nosocomial outbreaks of mucormycosis can occur in leukemic patients, although they are not as common as hospital-related *Aspergillus* infections.

The major risk factors for mucormycosis include uncontrolled diabetes mellitus and other forms of metabolic acidosis, treatment with corticosteroid drugs in organ or bone marrow transplantation, trauma and burns, malignant hematological disorders, and deferoxamine therapy to chelate aluminum or iron in dialysis patients. The underlying causes influence the clinical manifestation of the disease. For example, diabetics in ketoacidosis usually develop rhinocerebral mucormycosis, whereas patients with malignant hematological disease, lymphoma, severe neutropenia, or a history of deferoxamine therapy usually suffer from pulmonary mucormycosis. Both forms of disease are acquired through inhalation (Lueg et al, 1996; Ribes et al, 2000). Other routes of infection include direct skin contact, which results in cutaneous mucormycosis or ingestion of contaminated food, which leads to gastrointestinal mucormycosis. Cutaneous mucormycosis can occur in neonates, and trauma and burn patients. Gastrointestinal mucormycosis is nearly always limited to malnourished infants and transplant recipients.

Pathogenesis

The source of mucormycosis is exogenous and the organism usually gains entry into the host through the respiratory tract. Spores can also be introduced directly through abraded skin to cause primary cutaneous mucormycosis that can further proliferate and disseminate to other body organs.

Understanding of the pathogenesis of the disease is derived mainly from in vitro studies that investigated the ability of host defense constituents, such as neutrophils and macrophages to kill agents of mucormycosis. In addition, the development of animal models of mucormycosis has aided our understanding of pathogenesis. These models include mice or rabbits with mild diabetic ketoacidosis induced by streptosetozin or alloxan, cortisone-treated mice, neutropenic mice, and deferoxamine-treated animals. Inhalation of Mucorales spores by immunocompetent animals does not result in the development of mucormycosis (Waldorf et al, 1984). In contrast, when the animals are immunosupressed by corticosteroids or by induction of diabetes, the animals die from progressive pulmonary and hematogenously disseminated infection (Waldorf et al, 1984). The ability of inhaled spores to germinate and form hyphae in the host is critical for establishing infection. Bronchoalveolar macrophages harvested from lungs of immunocompetent mice are able to ingest and prevent germination of *R. oryzae* spores, thus preventing progression of the disease (Waldorf et al, 1984). However, these bronchoalveolar macrophages are unable to kill the organism because viable organisms can still be recovered from the phagolysosomes. In contrast, bronchoalveolar macrophages of immunosuppressed mice are unable to prevent germination of the spores in vitro or after infection induced by intranasal inoculation (Waldorf et al, 1984).

Severely neutropenic patients are at increased risk for developing mucormycosis, as well as other infections, whereas patients with AIDS are rarely infected with agents of Mucorales (Sugar, 2000). These findings suggest that neutrophils are critical for inhibiting fungal spore proliferation. Recruitment of neutrophils to sites of infection occurs in response to fungal constituents and activation of the alternative complement pathway (Diamond et al, 1978; Marx et al, 1982). Both mononuclear and polymorphonuclear phagocytes of normal hosts kill Mucorales by the generation of oxidative metabolites and the cationic peptides, defensins (Diamond et al, 1982; Waldorf et al, 1984; Waldorf, 1989). In the presence of hyperglycemia and low pH found in patients with diabetic ketoacidosis, these phagocytes are dysfunctional, and exhibit impaired chemotaxis and defective intracellular killing by both oxidative and non-oxidative mechanisms (Chinn and Diamond, 1982). The exact mechanisms by which ketoacidosis, diabetes, or steroids impair the function of these phagocytes remain unknown.

Phagocyte dysfunction alone cannot explain the high incidence of mucormycosis in patients with diabetic ketoacidosis because the incidence of this infection is increased much more than that of infections caused by other microbial pathogens (Kwon-Chung and Bennett, 1992; Richardson and Shankland, 1999; Ribes et al, 2000; Sugar, 2000). Therefore, Mucorales must possess virulence traits that enable the organism to survive in this subset of patients. One of these traits is the ability to acquire iron from the host (Artis et al, 1982; Boelaert et al, 1993). Iron is required by virtually all microbial pathogens for growth and virulence (Howard, 1999). In mammalian hosts, very little serum iron is available to microorganisms because it is highly bound to host carrier proteins such as transferrin (Artis et al, 1982). Sequestration of serum iron is a major host defense mechanism against Mucorales, because *Rhizopus* grows poorly in normal serum until exogenous iron is

added (Artis et al, 1982; Boelaert et al, 1993). Importantly, patients with elevated levels of available serum iron are uniquely susceptible to infection by Mucorales (Sugar, 2000). Patients who are treated with the iron chelator, deferoxamine, have a markedly increased incidence of invasive mucormycosis (Boelaert et al, 1994). Deferoxamine appears to predispose patients to *Rhizopus* infection by acting as a siderophore, which supplies previously unavailable iron to the fungus (Boelaert et al, 1993). The mechanism by which *Rhizopus* obtains iron from the iron-deferoxamine complex is believed to include binding of the iron-deferoxamine complex to the mould, followed by release of iron and subsequent transport of the reduced iron intracellularly (de Locht et al, 1994). This transport is likely mediated by iron permeases. Administration of deferoxamine worsens survival of guinea pigs infected with *Rhizopus* but not *Candida albicans* (Boelaert et al, 1993; Boelaert et al, 1994; de Locht et al, 1994). Additionally, in vitro studies of radiolabeled iron uptake from deferoxamine in serum show that *Rhizopus* is able to incorporate 8-fold and 40-fold more iron than are *Aspergillus fumigatus* and *C. albicans*, respectively (Boelaert et al, 1993).

As mentioned previously, patients with diabetic ketoacidosis are at high risk of developing rhinocerebral mucormycosis (Kwon-Chung and Bennett, 1992; Richardson and Shankland, 1999; Ribes et al, 2000; Sugar, 2000). These patients have elevated levels of available iron in their serum (Artis et al, 1982). Also, Artis and coworkers showed that sera collected from patients with diabetic ketoacidosis supported growth of *R. oryzae* at acidic pH (7.3–6.88) but not at alkaline pH (7.78–8.38) (Artis et al, 1982). Sera that did not support *R. oryzae* growth at acidic pH were found to have less available iron than sera that supported fungal growth. Furthermore, adding exogenous iron to sera allowed *R. oryzae* to grow profusely at acidic conditions but not at pH $\geq$ 7.4. Finally, simulated acidotic conditions decreased the iron-binding capacity of sera collected from normal volunteers, suggesting that acidosis temporarily disrupts the capacity of transferrin to bind iron (Artis et al, 1982). Therefore, the increased susceptibility of patients with diabetic ketoacidosis to mucormycosis is likely due in part to an elevation in available serum iron.

Fungi can obtain iron from the host using low molecular weight iron chelators (siderophores) or high-affinity iron permeases (Stearman et al, 1996; Howard, 1999). Because the siderophores of *Rhizopus* spp. are very inefficient at obtaining iron from serum (de Locht et al, 1994; Boelaert, 1993), it is believed that these siderophores contribute very little to the ability of this organism to grow in patients who are receiving deferoxamine or have diabetic ketoacidosis. The high affinity iron permeases are able to transport iron from serum intracellularly and therefore likely to be critical for the survival of the organism in susceptible hosts.

Other putative virulence factors include the ability of *R. oryzae* to adhere to the extracellular matrix proteins laminin and type IV collagen (Bouchara et al, 1996), and the secretion of aspartic proteinases (Farley and Sullivan, 1998). Additionally, *Rhizopus* species have an active ketone reductase system that may be an additional virulence factor by enhancing growth in the acidic and glucose-rich environment seen in ketoacidotic states (Anand et al, 1992). To date, none of these potential virulence factors have been proven to be essential for the development of mucormycosis, because the necessary molecular biology tools to construct mutants lacking a specific virulence factor have not yet been developed.

Clinical Manifestations

The clinical hallmark of mucormycosis is the rapid onset of tissue necrosis, with or without fever. This necrosis is the result of invasion of blood vessels and subsequent thrombosis. In most cases, the infection is relentlessly progressive and results in death unless treatment is promptly initiated. Based on clinical presentation and the involvement of a particular anatomic site, mucormycosis can be divided into at least six forms: *(1)* rhinocerebral, *(2)* pulmonary, *(3)* cutaneous, *(4)* gastrointestinal *(5)* disseminated, and *(6)* miscellaneous.

Rhinocerebral Mucormycosis. Rhinocerebral mucormycosis is the most common form of the disease representing between one-third to one-half of all cases (Pillsbury and Fischer, 1977). Approximately 70% of cases of rhinocerebral (occasionally referred to as craniofacial) mucormycosis are found in diabetic patients in ketoacidosis (McNulty, 1982) (See Color Fig. 15–2 in separate color insert). Rhinocerebral mucormycosis can also occur in patients who have received a solid organ transplant or who have prolonged neutropenia (Pillsbury and Fischer, 1977; Yanagisawa et al, 1977; Abedi et al, 1984; Peterson et al, 1997).

The initial symptoms are consistent with sinusitis, and include facial pain, unilateral headache, drainage, and soft tissue swelling. Fever is frequently present. The infection may rapidly extend into the contiguous tissues. Infected tissues are initially erythematous, and then become violaceous, and finally black as the blood vessels become thrombosed and tissue infarction occurs (See Color Fig. 15–2a in separate color insert). Infection can sometimes extend from the sinuses into the mouth and produce painful, necrotic ulcerations of the hard palate or from the sinuses on one side to the contralateral sinuses. If untreated, infection usually spreads from the ethmoid sinus to the orbit, resulting in loss of

extraocular muscle function and proptosis. Marked swelling of the conjunctiva may also be seen. Involvement of the optic nerve is manifested by blurred vision and eventually blindness. Cranial nerves five and seven may also be affected, resulting in ptosis, pupillary dilatation and occasionally, peripheral facial nerve palsy (See Color Fig. 15–2b in separate color insert). Cranial nerve findings represent extensive infection and signal a grave prognosis. Infection can also spread posteriorly from either the orbit or sinuses to the central nervous system. A bloody nasal discharge may be the first sign that infection has invaded through the terbinates and into the brain. Physicians should consider the possibility of mucormycosis of the central nervous system in patients with ketoacidosis who have altered mental status that persists even after metabolic abnormalities have been corrected. When there is extensive central nervous system involvement, the angioinvasive nature of the fungus may result in cavernous sinus and internal carotid artery thrombosis (Lowe and Hudson, 1975), and occasionally may lead to hematogenous dissemination of the infection (LeCompte and Meissner, 1947; Pillsbury and Fischer, 1977).

Previously, cases of rhinocerebral mucormycosis were usually fatal (LeCompte and Meissner, 1947). Although the mortality rate of rhinocerebral disease remains high, the infection can be cured when diagnosed early and treated with aggressive surgery and appropriate antifungal agents (Bullock et al, 1974; Parfrey, 1986). The nature of the underlying disease and the reversibility of the immune dysfunction are the most important determinants of survival. One study showed that 75% of patients with rhinocerebral disease who had no underlying immune compromise survived whereas 60% of those with diabetes and only 20% of patients with other immunocompromised states were cured (Blitzer et al, 1980).

Pulmonary Mucormycosis. Mucormycosis of this type occurs most commonly in leukemic patients who are receiving chemotherapy. These patients typically have severe neutropenia and are frequently receiving broad-spectrum antibiotics for unremitting fever. Patients with diabetic ketoacidosis can also develop pulmonary mucormycosis, although infections in these patients are less fulminant and follow a more subacute course than is typically seen in patients with neutropenia (Rothstein and Simon, 1986). Pulmonary mucormycosis may develop as a result of inhalation or by hematogenous or lymphatic spread. Symptoms include fever, dyspnea, and cough. Angioinvasion results in necrosis of tissue parenchyma, which may ultimately lead to cavitation and/or hemoptysis, which may be fatal if a major blood vessel is involved (Watts, 1983; Harada et al, 1992). If infection is not treated, hematogenous dissemination to the contralateral lung and other organs frequently occurs. Patients with untreated pulmonary mucormycosis usually die from disseminated disease before respiratory failure occurs (Tedder et al, 1994). The notable exception is the rare patient with massive hemoptysis (Murray, 1975; Pagano et al, 1995).

Cutaneous Mucormycosis. Patients who are at high risk of developing cutaneous mucormycosis are mainly those with burns or other forms of skin trauma, such as patients with open fractures or crash victims. In diabetic or immunocompromised patients, cutaneous lesions may arise at an insulin injection or catheter insertion site. A nationwide epidemic of cutaneous mucormycosis occurred in patients who had contaminated surgical dressings applied to their skin (Gartenberg et al, 1978; Mead et al, 1979).

Although cutaneous disease usually arises from primary inoculation of the infection site, it sometimes is due to disseminated disease. These two routes of infection have distinct clinical presentations. Primary infection produces an acute inflammatory response with pus, abscess formation, tissue swelling, and necrosis. The lesions may appear red and indurated, and often progress to black eschars. The necrotic tissue may slough, leaving large ulcers. Primary cutaneous disease, which may be polymicrobial, is generally rapidly aggressive even in the face of appropriate debridement and medical treatment. Occasionally, aerial mycelia may be visible on the surface of the cutaneous lesion. This form of cutaneous disease can be very invasive locally, and penetrate from the cutaneous and subcutaneous tissues into the adjacent fat, muscle, fascia, and even bone. Cutaneous and subcutaneous disease may lead to necrotizing fasciitis, which has a mortality approaching 80% (Patino et al, 1991). Secondary vascular invasion may also lead to hematogenously disseminated infection of the deep organs.

When cutaneous mucormycosis results from hematogenously disseminated infection, the lesion typically begins as an erythematous, indurated and painful cellulitis. It then progresses to an ulcer covered with a black eschar (See Color Fig. 15–3 in separate color insert).

Gastrointestinal Mucormycosis. Mucormycosis of the gastrointestinal tract is rare, mainly occurs in patients who are extremely malnurished (especially infants or children) and transplant recipients, and is thought to arise from ingestion of the organism. The stomach, colon, and ileum are the most commonly involved sites. Because this infection is acute and rapidly fatal, it is seldomly diagnosed during life. The symptoms are varied and depend on the site affected. Nonspecific abdominal pain and distention associated with nausea and vomiting are the most common symptoms. Fever and

hematochezia may also occur. The patient is often thought to have an intraabdominal abscess. The diagnosis may be made by biopsy of the suspected area during surgery or endoscopy.

Disseminated Mucormycosis. Hematogenously disseminated mucormycosis may originate from any primary site of infection. Pulmonary mucormycosis in severely neutropenic patients has the highest incidence of dissemination. Less commonly, dissemination can arise from the gastrointestinal tract, sinuses or cutaneous lesions, particularly in burn patients. The most common site of dissemination is the brain, but metastatic lesions may also be found in the spleen, heart, skin, and other organs. Cerebral infection following dissemination is distinct from rhinocerebral mucormycosis, and results in abscess formation and infarction. Patients present with sudden onset of focal neurological deficits or coma. The mortality associated with dissemination to the brain approaches 100% (Straatsma et al, 1962).

Miscellaneous Forms. Agents of Mucorales may cause infection in virtually any body site. Brain involvement in the absence of sinus infection, endocarditis, and pyelonephritis occurs occasionally, mainly in intravenous drug abusers (Virmani et al, 1982; Tuder, 1985; Woods and Hanna, 1986; Vesa et al, 1992). Other reports have described mucormycosis in bones (Maliwan et al, 1984; Pierce et al, 1987), mediastinum (Connor et al, 1979; Leong, 1978), and trachea (Andrews et al, 1997). Other unusual forms of mucormycosis include superior vena cava syndrome (Helenglass et al, 1981), and external otitis (Ogunlana, 1975). Although mucormycosis is not seen commonly in AIDS patients, there have been a number of case reports of this infection in this patient population.

Diagnosis
Diagnosis of mucormycosis almost always requires histopathologic evidence of fungal invasion of the tissues. Culture of organisms from a potentially infected site is rarely sufficient to establish the diagnosis of mucormycosis because the causative agent is ubiquitous, may colonize normal persons, and is a relatively frequent laboratory contaminant. Additionally, the organism may be killed during tissue grinding, which is routinely used to process tissue specimens for culture. Thus, a sterile culture does not rule out the infection. Furthermore, waiting for the results of the fungal culture may delay the institution of appropriate therapy. There is no reliable serologic test or skin test for mucormycosis. Therefore, the diagnosis should be made by biopsy of infected tissues. The biopsy specimen should demonstrate the characteristic wide, ribbon-like

aseptate hyphal elements that branch at right angles. The organisms are often surrounded by extensive necrotic debris (See Color Fig. 15–4 in separate color insert). Other fungi including *Aspergillus, Fusarium, or Scedosporium* spp. may look similar to the Mucorales on biopsy. However, these moulds have septae, are usually thinner, and branch at acute angles. The genus and species of the infecting organism may be determined by culture of the infected tissue. The organism is rarely isolated from cultures of blood, CSF, sputum, urine, feces, or swabs of infected areas.

While imaging techniques may be suggestive of mucormycosis, they are rarely diagnostic. In patients with rhinocerebral mucormycosis, computed tomography (CT) scanning of the sinuses may reveal mucoperiosteal thickening, air-fluid levels and bony erosion. Although evidence of infection of the soft tissues of the orbit may sometimes be seen by CT scan, magnetic resonance imaging (MRI) is more sensitive (Fatterpekar et al, 1999). Patients with early rhinocerebral mucormycosis may have a normal MRI, and surgical exploration with biopsy of the areas of suspected infection should always be performed in high-risk patients. The most common finding with CT of the orbit is thickening of the extraocular muscles. It is critically important to emphasize that if orbital mucormycosis is suspected, initial empiric therapy with a polyene antifungal should begin while the diagnosis is being confirmed, rather than waiting until a protracted series of diagnostic tests have been completed. A common clinical scenario is for the physician to make a presumptive diagnosis of orbital or rhinocerebral mucormycosis but to delay therapy for several days until diagnostic studies are completed.

The findings of pulmonary mucormycosis are often consistent with a bronchopneumonia caused by bacteria or infection with other fungi (particularly *Aspergillus* spp.). Early in the course of infection, focal or diffuse infiltrates are seen on chest X-rays; these then progress to consolidation, with or without cavitation (Tedder et al, 1994; McAdams et al, 1997). Wedge-shaped infarcts of the lung may also be seen, particularly following thrombosis of the pulmonary vessels due to fungal angioinvasion (Marchevsky et al, 1980). High-resolution chest CT scan is the best method of determining the extent of pulmonary mucormycosis, and may demonstrate evidence of infection before it is apparent on the chest X-ray.

The diagnosis of disseminated disease is difficult because patients are usually severely ill from multiple diseases and virtually always have negative blood cultures. If there is evidence of infarction in multiple organs, the diagnosis of mucormycosis should be considered. However, aspergillosis is commonly associated with an identical clinical picture. When disseminated mucormycosis is suspected, a careful search should be made for cutaneous lesions that can be biopsied for diagnostic purposes.

Treatment

Four factors are critical for eradicating mucormycosis: rapidity of diagnosis, reversal of the underlying predisposing factors (if possible), aggressive surgical debridement of infected tissue, and appropriate antifungal therapy. Early diagnosis is important because small, focal lesions can often be surgically excised before they progress to involve critical structures or disseminate. Correcting or controlling predisposing problems is also essential for improving the treatment outcome. In diabetic ketoacidotic patients, hyperglycemia and acidemia should be corrected. Discontinuation of iron chelation or immunosuppressive therapy, particularly steroids, should be strongly considered when the diagnosis of mucormycosis is made.

Mucormycosis is frequently rapidly progressive and antifungal therapy alone is often inadequate to control the infection. Thus, surgical debridement of the infected and necrotic tissue should be performed on an urgent basis. In rhinocerebral mucormycosis, early surgical excision of the infected sinuses and appropriate debridement of the retroorbital space can often prevent the infection from extending into the eye and obviate the need for enucleation. Repeated surgical exploration of the sinuses and orbit may be necessary to ensure that all necrotic tissue has been debrided and the infection has not progressed. In a retrospective study of patients with pulmonary mucormycosis, surgical treatment plus antifungal therapy greatly improved outcome compared to the use of antifungal therapy alone (Tedder et al, 1994). Cutaneous mucormycosis should also be treated by surgical debridement. Surgical debridement of necrotic tissue is frequently highly disfiguring; if the patient survives the acute phase of the disease, major reconstructive surgery may be necessary.

There have been no prospective randomized trials to define the optimal antifungal therapy for mucormycosis. Amphotericin B remains the only antifungal agent approved for the treatment of this infection (Kwon-Chung and Bennett, 1992; Richardson and Shankland, 1999; Ribes et al, 2000; Sugar, 2000). Because many Mucorales isolates are either relatively or highly resistant to amphotericin B, high doses of this drug are required. Amphotericin B deoxycholate should be administered at 1.0–1.5 mg/kg/day, however, this dose frequently causes nephrotoxicity. The lipid formulations of amphotericin B are significantly less nephrotoxic than amphotericin B deoxycholate and can be administered at higher doses for a longer period of time. Several case reports of patients with mucormycosis document successful treatment with up to 15 mg/kg/day of a lipid formulation of amphotericin B (Ericsson et al, 1993; Weng et al, 1998; Cagatay et al, 2001). However, the relative efficacy of the lipid formulations of amphotericin B versus the deoxycholate preparation as therapy for mucormycosis is unknown. Although many clinical mycologists believe that high doses of a lipid formulation should be used in patients who do not respond to initial amphotericin B deoxycholate, a consensus is developing in support of a lipid formulation of amphotericin B as the initial antifungal therapy for all patients with mucormycosis.

Itraconazole is the only marketed azole drug that has in vitro activity against Mucorales (Sun et al, 2002a). However, itraconazole has not been found to be effective for treating mucormycosis. Voriconazole, a recently approved second generation broad spectrum triazole, is not active against Mucorales in vitro (Sun et al, 2002a). However, posaconazole and ravuconazole, investigational triazoles, have promising in vitro activity against agents of mucormycosis, especially *Rhizopus* spp. (Sun et al, 2002a; Pfaller et al, 2002). In experimental animal models of disseminated mucormycosis, posaconazole was more efficacious than itraconazole, but less efficacious than amphotericin B (Sun et al, 2002b). Further data are needed to determine whether posaconazole or ravuconazole, alone or in combination with amphotericin B, may be useful for the treatment of mucormycosis.

Caspofungin, the first member of the novel echinocandin class of antifungal drugs to be marketed in the United States, has been approved for use in patients with invasive aspergillosis who are refractory to or intolerant of conventional therapy. This drug has minimal activity against agents of mucormycosis when tested in vitro by standard methods (Del Poeta et al, 1997; Espinel-Ingroff, 1998). While in vitro activity is not always predictive of a drug's activity in vivo, there are currently no in vivo data supporting the use of caspofungin for treatment of mucormycosis.

Some case reports have suggested that hyperbaric oxygen may be a beneficial adjunct to the standard surgical and medical antifungal therapy of mucormycosis, particularly for patients with rhinocerebral disease. In a small retrospective study of patients with rhinocerebral mucormycosis, 2 of 6 patients who received hyperbaric oxygen died, whereas 4 of 7 patients who received only standard debridement and amphotericin B died. The authors hypothesized that hyperbaric oxygen might be useful for treating mucormycosis in conjunction with standard therapy because higher oxygen pressure improves the ability of neutrophils to kill the organism (Couch et al, 1988). Additionally, high oxygen pressure inhibits the germination of fungal spores and growth of mycelia in vitro (Robb, 1966).

The overall survival rate of patients with mucormycosis is approximately 50%, although survival rates of up to 85% have been reported more recently. Much of the variability in outcome is due to the mix of patients in these studies. Rhinocerebral mucormycosis has a higher survival rate than does pulmonary or disseminated mucormycosis because rhinocerebral disease can frequently be diagnosed earlier and the most common underlying cause, diabetic ketoacidosis, can be readily treated (Parfrey, 1986). In contrast, pulmonary mucormycosis has a high mortality because it is difficult to diagnose, and frequently occurs in neutropenic patients. For example, in one large study, only 44% of patients with pulmonary mucormycosis were diagnosed premortem, and the overall survival rate was only 20% (Tedder et al, 1994). In a separate study in which 93% of the infections were diagnosed premortem, the survival rate was 73% (Parfrey, 1986). Mortality in patients with disseminated disease approaches 100%, in large part because surgical removal of infected tissues is not feasible.

ENTOMOPHTHORAMYCOSIS

Etiology

The order Entomophthorales includes two histopathologically similar, but clinically and mycologically distinct genera: *Basidiobolus* and *Conidiobolus* (Kwon-Chung and Bennett, 1992; Ribes et al, 2000; Sugar, 2000). Both basidiobolomycosis and conidiobolomycosis present mainly as subcutaneous infections in immunocompetent hosts. However, both of these infections occasionally disseminate in both immunocompetent and immuncompromised hosts (Ribes et al, 2000). Basidiobolomycosis is caused by *Basidiobolus ranarum*. Previous descriptions of this organism have used the synonyms *B. haptosporus*, *B. meristosporus*, or *B. heterosporus* (Ribes et al, 2000); however, *B. ranarum* is currently the preferred name. This organism predominantly infects the trunk and limbs. In contrast, conidiobolomycosis (also known as rhinophycomycosis, rhinoentomophthoromycosis, or nasofacial zygomycosis) is caused by *Conidiobolus coronatus* or *Conidiobolus incongruous*. Conidiobolomycosis primarily involves the nose and soft tissues of the face (Thakar et al, 2001).

Ecology and Epidemiology

Basidiobolomycosis is predominantly a disease of childhood and adolescence, and is only occasionally seen in adults (Kwon-Chung and Bennett, 1992). In contrast, conidiobolomycosis almost always afflicts adults (Martinson, 1971; Gugnani, 1992). Both diseases occur mainly in the tropical and subtropical regions of Africa and Southeast Asia. Rare cases have been seen in other parts of the world (Ribes et al, 2000). Although entomophthoramycosis occurs predominantly in healthy individuals, some cases have occurred in immunocompromised hosts (Dworzack et al, 1978; Walsh et al, 1994).

The agents of entomophthoramycosis are normal inhabitants of soil throughout the world. *Basidiobolus ranarum* is found in decaying vegetation, soil, and the gastrointestinal tracts of reptiles, fish, amphibians, and bats (Okafor et al, 1984). Similarly, *C. coronatus* is found in soil, decaying vegetation, insects, and in the gastrointestinal contents of lizards and toads (Dreschler, 1960; Rippon, 1982; Ribes et al, 2000). Although the agents of entomophthoramycosis are ubiquitous, this infection is rare. Only 150 cases were estimated to occur worldwide in 1991 (Costa et al, 1991). Therefore, it is possible that the individuals who develop this infection have a subtle defect in host immunity to this group of organisms.

The mode of transmission for *B. ranarum* is assumed to be through minor trauma and insect bites (Cameroon, 1990). Fungal spores are found in bristles of mites and are probably carried by other insects. Infected insects are ingested by reptiles and amphibians, which subsequently pass the spores in their excreta (Dreschler, 1956). *Basidiobolus ranarum* may be present on "toilet leaves" that are used for skin cleaning after a bowel movement. Thus, direct inoculation of the perineum may occur from these contaminated leaves. Consistent with this theory is the finding that the infection most commonly occurs on the buttocks, thighs, and perineum (Cameroon, 1990). *Basidiobolus ranarum* occasionally causes rhinocerebral infections in hyperglycemic patients, suggesting that this organism may also be acquired by inhalation (Dworzack et al, 1978).

Conidiobolomycosis occurs 8 times more frequently in males and is most common in individuals who work outdoors in the tropical and subtropical rain forests of Africa and Southeast Asia. The mode of transmission of conidiobolomycosis has not been clearly established. The predilection of the organism to infect the head and face suggests that the route of inoculation is via inhalation of spores or through minor trauma to the nose or face (Gugnani, 1992). This infection may be transmitted by insect bites (Thakar et al, 2001). Conidiobolomycosis also occurs in animals such as horses and mules (Thakar et al, 2001).

Clinical Manifestations

Basidiobolomycosis typically presents as a chronic infection of the subcutaneous tissue of the arms, legs, trunk, or buttocks (Goodman and Rinaldi, 1991), and is characterized by the presence of firm, painless nodular subcutaneous lesions that spread locally. The infection is slowly progressive if not treated but may heal

spontaneously (Bittencourt et al, 1991). Although dissemination usually does not occur (Chandler and Watts, 1987), invasion of the muscles deep beneath the subcutaneous infected areas has been reported (Kamalam and Thambiah, 1984). Additionally, *B. ranarum* occasionally infects the gastrointestinal track, predominantly the stomach, duodenum, and colon (Pasha et al, 1997). Symptoms of gastrointestinal basidiobolomycosis include fever, abdominal pain, diarrhea, constipation, weight loss, and sometimes chills and rigors. Angioinvasive disease similar to that in mucormycosis has been described (Kamalam and Thambiah, 1984).

Infections with *Conidiobolus* present most commonly as chronic sinusitis. The infection is initially manifest as a swelling of the inferior nasal turbinates. If untreated, infection subsequently extends to the adjacent facial and subcutaneous tissues, as well as the paranasal sinuses. Swelling of the nose, mouth, and perinasal tissue results in nasal congestion and drainage, sinus pain, and epistaxis (Onuigbo et al, 1975). Generalized facial swelling may be so severe that the patient is unable to open his eyes (Sugar, 2000). The presence of subcutaneous nodules in the eyebrows, upper lip, and cheeks may be quite disfiguring, especially if there is regional lymph node involvement and subsequent lymphedema (Ravisse et al, 1976). Occasionally, infection can involve the pharynx and larynx, resulting in dysphagia and airway obstruction. Unlike mucormycosis, conidiobolomycosis usually does not spread to the brain (Chandler and Watts, 1987). Disseminated infections are unusual, but have been reported in both immunocompetent and immunocompromised patients (Gugnani, 1992).

Diagnosis

In endemic areas of entomophthoramycosis, basidiobolomycosis and conidiobolomycosis can be distinguished from one another by the location of the infection and the age of the patient. The diagnosis is best made by biopsy of the infected subcutaneous or submucosal tissue. Both diseases have similar histopathology. The hyphae, which are broad, thin-walled, and occasionally septate, are best visualized with hematoxylin and eosin staining because of the presence of the Splendore-Hoeppli eosinophilic material (Chandler and Watts, 1987). Other stains such as periodic acid-Schiff and Gomori methenamine silver are less effective in staining the Entomophthorales (Pasha et al, 1997; Sugar, 2000). Hyphae are surrounded by eosinophils, as well as lymphocytes and plasma cells. Although the presence of eosinophils is an important histopathologic finding for entomophthoramycosis, eosinophilia can also occur with some parasitic infections. Angioinvasion with subsequent tissue necrosis and infarction is rarely seen in patients with entomophthoramycosis (Sugar, 2000). Because the agents of entomophthoramycosis cannot be identified at the species level by histopathology, specimens must be cultured.

Treatment and Prevention

No single drug has been proven to be effective in treating all cases of entomophthoramycosis. Potassium iodide (KI), trimethoprim-sulfamethoxazole, amphotericin B, azoles and a combination of these agents have been used with varying success. Because of the rarity of the infections, none of these treatment regimens have been directly compared. Furthermore, some cases of entomophthoramycosis may resolve without treatment. Potassium iodide has traditionally been used in the treatment of entomophthoramycosis, and both successes (Rippon, 1982; Bittencourt et al, 1982) and failures (Okafor and Gugnani, 1983) have been reported. The mechanism of action of KI is not known. To be efficacious, KI should be given for at least 3 months at 1.5–2.0 grams per day. Trimethoprim-sulfamethoxazole has fewer side effects than KI; however, the former drug must be administered for a long period of time (Drouhet and Dupont, 1983; Restrepo, 1994). Also, high concentrations of trimethoprim-sulfamethoxazole are required to inhibit the growth of the organism in vitro (Restrepo, 1994). Although fluconazole and itraconazole have been used to treat entomophthoramycosis, there is more experience with ketoconazole (Drouhet and Dupont, 1983; Costa et al, 1991; Thakar et al, 2001). Frequently, months of continuous treatment with ketoconazole or multiple courses of therapy have been required for resolution of the disease (Drouhet and Dupont, 1983; Thakar et al, 2001). Amphotericin B is usually not the first choice of treatment, but is often tried when other agents fail to cure the infection. Some isolates of B. ranarum and Conidiobolus spp. are susceptible to amphotericin B in vitro, while other isolates are resistant (Yangco et al, 1984). There are anecdotal reports of successful therapy with KI combined with trimethoprim-sulfamethoxazole (Gugnani, 1992), ketoconazole (Mukhopadhyay et al, 1995; Thakar et al, 2001), or fluconazole (Thakar et al, 2001), in patients in whom single-drug therapy had failed. The combination of amphotericin B and terbinafine has also been used (Foss et al, 1996). Experience with lipid formulations of amphotericin B is very limited.

In addition to antifungal therapy, surgical removal of accessible nodules and reconstruction of tissues that are grossly deformed by the chronic inflammatory process should be performed. Unfortunately, relapses of the infection after surgery often occur (Kwon-Chung and Bennett, 1992).

REFERENCES

Abedi E, Sismanis A, Choi K, Pastore P. Twenty-five years' experience treating cerebro-rhino-orbital mucormycosis. *Laryngoscope* 94:1060–1062, 1984.

Al-Asiri R H, Van Dijken P J, Mahmood M A, Al-Shahed M S, Rossi M L, Osoba A O. Isolated hepatic mucormycosis in an immunocompetent child. *Am J Gastroenterol* 91:606–607, 1996.

Anand V K, Alemar G, Griswold J A Jr. Intracranial complications of mucormycosis: an experimental model and clinical review. *Laryngoscope* 102:656–662, 1992.

Andrews D R, Allan A, Larbalestier R I. Tracheal mucormycosis. *Ann Thorac Surg* 63:230–232, 1997.

Artis W M, Fountain J A, Delcher H K, Jones H E. A mechanism of susceptibility to mucormycosis in diabetic ketoacidosis: Transferrin and iron availability. *Diabetes* 31:1110–1114, 1982.

Bearer E A, Nelson P R, Chowers M Y, Davis C E. Cutaneous zygomycosis caused by *Saksenaea vasiformis* in a diabetic patient. *J Clin Microbiol* 32:1823–1824, 1994.

Bittencourt A L, Arruda S M, de Andrade J A, Carvalho E M. Basidiobolomycosis: a case report. *Pediatr Dermatol* 8:325–328, 1991.

Bittencourt A L, Serra G, Sadigursky M, Araujo M G, Campos M C, Sampaio L C. Subcutaneous zygomycosis caused by *Basidiobolus haptosporus*: presentation of a case mimicking Burkitt's lymphoma. *Am J Trop Med Hyg* 31:370–373, 1982.

Blitzer A, Lawson W, Meyers B R, Biller H F. Patients survival factors in paranasal sinus mucormycosis. *Laryngoscope* 90:635–648, 1980.

Boelaert J R, de Locht M, Van Cutsem J, Kerrels V, Cantinieaux B, Verdonek A, Van Landuyt H W, Schneider Y J. Mucormycosis during deferoxamine therapy is a siderophore-mediated infection: In vitro and in vivo animal study. *J Clin Invest* 91:1979–1986, 1993.

Boelaert J R, Van Cutsem J, de Locht M, Schneider Y J, Crichton R R. Deferoxamine augments growth and pathogenicity of *Rhizopus*, while hydroxypyridinone chelators have no effect. *Kidney Int* 45:667–671, 1994.

Bouchara J P, Oumeziane N A, Lissitzky J C, Larcher G, Tronchin G, Chabasse D. Attachment of spores of the human pathogenic fungus *Rhizopus oryzae* to extracellular matrix components. *Eur J Cell Biol* 70:76–83, 1996.

Bullock J D, Jampol L M, Fezza A J. Two cases of orbital phycomycosis with recovery. *Am J Ophthalmol* 78:811–815, 1974.

Cagatay A A, Oncu S S, Calangu S S, Yildirmak T T, Ozsut H H, Eraksoy H H. Rhinocerebral mucormycosis treated with 32 gram liposomal amphotericin B and incomplete surgery: a case report. *BMC Infect Dis* 1:22, 2001.

Cameroon H M. Entomophthoromycosis, In: E S Mahgoub ed. *Tropical Mycoses*. Beerse, Belgium: Janssen Research Council, 186–198, 1990.

Chandler F W, Watts J C. Zygomycosis. In: Chandler F W, Watts J C, eds. *Pathologic Diagnosis of Fungal Infections*. Chicago, IL: ASCP Press, 85–95, 1987.

Chinn R Y, Diamond R D. Generation of chemotactic factors by *Rhizopus oryzae* in the presence and absence of serum: relationship to hyphal damage mediated by human neutrophils and effects of hyperglycemia and ketoacidosis. *Infect Immun* 38:1123–1129, 1982.

Cohen-Abbo A, Bozeman P M, Patrick C C. *Cunninghamella* infections: review and report of two cases of *Cunninghamella* pneumonia in immunocompromised children. *Clin Infect Dis* 17:173–177, 1993.

Connor B A, Anderson R J, Smith J W. *Mucor* mediastinitis. *Chest* 75:524–526, 1979.

Costa A R, Porto E, Pegas J R, dos Reis V M, Pires M C, Lacaz Cda S, Rodrigues M C, Muller H, Cuce L C. Rhinofacial zygomycosis caused by *Conidiobolus coronatus*. A case report. *Mycopathologia* 115:1–8, 1991.

Couch L, Theilen F, Mader J T. Rhinocerebral mucormycosis with cerebral extension successfully treated with adjunctive hyperbaric oxygen therapy. *Arch Otolaryngol Head Neck Surg* 114:791–794, 1988.

de Locht M D, Boelaert J R, Schneider Y-J. Iron uptake from feroxamine and from ferrirhizoferrin by germinating spores of *Rhizopus microsporus*. *Biochemical Pharmacol* 47:1843–1850, 1994.

Del Poeta M, Schell W A, Perfect J R. In vitro antifungal activity of pneumocandin L-743,872 against a variety of clinically important molds. *Antimicrob Agents Chemother* 41:1835–1836, 1997.

Del Valle Z A, Rubio S A, Mellado E P, Morales A C, Cabrera P E. Mucormycosis of the sphenoid sinus in an otherwise healthy patient. Case report and literature review. *J Laryngol Otol* 110:471–473, 1996.

Diamond R D, Haudenschild C C, Erickson N F 3rd. Monocyte-mediated damage to *Rhizopus oryzae* hyphae in vitro. *Infect Immun* 38:292–297, 1982.

Diamond R D, Krzesicki R, Epstein B, Jao W. Damage to hyphal forms of fungi by human leukocytes in vitro. A possible host defense mechanism in aspergillosis and mucormycosis. *Am J Pathol* 91:313–328, 1978.

Dreschler C. Supplementary development stages of *Basidiobolus ranarum* and *Basidiobolus haptosporus*. *Mycologia* 48:655–677, 1956.

Dreschler C. Two new species of *Conidiobolus* found in the plant detritus. *Am J Bot* 47:368–377, 1960.

Drouhet E, Dupont B. Laboratory and clinical assessment of ketoconazole in deep-seated mycoses. *Am J Med* 74:30–47, 1983.

Dworzack D L, Pollock A S, Hodges G R, Barnes W G, Ajello L, Padhye A. Zygomycosis of the maxillary sinus and palate caused by *Basidiobolus haptosporus*. *Arch Intern Med* 138:1274–1276, 1978.

Ericsson M, Anniko M, Gustafsson H, Hjalt C A, Stenling R, Tarnvik A. A case of chronic progressive rhinocerebral mucormycosis treated with liposomal amphotericin B and surgery. *Clin Infect Dis* 16:585–586, 1993.

Espinel-Ingroff A. Comparison of In vitro activities of the new triazole SCH56592 and the echinocandins MK-0991 (L-743,872) and LY303366 against opportunistic filamentous and dimorphic fungi and yeasts. *J Clin Microbiol* 36:2950–2956, 1998.

Farley P C, Sullivan P A. The *Rhizopus oryzae* secreted aspartic proteinase gene family: an analysis of gene expression. *Microbiol* 144:2355–2366, 1998.

Fatterpekar G, Mukherji S, Arbealez A, Maheshwari S, Castillo M. Fungal diseases of the paranasal sinuses. *Semin Ultrasound CT MR* 20:391–401, 1999.

Foss N T, Rocha M R, Lima V T, Velludo M A, Roselino A M. Entomophthoramycosis: therapeutic success by using amphotericin B and terbinafine. *Dermatol* 193:258–260, 1996.

Gartenberg G, Bottone E J, Keusch G T, Weitzman I. Hospital-acquired mucormycosis (*Rhizopus rhizopodiformis*) of skin and subcutaneous tissue: epidemiology, mycology and treatment. *N Engl J Med* 299:1115–1118, 1978.

Gonis G, Starr M. Fatal rhinoorbital mucormycosis caused by *Saksenaea vasiformis* in an immunocompromised child. *Pediatr Infect Dis J* 16:714–716, 1997.

Goodman N L, Rinaldi M G. Agents of zygomycosis. In: Balows A, Hausler W J, Herrmann K L, Isenberg H D, Shadoomy H J, eds. *Manual of Clinical Microbiology*, 5th ed. Washington DC: ASM Press, 674–692, 1991.

Gugnani H C. Entomophthoromycosis due to *Conidiobolus*. *Eur J Epidemiol* 8:391–396, 1992.

Harada M, Manabe T, Yamashita K, Okamoto N. Pulmonary mucormycosis with fatal massive hemoptysis. *Acta Pathol Japan* 42:49–55 1992.

Hay R J, Campbell C K, Marshall W M, Rees B I, Pincott J. Disseminated zygomycosis (mucormycosis) caused by *Saksenaea vasiformis*. *J Infect* 7:162–165, 1983.

Helenglass G, Elliott J A, Lucie N P. An unusual presentation of opportunistic mucormycosis. *Br Med J* (Clin Res Ed) 282:108–109, 1981.

Howard D H. Acquisition, transport, and storage of iron by pathogenic fungi. *Clin Microbiol Rev* 12:394–404, 1999.

Kamalam A, Thambiah A S. Muscle invasion by *Basidiobolus haptosporus*. *Sabouraudia* 22:273–277, 1984.

Kamalam A, Thambiah A S. Cutaneous infection by *Syncephalastrum*. *Sabouraudia* 18:19–20, 1980.

Kemna M E, Neri R C, Ali R, Salkin I F. *Cokeromyces recurvatus*, a mucoraceous zygomycete rarely isolated in clinical laboratories. *J Clin Microbiol* 32:843–845, 1994.

Kontoyianis D P, Vartivarian S, Anaissie E J, Samonis G, Bodey G P, Rinaldi M. Infections due to *Cunninghamella bertholletiae* in patients with cancer: report of three cases and review. *Clin Infect Dis* 18:925–928, 1994.

Kwon-Chung K J, Bennett J E. Mucormycosis. In: *Medical Mycology*. Philadelphia: Lea & Febiger, 524–559, 1992.

Kwon-Chung K J, Young R C, Orlando M. Pulmonary mucormycosis caused by *Cunninghamella elegans* in a patient with chronic myelogenous leukemia. *Am J Clin Pathol* 64:544–548, 1975.

LeCompte P M, Meissner W A. Mucormycosis of the central nervous system associated with hemochromatosis. *Am J Pathol* 23:673–676, 1947.

Leong A S Y. Granulomatous mediastinitis due to *Rhizopus* species. *Am J Clin Pathol* 70:103–107, 1978.

Lowe J T Jr, Hudson W R. Rhincerebral phycomycosis and internal carotid artery thrombosis. *Arch Otolaryngol* 101:100–103, 1975.

Lueg E A, Ballagh R H, Forte V. Analysis of the recent cluster of invasive fungal sinusitis at the Toronto Hospital for Sick Children. *J Otolaryngol* 25:366–370, 1996.

Lye G R, Wood G, Nimmo G. Subcutaneous zygomycosis due to *Saksenaea vasiformis*: rapid isolate identification using a modified sporulation technique. *Pathol* 28:364–365, 1996.

Maliwan N, Reyes C V, Rippon J W. Osteomyelitis secondary to cutaneous mucormycosis. Report of a case and a review of the literature. *Am J Dermatopathol* 6:479–481, 1984.

Marchevsky A M, Bottone E J, Geller S A, Giger D K. The changing spectrum of disease, etiology, and diagnosis of mucormycosis. *Human Pathol* 11:457–464, 1980.

Martinson F D. Chronic phycomycosis of the upper respiratory tract. *Rhinophycomycosis entomophthorae*. *Am J Trop Med Hyg* 20:449–455, 1971.

Marx R S, Forsyth K R, Hentz S K. Mucorales species activation of a serum leukotactic factor. *Infect Immun* 38:1217–1222, 1982.

McAdams H P, Rosado de Christenson M, Strollo D C, Patz E F Jr. Pulmonary mucormycosis: radiologic findings in 32 cases. *Am J Roentgenol* 168:1541–1548, 1997.

McNulty J S. Rhinocerebral mucormycosis: predisposing factors. *Laryngoscope* 92:1140–1143, 1982.

Mead J H, Lupton G P, Dillavou C L, Odom R B. Cutaneous *Rhizopus* infection. Occurrence as a postoperative complication associated with an elasticized adhesive dressing. *JAMA* 242:272–274, 1979.

Mukhopadhyay D, Ghosh L M, Thammayya A, Sanyal M. Entomophthoromycosis caused by *Conidiobolus coronatus*: clinicomycological study of a case. *Auris Nasus Larynx*. 22:139–142, 1995.

Murray H W. Pulmonary mucormycosis with massive fatal hemoptysis. *Chest* 68:65–68, 1975.

O'Connell M A, Pluss J L, Schkade P, Henry A R, Goodman D L. *Rhizopus*-induced hypersensitivity pneumonitis in a tractor driver. *J Allergy Clin Immunol* 95:779–780, 1995.

Ogunlana E O. Fungal air spora at Ibadan, Nigeria. *Appl Microbiol* 29:458–63, 1975.

Okafor B C, Gugnani H C. Nasal entomophthoromycosis in Nigerian Igbos. *Trop Geograph Med* 35:53–57, 1983.

Okafor J I, Testrake D, Mushinsky H R, Yangco B G. A *Basidiobolus* sp. and its association with reptiles and amphibians in southern Florida. *Sabouraudia* 22:47–51, 1984.

Onuigbo W I, Gugnani H C, Okafor B C, Misch K A. Nasal entomophthorosis in an Igbo from Nigeria. *J Laryngol Otol* 89:657–661, 1975.

Pagano L, Ricci P, Nosari A, Tonso A, Buelli M, Montillo M, Cudillo L, Cenacchi A, Savignana C, Melillo L. Fatal haemoptysis in pulmonary filamentous mycosis: an underevaluated cause of death in patients with acute leukaemia in haematological complete remission. A retrospective study and review of the literature. Gimema Infection Program (Gruppo Italiano Malattie Ematologiche dell'Adulto). *Br J Haematol* 89:500–505, 1995.

Parfrey N A. Improved diagnosis and prognosis of mucormycosis. A clinicopathologic study of 33 cases. *Medicine* 65:113–123, 1986.

Pasha T M, Leighton J A, Smilack J D, Heppell J, Colby T V, Kaufman L. Basidiobolomycosis: an unusual fungal infection mimicking inflammatory bowel disease. *Gastroenterol* 112:250–254, 1997.

Patino J F, Castro D, Valencia A, Morales P. Necrotizing soft tissue lesions after a volcanic cataclysm. *World J Surg* 15:240–247, 1991.

Peterson K L, Wang M, Canalis R F, Abemayor E. Rhinocerebral mucormycosis: evolution of the disease and treatment options. *Laryngoscope* 107:855–862, 1997.

Pfaller M A, Messer S A, Hollis R J, Jones R N. Antifungal activities of posaconazole, ravuconazole, and voriconazole compared to those of itraconazole and amphotericin B against 239 clinical isolates of *Aspergillus* spp. and other filamentous fungi: report from SENTRY Antimicrobial Surveillance Program, 2000. *Antimicrob Agents Chemother* 46:1032–1037, 2002.

Pierce P F, Wood M B, Roberts G D Jr *et al. Saksenaea vasiformis* osteomyelitis. *J Clin Invest* 25:933–935, 1987.

Pillsbury H C, Fischer N D. Rhinocerebral mucormycosis. *Arch Otolaryngol* 103:600–604, 1977.

Pritchard R C, Muir D B, Archer K H, Beith J M. Subcutaneous zygomycosis due to *Saksenaea vasiformis* in an infant. *Med J Aust* 145:630–631, 1986.

Ravisse P, Destombes P, Le Gonidec G. 10 new clinical cases of mycoses caused by Entomophorales in Cameroon. *Bull Soc Pathol Exot Filiales* 69:33–40, 1976.

Restrepo A. Treatment of tropical mycoses. *J Am Acad Dermatol* 31:S91–102, 1994.

Ribes J A, Vanover-Sams C L, Baker D J. Zygomycetes in human disease. *Clin Microbiol Rev* 13:236–301, 2000.

Richardson M D, Shankland G S. *Rhizopus, Rhizomucor, Absidia,* and other agents of systemic and subcutaneous zygomycoses. In: Murray P R, Baron E J, Pfaller M A, Tenover F C, Yolken R H eds. *Manual of Clinical Microbiology,* 7th ed. Washington, DC: ASM Press, 1242–1258, 1999.

Rippon J W. *Medical Mycology,* 2nd ed. Philadelphia: W. B. Saunders Co., 303–314, 1982.

Robb S M. Reactions of fungi to exposure to 10 atmospheres pressure of oxygen. *J Gen Microbiol* 45:17–29, 1966.

Rothstein R D, Simon G L. Subacute pulmonary mucormycosis. *J Med Vet Mycol* 24:391–394, 1986.

Stearman R, Yuan D S, Yamaguchi-Iwai Y, Klausner R D, Dancis A. A permease-oxidase complex involved in high-affinity iron uptake in yeast. *Science* 271:1552–1557, 1996.

Straatsma B R, Zimmerman L E, Gass J D M. Phycomycosis: a clinicopathologic study of fifty-one cases. *Lab Invest* 11:963–985, 1962.

Sugar A M. Agents of mucormycosis and related species. In: Mandell G L, Bennett J E, Dolin R eds. *Principles and Practice of Infectious Diseases,* 5th ed. Philadelphia: Churchill Livingstone, 2685–2695, 2000.

Sun Q N, Fothergill A W, McCarthy D I, Rinaldi M G, Graybill J R. In vitro activities of posaconazole, itraconazole, voriconazole, amphotericin B, and fluconazole against 37 clinical isolates of zygomycetes. *Antimicrob Agents Chemother* 46:1581–1582, 2002a.

Sun Q N, Najvar L K, Bocanegra R, Loebenberg D, Graybill J R. In vivo activity of posaconazole against *Mucor* spp. in an immunosuppressed-mouse model. *Antimicrob Agents Chemother* 46:2310–2312, 2002b.

Tedder M, Spratt J A, Anstadt M P, Hegde S S, Tedder S D, Lowe J E. Pulmonary mucormycosis: results of medical and surgical therapy. *Ann Thorac Surg* 57:1044–1050, 1994.

Thakar A, Baruah P, Kumar S, Sharma M C. Rhinophycomycosis. *J Laryngol Otol* 115:493–496, 2001.

Torell J, Cooper B H, Helgeson N G. Disseminated *Saksenaea vasiformis* infection. *Am J Clin Pathol* 76:116–121, 1981.

Tuder R M. Myocardial infarct in disseminated mucormycosis: case report with special emphasis on the pathogenic mechanisms. *Mycopathologia* 89:81–88. 1985.

Ventura G J, Kantarjian H M, Anaissie E, Hopfer R L, Fainstein V. Pneumonia with *Cunninghamella* species in patients with hematologic malignancies. A case report and review of the literature. *Cancer* 58:1534–1536, 1986.

Verweij P E, Voss A, Donnelly J P, de Pauw B E, Meis J F. Wooden sticks as the source of a pseudoepidemic of infection with *Rhizopus microsporus* var. *rhizopodiformis* among immunocompromised patients. *J Clin Microbiol* 35:2422–2423, 1997.

Vesa J, Bielsa O, Arango O, Llado C, Gelabert A. Massive renal infarction due to mucormycosis in an AIDS patient. *Infection* 20:234–236, 1992.

Virmani R, Connor D H, McAllister H A. Cardiac mucormycosis. A report of five patients and review of 14 previously reported cases. *Am J Clin Pathol* 78:42–47, 1982.

Waldorf A R, Ruderman N, Diamond R D. Specific susceptibility to mucormycosis in murine diabetes and bronchoalveolar macrophage defense against *Rhizopus. J Clin Invest* 74:150–160, 1984.

Waldorf A R. Pulmonary defense mechanisms against opportunistic fungal pathogens. *Immunol Ser* 47:243–247, 1989.

Walsh T J, Renshaw G, Andrews J, Kwon-Chung J, Cunnion R C, Pass H I, Taubenberger J, Wilson W, Pizzo P A. Invasive zygomycosis due to *Conidiobolus incongruus. Clin Infect Dis* 19:423–430, 1994.

Watts W J. Bronchopleural fistula followed by massive fatal hemoptysis in a patient with pulmonary mucormycosis. A case report. *Arch Intern Med* 143:1029–1030, 1983.

Weng D E, Wilson W H, Little R, Walsh T J. Successful medical management of isolated renal zygomycosis: case report and review. *Clin Infect Dis* 26:601–605, 1998.

Wimander K, Belin L. Recognition of allergic alveolitis in the trimming department of a Swedish saw mill. *Eur J Respir Dis* Suppl 107:163–167, 1980.

Woods K F, Hanna B J. Brain stem mucormycosis in a narcotic addict with eventual recovery. *Am J Med* 80:126–128, 1986.

Yanagisawa E, Friedman S, Kundargi R S, Smith H W. Rhinocerebral phycomycosis. *Laryngoscope* 87:1319–1335, 1977.

Yangco B G, Okafor J I, TeStrake D. In vitro susceptibilities of human and wild-type isolates of *Basidiobolus* and *Conidiobolus* species. *Antimicrob Agents Chemother* 25:413–416, 1984.

16

Hyalohyphomycoses (other than aspergillosis and penicilliosis)

HARRYS A. TORRES AND DIMITRIOS P. KONTOYIANNIS

Hyalohyphomycoses refer to human infections caused by soil-dwelling and plant saprophytic moulds (Ajello, 1986). Hyalohyphomycosis encompasses a loose artificial classification system since it does not refer to a specific taxonomic classification (Rippon, 1988a). Agents of hyalohyphomycosis include nonmelanin-producing, nondematiaceous moulds (Anaissie et al, 1989) whose typical appearance in histopathologic sections consists of colorless, hyaline, or light-colored septate hyphae. These hyphae are either branched or unbranched, and occasionally they are toruloid (Ajello, 1986; Anaissie et al, 1989; Liu et al, 1998).

Table 16–1 lists the fungal species reported to cause hyalohyphomycosis. Important human pathogens included in this group are *Aspergillus*, *Fusarium*, *Scopulariopsis*, *Pseudallescheria*, and *Scedosporium* (Ajello, 1986; Anaissie et al, 1989). The fungi are identified at the genus and species levels largely on the basis of morphology of their reproductive structures, including phialides (fertile cells), and conidia (spores) (Liu et al, 1998). The general characteristics of the heterogeneous group of fungi-causing hyalohyphomycosis are shown in Table 16–2.

Although several nondematiaceous moulds can cause opportunistic fungal infections in humans, this chapter focuses only on those that have been recognized as emerging pathogens. More common causes of hyalohyphomycosis, such as aspergillosis and penicilliosis, are discussed in Chapters 14 and 23, respectively.

SPECIFIC AGENTS OF HYALOHYPHOMYCOSIS

Fusarium Species

Epidemiology. *Fusarium* derives its name from its fusiform conidia (Young et al, 1978). Long been known as plant pathogens, these ubiquitous moulds are common in decomposing organic matter and soil (Anaissie et al, 1988; Walsh and Groll, 1999). *Fusarium* species cause fusariosis, an increasingly recognized life-threatening mycotic infection worldwide (Boutati and Anaissie, 1997; Walsh and Groll, 1999; Marr et al, 2002). Of note, the epidemiological distribution of fusariosis is not homogeneous, since 50% to 85% of the cases have been reported in the United States (Martino et al, 1994; Girmenia et al, 2000). It is unclear whether this reflects a unique ecological niche for these fungi or is at least partially due to the increased recognition of this infection in the United States. Outside the United States, most cases of fusariosis have been reported in the Mediterranean (e.g., France, Italy) or in tropical countries (e.g., Brazil) (Guarro and Gene, 1995; Girmenia et al, 2000). Similarly, a heterogeneous distribution of cases of fusariosis have been described in different cancer centers, with most cases reported from only a few centers within the United States (Girmenia et al, 2000). In fact, *Fusarium* species have emerged in some tertiary care cancer centers as the second most common filamentous fungal pathogen after *Aspergillus* (Walsh and Groll, 1999). Indeed, in a recent small study from a Brazilian cancer center, *Fusarium* species were identified as the most common mould associated with true fungemia in bone marrow transplant (BMT) recipients (Trabasso et al, 2001).

The portals of entry for *Fusarium* infection include the aerodigestive tract and the skin (via vascular catheters, periungual regions, or burns) (Richardson et al, 1988; Merz et al, 1988; Anaissie et al, 1989; Martino et al, 1994; Walsh and Groll 1999). The predominant mode of infection is inhalation into the lungs or upper airways (Fridkin and Jarvis, 1996). Therefore, not surprisingly, most cases of fusariosis are considered community acquired. However, *Fusarium* species can also cause nosocomial infections, such as postoperative endophthalmitis or peritonitis associated with dialysis catheters (Young et al, 1984; Fridkin and Jarvis, 1996). The water distribution system has been implicated recently as a reservoir of *Fusarium* species (Squier et al, 2000; Anaissie et al, 2001). In contrast, others have reported that the most likely source of *Fusarium* infection is the external environment rather than a nosomial source (Raad et al, 2002). More research is needed in this controversial area.

The genus *Fusarium* currently contains over 20 species. Among these, the most common human pathogens are *F. solani* (50%), *F. oxysporum* (14%), *F. verticilloides*

TABLE 16–1. *Agents of Hyalohyphomycosis*

Acremonium spp*	*Lecythophora* spp.
Aphanoascus spp.	*Microascus* spp.
Aspergillus spp.	*Myriodontium* spp.
Arthrographis spp.	*Paecilomyces* spp.*
Beauveria spp.	*Penicillium* spp.
Chrysosporium spp.*	*Pseudallescheria* spp.*
Colletotrichum spp.	*Scedosporium* spp.*
Coprinus spp.	*Schizophyllum* spp.
Cylindrocarpon spp.	*Scopulariopsis* spp.*
Fusarium spp.*	*Scytalidium* spp.
Geotrichum spp.	*Tritirachium* spp.
Gibberella spp.	*Trichoderma* spp.*
Gymnascella spp.	*Volutella* spp.

*Emerging pathogens discussed in this chapter.

(11%), *F. moniliforme* (10%), *F. proliferatum* (5%), and much less commonly *F. dimerum*, *F. chlamidosporum*, *F. nygamai*, *F. napiforme*, *F. semitectum*, and *F. equiseti* (Rabodonirina et al, 1994; Girmenia et al, 2000; Bodey et al, 2002; Letscher-Bru, et al, 2002). This uneven distribution of *Fusarium* species might be related to the relatively higher virulence of some species, such as *F. solani*, as evidenced by a murine animal model of fusariosis (Mayayo et al, 1999).

Pathogenesis. *Fusarium* species have the remarkable ability of being effective broad-spectrum pathogens against prokaryotic bacteria (e.g., *Pseudomonas*), plants, and mammals. The pathogenesis of infection by *Fusarium* species is related to the mould's ability to produce mycotoxins or to cause direct invasive disease (Nelson et al, 1994). Of note, like Zygomycetes and *Aspergillus* species, *Fusarium* species are highly angiotropic and angioinvasive, causing hemorrhagic in-

TABLE 16–2. *General Characteristics of Agents of Hyalohyphomycosis*

Ubiquitous, soil saprophytes

Port of acquisition: lung, skin, foreign bodies

Normally community-acquired but is sporadically acquired nosocomially

Rare causes of infection

Predominately cause localized infections in immunocompetent hosts, following traumatic inoculation

Uncommon causes of allergic sinusitis or asthma

Uncommon but emerging cause of severe and frequently fatal focal respiratory or disseminated opportunistic infections in severely compromised hosts

Resemble *Aspergillus* species in tissue (potential for misidentification)

Some organisms (e.g., *Fusarium* species, *Acremonium* species) can grow in blood cultures

Most organisms exhibit broad-spectrum resistance to existing antifungal drugs

farction and tissue necrosis, especially in pancytopenic hosts (Anaissie et al, 1988; Walsh and Groll, 1999).

The mycotoxins produced by *Fusarium* species include trichothecenes, e.g., T-2 toxin, fumonisins, zearalenones, fusaric acid, and apicidin (Pontón et al, 2000; Etzel, 2002). The molecular events that control the production of such toxins are unknown. The ability of *Fusarium* species to produce these toxins has been associated with crop destruction (Walsh and Groll, 1999), and with human or animal mycotoxicoses such as alimentary toxic aleukia (Nelson et al, 1994; Groll and Walsh, 2001). Furthermore, the ingestion of grains contaminated with these mycotoxins may cause allergic symptoms or be carcinogenic after long-term consumption (e.g., human esophageal cancer) (Nelson et al, 1994; Pitt, 2000; Pontón et al, 2000). In addition, exposure to fumonisin may play a role in human birth defects (Etzel, 2002). Several mycotoxins induce leukopenia and marrow destruction, and suppress platelet aggregation (Nelson et al, 1994). Whether their production also contributes to prolonged chemotherapy-induced myelosuppression remains unclear (Anaissie et al, 1988; Rabodonirina et al, 1994). Similarly, there are no data on whether mycotoxins are expressed in strains causing invasive human fusariosis (Nelson et al, 1994, Pontón et al, 2000).

Granulocytes and macrophages play essential roles in the immune defense against fusariosis. Granulocytes inhibit hyphal growth, while macrophages inhibit germination of conidia and growth of hyphae (Nelson et al, 1994; Walsh and Groll, 1999). Neutropenia seems to be the critical factor in the development of invasive fusariosis, and corticosteroids add to the immune-impaired state predisposing to invasive fusariosis (Walsh and Groll, 1999; Pontón et al, 2000). However, other host factors beside quantitative granulocytes counts could influence the development of fusariosis in immunocompromised patients. For example, patients with refractory aplastic anemia show a low incidence of *Fusarium* infection (Girmenia et al, 1999, 2000; Girmenia et al, 2000; Torres et al, 2003). Fusariosis is also distinctly uncommon in patients with chronic granulomatous disease (Cohen et al, 1981). Furthermore, *Fusarium* infections in immunosuppressed organ transplant recipients receiving a prolonged course of corticosteroids tend to remain localized; these patients also have a better outcome than do allogeneic BMT recipients who have graft-vs.-host disease (GVHD) and receive corticosteroids (Patel and Paya, 1997; Sampathkumar and Paya, 2001).

Finally, *Fusarium* species can adhere to silastic catheters, and infections of central venous catheters (CVCs), continuous ambulatory peritoneal dialysis (CAPD) catheters, and contact lenses have been reported (Nelson et al, 1994).

TABLE 16–3. *Clinical Manifestations of Fusariosis According to Underlying Condition*

Underlying Condition	Clinical Manifestations
Acute leukemia or other hematologic malignancy	FUO, sino-pulmonary infection, CVC-related fungemia, disseminated infection
Bone marrow transplant	Disseminated infection, pneumonia, sinusitis, meningoencephalitis
Solid organ transplant	Cutaneous infection, lung abscess, disseminated infection
Solid tumors	Onychomycosis, localized soft-tissue infection, disseminated infection (rare)
Severe burns	Burn-wound colonization or wound infection, necrotizing local infection, disseminated infection
Miscellaneous conditions*	Onychomycosis, invasive intranasal infection, endophthalmitis, disseminated infection
Immunocompetent host†	Osteomyelitis, keratitis, endophthalmitis

*Diabetes, myasthenia.
†Following trauma or surgery.
FUO, fever of unknown origin; CVC, central venous catheter.

Clinical Manifestations. *Fusarium* species can cause localized or disseminated infections (Fridkin and Jarvis, 1996). The clinical features of fusariosis are nonspecific (Anaissie et al, 1989), and host factors play a crucial role in determining the severity and type of infection. *Fusarium* infections in normal hosts are localized infections that frequently do not require any systemic therapy (Musa et al, 2000). A variety of clinical manifestations of fusariosis in the context of different underlying conditions are described in Table 16–3.

Fusarium species (especially *F. solani*) are the most frequent cause of fungal keratitis in the United States (Nelson et al, 1994). Endophthalmitis by contiguous extension to the anterior eye chamber is a feared complication of severe *Fusarium* keratitis (Goldblum et al, 2000). In addition, *Fusarium* species cause localized infections of the nails and skin (Anaissie et al, 1989; Fridkin and Jarvis, 1996). In fact, *Fusarium* has become increasingly recognized as a cause of paronychia in profoundly neutropenic patients (Walsh and Groll, 1999), and *Fusarium* onychomycosis can lead to disseminated fusariosis in immunocompromised patients (Girmenia et al, 1992; Nelson et al, 1994; Musa et al, 2000). *Fusarium* species are also a well-known cause of eumycetoma (Kontoyiannis, 2003), and they can cause infection in burn wounds, colonization in burn wounds (Wheeler et al, 1981), granulomas, ulcers, and panniculitis (Nelson et al, 1994). Recently, a case of intractable cutaneous fusariosis with erythematous facial plaques and deep dermal infiltrates in the absence of immunosuppression has been described (Assaf et al, 2000).

Fusarium species cause four patterns of infection in profoundly immunocompromised patients; refractory fever of unknown origin, sinopulmonary infection, disseminated infection, and a variety of focal single organ infections. The usual initial presentation of invasive fusariosis is a persistent fever in a profoundly neutropenic patient (Groll and Walsh, 2001). Pulmonary involvement with both nodular and cavitary lesions can also be observed (Boutati and Anaissie, 1997). Sinopulmonary fusariosis is clinically indistinguishable from the more common invasive aspergillosis. Pneumonia or other focal invasive infection due to *Fusarium* species can disseminate in the setting of continuous, profound immunosuppression. Almost any organ can be involved, including the skin, lung, kidney, spleen, liver, brain, bone marrow, heart, pancreas, eye, nose, palate, sinuses, or gastrointestinal tract (Merz et al, 1988; Richardson et al, 1988; Minor et al, 1989; Anaissie et al, 1989; El-Ani, 1990; Nelson et al, 1994; Mohammedi et al, 1995). Since *Fusarium* species are often resistant to antifungal agents, breakthrough fusariosis occurring during empiric or prophylactic therapy with amphotericin B, fluconazole, itraconazole, or ketoconazole in neutropenic patients is not uncommon (Freidank, 1995; Boutati and Anaissie, 1997; Fang et al, 1997; Segal et al, 1998; Walsh and Groll, 1999; Mattiuzzi et al, 2001).

Disseminated fusariosis represents the extreme end of the spectrum of the infection caused by *Fusarium* species. The first reported case of disseminated *Fusarium* infection was almost 30 years ago (Cho et al, 1973). Since then, the incidence of disseminated invasive fusariosis has increased significantly (Anaissie et al, 1988; Nelson et al, 1994; Pontón et al, 2000; Marr et al, 2002). Neutropenic patients with hematologic malignancies (especially acute leukemia), allogeneic BMT recipients, and patients with extensive burns are at increased risk of disseminated fusariosis (Anaissie et al, 1989; Martino et al, 1994; Rabodonirina et al, 1994; Freidank, 1995; Fang et al, 1997). In particular, patients with hematological malignancies, account for > 90% of the reported cases of disseminated fusariosis (Pontón et al, 2000). Infection typically occurs during a prolonged period of neutropenia, lasting up to 65 days (Merz et al, 1988; Rabodonirina et al, 1994; Boutati and Anaissie, 1997; Musa et al, 2000); *F. solani* causes disseminated fusariosis in almost half of the cases, followed by *F. oxysporum* and *F. moniliforme* (Nelson et al, 1994; Martino et al, 1994; Boutati and Anaissie, 1997).

As mentioned previously, the clinical setting and manifestations of severe fusariosis in immunosuppressed patients mimic those seen in patients with aspergillosis (Anaissie et al, 1989). However, some distinct differences can be seen, such as an increased incidence of skin and subcutaneous lesions and a positive blood culture, mainly in the first days of fever, for patients with disseminated fusariosis (Martino et al, 1994; Fridkin and Jarvis, 1996). These blood cultures are positive in disseminated fusariosis in 50% to 70% of the cases in contrast to invasive aspergillosis (Freidank, 1995; Perfect and Schell, 1996; Walsh and Groll, 1999). Skin lesions, the hallmark of disseminated fusariosis, occur in 60% to 90% of cases, compared with a rare occurrence (< 10%) of such lesions in disseminated aspergillosis (Warnock, 1998; Nelson et al, 1994; Bodey et al, 2002). Patients with neutropenia have a higher rate of disseminated skin lesions compared with nonneutropenic immunocompromised patients (Nucci and Anaissie, 2002). Subcutaneous nodules, palpable and nonpalpable purpura, red or gray macules, red or gray papules, macules or papules with progressive central necrosis with central, flaccid pustules, vesicles and hemorrhagic bullae are types of lesions seen in patients with disseminated fusariosis (Nelson et al, 1994, Musa et al, 2000; Bodey et al, 2002) (See Color Figs. 16–1a, 16–1b in separate color insert). These skin lesions can involve any site, with predominance on the extremities (Bodey et al, 2002; Nucci and Anaissie, 2002). The lesions, especially the subcutaneous nodules are often tender (Bodey et al, 2002) and most patients have lesions at various stages of evolution (Boutati and Anaissie, 1997; Bodey et al, 2002). The number of disseminated skin lesions is variable and ranges between 4 and more than 30 according to a recent report from our institution (Bodey et al, 2002). Skin lesions are an important potential source of diagnostic tissue in some patients with fusariosis (Nucci and Anaissie, 2002).

Other presentations of invasive fusariosis in compromised hosts include osteomyelitis, septic arthritis, myositis, foot abscesses, sinusitis, endocarditis, myocarditis, external otitis, peritonitis, brain abscesses, cystitis, meningoencephalitis, and chronic hepatic infection (Jakle et al, 1983; Young et al, 1984; Nuovo et al, 1988; Anaissie et al, 1988; Minor et al, 1989; Agamanolis et al, 1991; Nelson et al, 1994; Mohammedi et al, 1995; Girardi et al, 1999; Walsh and Groll, 1999, Rolston, 2001).

Laboratory Diagnosis. The pathological diagnosis of fusariosis is not easy because fusariosis is histopathologically similar to infections caused by other invasive moulds, most importantly *Aspergillus* species (Anaissie et al, 1989). Biopsy of lesions may reveal extensive necrosis surrounding the fungal elements, consisting of dichotomously branching, acutely angular septate hyphae, which are not reliably distinguishable from those of other hyaline moulds, including *Aspergillus* (Martino et al, 1994; Walsh and Groll, 1999; Sampathkumar and Paya, 2001). Therefore, culture is an important tool in diagnosing *Fusarium* infection. Immunohistologic staining of tissues has also been used successfully for diagnosing selected cases (Anaissie et al, 1989).

Definitive diagnosis of fusariosis relies on the recovery of *Fusarium* species from infected tissues or blood cultures (Anaissie et al, 1989; Groll and Walsh, 2001). *Fusarium* species are more readily isolated from blood cultures than are *Aspergillus* species (Fridkin and Jarvis, 1996; Kovacicova et al, 2001). While *Fusarium* species are a well-recognized cause of true fungemia, *Aspergillus* species recovered from blood cultures typically reflect pseudofungemia (Kontoyiannis et al, 2000). One explanation for the frequent presence of *Fusarium* species in the blood is that they can produce many dispersive conidia, a characteristic of yeasts but not of most common pathogenic moulds (Freidank, 1995). *Fusarium* species can also be recovered from urine in the setting of disseminated fusariosis (Richardson et al, 1988).

Microscopically, *Fusarium* colonies begin as a white patch, which quickly develops a pink, purple, or yellow center with a lighter periphery. *Fusarium* species may produce three types of spores called macroconidia, microconidia, and chlamydospores (Nelson et al, 1994). The morphology of the macroconidia (canoeshaped) is key for characterizing the genus *Fusarium* (See Color Fig. 16–2a in separate color insert) (Nelson et al, 1994; Segal et al, 1998). Identifying Fusarium species in a culture is difficult if macroconidia are not present, so confusion with other genera, such as *Acremonium*, *Cylindrocarpon*, or *Verticillium*, may occur (Freidank, 1995; Segal et al, 1998; Walsh and Groll, 1999). In addition to the morphology of the macroconidia, the presence of microconidia, the morphology of the conidiophores bearing the microconidia, and the presence of chlamydospores are also important in *Fusarium* taxonomy (See Color Fig. 16–2b in separate color insert) (Nelson et al, 1994). Other macroscopic and microscopic features, such as color of the colony, length and shape of the macroconidia and number, shape, and arrangement of microconidia, are key features for differentiating the various *Fusarium* species. However, differentiating species is difficult, because of their propensity for rapid morphologic change (Anaissie et al, 1988; El-Ani, 1990; Nelson et al, 1994). A reference laboratory is the best resource for identifying *Fusarium* species.

To enhance diagnostic potential, molecular methods such as polymerase chain reaction (PCR)-based techniques can be used to complement conventional isolation techniques, such as blood cultures. With the use of universal primers, genus-specific probes, or probes based on single-stranded conformational polymorphism, PCR techniques may detect *Fusarium* species, even to the species level, earlier in blood and bronchoalveolar lavage, and may distinguish these species from other filamentous fungi (Walsh et al, 1995; Hennequin et al, 1999). Polymerase chain reaction-based assays have the potential for use as an adjunct to conventional methods for the early detection and the assessment of the natural history of this fungal infection. However, as with all PCR diagnostic methods for invasive fungal infections, further studies are needed to define the sensitivity and specificity of this PCR assay for detecting *Fusarium* species (Van Burik et al, 1998).

Susceptibility In Vitro and In Vivo. Interpreting minimum inhibitory concentrations (MICs) of moulds have long been problematic (Rex et al, 2001), and applying in vitro susceptibility to hyalohyphomycetes is no exception to the rule. The methodology for determining in vitro susceptibility to antifungals is not currently standardized, even though progress is being made in this area (Espinel-Ingroff et al, 1997). Furthermore, there are no established breakpoints of susceptibility or resistance of moulds to various classes of antifungals. Therefore, moulds, including agents of hyalohyphomycosis, should not be routinely tested for susceptibility (Rex et al, 2001).

Fusarium species are one of the most drug-resistant fungi (Sampathkumar and Paya, 2001), and among them, *F. solani* is considered the most resistant (Rabodonirina et al, 1994; Capilla et al, 2001). The molecular mechanism of such resistance has not been studied (Kontoyiannis and Lewis, 2002). As is the case for other moulds, susceptibility testing of *Fusarium* is problematic and not standardized (Speeleveld et al, 1996; Segal et al, 1998). Recently, a standardized broth microdilution MIC method for testing the susceptibility of filamentous fungi, including *Fusarium* species, to antifungals has been proposed (Espinel-Ingroff et al, 1997). However, in vitro susceptibility or resistance to antifungal agents may not predict the clinical outcome of *Fusarium* infection (Nelson et al, 1994; Mohammedi et al, 1995).

Fusarium isolates are resistant to the antifungal agents miconazole, ketoconazole, 5-fluorocytosine, fluconazole, itraconazole, and nikkomycin Z (Merz et al, 1988; Richardson et al, 1988; Anaissie et al, 1989; Speeleveld et al, 1996; Marco et al, 1998; Johnson et al, 1999; Li and Rinaldi, 1999; Arikan et al, 2001; Capilla et al, 2001). Some of the newer triazoles, such as voriconazole, ravuconazole and posaconazole (SCH 56592), show variable activity in vitro and in animal models (Johnson et al, 1998; Marco et al, 1998; Arikan et al, 1999; Pfaller et al, 2002) (Table 16–4). However, these triazoles have no in vitro significant fungicidal effects on *F. solani*, unlike amphotericin B (Johnson et al, 1998; Marco et al, 1998). Other recent reports have shown that triazoles exhibit species-dependent fungistatic activity against *Fusarium* species, especially the non-*solani* *Fusarium* species; voriconazole appears to be the most potent of the three drugs (Huczko et al, 2001; Espinel-Ingroff et al, 2001; Paphitou et al, 2002). If considering *Fusarium* species as a group, the activity of voriconazole is not superior to that of amphotericin B (Espinel-Ingroff et al, 2001). However, the observation that voriconazole is efficacious in the treatment of fusariosis in experimental mouse models shows the potential of this new triazole for treating this refractory invasive fungal infection (Reyes et al, 2001).

TABLE 16–4. In Vitro *and* In Vivo *Susceptibility of Clinically Important Hyalohyphomycetes*

	Activity of Antifungal Agents	
Hyalohyphomycetes	In vitro activity	In vivo activity
Fusarium species	AmB, natamycin, terbinafine, posaconazole, ravuconazole,* voriconazole, AmB + rifampin, AmB + azithromycin, AmB + caspofungin	AmB deoxycholate or its lipid formulations, natamycin,[†] voriconazole, posaconazole
S. apiospermum	Miconazole, echinocandins, posaconazole, UR-9825. Variable to fluconazole, itraconazole, AmB, voriconazole	AmB, itraconazole,[‡] fluconazole, voriconazole, posaconazole, miconazole
S. prolificans	Ravuconazole, posaconazole, UR-9825, itraconazole + terbinafine, AmB + pentamidine Variable to itraconazole, voriconazole	None yet shown
Acremonium species*	AmB, fluconazole, itraconazole, and voriconazole	AmB deoxycholate or its lipid formulations[‡]
Scopulariopsis species	Voriconazole[§]	AmB, itraconazole[‡], terbinafine, voriconazole
Paecilomyces species	AmB, itraconazole, voriconazole	AmB, itraconazole[‡]
Trichoderma species	AmB, itraconazole, ketoconazole and miconazole	Few data available

*Susceptibility of this genus could be species-dependent.
[†]Local application.
[‡]Isolated reports of activity.
[§]Lower MICs than those with amphotericin B or itraconazole.
AmB, amphotericin B

New investigational azoles such as CS-758 are also active in vitro against *Fusarium* species (Fothergill et al, 2001) and further studies are warranted to determine if this activity is also present in vivo. Finally, terbinafine, a squalene epoxidase inhibitor, shows some in vitro activity against some isolates of non-*solani* *Fusarium* species (Speeleveld et al, 1996; Pontón et al, 2000).

Amphotericin B and natamycin are the most active agents against *Fusarium* species in vitro and in vivo (Anaissie et al, 1988; Anaissie et al, 1989; Martino et al, 1994; Johnson et al, 1998). Liposomal amphotericin B at high doses (10 to 20 mg/kg/day) significantly reduces tissue burden in the liver and spleen of immunocompetent mice infected with *F. verticillioides* (Ortoneda et al, 2002a).

Fusarium species are resistant to the recently introduced glucan synthesis inhibitors, caspofungin, anidulafungin, and micafungin (Espinel-Ingroff, 1998; Pfaller et al, 1998; Tawara et al, 2000; Arikan et al, 2001). One possible explanation is that *Fusarium* species may possess less 1,3-β-D-glucans than 1,6-β-glucan or other non-1,3-β-D-glucans (Tawara et al, 2000). Of note, despite the lack of activity of caspofungin alone, the in vitro combination of caspofungin and amphotericin B appears to be either synergistic or additive against some *Fusarium* isolates (Arikan et al, 2002; Kontoyiannis, unpublished data).

In view of the innate resistance of *Fusarium* species to antifungals alone in vitro, other combinations have been tried. In vitro synergy has been shown between amphotericin B and rifampin, for example (Stern, 1978), although this combination has been unsuccessful for treating fusariosis in humans (Minor et al, 1989). Interestingly, an in vitro additive interaction has been demonstrated between amphotericin B and azithromycin for treating *Fusarium* species, although azithromycin has no activity when tested alone (MIC > 128 mg/L) (Clancy and Nguyen, 1998). However, clinical data are needed to support the use of azithromycin in combination with amphotericin B.

Antifungal Therapy. In view of the relative rarity of human infections caused by *Fusarium* species, the human experience has been derived from uncontrolled case series. Furthermore, these reports have been confounded by other factors critical for response such as the recovery of neutrophil count. Therefore, the management of fusariosis is not well defined (Segal et al, 1998). The treatment of disseminated fusariosis in heavily immunosuppressed patients, in particular, has been disappointing; reported mortality and morbidity rates exceed 75% (Martino et al, 1994; Boutati and Anaissie, 1997; Musa et al, 2000). Relapse after subsequent episodes of neutropenia has also been reported (Bou-

TABLE 16–5. *Principles of Therapy in Fusariosis*

Early aggressive treatment with high doses of lipid amphotericin B

Low threshold for switching to a new triazole (e.g., voriconazole) with demonstrated preclinical and clinical activity against *Fusarium* species

Rapid tapering of steroids, if possible

Consideration for G-CSF-primed granulocyte transfusions

Long duration of antifungal therapy, which should be individualized

Remove catheter for CVC-related fungemia

Debridement of devitalized tissue of localized disease (e.g., onychomycosis, sinusitis, abscess)

tati and Anaissie, 1997). Some principles of therapy are depicted in Table 16–5.

The most important factors predicting the outcome of *Fusarium* infection are the extent of the infection and the recovery of immunosuppression of the host (Anaissie et al, 1989; Nelson et al, 1994; Boutati and Anaissie, 1997). An ominous outcome is expected in patients with disseminated multiple-organ infection, even when high doses (1.5 mg/kg/day) of amphotericin B deoxycholate are given (Anaissie et al, 1988). One of the most important clinical aspects of severe *Fusarium* infection is the relative lack of responsiveness of this fungus to either amphotericin B deoxycholate or a lipid formulation of amphotericin B in the setting of profound immunosuppression (Anaissie et al, 1988; Anaissie et al, 1992; Martino et al, 1994; Costa et al, 2000; Kovacicova et al, 2001). For that reason, amphotericin B deoxycholate at a dose of 1.5 mg/kg/day plus flucytosine at a dose of 25 mg/kg every 6 hours (adjusted to achieve maximal serum levels of < 60 mcg/ml) is sometimes used (Merz et al, 1988). However, the addition of flucytosine has not been proven more effective than high-dose amphotericin B as monotherapy. Higher doses of amphotericin B deoxycholate (1.0–1.5 mg/kg) or high-dose lipid formulations of amphotericin B (at least 5 mg/kg/day) have been administered to transiently stabilize fusariosis (Walsh and Groll, 1999). Walsh and coworkers reported 11 patients with fusariosis, including some with disseminated disease, with an 82% response rate (complete or partial) to amphotericin B lipid complex (5 mg/kg/day). However, confounding factors including neutrophil recovery, immunosuppressive tapering, and adjunctive surgical therapy were not specifically addressed in these patients (Walsh et al, 1988).

Since the new antifungal triazoles, specifically voriconazole, or posaconazole show preclinical activity against *Fusarium* species, they provide some hope in the management of this severe infection (McGinnis et al, 1998; Lozano-Chiu et al, 1999). However, in two pediatric patients with fusariosis treated with voriconazole a poor outcome was observed (Walsh el at, 2002). More experience is needed in order to evaluate the role of this second generation triazole against human fusariosis. The preliminary experience in our institution indicates that the response rate to posaconazole in patients with fusariosis refractory to or intolerant of standard therapy approaches 50% (Hachem et al, 2000).

Like a history of aspergillosis, a history of invasive fusariosis should not be an absolute contraindication to subsequent BMT, provided that evidence shows a response of the infection to antifungal therapy. The most important factors associated with a favorable outcome in the setting of BMT are the resolution of myelosuppression and the absence of severe GVHD (Boutati and Anaissie, 1997).

Topical therapy with natamycin is the mainstay of treatment for keratitis or corneal ulcers caused by *Fusarium* species (Reuben et al, 1989; Hirose et al, 1997). However failures are not uncommon (Sponsel et al, 2002). Novel antifungals given either systemically or topical might be of benefit in selected cases. In one patient with *F. solani* keratitis that progressed to fungal endophthalmitis, despite combined use of systemic amphotericin B and ketoconazole plus topical natamycin and amphotericin B, was successfully treated with amphotericin B lipid complex (total, 8.79 g) (Goldblum et al, 2000). In addition, another case has been recently reported of a patient with amphotericin B and natamycin-resistant *Fusarium solani* keratitis and endophthalmitis, who responded to systemic and topical posaconazole (Sponsel et al, 2002). Vitrectomy with intravitreal and intravenous administration of amphotericin B and oral flucytosine has been used to treat *Fusarium* endophthalmitis with various results (Rowsey et al, 1979; Gabriele and Hutchins, 1996; Glasgow et al, 1996). Some patients with mycetoma due to Fusarium respond to itraconazole (Restrepo, 1994). Interestingly, the application of high concentration of nystatin powder (6,000,000 units/g) can effectively halt the progression of invasive *Fusarium* infection in severely burned pediatric patients (Barret et al, 1999).

Adjunctive Therapy. In addition to topical treatment with natamycin, keratoplasty with removal of the contaminated lens should be part of the therapeutic regimen for *Fusarium* keratitis (Nelson et al, 1994). A few small uncontrolled series have shown that patients with either peritonitis following CAPD or with CVC-related fungemia have a good outcome when the catheter is removed (Anaissie et al, 1988; Nelson et al, 1994). Early recognition of *Fusarium* infections followed by early aggressive therapy or CVC removal if an indwelling venous port is colonized prevents systemic dissemination of the infection from these entry ports (Musa et al, 2000).

In immunocompetent patients, *Fusarium* onychomycosis should be treated with removal of the infected keratin and topical or systemic antimycotic therapy (Nelson et al, 1994; Gupta et al, 2000). Nail avulsion followed by the application of ciclopirox ointment and bifonazole ointment or 8% ciclopirox nail lacquer has been reported to be effective (Gupta et al, 2000). In patients with hematological malignancies, *Fusarium* onychomycosis should be treated aggressively, including nail removal and systemic antifungal therapy. Overall, surgical resection of infected necrotic tissue, when possible, is an important component of therapy against fusariosis (Nelson et al, 1994).

Other potentially beneficial adjuvant therapeutic strategies include shortening the duration of neutropenia with recombinant granulocyte-colony stimulating growth factors (G-CSF) and granulocyte-macrophage colony stimulating growth factors (GM-CSF) and performing granulocyte transfusion from G-CSF- and GM-CSF-stimulated donors (Boutati and Anaissie, 1997; Walsh and Groll, 1999). The use of GM-CSF and G-CSF has been associated with earlier recovery of neutropenia and survival in patients with invasive fungal infection, including fusariosis (Musa et al, 2000; Farmaki and Roilides, 2001). In profoundly neutropenic patients with fusariosis, granulocyte transfusion results in a favorable response rate of 33% to 50% (Martino et al, 1994; Rodriguez-Adrian et al, 1998). However, the presence of confounding factors such as achieving remission from an underlying malignancy, recovering of neutrophil counts, and extent of disease (localized instead of disseminated fusariosis) might cause the effects of this procedure to be overestimated. We and others (Segal et al, 1998) agree that the independent contribution of granulocyte transfusions is uncertain at the moment. Other potential adjuvant therapies include interferon-γ and interleukin-15 that enhance hyphal damage by neutrophils against *F. solani* and *F. oxysporum*, suggesting a positive effect of these cytokines on the immune response against fusariosis (Winn et al, 2001; Roilides et al, 2001).

Scedosporium apiospermum (*Pseudallescheria boydii*)

Epidemiology and Pathogenesis. *Scedosporium apiospermum* can be isolated from a wide variety of natural substrates, including water, sewage, soil, swamps, water-logged pastures, coastal tidelands, and poultry and cattle manure (Anaissie et al, 1989; Tadros et al, 1998). *Scedosporium apiospermum* is distributed worldwide (Rippon, 1988b) and causes localized and disseminated infections. The portal of entry is the lung, paranasal sinuses, or the skin following traumatic inoculation (Francis and Walsh, 1992; Tadros et al, 1998). *Pseudallescheria boydii* is a teleomorph or perfect stage of *S.*

apiospermum (Groll and Walsh, 2001). It is unknown whether the different in vivo characteristics of *P. boydii* and *S. apiospermum* are associated with different pathogenic behavior in vivo (Groll and Walsh, 2001). In animal models, T-lymphocyte-dependent immune processes play no major role in resistance to *S. apiospermum* (Corbel and Eades, 1976).

Clinical Manifestations. Scedosporiosis (pseudallescheriasis) comprises a spectrum of clinical diseases caused by *P. boydii*, a well-known causative agent of mycetoma, probably the most common manifestation of scedosporiosis. In fact, *S. apiospermum* (*P. boydii*) is the leading cause of eumycetoma in North America and Western countries (Francis and Walsh, 1992; Tadros et al, 1998; Kontoyiannis, 2003). Other presentations of scedosporiosis include corneal ulcers, keratitis, chorioretinitis, endophthalmitis, otitis, sinusitis, pneumonia, endocarditis, meningitis, cerebritis, arthritis, osteomyelitis, and skin, lung, and thyroid abscesses in both immunosuppressed and normal hosts (Travis et al, 1985; Rippon, 1988b; Kiratli et al, 2001; Wu et al, 2002; Kleinschmidt-DeMasters, 2002). *S. apiospermum* can also cause pneumonia, brain abscesses, and disseminated disease in victims of near drowning (Tadros et al, 1998).

Of note, *Scedosporium* infections may mimic more common infections in immunologically intact hosts; for example a lymphocutaneous presentation may mimic sporotrichosis (Rippon, 1988b) or chronic lymphadenitis may resemble tuberculous lymphadenitis (Kiraz et al, 2001). Bone and joint infections following puncture wounds of the extremities while gardening have also been associated to scedosporiosis (Patterson et al, 1990). Likewise, *S. apiospermum* arthritis is most often associated with puncture wounds, lacerations, bicycle injuries, and occurrence following podiatric surgery (Rippon, 1988b). Further, *Scedosporium apiospermum* is a cause of fungal infection in intravenous drug abusers (Armin et al, 1987).

In profoundly immunosuppressed patients, rapidly progressive severe sinopulmonary, sinoorbital or disseminated infection has been reported (Rippon, 1988b; Francis and Walsh, 1992; Groll and Walsh, 2001). Pulmonary colonization is more common than pulmonary scedosporiosis, and maxillary sinuses are the most common site of *S. apiospermum* sinusitis (Travis et al, 1985; Rippon, 1988b). In compromised hosts, especially in neutropenic patients, hematogenous dissemination as a complication of *S. apiospermum* pneumonia can involve almost any organ (Tadros et al, 1998). Manifestations include thyroid, brain or renal abscesses, meningitis, osteomyelitis, endophthalmitis, tenosynovitis, and skin and subcutaneous disease (Rippon, 1988b; Tadros et al, 1998; Patterson, 1999; Nesky et al, 2000).

Laboratory Diagnosis. Because *Scedosporium apiospermum*, like other agents of hyalohyphomycoses, is histologically similar to *Aspergillus* species, scedosporiosis cannot be distinguished from invasive aspergillosis on the basis of histopathology alone (Anaissie et al, 1989). However, procedures for diagnosing scedosporiosis are similar to those for diagnosing invasive aspergillosis (Groll and Walsh, 2001). Diagnosis is confirmed if cultures of biopsy specimens demonstrate masses of septate hyphae with terminal oval brown conidia (Francis and Walsh, 1992). True fungemia has been reported in the setting of scedosporiosis, especially in patients with disseminated infection (Raj and Frost, 2002).

Besides culture methods, serologic procedures, specifically counterimmunoelectrophoresis or immunodiffusion assays, have been reported to be reliable for both diagnosing and prognostically evaluating the various forms of scedosporiosis (Rippon, 1988b; Jabado et al, 1998). However, these techniques are not specific enough to diagnose *S. apiospermum* infection because cross-reactions with *Aspergillus* and other pathogens, as well as false-negative and false-positive results, are possible (Cimon et al, 2000; Jabado et al, 1998). Finally, PCR-based assays seem useful in the rapid diagnosis of infections caused by *S. apiospermum*, even before fungal cultures become positive (Hagari et al, 2002). However, further studies are needed to define the sensitivity and specificity of this assay for detecting *S. apiospermum*.

Susceptibility In Vitro and In Vivo. Antifungals including ketoconazole, fluconazole, itraconazole, amphotericin B and voriconazole have variable activity against *S. apiospermum* (Jabado et al, 1998; Espinel-Ingroff et al, 2001) (Table 16–4). Importantly, amphotericin B does not have fungicidal activity against *S. apiospermum*, with minimum lethal concentrations 50 (MLC$_{50}$) values of ≤ 2 mg/l and MLC$_{90}$ values of ≤ 4 mg/l (Johnson et al, 1998). In addition, poor inhibitory activity of liposomal nystatin and nystatin against this pathogen has been reported recently (Meletiadis et al, 2002). Itraconazole has been reported to have activity in vitro (MIC, 0.25–0.7 μg/ml) (Jabado et al, 1998; Kiraz et al, 2001), as has miconazole (Rippon, 1988b), and posaconazole (Marco et al, 1998). Fluconazole has been shown to produce 50% survival in an animal model of disseminated pseudallescheriasis, when administered in high doses (20 mg/kg) (Gonzalez et al, 2001). Of note, voriconazole and the new triazole Syn-2869 are more active than itraconazole against *S. apiospermum* in vitro (Johnson et al, 1998; Johnson et al, 1999). However, this activity does not appear to be fungicidal (Groll and Walsh, 2001). In a recent report of in vitro activity of itraconazole, fluconazole, amphotericin B, and posaconazole against 30 clinical isolates of *S. apiospermum*, posaconazole was the most active drug (Gonzalez et al, 2001). In addition, the investigational triazole UR-9825 seems to be effective in vitro against *S. apiospermum* (Meletiadis et al, 2002). In in vivo murine models of *S. apiospermum* infection, posaconazole is effective only at high doses (> 25 mg/kg), with a dose-related response and an approximately 75% survival rate (Gonzalez et al, 2001). Finally, echinocandins have been shown to have in vitro activity against *S. apiospermum*, but their antifungal efficacy in vivo has not been demonstrated (Groll and Walsh, 2001).

Antifungal Therapy.   Disseminated infection caused by *S. apiospermum* has a poor outcome. The virulence and antifungal drug resistance of this organism as well as the occurrence of infection during neutropenia contribute to the poor outcome (Marr et al, 2002; Raj and Frost, 2002). Because amphotericin B lacks in vitro activity against most *Scedosporium* isolates and results in poor in vivo therapeutic responses, it has been hypothesized that prior use of amphotericin B, by eliminating other more susceptible fungi, predisposes patients to *Scedosporium* infections (Jabado et al, 1998). *Scedosporium apiospermum* is probably best treated with an azole such as parenteral miconazole or itraconazole (Warnock, 1998). In fact, scedosporiosis is an indication for systemic miconazole therapy (Francis and Walsh, 1992; Jabado et al, 1998). However, the intravenous formulation is no longer available in the United States because of its significant toxicity.

In the neutropenic patient, high-dose amphotericin B may still be the preferred initial approach, with a low threshold for a second-line therapy based on itraconazole, voriconazole, or one of the investigational broad-spectrum triazoles (Groll and Walsh, 2001). Successful responses to itraconazole or voriconazole have been reported (Jabado et al, 1998; Nesky et al, 2000; Munoz et al, 2000; Walsh et al, 2002). Recently, one patient with multiple brain abscesses caused by *S. apiospermum* that progressed despite neurosurgical drainage and treatment with itraconazole, amphotericin B, and ketoconazole, was successfully treated with posaconazole alone (Mellinghoff et al, 2002).

For less severely immunocompromised or normal hosts, the triazoles may represent a valid alternative to amphotericin B (Kiraz et al, 2001; Groll and Walsh, 2001). Reversing the underlying cause of immunosuppression and performing aggressive surgical intervention are essential to survival for patients with invasive scedosporiosis (Groll and Walsh, 2001). In addition, adjunctive modalities such as surgery or use of interferon-γ have been reported as useful in treating S. apiospermum infections (Jabado et al, 1998).

Finally, *S. apiospermum* keratitis should be treated aggressively. Early detection and treatment likely improve visual outcome. Topical miconazole should be an important part of the regimen, which may include other antifungals such as natamycin and amphotericin B (Wu et al, 2002).

Scedosporium Prolificans

Epidemiology and Pathogenesis.   *Scedosporium prolificans* (formerly *Scedosporium inflatum*) is classified as an imperfect fungus, with a different teleomorph (*Petriella* species) than *S. apiospermum* (*P. boydii*) (Tadros et al, 1998; Revankar et al, 2002). The natural habitat of this fungus is the soil, although is occasionally detected in the air of hospitals undergoing reconstruction (Pontón et al, 2000). Interestingly, *S. prolificans* is not distributed worldwide; most cases have been reported in Spain and Australia, and sporadically in the United States (Spielberger et al, 1995; Kleinschmidt-DeMasters, 2002). The cause of this limited geographical distribution is unknown (Pontón et al, 2000; Barbaric and Shaw, 2001). *S. prolificans* can cause colonization of the external ear or the respiratory tract, mainly in patients affected with cystic fibrosis (Lopez et al, 2001; del Palacio et al, 2001). In addition, *S. prolificans* is an increasingly recognized human pathogen in both immunocompromised and normal hosts (Perfect and Schell, 1996; Patel and Paya, 1997; Groll and Walsh, 2001). Inhalation is the most likely route of acquisition, although the portal of entry for this fungus is unknown (Pontón et al, 2000). *S. prolificans* can enter the bloodstream through an indwelling CVC (Groll and Walsh, 2001).

Clinical Manifestations.   Most previous reports of infection caused by *S. prolificans* are localized infections complicating soil-contaminated wounds in immunocompetent individuals (Pontón et al, 2000; Groll and Walsh, 2001). *S. prolificans* has also been infrequently reported to cause posttraumatic osteomyelitis, septic arthritis, keratitis, keratouveitis, endocarditis, endophthalmitis, brain abscesses, meningoencephalitis, cerebritis, pneumonia, and peritonitis (Rippon, 1988b; Berenguer et al, 1997; Tadros et al, 1998; Maertens et al, 2000; Kleinschmidt-DeMasters, 2002). This fungus has recently emerged as a cause of severe opportunistic infections, mainly in profoundly neutropenic patients (Berenguer et al, 1997; Pontón et al, 2000), in whom rapidly fatal pneumonia and disseminated disease can occur (Maertens et al, 2000; Groll and Walsh, 2001). The lungs, brain, and kidneys are the organs most frequently involved in disseminated infections caused by *S. prolificans* (Berenguer et al, 1997). These invasive infections generally mimic those produced by more common moulds (Pontón et al, 2000; Carreter de

Granda et al, 2001). For example, cutaneous lesions may develop during fungemia and disseminated *S. prolificans* infection, mimicking fusariosis (Cuetara et al, 2000; Lopez et al, 2001). Because *S. prolificans* is resistant to currently used antifungals, it is not an uncommon cause of breakthrough infection occurring despite prophylactic, empiric, or targeted therapy with amphotericin B (Kontoyiannis, unpublished data). Similar to infections caused by *Fusarium* species, disseminated *S. prolificans* infections are commonly diagnosed antemortem since this fungus is frequently detected in blood cultures (Maertens et al, 2000; Barbaric and Shaw, 2001; Groll and Walsh, 2001).

Laboratory Diagnosis.   Blood cultures are positive for *S. prolificans* at a relatively high rate (70% to 80% of cases), especially in patients with disseminated infection (Berenguer et al, 1997; Maertens et al, 2000; Carreter de Granda et al, 2001; Revankar et al, 2002). *S. prolificans* is characterized by its inflated flask-shaped conidiogenous cells (Salkin et al, 1988) and can be easily differentiated from *Scedosporium apiospermum* because the latter has cylindrical, free, or intercalary conidiogenous cells (Pontón et al, 2000).

Susceptibility In Vitro.   *Scedosporium prolificans* is typically resistant to the currently available antifungal agents. Fluconazole, amphotericin B, and the new triazole Syn-2869 are all inactive in vitro against this fungus (Johnson et al, 1999; Espinel-Ingroff et al, 2001; Table 16–4) as are echinocandins. High MICs between 4 μg/ml and 12 μg/ml have been described for the echinocandins caspofungin and anidulafungin (Del Poeta et al, 1997; Espinel-Ingroff, 1998). Liposomal nystatin and nystatin were found to have poor activities against the *S. prolificans* (Meletiadis et al, 2002). Itraconazole and voriconazole have variable activity against *S. prolificans* (McGinnis et al, 1998; Johnson et al, 1999; Pontón et al, 2000; Huczko et al, 2001; Espinel-Ingroff et al, 2001; Carrillo and Guarro, 2001), and other new broad-spectrum triazoles, such as ravuconazole, posaconazole, the investigational triazole UR-9825 also show activity against this multiresistant fungus (Pontón et al, 2000; Huczko et al, 2001; Carrillo and Guarro, 2001; Meletiadis et al, 2002). A synergistic in vitro activity has been demonstrated for amphotericin B and pentamidine in 85% to 100% of *S. prolificans* strains (Afeltra et al, 2002). Other in vitro combination studies have demonstrated synergistic activity of itraconazole and terbinafine against 85% to 95% of *S. prolificans* isolates (Meletiadis et al, 2000); the MICs obtained with this combination are within levels achievable in plasma following the usual daily doses of the aforementioned drugs (Meletiadis et al, 2000) (Table 16–4).

Antifungal Therapy.   Since *S. prolificans* is resistant in vitro to currently available antifungals (Perfect and Schell, 1996; Warnock, 1998; Groll and Walsh, 2001), resistance in vivo is not surprising (Rippon, 1988b; Walsh et al, 2002). The prognosis depends largely on the host's immune status, the extent of infection, and the feasibility of surgical removal (Berenguer et al, 1997). Recovery from neutropenia is considered critical in cases of *S. prolificans* infection because this infection has poor outcome (mortality rate approach 100%) in persistently immunosuppressed patients despite aggressive systemic antifungal therapy (Barbaric and Shaw, 2001; Revankar et al, 2002). Early detection, surgical removal of infected tissue (if possible), and immunorestoration appear to be the major means of halting progression of this devastating infection (Rippon, 1988b; Perfect and Schell, 1996). In vitro, interferon-γ and GM-CSF can enhance neutrophil superoxide production, increasing the damage of *S. prolificans* hyphae by neutrophils and enhancing the fungicidal activity of macrophages-monocytes, thereby showing a positive immunomodulatory effect against this hyalohyphomycete (Groll and Walsh, 2001; Gil-Lamaignere et al, 2001). Finally, interleukin-15 also enhances hyphal damage by neutrophils, suggesting a differential effect of this cytokine on antifungal neutrophil activity against *S. prolificans* (Roilides et al, 2001). In in vivo murine models of *S. prolificans* infection, combined administration of liposomal amphotericin B and G-CSF has been reported to be effective (Ortoneda et al, 2002b).

Acremonium Species

Epidemiology and Pathogenesis.   *Acremonium* species (formerly *Cephalosporium* species) are ubiquitous fungi common in soil, plant debris, and rotting mushrooms (Guarro et al, 1997). These hyalohyphomycetes are distributed worldwide, found in Europe, Asia, Egypt, and North and Central America (Fridkin et al, 1996; Guarro et al, 1997). *Acremonium* species are primarily pathogens of plants and insects and only rarely cause invasive disease in humans (Schell and Perfect, 1996; Perfect and Schell, 1996). *Acremonium strictum*, *Acremonium kiliense* and *Acremonium falciforme* are the most common human pathogens (Fridkin et al, 1996; Anadolu et al, 2001; Nedret Koc et al, 2002). The skin, lungs, and gastrointestinal tract are the apparent portals of entry (Walsh and Groll, 1999). Most infections are community acquired; however, nosocomial transmission occurs sporadically. For example, an outbreak of *Acremonium kiliense* endophthalmitis occurred in patients who had undergone cataract surgery; the reservoir was determined to be a contaminated humidifier within the heating, ventilation, and air-conditioning system of the ambulatory surgical center (Fridkin et al, 1996).

Clinical Manifestations. Following traumatic inoculation, *Acremonium* species causes infections ranging from posttraumatic mycotic keratitis to mycetoma in normal hosts (Groll and Walsh, 2001). Indolent *Acremonium* skin infection has been also reported in immunocompetent patients (Anadolu et al, 2001). In heavily immunocompromised patients, fungemia and severe disseminated infection can be seen (Roilides et al, 1995; Schell and Perfect, 1996; Perfect and Schell, 1996; Patel and Paya, 1997; Groll and Walsh, 2001; Nedret Koc et al, 2002). *Acremonium* species have also been reported to cause hypersensitivity pneumonitis, sinusitis, arthritis, hemodialysis access graft infection, endocarditis, and cerebritis (Wetli et al, 1984; Rippon, 1988a; Fincher et al, 1991; Guarro et al, 1997; Tosti et al, 2000). The ability of *Acremonium* species to colonize soft contact lenses with subsequent ocular infection has also been demonstrated (Guarro et al, 1997).

Relatively few cases of disseminated *Acremonium* infections have been encountered, most of them in severely immunocompromised hosts (organ-transplant recipients, patients with myeloma or leukemia, and patients receiving prolonged corticoid therapy) (Brown et al, 1992; Jeffrey et all, 1993; Schell and Perfect, 1996). Disseminated cutaneous lesions may develop during fungemia and disseminated infection (Walsh and Groll, 1999). The failure rate of antifungal therapy is high (50%) (Guarro et al, 1997).

Laboratory Diagnosis. When *Acremonium* species invade tissue, not only do they produce hyphae, like *Fusarium* species, but also form adventitious structures within the infected tissue. Specifically, *Acremonium* species have been reported to form phialides, phialoconidia, and, budding yeast-like cells in tissue (Schell and Perfect, 1996). These small conidia-like structures can disseminate widely through the bloodstream, permitting frequent premorten diagnosis based on the recovery of *Acremonium* species from blood cultures of patients with disseminated disease or fungemia (Brown et al, 1992; Perfect and Schell, 1996; Liu et al, 1998; Groll and Walsh, 2001; Nedret Koc et al, 2002). The presence of adventitious forms has also been reported in infections with species of *Fusarium*, *Paecilomyces*, *Scedosporium*, and *Blastoschizomyces* (Schell and Perfect, 1996).

Acremonium species usually grow on Sabouraud agar within 5 days at 30°C (Fridkin et al, 1996). When grown in culture, they produce small conidia on slender phialides, resembling the early growth of *Fusarium* species. Further incubation, however, does not reveal the characteristic canoe-shaped macroconidia observed in *Fusarium* species (Walsh and Groll, 1999; Groll and Walsh, 2001).

Susceptibility In Vitro. *Acremonium* species commonly lack susceptibility to current antifungal agents (Groll and Walsh, 2001). Using nonstandardized methods of susceptibility testing, some studies consistently found amphotericin B to be more active than ketoconazole, fluconazole, or itraconazole against *Acremonium* isolates (Fincher et al, 1991; Guarro et al, 1997). However, the susceptibility of this genus to amphotericin B, fluconazole, itraconazole, and voriconazole could be species-dependent. In support of this, the MICs of all these agents are much lower against *A. alabamensis* than against *A. strictum* (Espinel-Ingroff et al, 2001). Promising in vitro data have recently been presented for the new triazoles, posaconazole, ravuconazole, and voriconazole (Pfaller et al, 2002).

Antifungal Therapy. Optimal treatment of *Acremonium* infections is not well defined (Nedret Koc et al, 2002). Some infections due to *Acremonium* species are refractory to conventional dosages of amphotericin B (Groll and Walsh, 2001). Patients that are unresponsive to amphotericin B deoxycholate therapy are candidates for treatment with lipid-formulations of amphotericin B or may be candidates for voriconazole and the investigational antifungal triazoles (Walsh and Groll, 1999; Groll and Walsh, 2001). Despite the in vitro resistance of these fungi to azole treatment alone, the combination of surgery and azole derivatives has occasionally been successful (Guarro et al, 1997). Several patients with endophthalmitis have been successfully treated with vitrectomy, repeated intravitreous administration of amphotericin B (5 µg to 7.5 µg), and oral fluconazole (200–400 mg/day) (Fridkin et al, 1996; Weissgold et al, 1996). The outcome of severe infections caused by *Acremonium* infections depends largely on the recovery of neutrophil counts (Guarro et al, 1997), as do the outcome of *Fusarium* infections.

Scopulariopsis Species

The genus *Scopulariopsis* has several species. *S. brevicaulis*, *S. brumptii*, *S. asperula*, *S. carbonaria*, *S. koningii*, and *S. fusca* are the most common pathogens. *Scopulariopsis* spp. are also common soil saprobes with a wide geographical distribution (Anaissie et al, 1989; Filipello Marchisio and Fusconi, 2001) and rare association either with localized invasive infections following traumatic or surgical injury or with serious infections in immunocompromised patients (Groll and Walsh, 2001).

Clinical Manifestations. A variety of infections caused by *Scopulariopsis* species have been described; onychomycosis, mycetoma, keratitis, and, occasionally, localized invasive infections following traumatic inoculation (Groll and Walsh, 2001). More severe manifestations such as pneumonia, endocarditis, brain abscesses, disseminated infection, invasive nasal septum infection, and recurrent multiple subcutaneous or skin lesions have also been described in immunocompromised hosts (Wheat et al, 1984; Wang et al, 1986; Neglia et al, 1987; Hagensee et al, 1994; Migrino et al, 1995; Tosti et al, 1996; Jabor et al, 1998; Sellier et al, 2000; Kouyoumdjian et al, 2001).

Susceptibility In Vitro. Limited data exist regard the susceptibility of this uncommon pathogen to currently available systemic antifungals (Table 16–4). As is the case for other hyalohyphomycetes, *Scopulariopsis* species appear to have inherently broad-spectrum resistance to different classes of antifungals. The MICs for amphotericin B, itraconazole, and voriconazole against *Scopulariopsis brumptii* have been shown to be > 2 μg/ml (Espinel-Ingroff et al, 2001). Terbinafine has shown to have fungicidal activity against *S. brevicaulis* (Petranyi et al, 1987).

Antifungal Therapy. To date, only a few cases of infection from *Scopulariopsis* species have been reported; they have occurred in immunocompromised patients, and only the minority have responded to antifungal treatment (Patel et al, 1994; Sellier et al, 2000). On the basis of very limited in vitro susceptibility data, therapeutic approaches have been designed to include amphotericin B or investigational triazoles. Combined surgery and long-term therapy with amphotericin B, itraconazole, and terbinafine can result in a favorable outcome in some *Scopulariopsis* species infections, although success has not been reported for *S. brevicaulis* infections in immunocompromised patients (Kriesel et al, 1994; Sellier et al, 2000).

Paecilomyces Species

Paecilomyces species are common environmental hyaline moulds that are seldom associated with severe invasive infections in immunocompromised patients (Rippon, 1988a; Walsh and Groll, 1999; Lovell et al, 2002; Safdar, 2002). This saprophytic fungus is found worldwide in soil and decaying vegetable matter and as airborne contaminants in clinical microbiology laboratories (Gutierrez-Rodero et al, 1999). Most infections occurred in immunocompromised patients or those with foreign bodies in place (Clark, 1999). The ability of *Paecilomyces* spp. to infect prosthetic implants and cause post surgical infection is increasingly recognized (Gutierrez-Rodero et al, 1999). In addition, diagnosis of acute leukemia, treatment with myeloablative chemotherapy or bone marrow transplantation,

and presence of neutropenia have also been associated with *P. lilacinus* infection (Orth et al, 1996). Of all *Paecilomyces* species, only *P. lilacinus*, *P. variotti*, *P. marquandii*, and *P. javanicus* have been associated with human mycotic infections (Gutiérrez-Rodero et al, 1999). The apparent portals of entry for this organism are the respiratory tract, indwelling catheters, and the skin (Tan et al, 1992; Walsh and Groll, 1999; Groll and Walsh, 2001).

Clinical Manifestations. Sinusitis, subcutaneous infection, cellulitis, endocarditis, peritonitis, pyelonephritis, endophthalmitis, keratitis, and orbital granuloma, caused by *Paecilomyces* species have been described in both immunocompetent and immunocompromised patients (Allevato et al, 1984; Rippon, 1988a; Castro et al, 1990; Perfect and Schell, 1996; Gucalp et al, 1996; Saberhagen et al, 1997; Kovac et al, 1998; Gutierrez-Rodero et al, 1999). However, most infections involve the skin or ocular structures (Perfect and Schell, 1996). Skin lesions erupt insidiously and are pleomorphic. They appear as discrete erythematous papules and molluscum contagiosum-like lesions similar to those seen in *Penicillium* (Orth et al, 1996). Also, erythematous macules, vesicles, pustules, and refractory nodular lesions are among the different cutaneous manifestations of such infection (Safdar, 2002). The lesions could also be similar in appearance to the hemorrhagic necrotizing papulovesicular and ecthyma gangrenosum-like eruptions seen in *Fusarium* infections and in disseminated aspergillosis (Orth et al, 1996). In immunocompromised hosts, invasive *Paecilomyces* infections may also manifest as fungemia, soft-tissue infections, pneumonia, or disseminated infection (Walsh and Groll, 1999).

Laboratory Diagnosis. Similar to *Fusarium*, *Scedosporium* species and *Acremonium* species, *Paecilomyces* species are recovered in blood cultures from patients with disseminated disease (Shing et al, 1996). Of note, *Paecilomyces* species in culture may be confused with *Penicillium* species owing to the similarity in the conidial structures of the two genuses (Saberhagen et al, 1997).

Susceptibility In Vitro. *Paecilomyces* species, especially *P. lilacinus*, typically show high MIC$_{90}$ values for all antifungal agents tested. MIC$_{50}$ values indicate good overall susceptibility, even though amphotericin B, itraconazole, and voriconazole show variable activity against the fungus, and fluconazole, flucytosine and nikkomycin Z have poor efficacy (Orth et al, 1996; Li and Rinaldi, 1999; Groll and Walsh, 2001; Espinel-Ingroff et al, 2001; Gottlieb and Atkins, 2001; Pfaller et al, 2002). Of note, it is important to distinguish the species of *Paecilomyces* because their susceptibility patterns appear to be species-dependent (Shing et al, 1996). For example, *P. lilacinus* is highly resistant in vitro to amphotericin B, flucytosine, and fluconazole, while *P. varioti* is usually susceptible to amphotericin B, and flucytosine in vitro (Shing et al, 1996; Aguilar et al, 1998). Susceptibility testing of *P. lilacinus* indicated possible borderline susceptibility to ketoconazole and miconazole (Orth et al, 1996), while the in vitro susceptibility of *P. lilacinus* to the new generation of triazoles (e.g., posaconazole, and ravuconazole) appears to be good (Safdar, 2002). A new azole, CS-758, appears to be an active in vitro against *P. lilacinus* (Fothergill et al, 2001). However, as is the case for mould infections in general, a correlation of susceptibility results on *Paecilomyces* species with clinical outcome has not been established, and therapy must be adjusted to clinical response (Das et al, 2000; Groll and Walsh, 2001).

Antifungal Therapy. While the management of localized *Paecilomyces* infections relies on the surgical resection of infected foci where feasible, the optimal agent for treating systemic infections has not been identified (Groll and Walsh, 2001). Agents reported to be useful against *Paecilomyces* include miconazole, griseofulvin, amphotericin B, ketoconazole, itraconazole, and terbinafine (Gucalp et al, 1996; Clark, 1999; Gutierrez-Rodero et al, 1999; Gottlieb and Atkins, 2001). The in vitro and in vivo multiresistance of *P. lilacinus* to amphotericin B, fluconazole, and itraconazole appears to correlate with poor outcome in BMT recipients (Walsh and Groll, 1999). However, the results of clinical treatment with amphotericin B vary (Shing et al, 1996; Chan-Tack et al, 1999; Das et al, 2000). Of interest, there may be synergism between amphotericin B and flucytosine (Aguilar et al, 1998).

By comparison, less compromised patients have responded to amphotericin B followed by itraconazole (Walsh and Groll, 1999). In a conservative approach, high-dose amphotericin B deoxycholate should be the initial therapeutic intervention; the lipid formulations of amphotericin B or investigational triazoles are reserved for patients refractory to or intolerant of deoxycholate amphotericin B (Groll and Walsh, 2001). The role of itraconazole and voriconazole as well as the investigational triazoles (i.e., posaconazole and ravuconazole) in the primary treatment of invasive *Paecilomyces* infections is unclear, especially in the setting of persistent neutropenia or immunosuppression (Hilmarsdottir et al, 2000; Groll and Walsh, 2001).

Triazoles in combination with either amphotericin B or flucytosine may also be effective in treating *Paecilomyces* infections; however, this is speculative owing to insufficient data (Das et al, 2000). A nonneu-

tropenic patient with progressive cutaneous infection due to *P. lilacinus* treated successfully with combination caspofungin and itraconazole has been reported recently (Safdar, 2002).

Less Common Agents of Hyalohyphomycosis
Localized infection, severe invasive infection, and disseminated infection caused by *Chrysosporium* and *Trichoderma* species have recently been reported, mainly in the setting of profound immunosuppression (Stillwell et al, 1984; Levy et al, 1991; Warwick et al, 1991; Munoz et al, 1997; Roilides et al, 1999; Wagoner et al, 1999). Less common agents of hyalohyphomycosis, such as *Lecythophora mutabilis* (formerly *Phialophora mutabilis*), *Geotrichum candidum*, *Arthrographis kalrae*, *Colletotrichum gloeosporioides*, *Beauveria bassiana*, and *Myriodontium keratinophilum*, have been reported to cause infections in either immunocompetent or immunocompromised patients (Maran et al, 1985; Ahmad et al, 1985; Rippon, 1988a; Jacobs et al, 1992; Degavre et al, 1997; Guarro et al, 1998; Farina et al, 1999; Kisla et al, 2000; Chin-Hong et al, 2001; Yamamoto et al, 2001; Henke et al, 2002).

Clinical Manifestations. *Trichoderma* species have been reported to cause sinusitis, pneumonia, brain or hepatic abscess, soft tissue, and disseminated infection in immunocompromised patients (Guarro et al, 1999; Groll and Walsh, 2001; Chouaki et al, 2002). In addition, *Trichoderma* species are frequently responsible for continuous ambulatory peritoneal dialysis-associated fungal peritonitis (Loeppky et al, 1983; Chouaki et al, 2002). Most *Trichoderma* infections are due to *Trichoderma longibrachiatum* and, rarely, *Trichoderma citrinoviride* (Loeppky et al, 1983; Munoz et al, 1997; Furukawa et al, 1998; Guarro et al, 1999; Richter et al, 1999; Hennequin et al, 2000; Chouaki et al, 2002). *Chrysosporium* species have been reported to cause keratitis, osteomyelitis, and severe invasive infection, including dissemination, in the setting of immunosuppression (Stillwell et al, 1984; Levy et al, 1991; Warwick et al, 1991; Roilides et al, 1999; Wagoner et al, 1999).

Laboratory Diagnosis. *Trichoderma* species appear as hyaline moulds indistinguishable from other hyalohyphomycetes in tissue (Groll and Walsh, 2001).

Susceptibility In Vitro and In Vivo. Most isolates of *Trichoderma* species show resistance to fluconazole, 5-flucytosine and nikkomycin Z in vitro and are either susceptible or intermediately resistant to amphotericin B, itraconazole, ketoconazole, and miconazole (Munoz et al, 1997; Li and Rinaldi, 1999; Chouaki et al, 2002). On the other hand, amphotericin B, itraconazole, posaconazole, ravuconazole and voriconazole appear to have activity against *Geotrichum* species (Pfaller et al, 2002).

Antifungal Therapy. A reasonable first-choice therapy in the rare case of infection caused by *Trichoderma* species is amphotericin B, either alone or in combination with itraconazole or ketoconazole (Chouaki et al, 2002). The appropriate duration for treatment is unclear; treatment should be individualized to each case according to the type and extent of the infection and to the underlying predisposing conditions (Munoz et al, 1997). The role of surgical resection is also uncertain; however, surgery may be considered for patients who do not respond to initial medical therapy (Munoz et al, 1997).

REFERENCES

Afeltra J, Dannaoui E, Meis J F, Rodriguez-Tudela J L, Verweij P E. In vitro synergistic interactino between amphotericin B and pentamidine against *Scedosporium prolificans*. *Antimicrob Agents Chemother* 46: 3323–3326, 2002.

Agamanolis D P, Kalwinsky D K, Krill C E Jr, Dasu S, Halasa B, Galloway P G. Fusarium meningoencephalitis in a child with acute leukemia. *Neuropediatrics* 22:110–112, 1991.

Aguilar C, Pujol I, Sala J, Guarro J. Antifungal susceptibilities of *Paecilomyces* species. *Antimicrob Agents Chemother* 42:1601–1604, 1998.

Ahmad S, Johnson R J, Hillier S, Shelton W R, Rinaldi M G. Fungal peritonitis caused by *Lecythophora mutabilis*. *J Clin Microbiol* 22:182–186, 1985.

Ajello L. Hyalohyphomycosis and phaeohyphomycosis: two global disease entities of public health importance. *Eur J Epidemiol* 2:243–51, 1986.

Allevato P A, Ohorodnik J M, Mezger E, Eisses J F. *Paecilomyces javanicus* endocarditis of native and prosthetic aortic valve. *Am J Clin Pathol* 82:247–252, 1984.

Anadolu R, Hilmioglu S, Oskay T, Boyvat A, Perksari Y, Gurgey E. Indolent *Acrimonium strictum* infection in an immunocompetent patient. *Internat J Dermatol* 40:451–453, 2001.

Anaissie E, Kantarjian H, Ro J, Hopfer R, Rolston K, Fainstein V, Bodey G. The emerging role of *Fusarium* infections in patients with cancer. *Medicine* 67:77–83, 1988.

Anaissie E J, Bodey G P, Rinaldi M G. Emerging fungal pathogens. *Eur J Clin Microbiol Infect Dis* 8:323–330, 1989.

Anaissie E J, Hachem R, Legrand C, Legenne P, Nelson P, Bodey G P. Lack of activity of amphotericin B in systemic murine fusarial infection. *J Infect Dis* 165:1155–1157, 1992.

Anaissie E J, Kuchar R T, Rex J H, Francesconi A, Kasai M, Muller F M, Lozano-Chiu M, Summerbell R C, Dignani M C, Chanock S J, Walsh T J. Fusariosis associated with pathogenic *Fusarium* species colonization of a hospital water system: a new paradigm for the epidemiology of opportunistic mold infections. *Clin Infect Dis* 33:1871–1878, 2001.

Arikan S, Lozano-Chiu M, Paetznick V, Nangia S, Rex J H. Microdilution susceptibility testing of amphotericin B, itraconazole, and voriconazole against clinical isolates of *Aspergillus* and *Fusarium* species. *J Clin Microbiol* 37:3946–3951, 1999.

Arikan S, Lozano-Chiu M, Paetznick V, Rex J H. In vitro susceptibility testing methods for caspofungin against *Aspergillus* and *Fusarium* isolates. *Antimicrob Agents Chemother* 45:327–330, 2001.

Arikan S, Lozano-Chiu M, Paetznick V, Rex J H. In vitro synergy of caspofungin and amphotericin B against *Aspergillus* and *Fusarium* spp. *Antimicrob Agents Chemother* 46:245–247, 2002.

Armin A R, Reddy V B, Orfei E. Fungal endocarditis caused by *Pseudallescheria* (*Petriellidium*) *boydii* in an intravenous drug abuser. *Texas Heart Institute Journal* 4:321–324, 1987.

Assaf C, Goerdt S, Seibold M, Orfanos C. Clinical picture. Cutaneous hyalohyphomycosis. *Lancet* 356:1185, 2000.

Barbaric D, Shaw P J. *Scedosporium* infection in immunocompromised patients: successful use of liposomal amphotericin B and itraconazole. *Med Pediatr Oncol* 37:122–125, 2001.

Barret J P, Ramzy P I, Heggers J P, Villareal C, Herndon D N, Desai M H. Topical nystatin powder in severe burns: a new treatment for angioinvasive fungal infections refractory to other topical and systemic agents. *Burns* 25:505–508, 1999.

Berenguer J, Rodriguez-Tudela J L, Richard C, Alvarez M, Sanz M A, Gaztelurrutia L, Ayats J, Martinez-Suarez J V. Deep infections caused by *Scedosporium prolificans*. A report on 16 cases in Spain and a review of the literature. *Scedosporium Prolificans* Spanish Study Group. *Medicine* 76:256–65, 1997.

Bodey G P, Boktour M, Mays S, Duvic M, Kontoyiannis D, Hachem R, Raad I. Skin lesions associated with *Fusarium* infection. *J Am Acad Dermatol* 47: 659–666, 2002.

Boutati E I, Anaissie E J. *Fusarium*, a significant emerging pathogen in patients with hematologic malignancy: ten years' experience at a cancer center and implications for management. *Blood* 90: 999–1008, 1997.

Brown N M, Blundell E L, Chown S R, Warnock D W, Hill J A, Slade R R. Acremonium infection in a neutropenic patient. *J Infect* 25:73–76, 1992.

Capilla J, Ortoneda M, Pastor F J, Guarro J. In vitro antifungal activities of the new triazole UR-9825 against clinically important filamentous fungi. *Antimicrob Agents Chemother* 45:2635–2637, 2001.

Carreter de Granda M E, Richard C, Conde E, Iriondo A, Marco de Lucas F, Salesa R, Zubizarreta A. Endocarditis caused by *Scedosporium prolificans* after autologous peripheral blood stem cell transplantation. *Eur J Clin Microbiol Infect Dis* 20:215–217, 2001.

Carrillo AJ, Guarro J. In vitro activities of four novel triazoles against *Scedosporium* spp. *Antimicrob Agents Chemother* 45:2151–2153, 2001.

Castro L G, Salebian A, Sotto M N. Hyalohyphomycosis by *Paecilomyces lilacinus* in a renal transplant patient and a review of human *Paecilomyces* species infections. *J Med Vet Mycol* 28:15–26, 1990.

Chan-Tack K M, Thio C L, Miller N S, Karp C L, Ho C, Merz W G. *Paecilomyces lilacinus* fungemia in an adult bone marrow transplant recipient. *Med Mycol* 37:57–60, 1999.

Chin-Hong P V, Sutton D A, Roemer M, Jacobson M A, Aberg J A. Invasive fungal sinusitis and meningitis due to *Arthrographis kalrae* in a patient with AIDS. *J Clin Microbiol* 39:804–807, 2001.

Chouaki T, Lavarde V, Lachaud L, Raccurt C P, Hennequin C. Invasive infections due to *Trichoderma* species: report of 2 cases, findings of in vitro susceptibility testing, and review of the literature. *Clin Infect Dis* 35:1360–1367, 2002.

Cho C T, Vats T S, Lowman J T, Brandsberg J W, Tosh F E. *Fusarium solani* infection during treatment for acute leukemia. *J Pediatr* 83:1028–1031, 1973.

Cimon B, Carrere J, Vinatier J F, Chazalette J P, Chabasse D, Bouchara J P. Clinical significance of *Scedosporium apiospermum* in patients with cystic fibrosis. *Eur J Clin Microbiol Infect Dis* 19:53–56, 2000.

Clancy C J, Nguyen M H. The combination of amphotericin B and azithromycin as a potential new therapeutic approach to fusariosis. *J Antimicrob Chemother* 41:127–130, 1998.

Clark N M. *Paecilomyces lilacinus* infection in a heart transplant recipient and successful treatment with terbinafine. *Clin Infect Dis* 28:1169–1170, 1999.

Cohen M S, Isturiz R E, Malech H L, Root R K, Wilfert C M, Gutman L, Buckley R H. Fungal infection in chronic granulomatous disease. The importance of the phagocyte in defense against fungi. *Am J Med* 71:59–66, 1981.

Corbel M J, Eades S M. The relative susceptibility of New Zealand black and CBA mice to infection with opportunistic fungal pathogens. *Sabouraudia* 14:17–32, 1976.

Costa A R, Valente N Y, Criado P R, Pires M C, Vasconcellos C. Invasive hyalohyphomycosis due to *Fusarium solani* in a patient with acute lymphocytic leukemia. *Int J Dermatol* 39:717–718, 2000.

Cuetara MS, del Palacio A, Sanchez-Godoy P, Wihelmi I, Calvo MT, Espinel-Ingroff A. Erythematous nodule in a hematology patient. *Enferm Infecc Microbiol Clin* 18:287–288, 2000.

Das A, MacLaughlin E F, Ross L A, Monforte H L, Horn M V, Lam G L, Mason W H. *Paecilomyces variotii* in a pediatric patient with lung transplantation. *Pediatr Transplant* 4:328–332, 2000.

Degavre B, Joujoux J M, Dandurand M, Guillot B. First report of mycetoma caused by *Arthrographis kalrae*: successful treatment with itraconazole. *J Am Acad Dermatol* 37:318–320, 1997.

del Palacio A, Garau M, Amor E, Martinez-Alonso I, Calvo T, Carrillo-Munoz A, Guarro J. Case reports. Transient colonization with *Scedosporium prolificans*. Report of four cases in Madrid. *Mycoses* 44:321–325, 2001.

Del Poeta M, Schell W A, Perfect J R. In vitro antifungal activity of pneumocandin L-743,872 against a variety of clinically important molds. *Antimicrob Agents Chemother* 41:1835–1836, 1997.

El-Ani A S. Disseminated infection caused by *Fusarium solani* in a patient with aplastic anemia. *N Y State J Med* 90:609–610, 1990.

Espinel-Ingroff A, Bartlett M, Bowden R, Chin N X, Cooper C Jr, Fothergill A, McGinnis M R, Menezes P, Messer S A, Nelson P W, Odds F C, Pasarell L, Peter J, Pfaller M A, Rex J H, Rinaldi M G, Shankland G S, Walsh T J, Weitzman I. Multicenter evaluation of proposed standardized procedure for antifungal susceptibility testing of filamentous fungi. *J Clin Microbiol* 35:139–143, 1997.

Espinel-Ingroff A. Comparison of in vitro activities of the new triazole SCH56592 and the echinocandins MK-0991 (L-743,872) and LY303366 against opportunistic filamentous and dimorphic fungi and yeasts. *J Clin Microbiol* 36:2950–2956, 1998.

Espinel-Ingroff A, Boyle K, Sheehan D J. In vitro antifungal activities of voriconazole and reference agents as determined by NCCLS methods: review of the literature. *Mycopathologia* 150:101–115, 2001.

Etzel RA. Mycotoxins. *JAMA* 287:425–427, 2002.

Fang C T, Chang S C, Tang I L, Hsueh P R, Chang Y L, Hung C C, Chen Y C. *Fusarium solani* fungemia in a bone marrow transplant recipient. *J Formos Med Assoc* 96:129–133, 1997.

Farina C, Vailati F, Manisco A, Goglio A. Fungaemia survey: a 10-year experience in Bergamo, Italy. *Mycoses* 42:543–548, 1999.

Farmaki E, Roilides E. Immunotherapy in patients with systemic mycoses: a promising adjunct. *Bio Drugs* 15:207–214, 2001.

Filipello Marchisio V, Fusconi A. Morphological evidence for keratinolytic activity of *Scopulariopsis* spp. isolates from nail lesions and the air. *Med Mycol* 39:287–294, 2001.

Fincher R M, Fisher J F, Lovell R D, Newman C L, Espinel-Ingroff A, Shadomy H J. Infection due to the fungus *Acremonium* (*Cephalosporium*). *Medicine* 70:398–409, 1991.

Fothergill A W, Rinaldi M G, Schwocho L R, Ohya S. Comparison of the investigational azole CS-758 (R-120758) to amphotericin B, fluconazole, and itraconazole against 250 mould fungi. Abstracts of the 41st Interscience Conference on Antimicrobial Agents and Chemotherapy, Chicago. Abstract J-822, 2001.

Francis P, Walsh T J. Approaches to management of fungal infections in cancer patients. *Oncology* 6:133–144, 1992.

Freidank H. Hyalohyphomycoses due to Fusarium spp.—two case reports and review of the literature. *Mycoses* 38:69–74, 1995.

Fridkin S K, Jarvis W R. Epidemiology of nosocomial fungal infections. *Clin Microbiol Rev* 9:499–511, 1996.

Fridkin S K, Kremer F B, Bland L A, Padhye A, McNeil M M, Jarvis W R. *Acremonium kiliense* endophthalmitis that occurred after cataract extraction in an ambulatory surgical center and was traced to an environmental reservoir. *Clin Infect Dis* 22:222–227, 1996.

Furukawa H, Kusne S, Sutton DA, Manez R, Carrau R, Nichols L, Abu-Elmagd K, Skedros D, Todo S, Rinaldi M G. Acute invasive sinusitis due to *Trichoderma longibrachiatum* in a liver and small bowel transplant recipient. *Clin Infect Dis* 26:487–489, 1998.

Gabriele P. Hutchins R K. *Fusarium* endophthalmitis in an intravenous drug abuser. *Am J Ophthalmology.* 122:119–121, 1996.

Gil-Lamaignere C, Maloukou A, Winn R M, Panteliadis C, Roilides E, The Eurofung Network. Effects of interferon-gamma and granulocyte-macrophage colony-stimulating factor on human neutrophil-induced hyphal damage of *Scedosporium* spp. Abstracts of the 41st Interscience Conference on Antimicrobial Agents and Chemotherapy, Chicago. Abstract J-469, 2001.

Girardi M, Glusac E J, Imaeda S. Subcutaneous *Fusarium* foot abscess in a renal transplant patient. *Cutis* 63:267–270, 1999.

Girmenia C, Arcese W, Micozzi A, Martino P, Bianco P, Morace G. Onychomycosis as a possible origin of disseminated *Fusarium solani* infection in a patient with severe aplastic anemia. *Clin Infect Dis* 14:1167, 1992.

Girmenia C, Iori A P, Boecklin F, Torosantucci A, Chiani P, De Fabriitis P, Taglietti F, Cassone A, Martino P. *Fusarium* infections in patients with severe aplastic anemia: review and implications for management. *Haematologica* 84:114–118, 1999.

Girmenia C, Pagano L, Corvatta L, Mele L, del Favero A, Martino P. The epidemiology of fusariosis in patients with haematological diseases. GIMEMA Infection Programme. *Br J Haematol* 111:272–276, 2000.

Glasgow B J, Engstrom R E Jr, Holland G N, Kreiger A E, Wool M G. Bilateral endogenous *Fusarium* endophthalmitis associated with acquired immunodeficiency syndrome. *Arch Ophthalmol* 114:873–877, 1996.

Goldblum D, Frueh B E, Zimmerli S, Bohnke M. Treatment of postkeratitis *Fusarium* endophthalmitis with amphotericin B lipid complex. *Cornea* 19:853–856, 2000.

Gonzalez G M, Tijerina R, Najvar L K, Bocanegra R, Rinaldi M G, Loebenberg D, Graybill J. Therapeutic efficacy of posaconazole in a murine *Pseudallescheria boydii* infection. Abstracts of the 41st Interscience Conference on Antimicrobial Agents and Chemotherapy, Chicago. Abstract J-1615, 2001.

Gottlieb T, Atkins BL. Case report. Successful treatment of cutaneous *Paecilomyces lilacinus* infection with oral itraconazole in an immune competent host. *Mycoses* 44:513–515, 2001.

Groll A H, Walsh T J. Uncommon opportunistic fungi: new nosocomial threats. *Clin Microbiol Infect* 7(Suppl 2):8–24, 2001.

Guarro J, Gene J. Opportunistic fusarial infections in humans. *Eur J Clin Microbiol Infect Dis* 14:741–754, 1995.

Guarro J, Gams W, Pujol I, Gene J. *Acremonium* species: new emerging fungal opportunists—in vitro antifungal susceptibilities and review. *Clin Infect Dis* 25:1222–1229, 1997.

Guarro J, Svidzinski T E, Zaror L, Forjaz M H, Gene J, Fischman O. Subcutaneous hyalohyphomycosis caused by *Colletotrichum gloeosporioides*. *J Clin Microbiol* 36:3060–3065, 1998.

Guarro J, Antolin-Ayala M I, Gene J, Gutierrez-Calzada J, Nieves-

Diez C, Ortoneda M. Fatal case of *Trichoderma harzianum* infection in a renal transplant recipient. *J Clin Microbiol* 37: 3751–3755, 1999.

Gucalp R, Carlisle P, Gialanella P, Mitsudo S, McKitrick J, Dutcher J. *Paecilomyces* sinusitis in an immunocompromised adult patient: case report and review. *Clin Infect Dis* 23:391–393, 1996.

Gupta AK, Baran R, Summerbell RC. *Fusarium* infections of the skin. *Curr Opin Infect Dis* 13:121–128, 2000.

Gutierrez-Rodero F, Moragon M, Ortiz de la Tabla V, Mayol M J, Martin C. Cutaneous hyalohyphomycosis caused by *Paecilomyces lilacinus* in an immunocompetent host successfully treated with itraconazole: case report and review. *Eur J Clin Microbiol Infect Dis* 18:814–818, 1999.

Hachem R, Raad I I, Afif C, Negroni R, Graybill J, Hadley S, Kantarjian H, Adams S, Mukwaya G. An open, non-comparative multicenter study to evaluate efficacy and safety of posaconazole (SCH 56592) in the treatment of invasive fungal infections refractory to or intolerant of standard therapy. *Abstracts of the 40th Interscience Conference on Antimicrobial Agents and Chemotherapy*, Toronto. Abstract J-1109, 2000.

Hagari Y, Ishioka S, Ohyama F, Mihara M. Cutaneous infection showing sporotrichoid spread caused by *Pseudallescheria boydii* (*Scedosporium apiospermum*): successful detection of fungal DNA in formalin-fixed, paraffin-embedded sections by semi-nested PCR. *Arch Dermatol* 138:271–272, 2002.

Hagensee M E, Bauwens J E, Kjos B, Bowden R A. Brain abscess following marrow transplantation: experience at the Fred Hutchinson Cancer Research Center, 1984–1992. *Clin Infect Dis* 19:402–408, 1994.

Henke MO, De Hoog GS, Gross U, Zimmermann G, Kraemer D, Weig M. Human deep tissue infection with an entomopathogenic *Beauveria* species. *J Clin Microbiol* 40:2698–2702, 2002.

Hennequin C, Abachin E, Symoens F, Lavarde V, Reboux G, Nolard N, Berche P. Identification of *Fusarium* species involved in human infections by 28S rRNA gene sequencing. *J Clin Microbiol* 37:3586–3589, 1999.

Hennequin C, Chouaki T, Pichon J C, Strunski V, Raccurt C. Otitis externa due to *Trichoderma longibrachiatum*. *Eur J Clin Microbiol Infect Dis* 19:641–642, 2000.

Hilmarsdottir I, Thorsteinsson S B, Asmundsson P, Bodvarsson M, Arnadottir M. Cutaneous infection caused by *Paecilomyces lilacinus* in a renal transplant patient: treatment with voriconazole. *Scand J Infect Dis* 32:331–332, 2000.

Hirose H, Terasaki H, Awaya S, Yasuma T. Treatment of fungal corneal ulcers with amphotericin B ointment. *Am J Ophthalmol* 124:836–838, 1997.

Huczko E, Minassian B, Washo T, Bonner D, Fung-Tomc J. In vitro activity of ravuconazole against Zygomycetes, *Scedosporium* and *Fusarium* isolates. Abstracts of the 41st Interscience Conference on Antimicrobial Agents and Chemotherapy, Chicago. Abstract J-810, 2001.

Jabado N, Casanova J L, Haddad E, Dulieu F, Fournet J C, Dupont B, Fischer A, Hennequin C, Blanche S. Invasive pulmonary infection due to *Scedosporium apiospermum* in two children with chronic granulomatous disease. *Clin Infect Dis* 27:1437–1441, 1998.

Jabor M A, Greer D L, Amedee R G. Scopulariopsis: an invasive nasal infection. *Am J Rhinol* 12:367–371, 1998.

Jacobs F, Byl B, Bourgeois N, Coremans-Pelseneer J, Florquin S, Depre G, Van de Stadt J, Adler M, Gelin M, Thys J P. *Trichoderma viride* infection in a liver transplant recipient. *Mycoses* 35:301–303, 1992.

Jakle C, Leek JC, Olson DA, Robbins DL. Septic arthritis due to *Fusarium solani*. *J Rheumatol* 10:151–153, 1983.

Jeffrey W R, Hernandez J E, Zarraga A L, Oley G E, Kitchen L W. Disseminated infection due to *Acremonium* species in a patient with Addison's disease. *Clin Infect Dis* 16:170, 1993.

Johnson E M, Szekely A, Warnock D W. In-vitro activity of voriconazole, itraconazole and amphotericin B against filamentous fungi. *J Antimicrob Chemother* 42:741–5, 1998.

Johnson E M, Szekely A, Warnock D W. In vitro activity of Syn-2869, a novel triazole agent, against emerging and less common mold pathogens. *Antimicrob Agents Chemother* 43:1260–1263, 1999.

Kiratli H, Uzun O, Kiraz N, Eldem B. Scedosporium apiospermum chorioretinitis. *Acta Ophthalmol Scand* 79:540–542, 2001.

Kiraz N, Gulbas Z, Akgun Y, Uzun O. Lymphadenitis caused by *Scedosporium apiospermum* in an immunocompetent patient. *Clin Infect Dis* 32:E59–E61, 2001.

Kisla T A, Cu-Unjieng A, Sigler L, Sugar J. Medical management of *Beauveria bassiana* keratitis. *Cornea* 19:405–406, 2000.

Kleinschmidt-DeMasters BK. Central nervous system aspergillosis: a 20-year retrospective series. *Hum Pathol* 33:116–124, 2002.

Kontoyiannis D P, Sumoza D, Tarrand J, Bodey G P, Storey R, Raad I I. Significance of aspergillemia in patients with cancer: a 10-year study. *Clin Infect Dis* 31:188–189, 2000.

Kontoyiannis DP, Lewis RE. Antifungal drug resistance of pathogenic fungi. *Lancet* 359:1135–1144, 2002.

Kontoyiannis D P. Mycetoma. In: Goldman L, Bennett JC, eds. *Cecil Textbook of Medicine*, 22nd ed. Philadelphia: W. B. Saunders Company, in press, 2003.

Kovac D, Lindic J, Lejko-Zupanc T, Bren AF, Knap B, Lesnik M, Gucek A, Ferluga D. Treatment of severe *Paecilomyces varioti* peritonitis in a patient on continuous ambulatory peritoneal dialysis. *Nephrol Dial Transplant* 13:2943–2946, 1998.

Kovacicova G, Spanik S, Kunova A, Trupl J, Sabo A, Koren P, Sulcova M, Mateicka F, Novotny J, Pichnova E, Jurga L, Chmelik B, Obertik T, West D, Krcery V Jr. Prospective study of fungaemia in a single cancer institution over a 10-y period: aetiology, risk factors, consumption of antifungals and outcome in 140 patients. *Scand J Infect Dis* 33:367–374, 2001.

Kouyoumdjian G A, Forstot S L, Durairaj V D, Damiano R E. Infectious keratitis after laser refractive surgery. *Ophthalmology* 108:1266–1268, 2001.

Kriesel J D, Adderson E E, Gooch W M 3rd, Pavia A T. Invasive sinonasal disease due to *Scopulariopsis candida*: case report and review of scopulariopsosis. *Clin Infect Dis* 19:317–319, 1994.

Letscher-Bru V, Campos F, Waller J, Randriamahazaka R, Candolfi E, Herbrecht R. Successful outcome of treatment of a disseminated infection due to *Fusarium dimerum* in a leukemia patient. *J Clin Microbiol* 40:1100–1102, 2002.

Levy F E, Larson J T, George E, Maisel R H. Invasive *Chrysosporium* infection of the nose and paranasal sinuses in an immunocompromised host. *Otolaryngol Head Neck Surg* 104:384–388, 1991.

Li RK, Rinaldi MG. In vitro antifungal activity of nikkomycin Z in combination with fluconazole or itraconazole. *Antimicrob Agents Chemother* 43:1401–1405, 1999.

Liu K, Howell D N, Perfect J R, Schell W A. Morphologic criteria for the preliminary identification of *Fusarium*, *Paecilomyces*, and *Acremonium* species by histopathology. *Am J Clin Pathol* 109:45–54, 1998.

Loeppky C B, Sprouse R F, Carlson J V, Everett E D. *Trichoderma viride* peritonitis. *South Med J* 76:798–799, 1983.

Lopez L, Gaztelurrutia L, Cuenca-Estrella M, Monzon A, Barron J, Hernandez JL, Perez R. Infection and colonization by *Scedosporium prolificans*. *Enferm Infecc Microbiol Clin* 19:308–313, 2001.

Lovell RD, Moll M, Allen J, Cicci LG. Disseminated *Paecilomyces lilacinus* infection in a patient with AIDS. *AIDS Read* 12:212–213,218,221, 2002.

Lozano-Chiu M, Arikan S, Paetznick V L, Anaissie E J, Loebenberg D, Rex J H. Treatment of murine fusariosis with SCH 56592. *Antimicrob Agents Chemother* 43:589–591, 1999.

Maertens J, Lagrou K, Deweerdt H, Surmont I, Verhoef G E, Verhaegen J, Boogaerts M A. Disseminated infection by *Scedosporium prolificans*: an emerging fatality among haematology patients. Case report and review. *Ann Hematol* 79:340–344, 2000.

Maran A G, Kwong K, Milne L J, Lamb D. Frontal sinusitis caused by *Myriodontium keratinophilum*. *Br Med J* 290(6463):207, 1985.

Marco F, Pfaller M A, Messer S A, Jones R N. In vitro activity of a new triazole antifungal agent, SCH 56592, against clinical isolates of filamentous fungi. *Mycopathologia* 141:73–77, 1998.

Marr KA, Carter RA, Crippa F, Wald A, Corey L. Epidemiology and outcome of mould infections in hematopoietic stem cell transplant recipients. *Clin Infect Dis* 34:909–917, 2002.

Martino P, Gastaldi R, Raccah R, Girmenia C. Clinical patterns of *Fusarium* infections in immunocompromised patients. *J Infect* 28 Suppl 1:7–15, 1994.

Mattiuzzi G N, Estey E, Rex J H, Lim J, Pierce S, Faderl S, Giles F, Thomas D, Cortes J, Kantarjian H. Intravenous itraconazole for prophylaxis of invasive fungal infections in patients with acute myelogenous leukemia and myelodysplastic syndrome. Abstracts of the 41st Interscience Conference on Antimicrobial Agents and Chemotherapy, Chicago, IL. Abstract J-831, 2001.

Mayayo E, Pujol I, Guarro J. Experimental pathogenicity of four opportunist *Fusarium* species in a murine model. *J Med Microbiol* 48:363–366, 1999.

McGinnis M R, Pasarell L, Sutton D A, Fothergill A W, Cooper C R Jr, Rinaldi M G. In vitro activity of voriconazole against selected fungi. *Med Mycol* 36:239–242, 1998.

Meletiadis J, Mouton J W, Rodriguez-Tudela J L, Meis J F, Verweij P E. In vitro interaction of terbinafine with itraconazole against clinical isolates of *Scedosporium prolificans*. *Antimicrob Agents Chemother* 44:470–472, 2000.

Meletiadis J, Meis JF, Mouton JW, Rodriquez-Tudela JL, Donnelly JP, Verweij PE. In vitro activities of new and conventional antifungal agents against clinical *Scedosporium* isolates. *Antimicrob Agents Chemother* 46:62–68, 2002.

Mellinghoff IK, Winston DJ, Mukwaya G, Schiller GJ. Treatment of *Scedosporium apiospermum* brain abscesses with posaconazole. *Clin Infect Dis* 34:1648–1650, 2002.

Merz W G, Karp J E, Hoagland M, Jett-Goheen M, Junkins J M, Hood A F. Diagnosis and successful treatment of fusariosis in the compromised host. *J Infect Dis* 158:1046–1055, 1988.

Migrino R Q, Hall G S, Longworth D L. Deep tissue infections caused by *Scopulariopsis brevicaulis*: report of a case of prosthetic valve endocarditis and review. *Clin Infect Dis* 21:672–674, 1995.

Minor R L Jr, Pfaller M A, Gingrich R D, Burns L J. Disseminated *Fusarium* infections in patients following bone marrow transplantation. *Bone Marrow Transplant* 4:653–658, 1989.

Mohammedi I, Gachot B, Grossin M, Marche C, Wolff M, Vachon F. Overwhelming myocarditis due to *Fusarium oxysporum* following bone marrow transplantation. *Scand J Infect Dis* 27:643–644, 1995.

Munoz F M, Demmler G J, Travis W R, Ogden A K, Rossmann S N, Rinaldi M G. *Trichoderma longibrachiatum* infection in a pediatric patient with aplastic anemia. *J Clin Microbiol* 35:499–503, 1997.

Munoz P, Marin M, Tornero P, Rabadan P M, Rodriquez-Creixems M, Gouza E. Successful outcome of *Scedosporium apiospermum* disseminated infection treated with voriconazole in a patient receiving corticosteroid therapy. *Clin Infect Dis* 31:1501–1503, 2000.

Musa M O, Al Eisa A, Halim M, Sahovic E, Gyger M, Chaudhri N, Al Mohareb F, Seth P, Aslam M, Aljurf M. The spectrum of *Fusarium* infection in immunocompromised patients with haematological malignancies and in non-immunocompromised patients: a single institution experience over 10 years. *Br J Haematol* 108:544–548, 2000.

Nedret Koc A, Erdem F, Patiroglu T. Case Report. *Acremonium falciforme* fungemia in a patient with acute leukaemia. *Mycoses* 45:202–203, 2002.

Neglia J P, Hurd D D, Ferrieri P, Snover D C. Invasive scopulariopsis in the immunocompromised host. *Am J Med* 83:1163–1166, 1987.

Nelson P E, Dignani M C, Anaissie E J. Taxonomy, biology, and clinical aspects of *Fusarium* species. *Clin Microbiol Rev* 7:479–504, 1994.

Nesky M A, McDougal E C, Peacock J E. *Pseudoallescheria boydii* brain abscess successfully treated with voriconazole and surgical drainage: case report and literature review of central nervous system pseudoallescheriosis. *Clin Infect Dis* 31:673–677, 2000.

Nucci M, Anaissie E. Cutaneous infection by *Fusarium* species in healthy and immunocompromised hosts: implications for diagnosis and management. *Clin Infect Dis* 35:909–920, 2002.

Nuovo M A, Simmonds J E, Chacho M S, McKitrick J C. *Fusarium solani* osteomyelitis with probable nosocomial spread. *Am J Clin Pathol* 90:738–741, 1988.

Orth B, Frei R, Itin PH, Rinaldi MG, Speck B, Gratwohl A, Widmer AF. Outbreak of invasive mycoses caused by *Paecilomyces lilacinus* from a contaminated skin lotion. *Ann Intern Med* 125:799–806, 1996.

Ortoneda M, Capilla J, Pastor FJ, Pujol I, Guarro J. Efficacy of liposomal amphotericin B in treatment of systemic murine fusariosis. *Antimicrob Agents Chemother* 46:2273–2275, 2002a.

Ortoneda M, Capilla J, Pujol I, Pastor FJ, Mayayo E, Fernandez-Ballart J, Guarro J. Liposomal amphotericin B and granulocyte colony-stimulating factor therapy in a murine model of invasive infection by *Scedosporium prolificans*. *J Antimicrob Chemother* 49:525–529, 2002b.

Paphitou N I, Ostrosky-Zeichner L, Paetznick V L, Rodriguez J R, Chen E, Rex J H. In vitro activities of investigational triazoles against *Fusarium* species: effects of inoculum size and incubation time on broth microdilution susceptibility test results. *Antimicrob Agents Chemother* 46:3298–3300, 2002.

Patel R, Gustaferro CA, Krom RA, Wiesner RH, Roberts GD, Paya CV. Phaeohyphomycosis due to *Scopulariopsis brumptii* in a liver transplant recipient. *Clin Infect Dis* 19:198–200, 1994.

Patel R, Paya C V. Infections in solid-organ transplant recipients. *Clin Microbiol Rev* 10:86–124, 1997.

Patterson T F, Andriole V T, Zervos M J, Therasse D, Kauffman C A. The epidemiology of pseudallescheriasis complicating transplantation: nosocomial and community-acquired infection. *Mycoses* 33:297–302, 1990.

Patterson J E. Epidemiology of fungal infections in solid organ transplant patients. *Transpl Infect Dis* 1:229–236, 1999.

Perfect JR, Schell WA. The new fungal opportunists are coming. *Clin Infect Dis* 22 Suppl 2:S112–S118, 1996.

Petranyi G, Meingassner JG, Mieth H. Activity of terbinafine in experimental fungal infections of laboratory animals. *Antimicrob Agents Chemother* 31:1558–1561, 1987.

Pfaller M A, Marco F, Messer S A, Jones R N. In vitro activity of two echinocandin derivatives, LY303366 and MK-0991 (L-743,792), against clinical isolates of Aspergillus, Fusarium, Rhizopus, and other filamentous fungi. *Diagn Microbiol Infect Dis* 30:251–255, 1998.

Pfaller M A, Messer S A, Hollis R J, Jones R N, and the SENTRY Participants Group. Antifungal activities of posaconazole, ravuconazole, and voriconazole compared to those of itraconazole and amphotericin B tested against 239 clinical isolates of Aspergillus spp. and other filamentous fungi: report from the SENTRY antimicrobial surveillance program, 2000. *Antimicrob Agents Chemother* 46:1032–1037, 2002.

Pitt JI. Toxigenic fungi: which are important? *Med Mycol* 38 Suppl 1:17–22, 2000.

Pontón J, Ruchel R, Clemons K V, Coleman D C, Grillot R, Guarro J, Aldebert D, Ambroise-Thomas P, Cano J, Carrillo-Munoz A J, Gene J, Pinel C, Stevens D A, Sullivan D J. Emerging pathogens. Med Mycol 38 Suppl 1:225–236, 2000.

Raad I, Tarrand J, Hanna H, Albitar M, Janssen E, Boktour M, Bodey G, Mardani M, Hachem R, Kontoyiannis D, Whimbey E, Rolston K. Epidemiology, molecular mycology, and environmental sources of Fusarium infection in patients with cancer. Infect Control Hosp Epidemiol 22:532–537, 2002.

Rabodonirina M, Piens M A, Monier M F, Gueho E, Fiere D, Mojon M. Fusarium infections in immunocompromised patients: case reports and literature review. Eur J Clin Microbiol Infect Dis 13:152–161, 1994.

Raj R, Frost AE. Scedosporium apiospermum fungemia in a lung transplant recipient. Chest 121:1714–1716, 2002.

Restrepo A. Treatment of tropical mycoses. J Am Acad Dermatol 1994 31:S91–102, 1994.

Reuben A, Anaissie E, Nelson P E, Hashem R, Legrand C, Ho D H, Bodey G P. Antifungal susceptibility of 44 clinical isolates of Fusarium species determined by using a broth microdilution method. Antimicrob Agents Chemother 33:1647–169, 1989.

Revankar SG, Patterson JE, Sutton DA, Pullen R, Rinaldi MG. Disseminated phaeohyphomycosis: review of an emerging mycosis. Clin Infect Dis 34:467–476, 2002.

Rex J H, Pfaller M A, Walsh T J, Chaturvedi V, Espinel-Ingroff A, Ghannoum M A, Gosey L L, Odds F C, Rinaldi M G, Sheehan D J, Warnock D W. Antifungal susceptibility testing: practical aspects and current challenges. Clin Microbiol Rev 14:643–658, 2001.

Reyes G H, Long L, Hossain M, Ghannoum M A. Evaluation of voriconazole efficacy in the treatment of murine fusariosis. Abstracts of the 41st Interscience Conference on Antimicrobial Agents and Chemotherapy, Chicago. Abstract J-1604, 2001.

Richardson S E, Bannatyne R M, Summerbell R C, Milliken J, Gold R, Weitzman S S. Disseminated fusarial infection in the immunocompromised host. Rev Infect Dis 10:1171–1181, 1988.

Richter S, Cormican M G, Pfaller M A, Lee C K, Gingrich R, Rinaldi M G, Sutton D A. Fatal disseminated Trichoderma longibrachiatum infection in an adult bone marrow transplant patient: species identification and review of the literature. J Clin Microbiol 37:1154–1160, 1999.

Rippon J W. Hyalohyphomycosis, pythiosis, miscellaneous and rare mycoses, and algoses. In: Rippon JW, ed. Medical Mycology, 3rd ed. Philadelphia: W. B. Saunders Company, 714–745, 1988a.

Rippon J W. Pseudallescheriasis. In: Rippon JW, ed. Medical Mycology, 3rd ed. Philadelphia: W. B. Saunders Company, 651–680, 1988b.

Rodriguez-Adrian L J, Grazziutti M L, Rex J H, Anaissie E J. The potential role of cytokine therapy for fungal infections in patients with cancer: is recovery from neutropenia all that is needed? Clin Infect Dis 26:1270–1278, 1998.

Roilides E, Bibashi E, Acritidou E, Trahana M, Gompakis N, Karpouzas J G, Koliouskas D. Acremonium fungemia in two immunocompromised children. Pediatr Infect Dis J 14:548–550, 1995.

Roilides E, Sigler L, Bibashi E, Katsifa H, Flaris N, Panteliadis C. Disseminated infection due to Chrysosporium zonatum in a patient with chronic granulomatous disease and review of non-Aspergillus fungal infections in patients with this disease. J Clin Microbiol 37:18–25, 1999.

Roilides E, Maloukou A, Gil-Lamaignere C, Winn R M, Panteliadis C, Walsh T J. Differential effects of interleukin 15 on hyphal damage of filamentous fungi induced by human neutrophils. Abstracts of the 41st Interscience Conference on Antimicrobial Agents and Chemotherapy, Chicago. Abstract J-468, 2001.

Rolston K V I. The spectrum of pulmonary infections in cancer patients. Curr Opin Oncol 13:218–223, 2001.

Rowsey J J, Acers T E, Smith D L, Mohr J A, Newsom D L, Rodriguez J. Fusarium oxysporum endophthalmitis. Arch Ophthalmol 97:103–5, 1979.

Saberhagen C, Klotz S A, Bartholomew W, Drews D, Dixon A. Infection due to Paecilomyces lilacinus: a challenging clinical identification. Clin Infect Dis 25: 1411–1413, 1997.

Safdar A. Progressive cutaneous hyalohyphomycosis due to Paecilomyces lilacinus: rapid response to treatment with caspofungin and itraconazole. Clin Infect Dis 34:1415–1417, 2002.

Salkin I F, McGinnis M R, Dykstra M J, Rinaldi M G. Scedosporium inflatum, an emerging pathogen. J Clin Microbiol 26:498–503, 1988.

Sampathkumar P, Paya C V. Fusarium infection after solid-organ transplantation. Clin Infect Dis 32:1237–1240, 2001.

Schell W A, Perfect J R. Fatal, disseminated Acremonium strictum infection in a neutropenic host. J Clin Microbiol 34:1333–1336, 1996.

Segal B H, Walsh T J, Liu J M, Wilson J D, Kwon-Chung K J. Invasive infection with Fusarium chlamydosporum in a patient with aplastic anemia. J Clin Microbiol 36:1772–1776, 1998.

Sellier P, Monsuez J J, Lacroix C, Feray C, Evans J, Minozzi C, Vayre F, Del Giudice P, Feuilhade M, Pinel C, Vittecoq D, Passeron J. Recurrent subcutaneous infection due to Scopulariopsis brevicaulis in a liver transplant recipient. Clin Infect Dis 30:820–823, 2000.

Shing M M, Ip M, Li C K, Chik K W, Yuen P M. Paecilomyces varioti fungemia in a bone marrow transplant patient. Bone Marrow Transplan 17:281–283, 1996.

Speeleveld E, Gordts B, Van Landuyt H W, De Vroey C, Raes-Wuytack C. Susceptibility of clinical isolates of Fusarium to antifungal drugs. Mycoses 39:37–40, 1996.

Spielberger R T, Tegtmeier B R, O'Donnell M R, Ito J I. Fatal Scedosporium prolificans (S. inflatum) fungemia following allogeneic bone marrow transplantation: report of a case in the United States. Clin Infect Dis 21:1067, 1995.

Sponsel WE, Graybill JR, Nevarez HL, Dang D. Ocular and systemic posaconazole(SCH-56592) treatment of invasive Fusarium solani keratitis and endophthalmitis. Br J Ophthalmol 86:829–830, 2002.

Squier C, Yu V L, Stout J E. Waterborne nosocomial infections. Curr Infect Dis Rep 2:490–496, 2000.

Stern G A. In vitro antibiotic synergism against ocular fungal isolates. Am J Ophthalmol 86:359–367, 1978.

Stillwell W T, Rubin B D, Axelrod J L. Chrysosporium, a new causative agent in osteomyelitis. A case report. Clin Orthop 184: 190–192, 1984.

Tadros T S, Workowski K A, Siegel R J, Hunter S, Schwartz D A. Pathology of hyalohyphomycosis caused by Scedosporium apiospermum (Pseudallescheria boydii): an emerging mycosis. Hum Pathol 29:1266–1272, 1998.

Tan T Q, Ogden A K, Tillman J, Demmler G J, Rinaldi M G. Paecilomyces lilacinus catheter-related fungemia in an immunocompromised pediatric patient. J Clin Microbiol 30:2479–2483, 1992.

Tawara S, Ikeda F, Maki K, Morishita Y, Otomo K, Teratani N, Goto T, Tomishima M, Ohki H, Yamada A, Kawabata K, Takasugi H, Sakane K, Tanaka H, Matsumoto F, Kuwahara S. In vitro activities of a new lipopeptide antifungal agent, FK463, against a variety of clinically important fungi. Antimicrob Agents Chemother 44:57–62, 2000.

Torres H A, Bodey G P, Rolston K V I, Kautarjian H M, Raad I I, Kontoyiannis D P. Infections in patients with aplastic anemia: experience at a tertiary care cancer center. Cancer, in press, 2003.

Tosti A, Piraccini B M, Stinchi C, Lorenzi S. Onychomycosis due to Scopulariopsis brevicaulis: clinical features and response to systemic antifungals. Br J Dermatol 135:799–802, 1996.

Tosti A, Piraccini B M, Lorenzi S. Onychomycosis caused by nondermatophytic molds: clinical features and response to treatment of 59 cases. *J Am Acad Dermatol* 42:217–224, 2000.

Trabasso P, Vigorito A C, De Souza C A, Moretti-Branchini M L. Invasive fungal infection in hematopoietic stem cell transplant recipients at a Brazilian university hospital. Abstracts of the 41st Interscience Conference on Antimicrobial Agents and Chemotherapy, Chicago, IL. Abstract K-1248, 2001.

Travis LB, Roberts GD, Wilson WR. Clinical significance of *Pseudallescheria boydii*: a review of 10 years' experience. *Mayo Clin Proc* 60:531–537, 1985.

Van Burik J A, Myerson D, Schreckhise R W, Bowden R A. Panfungal PCR assay for detection of fungal infection in human blood specimens. *J Clin Microbiol* 36:1169–1175, 1998.

Wagoner M D, Badr I A, Hidayat A A. *Chrysosporium parvum* keratomycosis. *Cornea* 18:616–620, 1999.

Walsh T J, Francesconi A, Kasai M, Chanock S J. PCR and single-strand conformational polymorphism for recognition of medically important opportunistic fungi. *J Clin Microbiol* 33:3216–3220, 1995.

Walsh T J, Hiemenz J W, Seibel N L, Perfect J R, Horwith G, Lee L, Silber J L, DiNubile M J, Reboli A, Bow E, Lister J, Anaissie E J. Amphotericin B lipid complex for invasive fungal infections: analysis of safety and efficacy in 556 cases. *Clin Infect Dis* 26:1383–1396, 1998.

Walsh T J, Groll A H. Emerging fungal pathogens: evolving challenges to immunocompromised patients for the twenty-first century. *Transpl Infect Dis* 1:247–261, 1999.

Walsh TJ, Lutsar I, Driscoll T, Dupont B, Roden M, Ghahramani P, Hodges M, Groll AH, Perfect JR. Voriconazole in the treatment of aspergillosis, scedosporiosis and other invasive fungal infections in children. *Pediatr Infect Dis J* 21:240–248, 2002.

Wang D L, Xu C, Wang G C. A case of mycetoma caused by *Scopulariopsis maduromycosis*. *Chin Med J* 99:376–378, 1986.

Warnock D W. Fungal infections in neutropenia: current problems and chemotherapeutic control. *J Antimicrob Chemother* 41 Suppl D:95–105, 1998.

Warwick A, Ferrieri P, Burke B, Blazar B R. Presumptive invasive *Chrysosporium* infection in a bone marrow transplant recipient. *Bone Marrow Transpl* 8:319–322, 1991.

Weissgold D J, Maguire A M, Brucker A J. Management of postoperative *Acremonium* endophthalmitis. *Ophthalmology* 103:749–756, 1996.

Wetli C V, Weiss S D, Cleary T J, Gyori E. Fungal cerebritis from intravenous drug abuse. *J Forensic Sci* 29:260–268, 1984.

Wheat L J, Bartlett M, Ciccarelli M, Smith J W. Opportunistic *Scopulariopsis* pneumonia in an immunocompromised host. *South Med J* 77:1608–1609, 1984.

Wheeler M S, McGinnis M R, Schell W A, Walker D H. *Fusarium* infection in burned patients. *Am J Clin Pathol* 75:304–311, 1981.

Winn R M, Maloukou A, Gil-Lamaignere C, Panteliadis C, Roilides E, The Eurofung Network. Interferon-gamma and granulocyte-macrophage colony stimulating factor enhance hyphal damage of *Aspergillus* and *Fusarium* spp by human neutrophils. Abstracts of the 41st Interscience Conference on Antimicrobial Agents and Chemotherapy, Chicago. Abstract J-134, 2001.

Wu Z, Ying H, Yiu S, Irvine J, Smith R. Fungal keratitis caused by *Scedosporium apiospermum*: report of two cases and review of treatment. *Cornea* 21:519–523, 2002.

Yamamoto N, Matsumoto T, Ishibashi Y. Fungal keratitis caused by *Colletotrichum gloeosporioides*. *Cornea* 20:902–903, 2001.

Young J B, Ahmed-Jushuf I H, Brownjohn A M, Parsons F M, Foulkes S J, Evans E G. Opportunistic peritonitis in continuous ambulatory peritoneal dialysis. *Clin Nephrol* 22:268–269, 1984.

Young N A, Kwon-Chung K J, Kubota T T, Jennings A E, Fisher R I. Disseminated infection by *Fusarium moniliforme* during treatment for malignant lymphoma. *J Clin Microbiol* 7:589–594, 1978.

17

Phaeohyphomycoses

JOHN R. PERFECT, WILEY A. SCHELL, AND GARY M. COX

Phaeohyphomycosis, which is a term first introduced by Ajello and colleagues (Ajello et al, 1974), has become a common clinical description for a series of infections produced by darkly pigmented moulds (Fader and McGinnis, 1988; Rinaldi, 1996). In its simplest definition, phaeohyphomycosis is an infection caused by fungi that are characterized by a brown to black color within the cell wall of vegetative cells, conidia, or both. Dark pigmentation of the moulds is caused by the cell wall deposition of dihydroxynaphthalene melanin that is formed through pentaketide metabolism. In most cases the brown–black coloration is observed within specimens of host tissue but at times it is revealed only when the fungus is grown in culture.

The term phaeohyphomycosis, which means "condition of fungi with dark hyphae," is not based on the name of a particular fungus but includes many genera and species. In addition, another descriptive term for these fungi is dematiaceous fungi. This term has gained clinical favor even though its Greek meaning of "bundle" does not reflect the pigmented structures that represent the unifying feature of these fungi (Revankar et al, 2002).

When phaeohyphomycoses are reviewed, two other clinicopathological conditions or descriptions should be considered. First, chromoblastomycosis is a chronic infection of skin and soft tissue characterized by the presence of muriform fungal structures, so-called sclerotic bodies, in the tissue. This histologically distinctive indolent soft tissue infection is observed frequently in tropical areas of the world. Second, eumycetoma is a chronic deep tissue infection that usually occurs in the lower extremities and is characterized by the presence of mycotic grains and sinus tracts. In its broadest clinical definition, phaeohyphomycosis includes these conditions and a wide range of other clinical presentations including superficial colonization of the skin, keratitis, subcutaneous cyst formation, allergic sinus disease, and fatal disseminated infections caused by dematiaceous fungi. A unifying theme for these fungi is their ability to produce melanin within their cell walls and form yeast and/or hyphal-like structures in host tissues. However, it should be emphasized that melanin is produced by some other pathogenic fungi, including the yeast, *Cryptococcus neoformans*, and several of the classic dimorphic fungi such as *Histoplasma capsulatum* and *Penicillium marneffei*. Thus, melanin production is not unique to the dematiaceous moulds. This chapter focuses on the broad group of phaeohyphomycoses, excluding, for the most part, eumycetoma and chromoblastomycosis, which are discussed in detail in Chapters 25 and 26, respectively.

TAXONOMY/ECOLOGY

Within our broad definition of phaeohyphomycosis there are over 100 dematiaceous fungi that have been reported to cause human colonization or disease (Dixon and Polak-Wyss, 1991). These fungi belong to different taxonomic classes including Hyphomycetes, Ascomycetes, Basidiomycetes, Coelomycetes, and Zygomycetes. As fungal taxonomy evolves in this era of molecular studies, some of the nomenclature that describes specific fungi continues to evolve and name changes should be expected. There is also a variation in the numbers of infections with various members of the dematiaceous fungal group. Some species are rare causes of disease with only an occasional case report documented in the literature and other species are associated with large series of reported human cases such as *Exophiala jeanselmei* and *Wangiella dermatitidis* for subcutaneous disease and *Cladophialophora bantiana* for cerebral disease.

Most dematiaceous fungi are ubiquitous and cosmopolitan saprobes of soil and decaying matter, and pathogens of plants. These fungi can be found in diverse environments such as greenhouses, showers, or even on pine needles, and occasionally can reach an infectious state in animals and humans when inoculated into host tissue.

Dematiaceous fungal infections occur worldwide. Although there has been no unique endemic area for most infections, cases can cluster under certain circumstances. For instance, there is some suggestion of a southern United States geographical bias in cases of allergic fungal sinusitis associated with dematiaceous fungi (Ferguson et al, 2000b). Similarly, chronic infections of the feet and legs are noted more commonly in tropical areas. In cases of localized skin and soft tissue infections, the mechanism for production of disease may be trauma with contaminated objects such as pine needles, thorns/splinters, or even medical instruments such as needles or catheters. Also, outbreaks of nosocomial dematiaceous fungal infections may be related to an environmental contamination of fluids, drugs, or medical equipment (*MMWR*, 2002).

Increased numbers of cases of phaeohyphomycosis have been observed in medical centers that care for a large immunocompromised patient population. For instance, solid organ transplantation patients are at a moderate risk for dematiaceous fungal infections and phaeohyphomycoses have been diagnosed at most transplant centers (Welty and Perfect, 1991; Vukmir et al, 1994; Singh et al, 1997; Clancy et al, 2000). The transplantation patient, exposed to constant invasive medical interventions combined with the thinning of the skin due to corticosteroids, is a particularly susceptible immunocompromised host for infection with these fungi. The most prevalent, severe immunosuppressive event in the world today is HIV infection, and phaeohyphomycosis does occur in AIDS patients (del Palacio-Hernanz et al, 1989; Perfect et al, 1993; Marriott et al, 1997). However, these infections are uncommon events in this special group of immunocompromised patients compared to other opportunistic fungal infections, e.g., cryptococcosis and penicilliosis.

HISTOPATHOLOGY/CULTURES

Tissue histopathology for phaeohyphomycosis is characteristic. The causative fungi can produce several forms in the tissue including budding yeasts, pseudohyphae, moniliform hyphae, regular or true hyphae, enlarged subglobose cells, or a combination of the above forms. In many cases, with the routine hematoxylin-eosin stain the fungal cells have a brown pigmented appearance. However, it should be noted that not all dematiaceous fungal structures appear brown in tissue with the hematoxylin-eosin stain. Species of the genera *Alternaria*, *Bipolaris*, and *Curvularia* often appear to be hyaline in tissue due to little formation of melanin in vivo. However, these fungi will turn brown or black on fungal culture plates. The presence of melanin within the fungus in tissue specimens can be confirmed by use of the Fontana-Masson stain. Other fungi such as *Aspergillus fumigatus* and *Coccidioides immitis* occasionally stain with Fontana-Masson but less consistently than the dematiaceous moulds.

Dematiaceous fungi can occur as contaminants of body surfaces and/or clinical specimens. In order to document infection, cultures should be obtained from sterile body sites or from tissue in which histopathology confirms fungal invasion. Specimens must not be allowed to become dessicated prior to processing, and tissue specimens should be minced rather than homogenized and then placed onto media. Standard fungal media will support growth of these fungi. Some dematiaceous fungi will be inhibited by cycloheximide, therefore a culture plate without this inhibitor should also be used when attempting to isolate a pigmented mould from a clinical specimen.

The identification of a dematiaceous fungus to genus and species levels is determined by its microscopic morphology with some appreciation of colony morphology and by physiological characteristics for a few species (Schell, 1997; Schell, 2003a; Schell et al, 2003b). Proper identification is important and expert mycological input may be necessary. The details for identification of each specific dematiaceous fungus producing human disease are beyond the scope of this chapter.

PATHOPHYSIOLOGY

Phaeohyphomycosis is a descriptive term that encompasses a wide variety of phylogenetically diverse pathogenic fungal species and it is not likely that there will be consistent unifying themes for the virulence potential of all these fungi. However, several common aspects of fungal pathogenesis can be emphasized. First, the presence of melanin has been implicated through genetic studies to be a virulence factor. A mutant strain of *Wangiella dermatitidis* that lacked melanin demonstrated reduced virulence by the measurement of survival in a mouse model of infection compared to the wild-type melanin-positive strain within certain inocula (Dixon et al, 1992; Dixon et al, 1989a). Further studies used molecular biology methods to specifically disrupt a gene involved in dihydroxynaphthalene melanin biosynthesis. The null melanin-negative mutants were found to be less resistant to neutrophil killing and concordantly less virulent in acute-infection animal models (Feng et al, 2001). Another study confirmed that melanin can protect a fungus from oxidative host cells such as neutrophils (Schnitzler et al, 1999) and may bind hydrolytic enzymes. However, it should be noted that nonmelanized fungal cells can persist in tissue and cause histopathology similar to the melanized cells (Dixon et al, 1992). Melanin also has been identified as a virulence factor in other fungi such as the rice blast fungus, *Magnaporthe grisea*, for the formation of appressoria that penetrate the plant tissue. In addition, melanin is a virulence factor for the basidiomycetous human pathogen *Cryptococcus neoformans*. Another area of molecular research on *W. dermatitidis* has been chitin biosynthesis. Null mutants made in several of the chitin synthase genes of *W. der-*

matitidis were less virulent than the wild-type strain both in immunocompetent and immunosuppressed murine models (Wang et al, 2001). Second, many of these dematiaceous fungi adapt locally to the harsh host tissue environment when introduced through trauma. This adaptive feature is seen in patients with fungal keratitis and those with subcutaneous nodules that likely represent direct inoculation into the skin and subcutaneous tissue. Added susceptibility to this localized fungal infection may be related to the thinning of skin structures and reduced host responses during corticosteroid therapy. Third, several of the dematiaceous fungi appear to have a tropism for brain tissue. For instance, brain abscesses are common clinical infections associated with *Cladophialophora bantiana, Dactylaria gallopava,* and *Ramichloridium mackenziei.* Fourth, these dematiaceous infections can occur in both immunocompetent and immunosuppressed patients and thus some of these fungi are considered both primary and/or secondary pathogens. However, the vast majority of disseminated infections with dematiaceous fungi, except those with brain infections, occur in immunosuppressed patients.

Understanding of the host immunology related to the phaeohyphomycoses remains rudimentary. Importance of both humoral and cell-mediated immunity has been demonstrated. For instance, humoral immunity studies have shown that purified rabbit IgG can inhibit the growth of *Fonsecaea pedrosoi* (Ibrahim-Granet et al, 1988). In the evaluation of cell-mediated immunity, a clinical study in patients with chromoblastomycosis demonstrated a normal response to bacterial antigens but a partial suppression of cell-mediated immune responses to fungal antigens at some time during infection (Fuchs and Pecher, 1992). Although risk factor analyses indicate that the host immune system plays an important role in phaeohyphomycotic infections, much work needs to be done to better characterize the components of the host responses to dematiaceous fungi.

RISK FACTORS

Dematiaceous fungi are not primarily equipped to invade the mammalian host as part of the fungal life-cycle; thus, in most cases the host presents with some risk factors that allow establishment and/or dissemination of fungal infection Table 17–1. In the era of increasing numbers of immunocompromised hosts, phaeohyphomycoses are emerging diseases (Perfect and Schell, 1996; Silveira and Nucci, 2001). Bone marrow and solid organ transplantation patients are at major risk for infection (Benedict et al, 1992; Singh et al, 1997; Clancy et al, 2000). The chronic use of corticosteroids that both thin the skin and predispose to a myriad of other immunodepressive actions increases the risk of infection for patients who commonly are exposed to dematiaceous fungi in an outpatient environment. Patients with skin or soft tissue trauma from contaminated vegetation (e.g., splinters), intravenous drug abuse (Vartian et al, 1985; Walz et al, 1997), and/or cardiothoracic surgery that introduces fungi at the time of surgery (Kaufman, 1971; Pauzner et al, 1997; Revankar et al, 2002) have been reported to develop phaeohyphomycosis. An occasional case of phaeohyphomycosis has been observed in AIDS patients (del Palacio-Hernanz et al, 1989; Perfect et al, 1993; Marriott et al, 1997), or in those receiving chronic ambulatory peritoneal dialysis (Kerr et al, 1983). These patient groups are at high risk for developing infections because of the combination of frequent exposures to dematiaceous fungi and their underlying immunosuppressive conditions.

CLINICAL MANIFESTATIONS

Although the dematiaceous fungi represent a phylogenetically diverse group of fungi, there are several well-described clinical syndromes produced by these fungi.

Superficial Phaeohyphomycosis

This category includes conditions known traditionally as tinea nigra and black piedra. Tinea nigra is a darkening of the skin due to growth in the stratum corneum of *Hortaea werneckii (Phaeoannellomyces werneckii).* Although the condition is harmless because only the stratum corneum is involved, tinea nigra can be mistaken for melanoma. Black piedra is colonization of the hair shaft by *Piedraia hortae,* which results in very hard knots of discrete fungal growth along the shaft.

TABLE 17–1. *Risk Factors for Dematiaceous Fungal Infections*

• Solid organ transplantation	• Long term indwelling catheter (e.g., continuous ambulatory peritoneal dialysis)
• Bone marrow transplantation	
• Corticosteroid therapy	
• Trauma	• HIV infection
• Intravenous drug abuse	• Cardiothoracic surgery
• Neutropenia	• Fresh water immersion
• Sinusitis	

Cutaneous Phaeohyphomycosis

This condition represents both initial colonization and then proliferation of the fungus within keratinized tissue, resulting in a chronic inflammatory reaction from tissue invasion (Welty and Perfect, 1991; Ronan et al, 1993). Examples include a dermatomycosis secondary to dematiaceous fungi like *Scytalidium* species or an onychomycosis with agents like *Scytalidium* or *Phyllosticta* species. Furthermore, under certain skin conditions, the dematiaceous fungi may simply colonize devitalized skin without invasion of viable tissue. Thus, treatment of the underlying condition or use of a simple antiseptic wash will remove these fungi from tissue. However, in severely immunosuppressed patients, some of these moulds may produce an aggressive soft tissue infection.

Mycotic Keratitis

Trauma to the cornea can provide a site for fungal organisms to lodge and grow. The fungus might be present on the instrument of trauma at impact or as airborne spores that contact an injured eye. The frequent use of steroid ophthalmic drops for corneal injuries may aid invasion of the cornea by these fungi. The dematiaceous fungi plus species of *Aspergillus*, *Fusarium*, and *Paecilomyces* are the main causes of fungal keratitis. Corneal infections have the potential to progress to endophthalmitis by spreading into internal ocular structures. Multiple dematiaceous moulds have caused ocular disease (Forster et al, 1975; Schell, 1986) but *Curvularia*, *Exophiala*, and *Exserohilum* species are the most common organisms (McGinnis et al, 1986).

Subcutaneous Phaeohyphomycosis

This form of phaeohyphomycosis is a relatively common presentation (Benedict et al, 1992; Sudduth et al, 1992; Ronan et al, 1993; Singh et al, 1997; Clancy et al 2000). Patients generally present with solitary, discrete, asymptomatic, subcutaneous lesions or cysts (See Color Figs. 17–1A, 17–B, and 17–C in separate color insert). Cysts can be misdiagnosed as ganglion cysts, epidermal inclusion cysts, Baker's cysts, or foreign body granulomas. Occasionally, deep subcutaneous ulcers develop and even satellite lesions, which might occur from autoinoculation. Cysts in the immunocompetent patient can be chronic, relatively asymptomatic, and can remain with little observable clinical change for years, but a fungus in tissue can be observed and cultured when the cyst is removed. Some of these resected cysts may contain the original wood splinter that introduced the fungus into the tissue. Among immunosuppressed patients these cysts are most commonly seen in solid organ transplant patients and those patients receiving chronic corticosteroids. Even among immunosuppressed patients, the majority of these skin lesions represent direct or primary inoculation into tissue rather than skin lesions that result from dissemination from another site of infection. The most common dematiaceous fungi to produce these cysts are *Exophiala jeanselmei*, *Wangiella dermatitidis*, and *Phialophora species*.

Foreign Body Phaeohyphomycosis

Various types of catheters in patients occasionally become colonized with dematiaceous fungi and sometimes these moulds will produce disease. Foreign body phaeohyphomycosis is most commonly seen in patients receiving chronic ambulatory peritoneal dialysis (CAPD) who develop fungal peritonitis (Kerr et al, 1983). This disease can also occur in patients with long indwelling subcutaneous intravenous catheters, likely related to a breech in sterile technique. While it is important to remove the foreign body in the treatment of these two infections, it is not yet clear whether these dematiaceous fungi produce a biofilm that enhances attachment to catheters leading to protection from host responses and antifungal drugs.

Fungal Sinusitis

Fungal sinus infections with dematiaceous fungi can present in three forms: first, allergic fungal sinusitis in which there is histopathologic evidence of inflammatory mucin with eosinophils and hyphae present within the mucin (Schell, 2000a); second, fungus ball/eumycetoma in the sinus cavity, which produces disease primarily by obstruction (there is no apparent fungal invasion into local soft tissue or bone in either of these two forms) (Corey et al, 1995); third, invasive fungal sinusitis manifested by extension of the infection into host tissue such as bone and even the brain (Washburn et al, 1988). *Aspergillus* species, zygomycetes, and dematiaceous moulds such as *Bipolaris*, *Curvularia*, and *Alternaria* species represent the primary etiological agents in the invasive fungal sinusitis syndrome (MacMillan et al, 1987; Gourley et al, 1990; Schell, 2000a; Schell, 2000b; Schell et al, 2003b).

Systemic Phaeohyphomycosis

Disseminated infection represents spread to distant organs from a local colonized or infected site. The fungus may have gained entry to the human host via contaminated surgery, trauma, or the lungs. Under certain circumstances infection will spread to distant sites such as the heart (endocarditis) (Kaufman, 1971) or brain (abscess) (Palaoglu et al, 1993; Horre and de Hoog, 1999). There has been a significant increase in cases of disseminated phaeohyphomycosis over the last decade. The vast majority of these cases (over 85%) are associated with some type of immunodeficiency, most commonly chemotherapy-induced neutropenia. However, there are occasional patients with disseminated phaeohyphomycosis who have no apparent risk factor(s) (See Color Figs. 17–2A and 17–2B in separate color insert) (Rohwedder et al, 1979; Flanagan and Bryceson, 1997; Khan et al, 2002). Disseminated disease has been associated with peripheral eosinophilia (Revankar et al, 2002), suggesting that certain patients with this infection have an ineffective TH2 immune response, which allows dissemination. Most patients with disseminated disease probably do not develop a proper immune response even when risk factors are not readily apparent.

The most commonly encountered dematiaceous fungi to produce disseminated disease include those that cause brain abscesses (See Color Fig. 17–2A in separate color insert) such as *Cladophialophora bantiana*, *Dactylaria gallopava*, and *Ramichloridium mackenziei* and meningitis such as *Scedosporium apiospermum* (Horre and de Hoog, 1999). *Scedosporium apiospermum* (teleomorph *Pseudallescheria boydii*) is a common cause of pneumonia or meningitis following near-drownings in fresh water, and is becoming a more common pathogen in severely immunosuppressed organ transplant recipients (Marr et al, 2002). *Scedosporium prolificans*, which is the most common cause of detectable bloodstream infections due to dematiaceous fungi, was originally encountered in bone and joint infections. Fungemia has been documented frequently as a complication of neutropenia and in patients with prosthetic heart valves. *Scedosporium prolificans* appears able to produce a steady stream of unicellular spores, and this phenomenon of adventitious sporulation appears to occur within invaded blood vessels (Schell, 1995; Liu et al, 1998). After surgical trauma, prolonged neutropenia, or in the presence of contaminated catheters, *Scedosporium*, *Bipolaris*, and *Wangiella* species most commonly produce a widely disseminated phaeohyphomycosis (Revankar et al, 2002).

ETIOLOGICAL AGENTS

Table 17–2 attempts to match the most common dematiaceous fungi with their primary clinical presentations. This list is not comprehensive since over 100 species have already been documented as etiologic agents and more dematiaceous moulds will be added to the list as the immunocompromised population expands. Also, this list emphasizes only the most common clinical presentations, but other manifestations may occur.

Several specific features about selected dematiaceous fungal infections deserve mention. First, virtually all cases of chromoblastomycosis are caused by three species, *Fonsecaea pedrosoi*, *Cladophialophora carrionii*, and *Phialophora verrucosa*. Second, the most clinically common group of dematiaceous fungi is comprised of *Alternaria* spp., *Bipolaris* spp., *Curvularia* spp., *Exophiala* spp., and *Wangiella dermatitidis*, which are associated with a myriad of clinical presentations. Third, the group of fungi that typically produce CNS infections includes *Cladophialophora bantiana*, *Dactylaria gallopava*, and *Ramichloridium mackenziei* (Bennett et al, 1973; Horre and de Hoog, 1999). In fact, *D. gallopava* has shown its innate potential for CNS infectivity by causing outbreaks of fungal encephalitis in turkeys (Georg et al, 1964) and occasional cases in humans (Sides et al, 1991). For this group of CNS pathogens, there is also some geographical limitation of infection. For example, *R. mackenziei* has been limited to infections in the Middle East (Kanj et al, 2001). Fourth, along with the known potential of *S. apiospermum* to cause meningitis in diabetics, patients receiving steroid therapy, or victims of fresh water near-drownings (Watanabe and Hironaga, 1981; Yoo et al, 1985; Dworzack et al, 1987), cases of meningitis have been caused by species of *Bipolaris*, *Exophiala*, *Alternaria* and *Sporothrix schenckii* (Perfect and Durack, 1997; Schell, 1997; Schell, 2003a). Fifth, although many different dematiaceous fungi have caused disease, there is clearly a spectrum of virulence potential. For example, species of genera such as *Cladosporium* or *Rhinocladiella* are environmentally common and more frequent colonizers of skin and airways than the more pathogenic dematiaceous fungi such as *F. pedrosoi*, *W. dermatitidis*, *D. gallopava*, and *C. bantiana*. Sixth, *S. schenckii*, which is a dematiaceous mould in culture, is generally considered a dimorphic fungus and sometimes classified within that group rather than under the dematiaceous mould group. Although the propensity of *S. schenckii* to produce soft tissue infections through traumatic inoculation does fit the common pattern of infection with dematiaceous fungi, see Chapter 22 for more information on Sporotrichosis.

The clinical syndromes associated with several of the most common dematiaceous mould genera are summarized herein. For a more comprehensive mycological description of these dematiaceous fungi, the reader is referred to reference books and monographs (Schell, 2003a; Schell et al, 2003b; Sigler, 2003).

Alternaria Species

The most common species is *Alternaria alternata* but in the clinical laboratory, identification generally is left at the genus level. This mould often causes local cutaneous infection (Viviani et al, 1986; Wiest et al, 1987). In addition, it may cause a sinonasal infection characteristically seen in immunosuppressed patients, which is similar to zygomycosis and does not commonly disseminate (Wiest et al, 1987; Morrison and Weisdorf, 1993).

TABLE 17–2. *Dematiaceous Fungi and Their Most Common Phaeohyphomycoses*

Etiologic Agent	Clinical Presentation	Frequency*	References
Alternaria spp. (*alternata*)	Osteomyelitis, cutaneous, sinusitis	++	Viviani et al, 1986; Schell, 2003a; Schell et al, 2003b;
Aureobasidium spp. (*pullulans*)	Peritonitis, cutaneous, spleen infection	±	Schell, 2003a; Schell et al, 2003b
Bipolaris spp. (*australiensis, hawaiiensis, spicifera*)	Meningitis, sinusitis, keratitis, peritonitis, endocarditis, disseminated infection	+++	Fuste et al, 1973; Rolston et al, 1985; Adam et al, 1986; McGinnis et al, 1986; Karim et al, 1993; Schell, 2003a; Schell et al, 2003b
Chaetomium spp (*atrobrunneum*) *Achaetomium* spp. (*strumarium*)	Fungemia, cutaneous, brain abscess	+	Sigler, 2003
Cladophialophora spp. (*bantiana, carrionii*)	Chromoblastomycosis, brain abscess	++	Bennett et al, 1973; Seaworth et al, 1983; Dixon et al, 1989b; Sekhon et al, 1992; Palaoglu et al, 1993; Schell, 2003a;
Cladosporium spp.	Colonizer, skin, keratitis	±	Schell, 2003a
Coniothyrium spp. (*fuckelii*)	Cutaneous, liver infection	±	Schell et al, 2003b
Curvularia spp (*lunata*)	Sinusitis, keratitis, endocarditis, subcutaneous cyst, pneumonitis	+++	Rohwedder et al, 1979; Monte and Hutchins, 1985; Yau et al, 1994; Fernandez et al, 1999; Schell, 2003a
Dactylaria spp. (*gallopava*)	Brain abscess, disseminated infection, pneumonitis	++	Sides et al, 1991; Vukmir et al, 1994; Schell, 2003a
Exophiala spp. (*jeanselmei*)	Subcutaneous cyst, eumycetoma, keratitis, meningitis/brain abscess, disseminated infection, peritonitis	++	Tintelnot et al, 1991; Sudduth et al, 1992; Gold et al, 1994; Schell, 2003a
Exserohilum spp. (*rostratum*)	Sinusitis, cutaneous, subcutaneous cyst, keratitis	+	McGinnis et al, 1986; Schell, 2003a
Fonsecaea spp. (*pedrosoi*)	Chromoblastomycosis, eumycetoma, pneumonitis	++	Morris et al, 1995; Schell, 1997; Schell, 2003a
Lasiodiplodia spp. (*theobromae*)	Keratitis	+	Sigler, 2003
Lecythophora spp. (*hoffmannii*)	Subcutaneous cyst, endocarditis, peritonitis	+	Sigler, 2003
Phaeoacremonium spp. (*parasiticum*)	Cutaneous, subcutaneous cyst	+	Schell, 2003a
Phaeoannellomyces spp. (*elegans, werneckii*)	Subcutaneous cyst	+	
Phialemonium spp. (*curvatum, obovatum*)	Subcutaneous cyst, endocarditis, peritonitis	+	Sigler, 2003
Phialophora spp. (*verrucosa, richardsiae*)	Chromoblastomycosis, eumycetoma, keratitis, osteomyelitis, endocarditis	++	Schell, 1997; Schell, 2003a; Schell et al, 2003b
Phoma spp.	Sinusitis, keratitis, subcutaneous cyst	+	Sigler, 2003
Ramichloridium spp. (*obovoideum, mackenziei*)	Brain abscess	+	Horre and de Hoog, 1999; Kanj et al, 2001
Rhinocladiella spp. (*aquaspersa, atrovirens*)	Colonizer, chromoblastomycosis, meningitis	++	del Palacio-Hernanz et al, 1989; Schell, 1997; Nucci et al, 2001; Sigler, 2003
Scedosporium spp. (*apiospermum, prolificans*)	Eumycetoma, meningitis, pneumonitis, fungemia, disseminated infection	+++	Watanabe and Hirogonga, 1981; Yoo et al, 1985; Dworzack et al, 1987; Berenguer et al, 1989; Berenguer et al, 1997; Maertens et al, 2002; Sigler et al, 2003
Scytalidium spp. (*dimidiatum*)	Cutaneous, nail, subcutaneous cyst	+	Sigler, 2003
Wangiella spp. (*dermatitidis*)	Cutaneous, subcutaneous cyst, keratitis, brain abscess, arthritis, disseminated infection	+++	Greer et al, 1979; Hiruma et al, 1993; Schell, 2003a

** + least common; +++ most common.
Source: adapted from Schell, 2003a.

Bipolaris Species

Three species cause the majority of disease: *B. australiensis, B. hawaiiensis,* and *B. spicifera.* This genus of brown/black moulds may infect many different organs of the body and cause meningitis, sinusitis, keratitis, peritonitis, soft tissue infections, and endocarditis (Rolston et al, 1985; Adam et al, 1986; McGinnis et al, 1986; Karim et al, 1993; Flanagan and Bryceson, 1997; Pauzner et al, 1997; Latham, 2000).

Cladophialophora Species

Species of this genus have undergone several taxonomic changes in the last several decades that can cause confusion in the clinical literature. For instance, *Cladophialophora bantiana* had previously been named *Cladosporium trichoides, Cladosporium bantianum* and *Xylohypha bantiana.* Despite controversy regarding the taxonomy, there is no clinical confusion about the ability of *C. bantiana* to cause central nervous system infection (Horre and de Hoog, 1999). Dozens of cases of cerebral phaeohyphomycosis have been reported making *C. bantiana* the most common dematiaceous mould to cause central nervous system infection (See Color Fig. 17–3 in separate color insert). Occasionally, *C. bantiana* causes soft tissue infection. Another species, *C. carrioni,* is a leading cause of chromoblastomycosis in Africa and Australia (Schell, 1997).

Cladosporium Species

The vast majority of clinical isolates of this genus represent colonization of nonsterile body sites (Schell, 2003a). Furthermore, *C. cladosporioides* and *C. sphaerospermum* are among the most common dematiaceous mould contaminants in the clinical microbiology laboratory. In order to conclude that infection is attributable to *Cladosporium* species, there must be histopathologic evidence of infection as well as a pure culture of the fungus, preferably obtained from a sterile body site.

Curvularia Species

Species of this genus are leading causes of dematiaceous fungal sinusitis and keratitis but like *Bipolaris* species, they can also produce other type infections such as soft tissue, endocarditis, and disseminated disease (Monte and Hutchens, 1985; Yau et al, 1994; Fernandez et al, 1999; Janaki et al, 1999). The most common species associated with clinical disease is *C. lunata.*

Exophiala Species

While species of this genus are a leading cause of subcutaneous phaeohyphomycosis, they can also cause peritonitis in CAPD patients and endocarditis as well as meningitis and brain abscess (Tintelnot et al, 1991; Sudduth et al, 1992; Gold et al, 1994). *Exophiala jeanselmei* is the major species producing clinical disease (See Color Figs. 17–1A, 17–B, and 17–C in separate color insert).

Fonsecaea Species

Fonsecaea pedrosoi is the most common cause worldwide of chromoblastomycosis (Schell, 1997). Occasionally, this species can cause invasive infection in severely immunosuppressed patients (Morris et al, 1995). Because of the pleomorphic structures of *F. pedrosoi,* it may be confused with *Rhinocladiella* and *Phialophora* species in culture. Thus, specimens need careful mycological evaluation (Schell et al, 2003b).

Phialophora Species

Species of this genus can produce a wide variety of infections ranging from chromoblastomycosis to opportunistic infections in AIDS patients and organ transplant recipients (Schell, 2003a; Schell et al, 2003b). Two of the most common species to infect humans are *P. verrucosa* and *P. richardsiae.*

Rhinocladiella Species

The only species regularly identified in the clinical laboratory is *Rhinocladiella atrovirens.* Because it can colonize nonsterile sites or appear in cultures as a contaminant, *R. atrovirens* requires other confirmation studies such as histopathology to support its significance when isolated from a nonsterile site. Although *R. atrovirens* has very little virulence potential, it has produced meningitis in severely immunosuppressed patients (del Palacio-Hernanz et al, 1989) and one reported case of a eumycetoma (Ndiaye et al, 2000). *Ramichloridium* is a genus that appears to be congeneric with *Rhinocladiella.* If the two genera are synonymous, *Rhinocladiella* would be the correct name based on nomenclature priority. Several brain infections have been caused by fungi identified as *Ramichloridium obovoideum* and *Ramichloridium mackenziei* (Horre and de Hoog, 1999; Kanj et al, 2001).

Scedosporium Species

Some mycologists have suggested *Scedosporium* species belong in the group of dematiaceous fungi because some isolates may appear as pale brown hyphae in unstained tissue or are positive for melanin with Fontana-Masson stain. However, current consensus places diseases caused by both *S. apiospermum* and *S. prolificans* within the hyalohyphomycoses. Thus, for a detailed discussion of scedosporiosis, see Chapter 16; here only a brief overview of scedosporiosis is provided. *Scedosporium apiospermum* is an anamorph of *Pseudallescheria boydii.* The necessity to have more than one name associated with this fungus occasionally can cause confusion. The rationale for multiple names being connected to a fungus is explained in detail elsewhere (Schell et al, 2003b). *Scedosporium apiospermum* can cause fungal eumycetoma, and also has the ability to produce disseminated disease including central nervous system involvement in patients with diabetes, receiving corticosteroids, and near-drowning victims (Berenguer et al, 1989). The common occurrence of *S. apiospermum* in the environment and the frequent use of empirical polyene drugs against which this fungus exhibits clinical resistance has enabled *S. apiospermum* to become an emerging pathogen in severely immunosuppressed patients. *Scedosporium prolificans* is another emerging pathogen (Berenguer et al, 1997; Maertens et al, 2002). Except for eumycetoma, it causes a range of infections similar to that of *S. apiospermum*. In patients with disseminated disease secondary to *S. prolificans*, blood cultures are likely to be positive as previously noted, probably due to the ability of this species to form unicellular spores in tissue (Liu et al, 1998; Schell, 1995). *Scedosporium prolificans* remains one of the most resistant fungi to presently available antifungal agents.

Wangiella *Species*

This mould can cause localized infection of skin, subcutaneous tissue, and also systemic infection involving the brain, joints and eye (Hiruma et al, 1993; Horre and de Hoog, 1999; Matsumoto et al, 1992). In the group of dematiaceous fungi, *W. dermatitidis* probably is the best-studied pathogen in terms of molecular biology, animal model experimentation, and virulence factors such as melanin.

LABORATORY STUDIES

It is important that dematiaceous fungi be identified correctly in the clinical laboratory. For instance, identification by genus and species may help predict the extent of infection and/or identify the pattern of drug susceptibility and thus help the clinician to choose the appropriate antifungal agent. The calcofluor-KOH procedure is extremely helpful in detecting the presence of dematiaceous fungi in specimens; however, it is not reliable for detecting the heavily melanized cells found in chromoblastomycosis. Diagnosis of phaeohyphomycosis relies on histopathology and culture. Identification of genera and species in the clinical laboratory is based almost exclusively on morphological study of macroscopic and microscopic features. In routine microbiology laboratories, there are no available serologic tests to diagnose infection with these fungi.

Blood cultures may be positive in cases of disseminated disease with *Scedosporium* species. In addition, nosocomial outbreaks of fungemia with *Exophiala* and *Rhinocladiella* species have been reported (Nucci et al, 2001). The presence of these particular fungi in blood

suggests a breech of aseptic technique during an invasive medical procedure or in the processing of blood cultures.

MANAGEMENT

With regard to the treatment of phaeohyphomycosis, the majority of clinical experience represents isolated cases or small series of infections with multiple different fungi. While evidence-based algorithms for treatment are not robust, there are several surgical and medical strategies that should be considered.

Surgery is an integral part of any treatment strategy. Primary treatment may require surgical debridement of selected skin and soft tissue, brain, and sinus fluid and structures. In soft tissue infections, the surgical approach varies. Best results for an ulcerative lesion or skin infection without a defined cyst are obtained with careful debridement and even use of Moh's procedure to identify borders of infection (Heinz et al, 1996). With surgery, lavage of residual tissue after surgery with an antiseptic agent is probably helpful, since fungal organisms might remain in the wound. For a subcutaneous cyst, complete removal of the encapsulated structure can be curative but care must be taken not to leak contents into the wound. Simple aspiration of cyst fluid is not optimal.

For single brain abscess, surgical debridement is probably essential for cure. While complete surgical removal of a brain abscess may not be possible, even partial debulking of the brain mass is helpful (Ferguson, 2000a). Occasionally infection may be spread with surgery (Shimosaka and Waga, 1983) and in the case of brain abscesses, it is probably wise to use adjunctive medical therapy. Although medical treatment of brain abscesses alone occasionally has been successful (Vukmir et al, 1994), there are many reported failures of medical treatment without combined medical–surgical therapy. Medical treatment alone should be reserved for patients with multiple abscesses and those for whom surgery is contraindicated.

In cases of sinus disease (eumycetoma), removal of the fungal mass through endoscopy may be curative. True eumycetoma in the extremities such as madura foot can be indolent and difficult to manage. Because of chronic scarring and fistulous tracts in soft tissue and possible bone involvement, obtaining disease free margins via surgery may be difficult. In these circumstances, medical therapy may be the best option.

Antifungal drugs have been used in the management of phaeohyphomycosis, with both in vitro and in vivo evidence for antifungal drug activity against these dematiaceous fungi (McGinnis et al, 1997; Espinel-Ingroff, 1998a; Espinel-Ingroff, 1998b; McGinnis and Pasarell, 1998). Because there are many genera and species included in the group of dematiaceous fungi, it is beyond the scope of this chapter to detail the antifungal activity against each genus or species. Nevertheless, several general comments on medical therapy are in order. First, polyene drugs show modest antifungal activity in vitro against dematiaceous fungi and have been used in treatment of some disseminated infections. However, polyenes are not consistently used as primary therapy for these infections. Second, flucytosine has in vitro antifungal activity against several dematiaceous fungi, but is most likely used in combination therapy because of rapid development of drug resistance when used alone. Third, the azole drugs are commonly chosen in treatment strategies for phaeohyphomycosis because these agents exhibit moderate to excellent in vitro antifungal activity against dematiaceous fungi and can be given safely for long periods of time. Among the older azoles, itraconazole has been best-studied, with a reported success rate of over 60% in one series (Sharkey et al, 1990). The newer triazoles, voriconazole, posaconazole, and ravuconazole, have moderate to excellent in vitro activity against dematiaceous moulds (McGinnis et al, 1997; Espinel-Ingroff, 1998a; Espinel-Ingroff, 1998b) and thus, are promising drugs for treatment of phaeohyphomycoses. In fact, most dematiaceous fungal infections in single case reports or small series have responded to these triazoles. Furthermore, in an animal model of cerebral *Ramichloridium* infection, posaconazole was found to be more effective than itraconazole or amphotericin B (Al-Abdely et al, 2000). It is likely that these extended-spectrum triazoles will become first-line therapy for phaeohyphomycosis. Fourth, echinocandins, a new class of antifungal agents which inhibit fungal β-glucan synthase, have inhibitory in vitro activity against many dematiaceous fungi (Del Poeta et al, 1997; Espinel-Ingroff, 1998b) but there has been no significant clinical experience with these agents. Finally, drug combinations in vitro commonly show either additive or synergistic activity against these dematiaceous fungi (McGinnis and Pasarell, 1998; Clancy et al, 2000; Meletiadis et al, 2000). For disseminated or intracranial disease with limited surgical options, two or three drug combinations, e.g., polyene, flucytosine, terbinafine, and/or newer triazole, may become the treatment regimen of choice.

There are several other aspects to the management of phaeohyphomycosis. First, immune modulation has been considered for treatment of some phaeohyphomycoses. In allergic fungal sinusitis, both corticosteroids for decreasing immune stimulation and immunotherapy to induce tolerance have their proponents but their precise value remains unclear (Corey et al, 1995; Ferguson, 1998). In patients with invasive dematiaceous fungal infections, control of the underlying disease and eliminating an immunosuppressive event, e.g., corticosteroids or neutropenia, should be a primary focus of management. Second, at present there is no approved standardized method for performing in vitro antifungal susceptibility testing against these moulds, but the NCCLS committee does have a proposed working protocol (National Committee for Clinical Laboratory Standards, 1998). In certain unique infections with dematiaceous fungi, an assessment of the in vitro activity of potentially useful antifungal agents may be reasonable. Third, disease caused by *Scedosporium apiospermum*, which is resistant to amphotericin B, frequently responds to the newer triazoles such as voriconazole and in some cases this azole has enabled dramatic clinical recoveries (Walsh et al, 2002). On the other hand, *Scedosporium prolificans* appears to be resistant to most classes of available antifungal drugs and only occasionally responds to the extended-spectrum triazoles. Thus, combinations of drugs have been tested for possible use against this fungus (Meletiadis et al, 2000). Finally, most cases of phaeohyphomycosis, even when surgery is performed and presumed curative, require drug treatment to eliminate any residual infection.

REFERENCES

Adam R D, Paquin M L, Peterson E A. Phaeohyphomycosis caused by the fungal genera *Bipolaris* and *Exserohilum*. A report of 9 cases and review of the literature. *Medicine* 65:203–217, 1986.

Ajello L, Georg L K, Steigbigel R T. A case of phaeohyphomycosis caused by a new species of *Phialophora*. *Mycologia* 66:490–498, 1974.

Al-Abdely H M, Najvar L, Bocanegra R, Fothergill A, Loebenberg D, Rinaldi M G, Graybill J R. SCH 56592, amphotericin B, or itraconazole therapy of experimental murine cerebral phaeohyphomycosis due to *Ramichloridium obovoideum* (*Ramichloridium mackenziei*). *Antimicrob Agents Chemother* 44:1159–1162, 2000.

Benedict L A, Kusne S, Torre-Cisneros J, Hunt S J. Primary cutaneous fungal infection after solid-organ transplantation. *Clin Infect Dis* 15:17–21, 1992.

Bennett J E, Bonner H, Jennings A E, Lopez R I. Chronic meningitis caused by *Cladosporium trichoides*. *Am J Clin Path* 59:398–407, 1973.

Berenguer J, Diaz-Mediavilla J, Urra D, Munoz P. Central nervous system infection caused by *Pseudallescheria boydii*: case report and review. *Rev Infect Dis* 11:890–896, 1989.

Berenguer J, Rodriquez-Tudela J L, Richard C. Deep infections caused by *Scedosporium prolificans*. A report on 16 cases in Spain and a review of the literature. *Medicine* 76:256–265, 1997.

Clancy C J, Wingard J R, Nguyen M H. Subcutaneous phaeohyphomycosis in transplant recipients: review of the literature and demonstration of in vitro synergy between antifungal agents. *Med Mycol* 38:169–175, 2000.

Corey J R, Delsupeke K G, Ferguson B J. Allergic fungal sinusitis: allergic, infectious or both? *Otolaryngol—Head Neck Surg* 113:110–119, 1995.

del Palacio-Hernanz A, Moore M K, Campbell C K, del Palacio-Perez-Medel A, del Castillo-Cantero R. Infection of the central nervous system by *Rhinocladiella atrovirens* in a patient with acquired immunodeficiency syndrome. *J Med Vet Mycol* 27:127–130, 1989.

Del Poeta M, Schell W A, Perfect J R. In vitro antifungal activity of pneumocandin L-743,872 against a variety of clinically important moulds. *Antimicrob Agents Chemother* 41:1835–1836, 1997.

Dixon D M, Polak A, Conner G W. Mel-mutants of *Wangiella dermatitidis* in mice: evaluation of multiple mouse and fungal strains. *J Med Vet Mycol* 27:335–341, 1989a.

Dixon D M, Walsh T J, Merz W G, McGinnis M R. Infections due to *Xylohypha bantiana* (*Cladosporium trichoides*). *Rev Infect Dis* 11:515–525, 1989b.

Dixon D M, Polak-Wyss A. The medically important dematiaceous fungi and their identification. *Mycoses* 34:1–18, 1991.

Dixon D M, Migliozzi J, Cooper C R, Jr., Solis O, Breslin B, Szaniszlo P J. Melanized and non-melanized multicellular form mutants of *Wangiella dermatitidis* in mice: mortality and histopathology studies. *Mycoses* 35:17–21, 1992.

Dworzack D L, Clark R B, Padgett P J. New causes of pneumonia, meningitis, and disseminated infections associated with immersion. *Infect Control Hosp Epidemiol* 1:615–633, 1987.

Espinel-Ingroff A. In vitro activity of the new triazole voriconazole UK 109,496 against opportunistic filamentous and dimorphic fungi and common and emerging yeast pathogens. *J Clin Microbiol* 36:198–202, 1998a.

Espinel-Ingroff A. A comparison of in vitro activities of the new triazole SCH56592 and the echinocandins MK 0991 L-743,872 and LY303366 against opportunistic filamentous and dimorphic fungi and yeasts. *J Clin Microbiol* 36:2950–2956, 1998b.

Fader R C, McGinnis M R. Infections caused by dematiaceous fungi: chromoblastomycosis and phaeohyphomycosis. *Infect Dis Clin North Am* 2:925–938, 1988.

Feng B, Wang X, Hauser M, Kauffman S, Jentsch S, Haase G, Becker J M, Szaniszlo P J. Molecular cloning and characterization of WdPks1, a gene involved in dihydroxynaphthalene melanin biosynthesis and virulence in *Wangiella* (*Exophiala*) *dermatitidis*. *Infect Immun* 69:1781–1794, 2001.

Ferguson B J. What role do systemic corticosteroids, immunotherapy, and antifungal drugs play in the therapy of allergic fungal rhinosinusitis? *Arch Otolaryngol—Head Neck Surg* 124:1174–1178, 1998.

Ferguson B J. Fungus balls of the paranasal sinuses. *Otolaryngol Clin North Amer* 33:389–398, 2000a.

Ferguson B J, Barnes L, Bernstein J M, Brown D, Clark C E, Cook P R, Dewitt W S, Graham S M, Gordon B, Javir A R, Krouse J H, Kuhn F A, Levine H L, Manning S C, Marple B F, Morgan A H, Osguthorpe J D, Skedros D, Rains B M, Ramadan H H, Terrell J E, Yonkers A J. Graphical variation in allergic fungal rhinosinusitis. *Otolaryngol Clin North Amer* 33:441–449, 2000b.

Fernandez M, Noyola D E, Rosemann S N, Edwards M S. Cutaneous phaeohyphomycosis caused by *Curvularia lunata* and a review of *Curvularia* infections in pediatrics. *Pediatr Infect Dis J* 18:727–731, 1999.

Flanagan K L, Bryceson A D. Disseminated infection due to *Bipolaris australiensis* in a young immunocompetent man: case report and review. *Clin Infect Dis* 25:311–313, 1997.

Forster R K, Rebell G, Wilson L A. Dematiaceous fungal keratitis: clinical isolates and management. *Br J Ophthalmol* 59:372–376, 1975.

Fuchs J, Pecher S. Partial suppression of cell mediated immunity in chromoblastomycosis. *Mycopathologia* 119:73–76, 1992.

Fuste F J, Ajello L, Threlkeld R, Henry J E, Jr. *Drechslera hawaiiensis*: Causative agent of a fatal fungal meningo-encephalitis. *Sabouraudia* 11:59–63, 1973.

Georg L K, Bierer B W, Cooke W B. Encephalitis in turkey poults due to a new fungus species. *Sabouraudia* 3:239–244, 1964.

Gold W L, Vellend H, Salit I E, Campbell I, Summerbell R, Rinaldi M, Simor A E. Successful treatment of systemic and local infections due to *Exophiala* species. *Clin Infect Dis* 19:339–341, 1994.

Gourley D S, Whisman B A, Jorgensen N L, Martin M E, Reid M J. Allergic *Bipolaris* sinusitis: clinical and immunopathologic characteristics. *J Allergy Clin Immunol* 85:583–591, 1990.

Greer K E, Gross G P, Cooper P H, Harding S A. Cystic chromomycosis due to *Wangiella dermatitidis*. *Arch Dermatol* 115:1433–1434, 1979.

Heinz T, Serafin D B, Schell W A, Perfect J R. Soft tissue fungal infections: surgical management of 12 immunocompromised patients. *Plastic Reconstr Surg* 97:1391–1399, 1996.

Hiruma M, Kawada A, Ohata H, Ohnishi Y, Takahashi H, Yamazaki M, Ishibashi A, Hatsuse K, Kakihara M, Yoshida M. Systemic phaeohyphomycosis caused by *Exophiala dermatitidis*. *Mycoses* 36:1–7, 1993.

Horre R, de Hoog G S. Primary cerebral infections by melanized fungi: a review. In: de Horre G S, ed. *Studies in Mycology #43: Ecology and Evolution of Black Yeasts and Their Relatives.* Baarn/Delft, The Netherlands: Centralbureau Voor Schimmel, 176–193, 1999.

Ibrahim-Granet O, de Bievre C, Jendoubi M. Immunochemical characterisation of antigens and growth inhibition of *Fonsecaea pedrosoi* by species-specific IgG. *J Med Microbiol* 26:217–222, 1988.

Janaki C, Sentamilselvi G, Janaki V R, Devesh S, Ajithados K. Eumycetoma due to *Curvularia lunata*. *Mycoses* 42:345–346, 1999.

Kanj S S, Amr S S, Roberts G D. *Ramichloridium mackenziei* brain abscess: report of two cases and review of the literature. *Med Mycol* 39:97–102, 2001.

Karim M, Sheikh H, Alam M, Sheikh Y. Disseminated *Bipolaris* infection in an asthmatic patient: case report. *Clin Infect Dis* 17:248–253, 1993.

Kaufman S M. *Curvularia endocarditis* following cardiac surgery. *Am J Clin Path* 56:466–470, 1971.

Kerr C, Perfect J R, Gallis H A, Craven P C, Drutz D J, Shelburne J, Gutman R. Fungal peritonitis in patients on chronic ambulatory peritoneal dialysis. *Ann Intern Med* 99:334–337, 1983.

Khan J A, Hussain S T, Hasan S. Disseminated *Bipolaris* infection in an immunocompetent host: an atypical presentation. *JAMA* 50:68–71, 2002.

Latham R H. *Bipolaris spicifera* meningitis complicating a neurosurgical procedure. *Scand J Infect Dis* 32:102–103, 2000.

Liu K, Howell D N, Perfect J R, Schell W A. Morphologic criteria for the preliminary identification of *Fusarium, Paecilomyces,* and *Acremonium* species by histopathology. *Am J Clin Path* 109:45–54, 1998.

MacMillan R H, III, Cooper P H, Body B A, Mills A S. Allergic fungal sinusitis due to *Curvularia lunata*. *Human Pathol* 18:960–964, 1987.

Maertens J, Lagrou K, Deweerdt H. Disseminated infection by *Scedosporium prolificans*: An emerging fatality among haematology patients. Case report and review. *Ann Hematol* 79:340–344, 2002.

Marr K A, Carter R A, Crippa R A, Wald A, Corey L. Epidemiology and outcome of mould infections in hematopoietic stem cell transplant recipients. *Clin Infect Dis* 34:909–917, 2002.

Marriott D J, Wong K H, Aznar E. *Scytalidium dimidiatum* and *Lecythophora hoffmannii*: unusual causes of fungal infections in a patient with AIDS. *J Clin Microbiol* 35:2949–2952, 1997.

Matsumoto T, Matsuda T, McGinnis M R, Ajello L. Clinical and mycological spectra of *Wangiella dermatitidis* infection. *Mycoses* 36:145–155, 1992.

McGinnis M R, Rinaldi M G, Winn R E. Emerging agents of phaeohyphomycosis: pathogenic species of *Bipolaris* and *Exserohilum*. *J Clin Microbiol* 24:250–259, 1986.

McGinnis M R, Pasarell R L, Sutton D A. In vitro evaluation of voriconazole against some clinically important fungi. *Antimicrob Agents Chemother* 41:1821–1834, 1997.

McGinnis M R, Pasarell L. In vitro evaluation of terbinafine and itraconazole against dematiaceous fungi. *Med Mycol* 36:243–246, 1998.

Meletiadis J, Mouton J W, Rodriquez-Tudela J L. In vitro interaction of terbinafine with itraconazole against clinical isolates of *Scedosporium prolificans*. *Antimicrob Agents Chemother* 44:470–472, 2000.

MMWR. *Exophiala* infection from contaminated injectable steroids prepared by a compounding pharmacy—United States, July–November, 2002. *Morbidity and Mortality Weekly Report MMWR* 51:1109–1112, 2002.

Monte S M D, Hutchens G M. Disseminated *Curvularia* infection. *Arch Path Lab Med* 109:872–874, 1985.

Morris A, Schell W A, McDonagh D, Chafee S, Perfect J R. *Fonsecaea pedrosoi* pneumonia and *Emericella nidulans* cerebral abscesses in a bone marrow transplant patient. *Clin Infect Dis* 21:1346–1348, 1995.

Morrison V A, Weisdorf D J. *Alternaria*: a sinonasal pathogen of immunocompressed hosts. *Clin Infect Dis* 16:265–270, 1993.

National Committee for Clinical Laboratory Standards V P. Reference method for broth dilution antifungal susceptibility testing of conidium-forming filamentous fungi; proposed standard. *National Committee for Clinical Laboratory Standards*, Villanova, PA :1–21, 1998.

Ndiaye B, Develoux M, Dieng M T, Kane A, Ndir O, Raphenon G, Huerre M. Current report of eumycetoma in Senegal: report of 109 cases. *J Mycol Med* 10:140–144, 2000.

Nucci M, Akiti T, Barreiros G, Silveira F, Revankar S G, Sutton D A, Patterson T F. Nosocomial fungemia due to *Exophiala jeanselmei* var. *jeanselmei* and *Rhinocladiella* species newly described causes of bloodstream infection. *J Clin Microbiol* 39:514–518, 2001.

Palaoglu S, Sau A, Yalcinlar Y, Scheithauer B W. Cerebral phaeohyphomycosis. *Neurosurg* 33:894–897, 1993.

Pauzner R, Goldschmied-Reouven A, Hay I, Vared Z, Ziskind Z, Hassin N, Farfel Z. Phaeohyphomycosis following cardiac surgery: case report and review of serious infection due to *Bipolaris* and *Exserohilum* species. *Clin Infect Dis* 25:921–923, 1997.

Perfect J R, Schell W A, Rinaldi M G. Uncommon invasive fungal pathogens in the acquired immunodeficiency syndrome. *J Med Vet Mycol* 31:175–179, 1993.

Perfect J R, Schell W A. The newer fungal opportunists are coming. *Clin Infect Dis* 22:112–118, 1996.

Perfect J R, Durack D T. Pathogenesis and management of fungal infections in the central nervous system. In: Scheld W M, Whitley R J, Durack DT eds. *Infections of the Central Nervous System*. New York: Lippincott-Raven, 721–738, 1997.

Revankar S G, Patterson J E, Sutton D A, Pullen R, Rinaldi M G. Disseminated phaeohyphomycosis: review of an emerging mycosis. *Clin Infect Dis* 34:467–476, 2002.

Rinaldi M G. Phaeohyphomycosis. *Dermatol Clin* 14:142–153, 1996.

Rohwedder J J, Simmons J L, Colfer H, Gatmaitan B. Disseminated *Curvularia lunata* infection in a football player. *Arch Intern Med* 139:940–941, 1979.

Rolston K V, Hopfer R L, Larson D L. Infections caused by *Drechslera* species: case report and review of the literature. *Rev Infect Dis* 7:525–529, 1985.

Ronan S G, Vzoaru I, Nadimpalli V, Guitart J, Manaligod J R. Primary cutaneous phaeohyphomycosis: report of seven cases. *J Cutan Pathol* 20:223–228, 1993.

Schell W A. Oculomycoses caused by dematiaceous fungi. *Proceedings of the VI International Conference on the Mycoses*. Pan American Health Organization, Washington, DC: Scientific Publication No. 470:105–109, 1986.

Schell W A. New aspects of emerging fungal pathogens. A multifaceted challenge. *Clin Lab Med* 15:365–387, 1995.

Schell W A. Agents of Chromoblastomycosis and Sporotrichosis. In: Ajello L, Hay R, eds. *Topley and Wilson's Microbiology and Microbial Infections, Vol. 4 Mycology*. London: Edward Arnold, 315–336, 1997.

Schell W A. Histopathology of fungal rhinosinusitis. *Otolaryngol Clin N Amer* 33:251–276, 2000a.

Schell W A. Unusual fungal pathogens in fungal sinusitis. *Otolarynol Clin North Amer* 33:367–373, 2000b.

Schell W A. Dematiaceous Hyphomycetes. In: Howard D H, ed. *Fungi Pathogenic for Humans and Animals*, second edition, revised and expanded. New York: Marcel Dekker, Inc: 565–636, 2003a.

Schell W A, Salkin I F, McGinnis J R. *Bipolaris, Exophiala, Scedosporium, Sporothrix* and Other Dematiaceous fungi. *In:* Murray P R, Baron E J, Jorgensen J H, Pfaller M A, Yolken R H, eds. *Manual of Clinical Microbiology*, 8th Ed. Washington DC: American Society for Microbiology: pp. 1820–1847, 2003b.

Schnitzler N, Peltroche-Llacsahuanga H, Bestier N, Zundorf J, Lutticken R, Haase G. Effect of melanin and carotenoids of *Exophiala* (*Wangiella*) *dermatitidis* on phagocytosis, oxidative burst, and killing by human neutrophils. *Infect Immun* 67:94–101, 1999.

Seaworth B J, Kwon-Chung C J, Hamilton J D, Perfect J R. Brain abscess caused by a variety of *Cladosporium trichoides*. *Am J Clin Path* 79:747–752, 1983.

Sekhon A S, Galbraith J, Mielke B W, Garg A K, Sheehan G. Cerebral phaeohyphomycosis caused by *Xylohypha bantiana*, with a review of the literature. *Eur J Epidemiol* 8:387–390, 1992.

Sharkey P K, Graybill J R, Rinaldi M G, Stevens D A, Tucker R M, Peterie J D, Hoeprich P D, Greer D L, Frenkel L, Counts G W, Goodrich J, Zellner S, Bradsher R W, van der Horst C M, Israel K, Pankey G A, Barranco C P. Itraconazole treatment of phaeohyphomycosis. *J Am Acad Dermatol* 23:577–586, 1990.

Shimosaka S, Waga S. Cerebral chromoblastomycosis complicated by meningitis and multiple fungal aneurysms after resection of a granuloma. Case Report. *J Neurosurg* 59:158–161, 1983.

Sides E H, Benson J D, Padhye A A. Phaeohyphomycotic brain abscess due to *Ochroconis gallopavum* in a patient with malignant lymphoma of a large cell type. *J Med Vet Mycol* 29:317–322, 1991.

Sigler L. Miscellaneous Opportunistic Fungi: Microascaceae and Other Ascomycetes, Hyphomycetes, Coelomycetes and Basidiomycetes. In: Howard D H, ed. *Fungi Pathogenic for Humans and Animals*, second edition, revised and expanded. New York: Marcel Dekker, Inc: 637–676, 2003.

Silveira F, Nucci M. Emergence of black moulds in fungal disease: epidemiology and therapy. *Cur Opin Infect Dis* 14:679–684, 2001.

Singh N, Chang F Y, Gayowski T, Marino I R. Infections due to dematiaceous fungi in organ transplant recipients: case report and review. *Clin Infect Dis* 24:369–374, 1997.

Sudduth E J, Crumbley A J, Farrar W E. Phaeohyphomycosis due to *Exophiala* species: clinical spectrum of disease in humans. *Clin Infect Dis* 15:639–644, 1992.

Tintelnot K, de Hoog G S, Thomas E, Steudel W I, Huebner K, Seeliger H P R. Cerebral phaeohyphomycosis caused by an *Exophiala* species. Mycoses 34:239–244, 1991.

Vartian C V, Shlaes D M, Padhye A A, Ajello L. *Wangiella dermatitidis* endocarditis in an intravenous drug user. *Am J Med* 78:703–707, 1985.

Viviani M A, Tortorano A M, Laria G, Giannetti A, Bignotti G. Two new cases of cutaneous alternariosis with a review of the literature. *Mycopathologia* 96:3–12, 1986.

Vukmir R B, Kusne S, Linden P, Pasculle W, Fothergill A W, Sheaffer J, Nieto J, Segal R, Merhav H, Martinez A J. Successful therapy for cerebral phaeohyphomycosis due to *Dactylaria gallopava* in a liver transplant recipient. *Clin Infect Dis* 19:714–719, 1994.

Walsh T J, Lutsar I, Driscoll T, Dupont B, Rhoden M, Gharamani P, Perfect J R. Voriconazole in the treatment of aspergillosis, scedosporiosis and other invasive fungal infections in children. *Pediatr Infect Dis J* 21:240–248, 2002.

Walz R, Bianchin M, Chaves M L, Cerski M R, Severo L C, Londero A T. Cerebral phaeohyphomycosis caused by *Cladophialophora bantiana* in a Brazilian drug abuser. *J Med Vet Mycol* 35:427–431, 1997.

Wang Z, Zheng L, Liu H, Wang Q, Hauser M, Kauffman S, Becker J M, Szaniszlo P J. WdChs2p, a class I chitin synthase, together with WdChs3p class III contributes to virulence in *Wangiella* (*Exophiala*) *dermatitidis*. *Infect Immun* 69:7517–7526, 2001.

Washburn R G, Kennedy D W, Begley M G, Henderson D K, Bennett J E. Chronic fungal sinusitis in apparently normal hosts. *Medicine Baltimore* 67:231–247, 1988.

Watanabe S, Hironaga M. An atypical isolate of *Scedoporium apiospermum* from a purulent meningitis in man. *Sabouraudia* 19:209–215, 1981.

Welty K E, Perfect J R. Cutaneous mycoses in solid organ transplants. *Clin Adv Treat Fungal Infect* 2:1–3, 1991.

Wiest P M, Wiese K, Jacobs M R, Morrissey A B, Abelson T I, Witt W, Lederman M M. *Alternaria* infection in a patient with acquired immune deficiency syndrome: case report and review of invasive *Alternaria* infections. *Rev Infect Dis* 9:799–803, 1987.

Yau Y C, de Nanassy J, Summerbell R C, Matlow A G, Richardson S E. Fungal sternal wound infection due to *Curvularia lunata* in a neonate with congenital heart disease: case report and review. *Clin Infect Dis* 19:735–740, 1994.

Yoo D, Lee W H S, Kwon-Chung K J. Brain abscess due to *Pseudallescheria boydii* associated with primary non-Hodgkin's lymphoma of the central nervous system: A case report and literature review. *Rev Infect Dis* 7:272–277, 1985.

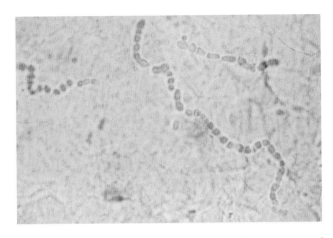

COLOR FIGURE 1–1. Unstained potassium hydroxide preparation of skin scrapings showing the presence of dermatophyte hyphae, which are fragmenting into arthrospores. (Reproduced by permission of Blackwell Science from *Slide Atlas of Fungal Infection: Superficial Fungal Infections*, MD Richardson, DW Warnock and CK Campbell, 1995.)

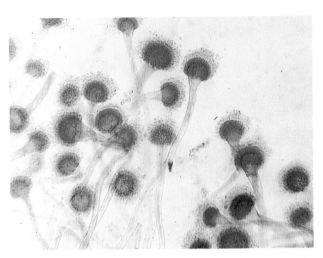

COLOR FIGURE 1–3. *Aspergillus fumigatus* conidiophores showing the characteristic pear-shaped vesicles on which are arranged a single layer of spore-producing cells termed phialides.

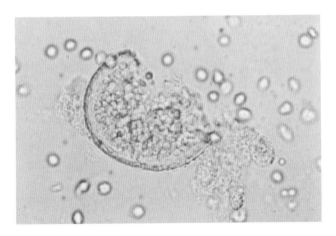

COLOR FIGURE 1–2. Unstained potassium hydroxide preparation of pus from a soft tissue abscess showing an open *Coccidioides immitis* spherule and released endospores. (Reproduced by permission of Bios Scientific Publishers from Verghese S, Arjundas D, Krishnakumari KC, Padmaja P, Elizabeth D, Padhye AA, Warnock DW. Coccidioidomycosis in India: report of a second imported case. *Med Mycol* 2002;40:307–309.)

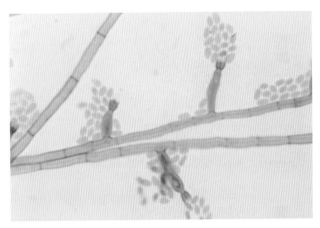

COLOR FIGURE 1–4. *Phialphora verrucosa* showing the characteristic small phialides with cup-shaped collarettes from which the conidia are being produced.

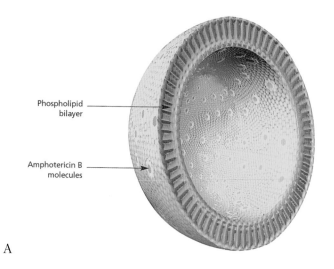

A

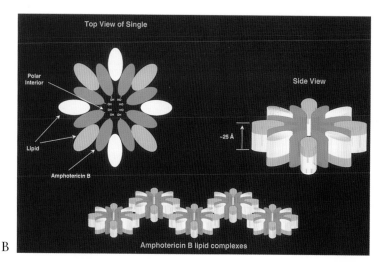

B

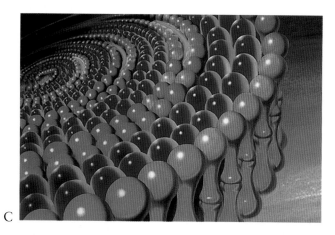

C

COLOR FIGURE 3–2. Amphotericin B lipid based formulations that have been approved by the U.S. Food & Drug Administration are represented in artistic drawings as follows: (*A*) liposomal amphotericin B (L-AmB); (*B*) amphotericin B lipid complex (ABLC); and (*C*) amphotericin B colloidal dispersion (ABCD).

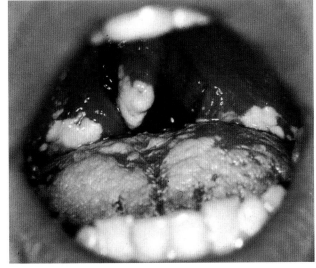

A

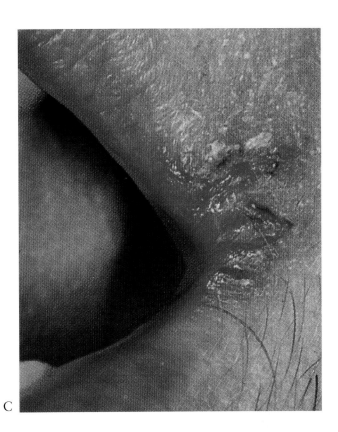

C

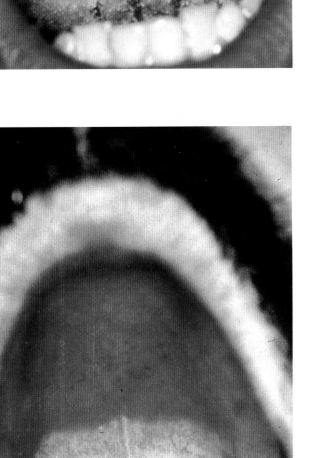

B

COLOR FIGURE 11–1. Oropharyngeal candidiasis demonstrating pseudomembranous type *(A)*, atrophic erythematous type associated with dentures *(B)*, and angular cheilitis *(C)*.

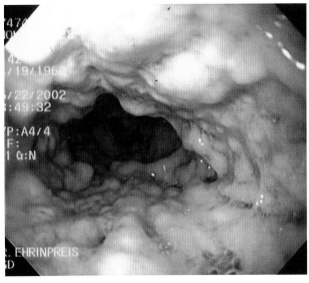

COLOR FIGURE 11–2. Type III esophageal candidiasis with confluent plaques.

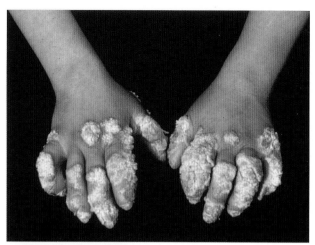

A

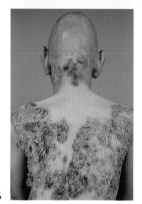

B

COLOR FIGURE 11–3. Chronic mucocutaneous candidiasis with crusting hyperkeratotic lesions on hands, trunk and scalp *(A and B)*.

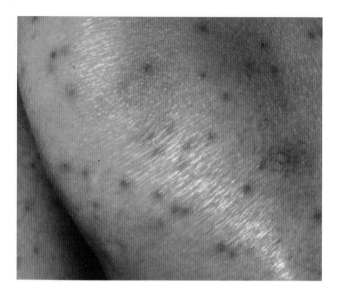

COLOR FIGURE 11–6. Metastatic papulopustular erythematous cutaneous candidiasis in a patient with leukemia.

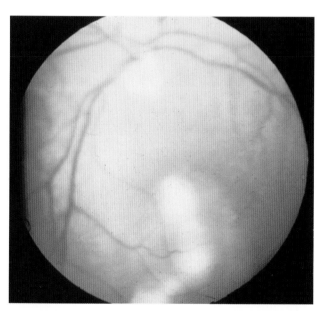

COLOR FIGURE 11–7. *Candida* chorioretinitis. Note white, cotton ball-like lesions.

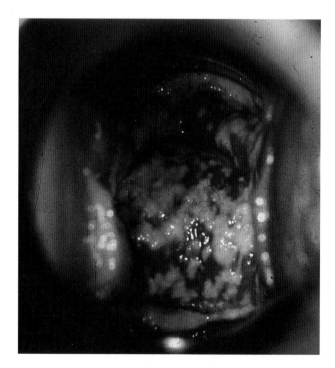

COLOR FIGURE 11–5. Vulvovaginal candidiasis with typical cottage cheese white clumpy vaginal discharge.

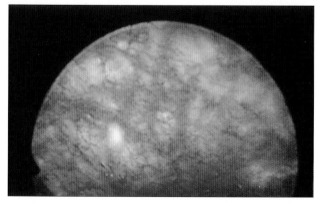

COLOR FIGURE 11–10. Snowstorm appearance of bladder in patient with cystitis due to *C. krusei*.

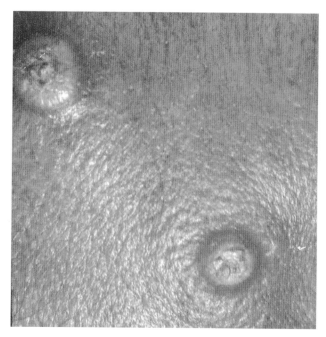

COLOR FIGURE 12–7. Molluscum contagiosum-like umbilicated papules in skin of an AIDS patient with disseminated cryptococcosis.

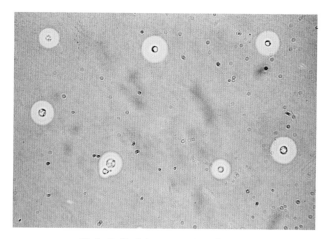

COLOR FIGURE 12–9. India ink preparation showing *Cryptococcus neoformans* in cerebrospinal fluid. Note budding yeast form and distinct outline of cell walls and surrounding capsules.

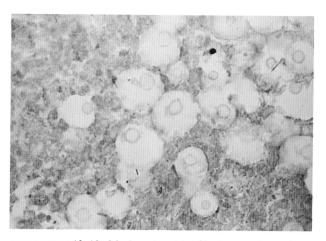

COLOR FIGURE 12–10. Mucicarmine stain of brain parenchyma showing numerous, densely-packed encapsulated cryptococci. Note variable size of capsule.

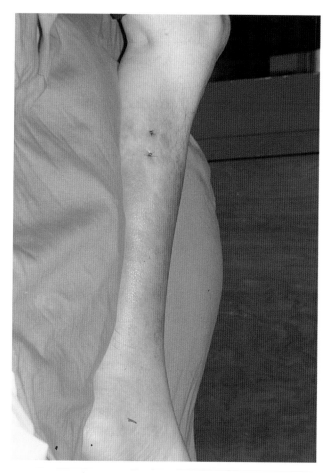

COLOR FIGURE 12–8. Cryptococcal cellulitis in corticosteroid treated renal transplant patient. Skin disease resembles Group A streptococcal cellulitis in appearance but has a more indolent course.

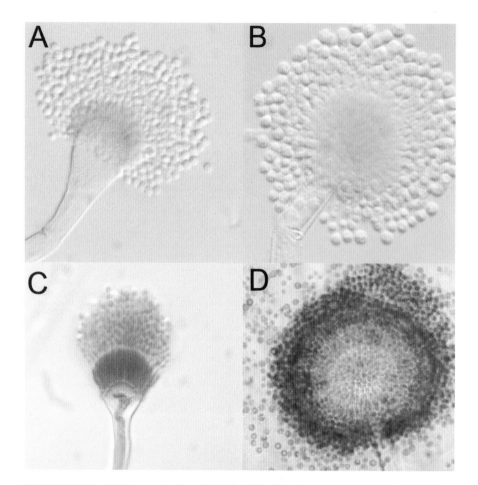

COLOR FIGURE 14–1. Microscopic characteristics of *Aspergillus* species fruiting structures. *(A) Aspergillus fumigatus; (B) Aspergillus flavus; (C) Aspergillus terreus; (D) Aspergillus niger.* (All magnifications 420×; photomicrographs kindly provided by Deanna Sutton.)

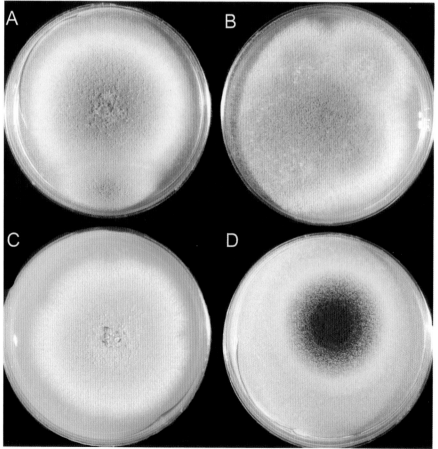

COLOR FIGURE 14–2. Colony morphology of *Aspergillus* species. *(A) Aspergillus fumigatus; (B) Aspergillus flavus; (C) Aspergillus terreus; (D) Aspergillus niger.* (Colony photographs kindly provided by Deanna Sutton.)

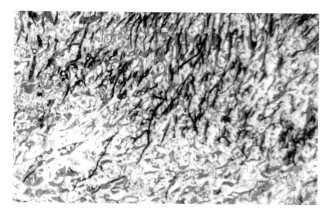

COLOR FIGURE 14–7. Lung tissue section showing thin, acutely branching hyphae on Gomori methenamine silver stain in patient with invasive pulmonary aspergillosis. (Original magnification ×420.)

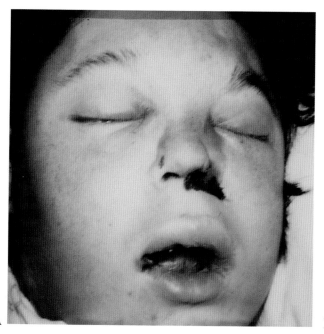

A

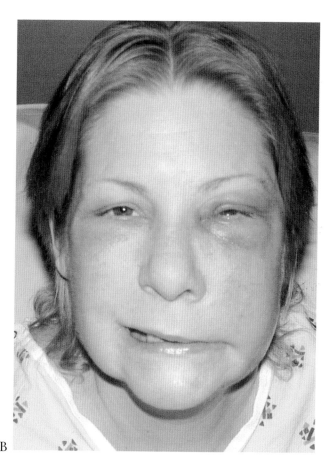

B

COLOR FIGURE 15–2. Rhinocerebral mucormycosis. (A) Pregnant patient with diabetic ketoacidosis. Note bilateral swelling and infarcted skin of nose and infranasal tissue. She also had naso-palatal fistula and gangrenous ulcer of palate. Patient died. (B) Patient with diabetic ketoacidosis. Note swelling, erythema, proptosis, ptosis, and peripheral left facial nerve palsy. Patient survived with aggressive medical–surgical therapy.

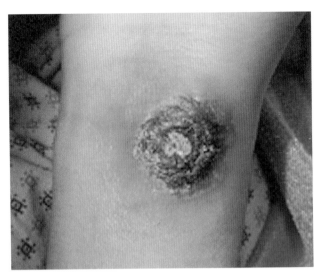

COLOR FIGURE 15–3. Cutaneous lesion (painful ulcer covered by black eschar surrounded by erythema) as manifestation of disseminated mucormycosis in patient with refractory leukemia. (Courtesy of Dimitrios P. Kontoyiannis.)

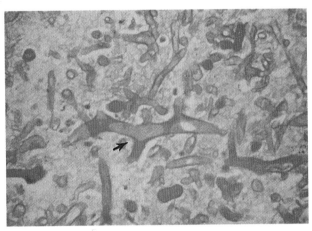

COLOR FIGURE 15–4. Periodic-acid Schiff stain of excised necrotic tissue from sinus. Note wide, ribbon-like, aseptate hyphae, branching at right angles, characteristic of Mucorales.

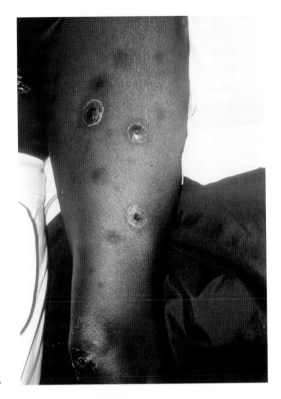

A

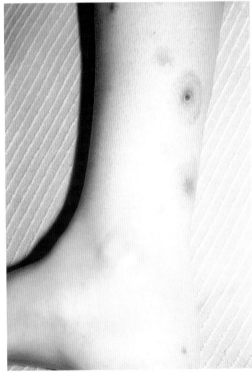

B

COLOR FIGURE 16–1. Characteristic skin lesions of disseminated fusariosis in neutropenic patients with hematological malignancies. Patients have tender subcutaneous nodules (A), macules or papules simultaneously showing various stages of evolution, and progressive central necrosis (B).

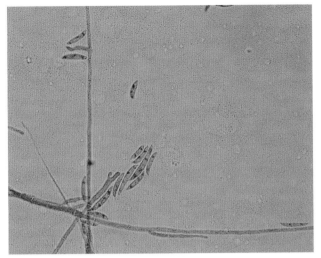

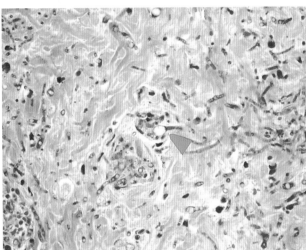

COLOR FIGURE 16–2. Microscopic features of *Fusarium* species show-ing (*A*) characteristic canoe-shaped morphology of the macroconidia (Lactophenol cotton blue stain; ×400), and (*B*) presence of chla-dmydospores in subcutaneous tissue (hematoxylin-eosin; ×400).

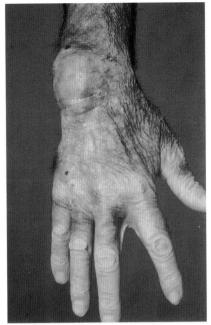

A

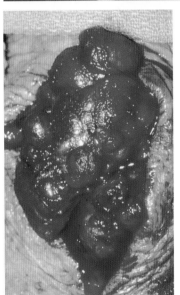

B

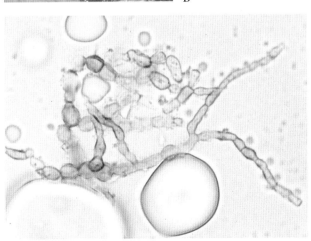

C

COLOR FIGURE 17–1. *(A)* Patient receiving long-term corticosteroid therapy developed cystic mass on dorsum of wrist; *(B)* exposure of the multiple cystic structures before surgical removal; *(C)* KOH preparation of cyst contents showing pigmented fungus, *Exophiala jeanselmei.*

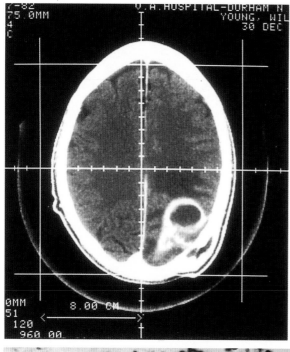

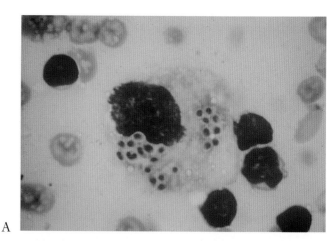

A

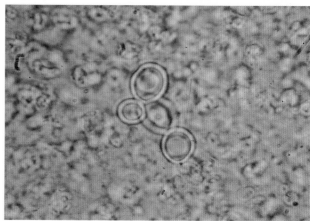

B

COLOR FIGURE 18–2. Yeast phase of *Histoplasma*. (*A*) Smear of lung biopsy specimen stained with Giemsa stain showing 2–4 μm yeasts within an alveolar macrophage, typical of *H. capsulatum* var. capsulatum; (*B*) KOH preparation of an aspirate taken from an abscess in bone showing large, thick-walled yeast forms typical of *H. capsulatum* var. *duboisii*.

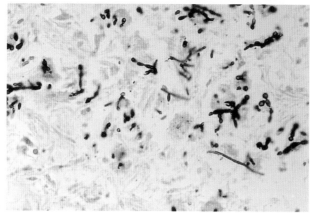

B

COLOR FIGURE 17–2. (*A*) An apparently normal patient with a visual field defect secondary to an occipital brain abscess shown on CT scan; (*B*) brain biopsy of lesion stained with hematoxylin-eosin shows pigmented fungal structures with both hyphal and yeast-like forms.

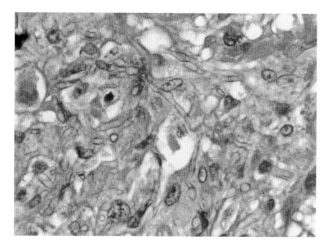

COLOR FIGURE 17–3. *Cladophialophora bantiana* in brain tissue (H and E stain).

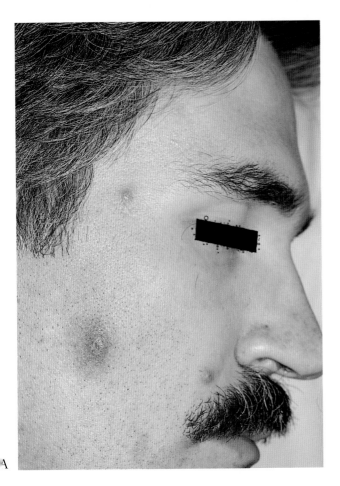

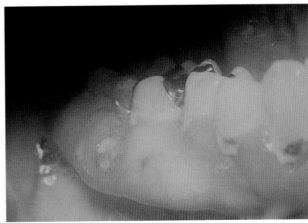

COLOR FIGURE 18–12. Painful, slowly enlarging gingival ulcer that was present for 4 months in an elderly man who had chronic progressive histoplasmosis.

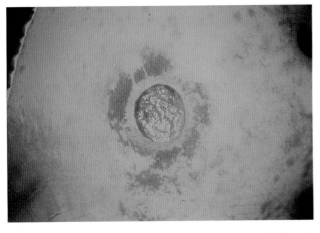

COLOR FIGURE 18–11. Skin lesions noted in patients with disseminated histoplasmosis (A) multiple papulopustules which appeared over the face and chest in a patient with HIV infection; (B) chronic ulcer on the thigh in an elderly man with chronic progressive disseminated histoplasmosis.

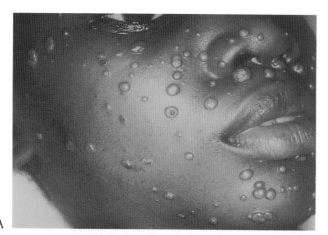

A

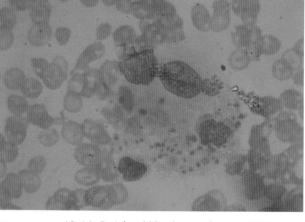

COLOR FIGURE 18–16. Peripheral blood smear from an AIDS patient who was severely ill with disseminated histoplasmosis; within neutrophils are seen multiple tiny yeasts typical of *H. capsulatum*.

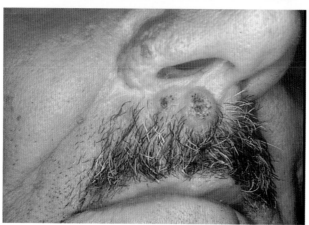

B

COLOR FIGURE 18–15. (*A*) Numerous molluscum-type skin lesions that appeared on the face of an African child with disseminated infection due to *H. duboisii*. (*B*) Solitary skin lesion typical of those seen with *H. duboisii*.

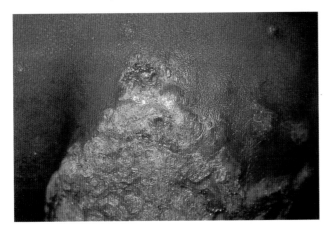

COLOR FIGURE 19-7. Verrucous lesion with subcutaneous abscesses on buttock caused by *B. dermatitidis*.

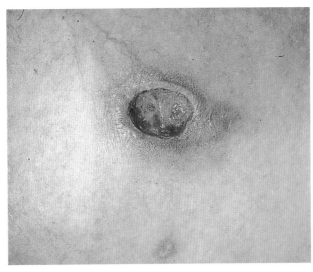

COLOR FIGURE 19-10. Ulcerative lesion on breast caused by *B. dermatitidis*. Note distinct and raised borders.

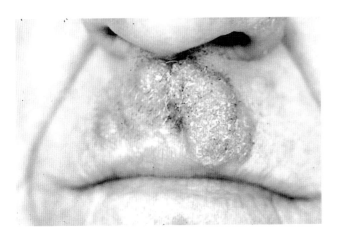

COLOR FIGURE 19-8. Verrucous lesion on upper lip due to *B. dermatitidis*. Note crusted, heaped-up, warty appearance and microabscesses manifested by black dots, peripherally located.

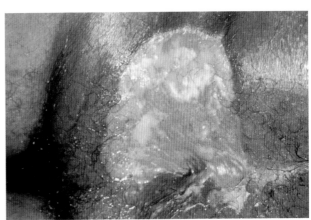

COLOR FIGURE 19-11. Extensive perirectal ulcerative lesion with overlying exudate in patient with multiorgan blastomycosis.

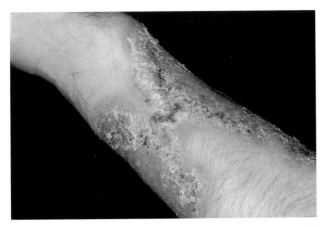

COLOR FIGURE 19-9. Healing verrucous lesion on arm in patient with pulmonary and cutaneous blastomycosis.

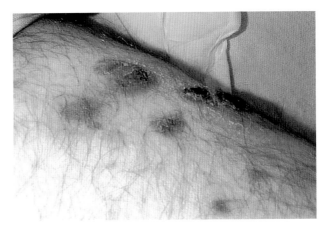

COLOR FIGURE 19-12. Blastomycotic subcutaneous nodules with superficial crusts on upper leg.

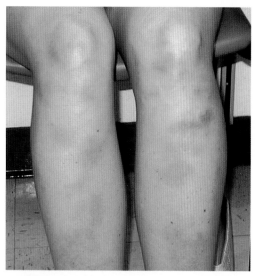

A

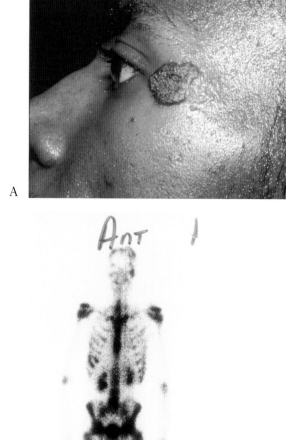

A

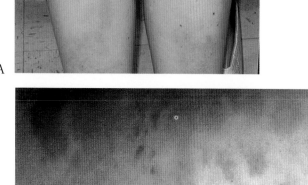

B

COLOR FIGURE 20–3. Erythema nodosum (A) and erythema multiforme (B) in patients with primary coccidioidal pneumonia.

B

COLOR FIGURE 20–8. Disseminated coccidioidomycosis in African American male: (A) verrucous skin lesion on face and (B) bone scan showing extensive disease involving shoulders, knees, ribs, vertebra, and pelvis.

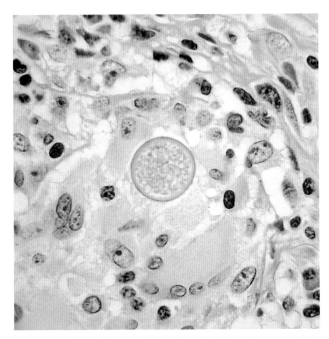

COLOR FIGURE 20–9. Hematoxylin-eosin stain of lung tissue containing coccidioidal spherule. Note surrounding inflammatory cells.

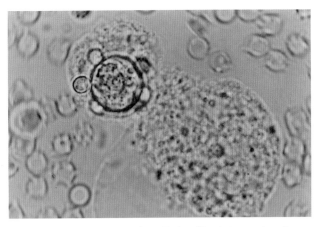

COLOR FIGURE 21–3. Macrophage-*P. brasiliensis* interaction. Ingestion of a multiple-budding yeast cell by a pseudopod (100×).

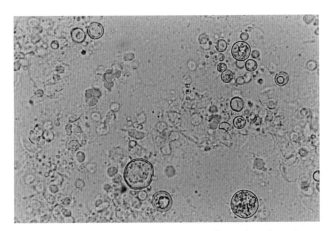

COLOR FIGURE 21–1. *P. brasiliensis* yeast cells in clinical specimen. Note round shape, thick refractile cell wall, intracytoplasmic vacuoles and differences in the size of yeast cells (40×).

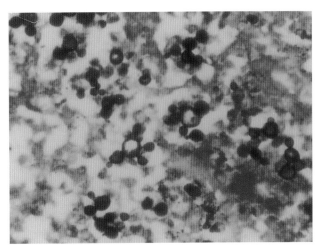

COLOR FIGURE 21–10. *P. brasiliensis* multiple budding yeast cells in a biopsy specimen. H and E plus Gomori methenamine-silver stain (40×).

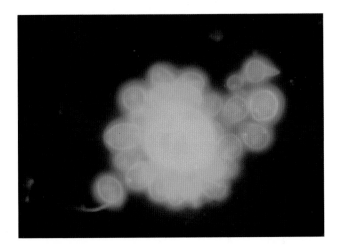

COLOR FIGURE 21–2. *P. brasiliensis* yeast cells from a 36°C culture. Note large mother cell with multiple buds. Calcofluor white (100×).

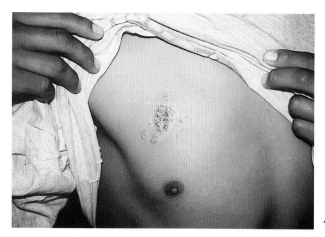

COLOR FIGURE 22–1. Plaque-like lesion due to *S. schenckii* on the anterior chest wall of an 18-year-old man.

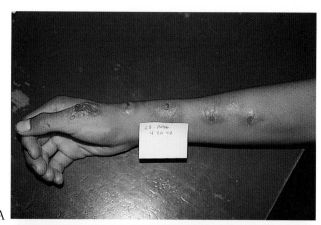

A

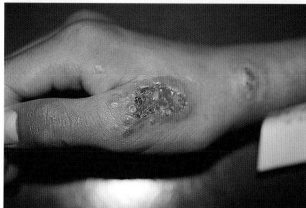

B

COLOR FIGURE 22–3. (*A*) Characteristic lesions of lymphonodular sporotrichosis involving the forearm in a 45-year-old man. (*B*) Primary lesion, which had become an ulcerated subcutaneous nodule.

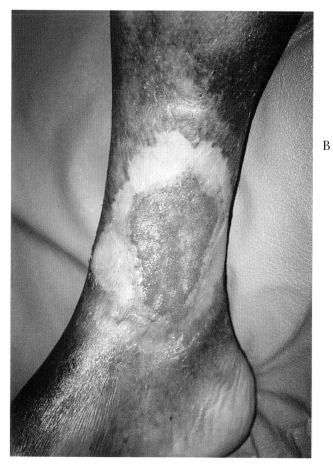

COLOR FIGURE 22–2. Fixed, chronic ulcerative lesion of sporotrichosis in a 58-year-old woman. The lesion had been present for 18 months.

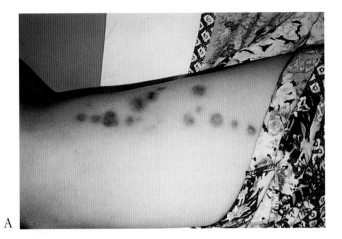

A

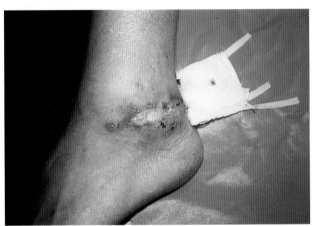

B

COLOR FIGURE 22–4. (*A*) Hyperpigmented lymphonodular sporotrichosis in a 28-year-old Peruvian woman. (*B*) Primary lesion for the patient in Figure 4A, a chronic ulceration overlying the lateral malleolus.

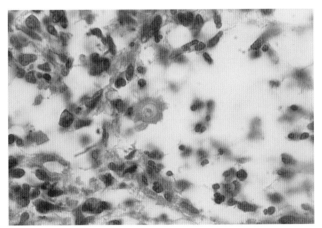

COLOR FIGURE 22–6. An asteroid body seen on H and E stain of tissue biopsy in patient with cutaneous sporotrichosis.

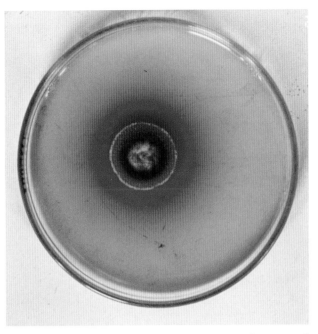

COLOR FIGURE 23–1. Mycelial (mould) form of *Penicillium marneffei* plated on Sabouraud dextrose agar and incubated for 5 days at 25°C, exhibiting soluble red pigment that has diffused into the medium.

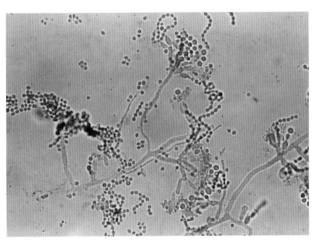

COLOR FIGURE 23–2. Photomicrograph of the mycelial (mould) form of *Penicillium marneffei* grown on Sabouraud dextrose agar at 25°C. Note the hyaline, septate, branched hyphae with branched conidiophores, or penicilli, and terminal conidia (magnification, ×600).

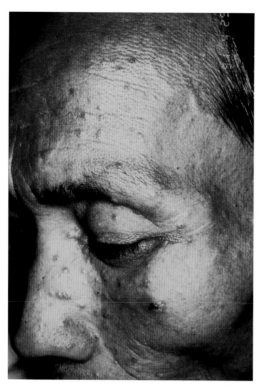

COLOR FIGURE 23–3. Patient with disseminated penicilliosis and small papular skin lesions with umbilication and early central necrosis.

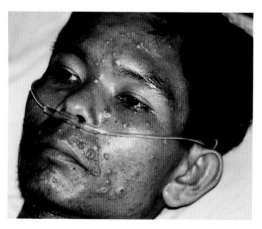

COLOR FIGURE 23–4. Patient with disseminated penicilliosis and papulo-umbilicated skin lesions of varying sizes.

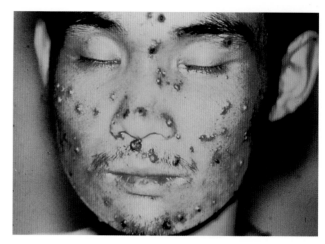

COLOR FIGURE 23–5. Patient with disseminated penicilliosis and papulonecrotic skin lesions.

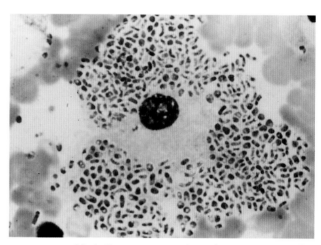

COLOR FIGURE 23–6. Bone marrow aspirate showing numerous basophilic bipolar intracellular and extracellular *P. marneffei* organisms. The organisms divide by fission (schizogony) and are 3–8 μm in diameter (Wright stain, ×400).

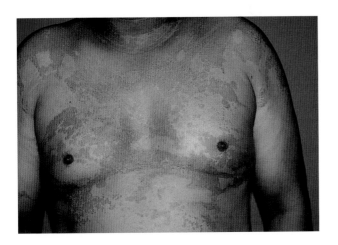

COLOR FIGURE 24–1. Typical appearance of tinea (pityriasis) versicolor.

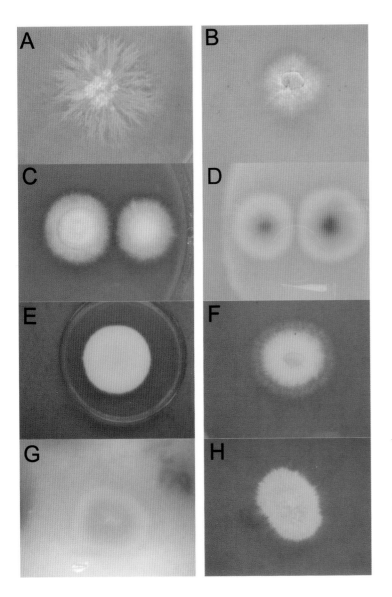

COLOR FIGURE 24–3. Typical colonial morphology of some common dermatophytes grown on potato dextrose agar at 30°C. *(A) M. canis; (B) E. floccosum; (C) T. rubrum* front view; *(D) T. rubrum* reverse view; *(E) T. mentagrophytes* var *interdigitale; (F) T. mentagrophytes* var *mentagrophytes; (G) T. tonsurans;* and *(H) M. gypseum.*

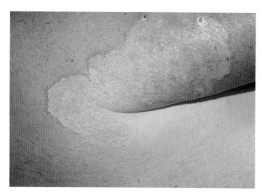

COLOR FIGURE 24–4. Tinea corporis on patient's upper arm and back demonstrating a well-demarcated plaque with slight scale typical of this infection.

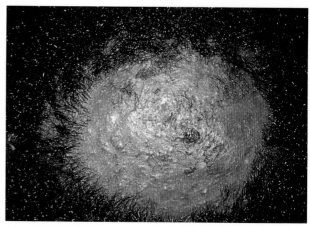

COLOR FIGURE 24–7. Inflammatory tinea capitis.

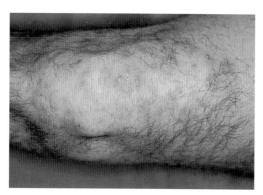

COLOR FIGURE 24–5. Majocchi's granuloma on the leg.

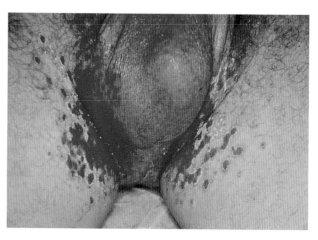

COLOR FIGURE 24–8. Candidal intertrigo. Note the bright red appearance, satellite lesions, and scrotal involvement.

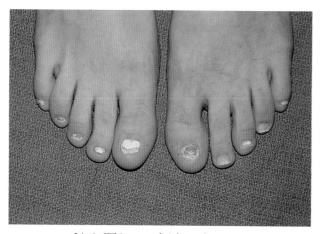

COLOR FIGURE 24–6. White superficial onychomycosis.

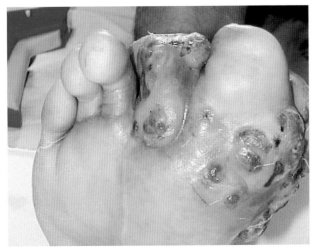

COLOR FIGURE 25–1. Foot eumycetoma caused by *Madurella myce-tomatis*.

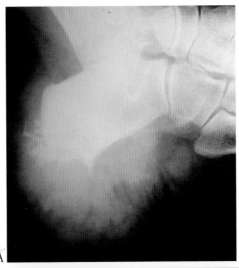

A

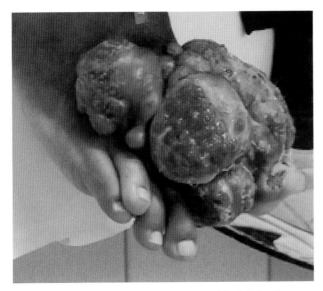

COLOR FIGURE 25–2. Foot eumycetoma caused by *Madurella myce-tomatis*.

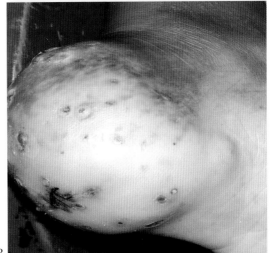

B

COLOR FIGURE 25–3. *(A)* Radiograph and *(B)* photo of a heel eu-mycetoma caused by *Madurella mycetomatis*, showing soft tissue swelling and osteolytic bone changes.

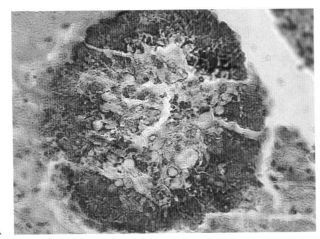

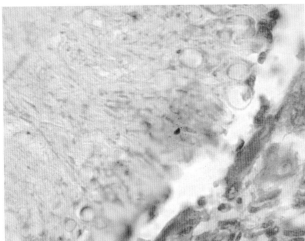

COLOR FIGURE 25–4. (A) Grain of *Madurella mycetomatis* (HE ×400). (B) Hyphae and peripheral chlamydoconidias in a grain (HE ×1000).

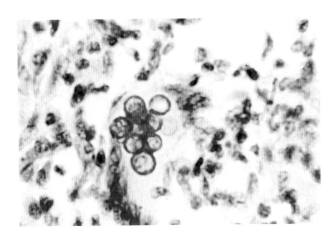

COLOR FIGURE 26–1. Hematoxylin-eosin stained tissue section showing sclerotic bodies (muriform cells) typical of chromoblastomycosis. (Courtesy of David W. Warnock.)

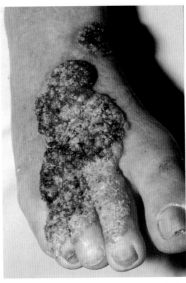

COLOR FIGURE 26–2. Nodular, cauliflower-like lesions of chromoblastomycosis in a patient from Brazil. (Courtesy of F. de Queiroz-Telles.)

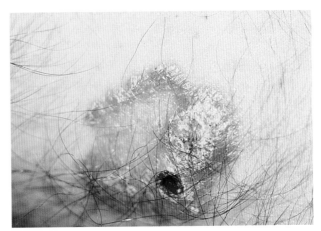

COLOR FIGURE 26–3. Plaque lesion of chromoblastomycosis of the arm in a farmer.

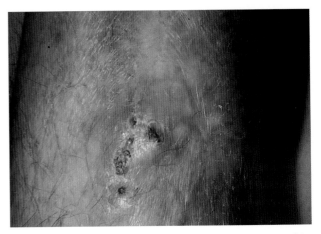

COLOR FIGURE 26–4. Cicatricial lesion of chromoblastomycosis of the leg with atrophic scarring.

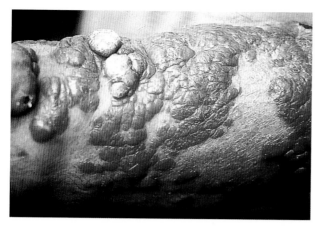

COLOR FIGURE 28–1. Multiple nodular, plaque-like lesions of the leg in a Peruvian patient with lobomycosis (Courtesy of Beatriz Bustamante).

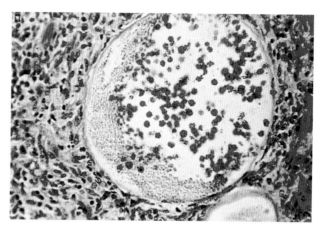

COLOR FIGURE 28–4. Hematoxylin-eosin stained section of nasal tissue demonstrating a sporangium of *Rhinosporidium seeberi*, containing numerous spores (Courtesy of David W. Warnock).

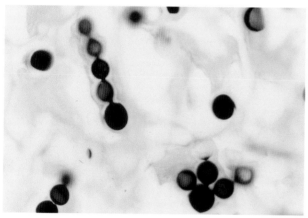

COLOR FIGURE 28–2. Gomori-methenamine silver stain showing characteristic chains of *L. loboi* cells and multiple buds (Courtesy of David W. Warnock).

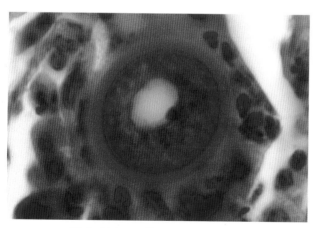

COLOR FIGURE 28–3. Hematoxylin-eosin stained section of lung tissue showing an adiaspore of *Emmonsia parva var. crescens* (Courtesy of David W. Warnock).

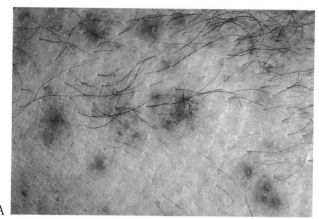

A

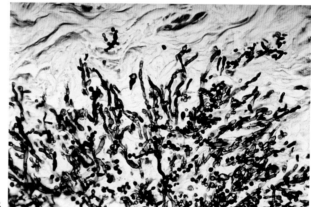

B

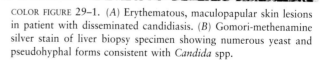

COLOR FIGURE 29–1. (*A*) Erythematous, maculopapular skin lesions in patient with disseminated candidiasis. (*B*) Gomori-methenamine silver stain of liver biopsy specimen showing numerous yeast and pseudohyphal forms consistent with *Candida* spp.

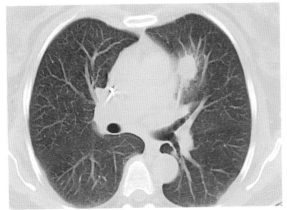

Day +8 post HSCT
T =38.6 C; ANC = 16

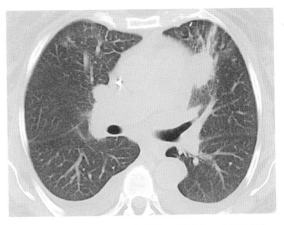

Day +18 post HSCT; ANC = 19,266

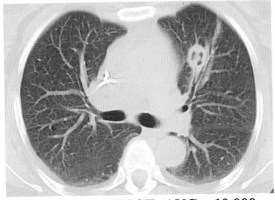

Day +38 post HSCT; ANC = 10,000

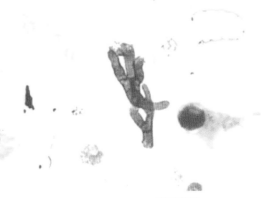

Day +15 post HSCT

COLOR FIGURE 29–3. Chest CT showing various manifestations of invasive pulmonary aspergillosis in neutropenic HSCT patient: (A)Nodular mass with "halo" sign—Day #8; (B) Enlarging mass with extension—Day #18; (C) Cavitary mass—smaller in size after therapy—Day #38; (D) BAL washings showing septate hyphae with dichotomous branching consistent with *Aspergillus* spp. HSCT = hematopoietic stem cell transplant; ANC = absolute neutrophil count.

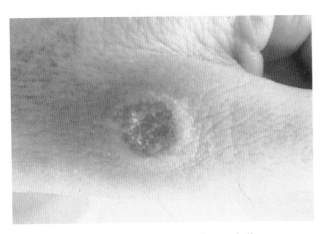

COLOR FIGURE 29–4. Nodular cutaneous lesion (bulls-eye appearance) of disseminated fusariosis.

V

MYCOSES CAUSED BY DIMORPHIC FUNGI

18

Histoplasmosis

CAROL A. KAUFFMAN

Histoplasmosis, the most common endemic mycosis in the United States, is caused by *Histoplasma capsulatum* var. *capsulatum*. *Histoplasma capsulatum* var. *duboisii* causes African histoplasmosis, which has different clinical manifestations. *Histoplasma capsulatum* is a thermally dimorphic fungus; in the environment and at temperatures below 35°C, it exists as a mould, and in tissues and at 35°–37°C, as a yeast. In the endemic area, along the Mississippi and Ohio River valleys in the United States, most persons are infected in childhood. The primary site of infection is the lungs following inhalation of the conidia from the environment. The severity of disease is related to the number of conidia inhaled and the immune response of the host; the primary host defense mechanism against *H. capsulatum* is cell-mediated immunity. Pulmonary infection is asymptomatic or only mildly symptomatic in most persons who have been infected; acute severe pneumonia and chronic progressive pulmonary infection also can occur. Asymptomatic dissemination of *H. capsulatum* to the organs of the reticuloendothelial system occurs in most infected individuals; however, symptomatic acute or chronic disseminated histoplasmosis, which is a life-threatening infection, occurs almost entirely in persons who have deficient cell-mediated immunity. Antifungal therapy is highly effective. For most patients with histoplasmosis, itraconazole, a triazole drug, is the treatment of choice.

ORGANISM

Histoplasmosis was first described and the organism given its name in 1904 by Samuel Darling, a physician working at the Canal Zone Hospital in Panama. He erroneously thought the organism, which in tissues resembled *Leishmania*, was a parasite. Within a few years it became clear that this organism was indeed a fungus. Several decades later it was shown that *H. capsulatum* was a thermally dimorphic fungus, and by 1949, an environmental reservoir for *H. capsulatum* had been proved by Emmons.

There are two varieties of *H. capsulatum* that are

pathogenic for humans, *H. capsulatum* var. *capsulatum* and *H. capsulatum* var. *duboisii*, which will mate in the laboratory and thus have been assigned varietal, rather than species status. At 25°–30°C, the organism exists in the mycelial form; the colony is white to tan in color. The aerial hyphae produce two types of conidia: macroconidia (tuberculate conidia) are thick-walled, 8–15 μm in diameter, and have distinctive projections on their surfaces, and microconidia are smooth-walled, 2–4 μm in diameter, and are the infectious form (Fig. 18–1). *H. capsulatum* var. *capsulatum* and *H. capsulatum* var. *duboisii* are indistinguishable in the mycelial phase.

At 37°C in tissues and in vitro, the organism undergoes transformation to the yeast phase. In vitro, the colony is cream-colored and becomes more gray with age. In the yeast phase in tissues, the two varieties of *H. capsulatum* differ in their appearance. *H. capsulatum* var. *capsulatum* appears as tiny 2–4 μm oval budding yeasts often found inside macrophages (See Color Fig. 18–2a in separate color insert). *Histoplasma capsulatum* var. *duboisii* is larger, 8–15 μm, thick-walled, may appear as short chains in tissues, and shows the "scar" from which its bud has been released at one end (Schwarz, 1970) (Fig. 18–2b).

In addition to the above two human pathogens, there is a third variety, *Histoplasma capsulatum* var. *farciminosum*, which is a pathogen of horses and mules. This organism causes lymphangitis in equines from the Middle East, northern Africa, central and southern Europe, Japan, the Philippines, and southern Asia (Gabal et al, 1983). The disease is characterized by multifocal suppurative lymphangitis and ulcerated cutaneous lesions that usually affect the head and forequarters; mucous membranes of the nares and oropharynx can also become ulcerated. Systemic infection does not occur.

In this chapter, *H. capsulatum* var. *capsulatum* is referred to simply as *H. capsulatum* and *H. capsulatum* var. *duboisii* as *H. duboisii*. Most of the chapter focuses on *H. capsulatum*, with additional comments, when relevant, regarding infection due to *H. duboisii*, which causes African histoplasmosis.

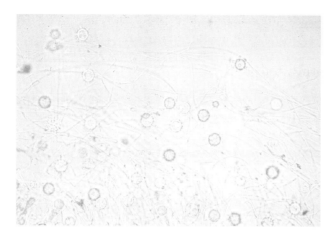

FIGURE 18–1. Mycelial phase of *H. capsulatum* grown at 25°C showing mostly tuberculate macroconidia and a few smaller microconidia.

ECOLOGY AND EPIDEMIOLOGY

Histoplasmosis occurs throughout the world, but is most common in North and Central America. Isolated cases have been reported from Southeast Asia and Africa and cases imported from endemic areas have been noted worldwide. In the United States, *H. capsulatum* is endemic in the Mississippi and Ohio River valleys and also exists in localized areas in many mideastern states (Fig. 18–3).

In the environment, *H. capsulatum* appears to have precise growth requirements related to humidity, acidity, temperature, and nitrogen content, but all of the specific conditions needed for growth in the soil have not been completely elucidated. What is known, however, is that soil containing large amounts of droppings from birds or bats supports luxuriant mycelial growth (Cano and Hajjeh, 2001). The soil under blackbird

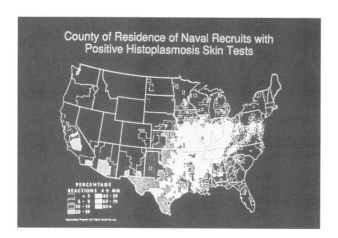

FIGURE 18–3. Histoplasmin reactivity in the continental United States among 275,558 white male naval recruits, ages 17–21 years (Edwards et al, 1969).

roosts and around chicken coops is especially likely to harbor *H. capsulatum* (Chick et al, 1981). Birds themselves are not infected with *H. capsulatum*, but can transiently carry the organism on beaks and feet and contribute to its spread. Once contaminated, soil yields *H. capsulatum* for many years after birds no longer roost in the area. Bats, in contradistinction to birds, can become infected with *H. capsulatum* and excrete the organism in their feces (Schwarz, 1981). Intestinal carriage by bats and their migratory patterns help to ensure expansion of geographic areas yielding *H. capsulatum*.

Infection with *H. capsulatum* results from passive exposure that occurs during typical day-to-day activities or from active exposure related to occupational or recreational activities. Most cases are sporadic, related to passive exposure, and not associated with a known source. Every year hundreds of thousands of individuals in the United States are infected with *H. capsulatum*; most of these individuals are not aware of this event. The two largest outbreaks ever reported were both associated with passive exposure of hundreds of thousands of people to *H. capsulatum* during urban construction projects in Indianapolis (Wheat et al, 1981; Sathapatayavongs et al, 1983; Wheat, 1997a). In other outbreaks, workers became infected after involvement in specific activities, such as cleaning bird or bat guano from bridges or heavy equipment or tearing down or cleaning out old buildings, especially chicken coops (Waldman et al, 1983; Jones et al, 1999). Other outbreaks have been associated with recreational pursuits, such as spelunking (Lottenberg et al, 1979), and ecological volunteer efforts (Brodsky et al, 1973).

The AIDS epidemic has had a significant effect on the epidemiology of histoplasmosis in the highly endemic areas. In the early 1990s in Kansas City, the rates of histoplasmosis in AIDS patients were as high as 12/100 patient-years, and in Houston were as high as 10/1000 AIDS patients (Dupont et al, 2000). This has decreased markedly with improved antiretroviral therapy. Currently most cases of histoplasmosis in AIDS patients are seen in those who have not received therapy for HIV infection, and in many cases, histoplasmosis is the AIDS-defining illness.

Histoplasma duboisii is more restricted in its geography, and occurs only in Africa between the Tropic of Cancer and the Tropic of Capricorn. Within these boundaries, most cases occur in Nigeria, Mali, Senegal, and Zaire; the disease has not been reported in East Africa. The exact ecological niche the organism occupies has not been determined, but cases have been described in association with bat guano (Schwarz, 1970; Gugnani et al, 1994). Cases of African histoplasmosis reported outside the endemic area have all been among African immigrants or travelers to other countries

(Shore et al, 1981, Nethercott et al, 1978). Although not common, *H. duboisii* has been reported to cause disseminated infection in patients with HIV infection (Manfredi et al, 1994).

PATHOGENESIS

The microcondia of the mycelial phase of *H. capsulatum* are 2–4 μm, a size that allows them to be easily aerosolized and inhaled into the alveoli of the host. At 37°C, the organism undergoes transformation to the yeast phase from the mycelial phase. Phagocytosis of either form (conidia or yeast) by alveolar macrophages and neutrophils occurs through binding of the organism to the CD18 family of adhesion promoting glycoproteins (Bullock and Wright, 1987). The yeast form of *H. capsulatum* is uniquely able to survive within the phagolysosomes of macrophages through several mechanisms, including the ability to resist killing by toxic oxygen radicals and to modulate the intraphagosomal pH (Fleischman et al, 1990; Eissenberg et al, 1993; Newman, 2001; Woods et al, 2001). Iron and calcium acquisition by the yeast are important survival tools, allowing growth within the macrophage (Woods et al, 2001). Surviving within the macrophage, *H. capsulatum* is transported to the hilar and mediastinal lymph nodes and subsequently disseminates hematogenously throughout the reticuloendothelial system in most cases of histoplasmosis.

Finally, after several weeks, specific T-cell immunity develops, macrophages become activated, and then killing of the organism ensues (Newman, 2001). At this point, long-lasting immunity to *H. capsulatum* occurs. Experimental animal models show the importance of CD4 cells in developing specific immunity to *H. capsulatum* (Deepe, 1988). Interferon-gamma produced by CD4 cells is probably the most important factor for activation of macrophages, but other cytokines (IL-12, TNF-alpha, GM-CSF) appear to also play a role, at least in the murine system (Newman, 2001). The clinical corollary in humans to the studies in the murine model is that most patients with severe infection with *H. capsulatum* are those with cellular immune deficiencies, especially those who have advanced HIV infection and low CD4 counts (Wheat, 1996; McKinsey et al, 1997). Of all the human mycoses, histoplasmosis appears to be the most pure example of the pivotal importance of the cell-mediated immune system in limiting the infection.

The extent of disease is determined both by the immune response of the host and the number of conidia that are inhaled. A healthy individual can develop severe life-threatening pulmonary infection if a large number of conidia are inhaled. This might occur during demolition or renovations on old buildings or as a result of spelunking in a heavily infested cave. Conversely, a small inoculum can cause severe pulmonary infection or progress to acute symptomatic disseminated histoplasmosis in a host whose cell-mediated immune system is unable to contain the organism.

Most persons who have been infected have asymptomatic dissemination; only rarely will this lead to symptomatic acute or chronic disseminated histoplasmosis (Schwarz, 1981). However, because dissemination is the rule, latent infection probably persists for a lifetime and reactivation can result if the host becomes immunosuppressed, presumably the mechanism by which persons who were born in the endemic area and had not returned for years develop histoplasmosis years later (Kauffman et al, 1978; Hajjeh, 1995).

Although uncommon, reinfection histoplasmosis can occur in persons who previously were infected (Dean et al, 1978), and is described most often after exposure to a heavily contaminated point source. Reinfection histoplasmosis is usually less severe than primary infection because there is residual immunity induced by the initial episode.

CLINICAL MANIFESTATIONS (TABLE 18–1)

Acute Pulmonary Histoplasmosis

The usual result of exposure of a normal host to *H. capsulatum* is asymptomatic infection. Depending on the endemic area, anywhere from 50%–85% of adults have been infected with *H. capsulatum*, and most have not had symptoms that were attributed to histoplasmosis. Symptomatic acute pulmonary histoplasmosis is most often manifested as a self-limited illness characterized by dry cough, fever, and fatigue. Approximately 5% of patients will develop erythema nodosum (Ozols and Wheat, 1981) and 5%–10% will develop myalgias and arthralgias/arthritis (Rosenthal et al, 1983). Joint involvement is usually polyarticular and symmetrical.

TABLE 18–1. *Classification of Clinical Manifestations of Histoplasmosis*

Acute pulmonary
  Sporadic
  Epidemic
Chronic cavitary pulmonary
Complications of pulmonary histoplasmosis
  Mediastinal granuloma
  Fibrosing mediastinitis
  Broncholithiasis
  Pericarditis
Disseminated
  Acute
  Chronic progressive
  Endocarditis
Focal organ system involvement
  Central nervous system
  Other organ systems

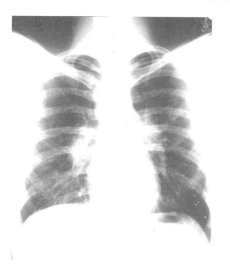

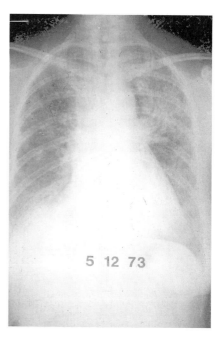

FIGURE 18–4. Acute pulmonary histoplasmosis. Note hilar adenopathy and mild lower lobe patchy pneumonitis.

FIGURE 18–5. Acute pulmonary histoplasmosis occurring in a kidney transplant recipient. Diffuse pulmonary infiltrates are present and the patient was markedly hypoxemic.

Chest radiographs usually show a patchy pneumonitis in one or more lobes often accompanied by hilar or mediastinal lymphadenopathy (Goodwin et al, 1981) (Fig. 18–4). Some patients have only hilar lymphadenopathy; when this is accompanied by arthralgias and erythema nodosum, the clinical picture mimics sarcoidosis (Thornberry et al, 1982). Improvement in several weeks is typical, but in some individuals fatigue may linger for months. Joint symptoms, when present, usually resolve over several weeks in response to antiinflammatory therapy.

Acute pulmonary histoplasmosis in patients who have cell-mediated immune defects is more severe than in normal hosts. Prostration, fever, chills, and sweats are prominent; marked dyspnea and hypoxemia can progress quickly to adult respiratory distress syndrome. Chest radiographs show diffuse bilateral infiltrates (Fig. 18–5).

When a person is exposed to a heavy inoculum of *H. capsulatum*, acute severe pulmonary infection, often termed epidemic histoplasmosis, can ensue (Goodwin et al, 1981; Cano and Hajjeh, 2001). Symptoms include high fever, chills, fatigue, dyspnea, cough, and chest pain. Acute respiratory failure and death may ensue. Chest radiographs show diffuse reticulonodular pulmonary infiltrates; mediastinal lymphadenopathy may or may not be present (Fig. 18–6). Most patients recover without treatment, but recovery is slow and most physicians prescribe an antifungal agent to hasten recovery. Over the ensuing months to years following resolution of the pneumonia, calcified nodules may develop throughout the lung fields (Gurney and Conces, 1996) (Fig. 18–7).

If a physician sees several cases that appear to be similar and that share a possible exposure or if the pa-

tient recounts that several of his or her associates have a similar illness, then the possibility of a fungal etiology is more likely to be entertained. Sporadic cases almost always are initially thought to be due to one of the usual causes of community-acquired pneumonia. Only after the patient fails to respond to several courses of antibiotics is the possibility of a fungal pneumonia raised. A history of activities in an endemic area likely to lead to exposure to *H. capsulatum* several weeks

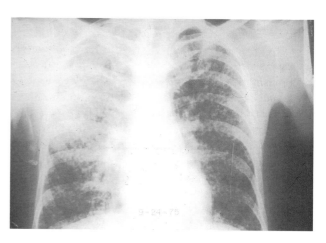

FIGURE 18–6. Acute "epidemic" pulmonary histoplasmosis occurring in a construction worker who cleaned bird and bat guano from a bridge prior to painting of the structure. The patient was severely ill, but responded quickly to amphotericin B therapy.

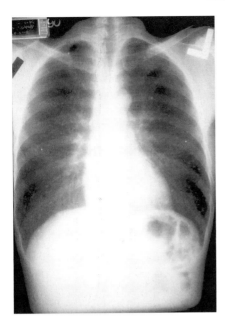

FIGURE 18–7. Diffuse calcified nodules throughout the lung fields in a patient who had acute "epidemic" pulmonary histoplasmosis 20 years earlier.

prior to the onset of symptoms should lead to further diagnostic tests for histoplasmosis. Included in the differential diagnosis of acute pulmonary histoplasmosis are acute pulmonary blastomycosis and pneumonias due to *Mycoplasma*, *Legionella*, and *Chlamydia*. Hilar or mediastinal lymphadenopathy, common with histoplasmosis, are uncommonly noted with pneumonia due to these other organisms.

Chronic Pulmonary Histoplasmosis

Chronic pulmonary histoplasmosis occurs almost entirely in older males with underlying chronic obstructive pulmonary disease (Goodwin et al, 1976; Wheat et al, 1984). The clinical manifestations include fatigue, fever, night sweats, chronic cough, sputum production, hemoptysis, dyspnea, and weight loss. This form of histoplasmosis is characterized by cavity formation in the upper lobes and progressive fibrosis in the lower lung fields (Fig. 18–8). The extensive scarring is thought to be related to the host's response to *H. capsulatum* antigens. Pleural involvement is uncommon. The disease is manifested by progressive respiratory insufficiency and if not treated is ultimately fatal in most patients (Furcolow, 1963; Parker et al, 1970; Goodwin et al, 1976). In many aspects, chronic cavitary pulmonary histoplasmosis mimics reactivation tuberculosis. The differential diagnosis of chronic pulmonary histoplasmosis also includes nontuberculous mycobacterial infections, blastomycosis, sporotrichosis, and coccidioidomycosis.

Complications of Pulmonary Histoplasmosis

Mediastinal Granuloma. Involvement of mediastinal lymph nodes is common during the course of acute pulmonary histoplasmosis. However, mediastinal granuloma, characterized by massive enlargement of mediastinal lymph nodes that frequently undergo caseation necrosis, is distinctly uncommon. These nodes can remain enlarged for months to years and can lead to impingement on airways or major vessels, displacement of the esophagus, or formation of fistulae between the nodes and adjacent structures in the mediastinum (Loyd et al, 1988). Compression of a bronchus can result in intermittent obstruction and pneumonia. In some cases, the nodes will spontaneously drain into adjacent soft tissues of the neck. Patients may be asymptomatic, have nonspecific systemic complaints of fatigue and not feeling well, or have symptoms, such as dyspnea, cough, or odynophagia related to the effects of the nodes on adjacent structures. Although it was initially thought that mediastinal granuloma progressed to fibrosing mediastinitis, current thinking is that these are two separate complications of pulmonary histoplasmosis (Davis et al, 2001).

Radiographs show only enlarged lymph nodes, sometimes with calcification noted. Computed tomography scans of the chest are more helpful, showing nodal enlargement, the presence of necrosis, and impingement on mediastinal structures (Gurney and Conces, 1996) (Fig. 18–9). Bronchoscopy or esophagoscopy can document extrinsic compression, traction diverticulae, or fistulae. Mediastinal granuloma as a complication of histoplasmosis must be differentiated from lymphoma and other tumors that cause mediastinal lymphadenopathy.

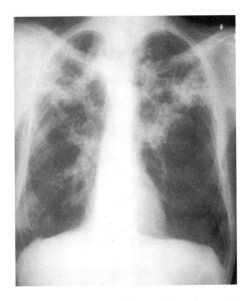

FIGURE 18–8. Chronic cavitary pulmonary histoplasmosis in an elderly man with severe underlying emphysema.

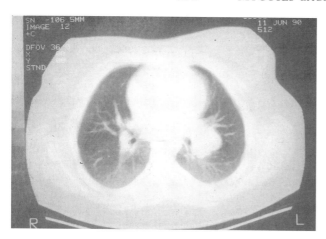

FIGURE 18–9. CT scan of a young woman who developed mediastinal granuloma due to *H. capsulatum*; the multiple enlarged mediastinal and left hilar lymph nodes had been present for at least 1 year at the time this scan was performed.

Fibrosing Mediastinitis. Fibrosing mediastinitis, an entity distinct from and much less common than mediastinal granuloma, is characterized by excessive fibrosis that progressively envelops the structures of the mediastinum (Goodwin et al, 1972; Loyd et al, 1988). The condition arises following infection with *H. capsulatum*, occurs mostly in young adults, and is presumably related to an abnormal fibrotic response to *H. capsulatum* in these individuals. The fibrosis can lead to obstruction of the superior vena cava or pulmonary arteries or veins; there may be occlusion of the bronchi. Rarely, the thoracic duct, recurrent laryngeal nerve, or right atrium are involved. Hemoptysis, dyspnea, and cough are common symptoms. Signs of superior vena cava syndrome or right heart failure may be prominent (Mathisen and Grillo, 1992).

Chest radiographs show subcarinal or superior mediastinal widening. Computed tomography scans reveal the extent of invasion of mediastinal structures, and angiography demonstrates invasion of the great vessels (Sherrick et al, 1994). Fibrosing mediastinitis is a progressive condition that culminates in death in a substantial number of those with the condition. There is no effective therapy for this progressive disease.

Broncholithiasis. Broncholithiasis occurs when calcified nodes or pulmonary granulomas erode into the bronchi. Ulceration into the bronchus with hemoptysis and expectoration of "stones" can ensue. Postobstructive pneumonia occurs if the node obstructs the bronchus. Computed tomography scans show the calcified node and its impingement on the bronchus, and bronchoscopy will usually confirm the diagnosis and rule out other endobronchial lesions (Conces et al, 1991).

Pericarditis. Pericarditis occurs in the setting of acute pulmonary histoplasmosis, is seen mostly in young persons, and is thought to be due to an inflammatory reaction to *H. capsulatum* in adjacent mediastinal nodes (Picardi et al, 1976; Wheat et al, 1983) (Fig. 18–10). Pericardial fluid is often hemorrhagic with a predominance of lymphocytes, and *H. capsulatum* cannot be grown from the fluid. Pleural effusions are also common in this setting, and the fluid is exudative and frequently bloody. The majority of patients exhibit no hemodynamic consequences; however, tamponade can occur and requires immediate drainage. Outcome is excellent; only rarely does acute pericarditis progress to constriction requiring a surgical procedure for relief of symptoms (Picardi et al, 1976; Wheat et al, 1983).

Disseminated Histoplasmosis

Although dissemination is common during the course of most infections with *H. capsulatum*, symptomatic dissemination occurs primarily in immunosuppressed patients and infants (Goodwin et al, 1980; Sathapatayavongs et al, 1983; Wheat et al, 1990b; Odio et al, 1999). In persons with HIV-1 infection and histoplasmosis, a CD4 count < 150/μL is associated with increased risk of disseminated histoplasmosis (McKinsey et al, 1997). A rapidly fatal course with diffuse involvement of multiple organs characterizes the infection in most immunosuppressed patients (Kauffman et al, 1978; Davies et al, 1978; Sathapatayavongs et al,

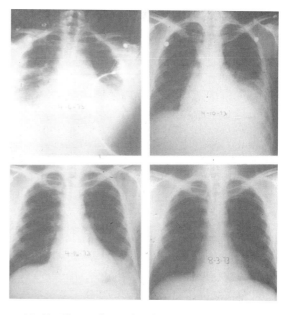

FIGURE 18–10. Chest radiographs of a young girl showing the natural course of pericarditis due to *H. capsulatum*. Initially a huge pericardial effusion, a modest left pleural effusion, and an infiltrate in the right lung were present; over the next 10 days, both the pericardial and pleural effusions decreased, and 4 months later, the heart size had returned to normal and the lung fields were clear.

1983; Odio et al, 1999). Patients often have dyspnea, renal failure, hepatic failure, coagulopathy, hypotension, and obtundation. Chest radiographs show diffuse interstitial or reticulonodular infiltrates, but may progress quickly to the findings associated with acute respiratory distress syndrome.

A chronic progressive course is typical of disseminated histoplasmosis in nonimmunocompromised middle-aged to older adults (Sarosi et al, 1971; Smith and Utz, 1972; Goodwin et al, 1980). This form of histoplasmosis is more common in men than women. A history of recent exposure often cannot be elicited, and overt defects in immune function have not been identified in these patients. However, because such patients are unable to eradicate the organism from their macrophages, it is presumed that they have a specific immune defect against *H. capsulatum* (Goodwin et al, 1980). Fever, night sweats, anorexia, weight loss, and fatigue are prominent. Pulmonary symptoms may or may not be present, but usually are not prominent.

In both acute and chronic disseminated histoplasmosis, hepatosplenomegaly, lymphadenopathy, and skin and mucous membrane lesions are frequently noted. A variety of different skin lesions, including papules, pustules, ulcers, and subcutaneous nodules, have been noted in patients with disseminated histoplasmosis (See Color Fig. 18–11A and 18–11B in separate color insert). Oropharyngeal ulcers or less commonly, nodules, can be found on the tongue, buccal and gingival mucosa, larynx, or lips in patients with either acute or chronic dissemination (See Color Fig. 18–12 in separate color insert). Patients with disseminated histoplasmosis can develop adrenal insufficiency as a result of destruction of the adrenal glands by infiltration with *H. capsulatum*. Addisonian crisis has been reported as the presenting manifestation of disseminated histoplasmosis. In addition, hypercalcemia has been associated with disseminated histoplsmosis, just as with other granulomatous diseases including tuberculosis, coccidioidomycosis and sardcoidosis (Murray and Heim, 1985).

Laboratory abnormalities noted with disseminated disease include an elevated erythrocyte sedimentation rate, pancytopenia, elevation of hepatic enzymes, especially alkaline phosphatase, and hyperbilirubinemia. Patients with adrenal insufficiency may have hyponatremia, hyperkalemia, and hypoglycemia. Abdominal CT scans show adrenal enlargement and sometimes necrosis in those with adrenal involvement (Wilson et al, 1984) (Fig. 18–13). Bone marrow, liver, and lymph node biopsy specimens often reveal granulomas.

Disseminated histoplasmosis must always be considered as a possible cause of fever of unknown origin in persons who have ever lived in the endemic area. Lymphomas, sarcoidosis, and mycobacterial infections must

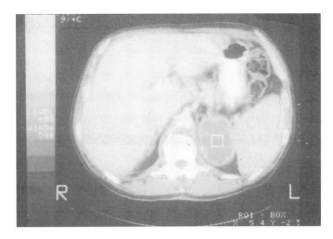

FIGURE 18–13. Abdominal CT scan showing adrenal enlargement with central necrosis in a patient with chronic progressive histoplasmosis complicated by Addison's disease.

be differentiated from disseminated histoplasmosis. Often such patients are treated inappropriately with corticosteroids without excluding active histoplasmosis. Although patients may initially appear to improve with corticosteroid treatment, they subsequently experience progressive illness and can die of overwhelming histoplasmosis (Gulati et al, 2000).

Endocarditis is an uncommon manifestation of disseminated histoplasmosis (Goodwin et al, 1980; Sathapatayavongs et al, 1983). Both native and prosthetic valve endocarditis have been reported (Bradsher et al, 1980; Gaynes et al, 1981; Kanawaty et al, 1991), as well as an infected left atrial myxoma (Rogers et al, 1978). The disease is manifest by major embolic episodes and poor outcome without surgical removal of the valve. *Histoplasma capsulatum* has also been described as a cause of infection of an aortofemoral prosthetic graft (Matthay et al, 1976).

Specific Organ System Involvement

Central nervous system involvement occurs either as one component of disseminated infection or as an isolated manifestation of infection with *H. capsulatum* (Wheat et al, 1990a). Most often, histoplasmosis of the central nervous system is manifested as subacute or chronic meningitis. Basilar meningeal involvement is typical and can lead to communicating hydrocephalus. Focal brain or spinal cord lesions can occur in those with meningitis or as isolated lesions without meningitis (Wheat et al, 1990a; Livas et al, 1995; Klein et al, 1999). In patients with meningitis, the typical CSF abnormalities include lymphocytic pleocytosis, elevated protein, and hypoglycorrachia; in those with focal lesions, the CSF findings are either within normal limits or show slight pleocytosis and elevated protein concentrations. Computed tomography or MRI scans show

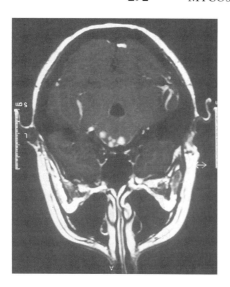

FIGURE 18–14. MRI scan of a woman with isolated CNS histoplasmosis; the scan shows meningeal enhancement as well as several enhancing lesions in the midbrain.

single or multiple enhancing brain lesions in those with focal infection and meningeal enhancement in those who have meningitis only (Fig. 18–14). *Histoplasma* meningitis must be differentiated from other causes of chronic lymphocytic meningitis, notably tuberculosis, coccidioidomycosis and less commonly blastomycosis, sporotrichosis, brucellosis, and sarcoidosis; mass lesions must be differentiated from other infectious processes as well as tumors (Klein et al, 1999).

Osteoarticular histoplasmosis is not common; typically, manifestations are those of chronic tenosynovitis and less commonly osteomyelitis and septic arthritris of a native joint or rarely, a prosthesis (Darouiche et al, 1992; Fowler et al, 1998). Infection of osteoarticular structures must be differentiated from the self-limited arthralgias and arthritis that are noted during the course of acute histoplasmosis and that are presumed secondary to the immune response to *H. capsulatum* (Rosenthal et al, 1983). Isolated infection of the GI tract is an uncommon manifestation of histoplasmosis. Diffuse infiltration of the bowel wall is usually noted; abdominal pain and diarrhea are prominent and malabsorption can result (Orchard et al, 1979; Lamps et al, 2000). In AIDS patients and perhaps more often in others than realized, GI tract involvement is commonly noted as one manifestation of disseminated histoplasmosis (Suh et al, 2001).

Genitourinary tract infection with *H. capsulatum* can be manifested as epididymal, testicular, or prostatic nodules (Kauffman et al, 1981; Schuster et al, 2000; Mawhorter et al, 2000). Other sites at which *H. capsulatum* has been reported to cause focal infection or involvement has been noted in association with widespread dissemination include kidneys, peritoneum, omentum, gallbladder, common bile duct, panniculus,

breast, thymus, sinuses, optic nerve, eyes, and ears (Schwarz, 1981).

Presumed Ocular Histoplasmosis

Ocular histoplasmosis is a diagnosis based on ophthalmological findings of discrete yellow-white lesions in the retina, so-called "histo spots"; these lesions are sight-threatening when they occur in the macula. However, there is little scientific evidence linking this syndrome to histoplasmosis (Schwarz, 1981). The association is based primarily on residence in an area endemic for histoplasmosis and positive histoplasmin skin tests and not by demonstration of fungus in the eye. Similar ophthalmological findings have been noted in patients who have never lived in the endemic area (Suttorp-Schulten al, 1997). Rarely, *H. capsulatum* can be recovered from the eye in patients with disseminated histoplasmosis, but the clinical and ophthalmological findings are not those described with ocular histoplasmosis (Specht et al, 1991).

African Histoplasmosis

Infection with *H. duboisii* differs from that due to *H. capsulatum* in that bone and skin are the two major organs affected (See Color Figs. 18–15a and 18–15b in separate color insert). Osteolytic lesions are often found in association with subcutaneous nodules and abscesses; skin nodules can ulcerate and drain. Lung involvement is more common than previously thought, and lymphadenopathy can be prominent. The infection is frequently indolent and not life-threatening, but in the exceptional patient, widespread visceral dissemination occurs and the disease resembles progressive disseminated histoplasmosis due to *H. capsulatum*.

DIAGNOSIS

Culture Methods

The definitive diagnostic test for histoplasmosis is growth of *H. capsulatum* from tissue or body fluids. For patients who have disseminated infection, samples taken from blood, bone marrow, liver tissue, skin, or mucosal lesions often yield *H. capsulatum*. The lysis-centrifugation (Isolator tube) system is more sensitive than automated systems for growing *H. capsulatum* from blood (Wilson et al, 1993). When sputum or bronchoalveolar lavage fluid is sent for culture, the laboratory should be informed that histoplasmosis is a possibility; use of a selective medium that uses ammonium hydroxide decreases the growth of commensal fungi and increases the yield of *H. capsulatum* (Smith and Goodman, 1975).

H. capsulatum may take as long as 6 weeks to grow at 30°C in the mould phase in vitro. The laborious task of converting the mould phase to the yeast phase in vitro is no longer required for definitive identification of *H. capsulatum*. As soon as growth of a mould has been detected, DNA probes for *H. capsulatum* can be used to rapidly confirm the identification of the organism. Cultures yield the organism in most cases of disseminated infection, chronic pulmonary histoplasmosis, and acute pulmonary histoplasmosis following a heavy-inoculum exposure. However, in most cases of acute pulmonary histoplasmosis and mediastinal granuloma and frequently in meningitis, cultures usually do not yield *H. capsulatum* (Wheat, 2001a).

Antigen Detection

Detection of circulating *H. capsulatum* polysaccharide antigen in urine and serum has proved extremely useful in patients, especially those with AIDS, who have disseminated infection with a large burden of organisms (Wheat et al, 1986b; Wheat et al, 1991; Wheat et al, 1992; Wheat, 2001a). Originally developed as a radioimmunoassay, antigen detection is now performed by enzyme immunoassay with greater ease and equivalent sensitivity and specificity (Durkin et al, 1997). The sensitivity for antigen detection is higher in urine than in serum. Antigen can be detected in the urine of approximately 90% and in the serum of approximately 50% of patients with disseminated infection (Wheat, 2001a). Antigen can be detected in urine of approximately 75% of patients with high-inoculum exposure acute pulmonary histoplasmosis within the first few weeks of illness; however, antigen is detected in only 10%–20% of patients with less severe and chronic pulmonary histoplasmosis. Antigen detection has also proved useful in bronchoalveolar lavage fluid from AIDS patients with diffuse pulmonary infiltrates due to histoplasmosis (Wheat et al, 1992a). Antigen can be detected in CSF from some patients with *Histoplasma* meningitis, but is less sensitive than assays for antibody in CSF (Wheat et al, 1985; Wheat et al, 1989).

False positive reactions have been noted in a majority of samples of urine and serum taken from patients with blastomycosis, paracoccidioidomycosis, or penicilliosis, but not with coccidioidomycosis (Wheat et al, 1997c). The major diagnostic dilemma in the United States is obviously with blastomycosis. Antigen detection also can be used to follow a patient's response to antifungal therapy. Levels should fall to below the level of detection with successful therapy; persistence implies continued active infection (Wheat et al, 1992b), and a rise in antigen levels is seen with relapse (Wheat et al, 1991).

Serological Tests

Serological tests play an important role in the diagnosis of several forms of histoplasmosis (Wheat, 2001a).

The standard assays for antibodies to *H. capsulatum* are the complement fixation (CF) test that uses two separate antigens, yeast and mycelial (or histoplasmin), and the immunodiffusion (ID) assay. A fourfold rise in CF antibody titer or a titer $\geq$ 1:32 is considered indicative of active histoplasmosis.

Antibodies frequently persist for years after infection; thus, the presence of a single low CF titer means little other than that the patient was exposed to *H. capsulatum* at some time. The CF test is less specific than the ID assay; moreover, cross-reactions with other fungal infections occur in only 5% of cases by ID, but in 18% of cases by CF (Wheat et al, 1986a).

The ID assay tests for the presence of M and H precipitin bands. An M band develops with acute infection, is often present in chronic forms of histoplasmosis, and persists for months to years after the infection has resolved. An H band is much less common, is rarely if ever found without an M band, and is indicative of chronic and progressive forms of histoplasmosis. Enzyme immunoassay methods are poorly standardized and are not recommended.

Serologic tests are most useful for patients with chronic pulmonary or disseminated histoplasmosis; in these forms of histoplasmosis, the chronicity of the infection ensures that sufficient time has elapsed for the patient to have developed antibodies. For acute pulmonary histoplasmosis, a rising antibody titer to *H. capsulatum* is diagnostic. Serological tests are less definitive in patients who have mediastinal lymphadenopathy and should always be confirmed by tissue biopsy. False positive CF tests occur in patients with lymphoma, tuberculosis, sarcoidosis, and other fungal infections, all of which may present as mediastinal masses. Because 2 to 6 weeks are required for appearance of antibodies, serological assays are less helpful in establishing a diagnosis in patients who have severe acute infection, and they are rarely useful in immunosuppressed patients, who mount a poor antibody response. A special use for antibody detection is in patients with *Histoplasma* meningitis. The presence of CF and/or ID antibodies against *H. capsulatum* in the CSF is adequate to make a diagnosis in the appropriate clinical setting and frequently is the only positive diagnostic test (Wheat et al, 1985).

Histopathological Examination

For the patient who is acutely ill, tissue biopsy should be done as soon as possible to look for *H. capsulatum*. Finding the distinctive 2–4 μm oval budding yeasts allows a presumptive diagnosis of histoplasmosis. Routine hematoxylin and eosin stains will not show the tiny yeasts; biopsy material must be stained with Gomori methenamine silver or periodic acid Schiff. Yeasts are typically found within macrophages, but also can be seen free in the tissues. In patients with disseminated infection, bone marrow, liver, skin, and mucocutaneous lesions usually reveal organisms, and in those with a large burden of organisms, routine peripheral blood smears may show yeasts within neutrophils (See Color Fig. 18–16 in separate color insert).

For patients with granulomatous mediastinitis, biopsy of nodes will often reveal caseous material, which may contain a few yeast-like organisms typical of *H. capsulatum*. It is unusual to find the yeasts of *H. capsulatum* on cytological examination of sputum or bronchoalveolar lavage fluid unless there is a large organism burden.

In histopathology specimens, the yeast phase of *H. duboisii* is distinctly different from that of *H. capsulatum*. Yeast forms of *H. duboisii* are approximately fourfold larger than *H. capsulatum* and may be seen as short chains in tissues. The distinction between these two varieties of *Histoplasma* is clinically relevant only for a small number of patients who could have either infection because they lived in areas of tropical Africa in which both organisms are found.

Skin Tests

Skin testing with histoplasmin antigen is not useful for diagnostic purposes. In the endemic area, most adults are skin test positive because of prior exposure to *H. capsulatum*. Cross-reactions occur with other fungal infections, especially blastomycosis, and placing a skin test can falsely elevate CF antibody titers. Patients who have severe histoplasmosis often are anergic.

TREATMENT

Most patients infected with *H. capsulatum* are asymptomatic or have mild, self-limited disease and, thus, do not need treatment with an antifungal agent. However, patients who have severe acute pulmonary, chronic pulmonary, or disseminated histoplasmosis do require treatment with an antifungal agent. Guidelines for the treatment of histoplasmosis have been published recently under the auspices of the Infectious Diseases Society of America and the Mycoses Study Group (Wheat et al, 2000).

Pulmonary Histoplasmosis

Acute Pulmonary Histoplasmosis. Most patients with acute pulmonary histoplasmosis do not require antifungal therapy; recovery occurs generally within a month without therapy. However, some patients do remain symptomatic for longer periods of time and should receive therapy. Oral itraconazole, 200 mg daily, for 6–12 weeks is recommended in such cases (Wheat et al, 2000).

Patients who have acute diffuse pulmonary histoplasmosis (epidemic histoplasmosis) should receive antifungal therapy. Although most patients will recover, deaths have occurred and recovery may be protracted. For those with only moderate illness, oral itraconazole, 200–400 mg daily can be used. For those who are severely ill, initial treatment should be with amphotericin B, 0.7 to 1.0 mg/kg daily. Corticosteroids, given as an intravenous bolus of methylprednisolone for several days or as 60 mg prednisone daily and tapered over 2 weeks, have proved to be helpful in patients with severe disease (Wheat et al, 2000). For most patients, antifungal treatment should continue for approximately 3 months.

Chronic Pulmonary Histoplasmosis. Treatment is indicated for all patients with chronic pulmonary histoplasmosis. Without therapy, inexorable progression to respiratory insufficiency is the rule (Furculow, 1963; Parker et al, 1970; Goodwin et al, 1976). For many years, amphotericin B, at a total dosage of 35 mg/kg, was the preferred agent, but it appears that itraconazole 200–400 mg daily is probably equally effective, much less toxic, and decidedly easier for patients to take. Ketoconazole, 400–800 mg daily, is effective, but associated with more side effects than itraconazole (NIAID, 1985; Dismukes et al, 1992). Fluconazole is less effective than itraconazole and should be considered second-line therapy (McKinsey et al, 1996). The total length of azole treatment is usually 12–24 months.

Complications of Pulmonary Histoplasmosis. It is not clear that antifungal agents alter the course of mediastinal granuloma. Some patients recover without treatment, and others continue to have symptoms, which usually leads to the use of antifungal agents. However, reports of successful therapy with either azoles or amphotericin B remain anecdotal. It seems reasonable to give oral itraconazole, 200–400 mg daily, for 6–12 months in patients who have symptoms. If the patient is severely ill with obstructive symptoms, amphotericin B should be given initially followed by itraconazole. Some patients benefit from surgical removal of obstructing nodes (Davis et al, 2001).

There is no known effective therapy for fibrosing mediastinitis. Frequently, however, oral itraconazole is tried because there is so little else that can be done. Use of corticosteroids and other antiinflammatory agents is not recommended. Surgery is controversial in the management of fibrosing mediastinitis; the operative mortality rates are high, and for many patients, the course of the disease is changed very little (Loyd et al, 1988; Mathisen and Grillo, 1992). For some patients, improvement occurs with placement of an intravascular stent to relieve obstruction or angiographic embolization of vessels identified as the source of hemoptysis.

Pericarditis is treated with nonsteroidal antiinflammatory agents and rarely corticosteroids. Antifungal agents are not recommended (Wheat et al, 2000). In the exceptional case associated with tamponade, pericardiocentesis and creation of a pericardial window are important therapeutic measures (Picardi et al, 1976).

Disseminated Histoplasmosis

Even though some patients with symptomatic disseminated histoplasmosis clear the infection themselves, as a general rule, all patients with this form of histoplasmosis should be treated with an antifungal agent (Wheat et al, 2000). Patients with severe acute disseminated infection should be treated initially with amphotericin B, 0.7–1.0 mg/kg daily. Data from a randomized, blinded comparative study in AIDS patients show that treatment with liposomal amphotericin B when compared with standard amphotericin B resulted in faster resolution of fever and improved survival (Johnson et al, 2002). However, it is not clear that all patients should receive this more costly antifungal agent for initial therapy based only on these data. The entire course of treatment can be given with amphotericin B; when standard amphotericin B is chosen, the total dosage should be 35 mg/kg. (Sarosi et al, 1971; Smith and Utz, 1972; Goodwin et al, 1980). This regimen is now uncommonly used. After clinical improvement is noted, which occurs within 2 weeks in most patients, therapy is usually changed to oral itraconazole, 200–400 mg daily.

Patients with less severe acute disseminated histoplasmosis and most patients with chronic progressive disseminated histoplasmosis can be treated with oral itraconazole, 200–400 mg daily (Dismukes et al, 1992; Wheat et al, 1995). In this group of patients, it is not known whether an initial course of induction therapy with amphotericin B should be given. The only data that address this question are from a retrospective laboratory evaluation of clearance of fungemia and antigenemia/antigenuria in AIDS patients enrolled in two separate trials of treatment with either liposomal amphotericin B or itraconazole. Patients who received liposomal amphotericin B had more rapid clearance of both fungemia and antigenemia/antigenuria than those who received itraconazole (Wheat et al, 2001b). These findings are more impressive when it is noted that patients in the liposomal amophotericin B trial were more severely ill than patients in the itraconazole trial. Fluconazole is less effective than itraconazole (McKinsey et al, 1996); this has been most clearly shown in AIDS patients, in whom relapse rates while receiving fluconazole were noted to be unacceptably high (Wheat et al, 1997b).

The length of therapy depends on the severity of the infection and the immune status of the host. The minimum period of treatment should be 6 months for the relatively healthy host; most patients probably will be treated for 12 months. Patients with chronic progressive dissemination may respond slowly to antifungal therapy; treatment is usually continued for 12–24 months in this group of patients. For patients with AIDS, lifelong maintenance therapy with 200 mg itraconazole has been the standard of therapy (Wheat et al, 1993), but use of highly active antiretroviral therapy has led some physicians to discontinue secondary itraconazole prophylaxis when CD4 counts are sustained at levels above 200 cells/μL (Dupont et al, 2000).

Histoplasma endocarditis should be treated with both surgical replacement of the valve and antifungal therapy (Bradsher et al, 1980; Gaynes et al, 1981; Kanawaty et al, 1991). Amphotericin B rather than an azole should be used for primary therapy. Lipid formulations of amphotericin B are clearly less toxic and would seem to be ideal for long-term treatment of this serious infection, but there is little experience reported for the treatment of *Histoplasma* endocarditis with any of the lipid formulations. If for any reason, surgical extirpation of the valve cannot be performed, lifelong suppression with itraconazole should be maintained.

Central Nervous System Histoplasmosis

Histoplasmosis involving the central nervous system is perhaps the most difficult treatment problem. Initial treatment should be with amphotericin B, and the total dosage usually administered is 35 mg/kg. Liposomal amphotericin B has been shown to achieve high concentrations in brain tissue in an experimental animal model of *Candida* infection (Groll et al, 2000). Whether this formulation would be more effective than standard amphotericin B is not known, but it seems reasonable to try liposomal amphotericin B in this circumstance. The most efficacious dosage is not known; 3–5 mg/kg daily has been recommended; the total dose that should be achieved is not known (Wheat et al, 2000).

Because the relapse rate is high, an azole should be given following initial therapy with amphotericin B. Itraconazole does not achieve adequate CSF levels, but has been used successfully for both cryptococcal and coccidioidal meningitis. On the other hand, fluconazole achieves higher CSF concentrations, but is less active against *H. capsulatum* than itraconazole. While neither azole drug is an ideal agent for treatment of *Histoplasma* meningitis, both drugs have been used for this indication (Tiraboschi et al, 1992; Bamberger, 1999). In the absence of comparative studies, either itraconazole, 200 mg twice daily or fluconazole, 800 mg daily, could be given for at least 12 months. Some patients, especially those who do not have normalization of CSF on therapy, should probably receive life-long suppressive therapy with an azole.

Enhancing mass lesions in the brain or spinal cord appear to respond to antifungal agents and do not require excision in most patients. Magnetic resonance imaging scans should be followed to assure resolution (Wheat et al, 1990a). In those patients who do not have meningitis, antifungal therapy can perhaps be stopped a few months after complete resolution of all lesions; careful follow-up is essential to assess possible relapse (Wheat et al, 2000).

Treatment of Infections Due to H. duboisii

Controlled trials have not been performed to determine the most efficacious treatment for *H. duboisii*. Anecdotal experience shows amphotericin B, ketoconazole, and more recently, itraconazole to be effective (Nethercott et al, 1978; Lortholary et al, 1999). There is no reason to doubt that the response to antifungal agents would be similar to that with *H. capsulatum*. Osteoarticular involvement, which is common in this form of histoplasmosis, will be slow to respond and requires long-term azole therapy.

PREVENTION

Persons who could be at risk for exposure to *H. capsulatum* through their occupation or leisure activities should be counseled to take appropriate precautions to prevent exposure (Lenhart et al, 1997). Workers should wear a respirator when dismantling known bird or bat roosts or chicken coops, refurbishing old structures that are found to have provided roosts for bats or birds, and moving large quantities of soil in areas known to be highly endemic for *H. capsulatum*. Soil or debris can be treated with formalin to inactivate the conidia prior to construction work, but this is rarely practical. Immunocompromised patients should be counseled to not undertake activities, such as spelunking or renovation projects, that might put them at risk for exposure to the conidia of *H. capsulatum*.

Prophylactic use of antifungal agents has been studied only in persons with AIDS. In the population with CD4 counts < 150 cells/μL, prophylaxis with itraconazole, 200 mg daily, is highly effective and should be considered in areas in which the rate of histoplasmosis exceeds 10 cases/100 patient years (McKinsey et al, 1999). However, prophylaxis with itraconazole does not appear to prolong survival in this patient population.

REFERENCES

Bamberger D M. Successful treatment of multiple cerebral histoplasmomas with itraconazole. *Clin Infect Dis* 28:915–916, 1999.
Bradsher R W, Wickre C G, Savage A M, Harston W E, Alford R H. *Histoplasma capsulatum* endocarditis cured by amphotericin B combined with surgery. *Chest* 78:791–795, 1980.
Brodsky A L, Gregg M B, Kaufman L, Mallison G F. Outbreak of histoplasmosis associated with the 1970 Earth Day activities. *Am J Med* 54:333–342, 1973.
Bullock W E, Wright S D. Role of the adherence-promoting receptors, CR3, LFA-1, and p150,95, in binding of *H. capsulatum* by human macrophages. *J Exp Med* 165:195–210, 1987.
Cano M, Hajjeh R A. The epidemiology of histoplasmosis: a review. *Sem Respir Infect* 16:109–118, 2001.
Chick E W, Compton S B, Pass T, Mackey B, Hernandez C, Austin E, Pitzer F R, Flanigan C. Hitchcock's birds, or the increased rate of exposure to *Histoplasma* from blackbird roost sites. *Chest* 80:434–438, 1981.
Conces D J, Tarver R D, Viz V A. Broncholithiasis: CT features in 15 patients. *AJR* 157:249–253, 1991.
Darouiche R O, Cadle R M, Zenon G J, Weinert M F, Hamill R J, Lidsky M D. Articular histoplasmosis. *J Rheumatol* 19:1991–1993, 1992.
Davies S F, Khan M, Sarosi G A. Disseminated histoplasmosis in immunologically suppressed patients. *Am J Med* 64:94–100, 1978.
Davis A M, Pierson R N, Loyd J E. Mediastinal fibrosis. *Sem Respir Infect* 16:119–130, 2001.
Dean A G, Bates J H, Sorrels C, Sorrels T, Germany W, Ajello L, Kaufman L, McGrew C, Fitts A. An outbreak of histoplasmosis at an Arkansas courthouse, with five cases of probable reinfection. *Am J Epidemiol* 108:36–46, 1978.
Deepe G S Jr. Protective imunity in murine histoplasmosis: functional comparison of adoptively transferrred T-cell clones and splenic T cells. *Infect Immun* 56:2350–2355, 1988.
Dismukes W E, Bradsher R W, Jr., Cloud G C, Kauffman C A, Chapman S W, George R B, Stevens D A, Girard W M, Saag M S, Bowles-Patton C, the NIAID Mycoses Study Group. Itraconazole therapy for blastomycosis and histoplasmosis. *Am J Med* 93:489–497, 1992.
Dupont B, Crewe Brown H H, Westermann K, Martins M D, Rex J H, Lortholary O, Kauffman C . Mycoses in AIDS. *Med Mycol* 38 (Suppl 1):259–267, 2000.
Durkin M M, Connolly P A, Wheat L J. Comparison of radioimmunoassay and enzyme-linked immunoassay methods for detection of *Histoplasma capsulatum* var. *capsulatum* antigen. *J Clin Microbiol* 35:2252–2255, 1997.
Edwards L B, Acquaviva S A, Livesay V T, Cross F W, Palmer C E. An atlas of sensitivity to tuberculin, PPD-B, and histoplasmin in the United States. *Ann Rev Resp Dis* 99(Part 2):1, 1969.
Eissenberg L G, Goldman W E, Schlesinger P H. *Histoplasma capsulatum* modulates the acidification of phagolysosomes. *J Exp Med* 177:1605–1611, 1993.
Fleischman J, Wu-Hsieh B, Howard D H. The intracellular fate of *Histoplasma capsulatum* in human macrophages is unaffected by recombinant human interferon-gamma. *J Infect Dis* 161:143–145, 1990.
Fowler V G Jr, Nacinovich F M, Alspaugh J A, Corey G R. Prosthetic joint infection due to *Histoplasma capsulatum*: case report and review. *Clin Infect Dis* 26:1017, 1998.
Furcolow M L. Comparison of treated and untreated severe histoplasmosis. *JAMA* 183:121–127, 1963.
Gabal M A, Hassan F K, Siad A A, Karim K A. Study of equine histoplasmosis farciminosi and characterization of *Histoplasma farciminosum*. *Sabouraudia* 21:121–127, 1983.
Gaynes R P, Gardner P, Causey W. Prosthetic value endocarditis caused by *Histoplasma capsulatum*. *Arch Intern Med* 141:1533–1537, 1981.
Goodwin R A, Nickell J A, des Prez R M. Mediastinal fibrosis complicating healed primary histoplasmosis and tuberculosis. *Medicine* (Baltimore) 51:227–246, 1972.
Goodwin R A Jr, Owens F T, Snell J D, Hubbard W W, Buchanan R D, Terry R T, Des Prez R M. Chronic pulmonary histoplasmosis. *Medicine* (Baltimore) 55:413–452, 1976.
Goodwin R A Jr, Shapiro J L, Thurman G H, Thurman S S, Des Prez R M. Disseminated histoplasmosis: clinical and pathologic correlations. *Medicine* (Baltimore) 59:1–33, 1980.

Goodwin R A, Loyd J E, Des Prez R M. Histoplasmosis in normal hosts. *Medicine* (Baltimore) 60:231–266, 1981.

Groll A H, Giri N, Petraitis V, Petraitiene R, Candelario M, Bacher J S, Piscitelli S C, Walsh T J. Comparative efficacy and distribution of lipid formulations of amphotericin B in experimental *Candida albicans* infection of the central nervous system. *J Infect Dis* 182:274–282, 2000.

Gugnani H C, Muotoe-Okafar F A, Kaufman L, Dupont B. Natural focus of *Histoplasma capsulatum* var. *duboisii* in a bat cave. *Mycopathologia* 127:151–157, 1994.

Gulati M, Saint S, Tierney L M. Clinical problem-solving. Impatient inpatient care. *N Engl J Med* 342:37–40, 2000.

Gurney J W, Conces D J. Pulmonary histoplasmosis. *Radiology* 199:297–306, 1996.

Hajjeh R A. Disseminated histoplasmosis in persons infected with human immunodeficiency virus. *Clin Infect Dis* 21(Suppl 1): S108–S110, 1995.

Johnson P C, Wheat L J, Cloud G A, Goldman M, Lancaster D, Bamberger D M, Powderly W G, Hafner R, Kauffman C A, Dismukes W E. The NIAID Mycoses Study Group. Safety and efficacy of liposomal amphotericin B compared with conventional amphotericin B for induction therapy of histoplasmosis in patients with AIDS. *Ann Intern Med* 137: 105–109, 2002.

Jones T F, Swinger G L, Craig A S, MsNeil M M, Kaufman L, Schaffner W. Acute pulmonary histoplasmosis in bridge workers: a persistent problem. *Am J Med* 106:480–482, 1999.

Kanawaty D S, Stalker M J B, Munt P W. Nonsurgical treatment of *Histoplasma* endocarditis involving a bioprosthetic valve. *Chest* 99:253–256, 1991.

Kauffman C A, Israel K S, Smith J W, White A C, Schwarz J, Brooks G F. Histoplasmosis in immunosuppressed patients. *Am J Med* 64:923–932, 1978.

Kauffman C A, Slama T G, Wheat L J. *Histoplasma capsulatum* epididymitis. *J Urology* 125:434–435, 1981.

Klein C J, Dinapoli R B, Temesgen Z, Meyer F B. Central nervous system histoplasmosis mimicking a brain tumor: difficulties in diagnosis and treatment. *Mayo Clin Proc* 74:803–807, 1999.

Lamps L W, Molina C P, West A B, Haggitt R C, Scott M A. The pathologic spectrum of gastrointestinal and hepatic histoplasmosis. *Am J Clin Pathol* 113:64–72, 2000.

Lenhart S W, Schafer M P, Singal M, Hajjeh R A. Histoplasmosis: protecting workers at risk. US Department of Health and Human Services, Cincinnati OH, 1997.

Livas I C, Nechay P S, Nauseef W M. Clinical evidence of spinal and cerebral histoplasmosis twenty years after renal transplantation. *Clin Infect Dis* 20:692–695, 1995.

Lortholary O, Denning D W, Dupont B. Endemic mycoses: a treatment update. *J Antimicrob Chemother* 43:321–331, 1999.

Lottenberg R, Waldman R H, Ajello L, Hoff G L, Bigler W, Zellner S R. Pulmonary histoplasmosis associated with exploration of a bat cave. *Am J Epidemiol* 110:156–161, 1979.

Loyd J E, Tillman B F, Atkinson J B, Des Prez R M. Mediastinal fibrosis complicating histoplasmosis. *Medicine* (Baltimore) 67:295–310, 1988.

Manfredi R, Mazzoni A, Nanetti A, Chiodo F. *Histoplasmosis capsulati* and *duboisii* in Europe: the impact of the HIV pandemic, travel, and immigration. *Eur J Epidemiol* 10:675–681, 1994.

Mathisen D J, Grillo H C. Clinical manifestations of mediastinal fibrosis and histoplasmosis. *Ann Thoracic Surgery* 54:1053–1058, 1992.

Matthay R A, Levin D C, Wicks A B, Ellis J H. Disseminated histoplasmosis involving an aortofemoral prosthetic graft. *JAMA* 235:1478–1479, 1976.

Mawhorter S D, Curley G V, Kursh E D, Farver C E. Prostatic and central nervous system histoplasmosis in an immunocompetent host: case report and review of the prostatic histoplasmosis literature. *Clin Infect Dis* 30:595–598, 2000.

McKinsey D S, Kauffman C A, Pappas P G, Cloud G A, Girard W M, Sharkey P K, Hamill R J, Thomas C J, Dismukes W E. Fluconazole therapy for histoplasmosis. *Clin Infect Dis* 23:996–1001, 1996.

McKinsey D S, Spiegel R A, Hutwanger L, Stanford J, Driks M R, Brewer J, Gupta M R, Smith D L, O'Connor M C, Dall L. Prospective study of histoplasmosis in patients infected with human immunodeficiency virus: incidence, risk factors, and pathophysiology. *Clin Infect Dis* 24:1195–1203, 1997.

McKinsey D S, Wheat L J, Cloud G A, Pierce M, Black J R, Bamberger D M, Goldman M, Thomas C J, Gutsch H M, Moskovitz B, Dismukes W E, Kauffman C A, NIAID Mycoses Study Group. Itraconazole prophylaxis for fungal infections in patients with advanced human immunodeficiency virus infection: randomized, placebo-controlled, double-blind study. *Clin Infect Dis* 28:1049–1056, 1999.

Murray J J, Heim C R. Hypercalcemia in disseminated histoplasmosis: aggravation by vitamin D. *Am J Med* 78:881–884, 1985.

National Institute of Allergy and Infectious Diseases (NIAID) Mycoses Study Group. Treatment of blastomycosis and histoplasmosis with ketoconazole: results of a prospective randomized clinical trial. *Ann Intern Med* 103:861–872, 1985.

Nethercott J R, Schachter R K, Givan K F, Ryder D E. Histoplasmosis due to *Histoplasma capsulatum* var. *duboisii* in a Canadian immigrant. *Arch Dermatol* 114:595–598, 1978.

Newman S L. Cell-mediated immunity to *Histoplasma capsulatum*. *Sem Respir Infect* 16:102–108, 2001.

Odio C M, Navarrete M, Carrillo J M, Mora L, Carranza A. Disseminated histoplasmosis in infants. *Pediatr Infect Dis J* 18:1065–1068, 1999.

Orchard J L, Luparello F, Brunskill D. Malabsorption syndrome occurring in the course of disseminated histoplasmosis. case report and review of gastrointestinal histoplasmosis. *Am J Med* 66:331–336, 1979.

Ozols I I, Wheat L J. Erythema nodosum in an epidemic of histoplasmosis in Indianapolis. *Arch Dermatol* 117:709–712, 1981.

Parker J D, Sarosi G A, Doto I L, Bailey R E, Tosh F E. Treatment of chronic pulmonary histoplasmosis. *N Engl J Med* 283:225–229, 1970.

Picardi J L, Kauffman C A, Schwarz J, Holmes J C, Phair J P, Fowler N O. Pericarditis caused by *Histoplasma capsulatum*. *Am J Cardiol* 37:82–88, 1976.

Rogers E W, Weyman A E, Noble R J, Bruins S C. Left artial myxoma infected with *Histoplasma capsulatum*. *Am J Med* 64:683–690, 1978.

Rosenthal J, Brandt K D, Wheat L J, Slama T G. Rheumatologic manifestations of histoplasmosis in the recent Indianapolis epidemic. *Arthr Rheum* 26:1065–1070, 1983.

Sarosi G A, Voth D W, Dahl B A, Doto I L, Tosh F E. Disseminated histoplasmosis: results of long-term follow-up. *Ann Intern Med* 75:511–516, 1971.

Sathapatayavongs B, Batteiger B E, Wheat J, Slama T G, Wass J L. Clinical and laboratory features of disseminated histoplasmosis during two large urban outbreaks. *Medicine* (Baltimore) 62:263–270, 1983.

Schuster T G, Hollenbeck B K, Kauffman C A, Chensue S W, Wei J T. Testicular histoplasmosis. *J Urology* 164:1652, 2000.

Schwarz J. African histoplasmosis, part 2. In: Baker R D, ed. *Human Infection with Fungi, Actinomycetes, and Algae.* New York: Springer-Verlag, 139–146, 1970.

Schwarz J. *Histoplasmosis.* Praeger Publishers, New York, 1981.

Sherrick A D, Brown L R, Harms G F, Myers J L. The radiographic findings of fibrosing mediastinitis. *Chest* 106:484–489, 1994.

Shore R N, Waltersdorff R L, Edelstein M V, Teske J H. African histoplasmosis in the United States. *JAMA* 245:734–735, 1981.

Smith C D, Goodman N L. Improved culture method for the isolation of *Histoplasma capsulatum* and *Blastomyces dermatitidis* from contaminated specimens. *Am J Clin Pathol* 63:276–280, 1975.

Smith J W, Utz J P. Progressive disseminated histoplasmosis: a prospective study of 26 patients. *Ann Intern Med* 76:557–565, 1972.

Specht C S, Mitchell K T, Bauman A E, Gupta M. Ocular histoplasmosis with retinitis in a patient with acquired immune deficiency syndrome. *Ophthalmology* 98:1356–1359, 1991.

Suh K N, Anekthananon T, Mariuz P R. Gastrointestinal histoplasmosis in patients with AIDS: case report and review. *Clin Infect Dis* 32:483–491, 2001.

Suttorp-Schulten M S A, Bollemeijer J G, Bos P J M, Rothova A. Presumed ocular histoplasmosis in the Netherlands—an area without histoplasmosis. *Br J Ophthalmol* 81:7–11, 1997.

Tiraboschi I, Casas Parera I, Pikielny R, Scattini G, Micheli F. Chronic *Histoplasma capsulatum* infection of the central nervous system successfully treated with fluconazole. *Eur Neurol* 32:70–73, 1992.

Thornberry D K, Wheat L J, Brandt K D, Rosenthal J. Histoplasmosis presenting with joint pain and hilar adenopathy. "pseudosarcoidosis". *Arthr Rheum* 25:1396–1402, 1982.

Waldman R J, England A C, Tauxe R, Kline T, Weeks R J, Ajello L, Kaufman L, Wentworth B, Fraser D W. A winter outbreak of acute histoplasmosis in northern Michigan. *Am J Epidemiol* 117:68–75, 1983.

Wheat L J, Slama T G, Eitzen H E, Kohler R B, French M L V, Biesecker J L. A large urban outbreak of histoplasmosis: clinical features. *Ann Intern Med* 94:331–337, 1981.

Wheat L J, Stein L, Corya B C, Wass J L, Norton J A, Grider K, Slama T G, French M L, Kohler R B. Pericarditis as a manifestation of histoplasmosis during two large urban outbreaks. *Medicine* (Baltimore) 62:110–119, 1983.

Wheat L J, Wass J, Norton J, Kohler RB, French M L V. Cavitary histoplasmosis occurring during two large urban outbreaks: analysis of clinical, epidemiologic, roentgenographic, and laboratory features. *Medicine* (Baltimore) 63:201–209, 1984.

Wheat J, French M, Batteiger B, Kohler R. Cerebrospinal fluid *Histoplasma* antibodies in central nervous system histoplasmosis. *Arch Intern Med* 145:1237–1240, 1985.

Wheat L J, French M L V, Kamel S, Tewari R P. Evaluation of cross-reactions in *Histoplasma capsulatum* serologic tests. *J Clin Microbiol* 23:493–499, 1986a.

Wheat L J, Kohler R B, Tewari R P. Diagnosis of disseminated histoplasmosis by detection of *Histoplasma capsulatum* antigen in serum and urine specimens. *N Engl J Med* 314:83–88, 1986b.

Wheat L J, Kohler R B, Tewari R P, Garten M, French M L V. Significance of *Histoplasma* antigen in the cerebrospinal fluid of patients with meningitis. *Arch Intern Med* 149:302–304, 1989.

Wheat L J, Batteiger B E, Sathapatayavongs B. *Histoplasma capsulatum* infections of the central nervous system: a clinical review. *Medicine* (Baltimore) 69:244–260, 1990a.

Wheat L J, Connolly-Stringfield P A, Baker R L, Curfman M F, Eads M E, Israel K S, Norris S A, Webb D H, Zeckel M L. Disseminated histoplasmosis in the acquired immune deficiency syndrome: clinical findings, diagnosis and treatment, and review of the literature. *Medicine* (Baltimore) 69:361–374, 1990b.

Wheat L J, Connolly-Stringfield P, Blair R, Connolly K, Garringer T, Katz B P. Histoplasmosis relapse in patients with AIDS: detection using *Histoplasma capsulatum* variety *capsulatum* antigen levels. *Ann Intern Med* 115:936–941, 1991.

Wheat L J, Connolly-Stringfield P, Williams B, Connolly K, Blair R,

Bartlett M, Durkin M. Diagnosis of histoplasmosis in patients with the acquired immunodeficiency syndrome by detection of *Histoplasma capsulatum* polysaccharide antigen in bronchoalveolar lavage fluid. *Am Rev Respir Dis* 145:1421–1424, 1992a.

Wheat L J, Connolly-Stringfield P, Blair R, Connolly K, Garringer T, Katz B P, Gupta M. Effect of successful treatment with amphotericin B on *Histoplasma capsulatum* variety *capsulatum* polysaccharide antigen levels in patients with AIDS and histoplasmosis. *Am J Med* 92:153–160, 1992b.

Wheat J, Hafner R, Wulfson M, Spencer P, Squires K, Powderly W, Wong B, Rinaldi M, Saag M, Hamill R, Murphy R, Connolly-Stringfield P, Briggs N, Owens S, NIAID Clinical Trials and Mycoses Study Group. Prevention of relapse of histoplasmosis with itraconazole in patients with the acquired immunodeficiency syndrome. *Ann Intern Med* 118:610–616, 1993.

Wheat J, Hafner R, Korzun AH, Limjoco M T, Spencer P, Larsen R A, Hecht F M, Powderly W, and AIDS Clinical Trial Group. Itraconazole treatment of disseminated histoplasmosis in patients with the acquired immunodeficiency syndrome. *Am J Med* 98:336–342, 1995.

Wheat J. Histoplasmosis in the acquired immunodeficiency syndrome. *Curr Topics Med Mycol* 7:7–18, 1996.

Wheat J. Histoplasmosis: experience during outbreaks in Indianapolis and review of the literature. *Medicine* (Baltimore) 76:339–354, 1997a.

Wheat J, MaWhinney S, Hafner R, McKinsey D, Chen D, Korzun A, Skahan K, Johnson P, Hamill R, Bamberger D, Pappas P, Stansell J, Koletar S, Squires K, Larsen R A, Cheung T, Hyslop N, Lai K K, Schneider D, Kauffman C, Saag M, Dismukes W, Powderly W, NIAID ACTG and Mycoses Study Group. Treatment of histoplasmosis with fluconazole in patients with acquired immunodeficiency syndrome. *Am J Med* 103:223–232, 1997b.

Wheat J, Wheat H, Connolly P, Kleiman M, Supparatpinyo K, Nelson K, Bradsher R, Restrepo A. Cross-reactivity in *Histoplasma capsulatum* variety *capsulatum* antigen assays of urine samples from patients with endemic mycoses. *Clin Infect Dis* 24:1169–1171, 1997c.

Wheat J, Sarosi G, McKinsey D, Hamill R, Bradsher R, Johnson P, Loyd J, Kauffman C A. Practice guidelines for the management of patients with histoplasmosis. *Clin Infect Dis* 30:688–695, 2000.

Wheat L J. Laboratory diagnosis of histoplasmosis: update 2000. *Sem Respir Infect* 16:131–140, 2001a.

Wheat L J, Cloud G, Johnson P C, Connolly P, Goldman M, Le Monte A, Fuller D E, Davis T E, Hafner R, ACTG, Mycoses Study Group of NIAID. Clearance of fungal burden during treatment of disseminated histoplasmosis with liposomal amphotericin B versus itraconazole. *Antimicrob Agents Chemother* 45:2354–2357, 2001b.

Wilson D A, Muchmore H G, Tisda R G, Fahmy A, Pitha J V. Histoplasmosis of the adrenal glands studied by CT. *Radiology* 150:779–783, 1984.

Wilson M L, Davis T E, Mirrett S, Reynolds J, Fuller D, Allen S D, Flint K K, Koontz F, Reller L B. Controlled comparison of the BACTEC high-blood-volume fungal medium, BACTEC plus 26 aerobic blood culture bottle, and 10-milliliter isolator blood culture system for detection of fungemia and bacteremia. *J Clin Microbiol* 31:865–871, 1993.

Woods J P, Heinecke E L, Luecke J W, Maldonado E, Ng J Z, Retallack D M, Timmerman M M. Pathogenesis of *Histoplasma capsulatum*. *Sem Respir Infect* 16:91–101, 2001.

19

Blastomycosis

ROBERT W. BRADSHER

Blastomycosis, one of the endemic mycoses in the United States, is caused by the dimorphic fungus, *Blastomyces dermatitidis*. The organism exists in nature in the mould or mycelial phase and converts to the parasitic or yeast phase at body temperature. The fungus may either produce epidemics of infection after a point-source exposure or cause disease in a sporadic manner in the endemic areas. *Blastomyces dermatitidis* can cause an infection with a subclinical illness and subsequent protection against progressive infection afforded by cellular immune mechanisms. By contrast, a patient may present with pneumonia or with extrapulmonary disease or both. Lung involvement in blastomycosis may mimic acute bacterial pneumonia, while chronic pulmonary presentations mimic lung cancer or tuberculosis. Skin disease, usually presenting as either verrucous or ulcerative lesions, is the most common extrapulmonary site followed by bone, prostate, and CNS disease. Diagnosis is often easily made by visualization of the yeast in smears, or in tissue specimens or by culture; recognition of *B. dermatitidis* by smear or culture provides a definitive diagnosis. Itraconazole has been shown to be the drug of choice for either pulmonary or extrapulmonary infection, except in cases of life-threatening infection when amphotericin B should be used.

Gilchrist first described blastomycosis in Baltimore in the 1890s as a skin infection caused by a protozoan organism (Gilchrist, 1894) and the illness was known for a time as Gilchrist's disease. There were some errors in the initial description. For example, blastomycosis is not common in the areas surrounding Baltimore, and infection of the skin occurs secondarily rather than primarily. Moreover, the organism is not a protozoan but a fungus. Gilchrist was the first to refute portions of his own descriptions when he isolated and named the fungus *B. dermatitidis* (Gilchrist et al, 1898). Because skin manifestations of blastomycosis are often very striking, the initial cases were perceived as mainly dermatologic in nature (Sarosi and Davies, 1979). The concept of primary pulmonary blastomycosis was not recognized until pathologic descriptions allowed the pathophysiologic mechanisms to be delineated (Witorsch and Utz, 1968). There are rare cases of cutaneous inoculation of *B. dermatitidis* in laboratory workers and veterinarians, but almost all cases of blastomycosis are considered to originate from a pulmonary portal of entry (Sarosi and Davis, 1979).

ORGANISM

Blastomyces dermatitidis is a round, budding, thick-walled yeast cell with a daughter cell forming a single bud that has a broad base (Fig. 19–1). Like *H. capsulatum*, this fungus is dimorphic, which means that it exists as a mycelial form in nature and a yeast form in tissue. *Blastomyces dermatitidis* grows in cultures as mycelia at 25°C and as a yeast at 37°C. The physiologic explanation for transformation from mycelia to yeast has been attributed to heat-related insults with resultant partial uncoupling of oxidative phosphorylation (Medoff et al, 1987). The perfect or sexual stage of the fungus is *Ajellomyces dermatitidis*, with the imperfect or conidial stage named the familiar *Blastomyces dermatitidis*. This imperfect stage grows as a fluffy white mould on fungal media at room temperature and as a brown, wrinkled, folded yeast at 37°C. It may be difficult to differentiate from other mycelia and that prompted workers to develop tests for differential exoantigen analysis of mycelial forms taken from cultures to discriminate early cultures of *H. capsulatum* and *B. dermatitidis* (Kaufman et al, 1983). The yeast varies in size from 5 to 15 μm and in the number of organisms found. Most are round and have a double cell wall appearance, which actually consists of the interior and exterior components of a thick cell surface. The yeast may be found inside or outside of macrophages in the pyogranulomatous tissue response. Unlike *Candida* or *Aspergillus*, colonization of the respiratory tract with *Blastomyces* does not occur. Consequently, detection of *Blastomyces* by smear, culture or histology secures a diagnosis of infection (Fig. 19–2).

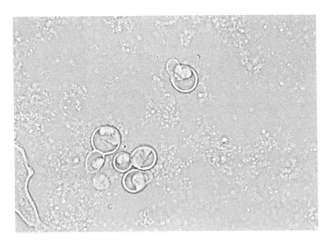

FIGURE 19–1. Exudate from sputum treated with KOH revealing *B. dermatitidis*.

EPIDEMIOLOGY AND IMMUNITY

Unlike many fungal infections which are opportunistic, blastomycosis is usually diagnosed in normal hosts. Otherwise, blastomycosis has a similar epidemiology to other endemic mycoses, i.e., histoplasmosis and coccidioidomycosis, although the latter two diseases are more common. Consequently, greater details are understood about their epidemiology. For example, histoplasmosis was once considered a rare but uniformly fatal infection (Parsons and Zaronfontis, 1945). However, utilizing *Histoplasma* skin testing within the histoplasmosis endemic areas, many persons without a history of clinical illness were found to be infected with *H. capsulatum* (Christie and Peterson, 1945).

The vast majority of patients with reported blastomycosis have had clinically recognized/diagnosed disease and are located within a fairly well-defined geographical area of the South and North Central United States. Many of these patients have a history of recre-

ational or occupational exposure to wooded areas and often to bodies of water, such as lakes or rivers. The incidence of blastomycosis depends on the reporting of clinically diagnosed cases of infection because there are no simple and reliable markers of previous infection, such as the histoplasmin skin test for histoplasmosis. However, it is becoming increasingly apparent that blastomycosis is similar to histoplasmosis with more and more patients with subclinical infection being discovered. Patients with acute blastomycosis who recovered without antifungal therapy have been reported; the majority of those cases, which are associated with point-source epidemics such as those at Big Fork, Minnesota (Tosh et al, 1974), and Eagle River, Wisconsin (Klein et al, 1986a) did not require antifungal therapy. In the Eagle River outbreak of blastomycosis, only 9 of the 44 patients with infection were treated with an antifungal agent (Klein et al, 1986a). None of the remaining 35 untreated patients had relapse or progressive infection. In addition, a group of patients has been reported who had surgical resection of a solitary pulmonary nodule that subsequently was found to be caused by *B. dermatitidis* (Edson et al, 1981). Since no other disease manifestation was present, surgical therapy alone was sufficient for cure (Edson and Keys, 1981).

In the Eagle River epidemic, not all of those with immune markers of infection (serology, antigen-induced lymphocyte transformation) had signs and symptoms characteristic of blastomycosis (Klein et al, 1986a). During experiments of specific immunity with cells from treated blastomycosis patients (Bradsher et al, 1985a; Bradsher et al, 1987a), two control persons with no history of blastomycosis had evidence of immunity. Cells from these two control subjects displayed lymphocyte responses to a *Blastomyces* antigen and macrophage inhibition of intracellular growth of the fungus similar to experiments using cells from persons with culture-proven infections and dissimilar to other control individuals with no history of exposure. Both controls had potential exposure as long-term avid hunters in the endemic region for blastomycosis (Bradsher et al, 1987a). This observation prompted studies of other persons who had comparable environmental exposures to patients with clinical blastomycosis, specifically, forestry workers in areas endemic for blastomycosis but not histoplasmosis (Northern Minnesota and Wisconsin) (Vaalar et al, 1990). Thirty percent of the workers had in vitro markers of immunity as evidence of subclinical infection with no question of cross-reactions due to prior infection with *Histoplasma capsulatum* (Vaalar et al, 1990). A mutant strain of *B. dermatitidis* (Wuthrich et al, 2000) has been demonstrated that does not cause systemic infection in animals but does induce cellular immunity. Subsequent challenge of the animals

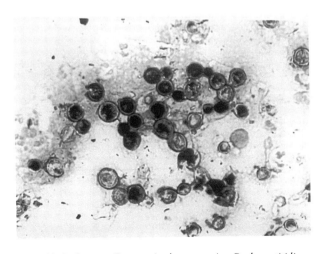

FIGURE 19–2. Sputum Gram stain demonstrating *B. dermatitidis*.

does not cause the lethal lung infection found in control animals (Wuthrich et al, 2000). Blastomycosis appears to have comparable patterns of subclinical infection with development of cellular immunity as the other, more extensively studied endemic mycoses, namely, histoplasmosis and coccidioidomycosis.

Endemic or sporadic cases account for the majority of reported cases of blastomycosis. The endemic area in North America includes the states bordering the Mississippi and Ohio Rivers, the Midwestern and Canadian provinces that border the Great Lakes, and a small area in New York and Canada along the St. Lawrence River (Sarosi and Davies, 1979). Most cases are reported from Arkansas, Mississippi, Alabama, Kentucky, Tennessee, and Wisconsin. Within these endemic regions are hyperendemic areas with unusually high rates of blastomycosis (Vaalar et al, 1990). Several epidemics of infection from point sources have also been described (Sarosi and Davies, 1979) including epidemics occurring in North Carolina, Minnesota, Illinois, Wisconsin, and Virginia.

Blastomycosis results from inhalation of spores from the soil. However, B. dermatitidis has been very difficult to isolate from soil, in contrast to the ease of growing H. capsulatum from soil. Blastomyces dermatitidis was recovered from soil and rotted wood in Georgia on three occasions (Denton and DiSalvo, 1964). Investigators isolated the yeast phase of the fungus from bird droppings (Sarosi and Serstock, 1976), and from a dirt floor in Canada (Bakerspigel et al, 1986). The organism was recovered without animal inoculation from a woodpile within a hyperendemic region in Wisconsin; several dogs in a nearby kennel had been diagnosed with blastomycosis (Baumgardener and Paretsky, 1999). Many other investigators have been unsuccessful in recovering the organism from soil including soil from highly suspicious areas based on epidemiologic clues to the location of the common-source exposure. However, B. dermatitidis was isolated from soil in association with epidemics in two separate reports (Klein et al, 1986a; Klein et al, 1987). The isolations were from wet earth containing animal droppings, proving that the fungus exists in microfoci in soil. In these epidemics, the isolation of the fungus was also noted to be associated with bodies of water. It has yet to be determined whether water is the primary factor or simply an explanation for greater exposure potential because of recreational activities in areas with wildlife or water (Bradsher, 1987b).

PATHOGENESIS

Infection with B. dermatitidis begins with inhalation of conidia into the lung followed by clearing of the organism by bronchopulmonary phagocytes. Alveolar macrophages have been shown to kill conidia (Sugar and Picard, 1991), which may explain why some persons are not infected even though they have the same exposure as an infected individual in an epidemic. As the fungus undergoes transition to yeast cells, growth occurs in the lung and the organisms can also spread to other organs by the bloodstream. With the development of immunity, inflammatory reactions occur, initially as a suppurative response with polymorphonuclear phagocytes, and subsequently influx of monocyte-derived macrophages. This pyogranulomatous response is distinctive of blastomycosis, although necrosis or fibrosis may also be found. Typically, the granuloma of blastomycosis does not caseate, as found in tuberculosis. In the skin lesions of this infection, the histologic changes may prompt an erroneous diagnosis of squamous cell carcinoma or keratoacanthoma [Bradsher et al, 1990]. Fungal stains would allow the correct diagnosis, but the misdiagnosis is usually discovered when a second distant site of infection is found. Despite spontaneous resolution of the pneumonia in some cases, endogenous reactivation may occur at either pulmonary or extrapulmonary sites even after previous therapy (Landis and Varkey, 1976).

CLINICAL MANIFESTATIONS

General

Frequently, initially blastomycosis is misdiagnosed because the clinical presentations are multiple and are similar to other more common conditions. Weight loss, fever, malaise, fatigue, and other nonspecific complaints are common but not helpful diagnostically. The stereotypical patient is a young to middle-aged male who either works in or visits outdoor areas in Arkansas, Mississippi, or another state in the endemic area. Dogs are in the same environment as humans and may get blastomycosis; a clinical clue to the diagnosis of blastomycosis in humans may be a history of a pet dog having been diagnosed with blastomycosis (Sarosi et al, 1983). Blastomycosis is not routinely transmitted from animal to human nor is infection typically spread from person to person. However, there are very rare reports of a dog with oral lesions transmitting infection to man via a bite (Gnann et al, 1983), or a man with penile blastomycotic lesions transmitting infection to a sexual partner (Farber et al, 1968).

In an outbreak of blastomycosis, women and children are as likely as males to be infected. Aside from an epidemic, only rarely are children diagnosed with blastomycosis (Steele and Abernathy, 1983). In endemic cases, the male-to-female ratio has been reported from 4:1 to 15:1 in various series (Bradsher, 1988). Some of these studies, however, were conducted in Vet-

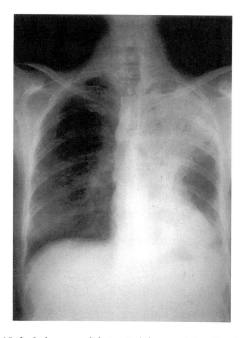

FIGURE 19–3. Lobar consolidation in left upper lobe of patient with pulmonary blastomycosis.

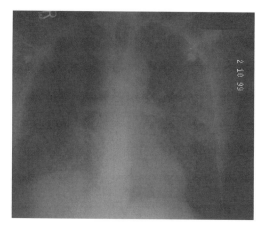

FIGURE 19–4. Acute left lung pneumonia due to *B. dermatitidis*.

erans Affairs Medical Centers, which obviously adds bias to the data. In an observational review of referrals of 135 patients over a 13-year period in Arkansas, 78 were male and 57 female (Bradsher, 1997). Extrapulmonary manifestations were found in 47% and 53% had only lung involvement. Women accounted for only 30% of the extrapulmonary cases while 47% of the pneumonia cases were in women (Bradsher, 1997). Greater numbers are required for confirmation, but men may be more likely than women to have extrapulmonary disease, just as occurs in paracoccidioidomycosis.

Since blastomycosis is not a common diagnosis in most clinical practices, a delay in diagnosis often occurs. The pulmonary manifestations may be diagnosed as acute bacterial community-acquired pneumonia on the one end of the spectrum or as tuberculosis or malignancy on the other. The skin lesions may be diagnosed as pyoderma gangrenosum or keratoacanthoma, while lesions in the larynx, central nervous system, skin, breast, lymph nodes, or essentially any organ are sometimes mistakenly diagnosed as cancer. Careful histologic investigation enables the correct diagnosis of blastomycosis in such cases.

Pulmonary Disease. The presentation of clinical blastomycosis for most patients is pneumonia with radiography revealing an alveolar or mass-like infiltrate (Fig. 19–3) as was seen in 16 of 17 patients with abnormal X-rays in one report (Halvorsen et al, 1984). In another series of 46 blastomycosis patients, 32% had a pulmonary mass lesion and 48% had an alveolar in-

filtrate on chest radiograph (Bradsher et al, 1985b). Miliary or reticulonodular types of presentations may also be seen. Hilar adenopathy and pleural effusions are uncommon (Brown et al, 1991). Although blastomycotic cavitary disease may occur, this pattern is not as commonly found as in chronic pulmonary histoplasmosis or reactivation tuberculosis.

Pulmonary blastomycosis includes acute pneumonia and chronic pneumonia. Acute pneumonia may present like acute bacterial pneumonia as with *Streptococcus pneumoniae*, causing fever, chills, and a productive purulent cough with or without hemoptysis (Fig. 19–4). Blastomycosis presenting as chronic pneumonia may cause weight loss, night sweats, fever, cough with sputum production, and chest pain, suggesting a diagnosis

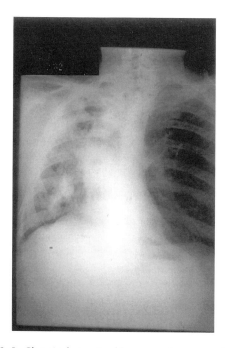

FIGURE 19–5. Chronic destructive blastomycotic pneumonia.

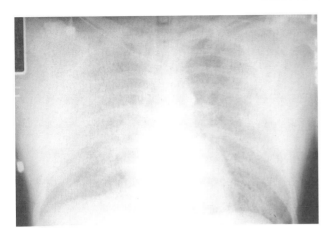

FIGURE 19–6. Diffuse alveolar opacities (acute respiratory distress syndrome) in lymphoma patient treated with corticosteroids.

of tuberculosis or lung cancer (Fig. 19–5). By contrast, blastomycosis patients with a pulmonary infiltrate may have no pulmonary symptoms at all; the diagnosis is made following routine X-rays with continued patient denial of pulmonary complaints even after extensive questioning. In one series of 26 pulmonary blastomycosis patients, 2 were asymptomatic, 16 had a chronic pneumonia picture, and 8 initially had acute pneumonia (Bradsher et al, 1985b).

Lung failure with the adult respiratory distress syndrome (ARDS) (Fig. 19–6) may be the presenting feature of blastomycosis in both immunocompetent and immunocompromised patients. Meyer and colleagues reported 10 patients with overwhelming ARDS caused by *B. dermatitidis*, and 5 of them died. Six of the patients had no underlying disease associated with altered immunity (Meyer et al, 1993). One patient with this syndrome reported by Evans and colleagues had a tracheal ulcer at the carina on bronchoscopy, prompting the speculation that a subcarinal lymph node ruptured into the trachea and spilled enough organisms into the lungs to cause ARDS (Evans et al, 1982). A number of cases of blastomycosis associated with ARDS have been described in immunocompromised hosts, especially corticosteroid treated patients (Pappas et al, 1993) and in AIDS patients (Pappas et al, 1992). In immunocompromised patients with ARDS, fulminant infection of the lungs relates to severe T cell dysfunction. Many patients with blastomycosis and the pattern of diffuse infiltrates, noncardiac pulmonary edema, and refractory hypoxemia die very quickly. Early therapy may improve survival; however, since blastomycosis is an extremely infrequent cause of ARDS, the diagnosis is usually not considered initially (Skillrud and Douglas, 1985).

Cutaneous Disease. Skin lesions are the most common manifestation of extrapulmonary blastomycosis

(Witorch and Utz, 1968; Sarosi and Davies, 1979). These lesions may be present with or without concomitant pulmonary lesions. Cutaneous lesions are either verrucous or ulcerative (Schwarz and Salfelder, 1977; Bradsher, 1988). The verrucous, or fungating, form has an irregular and raised border, often with crusting and exudate above an abscess in the subcutaneous tissue (See Color Figs. 19–7, 19–8, and 19–9 in separate color insert). Histologically, papillomatosis, downward proliferation of the epidermis with intraepidermal abscesses, and inflammatory cells in the dermis are features of the verrucous lesions (Schwarz and Salfelder, 1977; Sarosi and Davies, 1979). The cutaneous ulcerative form occurs when the subcutaneous abscess spontaneously drains; these ulcers demonstrate the same histologic changes as in the verrucous form of disease. The borders of the ulcer are usually raised and distinct (See Color Fig. 19–10 in separate color insert), and the base of the ulcer usually contains exudate (See Color Fig. 19–11 in separate color insert). Polymorphonuclear leukocytes are typically present on biopsy, even in those patients with little inflammation clinically apparent in the ulcer. Subcutaneous localization with formation of nodules, and only mild ulceration or verrucous appearance, may rarely be observed (See Color Fig. 19–12 in separate color insert). Such lesions are typically tender and may be confused with panniculitis or Weber-Christian disease (Maioriello and Merwin, 1970). Aspiration of the subcutaneous mass or biopsy will reveal *B. dermatitidis* organisms on microscopy and culture.

Skin lesions of blastomycosis may be confused with a number of alternative diagnoses, including basal cell carcinoma, squamous cell carcinoma, pyoderma gangrenosa, or keratoacanthoma. One patient was reported with what appeared to be condyloma acuminatum surrounding the anus (Bradsher et al, 1990). Only after postoperative suppurative drainage occurred was the histology reviewed and *B. dermatitidis* found.

Bone Disease. Bone infection due to *B. dermatitidis* infection is reported in as many as one-fourth of extrapulmonary cases and may be the reason the patient seeks medical attention (Moore and Green, 1982). Granuloma, suppuration, or necrosis may be found in the bone biopsy. The vertebrae, pelvis, sacrum, skull, ribs, or long bones are the most frequently reported sites of infection, but essentially any bone may be involved (Witorch and Utz, 1968; Saccente et al, 1998). The radiographic appearance of blastomycosis in bone is not specific and cannot be discriminated from that of other fungal, bacterial, or neoplastic disease. Debridement may be required for cure but most blastomycotic bone lesions resolve with antifungal therapy alone, unlike the usual bacterial osteomyelitis.

Joint Disease. Articular blastomycosis is much less common than osseous blastomycosis, and estimated to occur in approximately 3%–5% of cases (Bayer et al, 1979). Monoarthritis, especially involving the knee, is most common. The majority of patients with blastomycotic arthritis also have concurrent disease of the lungs and skin. Justa-articular osteomyelitis is less frequent. Microscopy or culture of synovial fluid is diagnostic in approximately 50% of cases.

Genitourinary Disease. The genitourinary (GU) system follows lung, skin and bone in frequency of involvement. Because men are more likely to have extrapulmonary blastomycosis, prostatitis and epididymoorchitis have been the more commonly reported forms of GU involvement (Witorch and Utz, 1968; Sarosi and Davies, 1979). Genitourinary involvement may be detected in urine collected after prostatic massage (Inoshita et al., 1983). As is the case with skin or bone infection, genitourinary blastomycosis will often be present at the same time as infection in the lung. Chest radiographs should be performed in every case of extrapulmonary blastomycosis, even in the patient without pulmonary complaints. Examples of female genital tract blastomycosis, which is less frequently diagnosed, include endometrial infection acquired by sexual contact with a man who had blastomycosis of the penis (Farber et al, 1968), tubo-ovarian abscess following hematogenous disseminaton (Murray et al, 1984), and tubo-ovarian abscess mimicking ovarian cancer (Mouzin and Beilke, 1996). Massive endometrial infection that caused uterine hemorrhage has also been described in one patient (Faro et al, 1987).

Central Nervous System Disease. Blastomycosis is reported to involve the nervous system in 5% to 10% of cases of disseminated disease. Meningitis, cerebral abscesses, or blastomycomas (granulomatous masses) are the usual manifestations of central nervous system blastomycosis (Roos et al, 1979; Kravitz et al, 1981). Whatever the form of disease, it is difficult to identify the organism. Radiographic imaging should direct the neurosurgeon to biopsy the cranial abscesses or blastomycoma, but identification of blastomycosis as the cause of meningitis is more problematic. Evaluation of lumbar CSF is less likely to be definitive for B. dermatitidis than ventricular fluid. In one series of 22 cases, CSF from lumbar puncture provided the diagnosis in only 2 patients, whereas ventricular CSF specimens were positive in 6 of 7 cases (Kravitz et al, 1981). A predominance of polymorphonuclear leukocytes in CSF is common in blastomycotic meningitis (Harley et al, 1994).

Other Clinical Manifestations. Blastomycosis may involve virtually any organ. Abscesses are most common in the subcutaneous tissue but, as already noted, may be found in the brain, skeletal system, prostate, or any other organ including the myocardium, pericardium, orbit, sinuses, and pituitary or adrenal gland (Witorch and Utz, 1968). The reticuloendothelial system has also been involved with reports of several cases of lymph node or hepatic disease (Sarosi and Davies, 1979; Bradsher et al, 1990; Bradsher, 1997). Splenic abscesses have likewise been documented (Dubuisson and Jones, 1983).

Lesions in the mouth and oropharyngeal area occur in blastomycosis but not as commonly as in disseminated histoplasmosis. Blastomycosis does seem to frequently involve the larynx (Suen et al, 1980; Dumich and Neal, 1983). Laryngeal biopsy reveals histologic features similar to those in the skin and the hyperplasia, acanthosis, and fungating appearance of laryngeal blastomycosis may be confused with squamous cell carcinoma. In some cases, fixation of the vocal cords secondary to fibrosis has led to radiation therapy or total laryngectomy due to an incorrect diagnosis of neoplasm.

Specific endocrine abnormalities may appear in patients with blastomycosis (Witorch and Utz, 1968). Adrenal insufficiency from gland destruction, thyroid infection, and hypercalcemia, as seen with other granulomatous diseases, have been reported. A single case of diabetes insipidus (Kelly, 1982) and another of hyperprolactinemia with galactorrhea and amenorrhea (Arora et al, 1989) are documented.

A number of other unusual clinical manifestations of blastomycosis have been described. Two cases in women with blastomycosis of the breast had abnormal mammograms with a strong clinical suspicion of carcinoma (Farmer et al, 1995). A computerized tomography scan that revealed partial destruction of a vertebral body consistent with metastatic disease caused one woman to be considered for cancer chemotherapy until a breast biopsy revealed B. dermatitidis on microscopy and subsequent culture. The breast mass in both patients resolved with antifungal therapy (Farmer et al, 1995). Other cases of blastomycosis of the breast have been reported (Seymour, 1982; Faro et al, 1987; Propeck and Scanlan, 1996). Seymour reported a patient with bilateral masses caused by B. dermititidis; one of these masses had an air fluid level (Seymour, 1982). A presumptive case of blastomycosis of the breast was reported when a skin lesion revealed blastomycosis and the unbiopsied breast mass resolved clinically and radiologically with antifungal therapy (Propeck and Scanlan, 1996).

Ocular involvement may assume several forms. A patient with a blastomycotic mass on the iris prompted a review of literature with the finding of 11 other cases of ocular blastomycosis, including iritis, uveitis, endophthalmitis and choroidal disease (Lopez et al, 1994). In a subsequent report, 2 more cases of choroidal blastomycosis were described (Gottlieb et al, 1995). Eyelid involvement has been reported to occur in patients with systemic blastomycosis (Vida and Moel, 1974; Bartley, 1995), but it is an infrequent occurrence in the experience of most experts. Ocular disease in canine blastomycosis, endophthalmitis in particular, is very common while blastomycosis involvement of the human eye is rare. The reason for this discrepancy is not understood but may be due to late diagnosis in dogs, allowing more dissemination of the infection.

Two cases of blastomycotic otitis media with cranial extension have been reported (Istorico et al, 1992). Both patients were cured with amphotericin B. One patient was described with *B. dermatitidis* infection in a presumed branchial cleft cyst infection (Bradsher et al, 1990). Surgical removal demonstrated lymphadenopathy and both suppurative and granulomatous inflammation with *B. dermatitidis* organisms. Sinusitis caused by *B. dermatitidis* is rare (Witzig et al, 1994a).

Blastomycosis in Special Population Groups
Several cases of blastomycosis have been reported during pregnancy (Ismail and Lerner, 1982; Tuthill et al, 1985; Daniel and Salit, 1989; MacDonald and Alguire, 1990; Maxson et al, 1992; Young and Schutze, 1995; Chakravarty et al, 1995), including, rarely, mothers who transmitted blastomycosis to the child via intrauterine transfer of the organisms (Tuthill et al, 1985; Maxson et al, 1992; Chakravarty et al, 1995).

Although blastomycosis may cause infections in immunocompromised patients, other endemic fungal infections such as histoplasmosis or coccidioidomycosis are much more likely to be opportunistic than blastomycosis. Immunosuppressed patients, including those with AIDS and sarcoidosis, transplantation recipients, and others receiving corticosteroids, usually develop blastomycosis following exposure in the environment or through subsequent reactivation, just as immunocompetent patients. *Blastomyces dermatitidis* has been reported as an opportunistic pathogen following infection with HIV in a relatively small number of cases (Pappas et al, 1992; Witzig et al, 1994b). When blastomycosis is seen in a patient with HIV, it may be widely disseminated and particularly severe.

Pappas and colleagues also described 34 non-HIV infected but otherwise immunosuppressed patients with blastomycosis. The immunocompromising conditions in these 34 patients were long-term glucocorticoid therapy in 12, hematologic malignancies in 10, cytotoxic chemotherapy in 4, solid organ transplant in 3, and miscellaneous other conditions in 5. These investigators found an increased frequency of cases of blastomycosis in this patient population from 1978 through 1991 as compared to an earlier period, 1956 through 1977 (Pappas et al, 1993). Although this change in frequency might be due to a bias in referral patterns of

patients, the authors speculated that this difference more likely reflected the continually expanding population of patients with complicated, immune compromising illnesses who have lived in the endemic area for blastomycosis (Pappas et al, 1993).

Blastomycosis may occur along with other infections or illnesses. Diabetes mellitus is suggested as a risk factor for blastomycosis but epidemiologic studies to compare the two illnesses are difficult to perform because of the relative lack of serologic or other markers of subclinical infection with *B. dermatitidis*. Blastomycosis has been described in association with tuberculosis, histoplasmosis and coccidioidomycosis (Causey and Campbell, 1992). Similarly, blastomycosis has been reported in association with idiopathic thrombocytopenic purpura and hemolytic anemia of unknown cause (Bradsher, 1997). Both patients were treated with corticosteroids for the hematologic conditions, while the blastomycosis was treated with antifungal agents. Steroids were rapidly tapered and the hematologic conditions did not recur after the blastomycosis was cured. Another patient with both sarcoidosis and blastomycosis was treated effectively with both corticosteroids and itraconazole with cure of the fungal infection (Bradsher et al, 1990). As long as effective antifungal chemotherapy is being given concurrently, steroid therapy may not have the deleterious result that has been described in undiagnosed or untreated blastomycosis. A similar observation has been made previously regarding other infectious diseases, particularly tuberculosis.

DIAGNOSIS

If suspected, *B. dermatitidis* is relatively easy to identify in tissue or exudates, and the organism is not difficult to culture within a 2- to 4-week incubation period. Either identifying the organism by histopathology or microscopy or growing *B. dermatitidis* in culture is necessary for a firm diagnosis. The fungus is most commonly identified on microscopy of exudate, sputum, or tissue following digestion of human cells with potassium hydroxide (Chapman, 2000a), but cytologic preparations can also be used for diagnosis (Sutliff and Cruthirds, 1973). Since the clinical picture of chronic pneumonia due to blastomycosis may mimic carcinoma of the lung, cytology specimens should be sent for cancer cytology. Identification of *B. dermatitidis* in expectorated sputum or BAL washings can diagnose the infection and thereby eliminate the need for surgical exploration.

Fortunately, diagnosis by smear, histopathology, or culture is reliable and relatively easy since serology is not as useful as in many other infectious diseases. There are no assays for antigen detection of blastomycosis such as with histoplasmosis or cryptococcosis or a polymerase chain reaction test as with tuberculosis. With blastomycosis, serologic diagnostic techniques, such as CF for antibodies, have been used as tools for epidemiologic assessments, but have not been helpful for clinical diagnosis. Cross reactivity to antigens of various fungi, in particular *B. dermatitidis* and *H. capsulatum*, limits specificity (Davies and Sarosi, 1987). For example, persons with culture-proven blastomycosis are just as apt to demonstrate CF antibodies against histoplasmin as against blastomycin (Sarosi and Davies, 1979). Immunodiffusion (ID) precipitin band testing of serum results in sensitivity rates of up to 80% while even better results have been reported with enzyme immunoabsorbant (EIA) techniques using a yeast-phase antigen (antigen A) (Klein et al, 1986b). In the largest outbreak of blastomycosis reported to date, Klein and coworkers described antibody detection by CF, ID, and EIA techniques in only 9%, 28%, and 77% of patients, respectively (Klein et al, 1986a). Consequently, the utility of current serologic tests for the diagnosis of blastomycosis is not helpful clinically.

Skin testing with blastomycin is even less useful than serology as a diagnostic study in individual patients with potential *B. dermatitidis* infection. In two series, 100% (Witorch and Utz, 1968) and 59% (Busey, 1964) of the culture-proven blastomycosis patients had negative blastomycin skin tests that could be explained only partially by anergy. Blastomycin, a mycelial-phase antigen, does not provide sufficient specificity or sensitivity for reliable patient assessment and is no longer available clinically. Although a commercially available EIA assay has been marketed recently based on studies showing high sensitivity and specificity (Bradsher and Pappas, 1995), visualization of the organism on smear or in tissue or a positive culture will likely remain the mainstay of diagnosis for the foreseeable future.

TREATMENT

The Infectious Diseases Society of America has published guidelines for the treatment of blastomycosis (Chapman et al, 2000b). The first consideration for the patient diagnosed with blastomycosis is whether or not to use an antifungal agent. Subclinical disease occurs with this infection just as with *H. capsulatum* and *Coccidioides immitis*. Sarosi and others reported patients infected in an outbreak in 1974 who did not receive amphotericin B but recovered (Tosh et al, 1974; Recht et al, 1979). In the largest epidemic of blastomycosis reported, Klein et al reported that only 9 of the 48 infected with the fungus received antifungal therapy (Klein et al, 1986a). Subclinical and untreated blastomycosis as detected by tests of cellular immunity (Bradsher, 1984; Bradsher et al, 1985a; Vaaler et al, 1990) suggest many infections resolve without antifungal therapy. In addition, there have been reports of endogenous reactivation of blastomycosis after a latency

period as long as 40 years (Landis and Varkey, 1976; Ehni, 1989). It is clear that many persons have infection with *B. dermatitidis* and recover without a diagnosis ever being made. Therefore, some patients with blastomycosis recover spontaneously without specific antifungal therapy just as occurs in the majority of cases of histoplasmosis and coccidioidomycosis.

The clinical presentation of the patient and the toxicity of antifungal agents are the major determinants of whether or not to observe the infection or use an antifungal agent. This approach of observation without therapy should be limited to mild pulmonary blastomycosis. If relapse of infection does occur, it may recur in the lung, but also may occur in a disseminated site such as skin, bone, central nervous system, or genitourinary system. Relapse has been discovered after the initial pulmonary infection either without or with treatment, so if therapy is not given the patient should be monitored for a prolonged period. If the patient has deterioration or progression of the primary pneumonia, antifungal therapy should be initiated. Observation alone may also be indicated in a patient who has already improved before the culture was identified as *B. dermatitidis*. The presence of pleural disease or any extrapulmonary manifestations during the course of illness requires antifungal treatment. With currently available antifungal agents that have less toxicity, observation without therapy is not as commonly done as formerly when only parenteral and toxic therapies, e.g., hydroxystilbamidine and amphotericin B, were available.

Effective therapy for blastomycosis has been available since the introduction of deoxycholate amphotericin B in 1956 (Chapman, 2000a). Intravenous amphotericin B in a total dosage of at least 1.0 g resulted in cure without relapse in five large series of patients with blastomycosis: in 77% (Busey, 1964), 84% (Witorch and Utz, 1968), 91% (Lockwood et al, 1969), 87% (Parker et al, 1969), and 90% (Seaburg and Dascomb, 1964). A total dosage of 2.0 g has been associated with cure rates of up to 97% (Abernathy, 1967). Relapse of blastomycosis following amphotericin B therapy appears to be dose-dependent and occurs only very rarely if a full course of drug is given. Relapse occurred in only 2 of 30 patients who received more than 1.5 g total dose of the drug, whereas 5 of 19 patients who received a smaller dose had relapse (Parker et al, 1969). Most cases of relapse of blastomycosis following amphotericin B occur shortly after completion of therapy. However, patients have had relapse of disease as long as 9 years following treatment (Landis and Varkey, 1976).

This high degree of antimycotic activity of amphotericin B is associated with a relatively large amount of toxicity. In a group of patients with blastomycosis (Abernathy, 1967), almost 75% experienced a decline in renal function and a number of other toxicities including anemia, anorexia, and nausea, fever, hypokalemia, and thrombophlebitis. Interruption of therapy during some point in the course was required in 41% of patients and termination of therapy with amphotericin B before reaching the desired total dose was mandatory because of toxicity in 14% of the patients (Abernathy, 1967). Therefore, the primary reason in the past for withholding or postponing treatment of blastomycosis was the toxicity of amphotericin B. Lipid formulations of amphotericin B which are less toxic than conventional amphotericin B have been used in anecdotal cases but not in comparative studies. The high cost of these lipid formulation drugs have limited their use in other endemic fungal diseases.

Azole antifungal agents have largely replaced amphotericin B as therapy of choice for most patients with blastomycosis, especially those with mild to moderate pulmonary or non-CNS disseminated disease. These drugs work by disrupting the cytoplasmic membranes as a consequence of inhibition of the synthesis of ergosterol, the major sterol of the fungal membrane (Como and Dismukes, 1994). Ketoconazole, itraconazole, and fluconazole are generally effective and well tolerated. Ketoconazole has rarely been described to cause sporadic cases of severe hepatocellular damage (Como and Dismukes, 1994). At higher dosages of the drug, hormonal abnormalities of gynecomastia, dysfunctional uterine bleeding and oligospermia may occur (Pont et al, 1984; Bradsher et al, 1985b). Ketoconazole may also cause common but less severe adverse effects including nausea and vomiting when the drug is taken without a meal, dizziness, pruritus, and headache. The absorption of ketoconazole and itraconazole capsules requires an acidic gastric content; consequently, concurrent antacids or acid suppression agents are contraindicated. Neither the oral solution of itraconazole or the various fluconazle formulations requires acidic gastric pH; as a result, these formulations do not have the same degree of poor absorption when used concurrently with acid suppressing agents (Como and Dismukes, 1994). Azole-drug interactions are a major concern, especially those related to itraconazole. Drugs such as rifampin, oral contraceptives, phenobarbital, and dilantin may be associated with reduced efficacy of itraconazole as a result of increased metabolism of the antifungal drug. Moreover, itraconazole may cause substantial increases in the blood levels of cyclosporine, digoxin, and several other drugs. Accordingly, careful review of all medications must be made when itraconazole therapy is planned (Como and Dismukes, 1994).

Ketoconazole has been effective for therapy of blastomycosis (NIAID, 1985; Bradsher et al, 1985a) but side effects prompted search for other agents. The mechanism of action and the pharmacokinetics of itra-

conazole are similar to that of ketoconazole (Como and Dismukes, 1994). The major theoretical advantage of itraconazole over ketoconazole was a lower rate of toxicity associated with itraconazole in investigational trials (Tucker et al, 1990). In addition, a higher efficacy rate was observed with itraconazole than with ketoconazole even though comparative clinical trials were not performed. In an open-label noncomparative trial, itraconazole capsules at a dose of 200 to 400 mg per day were evaluated by the NIAID Mycoses Study Group (Dismukes et al, 1992). Of the 40 patients with blastomycosis treated with itraconazole for > 2 months duration (median 6.2 months, range 3–24 months), 95% of were considered cured. In a second similar trial, itraconazole was used at a dose of 200 mg per day to treat 42 other patients with blastomycosis (Bradsher, 1992). While all of the patients showed a rapid initial response, 5 patients had a less than satisfactory overall response. Two had relapse successfully treated with another itraconazole course, 1 developed central nervous system disease and was switched to amphotericin B therapy, and 2 required amphotericin B therapy after relapse (Bradsher, 1992).

There has been limited experience in *B. dermatitidis* infections treated with fluconazole at doses of 200 to 800 mg per day (Pappas et al, 1995; Pappas et al, 1997). This agent, which is approved by the FDA only for cryptococcal and *Candida* infections, should not be considered equivalent to itraconazole for blastomycosis, but may be useful if itraconazole cannot be used because of significant azole-drug interactions. Another possible use of higher dose fluconazole (600–1000 mg/day) would be for central nervous system blastomycosis if amphotericin B cannot be used. Fluconazole penetrates well into the brain and cerebrospinal fluid while itraconazole does not.

While an intravenous formulation of itraconazole has been marketed, relatively few patients with blastomycosis have been treated with this form of the drug. Renal dysfunction is a contraindication for its use because of the cyclodextrin vehicle, which is cleared almost exclusively by the kidneys. For most patients with blastomycosis, current evidence does not suggest a major advantage of the intravenous formulation of itraconazole over the oral formulation. For the severely ill patient with blastomycosis, most authorities would initiate therapy with amphotericin B. For the rare patient who cannot tolerate amphotericin B and who cannot take oral therapy, intravenous itraconazole may be useful (Slain et al, 2001).

At least 6 months of oral therapy with azole antifungal agents has been recommended by most authorities, but there are no trials that have evaluated a shorter duration of therapy. Comparative lengths of therapy need to be studied to determine the optimal duration of therapy. Difficulties in designing suitable trials between intravenous amphotericin B and oral azole drugs have centered on the different routes of administration and the greater toxicity of amphotericin B versus the oral azoles.

The efficacy of oral itraconazole therapy of blastomycosis is impressive (Dismukes et al, 1992; Bradsher, 1992). However, in the very ill patient, amphotericin B 0.7–1.0 mg/kg/day remains the initial treatment of choice. After improvement of the patient with approximately 500 mg total dose of amphotericin B, a switch to oral itraconazole for the remainder of the treatment course is appropriate. One major disadvantage of oral therapy is the potential of patient noncompliance. For example, in earlier trials the majority of patients who failed ketoconazole treatment for blastomycosis had not taken the drug as instructed, a problem that is usually not encountered with intravenous therapy with amphotericin B. In addition, central nervous system blastomycotic infection may develop in patients receiving itraconazole or ketoconazole since penetration of these azoles into the brain parenchyma is minimal. For example, cases have been reported with clearing of cutaneous or pulmonary disease with ketoconazole but subsequent development of central nervous system disease (Bradsher et al, 1985a; Hebert et al, 1989; Pitrak and Andersen, 1989).

To summarize, based on available data and experience, itraconazole, at a dose of 200–400 mg per day for at least 6 months, is the therapy of choice for most patients with blastomycosis, especially those who are compliant and do not have overwhelming, life-threatening or CNS blastomycosis. Because of less toxicity despite a higher cost, itraconazole has replaced ketoconazole as first line therapy. For those persons with life-threatening manifestations of blastomycosis, such as adult respiratory distress syndrome or central nervous system disease, amphotericin B remains the initial treatment of choice (Chapman et al, 2000b).

PREVENTION

Since *B. dermatitidis* is an infrequent opportunistic pathogen in compromised hosts and since highly effective therapy for blastomycosis is available, prophylaxis regimens with antifungal drugs are not currently recommended. In addition, no vaccine against blastomycosis is currently available. However, efforts to develop a vaccine are ongoing. Mice vaccinated with an attenuated *B. dermatitidis* strain (mutation of WI-1 gene) demonstrated a cell-mediated host response but no clinical disease (Wuthrich et al, 2000). The potential target for such a vaccine would include those at high risk for developing blastomycosis, for example, certain laboratory workers, woodsmen, veterinarians,

and others living in the endemic area for *B. dermatitidis* who are at risk for complicated disease. Such persons include solid organ transplant recipients, HIV-infected patients, and other immunocompromised hosts.

REFERENCES

Abernathy R S. Amphotericin therapy of North American blastomycosis. *Antimicrob Agents Chemother* 3:208–211, 1967.

Arora N S, Oblinger M J, Feldman P S. Chronic pleural blastomycosis with hyperprolactinemia, galactorrhea and ammenorrhea. *Am Rev Respir Dis* 120:451–455,1989.

Bakerspigel A, Kane J, Schaus D. Isolation of *Blastomyces dermatitidis* from an earthen floor in Southwestern Ontario, Canada. *J Clin Microbiol* 24:890–891, 1986.

Bartley G B. Blastomycosis of the eyelid. *Ophthalmol* 102:2020–2023,1995.

Baumgardener D J, Paretsky K P. The in vitro isolation of *Blastomyces dermatitidis* from a woodpile in north central Wisconsin, USA. *Med Mycol* 37:163–168, 1999.

Bayer A S, Scott V J, Guze L B. Fungal arthritis. IV. Blastomycotic arthritis. *Sem Arthritis Rheum* 9:145–151, 1979.

Bradsher R W. Clinical features of blastomycosis. *Semin Respir Infect* 12:229–234,1997.

Bradsher R W. Development of specific immunity in patients with pulmonary or extrapulmonary blastomycosis. *Am Rev Respir Dis* 129:430–434, 1984.

Bradsher R W, Ulmer W C, Marmer D J, Towsend J W, Jacobs R F. Intracellular growth and phagocytosis of *Blastomyces dermatitidis* by monocyte-derived macrophages from previously infected and normal subjects. *J Infect Dis* 151:57–64, 1985a.

Bradsher R W, Rice D C, Abernathy R S. Ketoconazole therapy of endemic blastomycosis. *Ann Intern Med* 103:872–879, 1985b.

Bradsher R W, Balk R A, Jacobs R F. Growth inhibition of *Blastomyces dermatitidis* in alveolar and peripheral macrophages from patients with blastomycosis. *Am Rev Respir Dis* 135:412–417, 1987a.

Bradsher R W. Water and blastomycosis: Don't blame beaver. *Am Rev Respir Dis* 136:1324–1326, 1987b.

Bradsher R W. Blastomycosis. *Infect Dis Clin N Amer* 2:877–898, 1988.

Bradsher, R W, Martin M R, Wilkes T D, Waltman C, Bolyard K. Unusual presentations of blastomycosis: ten case summaries. *Infect Med* 7:10–19, 1990.

Bradsher R W. Fungal infections in normal hosts. Blastomycosis. *Clin Infect Dis* 14:S82–90,1992.

Bradsher R W, Pappas P G. Detection of specific antibodies in human blastomycosis by enzyme immunoassay. *South Med J* 88:1256–1259, 1995.

Brown L R, Swensen S J, Van Scoy R E, Prakash U B, Coles D T, Colby T V. Roentgenologic features of pulmonary blastomycosis. *Mayo Clin Proc* 66:29–38, 1991.

Busey J F. Blastomycosis: a review of 198 collected cases in VA hospitals. *Am Rev Respir Dis* 89:659–672,1964.

Causey W A, Campbell G D. Clinical aspects of blastomycosis. In: Al-Doory Y A, DiSalvo A F, eds. *Blastomycosis.* New York: Plenum Press, 165–88, 1992.

Chakravarty A, Saliga R, Mason E, Rajendran R, Muthuswamy P. Pneumonia and infraorbital abscess in a 29 year old diabetic pregnant woman. *Chest* 107:1752–1754, 1995.

Chapman S W. *Blastomyces dermatitidis*. In: Mandell G L, Bennett J E, Dolin R, eds. *Principles and Practice of Infectious Diseases.* New York: Churchill Livingstone, 2733–2746, 2000a.

Chapman S W, Bradsher R W, Campbell G D, Pappas P G, Kauffman C A. Practice guidelines for the management of patients with blastomycosis. *Clin Infect Dis* 30:679–683, 2000b.

Christie A, Peterson J C. Pulmonary calcifications in negative reactors to tuberculin. *Am J Public Health* 35:1131–1147, 1945.

Como J A, Dismukes W E. Systemic antifungal therapy: focus on oral azole drugs. *N Engl J Med* 330:263–272, 1994.

Daniel L, Salit I E. Blastomycosis during pregnancy. *Can Med Assoc J* 131:759–761,1989.

Davies S F, Sarosi G A. Serodiagnosis of histoplasmosis and blastomycosis. *Am Rev Respir Dis* 136:254–255, 1987.

Denton J F, DiSalvo A F. Isolation of *Blastomyces dermatitidis* from natural sites in Augusta, Georgia. *Am J Trop Med Hyg* 13:716–722, 1964.

Dismukes W E, Bradsher R W, Cloud G C, Kauffman C A, Chapman S W, George R B, Stevens D A, Girard W M, Saag M S, Bowles-Patton C, others in the NIAID Mycoses Study Group. Itraconazole therapy of blastomycosis and histoplasmosis. *Am J Med* 93:489–497, 1992.

Dubuisson R L, Jones T B. Splenic abscess due to blastomycosis: Scintigraphic, sonographic, and CT evaluation. *Am J Radiol* 140:66–68,1983.

Dumich P S, Neal H B, III. Blastomycosis of the larynx. *Laryngoscope* 93:1266–1270, 1983.

Edson R S, Keys T F. Treatment of primary pulmonary blastomycosis. *Mayo Clinic Proc* 56:683–685, 1981.

Ehni W. Endogenous reactivation in blastomycosis. *Am J Med* 86:831–832, 1989.

Evans M E, Haynes J B, Atkins J B, Atkinson J B, Delvaux T C Jr., Kaiser A. *Blastomyces dermatitidis* and the adult respiratory distress syndrome. *Am Rev Respir Dis* 126:1099–1102,1982.

Farber E R, Leahy M S, Meadows T R. Endometrial blastomycosis acquired by sexual contact. *Obstet Gynecol* 32:195–199,1968.

Farmer C, Stanley M W, Bardales R H, Korourian S, Shah H, Bradsher R, Klimberg V S. Mycoses of the breast: diagnosis by fine needle aspiration. *Diagn Cytopathol* 12:51–55,1995.

Faro S, Pastorek J G, Collins J, Spencer R, Greer D L, Phillips L E. Severe uterine hemorrhage from blastomycosis of the endometrium. *J Reprod Med* 32:247–249,1987.

Gilchrist T C. Protozoan dermatitis. *J Cutan Gen Dis* 12:496–499, 1894.

Gilchrist T C, Stokes W R. Case of pseudo-lupus vulgaris caused by *Blastomyces*. *J Exp Med* 3:53–78,1898.

Gnann J W, Bressler G S, Bodet C A, Avent K A. Human blastomycosis after a dog bite. *Ann Intern Med* 98:48–49, 1983.

Gonyea E F. The spectrum of primary blastomycotic meningitis: a review of central nervous system blastomycosis. *Ann Neurol* 3:26–39, 1978.

Gottlieb JL, McAllister IL, Guttman FA, Vine AK. Choroidal blastomycosis. *Retina* 15:248–252,1995.

Halvorsen RA, Duncan JD, Merten DF, Gallis HA, Putman CE. Pulmonary blastomycosis. *Radiology* 150:1–5,1984.

Harley W B, Lomis M, Haas D W. Marked polymorphonuclear pleocytosis due to blastomycotic meningitis: case report and review. *Clin Infect Dis* 18:816–818, 1994.

Hebert C A, King J, George R B. Late dissemination of pulmonary blastomycosis during ketoconazole therapy. *Chest* 95:240–242, 1989.

Inoshita T, Youngberg G A, Boelen L J, Langston J. Blastomycosis presenting with prostatic involvement: Report of 2 cases and review of the literature. *J Urol* 130:160–162,1983.

Ismail M A, Lerner S A. Disseminated blastomycosis in a pregnant woman. *Am Rev Respir Dis* 126:350–353,1982.

Istorico L J, Sanders M, Jacobs R F, Gillian S, Glasier C, Bradsher R W. Otitis media due to blastomycosis. *Clin Infect Dis* 14:335–338,1992.

Kaufman L, Standard P, Padhye A A. Exoantigen tests for the immuno-identification of fungal cultures. *Mycopathology* 82:3–12, 1983.

Kelly P M. Systemic blastomycosis with associated diabetes insipidus. *Ann Intern Med* 96:66–67,1982.

Klein B S, Vergeront J M, Weeks R J, Kumarum, Mathaig, Varkey B, Kaufman L, Bradsher R W, Stoebig J F, Davis J P. Isolation of *Blastomyces dermatitidis* in soil associated with a large outbreak of blastomycosis in Wisconsin. *N Engl J Med* 314:529–534, 1986a.

Klein B S, Kuritsky J N, Chappell W A, Kaufman L, Green J, Davies S F, Williams J E, Sarosi G A. Comparison of the enzyme immunoassay, immunodiffusion, and complement fixation tests in detecting antibody in human serum to the A antigen of *Blastomyces dermatitidis*. *Am Rev Respir Dis* 133:144–148, 1986b.

Klein B S, Vergeront J M, DiSalvo A F, Kaufman L, Davis J P. Two outbreaks of blastomycosis along rivers in Wisconsin: Isolation of *Blastomyces dermatitidis* from riverbank soil and evidence of its transmission along waterways. *Am Rev Respir Dis* 136:1333–1338, 1987.

Kravitz G R, Davies S F, Eckman M R, Sarosi G A. Chronic blastomycosis meningitis. *Am J Med* 71:501–505, 1981.

Landis F B, Varkey B. Late relapse of pulmonary blastomycosis after adequate treatment with amphotericin B. *Am Rev Respir Dis* 113:77–81, 1976.

Lockwood W R, Allison F Jr., Batson B E, Busey J F. The treatment of North American blastomycosis: Ten years' experience. *Am Rev Respir Dis* 100:314–320, 1969.

Lopez R, Mason J O, Parker J S, Pappas P G. Intraocular blastomycosis: case report and review. *Clin Infect Dis* 18:805–807, 1994.

MacDonald D, Alguire P C. Adult respiratory distress due to blastomycosis during pregnancy. *Chest* 98:1527–1528, 1990.

Maioriello R P, Merwin C F. North American blastomycosis presenting as an acute panniculitis and arthritis. *Arch Dermatol* 102:92–96, 1970.

Maxson S, Miller S F, Tryka F, Schutze G E. Perinatal blastomycosis: a review. *Pediatr Infect Dis J* 11:760–763, 1992.

Medoff G, Painter A, Kobayashi G S. Mycelial to yeast-phase transitions of the dimorphic fungi *Blastomyces dermatitidis* and *Paracoccidioides brasiliensis*. *J Bacteriol* 169:4055–4060, 1987.

Meyer K C, McManus E J, Maki D G. Overwhelming pulmonary blastomycosis associated with the adult respiratory distress syndrome. *N Engl J Med* 329:1231–1236, 1993.

Moore R M, Green N E. Blastomycosis of bone. *J Bone Joint Surg* 64:1094–1101, 1982.

Mouzin E L, Beilke M A. Female genital blastomycosis: case report and review. *Clin Infect Dis* 22:718–719, 1996.

Murray J J, Clark C A, Lands R H, Heim C R, Burnett L S. Reactivation blastomycosis presenting as a tubo-ovarian abscess. *Obstet Gynecol* 64:828–830, 1984.

National Institute of Allergy and Infectious Diseases (NIAID) Mycoses Study Group. Treatment of blastomycosis and histoplasmosis with ketoconazole. *Ann Intern Med* 103:861–872, 1985.

Pappas P G, Pottage J C, Powderly W G, Fraser V J, Stratton C W, McKenzie S, Tapper M L, Chmel H, Bonebrake F C, Blum R, Shafer R W, King C, Dismukes W E. Blastomycosis in patients with the acquired immunodeficiency syndrome. *Ann Intern Med* 116:847–853, 1992.

Pappas P G, Threlkeld M G, Bedsole G D, Cleveland K O, Gelfand M S, Dismukes W E. Blastomycosis in immunocompromised patients. *Medicine* 72:311–325, 1993.

Pappas PG, Bradsher RW, Chapman S W, Kauffman C A, Dine A, Cloud G A, Dismukes W E, and the NIAID Mycoses Study Group. Fluconazole therapy of blastomycosis. *Clin Infect Dis* 20:267–271, 1995.

Pappas P G, Bradsher R W, Kauffman C A, Cloud G A, Thomas C J, Campbell G D Jr., Chapman S W, Newman C, Dismukes W E, the National Institute of Allergy and Infectious Diseases Mycoses Study Group. Treatment of blastomycosis with higher doses of fluconazole. *Clin Infect Dis* 25:200–205, 1997.

Parker J D, Doto I L, Tosh F E. A decade of experience with blastomycosis and its treatment with amphotericin B. *Am Rev Respir Dis* 99:895–902, 1969.

Parsons R J, Zaronfontis C J D. Histoplasmosis in man: report of 7 cases and review of 71 cases. *Arch Intern Med* 75:1–23, 1945.

Pitrak D L, Andersen B R. Cerebral blastomycoma after ketoconazole therapy for respiratory tract blastomycosis. *Am J Med* 86: 713–714, 1989.

Pont A, Graybill J R, Craven P C, Galgiani J N, Dismukes W E, Reitz R E, Stevens D A. High-dose ketoconazole therapy and adrenal and testicular function in humans. *Arch Intern Med* 144: 2150–2153, 1984.

Propeck P A, Scanlan K A. Blastomycosis of the breast. *Am J Radiol* 166:726,1996.

Recht L D, Phillips J R, Eckman M R, Sarosi G A. Self-limited blastomycosis: a report of thirteen cases. *Am Rev Respir Dis* 120: 1109–1112, 1979.

Roos K L, Bryan J P, Maggio W W, Jane J A, Scheld W M. Intracranial blastomycoma. *Medicine* 66:224–235, 1979.

Saccente M, Abernathy R S, Pappas P G, Shah H R, Bradsher R W. Vertebral blastomycosis with paravertebral abscess: report of eight cases and review of the literature. *Clin Infect Dis* 26:413–418, 1998.

Sarosi G A, Serstock D S. Isolation of *Blastomyces dermatitidis* from pigeon manure. *Am Rev Respir Dis* 114:1179–1183, 1976.

Sarosi G A, Davies S F. Blastomycosis. State of the art. *Am Rev Respir Dis* 120:911–938, 1979

Sarosi G A, Eckman M R, Davies S F, Laskey W K. Canine blastomycosis as a harbinger of human disease. *Ann Intern Med* 98:48–49, 1983.

Schwarz J, Salfelder K. Blastomycosis: a review of 152 cases. *Curr Top Pathol* 65:165–200, 1977.

Seaburg J H, Dascomb H E. Results of the treatment of systemic mycosis. *JAMA* 188:509–513, 1964.

Seymour E Q. Blastomycosis of the breast. *Am J Radiol* 139:822–823, 1982.

Skillrud D M, Douglas W W. Survival in ARDS caused by blastomycosis infection. *Mayo Clin Proc* 60:266–269, 1985.

Slain D, Rogers P D, Cleary J D, Chapman S W. Intravenous itraconazole. *Ann Pharmacother* 35:720–729, 2001.

Steele R W, Abernathy R S. Systemic blastomycosis in children. *Pediatr Infect Dis* 2:304–307, 1983.

Suen J Y, Wetmore S J, Wetzel W J. Blastomycosis of the larynx. *Ann Otol* 89:563–566, 1980.

Sugar A M, Picard M. Macrophage-and oxidant-mediated inhibition of the ability of live *Blastomyces dermatitidis* conidia to transform to pathogenic yeast phase. *J Infect Dis* 163:371–375, 1991.

Sutliff W D, Cruthirds T P. *Blastomyces dermatitidis* in cytologic preparations. *Am Rev Respir Dis* 108:149–151, 1973.

Tosh F E, Hammerman K J, Weeks R J, Sarosi G A. A common source epidemic of North American blastomycosis. *Am Rev Respir Dis* 109:525–529, 1974.

Tucker R M, Haq Y, Denning D W, Stevens D A. Adverse events associated with itraconazole in 189 patients on chronic therapy. *J Antimicrob Chemother* 26:561–566, 1990.

Tuthill S W. Disseminated blastomycosis with intrauterine transmission. *South Med J* 78:1526–1527, 1985.

Vaaler A K, Bradsher R W, Davies S F. Evidence of subclinical blastomycosis in forestry workers in northern Minnestoa and northern Wisconsin. *Am J Med* 89:470–475, 1990.

Vida L, Moel S A. Systemic North American blastomycosis with orbital involvement. *Am J Ophthalmol* 77:240–242, 1974.

Winquist E W, Walmsley S L, Berinstein N L. Reactivation and dissemination of blastomycosis complicating Hodgkin's disease. *Am J Hematol* 43:129–132, 1993.

Witorsch P, Utz J P. North American blastomycosis: A study of 40 patients. *Medicine* 47:169–200, 1968.

Witzig R S, Quimosing E M, Campbell W L, Greer D L, Clark R A. *Blastomyces dermatitidis* infection of the paranasal sinuses. *Clin Infect Dis* 18:267–268, 1994a.

Witzig R S, Hoadley D J, Greer D L, Abriola K P, Hernandez R L. Blastomycosis and HIV. *South Med J* 87:715–719, 1994b.

Wuthrich M, Filutowicz H I, Klein B S. Mutation of the WI-1 gene yields an attenuated *Blastomyces dermatitidis* strain that induces host resistance. *J Clin Invest* 106:1381–1389, 2000.

Young L, Schutze G E: Perinatal blastomycosis: the rest of the story. *Pediatr Infect Dis J* 14:83, 1995.

20

Coccidioidomycosis

NEIL M. AMPEL

Coccidioidomycosis is a disease of the Western hemisphere caused by the dimorphic soil-dwelling fungus that until recently was recognized as the single species *Coccidioides immitis* (see TAXONOMY). First recognized as a clinical entity in Argentina in 1882, the first case associated with the San Joaquin Valley in California was reported soon after (Rixford and Gilchrist, 1896). Early cases presented with inflammatory lesions of the skin, bones, and joints that progressed to death despite attempts at treatment. By the turn of the century, the causative organism was identified as a mould despite its resemblance in tissue to a protozoan (Ophüls, 1905). For the first 40 years, coccidioidomycosis was thought to be a relatively rare but disfiguring and usually fatal disease. However, benign cases of pulmonary disease associated with erythema nodosum or erythema multiforme were increasingly observed (Dickson and Gifford, 1938). This form of illness, called Valley Fever, led to speculation that not all cases of coccidioidomycosis were fatal and that there was a wide spectrum of clinical manifestations of infection (Smith, 1940).

These observations ushered in a watershed period in the understanding of coccidioidomycosis led by Charles E. Smith and his colleagues. Smith developed the coccidioidin skin test, defined the incidence and prevalence of infection within the San Joaquin Valley, and described the relationship of skin-test reactivity to clinical disease (Smith et al, 1948). He also developed the coccidioidal serum antibody tests (Smith et al, 1950), variations of which are still in use today. However, there was no treatment for coccidioidomycosis until 1957, when Fiese reported the first use of amphotericin B to manage a case of disseminated disease (Fiese, 1957). Further strides in the therapy of coccidioidomycosis using amphotericin B were pioneered and described by Winn (Winn, 1959).

Since those times, much more has been elucidated about coccidioidomycosis, particularly with regard to immunology, treatment, identification of hosts at risk, and fungal antigen expression. However, it is astounding how much of the basic epidemiology, pathology, clinical expression, and mycology of coccidioidomycosis was established within the first 60 years of its recognition. This initial progress is eloquently reviewed in the monograph by Fiese (Fiese, 1958) and subsequently updated (Drutz and Catanzaro, 1978a,b). These early studies remain useful reading for anyone interested in coccidioidomycosis.

LIFE-CYCLE

Coccidioides is a soil-dwelling fungus in which man is an incidental and end-stage host. In the soil, the fungus exists as a mould with septate hyphae (Fig. 20–1). Intervening cells within the hyphal filaments degenerate. This arrangement allows for fragmentation of the hyphae with dislodgement of remaining intact cells, called arthroconidia, when disturbed. The barrel-shaped arthroconidia are approximately 2×5 μm, which makes airborne dispersal possible and increases the probability of reaching the small bronchi after inhalation into the lung of a susceptible host (Pappagianis, 1988).

Once inside the host, the fungus undergoes a profound morphological change in which the outer wall fractures, the inner wall thickens and the entire structure rounds up. Increased temperature, rise in CO_2 concentration (Klotz et al, 1984), decrease in pH, and interaction with professional phagocytes (Galgiani et al, 1982) facilitate this metamorphosis. The process can also be induced in vitro using a chemically defined medium (Converse, 1957). The resulting structure, called a spherule and unique among pathogenic fungi, internally segments into multiple uninucleate compartments while growing to a size of up to 120 μm. These structures, called endospores and 2–4 μm in diameter, are released into the surrounding tissue in packets if the spherule ruptures. After release, endospores can grow to become spherules themselves, repeating the cycle within the host (Sun and Huppert, 1976).

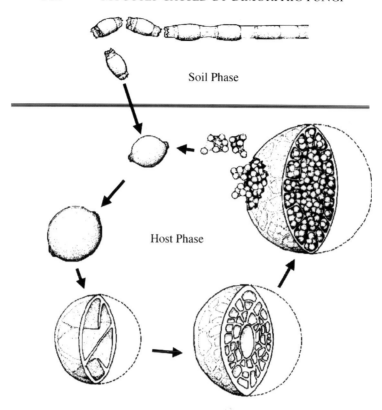

FIGURE 20–1. Life cycle of *Coccidioides*. Based on Kirkland and Fierer (1996).

ECOLOGY

The observation that *Coccidioides* was a soil-dwelling organism was first made when it was isolated from soil near a bunkhouse in association with an outbreak among farm workers (Stewart and Meyer, 1932). Since then, there have been several examples of identifying the organism in the soil in association with human cases (Winn et al, 1963; Wanke et al, 1999). Unfortunately, general soil sampling in the endemic area has not been very productive. Egeberg and Ely tested 500 soil samples obtained in and around animal burrows in the southern San Joaquin Valley and detected *Coccidioides* in only 35 (7%) (Egeberg and Ely, 1956). Overall, *Coccidioides* appears to prefer alkaline soils in relatively warm, dry climates (Maddy, 1965) and it preferentially grows in soils of high salt content, including borates, at higher temperatures (Egeberg et al, 1964). There are compelling data that *Coccidioides* is not uniformly distributed in the soil but is concentrated in animal burrows (Egeberg and Ely, 1956; Wanke et al, 1999) or in other soils containing increased nitrogenous waste, such as Amerindian middens (Lacy and Swatek, 1974). Better definition of the coccidioidal habitat is urgently needed to devise models for risk of acquisition (Kolivras et al, 2001).

TAXONOMY

The classification of *Coccidioides* remains uncertain but genetic analysis is clarifying this. Studies of 18S ribosomal DNA confirms that *Coccidioides* is within the class Ascomycetes and is closely related to the pathogenic fungi *Histoplasma capsulatum* and *Blastomyces dermatiditis* (Bowman et al, 1992). Among all organisms, it is most closely related to the nonpathogenic soil-dwelling fungus *Uncinocarpus reesii* (Pan et al, 1994). While taxonomic analysis has been hampered by the fact that no sexual stage for *Coccidioides* has been identified, Taylor and colleagues have found molecular evidence for sexual recombination (Burt et al, 1996). This group has also found genetic variability between clinical isolates from California, Arizona, and Texas (Burt et al, 1997) but has not linked these differences to differences in pathogenicity (Fisher et al, 2000). In contrast, *Coccidioides* in South America appears to have been derived from a single population from Texas and arrived in the continent from 9000 to 140,000 years ago, perhaps coincident with human migration into the area (Fisher et al, 2001). Recently, Taylor and colleagues have presented genetic evidence that *Coccidioides* consists of two distinct species, *C. immitis*, found only in California, and *C. posadasii*, found elsewhere (Fisher et al, 2002). Because there are no clear microbiological or clinical characteristics that distinguish these species, the genus term *Coccidioides* will be used throughout this chapter to refer to both organisms.

EPIDEMIOLOGY

The endemic regions of coccidioidomycosis coincide with areas in which the fungus inhabits the soil, between the latitudes of 40°N and 40°S in the Western Hemisphere. Within this general region, there is great variability in risk of infection. The endemic regions of coccidioidomycosis in North America have been associated with the Lower Sonoran Life Zone, a geoclimatic region characterized by hot summers, mild winters, rare freezes, and alkaline soil. Maddy has associated the local growth of the creosote bush (*Larrea tridentata*) as portending an increased risk of acquiring coccidioidomycosis (Maddy, 1958). However, there are exceptions to this association (Durry et al, 1997). In Central and South America, there are several geographic pockets where individuals have acquired coccidioidal infection (Pappagianis, 1988) including north-central Argentina, where the disease was first recognized. Recently, there are reports of cases acquired in northeast Brazil (Wanke et al, 1999). In general, these Central and South American areas are arid or semiarid.

The initial association of dust exposure and risk of coccidioidomycosis was made in a study of military personnel in the San Joaquin Valley (Smith et al, 1946b). The investigators also found a strong inverse association in the frequency of cases and precipitation. That is, the number of cases waxed during the dry central California summers and waned during the relatively wet winters. A similar association has been noted in Arizona, except that there are two periods of increased frequency of cases. The first occurs in the spring, after the winter rains, and the second occurs during the autumn, after the summer monsoon (Kerrick et al, 1985).

There are examples of epidemics of coccidioidomycosis when these patterns are exaggerated. For example, in December 1977, high-velocity winds over the lower San Joaquin Valley induced not only a local dust storm but also threw dust high into the atmosphere that blanketed regions to the north and west outside of the endemic zone, including the San Francisco Bay and Sacramento metropolitan regions. Within weeks of the storm, the number of cases of coccidioidomycosis in California was five times normal, with many cases reported from outside the endemic region (Flynn et al, 1979; Pappagianis and Einstein, 1978). Similarly, in January 1994, an earthquake-generated cloud of dust, emanating from the Santa Susana Mountains, dispersed over Ventura County, California, an area of low coc-

cidioidal endemicity. Within 2 weeks, increasing numbers of cases of coccidioidomycosis occurred in Simi Valley, a city located at the base of the mountains and in the plume of the dust cloud (Schneider et al, 1997). In the early 1990s, a nearly 10-fold increase in the number of cases of coccidioidomycosis was seen in the lower San Joaquin Valley. In this epidemic, drought, followed by heavy rains and then another drought, was climatologically associated with the marked increase in cases (Pappagianis, 1994).

There have also been several focal outbreaks of coccidioidomycosis associated with local conditions (Winn et al, 1963; Werner et al, 1972; Werner and Pappagianis, 1973; Larsen et al, 1985; Standaert et al, 1995; CDC, 2000; Cairns et al, 2000; CDC, 2001). These outbreaks share common traits. First, there was intense exposure to soil in a confined area, often in association with an archeological dig or other soil disturbance. In addition, those exposed were either young or not from the endemic region and so could be presumed to be nonimmune. These outbreaks are notable for their high attack rate and association with diffuse rash and extensive pulmonary infiltrates. When calculable, the incubation period between exposure and development of active disease was between 2 and 4 weeks. Because of this, the diagnosis was often established only after the individuals had returned to their homes outside the coccidioidal endemic area.

The prevalence and incidence of coccidioidomycosis in a region can be estimated using skin-test studies measuring delayed-type dermal hypersensitivity. A study of the prevalence of coccidioidin skin-test reactivity among naval recruits and others in 1957 did much to define the coccidioidal endemic area in the United States (Fig. 20–2) (Edwards and Palmer, 1957). In this study, highest prevalence was found in the southern San Joaquin Valley, in south-central Arizona, and along the western portion of the lower Rio Grande Valley in Texas. Regions of lesser endemicity included most of southwestern Arizona below the Mogollon Rim, southern Nevada and southwestern Utah, southern New Mexico and far western Texas.

In the past, rates of skin-test positivity were quite high in endemic regions. However, few recent studies exist. A recent analysis of skin-test responses in high-school students in the southern San Joaquin Valley found that the incidence of new skin-test reactions had decreased from greater than 10% each year in 1937–1939 to 2% in 1995 (Larwood, 2000). A study performed in 1985 in Tucson, Arizona found a prevalence of positive skin-test response of approximately 30% (Dodge et al, 1985), with an estimated yearly conversion rate of 3% each year. A third epidemiologic study of Torreon, a city in northeastern Mexico in the

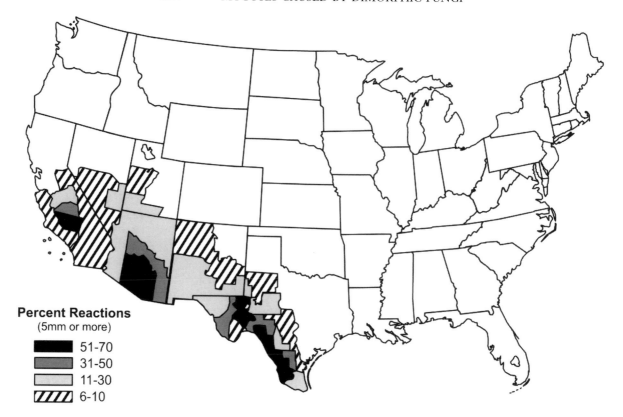

Percent Reactions
(5mm or more)

- 51–70
- 31–50
- 11–30
- 6–10

FIGURE 20–2. Endemic regions for coccidioidomycosis in the United States using response to dermal hypersensitivity testing. Increased intensity of shading indicates increased rates of positivity. Based on Edwards and Palmer, 1957.

state of Coahuila, described a prevalence of 40% (Padua y Gabriel et al, 1999). These data indicate that even in the coccidioidal endemic regions, most individuals have not acquired coccidioidomycosis and remain susceptible to infection.

Given the ability of arthroconidia to become airborne, it is not surprising that most cases of coccidioidomycosis are due to inhalation with the lung as the primary site of infection. However, there are occasional instances of primary cutaneous inoculation coccidioidomycosis. For the most part, these have occurred as traumatic injuries contaminated with soil or laboratory cultures containing *Coccidioides*; these skin lesions heal spontaneously in most cases (Carroll et al, 1977; O'Brien and Gilsdorf, 1986). Because disseminated disease so often presents with cutaneous lesions, Wilson and colleagues have outlined criteria for establishing primary inoculation as the route of infection (Wilson et al, 1953). These include development of a lesion within 1 to 3 weeks of a history of trauma or inoculation at the site, the rapid development of IgM but not IgG antibodies in the serum, development of a positive coccidioidin skin test after the diagnosis, and local but not distant adenopathy.

A variety of occupations have been associated with an increased risk of acquiring coccidioidomycosis. Not

unexpectedly, most of these are associated with working with soil or dust in endemic regions. These occupations include agricultural workers, excavators, military personnel (Johnson, 1981), and archeologists (Werner et al, 1972; Werner and Pappagianis, 1973). In addition, there are numerous cases of laboratory-acquired coccidioidomycosis (Looney and Stein, 1950; Fiese, 1958; Johnson et al, 1964; Johnson, 1981). The risk occurs because *Coccidioides* grows readily as a mould on a variety of artificial laboratory media. With time, fluffy aerial mycelia form that can easily become dislodged and airborne. The concentrations of airborne arthroconidia from artificial media are undoubtedly far higher than might be encountered naturally. Because of this, it is recommended that all laboratory procedures involving manipulation of known cultures of *Coccidioides* be performed inside a class II biological safety cabinet under BSL-3 containment. This procedure would also apply to soil and other environmental samples. Clinical specimens suspected of containing *Coccidioides* should be handled under BSL-2 containment (Warnock, 2000). Care should be taken to avoid percutaneous injury, since several laboratory instances of primary cutaneous coccidioidomycosis have also occurred (Johnson et al, 1964). Because of the potential of the mycelial phase for infectivity, *Coccidioides* is the only fungus listed by the U.S. government as a possible bioterrorist agent (Dixon, 2001).

There is no evidence for person-to-person transmission of coccidioidomycosis via aerosol spread. However, interhuman transmission has been reported to occur via a contaminated fomite. In this case, pulmonary coccidioidomycosis occurred in six health-care workers who changed the dressings and cast covering an area of draining osteomyelitis of a patient with disseminated coccidioidomycosis. Subsequent investigation revealed *Coccidioides* growing on the dressings and cast, which were dry at the time of removal. It was presumed that mycelial growth occurred on these objects and was the source of infection (Eckmann et al, 1964). Fomite transmission of coccidioidomycosis has been reported under a variety of other circumstances. The handling of raw cotton grown in the endemic area has been noted in several instances (Fiese, 1958; Gehlbach et al, 1973; Ogiso et al, 1997). Cleaning of dusty artifacts from an archeology site obtained from the coccidioidal endemic region also resulted in infection (Fiese, 1958). Recently, interhuman transmission has been documented to occur via transplant of *Coccidioides* infected organs to transplant recipients (See Section on SPECIAL HOSTS).

PATHOLOGY

Necrotizing granulomata surrounding coccidioidal spherules are the classic pathological manifestation of coccidioidomycosis and suggested to early investigators a similarity to the reaction seen in tuberculosis (Fiese, 1958). However, it was also recognized that an acute pyogenic response with polymorphonuclear leukocytes could occur, particularly in association with rapidly progressive lesions of disseminated disease. Some observers have suggested that this latter reaction is to endospores and not to spherules. In many instances, the two reactions are in close proximity (Huntington, 1980). The concept proposed is that with unrestrained fungal growth, endospores are released from the spherule, and there is an intense but nonprotective polymorphonuclear response. Soluble extracts of both mycelia and spherules are chemotactic for polymorphonuclear leukocytes and may play a role in initiating inflammation (Galgiani et al, 1978). This process may then evolve into a more protective granulomatous response surrounding the spherule in those individuals who are able to control their disease (Fiese, 1958). While in vitro data suggest that polymorphonuclear leukocytes can inhibit fungal growth (Galgiani et al, 1984), their role in controlling coccidioidal growth in vivo is unclear.

There have been numerous reports of tissue and peripheral blood eosinophilia in coccidioidomycosis. Peripheral blood eosinophilia during primary illness and eosinophils in CSF in coccidioidal meningitis are common enough in coccidioidomycosis to suggest the respective diagnoses (Ragland et al, 1993). Pulmonary eosinophilia due to coccidioidomycosis may resemble idiopathic eosinophilic pneumonia histologically except for the finding of spherules in tissue (Lombard et al, 1987). Extreme peripheral blood eosinophilia ($> 20\%$) has been associated with disseminated disease (Echols et al, 1982; Harley and Blaser, 1994). The pathologic finding of eosinophilic abscesses in coccidioidal-infected tissues has been associated with rupturing spherules with release of endospores.

The finding of the spherule in tissue is the sine qua non of coccidioidomycosis. The spherules may be of all sizes and sometimes can be shown to be rupturing and dislodging endospores. In addition, there have been several reports of mycelia within preexisting coccidioidal cavities (Putnam et al, 1975; Ragland et al, 1993), a report of mycelia being found in a coccidioidal empyema (Dolan et al, 1992), and another report of mycelia identified in the CSF in a severe case of coccidioidal meningitis (Kleinschmidt-DeMasters et al, 2000). The presumption in these cases is that local conditions allowed the fungus to revert to its saprophytic phase. There is no evidence that such patients are infectious.

Coccidioidomycosis may involve nearly any organ of the body. The most common symptomatic sites include the lungs, skin and subcutaneous soft tissue, bones and joints, and meninges. However, a variety of other organs may also be involved, often silently. These include the liver and spleen (Fiese, 1958), peritoneum (Chen, 1983a; Ampel et al, 1988), prostate (Chen and Schiff, 1985), epididymis (Chen, 1983b), urethra (Dunne et al, 1986), and female genital tract (Salgia et al, 1982; Bylund et al, 1986). Two recent reports describe pericarditis due to *Coccidioides*, both resulting in constrictive disease (Faul et al, 1999; Oudiz et al, 1995). Unlike histoplasmosis and tuberculosis, direct involvement of the gastrointestinal mucosa is extremely rare, if it exists at all (Fiese, 1958). However, there may be direct extension into the serosal surface of the gastrointestinal tract from an adjacent site (Kuntze et al, 1988). In addition, there are reports of direct infection of the tracheobronchial tree (Polesky et al, 1999). Eye involvement with coccidioidomycosis has been reported sparingly, mostly as asymptomatic chorioretinal scars (Rodenbiker et al, 1981) or as a scleritis or conjunctivitis associated with primary infection and erythema nodosum (Rodenbiker and Ganley, 1980). Active iridocyclitis and chorioretinitis have been reported, usually as part of overtly disseminated disease (Rodenbiker and Ganley, 1980).

While the most frequent pathological response to central nervous system infection by *Coccidioides* is a basilar granulomatous meningitis, a variety of other processes are seen, including parenchymal granulomata, and vasculitis (Mischel and Vinters, 1995). Intracranial coccidioidal abscesses have also been reported (Banuelos et al, 1996). Williams and colleagues have observed a CNS vasculitis of small and medium-sized arteries (Williams et al, 1992).

IMMUNE RESPONSE AND RELATION TO DISEASE

A strong cellular immune response is critical to the control of coccidioidal infection. For example, patients with defects in such defenses, such as those with HIV infection (Ampel et al, 1993), organ transplant recipients (Blair and Logan, 2001), and those on long-term corticosteroid therapy (Ampel et al, 1986), are at increased risk for developing severe symptomatic coccidioidomycosis. In addition, there is an association between the strength and type of the coccidioidal-specific immune response and the severity of clinical infection. Persons with self-limited pulmonary illness usually express a strong cellular immune response, manifested as a positive coccidioidin skin test reaction, and transiently produce low titer anticoccidioidal antibodies in their serum. On the other hand, those with disseminated coccidioidomycosis tend to lack a cellular immune response and have high and prolonged serum antibody titers (Drutz and Catanzaro, 1978a).

The dichotomous response seen in human coccidioidomycosis is suggestive of an immunological model in which the T helper lymphocyte response can be categorized as either Th1 (promoting cellular immunity and associated with production of the cytokines interferon-gamma [IFN-γ] and interleukin-2 [IL-2]), or as Th2 (promoting a humoral immune response and associated with production of IL-4, IL-5, and IL-10). Animal models of coccidioidomycosis support this concept. It is known that certain inbred mouse strains are relatively resistant to coccidioidal infection, while others are not. Magee and colleagues demonstrated that the resistant DBA/2 strain produces increased amounts of IFN-γ after pulmonary infection while its susceptible counterpart, BALB/c, produces predominantly IL-4. Moreover, when BALB/c mice are treated with recombinant IFN-γ or with antibody against IL-4, they are less susceptible to coccidioidal infection, while DBA/2 mice are rendered more susceptible if given antibody against IFN-γ (Magee and Cox, 1995).

Human in vitro immunological studies have confirmed the importance of the cellular immune response in coccidioidomycosis but have not been able to demonstrate a Th1/Th2 relationship. Peripheral blood mononuclear cells from subjects with disseminated coccidioidomycosis produce less IFN-γ in response to coc-

cidioidal antigen than do cells from healthy, immune donors (Corry et al, 1996; Ampel et al, 2001), but no IL-4 or IL-10 (Corry et al, 1996; Ampel et al, 2001). The addition of IFN-γ in vitro to cells from donors with disseminated disease does not increase the response (Ampel and Christian, 1997).

Clinically, the expression of delayed-type hypersensitivity (DTH) after skin testing with a coccidioidal antigen has been associated with an intact cellular immune response. The lack of such expression, called anergy, has been clearly associated with more severe, disseminated disease (Smith et al, 1946b; Drutz and Catanzaro, 1978a). This has led to the speculation that agents that could reverse coccidioidal anergy might serve as potential treatments for disseminated coccidioidomycosis. A recent report on the use of dendritic cells in human coccidioidomycosis holds promise (Richards et al, 2001).

Vaccination of mice with whole, formalin-killed spherules protects them from subsequent lethal challenge with *Coccidioides* (Levine et al, 1960). Unfortunately, the dose used proved to have a high incidence of local toxicity in humans (Williams et al, 1984). A double-blind, placebo-controlled study inoculating a lower dose of formalin-killed spherules in nonimmune people living in the coccidioidal endemic area showed a trend toward disease reduction in the vaccine group, but the differences were not statistically significant (Pappagianis, 1993). Since this trial, several laboratories have shown that immunization with fungal subunits may be protective in mice and could serve as human vaccine candidates in future studies. These include the 27K antigen preparation (Zimmermann et al, 1998), recombinant Ag2/PRA (Abuodeh et al, 1999; Jiang et al, 1999), and recombinant urease (Li et al, 2001).

CLINICAL MANIFESTATIONS OF COCCIDIOIDAL INFECTION

Primary Pulmonary Infection

Sixty percent of persons are completely asymptomatic at the time of initial pulmonary coccidioidal infection (Smith et al, 1948). Their only indication of infection is a positive reaction to a coccidioidal skin-test. The other 40% of those infected manifest a variety of symptoms, most commonly cough, usually dry but occasionally blood-tinged, fever, night sweats, pleuritic chest pain, and headache (Smith, 1951; Drutz and Catanzaro, 1978b). Fatigue may be prominent and profound. In some cases, there is an evanescent, diffuse, pruritic rash over the trunk and extremities early in the course of illness that may be confused with contact dermatitis or measles (Werner et al, 1972; Hobbs, 1989).

In up to one-quarter of cases, patients develop either erythema nodosum or erythema multiforme, usually a few days to weeks after the initial pulmonary symptoms. Erythema nodosum generally occurs as bright red, painful nodules on the lower extremities, while erythema multiforme tends to occur on the upper trunk and arms, often in a necklace distribution (See Color Fig. 20–3 in separate color insert). About one-third of these cases will also have arthralgias, most commonly of the ankles and knees, and called Desert Rheumatism (Fiese, 1958). Primary pulmonary coccidioidomycosis with erythema nodosum or erythema multiforme has a predilection for white females and is rarely seen in African American patients (Smith and Beard, 1946a). Smith correlated the onset of erythema nodosum with the development of coccidioidal skin-test reactivity (Smith, 1940). The development of either of these rashes during primary coccidioidomycosis is considered an indicator of a decreased risk for subsequent dissemination or chronic active infection (Fiese, 1958; Arsura et al, 1998).

There is great variability in the radiographic findings of primary pulmonary coccidioidomycosis (McGahan et al, 1981). Most frequently, a unilateral parenchymal infiltrate is present. The appearance may range from a subsegmental patchy alveolar process to a dense lobar infiltrate with atelectasis (Fig. 20–4). Ipsilateral or bilateral hilar adenopathy or mediastinal adenopathy is often present (Greendyke et al, 1970). A small pleural effusion ipsilateral to the pulmonary infiltrate occurs in approximately one-fifth of cases. Occasionally, large pleural effusions occur.

Not uncommonly, primary coccidioidal pneumonia may be confused with a community-acquired bacterial pneumonia. While at times difficult to distinguish, clues favoring a diagnosis of pulmonary coccidioidomycosis include persistent fatigue and headache, failure to improve with antibiotic therapy, hilar or mediastinal adenopathy on chest radiograph, and peripheral blood eosinophilia.

Pulmonary Sequelae of Primary Coccidioidal Pneumonia

In the vast majority of individuals with symptomatic primary coccidioidomycosis, the symptoms resolve spontaneously over a few weeks. However, radiographic abnormalities remain in approximately 5%. One of the most common is the coccidioidal nodule (Fig. 20–5). Nodules are benign residual lesions of coccidioidal pneumonia but are problematic because of their radiographic resemblance to pulmonary neoplasms. While usually single on plain chest radiograph, multiple lesions are frequently seen on CT of the chest. They range in size from a few millimeters to more than 5 cm in diameter and may be calcified. Currently, there is no radiographic way to clearly distinguish coccidioidal nodules from malignancies. Fine needle percutaneous aspirate with histological examination appears to be diagnostic in the majority of cases (Forseth et al, 1986; Chitkara, 1997).

Coccidioidal cavities occur when a pulmonary nodule excavates. In most cases, cavities are asymptomatic, between 2 and 4 cm in diameter, and their natural history is to slowly close over time (Hyde, 1968; Winn, 1968). Sputum cultures obtained from individuals with coccidioidal pulmonary cavities are frequently positive for *Coccidioides*. Radiographically, cavities are typically thin walled but may have a surrounding area of

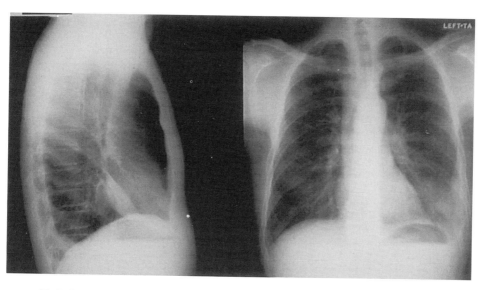

FIGURE 20–4. Primary coccidioidal pneumonia. Note the dense infiltrate with evidence of atelectasis and ipsilateral small pleura effusion.

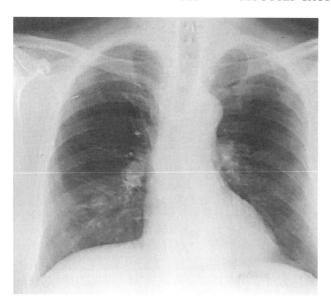

FIGURE 20–5. Right lower lobe coccidioidal nodule.

infiltration (Fig. 20–6). Their course can be complicated. One syndrome is persistent chest pain and cough, often associated with an air-fluid level within the cavity. The symptoms may be due to coccidioidal infection per se or to secondary bacterial or fungal infection within the cavity. Even *Coccidioides* itself has been found to secondarily infect coccidioidal cavities (Winn et al, 1994). Cavities have also been associated with

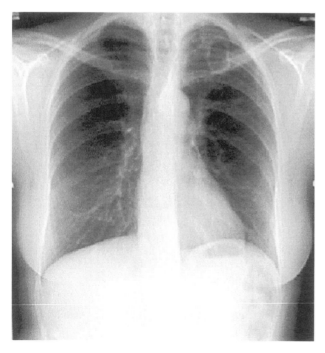

FIGURE 20–6. Left upper lobe coccidioidal cavity. Patient acquired infection while working on archeologic site 2 years previously and complained of persistent cough and chest pain.

significant hemoptysis. A unique complication is py-opneumothorax, due to rupture of a cavity into the pleural space. Patients complain of abrupt dyspnea and the chest radiograph reveals a collapsed lung with an ipsilateral pleural effusion that is inflammatory in nature (Edelstein and Levitt, 1983).

Coccidioidomycosis may result in chronic progressive pulmonary disease, often associated with bronchiectasis and fibrosis. The patient usually has persistent cough, fever, positive sputum cultures for *Coccidioides*, and persistently elevated coccidioidal serology. The chest radiograph may reveal biapical pulmonary fibrosis, similar to that seen in tuberculosis or histoplasmosis. Without therapy, the process is often chronic and progressive (Sarosi et al, 1970).

Finally, primary coccidioidomycosis may present as a diffuse pulmonary process, similar to miliary tuberculosis. There are two mechanisms. The first is overwhelming exposure among immunocompetent persons. Two such cases have been described in which apparent inhalation of a large inoculum of organisms resulted in a diffuse pneumonic process and respiratory failure (Larsen et al, 1985). In addition, other investigators recently reported their experience with diffuse pulmonary primary coccidioidomycosis among eight immunocompetent patients, who represented 1% of all patients hospitalized for coccidioidomycosis (Arsura and Kilgore, 2000). Diffuse pulmonary coccidioidomycosis may also be a manifestation of dissemination and is often associated with fungemia, usually occurring among immunocompromised patients. Mortality for this form of coccidioidomycosis is exceedingly high (Ampel et al, 1986).

Disseminated Coccidioidomycosis

Dissemination is defined as the spread of coccidioidal infection beyond the thoracic cavity. In most cases, disseminated disease portends a poorer prognosis than pulmonary coccidioidomycosis and is associated with a less vigorous cellular immune response to the fungus than occurs in those with pulmonary disease. Dissemination usually becomes clinically apparent within the first few months after pulmonary infection and may occur in individuals who are either symptomatic or asymptomatic at the time of initial infection. Indeed, in many individuals with disseminated disease, there is no evidence of the primary pulmonary infection. Disseminated coccidioidomycosis is estimated to occur in fewer than 1% of all those infected. Patients may have single or multiple sites of dissemination.

The skin is the most common site of extrathoracic dissemination. Reports of large, verrucous lesions, particularly of the face, were prominent in the earliest reports on coccidioidomycosis. However, skin lesions can take on a variety of forms, including papules, plaques, ulcers, draining sinuses, and subcutaneous abscesses (Hobbs, 1989). Early in the course of disease, skin lesions may appear to be particularly benign. Punch biopsies of any suspicious cutaneous lesion in a patient with coccidioidomycosis should be performed with material sent both for histopathological examination and for fungal culture.

Bones are also frequent sites of coccidioidal dissemination. The vertebrae are commonly affected (Kushwaha et al, 1996). The patient notes persistent back pain and, on examination, there is point tenderness and, in some cases, overlying soft tissue swelling. Plain radiography generally reveals a well-marginated lytic lesion (Zeppa et al, 1996). When a vertebral body is involved, there are usually one or more erosive lesions within the body with preservation of the body height and no involvement of the intervertebral disk. Magnetic resonance imaging reveals signal abnormalities within the vertebral body (Fig. 20–7) and often paravertebral and epidural soft tissue swelling (Olson et al, 1998). This mixture of bony and soft tissue inflammation can be very destructive and result in nerve root and spinal cord compression. Consequently, neurosurgical consultation is imperative.

Joints may be infected with or without underlying bone involvement. The knee is the most common site of coccidioidal synovitis. Patients present with chronic pain and swelling of the joint (Bayer and Guze, 1979). Magnetic resonance imaging reveals a thickened and enhanced synovium and occasional loss of underlying bone and cartilage (Lund et al, 1996). Arthocentesis demonstrates an inflammatory process but fungal culture is rarely positive. Synovial biopsy may be necessary to establish the diagnosis.

Meningitis usually manifests as severe and progressive headache and decreasing mental acuity. Lumbar puncture reveals a lymphocyte pleocytosis with an elevated protein and a markedly depressed CSF glucose concentration. A distinguishing characteristic is the presence of eosinophils in the CSF. Fungal culture is positive only occasionally. The diagnosis is usually established by the finding of anticoccidioidal antibodies in the CSF, although this test may be negative. Prior to the advent of antifungal therapy, coccidioidal meningitis was invariably fatal (Vincent et al, 1993). In one-half of patients, meningitis is the only clinically overt manifestation of coccidioidomycosis (Bouza et al, 1981). Coccidioidal meningitis should always be considered in the differential diagnosis of chronic lymphocytic meningitis, even outside the coccidioidal endemic region. A common complication is hydrocephalus, either communicating or noncommunicating, which may occur in the face of appropriate antifungal therapy. In all patients with coccidioidal meningitis, neuroradiography should be performed, with MR imaging the test of choice (Erly et al, 1999). Some patients may develop encephalitis or stroke, due to cerebral vasculitis (Williams, 2001).

SPECIAL HOSTS

Patients with conditions associated with depressed cellular immune function have been identified clearly as being at increased risk for developing severe and disseminated coccidioidomycosis. Included are those with underlying lymphoma or cancer chemotherapy (Deresinski and Stevens, 1975), those on chronic corticosteroids (Ampel et al, 1986), and those with immunosuppression due to HIV infection (Ampel et al, 1993). Because of improvement in antiretroviral therapy with subsequent immune reconstitution, the number of cases of active coccidioidomycosis in association with HIV infection appears to be declining (Woods et al, 2000).

There have been increasing reports of active coccidioidomycosis among those who have received allogeneic transplants (Hall et al, 1993; Blair and Logan, 2001). Most cases appear to be the result of reactivation of a previously acquired infection and emerge at a time of profound immunosuppression with resultant dissemination. Patients at risk usually have a history of prior active coccidioidomycosis or a positive coccidioidal serologic test just prior to transplantation. Antifungal prophylaxis with an azole appears to reduce sig-

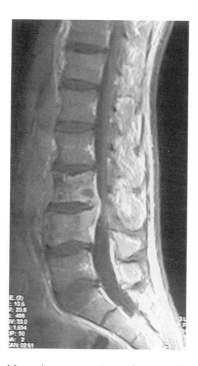

FIGURE 20–7. Magnetic resonance image demonstrating coccidioidal vertebral osteomyelitis. Note nonhomogeneous enhancement in L3 and L4 with lack of involvment of disk space.

nificantly the risk of active coccidioidomycosis among such patients (Blair and Logan, 2001). Recently, two patients developed fatal coccidioidomycosis after receiving a liver and kidney transplant from a single donor. A third recipient remained well. Retrospectively, the donor was found to have active coccidioidomycosis with positive coccidioidal serologies and evidence of meningitis (Wright et al, 2001). A case of fulminant pulmonary coccidioidomycosis due to transplant of an coccidioidal-infected lung has also been observed (Tripathy et al, 2002). These reports suggest that screening of potential organ donors as well as recipients for evidence of active coccidioidomycosis should be considered prior to organ transplantation.

Male sex and increasing age, particularly over 60 years, have been associated with increased risk of developing symptomatic coccidioidomycosis, but not necessarily disseminated disease (Arsura, 1997; Ampel et al, 1998; Gray et al, 1998; Leake et al, 2000). Diabetics may have an increased risk of severe pulmonary disease with cavitation (Pappagianis, 1988). Numerous studies have found that African American men are at markedly increased risk for the development of disseminated coccidioidomycosis when compared to other groups (Flynn et al, 1979; Williams et al, 1979; Ampel et al, 1998; Gray et al, 1998; Rosenstein et al, 2001). For these patients, the clinical presentation is often stereotypical, with widely disseminated disease typically involving the skin, subcutaneous tissue and vertebrae (See Color Fig. 20–8 in separate color insert). Filipino men have also been suggested to be at similar risk (Pappagianis, 1988).

Finally, women who acquire coccidioidomycosis during the second and third trimesters of pregnancy are at increased risk of developing severe, symptomatic, and often disseminated coccidioidomycosis (Wack et al, 1988; Caldwell et al, 2000). Women who have stable or asymptomatic coccidioidomycosis prior to pregnancy do not appear to develop worsening disease as pregnancy advances. Congenital anomalies have been observed in the newborns of women who received high-dose fluconazole for coccidioidal meningitis during their pregnancies (Pursley et al, 1996); thus, it is prudent to avoid high-dose azole therapy during pregnancy.

DIAGNOSIS

In almost all cases of coccidioidomycosis, some definitive laboratory test is required to establish the diagnosis. There are three mainstays for this: culture, histopathology, and serology. *Coccidioides* grows as a nonpigmented mould usually after 3 to 7 days of incubation at 35°C on a variety of artificial media, including blood agar. Any growth suspicious for *Coccidioides* can be formally identified using a commercially available chemiluminescent probe that hy-

bridizes with coccidioidal-specific DNA sequences. This methodology has a sensitivity and specificity of 99% and 100%, respectively (Stockman et al, 1993). Sputum or other respiratory secretions are frequently culture-positive in primary coccidioidomycosis, cavitary disease, and chronic or persistent pulmonary coccidioidomycosis. Biopsy specimens from disseminated sites are less likely to reveal growth. When coccidioidomycosis is suspected, cultures of fluid or tissue from involved sites should always be obtained. If positive, they provide absolute confirmation of the diagnosis. As previously mentioned, the growth of *Coccidioides* on artificial media represents a laboratory hazard and suspected samples should be handled accordingly (Warnock, 2000).

Histopathological identification of spherules is another method for establishing the diagnosis of coccidioidomycosis (See Color Fig. 20–9 in separate color insert). In some instances, such as biopsy of pulmonary nodules, identification of spherules appears to have greater sensitivity than culture (Forseth et al, 1986; Chitkara, 1997), while in other instances, such as evaluation of respiratory secretions, finding of spherules appears to be less sensitive (DiTomasso et al, 1994; Sarosi et al, 2001). For routine biopsies, the Gomori methenamine silver (GMS) stain or the periodic acid Schiff (PAS) stain is preferable to the hematoxylin-eosin method, because spherules can be readily identified in tissue with these stains. Microscopic examination of specimens treated with 10% potassium hydroxide (KOH) has been used in the past to identify spherules in respiratory fluids. However, this test has a very low sensitivity. The Papanicolaou stain is much more sensitive (Sarosi et al, 2001).

Serologic tests identifying anticoccidioidal antibodies were developed initially and their clinical use characterized by Smith and his colleagues nearly 50 years ago (Smith et al, 1956). They remain important today both in the diagnosis and the management of coccidioidomycosis (Pappagianis and Zimmer, 1990; Pappagianis, 2001). Because of changes in nomenclature and methodology, coccidioidal serologic tests can be confusing. A simple way of considering coccidioidal serology is to divide serologic tests into detection of IgM or IgG antibodies. IgM antibodies react with a heatstable polysaccharide antigen, occur soon after primary infection or relapse and then wane, are not useful in the diagnosis of meningitis, and do not predict severity of illness when quantified. IgM antibodies were first defined as tube precipitin (TP) antibodies because of their ability to produce a precipitate in a tube when combined with soluble antigen. If the test is performed in agar as a diffusion assay, it is termed an immunodiffusion tube precipitin (IDTP) test. Anticoccidioidal IgM antibodies can also be detected by latex agglutination (LA), but this test has a significant number of false positive results (Huppert et al, 1968). A commercially available enzyme immunoassay (EIA) also detects IgM anticoccidioidal antibodies (Zartarian et al, 1997).

IgG antibody can be detected by the ability of serum to fix complement when combined with coccidioidal antigen. This assay, which defined the original complement-fixing or CF antibody test, can also be performed by immunodiffusion (IDCF), with the advantage that it is not affected by anticomplementary serum. The CF antigen is heat-labile and has been identified as a chitinase (Zimmermann et al, 1996). EIA may also be used to detect IgG anticoccidioidal antibodies with comparable sensitivity to older tests (Zartarian et al, 1997), although the specificity may be less (Pappaginis, 2001). IgG antibodies are detected later than IgM antibodies but persist in those with continued active disease. Quantitation of CF antibody has prognostic significance. Patients with titers $\geq$ 1:16 are at greater risk of dissemination. Moreover, detection of IgG antibodies in the CSF supports the diagnosis of coccidioidal meningitis (Pappagianis and Zimmer, 1990).

THERAPEUTIC OPTIONS

Treatment alternatives for coccidioidomycosis must be tempered with the knowledge that there has never been a placebo-controlled trial of any antifungal agent in coccidioidomycosis and only one comparative trial. Amphotericin B, formulated with deoxycholate, has been used for the management of severe coccidioidomycosis for nearly 50 years (Winn, 1959). While no formal study has ever been done, review of published cases suggests that intravenous amphotericin B induces clinical improvement in up to 70% of patients treated (Hardenbrook and Barriere, 1982). Unfortunately, the well-known adverse events of amphotericin B have limited its usefulness. In addition, intravenous amphotericin is ineffective in coccidioidal meningitis, and intrathecal therapy is required. Because of these problems, the use of amphotericin B for the management of coccidioidomycosis has generally been supplanted by the oral azole antifungal drugs. However, many clinicians still prefer intravenous amphotericin B as initial therapy for severely ill patients. In addition, some patients will require amphotericin B if they fail to respond to azole antifungal drugs. There are several newer lipid formulations of amphotericin B. To date, none of these has been shown to have superior efficacy to the deoxycholate formulation in the treatment of coccidioidomycosis. At this time, these newer lipid formulations should be reserved for patients at risk for or with renal dysfunction.

Currently, there are three oral azole drugs available for the treatment of coccidioidomycosis: ketoconazole, fluconazole, and itraconazole. Only ketoconazole has been approved by the Food and Drug Administration for use in coccidioidomycosis. However, most experts prefer either fluconazole or itraconazole for the treatment of coccidioidomycosis because of the perception of increased efficacy and fewer toxicities compared to ketoconazole. Initial studies performed by the NIAID Mycoses Study Group and others suggested that the minimum azole dose should be 400 mg daily and that relapses are frequent once therapy is discontinued (Catanzaro et al, 1983; Graybill et al, 1990; Catanzaro et al, 1995). Recently, a comparative trial of fluconazole and itraconazole was completed among patients with pulmonary and nonmeningeal disseminated coccidioidomycosis. Results demonstrate that the two azole drugs were comparable in both efficacy (fluconazole 50% and itraconazole 63%, $p = 0.08$) and rate of relapse (fluconazole 28% and itraconazole 18%, $p > 0.2$). However, the response rate was higher with itraconazole in patients with bone disease, 52% vs. 26%, $p = 0.05$(Galgiani et al, 2000b).

Oral fluconazole and itraconazole have both demonstrated usefulness in the treatment of coccidioidal meningitis (Tucker et al, 1990; Galgiani et al, 1993), but fluconazole is the azole of choice. Ketoconazole should not be used to treat coccidioidal meningitis. Newer azole antifungal drugs, such as posaconazole and voriconazole, may have a place in the management of coccidioidomycosis, but comparative clinical studies are currently lacking (Catanzaro et al, 2000). Although antifungal susceptibility testing has gained credence as a useful technique for the management of some fungal infections, there is no standardized method for performing such an assay with *Coccidioides*. In fact, in an animal model of coccidioidomycosis, susceptibility testing failed to predict efficacy of antifungal agents (Gonzalez et al, 2001). Based on this study, such testing cannot be recommended at this time.

Newer classes of antifungals hold promise for the future. The 1,3-β-D-glucan synthase inhibitor caspofungin, an echinocandin, was found to have efficacy in the treatment of murine coccidioidomycosis (Gonzalez et al, 2001). Nikkomycins, chitin synthase inhibitors, also may find a use in the future treatment of coccidioidomycosis (Hector et al, 1990). While immunomodulating agents such as interferon-gamma would appear to be useful adjuncts in the management of severe coccidioidomycosis, there are no current data on use of these agents.

Although surgery plays a smaller role in the management of coccidioidomycosis then it did in the past, surgery still is vital as an adjunctive therapy in certain instances. It remains the major component of therapy in the management of pyopneumothorax and is required occasionally for extirpation of problematic pulmonary cavities. In addition, surgery is useful for drainage and debridement of extrapulmonary sites that fail to resolve with antifungal therapy and in the placement of shunt catheters in patients with hydrocephalus due to coccidioidal meningitis (Romeo et al, 2000). Finally, many patients with coccidioidal vertebral osteomyelitis require surgery in addition to chemotherapy (Wrobel et al, 2001).

TREATMENT STRATEGIES

Management of coccidioidomycosis is notoriously difficult because of the tremendous variability in course of illness among patients with similar types of disease and because of the multifarious nature of the disease in any given patient. In spite of these qualifiers, useful clinical guidelines have been published recently (Galgiani et al, 2000a).

Primary Pneumonia and Pulmonary Residua
The goal of therapy for primary pneumonia is to ameliorate symptoms. There are no data that such therapy will prevent dissemination. The vast majority of cases of primary pulmonary coccidioidomycosis do not require any therapy. However, it is prudent to follow all such patients for at least 1 year to document resolution of the initial process and to ensure that dissemination has not occurred. Therapy should be considered in those patients with severe symptoms including prostration, night sweats, and weight loss; in those with elevated serum CF titers (> 1:16); or in those with underlying conditions that increase their risk of severe coccidioidomycosis. If treatment is initiated, it should be continued for at least 3 to 6 months (Galgiani et al, 2000a). An oral azole, itraconazole or fluconazole, at a minimum daily dose of 400 mg, is recommended.

Management of pulmonary residua is more complex. Pulmonary nodules require no therapy. Most pulmonary cavities will also require no therapy, but antifungal therapy should be considered in those with persistent symptoms, including cough, chest pain, and hemoptysis. In cavities with an air-fluid level, treatment for a secondary bacterial infection is warranted. In rare cases, surgery may be required because of persistent hemoptysis or an enlarging cavity despite therapy. The mainstay of management of pyopneumothorax is surgical, but most clinicians would also use adjunctive antifungal therapy. For cases where treatment is indicated, oral azole therapy similar to that for primary pneumonia is appropriate.

Diffuse Pneumonia and Chronic Pulmonary Disease
Diffuse pulmonary coccidioidomycosis, whether due to high inoculum exposures or to fungemia in an immunocompromised host, should always be treated. Because of the severity of this manifestation of coccid-

ioidomycosis, most clinicians would begin with intravenous amphotericin B, 0.5–0.7 mg/kg/day, plus a concomitant azole drug, ≥ 400 mg/day, as initial therapy and then change to an oral azole antifungal alone once the patient is clinically stable. Antifungal therapy should be at least 1 year in duration and many clinicians would recommend lifelong therapy, particularly for the immunocompromised patient.

Chronic persistent coccidioidal pneumonia, consisting of cough, fevers, inanition and other symptoms for 6 weeks or more, also requires therapy. Treatment with an oral azole, itraconazole or fluconazole, at 400 mg daily is usually adequate. Therapy for months to years is the rule. Monitoring symptoms, periodically rechecking sputum cultures for growth of *Coccidioides*, and repeated assessment of serum CF titers is helpful in determining response. Similar therapy is also recommended for those patients with fibrocavitary disease. However, many of these patients will have minimal pulmonary symptoms. In such cases, in the absence of a positive sputum culture and elevated CF serologies, many authorities consider it appropriate to withhold antifungal therapy and observe the patient over time.

Disseminated Nonmeningeal Coccidioidomycosis
With rare exceptions, all forms of extrathoracic disseminated coccidioidomycosis require antifungal therapy. For nonmeningeal disseminated coccidioidomycosis, the type of antifungal therapy will depend on the clinical severity of disease. In those patients hospitalized because of coccidioidomycosis, intravenous amphotericin B, 0.5–0.7 mg/kg/day, should be initiated. Many clinicians experienced in the management of coccidioidomycosis would combine this at the outset with an oral azole, itraconazole or fluconazole, at 400 mg or more daily. While there is a theoretical risk of antagonism between two classes of drugs, polyenes and azoles (Sugar, 1995), this phenomenon has not been observed clinically in coccidioidomycosis. In fact, anecdotally, many patients appear to improve on such combined coverage. Once the patient has stabilized clinically, usually over 4 to 6 weeks, the amphotericin B can be stopped, leaving the patient on oral azole therapy only. However, some patients fail azole therapy after responding to amphotericin B. In such cases, reinstitution of amphotericin B will be required. Because relapse is frequent, particularly with oral azoles (Graybill et al, 1990; Catanzaro et al, 1995), azole therapy should be continued for a prolonged period, often years. Patients should be periodically monitored for evidence of disease activity at the site of dissemination, either through direct clinical observation or through imaging. In addition, CF serology should be obtained at 3- to 6-month intervals. Assessment of coccidioidal-specific cellular immunity at similar time points is help-

ful. There are no strict guidelines for discontinuing therapy in patients with disseminated nonmeningeal coccidioidomycosis and some patients may require life-long therapy. In a retrospective study, Oldfield and colleagues found that relapse was more frequent in those with a peak CF titer of ≥ 1:256 and in those who had persistently negative coccidioidal skin tests. End-of-therapy CF titer was not predictive (Oldfield et al, 1997). The risk of relapse is between 15% and 30% after azole therapy is discontinued. Relapses usually occur at the site of initial disease and within 1 year of stopping therapy (Graybill et al, 1990; Catanzaro et al, 1995; Galgiani et al, 2000b). It is reasonable to taper and then stop antifungal therapy in a patient with disseminated nonmeningeal coccidioidomycosis if there is minimal or no evidence of clinical disease; if the CF titer is < 1:2 when the peak CF titer was originally < 1:256; and if there is evidence of return of cellular immune response. Such patients should be followed at 3-month intervals to ensure that relapse does not occur.

Coccidioidal Meningitis

Intrathecal amphotericin B was the first effective treatment for coccidioidal meningitis (Einstein et al, 1961). Unfortunately, this method of administering the drug is associated with numerous adverse reactions, including discomfort due to repeated injections, arachnoiditis, myelitis, inadvertent brain stem puncture, and secondary bacterial infection. In 1993, a noncomparative study of oral fluconazole at 400 mg daily demonstrated a nearly 80% response rate to therapy, including subjects previously on intrathecal amphotericin B (Galgiani et al, 1993). In an earlier study, itraconazole also appeared to have efficacy (Tucker et al, 1990). Currently, the vast majority of patients receive an oral azole drug, preferably fluconazole, as their sole treatment for this form of disseminated coccidioidomycosis. Some clinicians will initiate therapy with doses > 400 mg daily and then reduce to 400 mg daily once the patient is stable (Galgiani et al, 2000a). Voniconazole has been used in a limited number of cases (Kortez et al, 2003). Current data suggest that the risk of relapse is exceedingly high if azole therapy is discontinued in patients with coccidioidal meningitis (Dewsnup et al, 1996). Therefore, therapy should be lifelong. If hydrocephalus occurs during treatment, a shunt is indicated but no change in medication is required (Galgiani et al, 2000a). Some clinicians feel that clinical cure may be possible with the combination of intrathecal amphotericin B (0.01–1.5 mg dosed daily to weekly) and oral azole (≥ 400 mg daily) therapy (Stevens and Shatsky, 2001). In addition, the colloidal dispersion formulation of amphotericin B (ABCD) may be less toxic than the deoxycholate formulation for intrathecal injection (Clemons et al, 2001). Unpublished data suggest that

intravenous infusion of liposomal amphotericin B may have efficacy in coccidioidal meningitis (personal communication, Paul Williams). Future studies should clarify these issues.

PREVENTION

Because coccidioidomycosis is usually acquired environmentally, there are no established methods to prevent infection within the endemic area. Measures that reduce dust, such as paving of roads or wetting soil at sites of construction, are probably helpful. Individuals who wish to reduce their risk of becoming infected should avoid activities that cause them to be exposed to soil. In addition, there have been recent efforts at attempting to predict when climatic conditions might increase the risk of coccidioidomycosis within certain areas (CDC, 2003).

As noted above, several antigens have been identified that have been demonstrated to protect animals from experimental coccidioidomycosis. In the future, these antigens could be used to develop a human vaccine.

REFERENCES

Abuodeh R O, Shubitz L F, Siegel E, Snyder S, Peng T, Orsborn K I, Brummer E, Stevens D A, Galgiani J N. Resistance to Coccidioides immitis in mice after immunization with recombinant protein or a DNA vaccine of a proline-rich antigen. Infect Immun 67:2935–2940, 1999.
Ampel N M, Ryan K J, Carry P J, Wieden M A, Schifman R B. Fungemia due to Coccidioides immitis. An analysis of 16 episodes in 15 patients and a review of the literature. Medicine (Baltimore) 65:312–321, 1986.
Ampel N M, White J D, Varanasi U R, Larwood T R, Van Wyck D B, Galgiani J N. Coccidioidal peritonitis associated with continuous ambulatory peritoneal dialysis. Am J Kidney Dis 11:512–514, 1988.
Ampel N M, Dols C L, Galgiani J N. Coccidioidomycosis during human immunodeficiency virus infection: results of a prospective study in a coccidioidal endemic area. Am J Med 94:235–240, 1993.
Ampel N M, Christian L. In vitro modulation of proliferation and cytokine production by human peripheral blood mononuclear cells from subjects with various forms of coccidioidomycosis. Infect Immun 65:4483–4487, 1997.
Ampel N M, Mosley D G, England B, Vertz P D, Komatsu K, Hajjeh R A. Coccidioidomycosis in Arizona: increase in incidence from 1990 to 1995. Clin Infect Dis 27:1528–1530, 1998.
Ampel N M Kramer L A, Kerekes K M, Johnson S M, Pappagianis D. Assessment of the human cellular immune response to T27K, a coccidioidal antigen preparation, by flow cytometry of whole blood. Med Mycol 39:315–320, 2001.
Aquet J, Stevens D A. Central nervous system abscesses due to Coccidioides species. Clin Infect Dis 22:240–250, 1996.
Arsura E L. The association of age and mortality in coccidioidomycosis. J Am Geriatr Soc 45:532–533, 1997.
Arsura E L, Kilgore W B, Ratnayake S N. Erythema nodosum in pregnant patients with coccidioidomycosis. Clin Infect Dis 27:1201–1203, 1998.

Arsura E L, Kilgore W B. Miliary coccidioidomycosis in the immunocompetent. *Chest* 117:404–409, 2000.

Banuelos A F, Williams P L, Johnson R H, Bibi S, Fredricks D N, Gilroy S A, Bhatti S U, Aguet J, Stevens D A. Central nervous system abscesses due to *Coccidioides* species. *Clin Infect Dis* 22: 240–250, 1996.

Bayer A S, Guze L B. Fungal arthritis. II. Coccidioidal synovitis: clinical, diagnostic, therapeutic, and prognostic considerations. *Semin Arthritis Rheum* 8:200–211, 1979.

Blair J E, Logan J L. Coccidioidomycosis in solid organ transplantation. *Clin Infect Dis* 33:1536–1544, 2001.

Bouza E, Dreyer J S, Hewitt W L, Meyer R D. Coccidioidal meningitis. An analysis of thirty-one cases and review of the literature. *Medicine (Baltimore).* 60:139–172, 1981.

Bowman B H, Taylor J W, White T J. Molecular evolution of the fungi: human pathogens. *Mol Biol Evol* 9:893–904, 1992.

Burt A, Carter D A, Koenig G L , White T J, Taylor J W. Molecular markers reveal cryptic sex in the human pathogen *Coccidioides immitis. Proc Natl Acad Sci U S A* 93:770–773, 1996.

Burt A, Dechairo B M, Koenig G L, Carter D A, White T J, Taylor J W. Molecular markers reveal differentiation among isolates of *Coccidioides immitis* from California, Arizona and Texas. *Mol Ecol* 6:781–786, 1997.

Bylund D J, Nanfro J J, Marsh W L, Jr. Coccidioidomycosis of the female genital tract. *Arch Pathol Lab Med* 110:232–235, 1986.

Cairns L, Blythe D, Kao A, Pappagianis D, Kaufman L, Kobayashi J, Hajjeh R. Outbreak of coccidioidomycosis in Washington state residents returning from Mexico. *Clin Infect Dis* 30:61–64, 2000.

Caldwell J W, Arsura E L, Kilgore W B, Garcia A L, Reddy V, Johnson R H. Coccidioidomycosis in pregnancy during an epidemic in California. *Obstet Gynecol* 95:236–239, 2000.

Carroll G F, Haley L D, Brown J M. Primary cutaneous coccidioidomycosis: a review of the literature and a report of a new case. *Arch Dermatol* 113:933–936, 1977.

Catanzaro A, Friedman P J, Schillaci R, Einstein H, Kirkland T N, Levine H B, Ross J B. Treatment of coccidioidomycosis with ketoconazole: an evaluation utilizing a new scoring system, *Am J Med* 74:64–69, 1983.

Catanzaro A, Galgiani J N, Levine B E, Sharkey-Mathis P K, Fierer J, Stevens D A, Chapman S W, Cloud G. Fluconazole in the treatment of chronic pulmonary and nonmeningeal disseminated coccidioidomycosis. NIAID Mycoses Study Group, *Am J Med* 98: 249–256, 1995.

Catanzaro A, Cloud G, Stevens D, Levine B, Williams P, Johnson R, Sanchez R, Perez L, Rendon A, Mirels L, Lutz J, Holloway M, Blum D, Murphy M, Galgiani J. Safety and tolerance of posaconazole (SCH 56592) in paients with nonmeningeal disseminated coccidioidomycosis. 40th Interscience Conference on Autimicrobial Agents and Chemotherapy, Toronto, Ontario. American Society for Microbiology. Abstract 1417, 2000.

Centers for Disease Control (CDC). Coccidioidomycosis in travelers returning from Mexico—Pennsylvania, 2000. *MMWR Morb Mortal Wkly Rep* 49:1004–1006, 2000.

Centers for Disease Control (CDC). Coccidioidomycosis in workers at an archeologic site—Dinosaur National Monument, Utah, June–July 2001. *MMWR Morb Mortal Wkly Rep* 50:1005–1008, 2001.

Centers for Disease Control (CDC). Increase in coccidioidomycosis—Arizona, 1998–2001. *MMWR Morb Mortal Wkly Rep* 52:109–111, 2003.

Chen K T. Coccidioidal peritonitis. *Am J Clin Pathol* 80:514–516, 1983a.

Chen K T. Coccidioidomycosis of the epididymis. *J Urol* 130:978–979, 1983b.

Chen K T, Schiff J J. Coccidioidomycosis of prostate. *Urology* 25; 82–84, 1985.

Chitkara Y K. Evaluation of cultures of percutaneous core needle biopsy specimens in the diagnosis of pulmonary nodules. *Am J Clin Pathol* 107:224–228, 1997.

Clemons K V, Sobel R A, Williams P L, Stevens D A. Comparative toxicities and pharmacokinetics of intrathecal lipid (amphotericin B colloidal dispersion) and conventional deoxycholate formulations of amphotericin B in rabbits. *Antimicrob Agents Chemother* 45:612–615, 2001.

Converse J L. Effect of surface active agents on endosporulation of *Coccidioides immitis* in a chemically defined medium. *J Bact* 74:106–107, 1957.

Corry D B, Ampel N M, Christian L, Locksley R M, Galgiani J N. Cytokine production by peripheral blood mononuclear cells in human coccidioidomycosis. *J Infect Dis* 174:440–443, 1996.

Deresinski S C, Stevens D A. Coccidioidomycosis in compromised hosts. Experience at Stanford University Hospital. *Medicine (Baltimore)* 54:377–395, 1975.

Dewsnup D H, Galgiani J N, Graybill J R, Diaz M, Rendon A, Cloud G A, Stevens D A. Is it ever safe to stop azole therapy for *Coccidioides immitis* meningitis?, *Ann Intern Med* 124:305–310, 1996.

Dickson E C, Gifford M A. Coccidioides infection (coccidioidomycosis). II. The primary type of infection. *Arch Intern Med* 62:853–871, 1938.

DiTomasso J P, Ampel N M, Sobonya R E, Bloom J W. Bronchoscopic diagnosis of pulmonary coccidioidomycosis. Comparison of cytology, culture, and transbronchial biopsy. *Diagn Microbiol Infect Dis* 18:83–87, 1994.

Dixon D M. *Coccidioides immitis* as a select agent of bioterrorism. *J Appl Microbiol* 91:602–605, 2001.

Dodge R R, Lebowitz M D, Barbee R, Burrows B. Estimates of *C. immitis* infection by skin test reactivity in an endemic community. *Am J Public Health* 75:863–865, 1985.

Dolan M J, Lattuada C P, Melcher G P, Zellmer R, Allendoerfer R, Rinaldi M G. *Coccidioides immitis* presenting as a mycelial pathogen with empyema and hydropneumothorax. *J Med Vet Mycol* 30:249–255, 1992.

Drutz D J, Catanzaro A. Coccidioidomycosis. Part I. *Am Rev Respir Dis* 117:559–585, 1978a.

Drutz D J, Catanzaro A. Coccidioidomycosis. Part II. *Am Rev Respir Dis* 117:727–771, 1978b.

Dunne W M, Jr, Ziebert A P, Donahoe L W, Standard P. Unexpected laboratory diagnosis of latent urogenital coccidioidomycosis in a nonendemic area. *Arch Pathol Lab Med* 110:236–238, 1986.

Durry E, Pappagianis D, Werner S B, Hutwagner L, Sun R K, Maurer M, McNeil M M, Pinner R W. Coccidioidomycosis in Tulare County, California, 1991: reemergence of an endemic disease. *J Med Vet Mycol* 35:321–326, 1997.

Echols R M, Palmer D L, Long G W. Tissue eosinophilia in human coccidioidomycosis. *Rev Infect Dis* 4:656–664, 1982.

Eckmann B H, Schaefer G L, Huppert M. Bedside interhuman transmission of coccidioidomycosis via growth on fomites. *Am Rev Respir Dis* 89:179–185, 1964.

Edelstein G, Levitt R G. Cavitary coccidioidomycosis presenting as spontaneous pneumothorax. *Am J Roentgenol* 141:533–534, 1983.

Edwards P Q, Palmer C E. Prevalence of sensitivity to coccidioidin, with special reference to specific and nonspecific reactions to coccidioidin and histoplasmin. *Dis Chest* 31:35–60, 1957.

Egeberg R O, Ely A F. *Coccidioides immitis* in the soil of the southern San Joaquin Valley. *Am J Med Sci* 231:151–154, 1956.

Egeberg R O, Elconin A E, Egeberg M C. Effect of salinity and temperature on *Coccidioides immitis* and three antagonistic soil saprophytes. *J Bact* 88:473–476, 1964.

Einstein H, Holeman C W, Sandidge L L, Holden D H. Coccidioidal meningitis. The use of amphotericin B in treatment. *Calif Med* 94:339–343, 1961.

Erly W K, Bellon R J, Seeger J F, Carmody R F. MR imaging of acute coccidioidal meningitis. *AJNR Am J Neuroradiol* 20:509–514, 1999.

Faul J L, Hoang K, Schmoker J, Vagelos R H, Berry G J. Constrictive pericarditis due to coccidiomycosis. *Ann Thorac Surg* 68:1407–1409, 1999.

Fiese M J. Treatment of disseminated coccidioidomycosis with amphotericin B: report of a case. *Calif Med* 86:119–120, 1957.

Fiese M J. *Coccidioidomycosis.* Springfield, IL: Charles C. Thomas, 1958.

Fisher M C, Koenig G L, White T J, Taylor J W. Pathogenic clones versus environmentally driven population increase: analysis of an epidemic of the human fungal pathogen *Coccidioides immitis. J Clin Microbiol* 38:807–813, 2000.

Fisher M C, Koenig G L, White T J, San-Blas G, Negroni R, Alvarez I G, Wanke B, Taylor J W. Biogeographic range expansion into South America by *Coccidioides immitis* mirrors New World patterns of human migration. *Proc Natl Acad Sci U S A* 98:4558–4562, 2001.

Fisher M C, Koenig G L, White T J, Taylor J W. Molecular and phenotypic description of *Coccidioides posadasii* sp. nov., previously recognized as the non-California population of *Coccidioides immitis. Mycologia* 94:73–84, 2002.

Flynn N M, Hoeprich P D, Kawachi M M, Lee K K, Lawrence R M, Goldstein E, Jordan G W, Kundargi R S, Wong G A. An unusual outbreak of windborne coccidioidomycosis. *N Engl J Med* 301:358–361, 1979.

Forseth J, Rohwedder J J, Levine B E, Saubolle M A. Experience with needle biopsy for coccidioidal lung nodules. *Arch Intern Med* 146:319–320, 1986.

Galgiani J N, Isenberg R A, Stevens D A. Chemotaxigenic activity of extracts from the mycelial and spherule phases of *Coccidioides immitis* for human polymorphonuclear leukocytes. *Infect Immun* 21:862–865, 1978.

Galgiani J N, Hayden R, Payne C M. Leukocyte effects on the dimorphism of *Coccidioides immitis. J Infect Dis* 146:56–63, 1982.

Galgiani J N, Payne C M, Jones J F. Human polymorphonuclear-leukocyte inhibition of incorporation of chitin precursors into mycelia of *Coccidioides immitis. J Infect Dis* 149:404–412, 1984.

Galgiani J N, Catanzaro A, Cloud G A, Higgs J, Friedman B A, Larsen R A, Graybill J R. Fluconazole therapy for coccidioidal meningitis. The NIAID-Mycoses Study Group. *Ann Intern Med* 119:28–35, 1993.

Galgiani J N, Ampel N M, Catanzaro A, Johnson R H, Stevens D A, Williams P L. Practice guideline for the treatment of coccidioidomycosis. Infectious Diseases Society of America. *Clin Infect Dis* 30:658–661, 2000a.

Galgiani J N, Catanzaro A, Cloud G A, Johnson R H, Williams P L, Mirels L F, Nassar F, Lutz J E, Stevens D A, Sharkey P K, Singh V R, Larsen R A, Delgado K L, Flanigan C, Rinaldi M G. Comparison of oral fluconazole and itraconazole for progressive, nonmeningeal coccidioidomycosis. A randomized, double-blind trial. Mycoses Study Group. *Ann Intern Med* 133:676–686, 2000b.

Gehlbach S H, Hamilton J D, Conant N F. Coccidioidomycosis. An occupational disease in cotton mill workers. *Arch Intern Med* 131:254–255, 1973.

Gonzalez G M, Tijerina R, Najvar L K, Bocanegra R, Luther M, Rinaldi M G, Graybill J R. Correlation between antifungal susceptibilities of *Coccidioides immitis* in vitro and antifungal treatment with caspofungin in a mouse model. *Antimicrob Agents Chemother* 45:1854–1859, 2001.

Gray G C, Fogle E F, Albright K L. Risk factors for primary pulmonary coccidioidomycosis hospitalizations among United States Navy and Marine Corps personnel, 1981–1994. *Am J Trop Med Hyg* 58:309–312, 1998.

Graybill J R, Stevens, D.A, Galgiani, J.N, Dismukes, W.E, Cloud G A. Itraconazole treatment of coccidioidomycosis. NAIAD Mycoses Study Group. *Am J Med* 89:282–290, 1990.

Greendyke W H, Resnick D L, Harvey W C. The varied roentgen manifestations of primary coccidioidomycosis. *Am J Roentgenol Radium Ther Nucl Med* 109:491–499, 1970.

Hall K A, Copeland J G, Zukoski C F, Sethi G K, Galgiani J N. Markers of coccidioidomycosis before cardiac or renal transplantation and the risk of recurrent infection. *Transplantation* 55:1422–1424, 1993.

Hardenbrook M H, Barriere S L. Coccidioidomycosis: evaluation of parameters used to predict outcome with amphotericin B therapy. *Mycopathologia* 78:65–71, 1982.

Harley W B, Blaser M J. Disseminated coccidioidomycosis associated with extreme eosinophilia. *Clin Infect Dis* 18:627–629, 1994.

Hector R F, Zimmer B L, Pappagianis D. Evaluation of nikkomycins X and Z in murine models of coccidioidomycosis, histoplasmosis, and blastomycosis. *Antimicrob Agents Chemother* 34:587–593, 1990.

Hobbs E R. Coccidioidomycosis. *Dermatol Clin* 7:227–239, 1989.

Huntington R W. Pathology of coccidioidomycosis. In: Stevens DA ed. *Coccidioidomycosis. A Text.* New York: Plenum Medical Book Company, 113–132, 1980.

Huppert M, Peterson E T, Sun S H, Chitjian P A, Derrevere W J. Evaluation of a latex particle agglutination test for coccidioidomycosis. *Am J Clin Pathol* 49:96–102, 1968.

Hyde L. Coccidioidal pulmonary cavitation. *Dis Chest* 54:Suppl 1:273–277, 1968.

Jiang C, Magee D M, Quitugua T N, Cox R A. Genetic vaccination against *Coccidioides immitis*: comparison of vaccine efficacy of recombinant antigen 2 and antigen 2 cDNA. *Infect Immun* 67:630–635, 1999.

Johnson J E III, Perry J E, Fekety F R, Kadull P J, Cluff L E. Laboratory-acquired coccidioidomycosis. *Ann Intern Med* 60:941–956, 1964.

Johnson W M. Occupational factors in coccidioidomycosis. *J Occup Med* 23:367–374, 1981.

Kerrick S S, Lundergan L L, Galgiani J N. Coccidioidomycosis at a university health service. *Am Rev Respir Dis* 131:100–102, 1985.

Kirkland T N, Fierer J. Coccidioidomycosis: a reemerging infectious disease. *Emerg Infect Dis* 2:192–199, 1996.

Kleinschmidt-DeMasters B K, Mazowiecki M, Bonds L A, Cohn D L, Wilson M L. Coccidioidomycosis meningitis with massive dural and cerebral venous thrombosis and tissue arthroconidia. *Arch Pathol Lab Med* 124:310–314, 2000.

Klotz S A, Drutz D J, Huppert M, Sun S H, DeMarsh P L. The critical role of CO2 in the morphogenesis of *Coccidioides immitis* in cell-free subcutaneous chambers. *J Infect Dis* 150:127–134, 1984.

Kolivras K N, Johnson P S, Comrie A C, Yool S R. Environmental variability and coccidioidomycosis (valley fever). *Aerobiologia* 17:31–42, 2001.

Kortez KJ, Walsh TJ, Bennett JE. Coccidioidal meningitis successfully treated with voriconazole. *Clin Infect Dis* 2003, in press.

Kuntze J R, Herman M H, Evans S G. Genitourinary coccidioidomycosis. *J Urol* 140:370–374, 1988.

Kushwaha V P, Shaw B A, Gerardi J A, Oppenheim W L. Musculoskeletal coccidioidomycosis. A review of 25 cases. *Clin Orthop* 332:190–199, 1996.

Lacy G H, Swatek F E. Soil ecology of *Coccidioides immitis* at Amerindian middens in California. *Appl Microbiol* 27:379–388, 1974.

Larsen R A, Jacobson J A, Morris A H, Benowitz B A. Acute respiratory failure caused by primary pulmonary coccidioidomycosis. Two case reports and a review of the literature. *Am Rev Respir Dis* 131:797–799, 1985.

Larwood T R. Coccidioidin skin testing in Kern County, California: decrease in infection rate over 58 years. *Clin Infect Dis* 30:612–613, 2000.

Leake J A, Mosley D G, England B, Graham J V, Plikaytis B D, Ampel N M, Perkins B A, Hajjeh R A. Risk factors for acute symptomatic coccidioidomycosis among elderly persons in Arizona, 1996–1997. *J Infect Dis* 181:1435–1440, 2000.

Levine B E, Cobb J M, Smith C E. Immunity to coccidioidomycosis induced mice by purified spherule, arthrospore, and mycelial vaccines. *Trans NY Acad Sci* 22:436–449, 1960.

Li K, Yu J J, Hung C Y, Lehmann P F, Cole G T. Recombinant urease and urease DNA of *Coccidioides immitis* elicit an immunoprotective response against coccidioidomycosis in mice. *Infect Immun* 69:2878–2887, 2001.

Lombard C M, Tazelaar H D, Krasne D L. Pulmonary eosinophilia in coccidioidal infections. *Chest* 91:734–736, 1987.

Looney J M, Stein T. Coccidioidomycosis. The hazard involved in diagnostic procedures, with report of a case. *N Engl J Med* 242:77–82, 1950.

Lund P J, Chan K M, Unger E C, Galgiani T N, Pitt M J. Magnetic resonance imaging in coccidioidal arthritis. *Skeletal Radiol* 25:661–665, 1996.

Maddy K T. The geographic distribution of *Coccidioides immitis* and possible ecologic implications. *Ariz Med* 15:178–188, 1958.

Maddy K T. Observations of *Coccidioides immitis* found growing naturally in soil. *Ariz Med* 22:281–288, 1965.

Magee D M, Cox R A. Roles of gamma interferon and interleukin-4 in genetically determined resistance to *Coccidioides immitis*. *Infect Immun* 63:3514–3519, 1995.

McGahan J P, Graves D S, Palmer P E, Stadalnik R C, Dublin A B. Classic and contemporary imaging of coccidioidomycosis. *Am J Roentgenol* 136:393–404, 1981.

Mischel P S, Vinters H V. Coccidioidomycosis of the central nervous system: neuropathological and vasculopathic manifestations and clinical correlates. *Clin Infect Dis* 20:400–405, 1995.

O'Brien J J, Gilsdorf J R. Primary cutaneous coccidioidomycosis in childhood. *Pediatr Infect Dis* 5:485–486, 1986.

Ogiso A, Ito M, Koyama M, Yamaoka H, Hotchi M, McGinnis M R. Pulmonary coccidioidomycosis in Japan: case report and review. *Clin Infect Dis* 25:1260–1261, 1997.

Oldfield E C, Bone W D, Martin C R, Gray G C, Olson P, Schillaci R F. Prediction of relapse after treatment of coccidioidomycosis. *Clin Infect Dis* 25:1205–1210, 1997.

Olson E M, Duberg A C, Herron L D, Kissel P, Smilovitz D. Coccidioidal spondylitis: MR findings in 15 patients. *AJR Am J Roentgenol* 171:785–789, 1998.

Ophüls W. Further observations on a pathogenic mould formerly described as a protozoan (*Coccidioides immitis*; *Coccidioides pyogenes*). *J Exp Med* 6:443–485, 1905.

Oudiz R, Mahaisavariya P, Peng S K, Shane-Yospur L, Smith C, Baumgartner F, Shapiro S. Disseminated coccidioidomycosis with rapid progression to effusive-constrictive pericarditis. *J Am Soc Echocardiogr* 8:947–952, 1995.

Padua y Gabriel A, Martinez-Ordaz V A, Velasco-Rodreguez V M, Lazo-Saenz J G, Cicero R. Prevalence of skin reactivity to coccidioidin and associated risks factors in subjects living in a northern city of Mexico. *Arch Med Res* 30:388–392, 1999.

Pan S, Sigler L, Cole G T. Evidence for a phylogenetic connection between *Coccidioides immitis* and *Uncinocarpus reesii* (Onygenaceae). *Microbiology* 140 (Pt 6):1481–1494, 1994.

Pappagianis D, Einstein, H. Tempest from Tehachapi takes toll or *Coccidioides* conveyed aloft and afar. *West J Med* 129:527–530, 1978.

Pappagianis D. Epidemiology of coccidioidomycosis. *Curr Top Med Mycol* 2:199–238, 1988.

Pappagianis D, Zimmer B L. Serology of coccidioidomycosis. *Clin Microbiol Rev* 3:247–268, 1990.

Pappagianis D. Evaluation of the protective efficacy of the killed *Coccidioides immitis* spherule vaccine in humans. The Valley Fever Vaccine Study Group. *Am Rev Respir Dis* 148:656–660, 1993.

Pappagianis D. Marked increase in cases of coccidioidomycosis in California: 1991, 1992, and 1993. *Clin Infect Dis* 19 Suppl 1:S14–18, 1994.

Pappagianis D. Serologic studies in coccidioidomycosis. *Semin Respir Infect* 16:242–250, 2001.

Polesky A, Kirsch C M, Snyder L S, LoBue P, Kagawa F T, Dykstra B J, Wehner J H, Catanzaro A, Ampel N M, Stevens D A. Airway coccidioidomycosis—report of cases and review. *Clin Infect Dis* 28:1273–1280, 1999.

Pursley T J, Blomquist I K, Abraham J, Andersen H F, Bartley J A. Fluconazole-induced congenital anomalies in three infants. *Clin Infect Dis* 22:336–340, 1996.

Putnam J S, Harper W K, Greene J F, Jr, Nelson K G, Zurek R C. *Coccidioides immitis*. A rare cause of pulmonary mycetoma. *Am Rev Respir Dis* 112:733–738, 1975.

Ragland A S, Arsura E, Ismail Y, Johnson R. Eosinophilic pleocytosis in coccidioidal meningitis: frequency and significance. *Am J Med* 95:254–257, 1993.

Richards J O, Ampel N M, Galgiani J N, Lake D F. Dendritic cells pulsed with *Coccidioides immitis* lysate induce antigen-specific naive T cell activation. *J Infect Dis* 184:1220–1224, 2001.

Rixford E, Gilchrist T C. Two cases of protozoon (coccidioidal) infection of the skin and other organs. *Johns Hopkins Hosp Rep* 1:209–268, 1896.

Rodenbiker H T, Ganley J P. Ocular coccidioidomycosis. *Surv Ophthalmol* 24:263–290, 1980.

Rodenbiker H T, Ganley J P, Galgiani J N, Axline S G. Prevalence of chorioretinal scars associated with coccidioidomycosis. *Arch Ophthalmol* 99:71–75, 1981.

Romeo J H, Rice L B, McQuarrie I G. Hydrocephalus in coccidioidal meningitis: case report and review of the literature. *Neurosurgery* 47:773–777, 2000.

Rosenstein N E, Emery K W, Werner S B, Kao A, Johnson R, Rogers D, Vugia D, Reingold A, Talbot R, Plikaytis B D, Perkins B A, Hajjeh R A. Risk factors for severe pulmonary and disseminated coccidioidomycosis: Kern County, California, 1995–1996. *Clin Infect Dis* 32:708–715, 2001.

Salgia K, Bhatia L, Rajashekaraiah K R, Zangan M, Hariharan S, Kallick C A. Coccidioidomycosis of the uterus. *South Med J* 75:614–616, 1982.

Sarosi G A, Parker J D, Doto I L, Tosh F E. Chronic pulmonary coccidioidomycosis. *N Engl J Med* 283:325–329, 1970.

Sarosi G A, Lawrence J P, Smith D K, Thomas A, Hobohm D W, Kelley P C. Rapid diagnostic evaluation of bronchial washings in patients with suspected coccidioidomycosis. *Semin Respir Infect* 16:238–241, 2001.

Schneider E, Hajjeh R A, Spiegel R A, Jibson R W, Harp E L, Marshall G A, Gunn R A, McNeil M M, Pinner R W, Baron R C, Burger R C, Hutwagner L C, Crump C, Kaufman L, Reef S E, Feldman G M, Pappagianis D, Werner S B. A coccidioidomycosis outbreak following the Northridge, Calif, earthquake. *JAMA* 277:904–908, 1997.

Smith C E. Epidemiology of acute coccidioidomycosis with erythema nodosum ("San Joaquin" or "Valley Fever"). *Am J Public Health* 30:600–611, 1940.

Smith C E, Beard R. Varieties of coccidioidal infection in relation to the epidemiology and control of the diseases. *Am J Public Health* 36:1394–1402, 1946a.

Smith C E, Beard R R, Rosenberger H G, Whiting E G. Effect of season and dust control on coccidioidomycosis. *JAMA* 132:833–838, 1946b.

Smith C E, Whiting E G, Baker E E, Rosenberger H G, Beard R, Saito M T. The use of coccidioidin. *Am Rev Tuberc* 57:330–360, 1948.

Smith C E, Saito M T, Beard R R, Kepp R M, Clark R W, Eddie B U. Serological tests in the diagnosis and prognosis of coccidioidomycosis. *Am J Hyg* 52:1–21, 1950.

Smith C E. Diagnosis of pulmonary coccidioidal infections. *Calif Med* 75:385–391, 1951.

Smith C E, Saito M T, Simons S A. Pattern of 39,500 serologic tests in coccidioidomycosis. *JAMA* 160:546–552, 1956.

Standaert S M, Schaffner W, Galgiani J N, Pinner R W, Kaufman L, Durry E, Hutcheson R H. Coccidioidomycosis among visitors to a *Coccidioides immitis*-endemic area: an outbreak in a military reserve unit. *J Infect Dis* 171:1672–1675, 1995.

Stevens D A, Shatsky S A. Intrathecal amphotericin in the management of coccidioidal meningitis. *Semin Respir Infect* 16:263–269, 2001.

Stewart R A, Meyer K F. Isolation of *Coccidioides immitis* (Stiles) from the soil. *Proc Soc Exp Biol Med* 29:937–938, 1932.

Stockman L, Clark K A, Hunt J M, Roberts G D. Evaluation of commercially available acridinium ester-labeled chemiluminescent DNA probes for culture identification of *Blastomyces dermatitidis*, *Coccidioides immitis*, *Cryptococcus neoformans*, and *Histoplasma capsulatum*. *J Clin Microbiol* 31:845–850, 1993.

Sugar A M. Use of amphotericin B with azole antifungal drugs. What are we doing? *Antimicrob Agents Chemother* 39:1907–1912, 1995.

Sun S H, Huppert M. A cytological study of morphogenesis in *Coccidioides immitis*. *Sabouraudia* 14:185–198, 1976.

Tripathy U, Yung G L, Kriett J M, Thistlethwaite P A, Kapelanski D P, Jamieson S W. Donor transfer of pulmonary coccidioidomycosis in lung transplantation. *Ann Thorac Surg* 73:306–308, 2002.

Tucker R M, Denning D W, Dupont B, Stevens D A. Itraconazole therapy for chronic coccidioidal meningitis. *Ann Intern Med* 112:108–112, 1990.

Vincent T, Galgiani J N, Huppert M, Salkin D. The natural history of coccidioidal meningitis: VA-Armed Forces cooperative studies, 1955–1958. *Clin Infect Dis* 16:247–254, 1993.

Wack E E, Ampel N M, Galgiani J N, Bronnimann D A. Coccidioidomycosis during pregnancy. An analysis of ten cases among 47,120 pregnancies. *Chest* 94:376–379, 1988.

Wanke B, Lazera M, Monteiro P C, Lima F C, Leal M J, Ferreira Filho P L, Kaufman L, Pinner R W, Ajello L. Investigation of an outbreak of endemic coccidioidomycosis in Brazil's northeastern state of Piaui with a review of the occurrence and distribution of *Coccidioides immitis* in three other Brazilian states. *Mycopathologia* 148:57–67, 1999.

Warnock D W. Mycotic agents of human disease. In: Fleming DO, Hunt DL, eds. *Biological Safety. Principles and Practices*. Washington, DC: ASM Press, 111–120, 2000.

Werner S B, Pappagianis D, Heindl I, Mickel A. An epidemic of coccidioidomycosis among archeology students in northern California. *N Engl J Med* 286:507–512, 1972.

Werner S B, Pappagianis D. Coccidioidomycosis in Northern California. An outbreak among archeology students near Red Bluff. *Calif Med* 119:10–20, 1973.

Williams P L, Sable D L, Mendez P, Smyth L T. Symptomatic coccidioidomycosis following a severe natural dust storm. An outbreak at the Naval Air Station, Lemoore, Calif. *Chest* 76:566–570, 1979.

Williams P L, Sable D L, Sorgen S P, Pappagianis D, Levine H B, Brodine S K, Brown B W, Grumet F C, Stevens D A. Immunologic responsiveness and safety associated with the *Coccidioides immitis* spherule vaccine in volunteers of white, black, and Filipino ancestry. *Am J Epidemiol* 119:591–602, 1984.

Williams P L, Johnson R, Pappagianis D, Einstein H, Slager U, Koster F T, Eron J J, Morrison J, Aguet J, River M E. Vasculitic and encephalitic complications associated with *Coccidioides immitis* infection of the central nervous system in humans: report of 10 cases and review. *Clin Infect Dis* 14:673–682, 1992.

Williams P L. Vasculitic complications associated with coccidioidal meningitis. *Semin Respir Infect* 16:270–279, 2001.

Wilson J W, Smith C E, Plunkett O A. Primary cutaneous coccidioidomycosis: criteria for diagnosis and a report of a case. *Calif Med* 79:233–239, 1953.

Winn R E, Johnson R, Galgiani J N, Butler C, Pluss J. Cavitary coccidioidomycosis with fungus ball formation. Diagnosis by fiberoptic bronchoscopy with coexistence of hyphae and spherules. *Chest* 105:412–416, 1994.

Winn W A. The use of amphotericin B in the treatment of coccidioidal disease. *Am J Med* 27:617–635, 1959.

Winn W A, Levine B E, Broderick J E, Crane R W. A localized epidemic of coccidioidal infection. *N Engl J Med* 268:867–870, 1963.

Winn W A. A long term study of 300 patients with cavitary-abscess lesions of the lung of coccidioidal origin. An analytical study with special reference to treatment. *Dis Chest* 54:Suppl 1:268+, 1968.

Woods C W, McRill C, Plikaytis B D, Rosenstein N E, Mosley D, Boyd D, England B, Perkins B A, Ampel N M, Hajjeh R A. Coccidioidomycosis in human immunodeficiency virus-infected persons in Arizona, 1994–1997: incidence, risk factors, and prevention. *J Infect Dis* 181:1428–1434, 2000.

Wright P, Pappagianis D, Taylor J, Moser S A, Louro A, Wilson M L, Pappas P G. Transmission of *Coccidioides immitis* from donor organs: a description of two fatal cases of disseminated coccidioidomycosis. 39th Annual Meeting of the Infectious Diseases Society of America. San Francisco, CA, Abstract 619, 2001.

Wrobel C J, Chappell E T, Taylor W. Clinical presentation, radiological findings, and treatment results of coccidioidomycosis involving the spine: report on 23 cases. *J Neurosurg* 95:33–39, 2001.

Zartarian M, Peterson E M, de la Maza L M. Detection of antibodies to *Coccidioides immitis* by enzyme immunoassay. *Am J Clin Pathol* 107:148–153, 1997.

Zeppa M A, Laorr A, Greenspan A, McGahan J P, Steinbach L S. Skeletal coccidioidomycosis: imaging findings in 19 patients. *Skeletal Radiol* 25:337–343, 1996.

Zimmermann C R, Johnson S M, Martens G W, White A G, Pappagianis D. Cloning and expression of the complement fixation antigen-chitinase of *Coccidioides immitis*. *Infect Immun* 64:4967–4975, 1996.

Zimmermann C R, Johnson S M, Martens G W, White A G, Zimmer B L, Pappagianis D. Protection against lethal murine coccidioidomycosis by a soluble vaccine from spherules. *Infect Immun* 66:2342–2345, 1998.

21

Paracoccidioidomycosis

ANGELA RESTREPO-MORENO

Paracoccidioidomycosis is an endemic fungal infection of pulmonary origin that disseminates to different sites, notably oral mucous membranes, adrenal glands, reticulo-endothelial system and skin; other organs may also be involved. The disease tends to run a chronic course with acute cases being rare; outbreaks have not been reported. Four clinical presentations are recognized: regressive subclinical infection, progressive disease that can be either chronic (adult-type), or acute/subacute (juvenile-type), and the residual form. This mycosis has certain peculiarities such as its restricted geographic distribution to Latin America, the predominance of male patients and the long periods of latency elapsing from the time of infection to the manifestations of overt disease. The etiologic agent is a thermally dimorphic fungus *Paracoccidioides brasiliensis* which at 35°C–37°C has a yeast form characterized by a mother cell surrounded by multiple blastoconidia resembling a pilot's wheel. At lower temperatures (< 28°C) the fungus grows as a mould that sporadically gives rise to conidia. The fungus microniche in nature has not yet been precisely defined. The disease can be successfully treated although fibrotic sequelae are common. A comprehensive review in 1994 describes the various aspects of the mycosis and its etiologic agent (Franco et al, 1994).

MICROBIOLOGY

Paracoccidioides brasiliensis is a dimorphic fungus that in host's tissues and in cultures at 36°C–37°C grows as a yeast (Y) whereas at lower temperatures (< 28°C), it develops as a mould (M). This eukaryotic microorganism is presently known only in its asexual (anamorph) state (Lacaz et al, 2002; Lacaz et al, 1998; Queiroz-Telles F, 1994).

Yeast colonies appear within a week of incubation at 36°C (range 28°C–37°C); they are soft, wrinkled and tan to cream. Microscopically, colonies reveal yeast cells of varying sizes (4–35 μm) and shapes but with predominance of round to oval structures. The most characteristic grouping is that a of mother cell surrounded by multiple buds of equal or different sizes resembling a pilot's wheel; the buds may present a con-

necting bridge with the mother cell. Sometimes single cells, with one bud or arranged in short chains can be observed; chalice-, balloon-shaped or broken cells are not infrequent. The yeast has a thick, refractile cell wall and contains prominent intracytoplasmic lipid vacuoles (See Color Figs. 21–1 and 21–2 in separate color insert.) (Lacaz et al, 2002; Lacaz et al, 1998; Brummer et al, 1993; Queiroz-Telles, 1994).

At temperatures ranging from 19°C to 28°C, *P. brasiliensis* grows as a mould; growth is rather slow, 15 to 30 days. It produces white to tan, irregularly shaped colonies with short hairy-looking mycelia; some isolates produce a brown pigment. Growth in solid media is often accompanied by cracks in the agar. Microscopic preparations from the mould, grown in the usual glucose-rich media, reveal only thin, septated hyphae with sparse terminal and intercalary chlamydospores. The latter are considered resistant structures and can also play a role in mycelial (M) to yeast (Y) transition by becoming yeast cells under the influence of temperature (Brummer et al, 1993; Lacaz et al, 2002; Lacaz et al, 1998). When grown under nutritional deprivation certain isolates produce conidia which vary from centrally bulging arthroconidia, single-celled to pear-shaped microconidia, all less than 5μm. Conidia respond to temperature changes, transforming either into yeast cells at 36°C or producing hyphae at 20°C–24°C. Furthermore, conidia are infectious for mice and produce a chronic, disseminated process (McEwen et al, 1987; Cock, 2000). *Paracoccidioides brasiliensis* conidia and yeast cells have been shown to produce melanin-like compounds, both in vitro and in vivo. This may explain pigmentation in culture and additionally, melanin may play a role in pathogenesis (Gómez et al, 2001).

Under the electron microscope the mycelium's cell wall is composed of two layers, the outermost made of β-1,3-glucan fibrils and the innermost, of rigid chitin fibrils. The septum comes from a deep invagination of the latter layer and of the cytoplasmic membrane; their growth towards the hyphal axis leaves a pore associated with Woronin bodies (Queiroz-Tellez, 1994). The yeast has a thicker cell wall composed mainly of α-1,3-

glucan that at its outermost layer has a slime surface of complex mucopolysaccharides (Queiroz-Tellez, 1994, San Blas and San Blas, 1994). Differences in cell wall glucose polymers in the two forms are important in the host-parasite interactions because macrophages do not have alpha glucanase and are unable to degrade the yeast cells (San Blas and San Blas, 1994; San Blas and Niño-Vega, 2000).

Woronin bodies tend to place *P. brasiliensis* in the subphylum *Ascomycotina*, series *Prototunicatae*, order *Onygenales* family Onygenaceae (Queiroz-Tellez, 1994). Molecular studies have confirmed this classification, placing *P. brasiliensis* close to *Blastomyces dermatitidis* and *Emmonsia parva* in the phylogenetic tree (Bialek et al, 2000a).

Paracoccidioides brasiliensis electrophoretic karyotype indicates a genome within a 45.7 to 60.9 Mbp size range. Each separate chromosomal band appears to be diploid (Cano et al, 1998; Montoya et al, 1999). *Paracoccidioides brasiliensis* M and Y forms are aerobic and require ample oxygen supply for their growth; however, in residual lesions, yeast cells tolerate oxygen restriction and can be recuperated only if cultured under microaerobic conditions (Brummer et al, 1993).

The host's hormones influence *P. brasiliensis* M to Y transition. The original studies, which arose in response to the observed predominance of male over female patients (ratio 14/1) (Brummer et al, 1993), revealed that in vitro *P. brasiliensis* secretes an estradiol-binding protein that attaches to the female hormone. Through regulation of protein expression, estradiol binding hinders the M to Y transformation (Restrepo et al, 1997). Other investigators have shown female mice at estrus (higher blood estrogen levels) cleared yeast from their tissues more efficiently (Sano et al, 1992). Aristizábal and coworkers infected male and female mice with conidia and observed different responses; in normal males conidia transformed into yeast cells and these multiplied actively resulting in progressive infection, whereas in normal females such transition was halted, fungal proliferation was inhibited and the infection was controlled (Aristizábal et al, 1998; Aristizábal et al, 2001). These results further support a role for 17β-estradiol in the innate resistance of females to paracoccidioidomycosis.

Isolates of *P. brasiliensis* are not equally virulent; furthermore they tend to lose virulence upon subculturing and regain it through animal passage (Brummer et al, 1993). Different *P. brasiliensis* isolates separated by random amplified polymorphic DNA analysis (RAPD) into two different patterns were used to inoculate mice. One RAPD group elicited a localized infection while the other gave rise to a disseminated infection (Molinari-Madlum et al, 1999). Virulence factors have not been completely defined but dimorphism and the yeast

non-degradable α-1,3-glucan cell wall polymer are important (San Blas and San Blas, 1994; San Blas and Niño-Vega, 2000). During the M to Y transition, an hsp70 gene is expressed differentially in the latter, indicating that this step is advantageous for the Y form as it increases resistance to environmental stress, a requirement for parasite survival in the mammalian host (Silva et al, 1999).

Isolates of *P. brasiliensis* from diverse geographical regions were studied by molecular biology tools (RAPD and RFLP). A dendogram showed high degree of similarity among strains with genetic differences expressed in clusters related to geographical origin. Five different groups were sorted, each of which was geographically distinct and corresponded to present country borders. The results support the concept that *P. brasiliensis* infections are acquired from exogenous sources and that this fungus occupies special niches within the natural environment (Niño-Vega et al, 2000).

GEOGRAPHIC DISTRIBUTION

Paracoccidioidomycosis is limited to Latin America where it is regularly reported from Mexico (23°N) downwards to Argentina (34°S), albeit not with the same frequency. Brazil is the country accounting for over 80% of all reports, followed at good distance by Venezuela, Colombia, Ecuador, and Argentina (Brummer et al, 1993; Blotta et al, 1999). No cases have been reported in Chile, Surinam, the Guyana, Nicaragua, or Belize. With rare exceptions (one case each in Trinidad, Grenada, and Guadaloupe), the Caribbean Islands appear free of the mycosis (Brummer et al, 1993; Restrepo, 1994; Wanke and Londero, 1994).

In countries reporting paracoccidioidomycosis, cases are diagnosed specifically in regions with significant rainfall, abundant forests, watercourses and limited temperature variations (17°C–24°C) (Restrepo, 1994). In a large series of Colombian cases, the municipalities implicated by the patients as their birth and permanent residence represented only 20.3% of the country's municipalities. Several ecological variables were studied at these sites and the incidence rate ratio was determined by multivariate analysis. The following ecological variables fitted the model: altitude from 1000 to 1499 meters above sea level, rainfall from 2000 to 2999 mm, presence of humid forests and coffee/tobacco crops (Calle et al, 2001).

The precise microniche of *P. brasiliensis* has not been ascertained and its isolation from nature has only been reported on six occasions (Franco et al, 2000). The fungus has also been cultured from an animal forage possibly contaminated with soil. Puzzling reports indicate isolation from bat guano and penguin feces (Franco et al, 2000). The recognition of the particular site where the fungus has its habitat has been hindered by the long latency periods recognized in patients reported in nonendemic areas, and by the lack of either epidemic outbreaks or acute cases (Franco et al, 1989; Brummer et al, 1993; Restrepo, l994; Restrepo, 2000).

Fifty-three cases of paracoccidioidomycosis have been reported from countries outside of the recognized endemic areas; 29 from Europe, l5 from the United States, 8 from Japan, and 1 from the Middle East (Brummer et al, 1993; Borgia et al, 2000; Manns et al, 1996; Giovanni et al, 2000; Restrepo, 2000). All of these patients had either lived or visited the Latin America endemic regions prior to the appearance of clinical manifestations. In 75% of these cases, the disease was diagnosed an average of 14 years (range 4 months–60 years) after departure from the endemic zones (Restrepo, 1994; Restrepo, 2000). In lymph node biopsies from patients with active and inactive (residual) lesions, intact and multiple budding yeast cells were found to be more numerous (49% and 33%) in active than in residual lesions (21% and 5%), with aberrant yeast cells predominating in the latter (76%). The low number of active cells remaining in walled-off lesions may have bearing on the prolonged latency of this infection (Restrepo, 2000).

This long latency clearly indicates that the patient can acquire the infection in a place different to the one where the diagnosis is made. Borelli postulated the concept of a reserved area (reservárea), a term that defines the site where the fungus has its natural habitat and the primary infection is acquired. By contrast, the endemic area is the site where the mycosis is diagnosed or reported (Borelli, 1972; Restrepo et al, 2001).

Ecology

Search for the habitat has been intense but unrewarding (Restrepo, 1994). It has been noticed that anthropic changes in endemic areas are important source of exposure (Restrepo, 2001). The records of 36 children diagnosed in the state of Rio de Janeiro were analyzed (Blotta et al, 1999). Most (44%) of these patients came from rural counties where appropriate environmental conditions were present (Rios-Gonçalves et al, 1998). These authors noticed that the abundant native forests had been gradually reduced over the years due to anthropic forces. In another study done in two Amazonian states where paracoccidioidomycosis had been rare, 13 childhood cases had been diagnosed. These children had lived permanently around forested areas where intense human colonization resulted in gradual destruction of the original ecosystem (Fonseca et al, 1999).

Paracoccidoidin skin testing reagents have not been standardized and they cross-react with *Histoplasma capsulatum*, a fungus well established in the paracoccidioidomycosis endemic regions. Nevertheless, skin tests have been useful in detecting subclinical infections (Naiff et al, 1988; Pereira, 1988; Restrepo, 1994). For instance, investigators used paracoccidioidin in places of birth and only residence of children with paracoccidioidomycosis. Logistic regression analyses showed that vicinity to certain water sources, contact with armadillos and work in orchards were associated with increased skin sensitivity (Cadavid and Restrepo, 1993). In Rio de Janeiro, Brazil, 34% of the children tested reacted to paracoccidioidin and their distribution by county of residence indicated that most (74%) inhabited the foothills around a particular sierra (Rios-Gonçalves et al, 1998).

In the Amazon River basin, positive paracoccidioidin skin test reactions were significantly higher (43.3%) in a particular tribe that had adopted novel agricultural practices (planting coffee) which required the felling of trees in the forest; this activity increased the likelihood of exposure to *P. brasiliensis* (Coimbra et al, 1994). Similar testing in residents of the Corrientes province, Argentina, where paracoccidioidomycosis had never been diagnosed, revealed 11.4% positive reactions. This province is close to the Brazilian Paraná's River dam where construction of a hydroelectric plant brought great anthropic changes (Mangiaterra et al, 1999). The above data indicate that disturbances in the reservarea constitute an important factor leading to *P. brasiliensis* infection.

The existence of naturally infected animals had not been proven to satisfaction until l986, when researchers working in the Brazilian jungles of Pará isolated *P. brasiliensis* from the organs of several nine-banded armadillos (Naiff et al, 1986). The corresponding isolates were shown by immunological and experimental animal studies to be identical with human *P. brasiliensis* isolates (Peraçoli et al, 1999; Silva-Vergara et al, 1999). Overall, 36% of 100 armadillos examined had *P. brasiliensis* in their lungs, spleens, livers and/or mesenteric lymph nodes (Bagagli et al, 1998; Silva-Vergara et al, 1999; Restrepo, 2001; Silva-Vergara et al, 2000). Recently, a seroepidemiologic study indicated that dogs can also be infected with this fungus as specific antibodies and skin test hypersensitivity to the dominant gp43 antigen were demonstrated (Ono et al, 2000).

EPIDEMIOLOGY

Paracoccidioidomycosis may occur as an infection or as a disease; the former is defined as an asymptomatic or subclinical infection occurring in normal individuals of the endemic areas in whom skin tests with paracoccidioidin prove reactive. The accidental demonstration of healed, residual *P. brasiliensis*-containing lesions in persons with no signs or symptoms of the mycosis documents the existence of the subclinical infection (Angulo and Pollak, 1971; Montenegro and Franco, 1994; Restrepo, 2000). By contrast, overt disease is characterized by an array of signs and symptoms (See Clinical Manifestations).

Since paracoccidioidomycosis is not a reportable disease, prevalence and incidence rates are difficult to assess. In Brazil annual incidence rates of 1 to 3 per 100,000 inhabitants and a mean mortality rate of 0.14 per 100,000 have been estimated (Coutinho et al, 2002; Wanke and Londero, 1994). In Colombia, lower but fluctuating incidence rates (0.05 to 0.22/100,000 inhabitants) have been recorded during a 30-year period (Torrado et al, 2000). Extrapolating these figures to the total Latin American population suggests that over 10 million persons may have been infected with the fungus. Considering that this mycosis afflicts mostly men in their productive years, the impact of paracoccidioidomycosis on the region's economy would be significant (Londero et al, 1988; Lacaz et al, 1991; Negroni, 1993; Wanke and Londero, 1994; Blotta et al, 1999).

Demographic Data

Age. Clinically manifest paracoccidioidomycosis is infrequent in children, adolescents and young adults who represent only 5% to 10% of all cases. Most (60%) patients are 30–50 years old. Subclinical infection measured by skin tests is also more common in adults although in certain areas, a significant number of children and youngsters have also been infected (Lacaz et al, 2002; Wanke and Londero, 1994; Londero et al, 1996; Blotta et al, 1999).

Gender. One of the most peculiar aspects of overt paracoccidioidomycosis is its distribution by gender. Although the average male to female ratio is 14:1, in Argentina, Colombia and Venezuela this ratio can be higher, 70:1 (Lacaz et al, 2002; Negroni, 1993; Restrepo et al, 1997, San Blas and Niño-Vega, 2000). Noteworthy, in children gender differences are not significant, nor does the frequency of subclinical infections vary according to gender, even in the adult population (Naiff et al, 1988; Pereira, 1988; Restrepo et al, 1997; Blotta et al, 1999).

Race. Due to the fact that interbreeding is common in Latin America, race influences are not apparent. Immigrants into endemic areas usually develop a severe disease indicative of their greater susceptibility to *P. brasiliensis* (Lacaz et al, 2002). The role of HLA antigens on this mycosis has been studied but no evidence of a specific association has emerged (Dias et al, 2000).

Occupation. Most (> 70%) patients with this mycosis have jobs centered in agriculture. In Uruguay, the disease is recognized as an occupational hazard as most cases occur in lumberjacks (Londero and Melo, 1988; Lacaz et al, 2002; Wanke and Londero, 1994).

Other Factors. Inadequate nutrition, smoking and alcoholism are considered predisposing conditions (Lacaz et al, 2002; Martinez and Moya, 1992; Negroni, 1993; Wanke and Londero, 1994).

HISTOPATHOLOGY

The early manifestations of paracoccidioidomycosis in man are not known as the time of exposure/infection cannot be determined. Data derived from animal models have delineated the initial steps and shown that few hours after challenge, polymorphonuclear leukocytes accumulate around fungal propagules. Within a day, mononuclear cells are noticed, increase progressively and gradually begin to transform into epithelioid cells. A week after challenge, granulomas form; epithelioid and giant cells surround *P. brasiliensis* and limited phagocytosis of the organism occurs. Granulomas increase in size and coalesce. Initially, granulomas are compact and contain only a few yeast cells as if the host's defenses had succeeded in restraining fungal multiplication. However, with progression of the infection, granulomas become loose and yeast cells enter into active multiplication. At this time, marked immunodepression can be demonstrated (McEwen et al, 1987; Singer-Vermes et al, 1993; Camargo and Franco, 2000; Cock et al, 2000). The epithelioid granuloma is the histological hallmark of paracoccidioidomycosis (Franco et al, 1994; Montenegro and Franco, 1994; Soares, 2000b; Diniz et al, 2001). In experimental animals the presence of loose granulomas composed of large mononuclear cells is associated with spleen hypoplasia and depressed immune responses (Soares et al, 2000a).

In animals the initial lung lesion occurs at the alveolar level and is exudative or granulomatous (Singer-Vermes et al, 1993; Lenzi et al, 1994; Burger et al, 1998; Cock et al, 2000). In humans, pneumonic foci exhibit acute alveolitis accompanied by proliferation of reticulin fibers and interstitial and peribronchial granulomatous inflammation surrounded by marked fibrosis (Angulo and Pollak, 1971; Tuder et al, 1985; Valle et al, 1992; Franco et al, 1994; Montenegro and Franco, 1994). Fibrosis is prominent in the perihilar region, the main bronchi, their branches and the large pulmonary vessels. Human autopsy and experimental animal studies have revealed that fibrosis is the result of an active, progressive pulmonary infection characterized by strong inflammatory responses centered on the granuloma. Collagen I and reticulin type fibers are visible and contribute to transformation of the lungs into a consolidated structure no longer capable of proper gaseous exchange.

In lymph nodes, cortical granulomas are formed initially but with time the inflammatory response involves the whole structure; in this case fistulae are formed. Involvement of the lymph node capsule facilitates coalescence of neighboring nodes with formation of large tumor-like masses. In the adrenal glands, lesions may be restricted or extensive; granulomas, necrosis and fibrosis cause marked enlargement and damage to the glands. Histopathology of the mucosa and skin shows epithelioid granulomas and intraepithelial abscesses; pseudoepitheliomatous hyperplasia is common, and central caseous necrosis may be present. In ulcerated skin lesions or ruptured lymph nodes, granulomas are associated with a mixed pyogenic infiltration (Angulo and Pollak, 1971; Mendes, 1994a; Montenegro and Franco, 1994).

PATHOGENESIS

Clinically, paracoccidioidomycosis may be cataloged as an infection or as a disease (Mendes, 1994a). Infection is contagion in the absence of clinical manifestations while disease is overt illness. Paracoccidioidomycosis is regressive if only mild pulmonary symptoms were experienced and required no medical treatment. The disease is progressive when clinical manifestations become apparent such as in the acute/subacute form (juvenile type) and the chronic adult-type disease. The acute/subacute form is characterized by predominant dissemination to the reticulo-endothelial system. Cell-mediated immunodepression is a regular feature of this form of disease. As implied by its name, the chronic form has a more prolonged course (months to years) and is manifested by important lung damage, as well as by extrapulmonary manifestations. Cellular immune responses are variable (Brummer et al, 1993; Negroni, 1993;

Mendes, 1994a; Bethlem et al, 1999). The residual form of disease is represented by the sequelae, e.g., pulmonary fibrosis and lymphatic obstruction, at the sites of formerly active lesions. (Londero, 1986; Mendes, 1994a; Montenegro and Franco, 1994) (Table 21–1).

In paracoccidioidomycosis, the host's immune response defines to a great extent the outcome of the infectious process. Both humoral and cellular immune responses play prominent roles.

Humoral Response

Almost all patients produce specific anti-*P. brasiliensis* antibodies and sometimes in abundance, as demonstrated by polyclonal activation and production of high levels of specific IgA and IgG isotype, as well as IgE antibodies (Mendes-Gianinni et al, 1994; Baida et al, 1999; Souza et al, 2000; Valle et al, 2000; Juvenale et al, 2001; Mamoni et al, 2001). Anti-idiotypic antibodies are detected in a large proportion of patients with the acute/subacute form of disease but not in chronic cases; these antibodies may play a part in the modulation of the immune response (Souza et al, 2000). Antibodies do not appear to play a role in host protection because high titers tend to parallel disease severity (Restrepo et al, 1983; Brummer et al, 1993; Blotta and Camargo, 1993; Del Negro et al, 2000; Valle et al, 2000; Juvenale et al, 2001). However, in high and low antibody responder mice infected with *P. brasiliensis*, the highest mortality and the most extensive dissemination were found in the low responder group (Soares et al, 2000b). Additionally, mice develop specific antibody recognition patterns during infection sug-

TABLE 21–1. *Paracoccidioidomycosis: Characteristics of the Clinical Forms*

Clinical Forms	Definition	Special Aspects	Host Immune Status	Immune Responses
Infection	Contagion with no clinical manifestations	Defined by positive skin test	Normal	Average positive skin reactions: 12%–20%
Disease subdivided in two broad categories	Presence of signs and symptoms	Male to female ratio = 14:1	Variable	Inbalance of the two arms of the immune response
1. Regressive (residual)	Mild pulmonary symptoms not requiring medical treatment	Goes unnoticed but is shown at autopsy in persons not known to have had disease	Normal and active	Host able to contain fungal infection
2. Progressive	Disseminated disease involving several organs/systems	Age and immune status influence clinical aspects	Abnormal	Humoral response is intense. Cellular immunity is depressed
2a. Acute/subacute or juvenile form	Significant involvement of the reticuloendothelial system	Common in children, adolescents and young adults	Significant immunodepression	High titers of antiidiotypic antibodies but CD4 cells are inactive
2b. Chronic or adult type form	• Unifocal • Multifocal Defined on number of organs affected	Often lungs are involved but respiratory symptoms may be minimum	Normal to depressed	Balance of the immune response tends to be preserved

gesting their interaction during progressive infection (Vaz et al, 1992). Circulating immune complexes have been detected in patients with depressed T-cell responses and appear to participate in cell-mediated immunodepression (Miura et al, 2000).

Cell-Mediated Response

Cellular immunity is crucial in disease control, explaining in part why patients with the acute/subacute progressive form are incapable of responding to mitogens and/or skin tests (Shikanai-Yasuda et al, 1992a; Musatti et al, 1994; Calich et al, 1998; Sugizaki et al, 1999; Karhawi et al, 2000; San Blas and Niño-Vega, 2000; Benard et al, 2001; Fornari et al, 2001). A correlation between high antibody titers, lack of T-cell lymphocyte responsiveness and severity of disease has become apparent. Adult patients with the progressive but less severe unifocal disease have low or undetectable anti-*P. brasiliensis* antibody titers and normal or slightly depressed cell mediated immune responses. This pattern is reversed in patients with progressive multifocal disease who exhibit high antibody levels and significant depression of cell mediated immune functions.

This disparity between humoral and cellular immune responses is dependent on the cytokines produced in response to fungal invasion, as initially demonstrated in experimental animal infections (Burger et al, 1998; Cano et al, 2000; Deepe et al, 2000; Kashino et al, 2000; Mendes-Gianinni et al, 2000; Soares et al, 2000a; Souto et al, 2000). In these models the predominance of a Th-2 cytokine pattern has been repeatedly demonstrated. Increased production of Th-2 cytokines (IL-10 IL-2, IL-4, and TNF-α) also occurs in severely ill patients whereas Th-1 cytokines, especially IL-2 and IFN-γ, decrease significantly (Musatti et al, 1994; Karhawi et al, 2000; Kurita et al, 2000; Benard et al, 2001; Diniz et al, 2001; Fornari et al, 2001). TH-2 cytokines appear to also influence the production of specific antibody isotypes. Thus, IgE and IgG4 production that depend on IL-4 for switching, are significantly higher in those patients with severe disease (Baida et al, 1999). Eosinophils are increased in some patients with the juvenile form of the mycosis, perhaps reflecting the Th-2 cytokine influence, as eosinophilia is related to IL-5 overproduction (Shikanai-Yasuda et al, 1992b)

The loss of immune balance observed in acute/subacute patients could also be influenced by the accelerated growth rate of *P. brasiliensis* in tissues as a heavy fungal load may down-regulate Th-1 responses, thereby favoring Th-2 cytokine expression (Musatti et al, 1994; Sugizaki et al, 1999; Diniz et al, 2001; Fornari et al, 2001). In support of this hypothesis, reduction of fungal load by antimycotic therapy is accompanied by restoration of the patient's immune capacity with delayed skin hypersensitivity, lymphocyte proliferative responses and production of Th-1 cytokines, especially INF-γ (Karhawi et al, 2000)

Experimental models mimic human paracoccidioidomycosis and allow modulation of the immune responses (Singer-Vermes et al, 1993; Calich et al, 1998; Cano et al, 2000; Deepe et al, 2000; Kashino et al, 2000; Soares et al, 2000b; Souto et al, 2000). Disruptions of the genes coding for certain cytokines (IL-4 and IL-12, INF-γ) have revealed that IL-12 and INF-γ are essential for protection while IL-4 may play a dual role. In patients, a lack of balance between IL-12 and IL-10 has also been associated with immunosuppression (Benard et al, 2001). Thus, active cellular immune responses can be correlated with an adequate control of the disease (Mussatti et al, 1994; Sugizaki et al, 1999; San Blas and Niño-Vega, 2000).

The macrophage is the most important effector cell in paracoccidioidomycosis but only if activated by IFN-γ. Otherwise the macrophage is permissive to fungal multiplication (See Color Fig. 21–3 in separate color insert). Once activated, peritoneal murine macrophages inhibit the conidia to yeast transition resulting in significant propagule destruction (Gónzalez et al, 2000). Killing is independent of oxygen-related mechanisms and is accomplished through nitric oxide and the L-arginine-nitric oxide pathway. By contrast, nitric oxide inhibitors arrest propagule transition, facilitating permissiveness of macrophages to intracellular fungal multiplication. Studies indicate that *P. brasiliensis* attaches to macrophages and facilitates its own uptake probably through cell wall components, among them the major glycoprotein (gp43) antigen (Almeida et al, 1998).

Polymorphonuclear neutrophils (PMNs) are also of great importance in the host–parasite interaction, especially during the initial stages. As shown in animal models, PMNs are the first and most prominent cells in the inflammatory infiltrate and participate actively in phagocytosis of the infecting propagules (Gónzalez and Cano, 2001; Kurita et al, 2000). PMNs inhibit and may even kill *P. brasiliensis* through the dual influence of several oxygen reactive intermediates and cytokines such as IL-1 beta and GM-CSF.

Development of fibrosis is another important facet of the host–parasite interaction. Fibrosis is mediated by fungal adherence to the extracellular matrix components. A tridimensional network of collagen, fibronectin, laminin and proteoglycans surrounds fungal cells in active multiplication. The ability of *P. brasiliensis* to bind to the extracellular matrix components activates growth factors and cytokines, reflecting the complexity of the host–parasite interactions (Lenzi et al, 1994; Burger et al, 1998; Cock et al, 2000; Mendes-Gianinni et al, 2000).

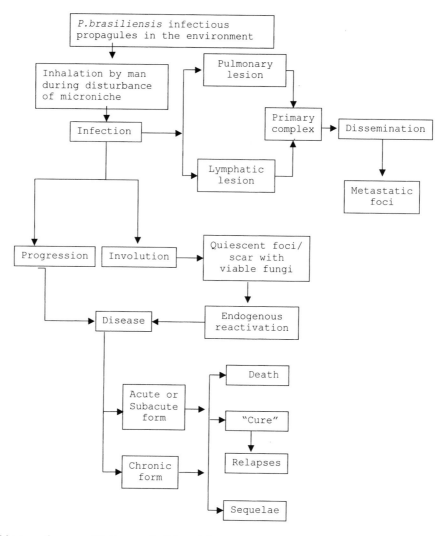

FIGURE 21–4. Natural history of paracoccidioidomycosis (Adapted from Montenegro and Franco, 1994).

CLINICAL MANIFESTATIONS

Paracoccidioidomycosis was first described in 1908 by Lutz in Brazil; Splendore studied more cases but mistook the disease for another fungal disease, namely, coccidioidomycosis. Years later, Almeida differentiated both fungi and gave *P. brasiliensis* its present name (Lacaz et al, 1991). All evidence indicates that infection is acquired by inhalation of the mycelium-derived propagules. For a number of years, many workers adhered to the original concept of traumatic implantation via contaminated plant materials (Franco et al, 1989; Lacaz et al, 1991). However, pathological and clinical data, as well as experimental studies, have made it clear that inhalation of infectious particles is the mode of transmission (Giraldo et al, 1976; Londero, 1986; Restrepo, 1994; Niño-Vega et al, 2000; Roldán et al, 2001). Figure 21–4 presents the natural history of paracoccidioidomycosis.

Overt paracoccidioidomycosis is a pleomorphic disease that may affect any organ or system and resemble other conditions, thus making diagnosis difficult in many patients. Almost all patients complain of constitutional symptoms such as malaise, weight loss, asthenia, and sometimes fever, plus an array of organ specific symptoms as described below. Delay in diagnosis results in progression of the disease and establishment of sequelae (Angulo and Pollak, 1971; Londero 1986; Franco et al, 1989; Lacaz et al, 2002; Negroni, 1993; Benard et al, 1994; Mendes, 1994a; Bethlem et al, 1999).

Lungs
The lungs are not only the primary site of infection but also the preferred fungal target. In 30% of the cases this is the only organ involved although at autopsy, over 90% of patients reveal lung pathology. The

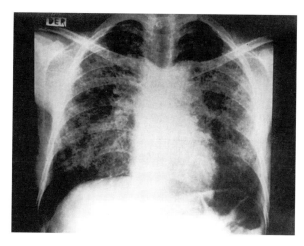

FIGURE 21–5. Chest X-ray from a patient with paracoccidioidomy-cosis. Bilateral infiltrates in central and lower lobes, with sparing of the apices. Note bullae at lung bases.

paucity of respiratory symptoms is remarkable even in patients with extensive radiographic findings. Physical examination may also be unrevealing, thus signaling the characteristic dissociation between scarcity of signs and symptoms and prominent radiographic abnormalities (Tuder et al, 1985; Londero, 1986; Londero and Melo, 1988; Restrepo et al, 1989; Valle et al, 1992; Mendes, 1994a; Tobón et al, 1995; Teixeira et al, 2000).

The most frequent respiratory symptom is productive cough (57%) and 11% of patients will have blood-tinged sputum. Chest pain is uncommon but dyspnea is a major complaint and its progression results in serious disability of the patient. Alteration of the normal respiratory sounds (rales, rhonchi, hypoventilation) are regularly detected. Plain chest X-rays reveal mostly infiltrative lesions of the alveoli or the interstitium although mixed lesions can also be observed; usually infiltrates are bilateral, symmetrical and preferentially located in the central and lower lobes (Figs. 21–5, 21–6). The apices are involved occasionally. In some patients the infiltrates are rather small in size and dispersed throughout the lungs.

Interstitial lesions may acquire a nodular or fibronodular character and persist even after proper treatment (Naranjo et al, 1990; Valle et al, 1992; Tobón et al, 1995). Cavities can be detected regularly by chest tomography (Fumari et al, 1999). Fibrosis is observed in approximately 60% of the cases and is characterized by honeycombing, often accompanied by bullae and emphysema (Tuder et al, 1985; Tobón et al, 1995; Fumari et al, 1999). Such lesions constitute the sequelae of an active mycotic process against which the host responded immunologically (Lenzi et al, 1994; Cock et al, 2000). Computerized tomography of the lungs re-

veals bilaterally symmetrical interstitial abnormalities such as interlobular septal thickness, confluent nodules, centrilobular and ground glass opacities, pericicatricial emphysema, and traction bronchiectasis, among others. Calcified lesions and hilar and mediastinal lymph node involvement, common in autopsy series, are also observed. The latter findings are infrequent in plain chest x-rays, probably due to masking by extensive parenchymal damage (Fumari et al, 1999; Teixeira et al, 2000).

Pulmonary function is altered with predominance of an obstructive pattern (Valle et al, 1992). Autopsies have revealed granulomas and fibrosis around the bronchi, with fibrous septa connecting such structures to other bronchi and to blood vessels as well (Angulo and Pollak, 1971; Tuder et al, 1985; Montenegro and Franco, 1994). Dissemination takes place through the lymphatic vessels, the blood and/or the bronchi reaching all pulmonary structures and thus causing significant damage and various degrees of respiratory incapacity that may lead to cor pulmonale (Angulo and Pollak, 1971; Tuder et al, 1985; Franco et al, 1989; Montenegro and Franco, 1994). Specific antifungal treatment is effective because it reduces alveolar damage, controls extrapulmonary lesions and decreases fungal load; however, therapy appears to have no effect on the interstitial disease which may improve independently of its stage at diagnosis (Naranjo et al, 1990; Valle et al, 1992; Mendes, 1994a; Tobón et al, 1995).

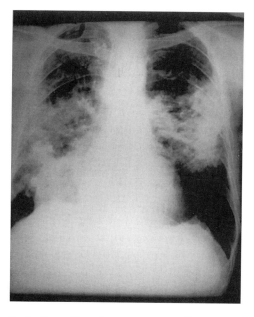

FIGURE 21–6. Chest X-ray from a patient with more severe pulmonary paracoccidioidomycosis. Infiltrates are extensive and coalesced into nodules. Note clear upper lobes.

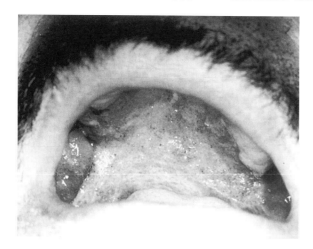

FIGURE 21–7. Mucous membrane lesion. Multiple infiltrative lesions of the palate with hemorrhagic dots (mulberry-like stomatitis).

Mucous Membranes

Lesions in the mucous membranes of the mouth, the oropharynx and the larynx are observed in approximately half of the patients; less common are lesions of the nasal and anal mucous membranes. Lesions are progressive, destructive and associated with pain and bleeding. Mucous membrane lesions which may mimic carcinoma are ulcerative, granulomatous, edematous and covered by small hemorrhagic dots (mulberry-like stomatitis) (Fig. 21–7). Involvement of the vocal cords, the epiglottis and the arytenoid and interarytenoid regions can also be observed. Lesions located in the mouth, larynx and/or pharynx produce hoarseness, dysphagia, dyphonia, sialorrhea, and gingival inflammatory changes resulting in tooth loosening (Lacaz et al, 2002; Negroni, 1993; SantAnna et al, 1999; Mendes, 1994a; Migliari et al, 1998; Bicalho et al, 2001). Many patients with oral mucosa lesions disregard their respiratory symptoms; however, clinical, laboratory and roentgenographic studies often reveal pulmonary involvement (Restrepo et al, 1989; Correa et al, 1991).

Skin

Skin lesions are detected in 12% to 32% of patients, are extremely diverse and may be single or multiple in number. Lesions are localized more frequently on the face and especially, in the perioral region. Lesions of the lower extremities are also observed frequently; other sites include the neck, trunk, upper extremities and in males, the external genitalia. Typically, lesions are ulcerative but ulcero-vegetative and nodular appearances are also seen (Fig. 21–8). Edema of the lips is frequent. In rare disseminated cases, multiple papulo-acneiform lesions may appear (Angulo and Pollak,

1971; Franco et al, 1989; Negroni, 1993; Marques, 1994a). Pulmonary involvement is seen in about 90% of patients with skin lesions (Correa et al, 1991).

In most cases, *P. brasiliensis* reaches the skin by hematogenous dissemination from the initial pulmonary focus. However, the skin may also be involved by extension of a previously established mucous membrane lesion or by the rupture of a contiguous lymph node (Angulo and Pollak, 1971; Marques, 1994a; Montenegro and Franco, 1994).

Lymph Nodes

Hypertrophied lymph nodes are frequent in children, adolescents and young adults who show extensive involvement of the reticulo-endothelial system (Fig. 21–9). The cervical lymph nodes are most commonly affected, followed by those in the supraclavicular and axillary regions. Mesenteric lymph node involvement may result in the formation of tumor-like lesions that exert undue pressure on abdominal organs. Lymph node involvement may be subclinical and demonstrable only by imaging and biopsy. Histopathology reveals architectural and functional alterations (Benard et al, 1994; Londero et al, 1996; Calegaro et al, 1997; Blotta et al, 1999; Castro et al, 1999).

Adrenal Glands

Dissemination to the adrenal glands may result in Addison's disease in 10% of the cases; minor dysfuction is observed in another 15%–40% of patients. The adrenals can be destroyed, resulting in permanent damage and requiring supportive corticosteroid therapy. However, recovery of gland function may follow specific treatment (Moreira et al, 1993; Tendrich et al, 1994).

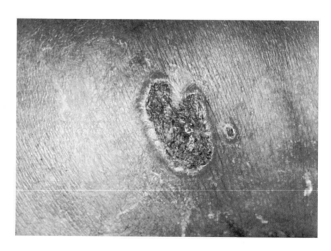

FIGURE 21–8. Ulcerative cutaneous lesion of the chest.

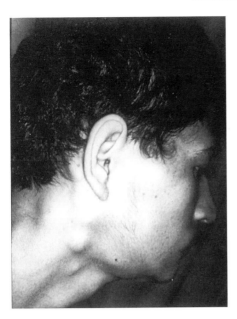

FIGURE 21–9. Enlarged cervical lymph nodes in patient with juvenile type disease.

Other Organs

The frequency of abdominal disease varies with the method of evaluation since focal lesions are usually asymptomatic; when endoscopy is utilized, 30% of patients will have ulcerative gastrointestinal lesions. Esophageal and gastric involvement is rare while lesions of the small and large intestine, sometimes simulating neoplastic processes, are more frequent (Mendes, 1994a; Valle et al, 1995; Chojniak et al, 2000). The spleen and liver are important sites of dissemination (20%); hepatosplenomegaly may occur and function may be impaired (Mendes, 1994a; Benard et al, 1994; Londero et al, 1996; Calegaro et al, 1997).

Central Nervous System

Involvement of the leptomeninges occurs more frequently than previously recognized. Chronic meningitis is the commonest manifestation but expanding, tumor-like lesions can also be observed (Nobrega, 1994; Silva et al, 2000; Villa et al, 2000). A brain imaging study should be performed when CNS disease is suspected.

Bone and Joint Lesions

Bone disease occurs mostly in younger patients; the osseous structures more frequently attacked are those of the upper extremities and chest. An intense osteolysis is seen on radiological examination (Mendes, 1994c; Amstalden et al, 1996; Doria and Taylor, 1997; Miranda-Aires et al, 1997; Nogueira et al, 2001).

Genital Tracts

Involvement of the genital tract is more frequent in males than in females. In both sexes, however, complications/dysfunction may result (Mendes, 1994a; Severo et al, 2000).

Sequelae

The most important sequelae of paracoccidioidomycosis are pulmonary fibrosis, adrenal destruction, vocal cord damage, tracheal stenosis and obstruction of lymphatic channels. Lung fibrosis results in cor pulmonale while lymphatic blockade produces untreatable ascites (Angulo and Pollak, 1971; Montenegro and Franco, 1994). Rarely, Leriche Syndrome may develop as a complication (Cherry et al, 1998).

Association with Other Diseases

In 10%–15% of the patients, paracoccidioidomycosis coexists with tuberculosis and this aggravates the patient's condition. The AIDS pandemic, although important in all P. brasiliensis endemic countries, has not increased incidence rates of this fungal disease. Approximately 60 patients with both disorders have been reported, although probably this number is much larger. Most patients with AIDS develop the progressive juvenile type of paracoccidioidomycosis associated with a high mortality (Marques and Shikanai-Yasuda, 1994b; Tobón et al, 1995; Cimerman et al, 1997; Santos et al, 1998; Benard and Duarte, 2000; Giovanni et al, 2000). A few cases of paracoccidioidomycosis, tuberculosis and AIDS have also been reported (Marques and Shikanai-Yasuda, 1994b; Nogueira et al, 1998). Paracoccidioidomycosis has also been diagnosed in patients with other immunosuppressive conditions, although rather infrequently (Marques and Shikanai-Yasuda, 1994b). Paracoccidioidomycosis thus differs from some other fungal diseases, e.g., cryptococcosis and candidiasis, which have a more marked opportunistic character.

It appears that the interaction of HIV and P. brasiliensis results in a somewhat new paradigm. In such patients, the manifestations of paracoccidioidomycosis correspond to the severe juvenile type disease, one that would have been acquired rather recently. The prediction would be that these patients should have been infected in the past, with their paracoccidioidomycosis representing endogenous reactivation of an old focus of infection and manifesting as the chronic adult form rather than the juvenile type of disease (Benard and Durante, 2000).

Differential Diagnosis

Depending on the site of lesions and the general condition of the patient, paracoccidioidomycosis can be confused with or misdiagnosed as one of several diseases including: tuberculosis, lymphoma, neoplastic processes, leprosy, leishmaniasis, sporotrichosis, and other mycoses (Londero and Melo, 1988; Franco et al, 1989; Mendes, 1994a).

MYCOLOGICAL DIAGNOSIS

Direct Examination and Histopathology
In clinical specimens P. brasiliensis appears as an oval to round yeast cell some provided with multiple peripheral buds (pilot wheel configuration). The cells possess a thick refractile wall (0.2 to 1 μm) and intracytoplasmic vacuoles (Fig. 21–1). Often yeast cells appear in chains and have single buds; bizarre yeast forms may also be observed (Lacaz et al, 2002; Brummer, 1993; Lacaz et al, 1998). Several procedures are adequate to visualize fungal elements, including fresh or KOH wet preparations, as well as calcofluor and immunofluorescence methods (Fig. 21–2) (Lacaz et al, 1991; Brummer et al, 1993; Lacaz et al, 1998). Sensitivity of the direct examinations varies from 85 to 100%.

Histopathologic preparations stained with hematoxylin and eosin, Gomori methenamine-silver, Papanicolaou or periodic acid-Schiff, as well as direct immunofluorescence stains, are very useful. These various methods reveal the multiple budding yeast elements, especially within granulomatous foci (See Color Fig. 21–10 in separate color insert). Short chains and cells with single buds also may be observed, and, in these cases, differentiation of P. brasiliensis from Cryptococcus neoformans, Blastomyces dermatitidis, and even Histoplasma capsulatum, must be made (Angulo and Pollak, 1971; Franco et al, 1989; Montenegro and Franco, 1994).

Cultures
Isolation of P. brasiliensis from clinical specimens requires a battery of selective and non-selective culture media and repeated samples. The addition of antibacterial drugs and mould inhibitors to the media has resulted in improved recovery rates, around 80% (Lacaz et al, 2002; Brummer et al, 1993). The use of digestion and concentration procedures for mucous specimens is also recommended. Modified Sabouraud's (Mycocel agar) and yeast extract agars incubated at room temperature (19°C–24°C) are the best media for isolation. In bacteria-free specimens (e.g., tissue biopsies, CSF, bone marrow), media without antibiotics, and incubated at 36°C can also be employed (Lacaz et al, 2002; Brummer et al, 1993).

At 18°C–24°C, growth is slow and takes 20–30 days. Microscopically, the mould shows only thin septate hyphae (3–4 μm in diameter) and intercallary chlamydospores (15–30 μm). However, in media with no carbohydrates and after prolonged incubation (> 2 months), the mould may also produce conidia. The mycelial form is not distinctive and consequently, dimorphism must be demonstrated by subculturing at 36°C. At this temperature, P. brasiliensis grows in 8–10 days as a cerebriform, cream-colored colony. Microscopically, oval to spherical yeast cells, 4 to 30 μm in diameter, can be observed. The large mother yeast cell bearing multiple buds (pilot's wheel) is characteristic of this fungus (Fig. 21–2) (Lacaz et al, 2002; Brummer et al, 1993; Castillo et al, 1994).

Serology
Various highly sensitive serological tests have been developed, especially for measurement of antibodies. The frequency of positive tests varies from 70%–95% depending on the test used and the severity of the disease process (Blotta and Camargo, 1993; Brummer et al, 1993; Castillo et al, 1994; Mendes-Giannini et al, 1994; Camargo and Franco, 2000; Del Negro et al, 2000; Valle et al, 2000).

Due to the fact that antigens prepared from P. brasiliensis vary greatly in quality depending on fungal isolate (strain B339 seems the most useful) and many other factors, attempts have been made to obtain purified fractions. A specific gp43-kDa glycoprotein fraction, considered the dominant P. brasiliensis antigen, has been sequenced and cloned but its expression has proven difficult (Travassos, 1994). A 27-kDa recombinant antigen has also been produced and when tested by enzyme-linked immunosorbent assay (ELISA), the sensitivity was 73% and specificity varied from 59 to 87%; the positive predictive value was 90% (Ortiz et al, 1998). Both a 7-day crude gp43 exoantigen and a 3-day gp43 antigen washed from the surface of fungal agar cultures (cell-free antigen) display sensitivity and specificity similar to that of the purified antigen (Mendes-Giannini et al, 1994; Camargo and Franco, 2000). Immunoblotting techniques have been used to determine the antigens most frequently recognized by patient's sera. Besides the 43-kDa glycoprotein that was recognized by 100% of patients' sera, a 70-kDa glycoprotein also showed high reactivity (96%); antibodies to both glycoproteins are considered to be markers of human paracoccidioidomycosis (Camargo and Franco, 2000; Valle et al, 2000).

Various studies have reinforced the importance of immunodiffusion, counterimmuno-electrophoresis, complement fixation, indirect immunofluorescence and ELISA techniques for antibody detection in the diagnosis and follow-up of patients with paracoccidioidomycosis. Patients with severe forms of the disease (chronic multifocal disseminated and juvenile) show significantly higher antibody levels than patients with less extensive disease. Only chronic patients with limited dissemination cleared their antibodies after 1 year of follow-up while those with more severe disease needed over 2 years (Camargo and Franco, 2000; Del Negro et al, 2000).

Antigen detection may be preferred for early diagnosis in immunocompromised individuals or when antibody detection is nonconclusive. Monitoring circulating antigens may also be important as a criterion of cure. An inhibition ELISA was developed via the production of monoclonal antibodies against a 87-kDa antigenic fraction; test sensitivity was 80% and even higher in severe forms of the disease (Gómez et al, 1997). In patients with severe juvenile disease, follow-up studies during and after itraconazole therapy indicated that antigen titers dropped significantly after 20 weeks on therapy. In contrast, in those patients who had the same clinical form of disease but were also HIV positive, antigenemia persisted at elevated titers even after 68 weeks of treatment. Patients with chronic multifocal or chronic unifocal disseminated disease had significant decreases in antigen titers after 28 and 40 weeks on treatment, respectively. Antigen decreases correlated with clinical improvement (Gómez et al, 1998). Parallel testing for antibody levels in the same patients revealed that antibody titers were rather unpredictable.

Attempts at determining the levels of both specific gp43 antigen and antibodies in saliva, as well as immune complexes, revealed that IgG antibody levels were elevated in saliva and serum but detection of immune complexes failed to differentiate patients from controls. Specific IgA antibodies were also detected in saliva, suggesting a role at the mucosal surface (Miura et al, 2000). Detection of circulating antigens (70-kDa and 43-kDa) in urine samples by use of a polyclonal anti-*P. brasiliensis* antibody has also been done. Ninety-one percent of patients had detectable urinary antigen by ELISA and 75% by immunoblot testing. Both tests appeared to be specific as neither antigen was detected in control samples. In specimens collected during clinical recovery there was a decrease in reactivity, while the 43-kDa antigen persisted or increased in patients who relapsed (Salina et al, 1998).

Skin Testing

During therapy, conversion from a non-reactive to a reactive paracoccidioidin skin test signals a good prognosis (Brummer et al, 1993; Negroni, 1993). Nevertheless, as a diagnostic tool, the skin test has no value. However, the test can be used to determine subclinical infection in the general population of endemic areas (Naiff et al, 1988; Pereira, 1988; Rios-Gonçalves et al, 1998).

Gene Probes

DNA probe assays have been prepared for the rapid identification of *P. brasiliensis* mycelial or yeast cultures (Sandlu et al, 1997). In addition, several authors have made use of molecular biology tools, especially PCR, to detect the presence of *P. brasiliensis* DNA in tissues. Results have indicated that the gene probes are highly specific and useful in diagnosis (Bialek et al, 2000b; Gomes et al, 2000; Lindsley Hirst et al, 2001; Sano et al, 2001).

TREATMENT

Paracoccidioidomycosis was considered fatal up to l940 when Ribeiro tried sulfonamide therapy; today it can be effectively treated with a variety of antifungal drugs plus support via other measures such as adequate nutrition, control of anemia, and concurrent use of antiparasitic medications (Naranjo et al, 1990; Mendes et al, 1994b). Present therapies utilize fungistatic rather than fungicidal medications and consequently, an intact host immune response is required. Treatment options include sulfonamides, amphotericin B and azole derivatives (Table 21–2). *Paracoccidioides brasiliensis* is remarkably susceptible to these drugs (Hahn and Hamdan, 2000). Treatment has two phases, attack and maintenance.

Sulfonamides

This class of drugs continues to be used by some physicians due to low cost, facility of administration, and lack of major toxicity. Among the various sulfonamides, the rapidly excreted sulfadiazine is preferred by many; sulfamethoxypyridazine, a slowly excreted compound, is also employed. The dosages, duration of treatment, side effects and other pertinent information are presented in Table 21–2. Approximately 70% of patients on sulfonamide therapy respond to the initial course; however, relapses are frequent (25%) during maintenance therapy, with acquired resistance appearing in l5% of such cases. After clinical and mycological improvement, the initial daily dose should be reduced by half. Prolonged follow-up has demonstrated high morbidity (43%) in spite of sulfonamide treatment. The recommended period for maintenance treatment is 2–3 years, a shortcoming because such a prolonged period hinders patient compliance. Sulfonamide levels should be monitored to determine dose and frequency of administration (Mendes et al, 1994b).

Improvement of outcomes (associated with both initial therapy and rate of relapse) has been obtained with the combination drug trimethoprim-sulfamethoxazole (cotrimoxazole)or the combination drug trimethoprim-sulfadiazine (cotrimazine). For adults, one double-

TABLE 21–2. *Treatment of Paracoccidioidomycosis**

Drug (Route of Administration)	Duration of Treatment (Months)	Adult Dose Per Day	Major Side Effects	Response (%)	Relapse (%)
Sulfonamides					
Sulfadiazine (po)	≥ 36	4.0–6.0 g/day in 4 doses	Crystalluria Hypersensitivity reactions	69	25
Sulfamethoxy-pyridazine (po)	≥ 36	1.0–2.0 g/day Reduce dose by half after clinical and mycological improvement	Crystalluria Hypersensitivity reactions	60–69	25
Trimethoprim (TMP) plus sulfamethoxazole (SMX): TMP/SMX (po, im, iv)	> 6	160 mg TMP and 800 mg SMX per tablet. 1 tab bid. for adults, iv 250 ml in 5% glucose	Same	80	20
Trimethoprim plus sulfadiazine: Cotrimazine (CT) (po)	> 6	410 mg CT bid	Same	80	20
Polyene					
Amphotericin B (iv)	Should be followed by prolonged maintenance treatment with azole or sulfa drug	0.5–0.75 mg/kg/day Total cumulative dose 1.0–2.0 g	Nephrotoxicity. hypokalemia, nausea, vomiting, headache, fever	70	25
Azoles					
Ketoconazole (po)	6–24 (mean 12)	400 mg/day (attack) 200 mg/day (maintenance)	Hepatotoxicity endocrine problems, nausea, vomiting	90	11
Itraconazole (po)	3–12 (mean 6)	200 mg/day (attack) 100 mg/day (maintenance)	Hepatotoxicity, azole-drug interactions	98	< 5
Fluconazole (po, iv)	12–24	Up to 600 mg/day	Minor toxicity	60	45 (not recommended)

*Treatment should not be rigid but tailored according to an individual patient's needs.
Bid, twice daily; po, oral; iv, intravenous; im, intramuscular.

strength cotrimoxazole (160 mg of trimethoprim and 800 mg of sulfamethoxazole per tablet) given every 12 hours has proven adequate. Children should be given half the dose prescribed to adults (Mendes et al, 1994b). Cotrimoxazole can be administered by the oral, intravenous or intramuscular routes (Mendes et al, 1994b).

Amphotericin B

This polyene drug is considered by some as the drug of choice for patients with severe forms of paracoccidioidomycosis and also for those resistant to sulfonamides. However, initial treatment with amphotericin B should be followed by sulfonamide or azole maintenance therapy (Mendes et al, 1994b). The need for intravenous administration of amphotericin B and the known toxic effects of this polyene represent negative features. Relapses have been observed in 15%–25% of patients even with appropriate treatment (Mendes et al, 1994b). The use of the combined amphotericin B-sulfonamide or azole regimen should consist of initial therapy with 1.0–2.0 g cumulative dose of amphotericin B, followed by maintenance therapy with a sulfa or an azole drug. With this drug combination, clinical improvement can be achieved in about 75% of patients; about 10% fail to respond and the remaining die during treatment. Amphotericin B lipid formulations have been used sporadically in patients with the juvenile form of disease with conflicting results (Dietze et al, 1999).

Azoles

Undoubtedly, the introduction of antifungal azole drugs for treatment of paracoccidioidomycosis has not only improved patients' prognosis but has also greatly facilitated therapy and compliance (Table 21–2). Ketoconazole, itraconazole and fluconazole are highly active in vitro against *P. brasiliensis* with minimal inhibitory concentrations of 0.0009–0.015 μg/ml (ketoconazole), 0.0009–0.5 μg/ml (itraconazole), and 0.125–0.5 μg/ml (fluconazole) (Hahn and Hamdan, 2000). Ketoconazole, an imidazole, is effective in 90% of patients at a dose of 200 to 400 mg/day given for a mean period of 12 months, depending on illness severity and patient response (Restrepo et al, 1983). Approximately 8% of the cases do not improve due to inadequate absorption and lack of gastric acidity, or low blood levels secondary to simultaneous administration of ketoconazole and drugs such as rifampin that accelerate the metabolism of ketoconazole. Relapses occur in 11% of the cases. Toxicity is relatively low at the indicated doses although endocrine disturbances, e.g., gynecomastia and decreased libido, gastrointestinal symptoms and hepatotoxicity, have been reported (Restrepo et al, 1983). Ketoconazole is the least expensive of the azole drugs.

The triazole derivative, itraconazole, was first used in 1982 (Naranjo et al, 1990; Tobón et al, 1995). Patients receive 400 mg as the loading dose, followed by 200 mg per day for periods of 3 to 12 months (average 6 months). Efficacy has been observed in 98% of the cases, including patients with severe, juvenile-type disease. The relapse rate is low, less than 5%. Side effects are few and consist of transitory elevation of hepatic enzymes and some gastrointestinal disturbances; no significant endocrine disturbances have been reported. In spite of this low toxicity profile, itraconazole has some problems related to its requirement for an acid gastric pH, attendant erratic blood levels, and frequent drug interactions which either hinder absorption of itraconazole or result in toxicity of other concurrently administered drugs. The relative high cost of itraconazole is also an important issue. Even so, itraconazole is the drug of choice for most patients with paracoccidioidomycosis (Naranjo et al, 1990; Mendes et al, 1994b; Tobón et al, 1995). A new liquid solution formulation of itraconazole with enhanced absorption and improved pharmacological profile is now available (Stevens, 1999).

Fluconazole, another triazole, has been used in some patients but high doses (400–600 mg /day) and long treatment periods (over 12 months) are needed to avoid relapses. Accordingly, fluconazole is not recommended over ketoconazole or itraconazole (Mendes et al, 1994b). Other compounds such as terbinafine have been used infrequently (Ollague et al, 2000).

In addition, immunomodulation has been tried in both humans and experimental models and the results are encouraging (San Blas and Niño-Vega, 2000). A group in Brazil has used glucan as a stimulant in patients with severe paracoccidioidomycosis with apparent good results (Meira et al, 1996).

PREVENTION

Immune protection in mice using a DNA vaccine originating in the gp43 gene is presently under development (Pinto et al, 2000). Since the precise niche of *P. brasiliensis* has not been established and since many patients do not develop clinical disease until years after exposure in the endemic area (prolonged latency period), no environmental or occupational preventive strategies have been proposed.

REFERENCES

Almeida S R, Unterkircher C S, Camargo Z P. Involvement of the major glycoprotein (gp43) of *Paracoccidioides brasiliensis* in attachment to macrophages. *Med Mycol* 36:405–411, 1998.

Amstalden E M, Xavier R, Kattapuran S V, Bertolo M B, Swartz M H, Rosenberg A. Paracoccidioidomycosis of bone and joints. *Medicine* 75:212–225, 1996.

Angulo A, and Pollak L. Paracoccidioidomycosis. In: Baker R D, ed. *The Pathologic Anatomy of the Mycoses: Human Infections with Fungi, Actinomycetes and Algae*. Berlin: Springer Verlag, 507–576, 1971.

Aristizábal B H, Clemons K V, Stevens D A, Retrepo A. Morphological transition of *Paracoccidioides brasiliensis* conidia to yeast cells: In vivo inhibition in females. *Infect Immun* 66:5587–5591, 1998.

Aristizábal B H, Clemons, K V, Cock A M, Restrepo A, Stevens D A. Experimental *Paracoccidioides brasiliensis* infection in mice: influence of the hormonal status of the host on tissue responses. *Med Mycol* 40:169–178, 2002.

Bagagli E, Sano A, Coelho KI, Alquati S, Miyahi M, Camargo Z P, Gomes G M, Franco M, Montenegro R M. Isolation of *Paracoccidioides brasiliensis* from armadillos (*Dasypus novemcinctus*) captured in an endemic area of paracoccidioidomycosis. *Am J Trop Med Hyg* 58:505–512, 1998.

Baida H, Biselli P J, Juvenale M, del Negro G M B, Mendes-Giannini M J, Duarte A J, Benard G. Differential antibody isotype expression to the major *Paracoccidioides brasiliensis* antigen in juvenile and adult form paracoccidioidomycosis. *Microb Infect* 1:273–278, 1999.

Benard G, Ori N W, Marques H H S, Mendoça M, Aguirre M Z, Camos A E, Del Negro G M. Severe acute paracoccidioidomycosis in children. *Pediatr Infect Dis* 13:510–515, 1994.

Benard G, Mendes-Giannini M J, Juvenale M, Miranda E T, Duarte A J. Immunosuppression in paracoccidioidomycosis: T cell hyporesponsiveness to two *Paracoccidioides brasiliensis* glycoproteins that elicit strong humoral immune response. *J Inf Dis* 175:1263–1267, 1997.

Benard G, Duarte A J S. Paracoccidioidomycosis: A model for evaluation of the effects of human immunodeficiency virus infection on the natural history of endemic tropical diseases. *Clin Infect Dis* 31:1032–1039, 2000.

Benard G, Romano C C, Cacere C R, Juvenale M, Mendes-Gianni M J, Duarte A J S. Imbalance of IL-2, IFN-gamma and IL-10 secretion in the immunosuppression associated with human paracoccidioidomycosis. *Cytokine* 13: 248–252, 2001.

Bethlem E P, Capone D, Maranhao B, Carvalho C R, Wanke B. Paracoccidioidomycosis. *Curr Opin Pulm Med* 5:319–325, 1999.

Bialek R, Ibrecevic A, Fothergill A, Begerow D. Small subunit ribosomal DNA sequences shows *Paracoccidioioides brasiliensis* closely related to *Blastomyces dermatitidis*. *J Clin Microbiol* 38: 3190–3193, 2000a.

Bialek R, Ibricevic A, Aepinus C, Najvar L K, Fothergill A W, Knobloch J, Graybill J R. Detection of *Paracoccidioides brasiliensis* in tissue samples by a nested PCR assay. *J Clin Microbiol* 38:2940–2942, 2000b.

Bicalho R N, Espírito Santo M F, Aguiar M C F, Santos V R. Oral paracoccidioidomycosis: a retrospective study of 62 Brazilian patients. *Oral Diseases* 7:56–60, 2001.

Blotta M H S L, Camargo Z P. Immunological response to cell-free antigens of *Paracoccidioides brasiliensis*: relationship with clinical forms of paracoccidioidomycosis. *J Clin Microbiol* 31:671–676, 1993.

Blotta M H, Mamoni R L, Oliveira S J, Nouer S A, Papaiordanou P M, Goveia A, Camargo Z P. Endemic regions of paracoccidioidomycosis in Brazil: a clinical and epidemiologic study of 584 cases in the southeast region. *Am J Trop Med Hyg* 61:390–394, 1999.

Borelli D. Some ecological aspects of paracoccidioidomycosis. In: *Proc Panam Symp Paracoccidioidomycosis*, Washington DC, Pan American Health Organization Scientific Publication 254:59–64, 1972.

Borgia G, Raynaud L, Cerrini R, Ciampi R, Schioppa O, Dello Ruso M, Gentile I, Piazza M. A case of paracoccidioidomycosis: experience with long term therapy. *Infection* 28:119–120, 2000.

Brummer E, Castañeda E, Restrepo A. Paracoccidioidomycosis: An update. *Clin Microbiol Rev* 6:89–117, 1993.

Burger E, Miyahi M, Sano A, Calich V L, Nishimura K, Lenzi H L. Histopathology of paracoccidiomycotic infection in athymic, euthymic mice: a sequential study. *Am J Trop Med Hyg* 55:235–242, 1998.

Cadavid D, Restrepo A. Factors associated with *Paracoccidioides brasiliensis* infection among permanent residents of 3 endemic areas in Colombia. *Epidemiol Infect* 111:121–133, 1993.

Calegaro J U, Gomes E F, Rodah J E. Paracoccidioidomicose infantil. Relato de dos casos estudados por galio[67] (^{67}Ga). *Radiol Bras* 30:343–346, 1997.

Calle D, Rosero S, Orozco L C, Camargo D, Castañeda E, Restrepo A. Paracoccidioidomycosis in Colombia: an ecological study. *Epidemiol Infect* 126:309–315, 2001.

Calich V L G, Vaz C A C, Burger E. Immunity to *Paracoccidioides brasiliensis* infection. *Res Immunol* 149: 407–416, 1998.

Camargo Z P, Franco M F. Current knowledge on pathogenesis and immunodiagnosis of paracoccidioidomycosis. *Rev Iberoam Micol* 17:41–48, 2000.

Cano M I, Cisalpino P S, Galindo I, Ramirez J L, Mortara R A, Silveria J F. Electrophoretic karyotypes and genome sizing of the pathogenic fungus *Paracoccidioides brasiliensis*. *J Clin Microbiol* 36:742–747, 1998.

Cano L E, Singer-Vermes T A, Costa T A, Mengel J O, Xidieh C F, Arruda D C, Andrade C A, Vaz C A, Burger E, Calich V L. Depletion of CD8+ cells in vivo impairs host-defense of mice resistant and susceptible to pulmonary paracoccidioidomycosis. *Infect Immun* 68:3532–359, 2000.

Castillo J, Ordóñez N, López S, Castañeda E. Paracoccidioidomicois: diagnóstico por el laboratorio de 333 casos. *Biomédica* 14:230–239, 1994.

Castro C C, Benard G, Ygaki Y, Cerrig J. MRI of head and neck paracoccidioidomycosis. *Br J Radiol* 72:717–22, 1999.

Cherri J, Freitas M A, Llorach-Velludo M A, Piccinato C E. Paracoccidioidomycosis aortitis with embolization to the lower limbs. Report of a case and review of the literature. *J Cardiovasc Surg (Torino)* 39:573–576, 1998.

Chojniak R, Viera R A, Lopez A, Silva J C, Godoy C E. Intestinal paracoccidioidomycosis simulating colon cancer. *Rev Soc Bras Med Trop* 33:309–312, 2000.

Cimerman S, Bacha H A, Ladeira M C T, Silveira O S, Colombo A I. Paracoccidioidomycosis in a boy infected with HIV. *Mycoses* 40:434–344, 1997.

Cock A M, Cano L E, Vélez D, Aristizábal B, Trujillo J, Restrepo A. Fibrotic sequelae in pulmonary paracoccidioidomycosis: Histopathological aspects in BALB/C mice infected with viable and non-viable propagules. *Rev Inst Med Trop S Paulo* 42:59–66, 2000.

Coimbra C E A, Wanke B, Santos R V, Valle A C F D, Costa R I

B, Zancope-Oliveria R M. Paracoccidioidin and histoplasmin sensitivity in the Tupí-Mondé Amerindian populations from Brazilian Amazonia. *Ann Trop Med Parasitol* 88:197–207, 1994.

Correa A L, Franco L, Restrepo A. Paracoccidioidomicosis: Coexistencia de lesiones pulmonares y patología pulmonar silente. descripción de 64 pacientes. *Acta Med Col* 16: 304–308, 1991.

Coutinho Z, Silva D, Lazera M, Petri V, Oliveira R M, Sabroza P C, Wanke B. Paracoccidioidomycosis mortality in Brazil (1980–1995). *Cad Saude Publica* (Brazil) 18:1441–1454, 2002.

Deepe G S, Romani L, Calich V L G, Huffnagle G, Arruda E E, Molinari-Maldlum E E, Perfect J R. Knockout mice as experimental models of virulence. *Med Mycol* 38 (Suppl 1):87–98, 2000.

Del Negro G M B, Pereira C N, Andrade H F, Palacios S A, Vidal M M, Chartbel C, Benard G. Evaluation of tests for antibody response in the follow-up of patients with acute and chronic forms of paracoccidioidomycosis. *J Med Microbiol* 49:37–46, 2000.

Dias M F, Pereira A C, Pereira A, Alves M S. The role of HLA antigens in the development of paracoccidioidomycosis. *J Eur Acad Dermatol Venereol* 14:166–171, 2000.

Dietze R, Fowler V G, Steiner T S, Pencanna P M, Corey G R. Failure of amphotericin B colloidal dispersion in the treatment of paracoccidioidomycosis. *Am J Trop Med Hyg* 60:837–839, 1999.

Diniz S N, Cisalpino P S, Freire A T, Silva-Teixeira D N, Contigli C, Rodriguez J V, Goes A M. In vitro granuloma formation, NO production and cytokines profile from human mononuclear cells induced by fractionated antigens of *Paracoccidioides brasiliensis*. *Hum Immunol* 62:299–808, 2001.

Doria A S, Taylor G A. Bony involvement in paracoccidioidomycosis. *Pediatr Radiol* 27:67–69, 1997.

Fonseca E R, Pardal P P, Severo L C. Paracoccidioidomicose em crianças em Belém do Pará. *Rev Soc Bras Med Trop* 32:31–33, 1999.

Fonseca L C, Mignone C. Paracoccidioidomicose do intestino delgado, aspectos anatomo-clínicos e radiológicos de 125 casos. *Rev Hosp Clin Fac Med S Paulo* 31:199–207, 1976.

Fornari M C, Bava A J, Guereno M T, Berardi V E, Silaf M R, Negroni R, Diez R A. Hig serum interluekin-10 and tumor necrosis factor in chronic paracoccidioidomycosis. *Clin Diag Lab Immunol* 8:1036–1038, 2001.

Franco M, Mendes R P, Moscardi-Bacchi M M, Rezkallah-Iwasso M, Montenegro M R. Paracoccidioidomycosis. *Bailliere's Clin Trop Med Comm Dis* 4:185–220, 1989.

Franco M, Lacaz C S, Restrepo A, Del Negro G, eds. *Paracoccidioidomycosis*. Boca Raton, FL: CRC Press, 1994.

Franco M, Bagagli E, Scapolio S, da Silva Lacaz C. A critical analysis of isolation of *Paracoccidioides brasiliensis* from soil. *Med Mycol* 38:185–191, 2000.

Fumari K, Kavakama J, Shikanai-Yasuda M A, Castro L G, Benard G, Rocha M S, Cedrri C G, Müller N I. Chronic pulmonary paracoccidioidomycosis (South American Blatomycosis): high resolution CT findings in 41 patients. *Am J Roentgenol* 173:59–64, 1999.

Giovanni E M, Mantessi A, Loducca S V L, Magalhaes M H C G, Paracoccidioidomycosis in an HIV-positive patient: a case report with gingival aspects. *Oral Dis* 6: 327–329, 2000.

Giraldo R, Restrepo A, Gutierrez F, Robledo M, Londoño F, Hernandez H, Sierra F, Calle G. Pathogenesis of paracoccidioidomycosis: A model based on the study of 46 patients. *Mycopathol* 58:63–70, 1976.

Gomes G M, Cisalpino P S, Taborda C P, Camargo Z P. PCR for diagnosis of paracoccidioidomycosis. *J Clin Microbiol* 38: 3478–3480, 2000.

Gómez B L, Figueroa J, Hamilton A, Ortiz B, Robledo M A, Hay R J, Restrepo A. Use of monoclonal antibodies in the diagnosis of paracoccidioidomycosis: New strategies for the detection of circulating antigens. *J Clin Microbiol* 35:3278–3283, 1997.

Gómez B L, Figueroa J I, Hamilton A J, Díez S, Rojas M, Tobón A M, Hay R J, Restrepo A. Antigenemia in patients with paracoccidioidomycosis: Detection of the 87 kDa determinant during and after antifungal therapy. *J Clin Microbiol* 36:3309–3316, 1998.

Gómez B L, Nosanchuk J, Díez S, Youngchim S, Aisen P, Cano L E, Restrepo A, Casadevall A, Hamilton A J. Detection of melanin-like pigments in the dimorphic fungal pathogen *Paracoccidioides brasiliensis* In vitro and during Infection. *Infect Immun* 69:5760–5767, 2001.

González A, de Gregory W, Vélez D, Restrepo A, Cano L E. Nitric oxide participation in the fungicidal mechanims of gamma interferon-activated murine macrophages against *P. brasiliensis* conidia. *Inf Immun* 68:2546–2552, 2000.

Gonzalez A, Cano L E. Participación del polimorfonuclear neutrófilo en la respuesta inmune contra *Paracoccidioides brasiliensis*. Revisión de tema. *Biomédica* 21: 264–274, 2001.

Hahn R C, Hamdan J S. Effects of amphotericin B and three azole derivatives on the lipids of yeast cells of *Paracoccidioides brasiliensis*. *Antimicrob Agents Chemother* 44:1997–2000, 2000.

Juvenale M, Del Negro G M B, Duarte A J, Benard G. Antibody isotypes to a *Paracoccidioides brasiliensis* somatic antigen in subacute and chronic form paracoccidioiomycosis. *J Med Microbiol* 50:127–134, 2001.

Karhawi A S, Colombo A L, Salom,,o R. Production of IFN-gamma is impaired in patients with paracoccidioidomycosis during active disease and is restored after clinical remission. *Med Mycol* 38:225–229, 2000.

Kashino S S, Fazioli R A, Cafalli-Favati C, Fazioli R A, Caballi-Farati C, Meloni-Bruneri L H, Vaz C A, Beuger E, Singer M L, Calich V. Resistance to *Paracoccidioides brasiliensis* infection is linked to a preferential Th1 immune response, whereas susceptibility is associated with absence of IFN-gamma production. *J Interf Cytok Res* 20:89–97, 2000.

Kurita N, Oarada M, Miyaji M, Ito E. Effect of cytokines on antifungal activity of human polymorphonuclear leucocytes against yeast cells of *Paracoccidioides brasiliensis*. *Med Mycol* 38:177–182, 2000.

Lacaz C S, Porto E, Martins J E C, Heins-Vaccari E, de Melo N T. Paracoccidioidomicose. In: Lacaz C S, Porto E, Martins J E C, eds. *Tratado de Micologia Medica Lacaz*. Sâo Paulo: Sarvier Publishers, 639–729, 2002.

Lacaz C S, Porto E, Heins-Vaccari E M, Melo N T. Fungos, Actinomicetos, Algas de Interesse Médico. Sao Paulo: Sarvier Publishers, 277–281, 1998.

Lenzi H L, Calich V L, Miyahi M, Sano A, Nishimura K, Burger E. Fibrosis patterns of lesions developed by athymic and euthymic mice infected with *Paracoccidioides brasiliensis*. *Braz J Med Biol Res* 27:2301–2308, 1994.

Lindsley Hirst S F, Iqbal N J, Morrison C J. Rapid identification of dimorphic yeast-like fungal pathogens using specific DNA probes. *J Clin Microbiol* 39:3505–3511, 2001.

Londero A T. Paracoccidioidomicose: Patogenia, formas clinicas, manifestacões pulmonares e diagnostico. *J Pneumol (Brazil)* 12: 41–57, 1986.

Londero A T, Melo I S. Paracoccidioidomicose. *J Bras Med* 55:96–111, 1988.

Londero A T, Rios-Gonçalves A J, Terra G M, Nogueira S A. Paracoccidioidomycosis in Brazilian children. A critical review (1911–1994). *Arq Bras Med* 70:197–203, 1996.

Mangiaterra M L, Giusiano G E, Alonso J M, Gorodner J O. *Paracoccidioides brasiliensis* infection in a subtropical region with important environmental changes. *Bull Soc Pathol Exot* 92:173–176, 1999.

Mamoni R L, Rossi C L, Camargo Z P, Blotta M H. Capture enzyme-linked immunosorbent assay to detect specific immuno-

globulin E in sera of patients with paracoccidioidomycosis. *Am J Trop Med Hyg* 65:237–241, 2001.

Manns B J, Baylis B W, Urbanski S J, Gibb A S, Rabin H R. Paracoccidioidomycosis: case report and review. *Clin Infect Dis* 23:1026–1032, 1996.

Marques S A. Cutaneous lesions. In: Franco M, Lacaz C S, Restrepo A, Del Negro G, eds. *Paracoccidioidomycosis*. Boca Raton, FL: CRC Press, 259–266, 1994a.

Marques S A, Shikanai-Yasuda M A. Paracoccidioidomycosis associated to immunosuppression, AIDS, and cancer. In: Franco M, Lacaz C S, Restrepo A, Del Negro G, eds. *Paracoccidioidomycosis*. Boca Raton, FL: CRC Press, 393–405, 1994b.

Martinez R, Moya M J. The relationship between paracoccidioidomycosis and alcoholism. *Rev Saúde Públ São Paulo* 26:12–16, 1992.

McEwen J G, Bedoya V, Patiño M M, Salazar ME, Restrepo A. Experimental murine paracoccidioidomycosis induced by the inhalation of conidia. *J Med Vet Mycol* 25:165–175, l987.

Meira D A, Pereira P C, Marcondes-Machado J. Mendes R P, Barraviera B, Pellegrino J, Rezkallah-Iwasso M T, Peraçoli M T S, Castilho L M, Tomazini I, Silva C L, Tiraboshi N P, Curi P R. The use of glucan as immunostimulant in the treatment of paracoccidioidomycosis. *Am J Trop Med Hyg* 55:496–503, 1996.

Mendes R P M. The gamut of clinical manifestations. In: Franco M, Lacaz C S, Restrepo A, Del Negro G, eds. *Paracoccidioidomycosis*. Boca Raton, FL: CRC Press, 233–258, 1994a.

Mendes R P, Negroni R, Arachevala A. Treatment and control of cure. In: Franco M, Lacaz C S, Restrepo A, Del Negro G, eds. *Paracoccidioidomycosis*. Boca Raton, FL: CRC Press, 373–392, 1994b.

Mendes R P. Bone and joint lesions. In: Franco M, Lacaz C S, Restrepo A, Del Negro G, eds. *Paracoccidioidomycosis*. Boca Raton, FL: CRC Press, 331–338, 1994c.

Mendes-Gianinni M J S, Del Negro G B, Siquiera A M. Serodiagnosis. In: Franco M, Lacaz C S, Restrepo A, Del Negro G, eds. *Paracoccidioidomycosis*. Boca Raton, FL: CRC Press, 345–363, 1994.

Mendes-Giannini M J S, Taylor M L, Bouchara J B, Burger E, Calich V L G, Escalante E D, Hanna S A, Lenzi H L, Machado M P, Miyahi M, Silva J L M, Mota E M, Restrepo A, Restrepo S, Tronchini G, Vincenzi L R, Xidieh C F, Zenteno E. Pathogenesis II: Fungal responses to host responses: interaction of host cells with fungi. *Med Mycol* 38(Suppl 1):113–123, 2000.

Migliari D A, Sugaya N N, Mimura M A, Cuce L C. Periodontal aspects of the juvenile form of paracoccidioidomycosis. *Rev Inst Med Trop S Paulo* 40:15–18, l998.

Miranda-Aires E, Costa Alves C A, Ferreira A V, Moreira, I M, Pappalardo M C, Peluso, D, Silva R J. Bone paracoccidioidomycosis in an HIV-positive patient. *Braz J Infect Dis* 1:260–265, 1997.

Miura C S N, Estevão D, Lopes J D, Itano E N. Levels of specific antigen (gp43), specific antibodies, and antigen-antibody complexes in saliva and serum of paracoccidioidomycosis patients. *Med Mycol* 39:423–428, 2000.

Molinari-Madlum E E, Felipe M S, Soares C M. Virulence of *Paracoccidioides brasiliensis* can be correlated to groups defined by by random amplified polymorphic DNA analysis (RAPD). *Med Mycol* 36:269–276, 1999.

Montenegro M R, Franco M. Pathology. In: Franco M, Lacaz C S, Restrepo A, Del Negro G, eds. *Paracoccidioidomycosis*. CRC Press, Boca Raton, FL: 131–150, 1994.

Montoya A E, Alvarez A L, Moreno M N, Restrepo A, McEwen J G. Electrophoretic karyotype of environmental isolates of *Paracoccidioides brasiliensis*. *Med Mycol* 37:219–222, 1999.

Moreira A, Martínez R C, Castro M, Elias L K. Adrenocortical dysfunction in paracoccidioidomycosis: comparison between plama β lipotrophin/adreno-corticotrophin levels and adrenocortical tests. *Clin Endocrinol* 36:545–550, 1993.

Musatti C C, Peracoli M T, Soares A M V C, Rezkallah-Iwso M T. Cell-mediated immunity in patients with paracoccidioidomycosis. In: Franco M, Lacaz C S, Restrepo A, Del Negro G, eds. *Paracoccidioidomycosis*. Boca Raton, FL: CRC Press, 175–186, 1994.

Naiff R, Ferreira L, Barrett T, Naiff M, Arias J. Enzootic paracoccidioidomycosis in armadillos (*Dasypus novemcinctus*) in the State of Para. *Rev Inst Med Trop S Paulo* 28:19–27, 1986.

Naiff R D, Barret T V, Arias J R, Naiff M F. Encuesta epidemiológica de histoplasmosis, paracoccidioidomicosis y leishmaniasis mediante pruebas cutáneas. *Bol Of Sanit Panam* 104:35–50, 1988.

Naranjo M S, Trujillo M, Múnera M, Gomez I, Restrepo A. Treatment of paracoccidioidomycosis with itraconazole, *J Med Vet Mycol* 28:67–76, 1990.

Negroni R. Paracoccidioidomycosis (South American blastomycosis, Lutz mycosis). *Int J Dermatol* 12:847–859, 1993.

Niño-Vega G A, Calgano A M, San Blas G, San Blas F, Gooday G W, Gow N A. RFLP analysis reveals marked geographical isolation between strains of *Paracoccidioides brasiliensis*. *Med Mycol* 38:437–441, 2000.

Nóbrega J P S. Neuroparacoccidioidomycosis. In: Franco M, Lacaz C S, Restrepo A, Del Negro G, ed. *Paracoccidioidomycosis*. Boca Raton, FL: CRC Press, 321–330, 1994.

Nogueria S A, Caiuby M J, Vasconcellos V, Halpern M, Gouveia C, Thorpe B, Ramparina C, Macicira J M P, Lambert J S. Paracoccidioidomycosis and tuberculosis in AIDS patients: Report of two cases in Brazil. *Int J Infect Dis* 2:168–172, 1998.

Nogueira S A, Guedes A L, Wanke B, Capella S, Rodrigues K, Abreu T F, Morais J C, Lambert J S. Osteomyelitis caused by *Paracoccidioides brasiliensis* in a child from the metropolitan area of Rio de Janeiro. *J Trop Pediatr* 47:311–315, 2001.

Ollague J M, de Zurita A M, Calero G. Paracoccidioidomycosis (South American blastomycosis) successfully treated with terbinafine: first case report. *Br J Dermatol* 143:188–191, 2000.

Ono M A, Bracarense A P F R L, Morais H A S, Trapp S M, Belitardo D R, Camargo Z P. Canine paracococcidioidomycosis: a seroepidemiologic study. *Med Mycol* 39:277–282, 2000.

Ortiz B, Díez S, Urán M E, Rivas J M, Caicedo V, Restrepo A, McEwen J G. Use of the 27 kDa recombinant protein from *Paracoccidioides brasiliensis* and its use in the serodiagnosis of paracoccidioidomycosis. *Clin Diag Immunol* 5:826–830, 1998.

Peraçoli M T S, Sugizaki M F, Mendes R P, Naiff R, Montenegro M R. *Paracoccidioides brasiliensis* isolated from armadillos is virulent to Syriam hamsters. *Mycopathologia* 148:123–130, 1999.

Pereira A J C S. Inquérito intradérmico para paracoccidioidomicose em Goiânia. *Rev Pat Trop* 17:157–186, 1988.

Pinto A R, Oucia R, Diniz S N, Franco M F, Taravasso L R. DNA-based vaccination against murine paracoccidioidomycosis using *gp43* gene from *Paracoccidioides brasiliensis*. *Vaccine* 18:3050–3058, 2000.

Queiroz-Telles F. *Paracoccidioides brasiliensis*: Ultrastructural findings. In: Franco M, Lacaz C S, Restrepo A, Del Negro G, eds. *Paracoccidioidomycosis*. CRC Press, Boca Raton, FL: 27–48, 1994.

Restrepo A, Gomez I, Cano L E, Arango MD, Gutierrez F, Sanin A, Robledo M A. Treatment of paracoccidioidomycosis with ketoconazole. A three years experience. *Am J Med* 74(Suppl. B):48–52, 1983.

Restrepo A, Trujillo M, Gómez I. Innapparent lung involvement in patients with the subacute juvenile type of paracoccidioidomycosis. *Rev Inst Med Trop S Paulo* 31:18–22, 1989.

Restrepo A. Ecology of *Paracoccidioides brasiliensis*. In: Franco M, Lacaz C S, Restrepo A, Del Negro G, eds. *Paracoccidioidomycosis*. Boca Ratón, FL: CRC Press, 121–130, 1994.

Restrepo A, Salazar M E, Clemons K V, Feldman D, Stevens D A.

Hormonal Influences in the host-interplay with *Paracoccidioides brasiliensis*. In: Stevens D A, Vanden Bosche H, Odds F, eds. *Topics on Fungal Infections*. National Foundation for Infectious Diseases, 125–133, 1997.

Restrepo A. Morphological aspects of *Paracoccidioides brasiliensis* in lymph nodes: implications for the prolonged latency of paracoccidioidomycosis? *Med Mycol* 38:317–322, 2000.

Restrepo A, McEwen J G, Castañeda E. The habitat of *Paracoccidioides brasiliensis*: How far from solving the riddle? *Med Mycol* 39:233–241, 2001.

Rios-Gonçalves A J, Londero A T, Terra G M F, Rozenbaum R, Abreu T F, Nogueira S A. Paracoccidioidomycosis in children in the state of Rio de Janeiro (Brazil). Geographic distribution and the study of a "reservarea". *Rev Inst Med Trop S Paulo* 40:11–13, 1998.

Roldán J C, Tabares A M, Gómez B L, Aristizábal B E, Cock A M, Restrepo A. The oral route in the pathogenesis of paracoccidioidomycosis: An experimental study in BALB/c mice infected with *P. brasiliensis* conidia. *Mycopathologia* 151:57–62, 2001.

Salina M A, Shikanai-Yasuda M A, Mendes R P, Barraviera B, Mendes-Giannini M J. Detection of circulating antigen in urine of paracocciodiomycosis patients before and during treatment. *J Clin Microbiol* 36:1723–1728, 1998.

San Blas G, San Blas F. Biochemistry of *Paracoccidioides brasiliensis* dimorphism. In: Franco M, Lacaz C S, Restrepo A. and Del Negro G, eds. *Paracoccidioidomycosis*. Boca Raton, FL: CRC Press, 49–66, 1994.

San Blas G, Niño-Vega G. *Paracoccidioides brasiliensis*: virulence and host response. In: Cihlar R L, Caldernone R A, eds. *Fungal Pathogenesis: Principles and Clinical Applications*. New York: Marcel Dekker, Inc., 205–226, 2001.

Sandlu G S, Aleff R A, Kline B C, Lacaz C S. Molecular detection and identification of *Paracoccidioides brasiliensis*. *J Clin Microbiol* 35:1894–1896, 1997.

Sano A, Miyaji M, Nishimura K. Studies on the relationship between the estrous cycle of BALB/c mice and their resistance to *P. brasiliensis* infection. *Mycopathologia* 119:141–145, 1992.

Sano A, Yokoyama K, Tamura M, Mikami Y, Takahashi I, Fukushima K, Miyahi M, Nishimura K. Detection of gp43 and ITS1-5.8S-ITS2 ribosomal RNA genes of *Paracoccidioides brasiliensis* in paraffin embedded tissues. *Nippo Ishinkin Gakkai Zassh* 42:23–27, 2001.

Santos J W A, Costa J M, Cechella M, Michel G T, Figereido C W C, Londero A T. An unusual presentation of paracoccidioidomycosis in an AIDS patient. *Mycopathol* 142:139–142, 1998.

SantAnna G D, Mauri M, Arrarte J L, Camargo H. Laryngeal manifestations of paracoccidioidomycosis (South American Blastomycosis). *Arch Otolatyngol Head Neck Surg* 125:1375–1378, 1999.

Severo L C, Kauer C L, Oliveira F D, Rigatti R A, Hartman A A, Londero A T. Paracoccidioidiomycosis of the male genital tract. Report of eleven cases and review of the Brazilian literature. *Rev Inst Med Tropical S Paulo* 42:38–40, 2000.

Shikanai-Yasuda M A, Segurado A A C, Pinto W P, Segurado A L, Ponto W P, Nicodemo A C, Sato M, Duarte AJ, Del Negro G M, Hutzer RH. Immunodeficiency secondary to juvenile paracoccidioidomycosis. *Mycopathologia* 120:23–28, 1992a.

Shikanai-Yasuda M A, Higaki Y, Uip D E, Mori N S, Del Negro G, Melo N T, Hutzler R U, Amato Neto V. Comprometimiento da medula ossea e eosinofilia na paracoccidiodiomicose. *Rev Inst Med Trop S Paulo* 34:85–90, 1992b.

Silva S P, Borges-Walmsley M I, Pereira I S, Soares C M, Walmsley A, Felipe M S. Differential expression of an hsp70 gene during transition from the mycelial to the infective yeast form of the human pathogenic fungus *Paracoccidioides brasiliensis*. *Mol Microbiol* 31:1039–1050, 1999.

Silva C E, Cordeiro A F, Gollner A M, Cupolilo S M, Quesada-Filguerias M, Curzio M F. Paracoccidioidomycosis of the central nervous system: case report. *Arq Neurosiquiatr* 58:741–747, 2000.

Silva-Vergara M L, Martinez R. Role of the armadillo *Dasypus novemcinctus* in the epidemiology of paracoccidioidomycosis. *Mycopathologia* 144:131–133, 1999.

Silva-Vergara M L, Martínez R, Camargo Z P, Malta M H B, Maffei C M L, Chadu J B. Isolation of *Paracoccidioides brasiliensis* from armadillos (*Dasypus novemcinctus*) in areas where the fungus was recently isolated from soil. *Med Mycol* 38:193–199, 2000.

Singer-Vermes L M, Burger E, Russo M, Vaz C, Calich V L G. Advances in experimental paracoccidioidomycosis using an isogenic murine model. *Arch Med Res* 24:239–245, 1993.

Soares A M V, Peraçoli M T S, Santos R R D. Correlation among immune response, morphogenesis of the granulomatous reaction and spleen lymphoid structure in murine experimental paracoccidioidomycosis. *Med Mycol* 38:371–377, 2000a.

Soares A M, Rezkallah-Iwasso M T, Oliveira S L, Peraçoli M T, Montenegro M R, Musatti C C. Experimental paracoccidioidomycosis in high and low antibody responder mice. *Med Mycol* 38:309–15, 2000b.

Souto J T. Figueireido F, Furlanetto A, Pfeffer K, Rossi M A, Silva J S. Interferon-γ and tumor necrosis factor-α determine resistance to *Paracoccidioides brasiliensis* infection in mice. *Am J Pathol* 156:1811–1820, 2000.

Souza A R, Gesztesi J L, Negro G M B, Benard G, Sato J, Santos M V B, Abrahão T B, Lopes J D. Anti-idiotypic antibodies in patients with different clinical forms of paracoccidioidomycosis. *Clin Diagn Lab Immunol* 7:175–181, 2000.

Stevens D A. Itraconazole in cyclodextrin solution. *Pharmacother* 19:603–611, 1999.

Sugizaki M F, Peraçoli M T S, Mendes-Giannini M J, Soares A M V C, Kurokawa C S, Mendes R P, Marques S A, Freire-Maia D V. Correlation between antigenemia of *Paracoccidioides brasiliensis* and inhibition effect of plasma in patients with paracoccidioidomycosis. *Med Mycol* 37:277–284, 1999.

Teixeira A B, Echtbehere E C, Lima M C, Santos A O, Pires B C, Valencia J T, Ramos C D, Camargo E E. Gallium-67 imaging in a patient with paracoccidioidomycosis. *Rev Inst Med Trop S Paolo* 42:167–170, 2000.

Tendrich M, Wanke B, Del Negro G, Wajchenberg B L. Adreno-cortical involvement. In: Franco M, Lacaz C S, Restrepo A, Del Negro G, eds. *Paracoccidioidomycosis*. Boca Raton, FL: CRC Press, 303–312, 1994.

Tobón AM, Gómez I, Franco L, Restrepo A. Seguimiento post-terapia en pacientes con paraoccidioidomicosis tratados con itraconazol. *Rev Colomb Neumol* 7:74–78, 1995.

Tobón A M, Orozco B, Estrada S, Jaramillo E, de Bedout C, Arango M, Restrepo A. Paracoccidioidomycosis and AIDS: report of the two Colombian cases. *Rev Inst Med Trop* 40: 377–381, 1998.

Torrado E, Castañeda E, de la Hoz F, Restrepo A. Paracoccidioidomicosis: definición de las áreas endémicas de Colombia. *Biomédica* 20:327–334, 2000.

Travassos L R. Immunochemistry of *Paracoccidiodes brasiliensis* antigens. In: Franco M, Lacaz C S, Restrepo A, Del Negro G, eds. *Paracoccidioidomycosis*. Boca Raton, FL: CRC Press, 67–86, 1994.

Tuder R M, El Ibrahim R, Godoy C E, de Brito T. Pathology of the pulmonary paracoccidioidomycosis. *Mycopathologia* 92:179–188, 1985.

Valle A C F, Guimarães R R, Lopes D J, Capone D. Aspectos radiológicos torácicos na paracoccidioidomicose. *Rev Inst Med Trop S Paulo* 34:107–115, 1992.

Valle A C F, Aprigliano F F, Moreira J S, Wake B. Clinical and endoscopic findings of the upper respiratory and digestive tracts in post-treatment follow-up of paracoccidioidomycosis patients. *Rev Inst Med Trop S Paulo* 27:407–413, 1995.

Valle A C F, Costa R L B, Montero P C F, Heldern J V, Muniz M M, Zancopé-Oliveira R M. Interpretation and clinical correlation of serological tests in paracoccidioioimycosis. *Med Mycol* 39:373–377, 2000.

Vaz C A C, Mackenzie D W R, Hearn V M, Camargo Z P, Singer Vermes L M, Burger E, Calich V L G. Specific recognition pattern of IgM and IgG antibodies produced in the course of experimental paracoccidioidomycosis. *Clin Exp Immunol* 88:119–123, 1992.

Villa L A, Tobón A M, Restrepo A, Calle D, Rosero S, Gómez B L, Restrepo A. Central nervous system paracoccidioidomycosis. Report of a case successfully treated with itraconazole. *Rev Inst Med Trop S Paulo* 42:231–234, 2000.

Wanke B, Londero A T. Epidemiology and paracoccidioidomycosis infection. In: Franco M, Lacaz C S, Restrepo A, Del Negro G, eds. *Paracoccidioidomycosis*. Boca Raton, FL: CRC Press, 109–120, 1994.

22

Sporotrichosis

PETER G. PAPPAS

Sporotrichosis is a chronic pyogranulomatous infection caused by the thermally dimorphic fungus *Sporothrix schenckii*. Infection is usually limited to the skin and subcutaneous tissues, but can involve virtually any organ in its disseminated form. Less common localized forms of sporotrichosis include arthritis, osteomyelitis, meningitis, chronic pulmonary infection, and ocular disease.

Schenck originally described sporotrichosis in 1898 in a 36-year old man who presented with several discrete indurated lesions extending along the lymphatics from the index finger proximally to the forearm. The organism obtained from cultures of the purulent drainage from one of these lesions revealed heavy growth of a moderately rapidly growing fungus that he designated as possibly related to *Sporotrichum* spp. (Schenck, 1898). Subsequently, investigators reported a second case of sporotrichosis in a 5-year-old boy with chronic ulceration of the index finger and associated nodular lymphangitis of the forearm (Hektoen and Perkins, 1900). Treatment entailed serial incision and drainage of each subcutaneous nodule followed by local wound care resulting in eventual full recovery. The fungus isolated from this young patient was referred to as *Sporothrix schenckii*. However, the more common designation, *Sporotrichum schenckii*, was used through the late 1960s until Carmichael's observation that the organism had a different manner of sporulation when compared to *Sporotrichum* spp., and the name *Sporothrix schenckii* was officially readopted (Carmichael, 1962).

After the initial description of sporotrichosis, most early cases were reported from France. One of the case reviews from France involved approximately 250 patients with sporotrichosis and remains one of the largest reports of this condition to date (de Beurman and Gougerot, 1912). As knowledge of the disease became more widespread, fewer cases were identified in Europe and cases of sporotrichosis began to be reported worldwide, with the abundance of cases emerging from the United States, Mexico, and South America.

Sporotrichosis was originally considered a sporadic infection, though clusters of cases and larger epidemics were occasionally observed. In the largest of these outbreaks, almost 3000 cases of sporotrichosis occurred among South African gold miners between 1941 and 1944. The cause of the initial outbreak was discovered to be infected mining timbers, and the epidemic was brought under control by spraying these timbers with fungicidal agents (Transvaal Mine Medical Officers' Association Symposium, 1947). Since the report of the large South African outbreak, many smaller epidemics have been reported, mostly occurring in North and South America and Japan (Ellner, 1960; D'Alessio et al, 1965; Powell et al, 1978; Itoh et al, 1986; Centers for Disease Control, 1988; Kushuhara et al, 1988; Kwon-Chung and Bennett, 1992; Barile et al, 1993; Hajjeh et al, 1997).

MYCOLOGY

Sporothrix schenckii demonstrates thermal dimorphism, growing as a mould at room temperature (25°C–28°C), and as a yeast at 35°C–37°C (Kwon-Chung and Bennett, 1992). There is evidence to suggest that isolates from fixed dermatologic lesions are less tolerant to higher temperatures, growing well at 35°C, but either failing to grow or growing only very slowly at 37°C (Kwon-Chung, 1979). In contrast, isolates from lung, synovial tissue, or lymphocutaneous lesions and other deep tissues usually grow well at body temperature. Not all investigators have been able to reproduce these observations (Mackinnon and Conti-Diaz, 1962; Mackinnon et al, 1964; Albornoz et al, 1986).

Colonies grow within a few days to 2 weeks when incubated on Sabouraud's dextrose agar at 25°C–28°C. The initial colony is moist and whitish. Within 10 to 14 days, most colonies develop a black or brown pigmentation around the periphery of the colony (Kwon-Chung and Bennett, 1992). The identification of *S. schenckii* is based on its colonial and microscopic morphology in the mould phase and its conversion to yeast phase at 35°C–37°C. The yeast phase of *S. schenckii*, while rarely seen in clinical specimens, is acapsular and has a distinctive oval to cigar-shaped appearance. Distinction between *S. schenckii* and a much less common pathogen, *S. cyanescens*, can be difficult, though the colonies of *S. cyanescens* produce a water-soluble purplish pigment and thermodimorphism is less readily demonstrated in this species (Kwon-Chung and Bennett, 1992). *Sporothrix schenckii* variety *luriei* has a distinctive morphologic appearance with a yeast form that is large, thick-walled, and demonstrates budding. In addition, the organism can survive as a yeast at 25°C (Alberici et al, 1989).

Virulence factors for *S. schenckii* have not been elucidated completely. It is clear that the organism is not very virulent in many animal models including the guinea pig, rabbit, mouse, and hamster (Mackinnon et al, 1964; Dixon et al, 1992; Tachibani et al, 2001). The organism produces melanin, which is a virulence factor for other yeasts including *Cryptococcus neoformans* (Romero-Martinez et al, 2000). The organism also produces extracellular proteins, which could possibly play a role in virulence. In addition, *S. schenckii* contains the unique substance, L-rhamnose, which complexes with other glycoproteins to form rhamnomannans, which are not found in other fungal cell walls. The potential role of the rhamnomannans as a virulence factor is not well understood (Kauffman, 1999).

Conditions of growth may also play an important role in virulence. Recently, Fernandes and colleagues, using a mouse model, observed that conidia grown for 4 days demonstrated more virulence than conidia grown for 10–12 days (Fernandes et al, 1999). Thermotolerance is also probably an important virulence factor among selected strains of *S. schenckii* causing visceral or lymphonodular disease, as these organisms tend to multiply at 37°C whereas organisms that are less thermotolerant tend to be less invasive and cause chronic fixed cutaneous lesions (Mackinnon and Conti-Diaz, 1962; Mackinnon et al, 1964; Mackinnon et al, 1969; Kwon-Chung and Bennett, 1992).

EPIDEMIOLOGY

In recent decades, most cases of sporotrichosis have been reported from the United States, Central and South America, Africa, and Japan (Ellner, 1960; D'Allessio et al, 1965; Ochoa et al, 1970; Velasco-Castrejon and Gonzalez-Ochoa, 1976; Powell et al, 1978; Itoh et al, 1986; Centers for Disease Control, 1988; Kushuhara et al, 1988; Barile et al, 1993; Hajjeh et al, 1997; Pappas et al, 2000). The majority of cases are sporadic, occurring after direct inoculation through the skin from an infectious source. There is a predominance of males among reported cases of sporotrichosis, probably reflecting occupational exposure. Occupational risk factors include gardening or farming, forestry, nursery workers, outdoor laborers,

and other activities that involve exposure to *S. schenckii* contaminated material such as sphagnum moss, roses, or other vegetation (Powell et al, 1978; Centers for Disease Control, 1982; Centers for Disease Control, 1988; Coles et al, 1992).

The incidence of sporotrichosis varies widely from country to country based on observational data and case reports. Few countries have national surveillance or reporting systems for the deep mycoses, consequently only crude estimates of disease incidence are generally available. Surveillance data notwithstanding, the disease appears to have become extremely rare in Western Europe, with the exception of Italy, where sporadic cases are still reported (Barile et al, 1993). In the Unites States, the incidence is less than one case per 100,000 and probably more accurately approximates one case per million persons (Hajjeh et al, 1997). Data from Japan suggest a similar incidence (Itoh et al, 1986; Kushuhara et al, 1988). The countries of Central and South America appear to have the heaviest burden of disease based on scattered reports and few prospective studies. Observations from some hyperendemic regions in the Andean highlands of South America suggest that the incidence of disease is highest among children and adolescents in rural villages, approximating 1 case per 1000 in some regions (Pappas et al, 2000). Among these children there appears to be no male predominance in reported disease.

Transmission of *S. schenckii* usually occurs through a traumatic break in the skin and exposure to infectious material. A primary lesion usually occurs at the site of inoculation, and this may be followed by local lymphangitic spread or the development of a fixed cutaneous lesion. Extracutaneous sporotrichosis may occur as a result of direct inoculation such as penetrating trauma into a joint or the eye, or through dissemination from another site such as the skin or lungs. Patients with pulmonary sporotrichosis probably acquire disease through inhalation, as these patients usually provide no history consistent with cutaneous disease (Pluss and Opal, 1986).

Several cases of laboratory-acquired sporotrichosis have been reported (Thompson and Kaplan, 1977; Cooper et al, 1992). These cases have occurred typically among persons working with infected laboratory animals or other contaminated material, with direct inoculation to the upper extremities. In two cases, direct inoculation into the conjunctivae occurred when a suspension of *S. schenckii* mycelial elements was spattered into the eyes (Thompson and Kaplan, 1977). Person-to-person transmission, if it occurs, is exceedingly rare. There are, however, several reports of sporotrichosis occurring in family members or persons living in the same household (Garrett and Robbins, 1960; Yamada et al, 1990). In most of these instances, disease was felt to be due to a common source rather than person-to-person spread. Sporotrichosis as result of zoonotic exposure to domestic and wild animals has also been well described (Caravalho et al, 1991; Reed et al, 1993; Saravanakumar et al, 1996; de Lima Barros et al, 2001; Fleury et al, 2001). Clinical sporotrichosis may occur in birds, dogs, squirrels, horses, rats, and cats; thus veterinarians and pet owners are at relatively increased risk for acquiring infection. Recently, several well-documented cases of feline-transmitted sporotrichosis have been reported in the United States and Brazil (Caravalho et al 1991; Fleury et al, 2001).

Most cases of sporotrichosis are sporadic, though many outbreaks of sporotrichosis have been reported. Most outbreaks have been traced to occupational exposure such as workers handling plants, contaminated sphagnum moss or soil. Forrester was among the first to suggest an occupational predisposition to sporotrichosis in his review of 14 tree nursery workers with sporotrichosis from Wisconsin in 1926 (Forrester, 1926). More recent epidemics in the United States in Wisconsin, Florida, Vermont, Mississippi, and a large multistate outbreak have been reported following exposure to seedlings, other plants, and sphagnum moss (Ellner, 1960; D'Alessio et al, 1965; Powell et al, 1978; Centers for Disease Control, 1982). In the largest of these epidemics, 84 cases of cutaneous sporotrichosis occurred in persons handling conifer seedlings that had been packed with sphagnum moss harvested in Wisconsin (Centers for Disease Control, 1988; Coles et al, 1992). Cases were confirmed in 14 states in this multistate outbreak.

The most recently documented outbreak of sporotrichosis in the United States occurred among nine tree nursery workers from one nursery in Florida in 1994 (Hajjeh et al, 1997). A case-control study conducted in parallel with this epidemic suggested that occupational inexperience and handling sphagnum moss were independently associated with an increased risk, whereas longer work experience and wearing gloves were associated with decreased risk of sporotrichosis (Hajjeh et al, 1997).

CLINICAL MANIFESTATIONS

Lymphocutaneous

Lymphocutaneous lesions are the hallmark of sporotrichosis. Disease typically arises at a site of minor trauma and may begin as a erythematous papule that enlarges over days or weeks. The lesion may become a fixed subcutaneous nodule or plaque, or may develop into a chronic nonhealing ulcerative lesion (See Color Figs. 22–1 and 22–2 in separate color insert). These lesions are usually painless and systemic symptoms of fever,

malaise, weight loss, and chills are usually absent. Classically, a "sporotrichoid" eruption of similar-appearing subcutaneous nodules develops along the lymphatic system of the involved anatomic site (See Color Figs. 22–3a, 22–3b, 22–4a, and 22–4b in separate color insert). Lesions are typically erythematous or violaceous, and the intervening skin is usually normal. Over time, these nodules may undergo suppuration, drainage and ulcer formation, similar to the primary lesion. Secondary lymphadenopathy may occur, although lymph nodes are not usually involved directly with *S. schenckii* infection, and most cases of enlarged nodes represent reactive lymphadenopathy.

Some patients present with a fixed ulceration or a proliferative, plaque-like lesion. These lesions can be chronic for many months or years, remaining more or less unchanged (Kauffman, 1999). The propensity for these lesions to evolve into progressive nodular lymphangitis or disseminated disease is very low and may relate to the observation that many of these *S. Schenckii* organisms are less thermotolerant than more invasive strains (Kwon-Chung, 1979).

Disseminated cutaneous lesions involving multiple extremities, the face, trunk, and abdomen may occur in normal individuals after either intense exposure to the organism, significant autoinoculation, or rarely, hematogenous dissemination. Patients with disseminated skin lesions secondary to hematogenous spread are virtually all severely immunocompromised as a consequence of advanced HIV disease, organ transplantation, or another significant underlying disorder (Ware et al, 1999).

Osteoarticular

Osteoarticular sporotrichosis is usually manifest as a slowly progressive, indolent process involving a major peripheral joint, typically the knee, elbow, ankle, or wrist (Altner and Turner, 1970; Crout et al, 1977; Yao et al, 1986; Chowdhary et al, 1991). Occasionally, metacarpal or metatarsal joints may be involved either as a manifestation of dissemination or direct extension from a cutaneous lesion. Arthritis has also been reported to follow a penetrating joint injury. Frank bony involvement is a frequent concomitant of sporotrichoid arthritis, usually at a contiguous periarticular site (Altner and Turner, 1970; Yao et al, 1986). Patients with osteoarticular sporotrichosis often present with localized pain and swelling without significant fever or other systemic symptoms. Untreated, the process inevitably progresses until the joint is destroyed and/or function significantly impaired.

Sporothrix schenckii is also a cause of granulomatous tenosynovitis, usually presenting in the wrist with painless swelling and limitation of range of motion. In severe cases, neurologic or musculoskeletal symptoms due to entrapment of the median nerve or tendon rupture can be seen (Stratton et al, 1981; Schwartz, 1989). Surgical intervention is necessary for decompression, debridement, and repair of damaged tendons. At surgery, the finding of "rice bodies" in the synovial space is a nonspecific finding consistent with sporotrichosis, but can also be seen in cases of granulomatous tenosynovitis due to other organisms such as mycobacteria.

Pulmonary

Pulmonary sporotrichosis is a rare disorder. In the largest review of this topic, Pluss and Opal reviewed 51 cases, of which the vast majority were middle-aged white males presenting with cough, low-grade fever, weight loss, and upper lobe cavitary disease (Pluss and Opal, 1986). Preexisting lung disease was common. Hemoptysis occurred in fewer than 20%, but could be significant if present.

Chest roentgenographic findings associated with pulmonary sporotrichosis are nonspecific. Cavitary lung lesions, which are common with pulmonary sporotrichosis, are usually single and often involve the upper lobes (Wilson et al, 1967; Pluss and Opal, 1986). There may be extensive surrounding fibrosis, which is indistinguishable from the fibrosis associated with other causes of chronic necrotizing pneumonia (Fig. 22–5). The classic single thin-walled cavity associated with pulmonary sporotrichosis and coccidioidomycosis is relatively uncommon (Pluss and Opal, 1986).

Among patients with pulmonary sporotrichosis, disease is usually limited to the lungs, although multiple organ involvement can occur. Untreated, pulmonary sporotrichosis leads to slow and inexorable clinical deterioration; spontaneous remission is rare.

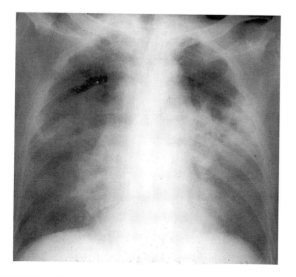

FIGURE 22–5. Chest roentgenogram from a patient with chronic fibrocavitary pulmonary sporotrichosis.

Disseminated

Sporotrichosis can involve virtually any organ, manifesting as disseminated disease in either of two forms: (1) disseminated cutaneous disease and (2) disseminated visceral disease (Lurie, 1963; Wilson et al, 1967; Donabedian et al, 1994; Castrejon et al, 1995). Both of these disease presentations result from hematogenous dissemination. In the first form, multiple skin lesions may occur spontaneously on the extremities, trunk, abdomen, and head and neck. These lesions are often small pustules on an erythematous base and not particularly distinctive. They can be mistaken for the skin lesions of varicella, disseminated bacterial infection, or another disseminated fungal infection. The CNS and the peripheral joints are probably the most common sites for disseminated visceral disease (Wilson et al, 1967). Clinically, CNS disease is usually associated with chronic indolent meningitis, focal cranial nerve abnormalities, and hydrocephalus. Cerebrospinal fluid analysis usually reveals evidence of chronic inflammation with hypoglycorrhachia, elevated CSF protein, and mononuclear cell pleocytosis (Wilson et al, 1967; Donabedian et al, 1994). Endophthalmitis due to S. schenckii may occur either as an extension of a CNS infection, or independently as a consequence of hematogenous dissemination or directly from penetrating trauma (Kurosawa et al, 1988; Cartwright et al, 1993).

Special Populations

Children. Unlike cryptococcosis and blastomycosis, sporotrichosis is not uncommon in children (Gluckman, 1965; Chandler et al, 1968; Orr and Riley, 1971; Burch et al, 2001). Indeed, in some populations the highest incidence of disease is among preadolescent children (Pappas et al, 2000). Disease manifestations are similar to those in adults, although multiple cutaneous sites and facial lesions are more common in children with sporotrichosis, possibly due in part to autoinoculation (Gluckman, 1965; Chandler et al, 1968; Orr and Riley, 1971; Pappas et al, 2000; Burch et al, 2001). For unclear reasons, extracutaneous and hematogenously disseminated cutaneous disease are particularly uncommon among children.

Immunocompromised Patients. A growing number of patients with sporotrichosis and HIV/AIDS or other significant underlying immune disorders have been reported (Kurosawa et al, 1988; Keiser and Whittle, 1991; Donabedian et al, 1994; al-Tawfiq and Wools, 1998; Ware et al, 1999; Edwards et al, 2000). Patients with these disorders are much more likely to present with hematogenously disseminated disease, and a disproportionate number of these patients develop complicated S. schenckii infections, including fungemia, meningitis, endophthalmitis, and multiorgan disease (Kurosawa et al, 1988; Keiser and Whittle, 1991; Donabedian et al, 1994; al-Tawfiq and Wools, 1998; Edwards et al, 2000). Whereas mortality associated with sporotrichosis among non-immunocompromised patients is very low, disseminated disease in the immunocompromised patient can be rapidly fatal if unrecognized and untreated.

DIAGNOSIS

The clinical diagnosis of lymphocutaneous sporotrichosis can be misleading because sporotrichosis is clinically indistinguishable from other common causes of nodular lymphangitis (Kostman and DiNubile, 1993). Lymphonodular sporotrichosis may appear identical to cutaneous nocardiosis, mycobacterial infections, especially due to *Mycobacterium marinum* and *Mycobacterium chelonae*, tularemia resulting from direct cutaneous inoculation, and cutaneous leishmaniasis (Kostman and DiNubile, 1993). Less common causes of a lymphonodular sporotrichoid eruption include *Mycobacterium avium* complex, other mycobacteria, *C. neoformans*, *B. dermatitidis*, and rarely, *C. immitis*.

The diagnosis of sporotrichosis is confirmed by a positive culture for *S. schenckii* from an involved site (tissue or body fluid). The organism is not considered a colonizer; thus, its isolation from a clinical specimen is virtually always considered diagnostic. Optimally, clinical specimens for culture should be collected from purulent cutaneous lesions. Alternatively, a skin biopsy of a suspicious area is usually sufficient. For patients with suspected pulmonary sporotrichosis, expectorated purulent sputum can be a source for culture; otherwise, a bronchoalveolar lavage or a transbronchial biopsy specimen is necessary (Pluss and Opal, 1986; Farley et al, 1991). For patients with osteoarticular disease, the organism is readily recovered from synovial fluid or involved boney or synovial tissue. Isolation of *S. schenckii* from blood and other body fluids, including cerebrospinal fluid, is unusual even among patients with disseminated disease (Scott et al, 1987).

Direct examination of clinical specimens is usually unsuccessful in a search for specific histopathologic evidence of sporotrichosis. Owing to the relative paucity of organisms, yeast forms are seen uncommonly on biopsy specimens using Gram stain, KOH or other special stains. The fungal cell may have a very pleomorphic appearance ranging from spherical to elongated. However, the typical ovoid cigar-shaped yeast forms, which are most suggestive of the diagnosis, are uncommonly seen. Similarly, the classic finding of asteroid bodies in tissue specimens is uncommon (See Color Fig. 22–6 in separate color insert). Serologic assays for the detection of antibodies to *Sporothrix schenckii* are neither readily available nor appropriately standardized; thus, this method of diagnosis is not generally useful, although assay of CSF for antibody has been advocated for patients with suspected *Sporothrix* meningitis (Scott et al, 1987).

In many countries, a skin test (sporotrichin test) is available to detect exposure to *S. schenckii*. The skin test antigen, which consists of an extract from laboratory-cultured strains of *S. schenckii*, is not standardized. The test is used as an adjunct to the diagnosis of cutaneous sporotrichosis among patients with clinically compatible lesions before culture data are available or in whom cultures are negative. Although a positive skin test is generally regarded as evidence of recent exposure to *S. schenckii*, this diagnostic modality remains of questionable value, even in areas of the world where it is readily available. At present, the sporotrichin skin test is not available commercially within the United States.

TREATMENT

Supersaturated Solution of Potassium Iodide
Effective therapy for cutaneous sporotrichosis has been available for almost a century. In the early 1900s, de-Beurmann noted that iodides were effective in the treatment of this form of sporotrichosis, though the mechanism by which iodides act is still not understood almost 100 years later (Urabe and Nagashima, 1969; Sterling and Heymann, 2000). Supersaturated solution of potassium iodide (SSKI) does not inhibit or kill *S. schenckii* directly nor does it enhance killing of the organism when combined with neutrophils (Rex and Bennett, 1990). Nonetheless, a large amount of clinical experience and published data indicate that SSKI is an acceptable and very effective treatment for uncomplicated cutaneous sporotrichosis.

For patients undergoing treatment with SSKI, it is recommended to begin with 5 drops SSKI in water or juice 3 times daily, gradually increasing each dose by 5 drops weekly to a maximum of 40 or 50 drops SSKI 3 times daily as tolerated. Administration usually continues until active lesions have disappeared for at least 4 weeks. Therapy is rarely continued beyond 6 months, in part because of poor patient tolerance and difficulty in administration. Recognizing these problems, Cabezas and colleagues, studying a group of Andean natives in Peru, found that once daily dosing with SSKI was equivalent to standard dosing at 2 to 3 times daily, thereby demonstrating that this was an effective approach to treatment for many patients with cutaneous sporotrichosis (Cabezas et al, 1996).

Adverse effects, which are common with SSKI especially at higher doses, include anorexia, nausea, a metallic taste, swelling of the salivary glands, rash, and fever (Kauffman, 1995). Despite these obvious obstacles to good compliance, SSKI remains the least expensive and widely used therapy for sporotrichosis. Given that sporotrichosis primarily occurs in regions of the world where antifungal therapy with azole drugs is generally not affordable, SSKI remains the treatment of choice for individuals in these regions with uncomplicated lymphocutaneous sporotrichosis. Response to therapy among compliant patients with uncomplicated disease is in excess of 90%. Supersaturated solution of potassium iodide is not effective for visceral sporotrichosis.

Hyperthermia

Hyperthermia has been used successfully in the treatment of lymphocutaneous sporotrichosis based on an observation made originally in 1951 (Thomas et al, 1951). Most of the recent work on hyperthermic therapy for sporotrichosis has been conducted in Japan, utilizing hot baths, hot compresses, and hand-held heating devices. Hiruma and colleagues reported that 18 of 21 patients were cured when using pocket warmers directly applied over a fixed lesion for 40 to 60 minutes daily for an average of 8 weeks. Additional studies evaluating infrared therapy have been done, but have been limited due to the potential for phototoxicity (Hiruma et al, 1992).

The mechanism by which hyperthermia leads to improvement in sporotrichosis remains unknown, but probably relates to the limited thermotolerance of *S. schenckii*. Over 2 decades ago, Kwon Chung demonstrated the inability of *S. schenckii* obtained from fixed cutaneous lesions to survive at temperatures of 37°C or higher (Kwon-Chung, 1979). Additionally, Hiruma and Kagawa demonstrated that *S. schenckii* germination was markedly decreased when organisms were heated to $\geq 40°C$ (Hiruma and Kagawa, 1983). Despite clinical evidence to support its use, the role of hyperthermia as therapy for sporotrichosis remains very limited and probably should be restricted to patients with fixed cutaneous lesions who cannot afford or tolerate existing oral therapies.

Azoles

The azole antifungal drugs have become the mainstay of therapy for most patients with lymphocutaneous sporothrichosis. Of the three available oral azoles, itraconazole is the drug of choice with a success rate exceeding 90% (Restrepo et al, 1986; Sharkey-Mathis et al, 1993; Kauffman et al, 2000). Itraconazole should be administered orally at doses of 100 to 200 mg daily for at least 1 month beyond resolution of symptoms and signs. Fluconazole is generally less effective than itraconazole at similar doses and should be considered a second line therapy for sporotrichosis among patients

who either have no access to or can not tolerate itraconazole, or for whom itraconazole is contraindicated due to drug–drug interactions (Kauffman et al, 1996). Fluconazole should be administered orally starting at doses of 400 mg daily. Higher doses may be more effective but are unapproved for this purpose. Ketoconazole is the least effective of the available oral azoles and should only be used when access to the other two agents is limited (Calhoun et al, 1991). If therapy with ketoconazole is necessary, initial dosing is 400 mg daily, increasing to 600 mg and 800 mg daily as clinically indicated for unresponsive cases. All of the azole drugs are better tolerated than SSKI.

For patients with extracutaneous disease, especially those with osteoarticular disease, itraconazole 200 mg bid provides a good alternative to amphotericin B (Sharkey-Mathis et al, 1993; Kauffman et al, 2000). There has been less experience with fluconazole for this purpose (Kauffman et al, 1996). Ketoconazole is generally not recommended for the treatment of patients with extracutaneous sporotrichosis (Kauffman et al, 2000). Among patients with nonlife-threatening pulmonary disease, itraconazole provides a reasonable alternative to amphotericin B. For central nervous system and other forms of disseminated sporotrichosis, there is little role for initial therapy with any of the azoles, although they may play a role as chronic suppressive therapy among those who demonstrate an initial response to amphotericin B (Kauffman et al, 2000).

Terbinafine

Terbinafine, a recently licensed allylamine antifungal agent in the United States, has good activity against *Sporothrix schenckii* in vitro and in vivo, and there is a moderate amount of clinical data supporting its usefulness for the treatment of lymphocutaneous sporotrichosis (Hull and Vismer, 1992; Hull and Vismer, 1997; Pappas et al, 2001). In a recently completed randomized, double-blinded study involving 63 patients, two different regimens of terbinafine were compared among patients with uncomplicated lymphocutaneous sporotrichosis. Patients received either terbinafine 500 mg or 1000 mg daily for up to 24 weeks. A much better response was noted among the group receiving higher dose terbinafine (87% vs. 52%), and the percent success rate in the higher dose group was similar to that seen in patients treated with itraconazole (Pappas et al, 2001). While not approved for this purpose, terbinafine appears to be a safe, well tolerated, and reasonable alternative to itraconazole for patients with lymphocutaneous disease. Because there are little data concerning the use of terbinafine in the treatment of extracutaneous sporotrichosis, it is not recommended in this setting.

Amphotericin B

Amphotericin B, 1.0–2.0 grams total dose, remains the mainstay of therapy for patients with disseminated or life-threatening sporotrichosis, including those patients with CNS disease and moderate to severe pulmonary sporotrichosis (Kauffman et al, 2000). It is also the most appropriate initial therapy for immunocompromised patients with disseminated disease. There are little data comparing amphotericin B to other forms of therapy, especially for more serious complications of sporotrichosis such as pulmonary and CNS disease; however, the seriousness of these manifestations generally merit a more aggressive therapeutic approach. Thus, the recently published treatment guidelines for sporotrichosis suggest amphotericin B be used as initial therapy for patients with either meningeal or life-threatening disease until the condition has been clinically stabilized (Kauffman et al, 2000).

Notably, there are no comparative trials between different agents for the treatment of sporotrichosis. The largest trials involve pilot studies or dose-ranging studies to determine a range of efficacy and optimal dosing of a single agent. Furthermore, there are no studies of combinations of antifungal agents. Limitations to the study of the treatment of sporotrichosis relate to its rarity in the developed world.

Surgery

The role of surgery in the treatment of sporotrichosis is unclear. Among patients with pulmonary sporotrichosis involving a well-defined anatomic area and no more than one lobe, surgery may be a reasonable option provided there are no contraindications to surgery and there is no evidence of sporotrichosis involving the other lung or other extracutaneous sites (Pluss and Opal, 1986; Kwon-Chung and Bennett, 1992). The only other role for surgery is its use in the debridement of involved synovial spaces, particularly for synovitis involving the wrist (Stratton et al, 1981; Schwartz, 1989). The role of synovectomy in this setting is difficult to assess since most of these patients have received concomitant antifungal therapy. However, in many instances surgery is performed to preserve or improve function that has been lost due to progressive destruction of bones and joints.

PREVENTION

There is no vaccine for sporotrichosis; thus, prevention of the disease involves avoidance of exposure to the organism among individuals involved in high-risk activities. In particular, gardeners, nursery workers, foresters, veterinarians, and construction workers are at increased risk of developing sporotrichosis as a consequence of direct cutaneous inoculation. Avoidance of

exposure requires the wearing of gloves. There is no evidence that wearing a mask prevents airborne transmission of the organism. Perhaps the greatest potential role for prevention is in developing countries where sporotrichosis remains a significant regional public health threat. In those settings where lack of sanitation, poverty, and poor personal hygiene are common problems, efforts to expand awareness of the disease and improve personal hygiene might lessen morbidity associated with *S. schenckii* infection.

REFERENCES

Alberici F, Paties C T, Lombardi G, Ajello L, Daufman L, Chandler F. *Sporothrix schenckii var luriei* as the cause of sporotrichosis in Italy. *Eur J Epidemiol* 5:173–177, 1989.

Albornoz M B, Mendoza M, Torres E D. Growth temperatures of isolates of *Sporothrix schenckii* from disseminated and fixed cutaneous lesions of sporotrichosis. *Dermatologica* 95:81–83, 1986.

al-Tawfiq J A, Wools K K. Disseminated sporotrichosis and *Sporothrix schenckii* fungemia as the initial presentation of human immunodeficiency virus infection. *Clin Infect Dis* 26:1403–1406, 1998.

Altner P C, Turner R R. Sporotrichosis of bones and joints: review of the literature and report of six cases. *Clin Orthop* 68:138–148, 1970.

Barile F, Mastrolonardo M, Loconsole F, Rantuccio F. Cutaneous sporotrichosis in the period 1978–1992 in the province of Bari, Apulia, Southern Italy. *Mycoses* 36:182–185, 1993.

Burch J M, Morelli J G, Weston W L. Unsuspected sporotrichosis in childhood. *Pediatr Infect Dis J* 20:442–445, 2001.

Cabezas C, Bustamante B, Holgado W, Begue R E. Treatment of cutaneous sporotrichosis with one daily dose of potassium iodide. *Pediatri Infect Dis J* 15:352–354, 1996.

Calhoun D L, Waskin H, White M P, Bonner J R, Mulholland J H, Rumans L W, Stevens D A, Galgiani J N. Treatment of systemic sporotrichosis with ketoconazole. *Rev Infect Dis* 13:47–51, 1991.

Caravalho J, Caldwell J B, Radford B L, Feldman A R. Feline-transmitted sporotrichosis in the Southwestern United States. *West J Med* 154:462–465, 1991.

Carmichael J W. *Chrysosporium* and some other aleuriosporic hyphomycetes. *Can J Bot* 40:1137–1173, 1962.

Cartwright M J, Promersberger M, Stevens G A. *Sporothrix schenckii* endophthalmitis presenting as granulomatous uveitis. *Brit J Ophthalmol* 77:61–62, 1993.

Castrejon O V, Robles M, Zubieta Arroyo O E. Fatal fungaemia due to *Sporothrix schenckii*. *Mycoses* 38:373–376, 1995.

Centers for Disease Control. Sporotrichosis associated with Wisconsin sphagnum moss. *MMWR* 31:542–544, 1982.

Centers for Disease Control. Multistate outbreak of sporotrichosis in seedling handlers, 1988. *MMWR* 37:652–653, 1988.

Chandler J W, Kriel R L, Tosh F E. Childhood sporotrichosis. *Amer J Dis Child* 115:368–372, 1968.

Chowdhary G, Weinstein A, Klein R, Mascarenhas B R. Sporotrichal arthritis. *Ann Rheum Dis* 50:112–114, 1991.

Coles F B, Schuchat A, Hibbs J R, Kondracki S F, Salkin I F, Dixon D M, Chang H G, Duncan R A, Hurd N J, Morse D L. A multistate outbreak of sporotrichosis associated with sphagnum moss. *Am J Epidemiol* 136:475–487, 1992.

Cooper D R, Dixon D M, Salkin I F. Laboratory-acquired sporotrichosis. *J Med Vet Mycol* 30:169–191, 1992.

Crout J E, Brewer N S, Tompkins R B. Sporotrichosis arthritis: clinical features in seven patients. *Ann Intern Med* 86:294–297, 1977.

D'Alessio D J, Leavens L J, Strumpf G B, Smith C D. An outbreak of sporotrichosis in Vermont associated with sphagnum moss as the source of infection. *N Engl J Med* 272:1054–1058, 1965.

de Beurmann L, Gougerot H. *Les Sporotrichoses.* Paris: Felix Alcan, 1912.

de Lima Barros M B, Schubach T M, Galhardo M C, Schubach A D, Monteiro P C, Reis R S, Mancope-Oliveira R M, Dos Santos Lazera M, Cuzzi-Maya T, Blanco T C, Marzochi K B, Wanke B, Do Valle A C. Sporotrichosis: an emergent zoonosis in Rio de Janeiro. *Memorias do Instituto Oswaldo Cruz* 96:777–779, 2001.

Dixon D M, Duncan R A, Hurn N J. Use of a mouse model to evaluate clinical and environmental isolates of *Sporothrix* spp. from the largest U.S. outbreak of sporotrichosis. *J Clin Microbiol* 30:951–951, 1992.

Donabedian H, O'Donnell E, Olszewski C, MacArthur R D, Budd N. Disseminated cutaneous and meningeal sporotrichosis in an AIDS patient. *Diag Microbiol Infect Dis* 18:111–115, 1994.

Edwards C, Reuther W L, Greer D L. Disseminated osteoarticular sporotrichosis: treatment in a patient with acquired immunodeficiency syndrome. *So Med J* 93:803–806, 2000.

Ellner P D. An outbreak of sporotrichosis in Florida. *JAMA* 173:113–117, 1960.

Farley M L, Fagan M F, Mabry L C, Wallace R J. Presentation of *Sporothrix schenckii* in pulmonary cytology specimens. *Acta Cytologica* 35:389–395, 1991.

Fernandes K S, Mathews H L, Lopes Bezerra L M. Differences in virulence of *Sporothrix schenckii* conidia related to culture conditions and cell-wall components. *J Med Microbiol* 48:195–203, 1999.

Fleury R N, Taborda P R, Gupta A K, Fujita M S, Rosa P S, Weckwerth A C, Negrao M S, Bastazini I. Zoonotic sporotrichosis. Transmission to humans by infected domestic cat scratching: report of four cases in Sao Paulo, Brazil. *Int J Dermatol* 40:318–322, 2001.

Forrester H R. Sporotrichosis, an occupational dermatosis. *JAMA* 87:1605–1609, 1926.

Garrett H D, Robbins J B. An unusual occurrence of sporotrichosis: eight cases in one residence. *Arch Dermatol* 82:570–571, 1960.

Gluckman I. Sporotrichosis in children. *S Afr Med J* 39:991–1002, 1965.

Hajjeh R, McDonnell S, Reef S, Licitra C, Hankins M, Toth B, Padhye A, Kaufman L, Pasarell L, Cooper C, Hutwagner L, Hopkins R, McNeil M. Outbreak of sporotrichosis among tree nursery workers. *J Infect Dis* 176:499–504, 1997.

Hektoen L, Perkins C F. Refractory subcutaneous abscesses caused by *Sporothrix schenckii*. A new pathogenic fungus. *J Exp Med* 5:77–89, 1900.

Hiruma M, Kagawa S. The effects of heat on *Sporothrix schenckii in vitro* and *in vivo*. *Mycopathologica* 84:21–30, 1983.

Hiruma M, Kawada A, Noguchi H, Ishibashi A, Conti Diaz I A. Hyperthermic treatment of sporotrichosis: experimental use of infrared and far infrared rays. *Mycoses* 35:293–299, 1992.

Hull P R, Vismer H F. Treatment of cutaneous sporotrichosis with terbinafine. *Brit J Dermatol* 39:51–55, 1992.

Hull P R, Vismer H F. Potential use of terbinafine in the treatment of cutaneous sporotrichosis. *Rev Contemp Pharmacother* 8:343–347, 1997.

Itoh M, Okamoto S, Kariya H. Survey of 200 cases of sporotrichosis. *Dermatologica* 172:209–213, 1986.

Kauffman C A. Old and new therapies for sporotrichosis. *Clin Infect Dis* 21:981–985, 1995.

Kauffman C A, Pappas P G, McKinsey D S, Greenfield R A, Perfect J R, Cloud G A, Thomas C J, Dismukes W E. Treatment of lymphocutaneous and visceral sporotrichosis with fluconazole. *Clin Infect Dis* 22:46–50, 1996.

Kauffman C A. Sporotrichosis. *Clin Infect Dis* 29:231–237, 1999.

Kauffman C A, Hajjeh R, Chapman S W for the Mycoses Study Group. Practice guidelines for the management of patients with sporotrichosis. *Clin Infect Dis* 30:684–687, 2000.

Keiser P. Whittle D. Sporotrichosis in human immunodeficiency virus-infected patients: report of a case. *Rev Infect Dis* 13:1027–1028, 1991.

Kostman J R, DiNubile M J. Nodular lymphangitis: a distinctive but often unrecognized syndrome. *Ann Intern Med* 118:883–888, 1993.

Kurosawa A, Pollock S C, Collins M P, Kraff C R, Tso M O. *Sporothrix schenckii* endophthalmitis in a patient with human immunodeficiency virus infection. *Arch Ophthalmol* 106:376–380, 1988.

Kushuhara M, Hachisuka H, Sasai Yoichiro. Statistical survey of 150 cases with sporotrichosis. *Mycopathologia* 102:129–133, 1988.

Kwon-Chung K J. Comparison of isolates of *Sporothrix schenckii* obtained from fixed cutaneous lesions with isolates from other types of lesions. *J Infect Dis* 139:424–431, 1979.

Kwon-Chung K J, Bennett J E. Sporotrichosis. In: Kwon-Chung K J, Bennett J E, eds. *Medical Mycology*. Philadelphia: Lea & Febiger, 707–729, 1992.

Lurie H I. Five unusual cases of sporotrichosis from South Africa showing lesions in muscles, bones, and viscera. *Brit J Surg* 50:585–591, 1963.

Mackinnon J E, Conti-Diaz I A. The effect of temperature on sporotrichosis. *Sabouraudia* 2:56–59, 1962.

Mackinnon J E, Conti-Diaz I A, Yarzabal L A. Experimental sporotrichosis, ambient temperature and amphotericin B. *Sabouraudia* 3:192–194, 1964.

Mackinnon J E, Conti-Diaz I A, Gezuele E, Civila E, DaLuz S. Isolation of *Sporothrix schenckii* from nature and considerations on its pathogenicity and ecology. *Sabouraudia* 7:38–45, 1969.

Ochoa A G, Ricoy E, Velasco O, Lopez R, Navarrete F. Valoracion comparativa de los antigenos polisacarido y celllar de *Sporothrix schenckii*. *Rev Invest Salud Publ Mex* 30:303–315, 1970.

Orr E R, Riley H D. Sporotrichosis in childhood: report of ten cases. *J Pediatrics* 78:951–957, 1971.

Pappas P G, Tellez I, Deep A A, Nolasco D, Holgado W, Bustamante B. Sporotrichosis in Peru: description of a hyperendemic area. *Clin Infect Dis* 30:65–70, 2000.

Pappas P G, Bustamante B, Nolasco D, Restrepo A, Toban A, Tiraboschi Foss N, Dietze R, Fothergill A, Perez A, Felser J. Treatment of lymphocutaneous sporotrichosis with terbinafine: results of randomized double-blind trial. 39th Annual Infectious Diseases Society of America Meeting, San Francisco, CA. Abstract #648, 2001.

Pluss J L, Opal S M. Pulmonary sporotrichosis: review of treatment and outcome. *Medicine* 65:143–153, 1986.

Powell K E, Taylor A, Phillips B J, Durward L B, Campbell G D, Kaufman L, Kaplan W. Cutaneous sporotrichosis in forestry workers: epidemic due to contaminated sphagnum moss. *JAMA* 240:232–235, 1978.

Reed K D, Moore F M, Geiger G E, Stemper M E. Zoonotic transmission of sporotrichosis: case report and review. *Clin Infect Dis* 16:384–387, 1993.

Restrepo A, Robledo J, Gomez I, Tabares A M, Gutiérrez R. Itraconazole therapy in lymphangitic and cutaneous sporotrichosis. *Arch Dermatol* 122:413–417, 1986.

Rex J H, Bennett J E. Administration of potassium iodide to normal volunteers does not increase killing of *Sporothrix schenckii* by their neutrophils or monocytes. *J Med Vet Mycol* 28:158–189, 1990.

Romero-Martinez R, Wheeler M, Guerrero-Plata A, Rico G, Torres-Guerrero H. Biosynthesis and functions of melanin in *Sporothrix schenckii*. *Infect Immun* 68:3696–3703, 2000.

Saravanakumar P S, Eslami P, Zar F A. Lymphocutaneous sporotri-

chosis associated with a squirrel bite: case report and review. *Clin Infect Dis* 23:647–648, 1996.

Schenck B R. Refractory subcutaneous abscesses caused by a fungus possibly related to the sporotricha. *Johns Hopkins Hosp Bull* 9: 286–290, 1898.

Schwartz D A. *Sporothrix* tenosynovitis—differential diagnosis of granulomatous inflammatory disease of the joints. *J Rheumatol* 16:550–553, 1989.

Scott E N, Kaufman L, Brown A C, Muchmore H G. Serologic studies in the diagnosis and management of meningitis due to *Sporothrix schenckii. N Engl J Med* 317:935–938, 1987.

Sharkey-Mathis P K, Kauffman C A, Graybill J R, Stevens D A, Hostetler J S, Cloud G, Dismukes W E. Treatment of sporotrichosis with itraconazole. *Am J Med* 95:279–285, 1993.

Sterling J B, Heymann W R. Potassium iodide in dermatology: a 19th century drug for the 21st century-users, pharmacology, adverse effects, and contraindications. *J Am Acad Dermatol* 43:691–697, 2000.

Stratton C W, Lichtenstein K A, Lowenstein S R, Phelps D B, Reller L B. Granulomatous tenosynovitis and carpal tunnel syndrome caused by *Sporothrix schenckii. Am J Med* 71:161–164, 1981.

Tachibani T, Matsuyama T, Ito M, Mitsuyama M. *Sporothrix schenckii* thermo-intolerant mutants losing fatal visceral infectivity but retaining high cutaneous infectivity. *Med Mycol* 39:295–298, 2001.

Thomas C L, Pierce H E, Babiner G W. Sporotrichosis responding to fever therapy. *JAMA* 147:1342–1343, 1951.

Thompson D W, Kaplan A W. Laboratory-acquired sporotrichosis. *Sabouraudia* 15:167–170, 1977.

Transvaal Mine Medical Officers' Association. Sporotrichosis infection in mines of the Witwatersrand: a symposium. Johannesburg, Transvaal Chamber of Mines, 1947.

Urabe H, Nagasthima T. Mechanism of antifungal action of potassium iodide on sporotrichosis. *Dermatol Int* 1:36–38, 1969.

Velasco-Castrejón O, Gonzalez-Ochoa Y A. La esporotricosis en un peque o poblado de la Sierra de Puebla. *Rev Invest Salud Publ Mex* 36:133–137, 1976.

Ware A J, Cockrell C J, Skiest D J, Kussman H M. Disseminated sporotrichosis with extensive cutaneous involvement in a patient with AIDS. *J Am Acad Dermatol* 40:350–355, 1999.

Wilson D E, Mann J J, Bennett J E, Utz J P. Clinical features of extracutaneous sporotrichosis. *Medicine* (Baltimore) 46:265–279, 1967.

Yamada Y, Dekio S, Jidoi, J, Ozasa S, Tohgi K. A familial occurrence of sporotrichosis. *J Dermatol* 17:255–259, 1990.

Yao J, Penn R G, Ray S. Articular sporotrichosis. *Clin Orthop* 204:207–214, 1986.

23

Penicilliosis

KENRAD E. NELSON AND THIRA SIRISANTHANA

More than 200 species of the *Penicillium* genus have been described. *Penicillium* organisms are abundant in nature and are common laboratory contaminants. However, *Penicillium marneffei* is the only dimorphic species. The organism is commonly responsible for disseminated invasive infections in humans with HIV infection or AIDS in the endemic areas of Southeast Asia and southern China. *Penicillium marneffei* has also been found to cause natural infections in several species of rodents in the endemic areas and rodents can be infected experimentally.

HISTORY

Penicillium marneffei was originally isolated from the liver of a bamboo rat (*Rhizomys sinensis*) at the Pasteur Institute in Dalat, Viet Nam in 1956. Capponi and colleagues observed the death of bamboo rats due to disseminated infections with *P. marneffei* involving their reticuloendothelial system (Capponi et al, 1956). These investigators passed the newly discovered organism experimentally in mice, and it was sent to the Pasteur Institute in Paris for further study. At the Pasteur Institute, the fungus was characterized by Segretain and named *Penicillium marneffei* in honor of Dr. Hubert Marneffe, the Director of the Pasteur Institute of Indochina (Segretain, 1959a). Subsequently, Segretain became the first known human to be infected with the organism in 1959 when he accidentally stuck his finger with a needle he was using to inoculate a hamster. The clinical manifestations of his infection were a subcutaneous nodule at the site of the inoculation and lymphadenitis involving the draining auxiliary lymph nodes. The infection responded to treatment with high doses of oral nystatin.

The first natural human infection with *P. marneffei* was reported in 1973 in a 61-year-old U.S. missionary who was suffering from Hodgkin's disease. His infection was discovered when he underwent a staging splenectomy for Hodgkin's disease (Di Salvo et al, 1973). The missionary had visited Southeast Asia after Hodgkin's disease had been diagnosed 1 year prior to

the splenectomy. At surgery the excised spleen contained a tan nodular mass, 9 cm in diameter with a necrotic center, which grew *P. marneffei* when cultured on Sabouraud dextrose agar at 25°C. The patient survived after being treated with amphotericin B.

The second case of penicilliosis was reported in 1984 in a 59-year-old man who had traveled in Southeast Asia (Pautler et al, 1984). He had recurrent episodes of hemoptysis and *P. marneffei* organisms were isolated from his sputum. Also in 1984, five additional cases who had been seen at Ramathibodi Hospital in Bangkok, Thailand between 1974 and 1982 were reported (Jayanetra et al, 1984). Eight cases of *P. marneffei* infection were reported from Guangxi province in southern China that had occurred between 1964 and 1983 (Deng et al, 1985). Additional cases were recognized from 1985 to 1991 in southern China (Li et al, 1985; Wang et al, 1989; Li et al, 1991). These patients were not immunocompromised. All cases had occurred prior to the AIDS epidemic in Southeast Asia.

In the late 1980s and early 1990s several reports of disseminated penicilliosis in HIV-infected patients were published; these included patients who were infected in Southeast Asia but whose infections were diagnosed after they returned to the United States or Europe (Piehl et al, 1988; Peto, et al, 1988; Hulshof et al, 1990; Jones and See 1992; Viviani et al, 1993; Hilmarsdottir et al, 1993; Kronauer et al, 1993; Sobotta et al, 1996). An HIV-positive Congolese physician developed disseminated penicilliosis while he was working at the Pasteur Institute in Paris (Hilmarsdottir et al, 1994). The organism had not been handled directly by the physician, but organisms were being cultured in the building where he was attending a course. This case illustrates the potential hazard of laboratory acquired infection and suggests an airborne route of infection.

As the HIV/AIDS pandemic has spread in Southeast Asia, *P. marneffei* infection has become a very common opportunistic infection in HIV-infected patients in the region (Supparatpinyo et al, 1992a; Supparatpinyo et al, 1994; Nelson et al, 1999). Infection with this organism is now the fourth most common opportunistic infection in AIDS patients in northern Thailand, exceeded only by tuberculosis, *Pneumocystis carinii* pneumonia, and cryptococcosis (Supparatpinyo et al, 1994). A total of 550 cases of penicilliosis and 793 cases of cryptococcosis were diagnosed at Chiang Mai University hospital in northern Thailand, between 1991 and 1994. Nearly all of these patients were HIV positive (Chariyalertsak et al, 1996). The endemic area includes Thailand, Southern China, Hong Kong, Taiwan, Burma, Laos, Vietnam, Malaysia, and northeast India.

EPIDEMIOLOGY

The natural reservoir of *P. marneffei* is almost certainly the soil. However, the organism was first isolated from Chinese bamboo rats, *R. sinensis*, in Vietnam in 1956 (Capponi et al, 1956). Since the original isolation, several investigators in China and Southeast Asia have cultured rodents and environmental samples in order to better understand the reservoir. The organism has been isolated from the internal organs of four species of bamboo rats in Asia (Table 23–1). Two investigators reported data from bamboo rats collected from the Guangxi province of China. Deng and colleagues isolated *P. marneffei* from the internal organs of 18 of 19 *R. pruinosus* rats (Deng et al, 1986) and Li and colleagues found the organism in 15 of 16 *R. pruinosus* rats (Li et al, 1989). These infected animals showed no signs of illness. However, fatal infections had been observed in bamboo rats that were experimentally infected in Vietnam in 1956 (Capponi et al, 1956; Segretain, 1959b). In another survey in Guangxi province in China, workers isolated *P. marneffei* from 39 of 43 bamboo rats (37 of 41 *R. pruinosus* and 2 of 2 *R. sinensis*) (Deng et al, 1988). They were also able to isolate *P. marneffei* from soil samples taken from 3 burrows of *R. pruinosus* rats and from the feces of 3 animals. Another survey in Southern China isolated *P. marneffei* from 114 of 179 (63.7%) *R. pruinosus* rats (Wei et al, 1987). A study of the prevalence of *P. marneffei* infections in bamboo rats in central Thailand was done

in 1987 and *P. marneffei* was isolated from 6 of 8 (75%) *R. pruinosus* rats and 6 of 31 (19%) *Cannomys badius* rats (Ajello et al, 1995). Organisms were cultured from the lungs (83%), liver (33%), and pancreas (33%) of these animals.

The prevalence of *P. marneffei* in bamboo rats from northern Thailand was studied in 75 bamboo rats; *P. marneffei* was isolated from the internal organs of 13 of 14 (92.8%) large bamboo rats, *R. sumatrensis*, and 3 of 10 (30%) reddish-brown small bay bamboo rats, *Cannomys badius* (Chariyalertsak et al, 1996). All 51 grayish black *C. badius* rats were negative on culture. Among the *R. sumatrensis* rats, the fungus was most commonly isolated from lungs (86%), spleen (50%), and liver (29%). The investigators also studied 28 soil samples and 67 environmental samples, which had been collected from the residential areas of patients with clinical *P. marneffei* infection. These samples were evaluated using a modified flotation method combined with mouse inoculation to isolate the fungus from the environmental samples (Vanittanakom et al, 1995). *Penicillium marneffei* was isolated from one soil sample obtained from a burrow of *R. sumatrensis* rats using this method (Chariyalertsak et al, 1996). The other environmental samples were negative.

It is somewhat curious that the prevalence of *P. marneffei* infection among bamboo rats is very high in the numerous surveys that have been reported in the literature, yet the fungus has not been isolated from any other animal in nature. This observation might reflect the animals that are selected for study, since negative results have not been reported from other species. However, in part, this finding might also reflect the fact that the range of the two genera of bamboo rats, *Rhizomys* and *Cannomys*, coincide with the environmental soil reservoir of *P. marneffei* (Corbet et al, 1992). Furthermore, bamboo rats inhabit remote mountainous areas and have extensive soil contact when they burrow. The common isolation of *P. marneffei* from the lungs of infected animals and the rarity of recovery of the organism from the gastrointestinal tract sug-

TABLE 23–1. *Prevalence of* Penicillium marneffei *Infection in Trapped Bamboo Rats in Asia*

Species	Positive/Tested (%)	Country	References
Rhizomys sinensis	1/1 (100)	Vietnam	Capponi et al, 1956
(Chinese bamboo rat)	2/2 (100)	China	Deng et al, 1988
Rhizomys pruinosus	37/41 (90)	China	Deng et al, 1988
(Hoary bamboo rat)	15/16 (94)	China	Li et al, 1988
	114/179 (64)	China	Wei et al, 1987
	6/8 (75)	Thailand	Ajello et al, 1995
Cannomys badius	6/31 (19)	Thailand	Ajello et at, 1995
(Bay bamboo rat or lesser bamboo rat)	3/61 (5)	Thailand	Chariyalertsak et al, 1996a
Rhizomys sumatrensis	13/14 (93)	Thailand	Chariyalertsak et al, 1996a
(Sumatran bamboo rat)			

gests that *P. marneffei* infection is commonly acquired by these animals by inhalation of conidia rather then by ingestion.

A case-control study compared patients with AIDS who had *P. marneffei* infections to AIDS patients with negative *P. marneffei* cultures in order to help understand the risk factors associated with infection (Chariyalertsak et al, 1997). This study included 80 patients with penicilliosis and 160 control AIDS patients who were admitted to Chiang Mai University Hospital in northern Thailand between December 1993 and October 1995. The main risk factor was occupational soil exposures, especially during the rainy season. Both cases and controls often were familiar with and had seen bamboo rats; 31.3% of cases and 28.1% of controls had eaten bamboo rats but these differences were not significant. The most tenable hypothesis at present is that *P. marneffei* infections, both in humans and bamboo rats, are acquired from a common soil reservoir.

Disseminated *P. marneffei* infections in northern Thailand have been markedly seasonal with a doubling of cases during the rainy season (Chariyalertsak et al, 1996b). This seasonality contrasts with *C. neoformans* infection in AIDS patients, which has shown a steady increase during the 1990s as the number of AIDS cases has increased, but is not associated with seasonality. This seasonality suggests that many *P. marneffei* infections in AIDS patients may be acquired recently. Also, the environmental reservoir for *P. marneffei* appears to expand during the rainy season. Penicilliosis, while occurring in AIDS patients throughout Thailand, is much more common in the upper northern areas of the country (Chariyalertsak et al, 2001). Whereas penicilliosis accounted for nearly 7.0% of AIDS-defining illnesses in northern Thailand, penicilliosis was seen in only 0.4%–1.0% of AIDS patients in other regions of the country.

MYCOLOGY

Penicillium marneffei grows as a mould on Sabouraud dextrose agar at 25°C. The mycelial form of the organism is quite variable with green/yellow color with a reddish center. The reverse side of the colony becomes red-brown and a soluble red pigment diffuses into the agar (See Color Fig. 23–1 in separate color insert). Microscopic examination of the mycelial colony reveals hyaline, septate, branched hyphae with branched conidiophores, or penicilli (See Color Fig. 23–2 in separate color insert). The conidiophores consist of basal stripes with terminal verticils of 3 to 5 metulae. Each metula has 3 to 16 phialides. The conidia are oval, smooth-walled, and are 3 μm $\times$ 2 μm. They are formed basipetally in chains from each phialide. When the or-

ganism is transferred to brain–heart infusion agar and incubated at 37°C, white to tan-colored colonies of the yeast form develop; no diffusible pigment is produced. Under the microscope the yeasts are unicellular, pleomorphic, elliptical to rectangular cells, which are approximately 2 μm $\times$ 6 μm in diameter and divide by fission. One or sometimes two septae are seen in the yeast cells.

The organism was first studied in 1959 (Segretain, 1959a). *Penicillium marneffei* was originally classified among *Penicillium* species in the section Asymmetrica, subsection of Divaricata in Raper and Thom's taxonomic classification of *Penicillium* species (Raper and Thom, 1949). Pitt later placed *P. marneffei* in the subgenus *Biverticillium* (Pitt, 1979). Recent phylogenetic analysis of nucleotide sequences of nuclear and michondrial ribosomal DNA has found that *P. marneffei* is closely related to species of *Penicillium* subgenus *Biverticillium* and sexual *Talaromyces* species with asexual biverticillate states (LoBuglio and Taylor, 1995). This genetic analysis allowed the design of unique oligonucleatide primers for the specific amplification of *P. marneffei* DNA.

Penicillium marneffei requires an organic source of nitrogen for mycelial growth. Casein hydrolysate, peptone, and asparagine are utilized whereas NaNO$_3$ and (NH$_4$)$_2$ PO$_4$ are not. Glucose, lactose, xylose, maltose, laevulose, and mannitol are used as carbon sources. The organism is sensitive to cycloheximide (Sekhon et al, 1982). Investigators have biotyped 32 clinical isolates of *P. marneffei* and found 17 different biotypes (Wong et al, 2001). However, none of the biotypes correlated with the clinical characteristics of the infection.

PATHOLOGY AND PATHOGENESIS

Penicillium marneffei infection results from the inhalation of infectious spores (arthroconidia) from the mould form of the organism. At body temperatures (35°C–37°C), the fungus converts to the yeast form which is disseminated by hematogenous means. The organism primarily infects the reticuloendothelial system, commonly involving liver, spleen, lymph nodes, bone marrow, bone, skin, and lungs. Similar to other pathogenic dimorphic fungi, the initial host response to *P. marneffei* is histiocytic in nature. The infected histiocytes contain a few to many globose to oval yeast cells of *P. marneffei* of fairly uniform size. In the immunocompetent host, the immune response leads to the formation of granulomata including histiocytes, lymphocytes, plasma cells, and multinucleated giant cells. In patients whose cellular immunity is compromised, tissue necrosis occurs with little or no granuloma formation. Necrotic lesions are surrounded by histiocytes containing yeast cells. Also many extracellular yeasts are present, which are longer and may be irregular in shape, compared to intracellular organisms. This histopathologic appearance is common in patients with disseminated penicilliosis. As the infection progresses, the intracellular fungi are released after cellular disruption and abscess formation and necrosis may occur.

In histologic specimens, neither the cell wall nor the cytoplasm of *P. marneffei* cells take up the hematoxylin-eosin stain well. Thus, in H and E stained sections, the organisms may appear to be encapsulated. However, the cell walls and septa are readily stained with Gomori methenamine-silver or periodic-acid Schiff stains. The *P. marneffei* organisms in histiocytes may resemble *H. capsulatum var capsulatum*. However, when found extracellularly, *P. marneffei* is usually considerably larger than *H. capsulatum*. The extracellular *P. marneffei* organisms are elongated, sometimes curved, and measure up to 8 to 13 μm in length. In contrast, yeast cells of *H. capsulatum var capsulatum* are smaller in size, measuring 2–4 μm. By contrast, *H. capsulatum var duboisii* cells are larger, measuring 8–15 μm. *Penicillium marneffei* organisms characteristically contain a single transverse septum and divide by schizogony (fission), whereas *Histoplasma* divide by budding (Table 23–2).

Chronic latent infections with *P. marneffei* are likely common among persons exposed in areas where the organism is endemic. This hypothesis is supported, in part, by analogy with histoplasmosis pathogenesis and by the long latent periods in some patients between exposure in an endemic area and the onset of clinical infection subsequent to immunosuppression from HIV infection (Jones and See, 1992; Hilmarsdottir et al, 1993). However, no laboratory methods have been reported to detect latently infected individuals. The development of a skin test, or other methods, to detect delayed type hypersensitivity has not been reported for *P. marneffei*. The normal host develops a cell-mediated immune response to *P. marneffei* (Deng et al, 1988). The role of T lymphocytes in host defenses against *P. marneffei*

has been evaluated in mice experimentally depleted of CD4+ T lymphocytes (Viviani et al, 1993). These mice developed disseminated infections similar to those seen in AIDS patients. In addition, the in vitro interaction of *P. marneffei* with human leukocytes demonstrated that monocyte-derived macrophages recognize and phagocytose *P. marneffei* even in the absence of opsonization (Rongruagruang and Levitz, 1999). However, serum factors are required to stimulate TNF-a production. Additional research on the sequence of phagocytosis and killing or persistence of *P. marneffei* is needed in order to better understand the natural history and pathogenesis of this infection.

CLINICAL FEATURES

Clinically apparent infection with *P. marneffei* occurs most frequently in patients who are severely immunocompromised from an HIV infection. However, infections may also occur in healthy persons or in those immunocompromised for reasons other than HIV/AIDS. Serologic evidence of subclinical infection in a laboratory technician working with the organism has been demonstrated (Vanittanakom et al, 1997b). It is likely that subclinical infections may occur commonly in persons living in endemic areas who are exposed to the organism in nature. However, there is no method to document subclinical infections at present. Disseminated infections have been documented among individuals who have not had contact with areas where the organism is endemic for more than a decade (Jones and See, 1992).

Typical symptoms and signs of disseminated penicilliosis include fever, malaise, marked weight loss, generalized lymphadenopathy, hepatosplenomegaly, and cough (Supparatpinyo et al, 1994; Nelson et al, 1999) (Table 23–3). These nonspecific symptoms are commonly experienced by patients with other chronic infections, such as tuberculosis and other disseminated mycoses. In addition, over 70% of HIV-infected pa-

TABLE 23–2. *Microbiologic Characteristics of* P. marneffei *and* H. Capsulatum

Characteristic	P. marneffei	H. capsulatum
Morphologic features	Biphasic (mould form at 25°C–30°C, yeast form at 35°C–37°C	Biphasic (mould form at 25°C–30°C, yeast form at 35°C–37°C)
Distribution	Southern China and Southeast Asia	Worldwide (N. America, S. America, Asia, Africa (H. duboisii)
Tissue form	Yeast	Yeast
Size; intracellular (Macrophages)	2–3 × 2–6 μm	2–3 × 2–3 μm
Extracellular	2–3 × 8–13 μm, elongated, curved Septae visible with GMS stain	Smaller 3–4 μm, diameter (H. duboisii larger, 6–17 μm diameter) No septae
Cell division	Schizogony (fission)	Budding
Specific exoantigen	Positive	Positive

TABLE 23–3. *Signs and Symptoms in 80 HIV-infected Patients with Disseminated* Penicillium marneffei *Infection in N. Thailand*

Symptoms	Number	(%)
Fever	74	(93)
Skin Lesions	54	(68)
Cough	39	(49)
Diarrhea	25	(31)
Signs		
Elevated temp ≥ 38.3°C	79	(99)
Marked weight loss	61	(76)
Anemia	62	(78)
Oral candidiasis	59	(74)
Skin lesions	57	(71)
Generalized lymphadenopathy	46	(58)
Hepatomegaly	41	(51)
Splenomegaly	13	(16)
Genital ulcer	5	(6)

Source: Supparatpinyo et al, Lancet 344:110–113, 1994.

tients with disseminated *P. marneffei* infections present with skin lesions, which are typically symmetrical lesions on the face, chest, and extremities. They appear originally as papules and subsequently become umbilicated, and may become necrotic (See Color Figs. 23–3, 23–4, and 23–5 in separate color insert). Some patients may have smaller, nearly confluent papules, which resemble acne vulgaris or seborrhea. Although skin lesions are more common in patients with *P. marneffei* infection than in those with histoplasmosis or cryptococcosis, the appearance of these lesions is not sufficiently characteristic to be diagnostic. However, a diagnosis can be made by examining a Wright's stain of a skin biopsy or skin smear. Patients with HIV infection who have disseminated penicilliosis are usually severely immunosuppressed with CD4+ cell counts below 100 cells/μl; the mean CD4+ cell count in one series of cases was 63.8 cells/μl (Vanittankom et al, 1997c). Disseminated penicilliosis infections have been reported in children with AIDS who lived in an endemic area. However, the incidence appears to be lower in pediatric than in adult AIDS cases, probably because of less frequent exposure to an environmental reservoir among children. One study reported 5 cases of penicilliosis among 157 pediatric AIDS cases diagnosed in northern Thailand (Sirisanthana et al, 1995).

UNUSUAL CLINICAL MANIFESTATIONS

As the pandemic of HIV/AIDS spreads in Asia and penicilliosis is more widely appreciated, an increasing number of patients have been reported with unusual manifestations of *P. marneffei* infections. Patients with chronic lymphadenopathy resembling tuberculous lymphadenopathy have been reported from Hong Kong (Yuen et al, 1986). Osteomyelitis has been reported in

infected adults and may be more common in pediatric patients infected with *P. marneffei* (Chan and Woo, 1990; Sirisanthana et al, 1995). Some patients have prominent pulmonary symptoms, including localized bronchopulmonary disease, bronchopneumonia, cavitary lung disease, and pleural effusions (Chan et al, 1989; Supparatpinyo et al, 1994), and a retropharyngeal abscess with upper airway obstruction has been observed (Ko, 1994). One patient had reactive hemophagocytic syndrome characterized by the proliferation of activated histiocytes throughout the reticuloendothelial system (Chim et al, 1998), and *P. marneffei* has been noted rarely to cause oral (Tong et al, 2001) and genital ulceration (Supparatpinyo et al, 1994).

PENICILLIOSIS IN HIV-NEGATIVE PATIENTS

Although most patients with disseminated penicilliosis infection are severely immunocompromised due to AIDS, some patients are HIV negative. Cooper and Haycocks reviewed 63 penicilliosis cases that had been reported in HIV-negative patients. Twenty-four of the 63 patients (38%) had other conditions predisposing them to a systemic fungal infection. The response to antifungal therapy did not differ substantially by whether or not the patients were HIV infected; patients who were untreated had very high mortality rates irrespective of their HIV status (Cooper and Haycocks, 2000).

Investigators from Hong Kong compared the clinical and laboratory features of 8 HIV-positive and 7 HIV-negative patients with penicilliosis (Wong et al, 2000). Most of the HIV-negative patients (85.2%) had underlying diseases including hematologic malignancies or had received corticosteroids or cytotoxic drugs. The clinical features were not greatly different in the two groups of patients. However, HIV-infected patients had a higher prevalence of fungemia. The investigators, utilizing a *P. marneffei*-specific mannoprotein, Mp1 EIA, found that serum antigen titers were higher in HIV-positive patients, whereas serum antibody levels were higher in HIV-negative patients.

DIAGNOSIS

The diagnosis of penicilliosis rests on the demonstration of the organism in the tissues or the isolation of the organism in cultures from infected patients. The organism grows readily on routine mycological media, such as Sabouraud dextrose agar or inhibitory mould agar. When cultures are incubated at 25°C–30°C, *P. marneffei* grows as a mould with typical filamentous reproductive structures of the genus *Penicillium*. The mould form produces a pink or rose-red pigment that diffuses into the medium (See Color Fig. 23–1 in separate color insert). Other *Penicillium* species may also produce a pigment (Viviani and Tortorano, 1998). Therefore, conversion of an organism to the yeast form is required before concluding the isolate is *P. marneffei*. The organism grows as a yeast when incubated at 35°C–37°C. This form does not produce a red pigment. When incubated at this temperature, the organism undergoes transition into the yeast phase after 12–24 hours or so of incubation. The conidia swell and develop into septate hyphae. These hyphae fragment and develop single cells that divide by schizogony (fission). The conversion of the mycelial phase of the organism into the fission yeast phase at higher incubation temperatures is diagnostic of *P. marneffei*. No other *Penicillium* converts to the yeast phase when incubated at 35°C–37°C. In addition, an exoantigen test for *P. marneffei* has been described, which can also be used to identify cultures of the organism (Sekhon et al, 1982a).

The organism has been isolated from several sites including skin, blood, bone marrow, lymph nodes, and sputum (Table 23–4). In a population of patients in northern Thailand with disseminated penicilliosis, the organism was isolated from the blood cultures of 76% of 78 patients (Supparatpinyo et al, 1992a). However, the blood cultures were positive for gram negative bacilli (*Salmonella choleraesuis*, *S. enteritidis* and *Shigella flexneri*) in 9 of the 19 patients whose cultures did not yield *P. marneffei*. Since these gram negative organisms grow more rapidly, they could have outgrown the fungus and been responsible for a false negative culture for *P. marneffei*.

Detection of the organism in biopsies or touch smears of skin lesions or bone marrow aspirates is often possible. A presumptive diagnosis can be made if microscopic examination of a Wright or Giemsa-stained specimen discloses intracellular or extracellular basophilic, spherical, oval, and elliptical yeast-like organisms that are 3–8 μm in diameter, and if the organisms have a clear central septation and are dividing by schizogony (fission) (See Color Fig. 23–6 in separate color insert). *Histoplasma capsulatum* can resemble *P. marneffei* but *H. capsulatum* divides by budding and is usually

smaller in size (Table 23–2). Occasionally *P. marneffei* can be detected in stained smears of peripheral blood (Supparatpinyo et al, 1994b).

Immunohistochemical and Serologic Diagnosis
The use of an exoantigen test has been described for the identification of *P. marneffei* and its differentiation from other species of *Penicillium* (Sekhon et al, 1982; Sekhon et al, 1989). However, the test is not widely used because commercial reagents are not available. Investigators have described the use of a monoclonal antibody in formalin-fixed tissues to detect a specific galactomannan that has an epitope common to *P. marneffei* and *Aspergillus* species (Estrada et al, 1992). The two invasive fungi must then be differentiated using morphologic criteria. Workers have also reported the use of a specific fluorescent antibody, which will differentiate *P. marneffei* from other dimorphic fungi in tissue sections (Kaufman et al, 1995).

Several investigators, using different methodologies, have reported the detection of antibodies to *P. marneffei*-antigens in infected patients. A study in an HIV-infected patient found *P. marneffei* antibodies in serum specimens using immunodiffusion methods with a mycelial phase culture filtrate as antigen (Viviani et al, 1993). Similar antibodies were found in immunocompetent patients infected with *P. marneffei* (Sekhon et al, 1994). Immunodiffusion has been used to detect antibodies to specific fission arthroconidial filtrate antigens. However, only 2 of 17 *P. marneffei*-infected patients had antibody responses with this assay (Kaufman et al, 1996). An indirect fluorescent antibody test for *P. marneffei* successfully detected antibodies in 8 infected patients and was negative in uninfected controls (Yuen et al, 1994). Serum antibodies were detected by ELISA to a purified recombinant mannoprotein of *P. marneffei* in 14 of 17 (82%) HIV-infected patients with documented infection (Cao et al, 1998). No false-positive results were found in 90 healthy blood donors, 20 patients with typhoid fever, or 55 patients with tuberculosis. The protein antigens of yeast and mould phases of *P. marneffei* have been studied by gel electrophoresis and immunoblot assays (Vanittanakom et al, 1997a). More than 20 yeast phase proteins were detected, of which 10 reacted with IgG in the pooled sera of 28 AIDS patients with *P. marneffei* infection. Four immunogenic proteins of 200, 88, 54, and 50 kDA size were produced in large quantity by cultures in the early stationary growth phase. Antibodies to 2 of these proteins, 54 and 50 kDA, were detected by immunoblot in about 60% of *P. marneffei*-infected AIDS patients but rarely (< 5%–10%) in AIDS patients without penicilliosis or other controls. One patient's sera was strongly positive 2 months prior to a clinical *P. marneffei* infection and one asymptomatic laboratory

TABLE 23–4. *Tissue or Body Fluid Sources of Isolates of* P. marneffei *in 80 HIV-infected Patients with Penicilliosis From N. Thailand*

Specimen	Number	Positive (%)
Blood culture	78	59 (76)
Skin	52	47 (90)
Bone marrow	26	26 (100)
Sputum	41	14 (34)
Lymph node	9	9 (100)
Cerebrospinal fluid	20	3 (15)
Pleural fluid	20	1 (5)

Source: Supparatpinyo et al, Lancet 344:110–113, 1994a.

worker working with *P. marneffei* cultures was antibody positive. Further studies of these proteins and a 61-kDA antigen after purification found that 86% of sera from 21 *P. marneffei*-infected patients recognized the 61-kDA and 71% and 48% recognized the 54 kDA and 50-kDA antigens, respectively (Jeavons et al, 1998). Other investigators have identified a 38 kDA antigen from *P. marneffei* that was recognized by 45% of sera from AIDS patients with penicilliosis (Congtrakool et al, 1997).

Antigen Detection

Several investigators have described methods to detect *P. marneffei* antigens in serum or urine of infected patients as a method to confirm the diagnosis prior to the isolation of the organism in culture. Evaluation of immunodiffusion and latex agglutination tests to detect antigenemia in 17 *P. marneffei*-infected patients yielded positive results in 58.8% of infected patients with the immunodiffusion test and 76.5% of patients with the latex agglutination test (Kaufman et al, 1996). Fifteen controls and six patients with cryptococcosis and histoplasmasis were nonreactive. A solid-phase enzyme immunoassay utilizing antibody to *H. capsulatum var capsulatum* to detect *H. capsulatum* antigen in the urine of actively infected patients was cross reactive with *P. marneffei* in 17 of 18 patients (Wheat et al, 1997). This assay also was commonly positive in patients with *Blastomyces dermatitidis* and *Paracoccidioides brasiliensis* infections. Desakorn and colleagues reported the development of a method for the quantitation of *P. marneffei* antigen in the urine using fluorescein isothiocyanate-labelled purified rabbit hyperimmune immunoglobulin G in an enzyme immunoassay (Desakorn et al, 1999). These investigators studied 33 patients with culture proven *P. marneffei* infection and 300 controls, including 52 healthy subjects and 248 hospitalized patients in northeast Thailand with a variety of other infections, including melioidosis (N = 168), other septicemias (N = 12), other fungal infections (N = 34) and miscellaneous conditions (N = 34). All of the patients with penicilliosis had measurable antigen in the urine, and in all but two patients, the titers were over 1:40; and the median titer was 1:20,480. Whereas 27% of the hospitalized controls and 6% of healthy subjects were positive, the titers were usually below 1:40 in these control groups, leading the investigators to propose a diagnostic cut-off titer of 1:40, which yielded an assay that was 97% sensitive and 98% specific and had a positive predictive value of 84.2% and a negative predictive value of 99.7%.

Vanittanakom and coworkers have reported the development of a polymerase chain reaction/hybridization technique for the rapid detection of *P. marneffei* DNA in patient serum or environmental samples (Vanittanakom et al, 1997b). This PCR test was positive in 5 of 10 patients who had been treated for 1–7 days with amphotericin B. Further evaluation of the sensitivity of this PCR test in untreated patients and to monitor responses to treatment is needed.

Finally, several investigators have reported methods using restriction enzymes to subtype *P. marneffei* isolates. The use of *Hae*III restriction enzymes to digest *P. marneffei* DNA yielded two DNA profiles (RFLP types I and II) (Vanittanakom et al, 1996). More recently, the use of *Not*I and pulsed-field gel electrophoresis (PFGE) was used to study the genomic DNA of 64 *P. marneffei* isolates from patients in Thailand (Trewatcharegon et al, 2001). A total of 54 distinct macrorestriction profiles were identified in these patients. Antifungal sensitivity tests, restriction fragment-length polymorphism, and randomly amplified polymorphic DNA patterns in combination have been utilized to subtype 24 strains isolated between 1987 and 1998 from patients in Taiwan (Husch et al, 2000). The investigators identified 8 highly related patterns and found increased numbers and diversity of strains isolated between 1996 and 1998 compared to those isolated prior to 1996.

TREATMENT

Disseminated penicilliosis is usually fatal if not treated with appropriate antifungal drugs. However, with early diagnosis and institution of appropriate therapy the mortality can be reduced to 10%–20% or lower, even among patients with AIDS. Relapse is commonly seen after clinical response among immunocompromised patients unless suppressive doses of antifungal agents are continued.

The in vitro susceptibility of *P. marneffei* to antifungal agents has been evaluated by several investigators (Table 23–5). A study of 30 clinical isolates from Thailand found that all were susceptible to itraconazole, ketoconazole, and miconazole (Supparatpinyo et al, 1993). The organism was intermediately susceptible to amphotericin B, and least susceptible to fluconazole. Some strains were resistant to fluconazole. Clinical responses to therapy correlate with in vitro susceptibility. Amphotericin B has been shown to be effective in the treatment of disseminated penicilliosis (Supparatpinyo et al, 1992a). However, the drug needs to be continued for at least 6–8 weeks. Itraconazole is also effective clinically but clearance of positive fungal cultures is often delayed for 8 weeks or more (Supparatpinyo et al 1992b).

Based upon these clinical results and in vitro data on the antifungal susceptibility of *P. marneffei*, an open label noncomparative study was done to evaluate the combination of amphotericin B given intravenously for

TABLE 23–5. *In Vitro Drug Susceptibility (MIC, Range) of* Penicillium marnefffei

References	Number of Isolates	Amb	Flu	Itra	Keto	5-Fc
Jayanetra et al, 1984	3	0.78–3.12	ND	ND	ND	ND
Sekhon et al, 1992	10	< 0.195–1.56	0.195–100	< 0.195	0.195–0.39	ND
Drouhet, 1993	10	0.04–1.6	50	≤ 0.04	≤ 04	≤ 0.04
Supparatpinyo et al, 1993	30	0.25–4.0	≤ 0.313–20	≤ 0.02–0.078	0.002–0.078	0.02–0.9
Imwidthaya et al, 2001	30	0.125–0.5	4.0–8.0	< 0.032	< 0.125	ND

Amb, amphotericin B; Flu, fluconazole; Itra, itraconazole; Keto, ketoconazole; 5-Fc, flucytosine; ND, not done.

2 weeks at 0.6 mg/kg/day followed by itraconazole 400 mg/day taken orally for 10 weeks. This regimen was evaluated in the hope of minimizing the duration and toxicity associated with parenteral amphotericin B while concurrently clearing the fungal cultures more rapidly than with oral itraconazole alone (Sirisanthana et al, 1998). Of 74 HIV positive patients with disseminated penicilliosis treated with this regimen, 72 (97.3%) responded. No serious adverse drug effects were observed. After 2 weeks of therapy, 12 patients remained febrile and 11 patients still had skin lesions; by the 4th week of therapy, all patients were afebrile and had resolved their skin lesions. Fungemia was cleared after 2 weeks of treatment in the 65 patients who had a positive blood culture at baseline (Sirisanthana et al, 1998).

Despite the favorable initial responses to therapy with amphotericin B and itraconazole, relapses are common after antifungal therapy is discontinued in patients with AIDS (Supparatpinyo et al, 1993; Supparatpinyo et al, 1992b). Therefore, continued suppressive therapy is required to prevent relapse in AIDS patients with disseminated penicilliosis who respond to initial therapy. Suppressive therapy is probably required in AIDS patients for as long as significant immunocompromise persists. In a controlled trial of 71 HIV-infected patients with penicilliosis in Thailand, 20 (57%) of 35 patients assigned to the placebo group relapsed whereas none of 36 patients given suppressive itraconazole 200 mg once daily relapsed ($p < 0.001$) (Supparatpinyo et al, 1998). The therapy was well tolerated and the patients in this trial were very compliant with treatment.

In areas where systemic fungal infections, such as *P. marneffei*, *H. capsulatum*, *C. neoformans* and other fungal infections, are common AIDS-associated opportunistic infections, primary prophylaxis against these infections should be considered. In northern Thailand, HIV infections are common, involving 2%–3% of the general population. Moreover, disseminated fungal infections, especially those due to *P. marneffei*, *C. neoformans*, and *H. capsulatum* are also common, accounting for over a third of the reported AIDS defining illnesses in this population (Chariyalertsak et al, 2001). In order to evaluate the efficacy of primary prophylaxis to prevent systemic fungal infection in this population, a clinical trial was done in 129 patients who were HIV positive, had CD4+ cell counts < 200 cells/μl, and had not experienced a systemic fungal infection. Patients were randomized to receive oral itraconazole (200 mg/day) or a matched placebo (Supparatpinyo et al, 1998). Systemic fungal infections developed in 1 (1.6%) of 63 patients assigned to itraconazole and 11 (16.7%) of 66 patients assigned to placebo ($p = .003$). In the placebo group, 7 patients developed cryptococcosis and 4 had penicilliosis. The one patient in the itraconazole group who became infected developed penicilliosis.

SUMMARY

Much remains to be learned about the epidemiology, ecology, and natural history of *P. marneffei* infections in humans. The environmental reservoir in nature is not well understood. Understanding the factors related to latent infection and developing methods for the detection of latent infection in humans are important challenges for the future. The unique susceptibility to *P. marneffei* infection among several species of bamboo rats and humans with HIV infection is also not well understood. Undoubtedly, future research will lead to a better understanding of these important characteristics of this emerging infection.

REFERENCES

Ajello L, Padhye A A, Sukroongreung S, Nilakul CH, Tantimavanic S. Occurrence of *Penicillium marneffei* infections among wild bamboo rats in Thailand. *Mycopathology* 131:1–8, 1995.

Cao L, Chen D L, Lee C, Chan C M, Chan K M, Vanittanakom N, Tsang D N C, Yuen K Y. Detection of specific antibodies to an antigenic mannoprotein for diagnosis of *Penicillium marneffei*: Penicilliosis. *J Clin Microbiol* 36:3028–3031, 1998.

Capponi M, Sureau P, Segretain G. Penicilliose de *Rhizomys sinensis*. *Bull Soc Pathol Exot* 49:418–421, 1956.

Chan J K C, Tsang D N C, Wong D K K. *Penicillium marneffei* in bronchoalveolar lavage Fluid. *Acta Cytol* 33:523–526, 1989.

Chan Y F, Woo K C. *Penicillium marneffei* osteomyelitis. *J Bone Joint Surg* 72 (Br), 500–503, 1990

Chariyalertsak S, Vanittanakom P, Nelson K E, Sirisanthana T, Vanittanakom N. *Rhizomys sumatrensis* and *Cannomys badius*, new natural animal hosts of *Penicillium marneffei J. Med Vet Mycol* 34:105–110, 1996a.

Chariyalertsak S, Sirisanthana T, Supparatpinyo K, Nelson KE. Seasonal variation of disseminated *Penicillium marneffei* infection in northern Thailand: a clue to the reservoir. *J Infect Dis* 173:1490–1493, 1996b.

Chariyalertsak S, Sirisanthana T, Supparatpinyo K, Praparattanapan J, Nelson K E. A case-control study of risk factors for *P. marneffei* infections in human immunodeficiency virus-infected patients in Northern Thailand. *Clin Infect Dis* 24:1080–1086, 1997.

Chariyalertsak S, Sirisanthana T, Saengwonloey O, Nelson K E. Clinical presentation and risk behaviors of patients with acquired immunodeficiency syndrome in Thailand, 1994–1998: regional variation and temporal trends. *Clin Infect Dis* 32:955–962, 2001.

Chim C S, Fong C Y, Ma S K, Wong S S, Yuen K Y. Reactive hemophagocytic syndrome associated with *Penicillium marneffei* infection. *Am J Med* 196–197, 1998.

Chongtrakool P, Chaiyaroj S C, Vithayasai V, Trawatcharegon S, Teanpaisan R, Kalnawakul S, Sirisinha S. Immunoreactivity of a 38-kilodalton *Penicillium marneffei* antigen with human immunodeficiency virus-positive sera. *J Clin Microbiol* 35:2220–2223, 1997.

Cooper C R, Haycocks N G. *Penicillium marneffei*: An insurgent species among the *Penicillia*. *J Eukaryot Microbiol* 47:24–28, 2000.

Corbet G B, Hill J E. Subfamily *Rhizomyinae*: bamboo rats. In: *The Mammals of the Indo Malaya Region: A Systematic Review*. Oxford, UK: Oxford University Press, 404–407, 1992.

Deng Z, Connor D H. Progressive disseminated penicilliosis caused by *Penicillium marneffei*: Report of eight cases and differentiation of causative organism from *Histoplasma capsulatum*. *Am J Clin Pathol* 84:323–327, 1985.

Deng Z L, Ribas J L, Gibson DW, Connor D H. Infections caused by *Penicillium marneffei* in China and Southeast Asia: Review of eighteen published cases and report of four more Chinese cases. *Rev Infect Dis* 10:640–652, 1988.

Deng Z L, Yun M, Ajello L. Human *Penicilliosis marneffei* and its relation to the bamboo rat (*Rhizomys pruinosus*). *J Med Vet Mycol* 24:383–389, 1986.

Desakorn V, Smith M D, Walsh A L, Simpson A J H, Sahassananda D, Rajanuwong A, Wuthiekienum V, Howe P, Angus B J, Suntharasamai P, White N J. Diagnosis of *Penicillium marneffei* infection by quantitation of urinary antigen by using an enzyme immunoassay. *J Clin Microbiol* 37:117–121, 1999.

Di Salvo A F, Fickling A M, Ajello L. Infection caused by *Penicillium marneffei*: A description of first natural infection in man. *Am J Clin Pathol* 60:259–263, 1973.

Drouhet E. Penicilliosis due to *Penicillium marneffei*: A new emerging systemic mycosis in AIDS patients traveling or living in Southeast Asia, Review of 44 cases reported in HIV infected patients during the last 5 years compared to 44 cases of non AIDS patients reported over 20 years. *J Mycol Med* (Paris) 4:195–224, 1993.

Estrada J A, Stynen D, Cutsem J V, Pierard-Franchimont C, Pierard G E. Immunohistochemical identification of *Penicillium marneffei* by monoclonal antibody. *Dermatol* 31:410–412, 1992.

Hilmarsdottir I, Meynard J L, Rogeaux O, Guermonprez G, Datry A, Katlama C, Brucker G, Coutellier A, Danis M, Gentilini M. Disseminated *Penicillium marneffei* infection associated with human immunodeficiency virus: a report of two cases and a review of 35 published cases. *J Acquir Immune Defic Syndr* 6:466–471, 1993.

Hilmarsdottir I, Coutellier A, Elbaz J, Klein J M, Datry A, Gueho E, Herslon S. A French case of laboratory-acquired disseminated *Penicillium marneffei* infection in a patient with AIDS (letter). *Clin Infec Dis* 19:357–358, 1994.

Hulshof C M J, van Zanten R A, Sluiters J F, van der Ende M E, Samson R S, Zondervan P E, Wagenvoort J H. *Penicillium marneffei* in an AIDS patient (letter) *Eur J Clin Microbiol Infect Dis* 9:370, 1990.

Husch P R, Teng L J, Hung C C, Hsu J H, Yang P, Ho S W, Luh K T. Molecular evidence for strain dissemination of *Penicillium marneffei*: an emerging pathogen in Taiwan. *J Infect Dis* 181:1706–1712, 2000.

Imwidthaya P, Thipsuvan K, Chaiprasert A, Danchaivijitra S, Sutthent R, Jearanaisilavong J. *Penicillium marneffei*: types and drug susceptibility. *Mycopathologia* 149:109–115, 2001.

Jayanetra P, Nitiyanant P, Ajello L, Padhye A A, Lolekha S, Atichartakan V, Vathesatogit P, Sathaphatayavongs B, Prajaktam R. *Penicilliosis marneffei* in Thailand: report of five human cases. *Am J Trop Med Hyg* 33; 637–44, 1984.

Jeavons L, Hamilton A J, Vanittanakom N, Ungpakorn R, Evans E G V, Sirisanthana T, Hay R J. Identification and purification of specific *Penicillium marneffei* antigens and their recognition by human immune sera. *J Clin Microbiol* 36:949–954, 1998.

Jones P D, See J. *Penicillium marneffei* infection in patients infected with human immunodeficiency virus: Late presentation in an area of nonendemicity (letter). *Clin Infect Dis* 15:744, 1992.

Kaufman L, Standard P G, Anderson S A, Jalbert M, Swisher B L. Development of specific fluorescent antibody test for tissue form of *Penicillium marneffei*. *J Clin Microbiol* 33:2136–2138, 1995.

Kaufman L, Standard P G, Jalbert G, Kantipong D, Limpakarajanarat K, Mastro T D. Diagnostic antigenemia tests for *Penicillium marneffei*. *J Clin Microbiol* 34:2503–2505, 1996.

Ko K F. Retropharyngeal abscess caused by *Penicillium marneffei*: An unusual cause of upper airway obstruction. *Otolaryngol Head Neck Surg*, 110:445–446, 1994.

Kronauer C M, Schar G, Barben M, Buhler H. HIV-associated *Penicillium marneffei* infection. *Schweiz med Wochenschr* 123:385–390, 1993.

Li J S, Pan L Q, Deng Z L, Yoo C L. A case report on *Penicillium marneffei*. *J Clin Dermatol* (China) 14:24–26, 1985.

Li J S, Pan L Q, Wu S X. Mycologic investigation on *Rhizomys pruinosus senex* in Guangxi as natural carrier with *Penicillium marneffei*. *Clin Med J* (Engl) 102:477–485, 1989.

Li J S, Pan Q, Wu S X, Su S X, Su S B, Shan J H. Disseminated *Penicilliosis marneffei* in China: Report of three cases. *Clin Med J* 104:247–251, 1991.

LoBuglio K F and Taylor J W. Phylogeny and PCR identification of the human pathogenic fungus *Penicillium marneffei*. *J Clin Microbiol* 33:85–89, 1995.

Nelson K E, Kaufman L, Cooper C R, Merz W G. *Penicillium marneffei*: An AIDS-related illness from Southeast Asia. *Infect Med* 16:118–121, 1999.

Pautler K B, Padhye A A, Ajello L. Imported *Penicilliosis marneffei* in the United States: report of a second human infection. *Sabouraudia* 22:433–438, 1984.

Peto T E, Bull R Millard P R, Mackenzie D W, Campbell C K, Haines M E, Mitchell R G. Systemic mycosis due to *Penicillium marneffei* in a patient with antibodies to human immunodeficiency virus. *J Infect* 16:285–290, 1988.

Piehl M R, Kaplan R I, Haber M H. Disseminated penicilliosis in a patient with acquired immunodeficiency syndrome. *Arch Pathol Lab Med* 112:1262–1264, 1988.

Pitt J I. The genus *Penicillium* and its teleomorphic states *Eupenicillium* and *Talaromyces*, Academic Press Inc, New York, 1979.

Raper K B, Thom C. *A Manual of the Penicillia*. Baltimore: The Williams and Wilkins Co, 1949.

Rongruagruang Y, Levitz SM. Interaction of *Penicillium marneffei* with human leukocytes in vitro. *Infect Immun* 67:4732–4736, 1999.

Segretain G, *Penicillium marneffei* n.sp. agent d'une mycose du système reticuloendothelial. *Mycopath Mycologia Appl* 11:327–353, 1959b.

Segretain G. Description d'une nouvelle espiece de pencillium: *Peni-*

cillium marneffei n. sp. *Bull Société Mycologique France* 75:412–416, 1959a.

Sekhon A S, Li J S K, Garg A K. *Penicilliosis marneffei* serological exoantigen studies. *Mycopathologia* 77:51–57, 1982.

Sekhon A S, Garg A K, Padhye A A. Antigenic relationship of *Penicillium marneffei* to *P. primulinum*. *J Med Vet Mycol* 27:105–112, 1989.

Sekhon A S, Padhye AA, Garg A K. In vitro sensitivity of *Penicillium marneffei* and *Pythium insidiosum* to various antifungal agents. *Eur J Epidemiol* 8:427–432, 1992.

Sekhon A S, Stein L, Garg A K, Black W A, Glezos J Q, Wong C. Pulmonary *Penicilliosis marneffei*: Report of the first imported case in Canada. *Mycopathologia* 128:3–7, 1994.

Sirisanthana V, Sirisanthana T. Disseminated *Penicillium marneffei* infection in human immunodeficiency virus-infected children. *Pediatr Infect Dis J* 14:935–940, 1995.

Sirisanthana T, Supparatpinyo K, Periens T, Nelson K E. Amphotericin B and itraconazole for treatment of disseminated *Penicillium marneffei* infection in human immunodeficiency virus-infected patients. *Clin Infect Dis* 26:1107–1110, 1998.

Sobotta I, Albrecht H, Mack D, Mack D, Stellbrink H J, van Lunzen J, Tintelnot H, Laufs R. Systemic *Penicillium marneffei* infection in a German AIDS patient. *Eur J Clin Microbiol Infect Dis* 15:256–259, 1996.

Supparatpinyo K, Chiewchanvit S, Hirunsri P, Uthammachai C, Nelson K E, Sirisanthana T. *Penicillium marneffei* infection in patients infected with human immunodeficiency virus. *Clin Infect Dis* 14:871–874, 1992a.

Supparatpinyo K, Chiewchanvit S, Hirunsri P, Baosung V, Uthammachai C, Chaimongkol B, Sirisanthana T. An efficacy study of itraconazole in the treatment of *Penicillium marneffei* infection. *J Med Assoc Thailand* 75:688–691, 1992b.

Supparatpinyo K, Nelson K E, Merz W G, Breslin B J, Cooper C R, Kamwan C, Sirisanthana T. Response to anti-fungal therapy by human immunodeficiency virus infected patients with disseminated *Penicillium marneffei* infections and in vitro susceptibilities of isolates from clinical specimens. *Antimicrob Agents Chemother* 37:2407–2411, 1993.

Supparatpinyo K, Khamwan C, Baosoung V, Nelson K E, Sirisanthana T. Disseminated *Penicillium marneffei* infection in southeast Asia. *Lancet* 344:110–113, 1994a.

Supparatpinyo K, Sirisanthana T. Disseminated *Penicillium marneffei* infection diagnosed on examination of a peripheral blood smear of a patient with human immunodeficiency virus infection. *Clin Infect Dis* 18:246–247, 1994b.

Supparatpinyo K, Perriens J, Nelson K E, Sirisanthana T. A controlled trial of itraconazole to prevent relapse of *Penicillium marneffei* infection in patients infected with the human immunodeficiency virus. *N Engl J Med* 339:1739–1743, 1998.

Tong A C, Wong M H, Smith N H T. *Penicillium marneffei* infection presenting as oral ulcerations in a patient infected with human immunodeficiency. *J Oral Maxillofac Su*rg 59:953–956, 2001.

Trewatcharegon S, Sirisinha S, Romsai A, Eampokalap B, Teanpaisan R, Chaiyaroj S. Molecular typing of *Penicillium marneffei* isolates from Thailand by NotI macrorestriction and pulsed-filed gel electrophoresis. *J Clin Microbiol* 39:4544–4548, 2001.

Vanittanakom N, Mekaprateep M, Sriburee P, Vanittanakom P, Khanjanasthiti. Efficiency of the flotation method in the isolation of *Penicillium marneffei* from seeded soil. *J Med Vet Mycol* 33:271–273, 1995.

Vanittanakom N, Cooper C R, Chariyalertsak S, Youngchin S, Nelson K E, Sirisanthana T. Restriction endonuclease analysis of *Penicillium marneffei*. *J Clin Microbiol* 34:1834–1836, 1996.

Vanittanakom N, Mekaprateep M, Sittisombut N, Supparatpinyo K, Kanjanasthiti P, Nelson K E, Sirisanthana T. Western immunoblot analysis of protein antigens of *Penicillium marneffei*. *J Med Vet Mycol* 35:123–131, 1997a.

Vanittanakom N, Merz W G, Nelson K E, Sirisanthana T. Rapid detection of *Penicillium marneffei* by polymerase chain reaction/hybridization technique. 13th Congress of International Society for Human and Animal Mycology, Parma, Italy, June 8–13, 1997b.

Vanittanakom N, Sirisanthana T. *Penicillium marneffei* infection in patients infected with human immunodeficiency virus. *Curr Topics in Med Mycol* 8:35–42, 1997c.

Viviani M A, Hill J O, Dixon D M. *Penicillium marneffei*: dimorphism and treatment. In: Vanden Bossche H, Odds F, Kerridge D, eds. *Dimorphic Fungi in Biology and Medicine*. New York: Plenum Press, 413–22, 1993a.

Viviani M A, Tortorano A M, Rizzardini G, Quirino T, Kaufman L, Padhye A A, Ajello L. Treatment and serological studies of an Italian case of *Penicilliosis* marneffei contracted in Thailand by a drug addict infected with the human immunodeficiency virus. *Eur J Epidemiol* 9:79–85, 1993b.

Viviani M A, Tortorano A M. *Penicillium marneffei*. In: Ajello L, Hay R J, eds. *Topley and Wilson's Microbiology and Microbial Infections*, 9th Ed, Vol 4. London, UK: Arnold Press, 409–419, 1998.

Wang I L, Yeh H P, Chang S C, Chin J S. Penicilliosis due to *Penicillium marneffei*: A case report. *Derm Sinica* 7:19–22, 1989.

Wei X G, Ling Y M, Li C, Zhang F S. Study of 179 bamboo rats carrying *Penicillium marneffei* (in Chinese). *China J Zoonoses* 3:34–35, 1987.

Wheat J, Wheat H, Connolly P, Kleiman M, Supparatpinyo K, Nelson K E, Bradsher R, Restrepo A. Cross-reactivity in *Histoplasma capsulatum* variety *capsulatum* antigen assays of urine samples from patients with endemic mycoses. *Clin Infect Dis* 24:1169–1171, 1997.

Wong S S, Wong K H, Hui T, Lee S S, Lo J Y, Cao L, Yuen K Y. Differences in clinical and laboratory diagnostics characteristics of *Penicilliosis marneffei* in human immunodeficiency virus (HIV)- and non-HIV infected patients. *J Clin Microbial* 39:4534–4540, 2000.

Wong S S Y, Ho T Y C, Nagan A H Y, Woo P C Y, Que T-L, Yuen K-y. Biotyping of *Penicillium marneffei* reveals concenration-dependent growth inhibiton by galactose. *J Clin Microbiol* 39: 1416–1421, 2001.

Yuen K, Wong S S, Tsang D N, Cau P Y. Serodiagnosis of *Penicillium marneffei* infection. *Lancet* 344:444–445, 1994.

Yuen W C, Chan Y F, Loke S L, Seto W H, Poon G P, Wong K K. Chronic lymphadenopathy caused by *Penicillium marneffei*: a condition mimicking tuberculous lymphadenopathy. *Br J Surg* 73:1007–1008, 1986.

VI

MYCOLOGY INVOLVING SKIN AND SUBCUTANEOUS TISSUES

24

Superficial cutaneous fungal infections

JEFF WEEKS, STEPHEN A. MOSER, AND BONI E. ELEWSKI

In this chapter, we review cutaneous diseases caused by a variety of fungal pathogens infecting the skin, hair, and nails. These diseases are divided into the following classification based on level of invasion, host inflammatory response, and pathogen: *(1)* superficial mycoses, *(2)* dermatophytoses, *(3)* cutaneous disease caused by nondermatophyte moulds, and *(4)* cutaneous candidiasis. Superficial mycoses are characterized by fungal invasion into the superficial stratum corneum with little to no inflammatory response. Dermatophytoses are caused by dermatophytes, which are a closely related group of fungi that invade the full thickness of the stratum corneum and result in a host-mediated immune response. Several nondermatophyte moulds produce infections that mimic dermatophytoses. Cutaneous candidiasis results from invasion of deep layers of the skin by members of the *Candida* genus.

SUPERFICIAL MYCOSES

Definition

Superficial mycoses are fungal infections of the skin and hair that invade only the most superficial layers and cause little or no inflammatory response. These mycoses include the malasseziores, tinea nigra, black piedra, and white piedra. Superficial invasion of the nail plate, so-called white superficial onychomycosis, is discussed in the Dermatophytoses section.

Etiology and Epidemiology

Current information indicates that the malassezioses are caused by members of *Malassezia* genus of which there are seven recognized species including *M. furfur*, *M. globosa*, *M. obtusa*, *M. slooffiae*, *M. sympodialis*, *M. pachydermatis*, and *M. restricta*. *Malassezia globosa* (formerly serovar B of *M. furfur*) correlates best with the origial description of *Pityrosporum orbiculare* and appears to be the causative fungal agent of tinea versicolor. Seborrheic dermatitis and dandruff are most often associated with *M. restricta* (formerly serovar C of *M. furfur*) (Gemmer et al, 2002). These fungal organisms are part of the normal skin flora. Disease is widespread but more common in patients living in warm, humid climates. The other causative organisms of superficial mycoses are found in the humid, tropical climates of Central and South America, Africa, and Asia. *Hortaea (Exophiala) werneckii* is the cause of tinea nigra, whereas black piedra is caused by *Piedraia hortae* and white piedra by *Trichosporon* species.

Pathogenesis

Malassezia yeasts, previously called *Pityrosporum ovale* and *Pityrosporum orbiculare*, are dimorphic fungi that can be isolated from the skin of 97% of healthy adults (Hoeprich et al, 1994). Certain conditions, such as tropical ambient temperatures and humidity, predispose to malasseziosis in genetically susceptible persons. The organism exists normally in the round blastophore form and becomes pathogenic after transformation to the mycelial form. The host's cell-mediated immunity may influence the clinical presentation and T-cell deficiencies are associated with extensive disease.

Unlike *Malessezia*, *Hortaea werneckii* and *Piedraia hortae* are pathogens acquired from the environment. *Trichosporon* species (including *T. ovoides*, *T. mucoides*, and *T. inkiu*) are also acquired environmentally, but may be part of the normal skin flora, particularly in the axillae and genital areas.

Clinical Presentations

Malasseziores. *Malassezia* species cause three clinical forms of disease. Pityriasis (tinea) versicolor presents as hypo- to hyperpigmented macules or patches with slight scales on the upper trunk, neck, and upper arms (See Color Fig. 24–1 in separate color insert). Occasionally, the lesions may be papular, erythematous, or pruritic. *Malassezia* folliculitis is characterized by pruritic, follicular papules, and pustules on the upper back, chest, shoulders, and less commonly, the face and neck. Seborrheic dermatitis presents as pruritic red patches with greasy scales on the scalp, eyebrows, nasolabial folds, ears, presternal area, axilla, and groin. In infancy, seborrheic dermatitis on the scalp is called cradle cap.

Tinea Nigra. Although this condition is caused by *Hortaea (Exophiala) werneckii,* which is not a dermatophyte, it is called *tinea* by convention. *Tinea nigra* is characterized by asymptomatic, nonscaly, coin-sized, brown to gray patches on the palms and soles of young adults. Confirmation of this diagnosis is easily obtained by the presence of pigmented hyphae on a potassium hydroxide preparation.

Black Piedra. Piedra is the Spanish word for stone. In black piedra, superficial infection of hair shafts by *Piedraia hortae* results in asymptomatic, stone-like concretions on scalp and facial hair. Alopecia does not occur but hairs may break at the site of infection.

White Piedra. *Trichosporon* species including *T. ovoides* cause another superficial infection of hair shafts called white piedra. Concretions in this disease are white to tan and are found on facial, axillary, and pubic hair. Infection of perianal hair occurs with increased frequency in HIV-infected patients.

Diagnosis

Malasseziones. The genus *Malassezia* is comprised of the *M. furfur*-complex, a group of related lipophilic yeasts, and *M. pachydermatis.* The *M. furfur*-complex includes *M. furfur, M. sympodialis, M. globosa, M. restricta, M. slooffiae,* and *M. obtusa,* all of which are dependent upon lipids for growth. In practice, referring to these as *M. furfur* complex is adequate. *M. pachydermatis* is a distinct species, and is also lipophilic but does not have an absolute requirement for lipids (Marcon and Powell, 1992).

Skin scrapings examined with KOH-Calcofluor white will reveal short, septate, occasionally branching filaments, 2.5–4 μm in diameter of varying lengths, and clusters of small, unicellular oval, or round budding yeast cells (4–8 μm). Referred to by some as "spaghetti and meat balls," this finding is considered diagnostic in this setting. The inexperienced examiner must be careful not to confuse *M. furfur* complex with *Candida* spp., which can be differentiated by the presence of pseudohyphae.

Culture from skin scrapings is not necessary if a diagnosis is made from direct microscopic examination. However, if the microscopic appearance is atypical or if species identification is required, then culture on media containing antibacterial agents and cycloheximide overlaid with sterile olive oil incubated at 30°C is required. When *M. furfur* is the agent of catheter-associated fungemia, scant growth on initial subculture from blood culture bottles onto media without lipid supplement may occur. *Malassezia pachydermatis* lacks the requirement for lipid supplement. Colonies in culture develop slowly and are cream colored and raised,

consisting of mostly yeasts cells. Microscopically this yeast is distinguished by the presence of a collarette between mother and daughter cells.

Tinea Nigra. *Hortaea werneckii,* the primary cause of tinea nigra, is found most commonly in the tropical areas of Central and South America, Asia, and Africa (Kwon-Chung and Bennett, 1992). Diagnosis can be made by examination of skin scale with KOH demonstrating the brown-pigmented hyphae and budding yeast cells. Growth on Saboraud's dextrose agar is slow, initially black and yeast-like, and upon extended incubation may produce gray–black aerial mycelium. However, the yeast form remains the predominant morphologic feature.

Black Piedra. *Piedraia hortae,* the etiologic agent of black piedra, is found in tropical South and Central American, Southeast Asia, and Africa. Hairs with visible nodules should be plucked, treated with KOH and examined under the microscope. The nodule should be crushed, taking care not to break the coverslip. The finding of septate brown hyphae, asci, and fusiform ascospores confirms the diagnosis. Culture if done should be on media with antibacterial agents, as well as media with both antibacterial agents and cycloheximide.

White Piedra. The etiologic agent of white piedra is *Trichosporon* species, yeast-like organisms that form true hyphae, arthroconidia, and blastoconidia. Direct microscopic examination of hair nodules revealing these characteristics should be sufficient for diagnosis. If culture is performed, colonies appear rapidly (1–2 days) at 30°C on selective agar containing antibacterial agents. Species identification can be accomplished using commercially available assimilation kits, but should be used in conjunction with morphologic criteria (e.g., formation of arthroconidia and blastoconida). Diagnosis can be easily confirmed by direct microscopic examination of KOH mounted scrapings of involved skin or hair. Pityriasis versicolor can be confirmed when both round, budding yeast cells and short fat hyphae ("spaghetti and meatballs") are observed. Wood's light examination may reveal bright yellow fluorescence. Fungal culture is not helpful because the organism may occur in normal skin. Pigmented, irregular, septate hyphae are observed in tinea nigra. Hair shafts from black piedra show masses of intertwined pigmented hyphae and occasional ascospores. In white piedra, there are masses of hyphae with numerous septa along with plentiful blastoconidia and arthroconidia.

Differential Diagnosis

Although the superficial mycoses all have distinctive clinical presentations, there are some important dis-

TABLE 24–1. *Treatment of Malassezioses*

Tinea Versicolor	Seborrheic Dermatitis	*Malassezia* Folliculitis
Topical Agents	**Topical Agents**	**Topical Agents**
• Selenium sulfide 2.5% shampoo* • Ketoconazole 2% shampoo* or cream • Ciclopirox 0.1% solution • Terbinafine 1% cream • Zinc pyrithione shampoo*	• Ketoconazole 1%–2% shampoo at least twice weekly • Zinc pyrithione shampoo qd • Selenium sulfide shampoo qd • Mild topical steroids (hydrocortisone 1%, desonide 0.05%, etc.) bid	• Azole cream or shampoo bid • Selenium sulfide shampoo qd **Oral Drugs** • Ketoconazole • Itraconazole
Oral Drugs • Ketoconazole 200 mg/day for 5–7 days • Fluconazole 400 mg once, repeated in 1 week • Itraconazole 200 mg/day for 5–7 days		

*Shampoos should be applied to affected areas once daily for 2 weeks, left on 5 to 10 minutes, then rinsed off.

eases to consider in the differential diagnosis. Vitiligo, pityriasis alba, pityriasis rosea, cutaneous T-cell lymphoma, and even secondary syphilis may resemble pityriasis versicolor. The red papules and pustules of *Malassezia* folliculitis may mimic bacterial or candidal folliculitis. It is sometimes difficult to distinguish seborrheic dermatitis from atopic dermatitis and psoriasis. Tinea nigra may resemble lentigo, pigmented seborrheic keratosis, nevus, or melanoma but is easily identified with a KOH examination.

Treatment (Table 24–1)

Malassezioses. Numerous topical products are used in the treatment of pityriasis versicolor (Table 24–1). Apply selenium sulfide 2.5% or ketoconazole 2% shampoo liberally over and beyond the affected areas for 10 minutes once daily for a 2-week period and repeat once or twice monthly to minimize recurrence. Topical azole antifungal creams have also been proven effective against pityriasis versicolor, as has ciclopirox 0.1% solution (Corte et al, 1991) and zinc pyrithione shampoo (Faergemann and Fredriksson, 1980). When extensive lesions are present or when topical creams have been ineffective, systemic therapy may be indicated. Options include: oral ketoconazole 200 mg per day for 5 to 7 days (Hay and Midgeley, 1984), fluconazole 400 mg once, repeated in 1 week, and itraconazole 200 mg per day for 5 to 7 days (Delescluse, 1990). The newer antimycotic drugs have a favorable safety profile. Prophylactic usage may decrease the rate of recurrence (60% in 1 year).

Topical antifungal drugs are generally very effective in seborrheic dermatitis, which led to the current belief that *Malassezia* is implicated in the pathogenesis. Ketoconazole 2% shampoo applied at least twice weekly has been very successful on the scalp (Faerge-

mann and Fredriksson, 1990). Shampoos containing zinc pyrithione (Marks et al, 1985) or selenium sulfide (Shuster, 1984) also work well. Topical steroids may be effective. However, seborrheic dermatitis often recurs quickly after discontinuation of therapy.

Malassezia folliculitis responds well to both topical and systemic antimycotic therapy. Topical treatment with an azole cream or shampoo or selenium sulfide is often sufficient (Ford et al, 1982; Back et al, 1985). Oral ketoconazole and itraconazole have been used successfully in those patients not responding to topical therapy (Ford et al, 1982). As in all malassezioses, recurrence is likely and a prophylactic treatment schedule is necessary.

Tinea Nigra. Topical therapy with an azole such as miconazole, clotrimazole, econazole, or ketoconazole is usually effective. Other effective topical agents include naftifine, terbinafine, and Whitfield's ointment. Oral therapy is rarely needed and griseofulvin is ineffective.

Piedras. Both black and white piedras may be treated with 2% ketoconazole shampoo. Alternative therapy includes shaving or clipping off infected hairs.

Prevention

Presence of *Malassezia* species as part of the normal skin flora may explain the high recurrence rate. Consequently, prophylactic therapy is generally required. Oral ketoconazole, fluconazole, and itraconazole, dosed once or twice monthly, offer one option. Topical medications can also be intermittently applied, but compliance issues often develop.

Prevention of infection or reinfection by *H. werneckii, P. hortae,* and *T. ovoides* is dependent upon avoidance of endemic sites.

DERMATOPHYTOSES

Fungi that are able to subsist within the keratinous elements of living skin are called dermatophytes, which belong to one of three genera, *Epidermophyton*, *Microsporum*, and *Trichophyton*. Among these genera, there are 10 common species and greater than 20 other species that occasionally cause disease. The distribution of some species is worldwide while others are restricted to certain geographic locations. The morphology and pathogenicity of the species are similar. Tinea, an adjective used to describe infections caused by dermatophytes, is used as a preface to the Latin designation of the affected body part. For example, tinea corporis is an infection of the glabrous skin.

Epidemiology

Dermatophytes are often classified according to the source of infection. Arthropophilic organisms are acquired from other humans. Infections due to these pathogens are usually relatively noninflammatory. Geophilic organisms are acquired from the soil. Infections due to zoophilic organisms are acquired from animals and tend to be inflammatory. The epidemiology and etiology of the most common dermatophytoses are discussed separately.

Mycology

Collection and Transport of Specimens. Depending upon the body site involved, hair, skin, or nail scrapings are collected for both direct microscopic examination and culture. Lesions of the skin, scalp, and nail should be cleaned with 70% alcohol before samples are collected to reduce the amount of bacterial contamination, which may mask the presence of a fungus in culture. Specimens should be collected into folded squares of stiff black paper, which allows for easy visualization of the specimen and helps to keep the specimen dry until processing. If sending the specimen to a reference laboratory, it can be contained by folding the paper and mailing in an envelope. There are commercially available collection and mailing kits that facilitate this process (Dermapac, Key Scientific Products, Round Rock, TX).

SKIN. In glabrous (smooth and bare) skin, the advancing edge of the lesion provides the highest probability of finding diagnostic material. Material should be collected by scraping the edge of the lesion with the blunt edge of a scalpel. For infection of the toe webs, the soggy skin should be peeled away, and if vesicles are present, the whole top of the lesion should be removed.

SCALP. Hair from areas of suspected infection must be submitted with the root end attached, e.g., plucked not clipped. Hair samples can also be obtained by brushing the hair and culturing the material directly. In 'black-dot' tinea capitis lesions, the hair becomes fragile and breaks off at the skin surface. In these cases, collection should be by scraping with a scalpel as noted above.

NAIL. The affected nail should be clipped as proximally as possible through the entire thickness of the nail, obtaining the maximum amount of crumbly material, which is concentrated on the underside of the nail. The use of a pincer-type nail clipper is the most effective method. If nail dystrophy is wholly proximal, a scraping can be taken from the affected portion of the nail by scraping with a scalpel blade.

Fungal elements may not be numerous or equally distributed; therefore the quantity as well as the quality of the specimen is important. As a rule, attempts should be made to obtain 10–15 mm² of skin, about twice this amount of nail, and 4–6 hairs. This will allow for satisfactory microscopic examination and culture.

Microscopic Examination. Rapid detection of fungal elements in specimens from suspected dermatophytoses can be accomplished using microscopy. Material (scrapings or hair) is placed on a glass slide; a strong base is added (20% KOH) and overlaid with a cover slip. The KOH will digest the host material (the process is speeded up by gently heating) and reveal the presence of fungal hyphae, arthroconidia, or yeast cells. Small numbers of fungal elements may be present and the addition of Calcofluor white, which binds to the cell wall of fungi and fluoresces when observed under ultraviolet light, will increase the sensitivity of the procedure.

Culture Methods. Culture, a necessary adjunct to microscopic examination of specimens, is important from both a therapeutic and epidemiological standpoint. Although the majority of etiologic agents are dermatophytes, other filamentous fungi can be the causative agents of skin and nail infections and require a different therapeutic approach. In addition, determining the identity of the etiologic agent will allow determination of the possible source of the infection, e.g., zoophilic or anthropophilic organisms.

The choice of media for primary isolation should include both selective and nonselective media. Optimal isolation of dermatophytes occurs on selective media containing antibiotics to suppress bacterial growth and cycloheximide to suppress contaminating saprophytic moulds. However, some moulds that may be etiologic agents are inhibited by cycloheximide. Therefore, use of a general medium is necessary in the case of nail, palm, and sole lesions in which nondermatophytes such as *Scytalidium* spp. may be involved.

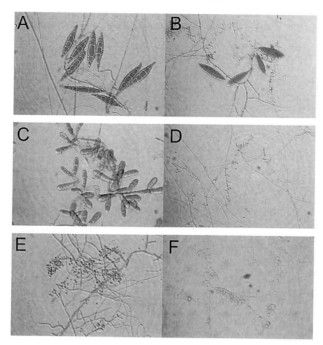

FIGURE 24–2. Examples of the microscopic morphology of common dermatophytes. A: *M. canis* macroconidia; B: *M. gypseum* macroconidia and microcondida; C: Clusters of *E. floccosum* macroconidia; D: *T. rubrum* en terse microconidia; E: *T. mentagrophytes* var *mentagrophytes* en grappe microcondidia; F: *T. tonsurans* characteristic "balloon" microconidia and a macroconidium. Magnifications approximately 400×.

Etiologic Agents

The etiologic agents of dermatophytoses are collectively referred to as dermatophytes and include members of the genera *Microsporum*, *Epidermophyton*, and *Trichophyton*. Both asexual (anamorph) and sexual (teleomorph) stages have been described. Those that demonstrate a sexual stage are classified in the genus *Arthroderma*. From a practical standpoint only the asexual forms are encountered in the diagnostic mycology laboratory. A summary of the major characteristics of the most common dermatophytes follows. Detailed descriptions of these and other related fungi can be found elsewhere (Kane and Summerbell, 1999).

Microsporum. This genus differs from other dermatophytes by the rough (echinulate) surface of the macroconidia, which may be an especially prominent feature as in *M.canis* (Fig. 24–2A) or more subtle requiring close examination with oil immersion objective. *Microsporum* species sporulate profusely, producing numerous macroconidia as well as lesser numbers of clavate microconidia (Fig. 24–2B). A notable exception is *M. audouinii*, which rarely sporulates. Macroconidia, when formed, are usually borne singularly on coni-

diophores, are multiseptate (1–15 septa), typically fusiform but range from obovate (*M. nanum*) to cylindrofusiform (*M. vanbreuseghemii*), are thin or thick walled, and range from 6 to 160 μm in length and 6 to 25 μm in width.

M. audouinii: This species may be difficult to identify due to the lack of sporulation. Colonies on Saboraud's dextrose agar are gray–white, cream to tan with a red–brown pigment on the reverse side of the culture plate. The most distinctive microscopic finding is apiculate terminal chlamydospores. Growth on rice grains is scant and characterized by a brown discoloration of the rice.

M. canis: This rapidly growing organism is characterized by a granular appearance, buff in color and a yellow–orange to orange–brown on the reverse side (See Color Fig. 24–3A in separate color insert) differentiating it from another closely related *Microsporum*, *M. gypseum* (See Color Fig. 24–3H in separate color insert). Most strains make abundant fusiform, echinulate, thick-walled multiseptate macroconidia and few microconidia (Fig. 24–2A). Occasional isolates may not sporulate well or are atypical, (*M. canis* var. *distortum*) and additional tests are required for identification. These tests include the hair perforation and sporulation when grown on rice grains.

Epidermophyton. The single pathogenic species, *E. floccosum*, is distinguished by the formation of obovate to broadly clavate multicell (1–9 septa) macroconidia (20–60 μm by 4–13 μm) with smooth walls and by the absence of microconidia (Fig. 24–2C). Colonies develop slowly, are frequently grainy, and develop folds, suede-like in texture, and range from olive to yellow or yellow–brown (See Color Fig. 24–3B in separate color insert).

Trichophyton. The macroconidia of this genus are multicell (1–12 septa), smooth walled, variable in shape (clavate, cylindrical, cylindrofusiform), and formed singularly or in clusters on conidiophores. They may be abundant, rare, or absent depending on the species or strain and culture conditions.

T. RUBRUM. The macroscopic colony appearance can be variable. Typical colonies are white to buff in color, with or without a wine red color on the reverse side (See Color Figs. 24–3C and 24–3D in separate color insert). Some are granular while others are downy in appearance. The main identifying characteristics are the presence of club-shaped microconidia arranged along the hyphae (Fig. 24–2D), smooth-walled macroconidia, inability to perforate hair in vitro, and lack of urease production.

T. mentagrophytes complex. Both zoophilic (var. *interdigitale*) and anthropophilic (var. *mentagrophytes*) strains have been described. Zoophilic strains produce colonies that are granular, off-white color (See Color Fig. 24–3E in separate color insert), while anthropophilic strains are white and fluffy (See Color Fig. 24–3F in separate color insert). Pigment on the reverse side may be present and may resemble that produced by *T. rubrum*. The main identifying characteristics of *T. mentagrophytes* complex are the production of rounded microconidia arranged along the hyphae (Fig. 24–2E) and in grape like clusters, smooth-walled macroconidia, spiral hyphae, positive test for in vitro hair perforation, and production of urease.

T. TONSURANS. Colonies appear powdery or grainy, usually with a brown to tan color that may be lost upon subculture (See Color Fig. 24–3G in separate color insert). The reverse pigment if present has a yellow–brown or red appearance. The main identifying characteristics include the production of abundant microconidia of varying shapes, club, or elongated or balloon-like (Fig. 24–2F). Some strains make abundant arthroconidia and chlamydospores. Growth is stimulated in the presence of thiamin.

T. VIOLACEUM. Growth is slow, producing colonies that are heaped and convoluted, with a violet or lavender surface and a purple color on the reverse side. The main identifying characteristics are the rate of growth, colony appearance, lack of micro- and macroconidia, and stimulation of growth by thiamin.

T. SCHOENLEINII. Growth is slow, producing white to tan, heaped, and convoluted colonies without any color on the reverse side. Main identifying characteristics include lack of both micro- and macroconidia, and the formation of "favic chandeliers," which are antler-like structures at the tips of hyphae.

T. CONCENTRICUM. Growth is slow, producing beige to brown or reddish colonies that are convoluted, becoming glabrous. Main identifying characteristics are the lack of sporulation, stimulation by thiamin (50% of strains), the geographic location, and the clinical picture.

Pathogenesis

Dermatophytes are primary cutaneous pathogens and comprise the largest group of fungi that cause skin disease. These fungi appear to be uniquely qualified to invade hair, nails, and skin, in part due to their ability to produce keratinases, which are enzymes that digest keratin in vitro. Another factor that may enhance their pathogenicity is the production of mannans, cell wall components that are immunoinhibitory in vitro (Blake et al, 1991). Mannans may also be able to prevent elimination of the dermatophyte from the host by suppressing cell-mediated immunity in vivo. Infection is enhanced by damage to the skin surface. For example, tinea cruris and interdigital tinea pedis frequently occur in areas that have become macerated secondary to occlusion. Human genetics also appears to play a role in the pathogenicity of some dermatophytes. Tinea unguium (onychomycosis) may be an autosomal dominant trait in some families. Tinea imbricata, which is caused by *Trichophyton concentricum* and thought to be inherited in an autosomal recessive fashion, is a variant of tinea corporis.

Several host-mediated factors limit invasion by dermatophytes. Progesterone has been shown to inhibit growth in vitro (Heoprich et al, 1994), which may explain the increased incidence of some dermatophytoses in men. Unsaturated fatty acids found in sebum also inhibit dermatophyte growth in vitro. The production of sebum by adult scalps may be responsible for the infrequency of adult tinea capitis. Conversely, the absence of sebum on the palms and soles could explain the persistence of dermatophyte infection at these sites. Immunodeficient patients are more likely to have deep localized dermatophyte invasion.

Tineas

Tinea Corporis

DEFINITION. Tinea corporis is defined as dermatophytosis of the glabrous skin of the face (excluding the beard), trunk, and limbs (including the dorsal hands and feet).

SYNONYMS. Dermatophytosis of the glabrous skin, ringworm, tinea circinata, tinea glabrosa (Demis, 1999).

INCIDENCE AND EPIDEMILOGY. Tinea corporis is a very common disease that, although present worldwide, is more prevalent in persons living in warm, humid climates. Unlike some other superficial fungal infections, tinea corporis shows no preference for certain age groups, races or ethnicities. Patients with systemic diseases such as diabetes mellitus, Cushing syndrome, or HIV infection, and those immunocompromised for other reasons are predisposed to tinea corporis (Mandel, 1961; Callaway, 1962). Those patients with chronic dermatophyte infections at other sites such as scalp, hands, feet, or nails are at risk of having the infection spread to glabrous skin (Geary, 1960; Rippon, 1988). Other risk factors include outdoor occupations, close association with animals, and contact sports.

Any of the dermatophyte species are capable of causing tinea corporis. Worldwide, the anthropophilic species, *T. rubrum,* is the most common pathogen (Rippon, 1988; Elewski and Hazen, 1989). In children, especially those with a personal or household history of tinea capitis, *T. tonsurans* is often the culprit. Persons with frequent contact with animals, especially kittens, puppies, horses, cattle, rodents, and fowl, may be exposed to zoophilic organisms such as *M. canis* and *T. mentagrophytes* var. mentagrophytes. Geophilic species, most often *M. gypseum*, are more likely to infect gardeners or other persons in contact with the soil.

CLINICAL PRESENTATIONS. The clinical presentations of tinea corporis vary widely from noninflammatory, scaly plaques to inflammatory pustules. This variation is somewhat dependent on the infecting organism. The anthropophilic pathogens are more likely to produce the classical annular plaque with advancing scale and central clearing (See Color Fig. 24–4 in separate color insert). Other noninflammatory lesions may be oval, circinate, and may or may not have erythema. Geophilic and zoophilic species are more apt to cause inflammatory lesions that can range from vesicles and pustules to bulla. All lesions of tinea corporis are usually pruritic.

Invasion of hair follicles results in perifollicular pustules that may resemble a bacterial folliculitis. This may eventually result in penetration of follicle walls and granuloma formation (Majocchi's granuloma) around fragments of hair or keratin (See Color Fig. 24–5 in separate color insert). Majocchi's granuloma is most often seen in women with onychomycosis or tinea pedis who shave their legs (Wilson et al, 1954).

Infection by the zoophilic organism, *T. verrucosum*, also usually causes an exuberant inflammatory response. Follicular pustules with surrounding erythema present a kerion-like appearance (Powell and Muller, 1982). These lesions frequently cause hair loss and scarring.

Tinea profunda, which is another intense inflammatory reaction of the glabrous skin that resembles scalp kerions, is a rare presentation and more likely to occur in patients with suppressed cellular immunity. The verrucous lesions of tinea profunda may resemble those of North American blastomycosis (Demis, 1999).

DIAGNOSIS. Whenever tinea corporis is suspected, the diagnosis can be confirmed easily with a microscopic examination of scale mounted in KOH. Collect the scale on a glass slide by scraping outward from the advancing raised edge of the lesion with a scalpel blade held perpendicular to the skin, and cover the scale with one or two drops of 10% to 20% KOH and a cover slip. The KOH breaks down the epithelial cells but leaves the fungal elements unharmed. Fungal stains, such as chlorazole Black E or Parker blue–black ink may be added to the KOH to enhance the visibility of the hyphae.

The hyphae of all dermatophytes look the same under direct microscopic examination with KOH. Cultures are necessary to identify the particular pathogen. Collect skin scrapings as detailed above. Commercial collection packages and mailing envelopes are available for this purpose. Alternatively, scrapings may be collected in squares of stiff black paper, which are folded and secured with paper clips. Features of colonies, combined with microscopic examination of the microconidia and macroconidia allow identification of the genus and species.

DIFFERENTIAL DIAGNOSIS. Multiple conditions should be included in the differential diagnosis of tinea corporis. The scaly, less inflammatory lesions must be distinguished from those of psoriasis, seborrheic dermatitis, secondary syphilis, tinea versicolor, and discoid lupus erythematosus. Annular lesions may resemble the herald patch of pityriasis rosea, nummular eczema, or erythema annulare centrifugum. Majocchi's granuloma and other inflammatory lesions involving hair follicles can be confused with bacterial pyodermas, deep fungal infections, and tuberculosis (Powell and Muller, 1982).

TREATMENT. Therapy with topical antimycotic agents is usually sufficient for cure of tinea corporis (Drake et al, 1996a) (Table 24–2). These medications are applied to the lesion and to at least a 2.5 cm border of adjacent clinically uninvolved skin, once or twice daily as directed by the manufacturer. Therapy should continue for 1 to 2 weeks after all signs of infection are cleared. Most commercially available topical drugs are effective in tinea corporis. However, nystatin and topical am-

TABLE 24–2. *Selected Topical Antimycotic Drugs for Tinea Corporis*

Drug	Frequency of Dosing
Allylamines	
Butenafine	Once daily
Naftifine	Once daily
Terbinafine	Once daily
Imidazoles	
Clotrimazole	Twice daily
Econazole	Once daily
Ketoconazole	Once or twice daily
Miconazole	Twice daily
Oxiconazole	Once or twice daily
Sulconazole	Once or twice daily
Substituted Pyridones	
Ciclopirox	Twice daily
Other	
Tolnaftate	Twice daily

TABLE 24–3. *Oral Antimycotic Drugs for Tinea Corporis*

Drug	Dose	Duration of Therapy
Griseofulvin	Microsize 20 mg/kg/day Ultramicrosize 15mg/kg/day	2 to 4 weeks
Fluconazole	150–300 mg once weekly	2 to 4 weeks
Itraconazole	200 mg/day	1 week
Terbinafine	250 mg/day	1 week

photericin B do not control dermatophytes and should not be used (Lescher, 1996).

Clinical experience argues against use of topical steroids for tinea corporis (Drake et al, 1996a). Although they may initially reduce itching and other symptoms through their antiinflammatory effects, continued use of topical steroids may suppress the cellular response to infection and result in extensive disease. Topical steroids may also change the clinical appearance of the lesion, resulting in "tinea incognito." Likewise, products combining topical antimycotics and steroids should be avoided.

In some cases, topical antimycotic agents are insufficient for the treatment of tinea corporis. Patients who have failed topical therapy, those with inflammatory infections, those with extensive disease, and those immunocompromised by therapy or disease, require oral antifungal therapy. Suitable medications include griseofulvin, fluconazole, itraconazole, and terbinafine (Table 24–3).

PREVENTION. In general, treatment of tinea corporis with effective medications results in a permanent cure. However, the ubiquitous nature of the fungal infectious agents makes reexposure and reinfection a constant possibility. Moist, damp environments such as those in locker rooms are likely to have high loads of fungal elements and should be avoided. It also is possible for infected persons to transmit the pathogens to other persons by close physical contact. Thus, it is important to identify and treat these patients. If zoophilic organisms are identified by culture, the infected animals should be identified and taken to a veterinarian for treatment. When geophilic pathogens are isolated, contact with the infected soil should be avoided.

Tinea Barbae

DEFINITION. Tinea barbae is dermatophytosis of the facial beard area of men.

SYNONYMS. Barbers' itch, ringworm of the beard, tinea sycosis, trichophytosis barbae (Demis, 1999).

INCIDENCE AND EPIDEMIOLOGY. Historically, tinea barbae was a fairly common condition often transmitted by contaminated razors at barbershops (Rippon, 1988). This dermatophytosis is now seen rarely and most often acquired from animal sources, explaining the increased prevalence in rural areas. Two of the most common causative agents are *Trichophyton mentagrophytes* and *T. verrucosum*. Both species are usually acquired from animals. *Microsporum canis* is another zoophilic pathogen that can rarely cause tinea barbae. Anthropophilic dermatophytes that may cause this disease include *T. rubrum*, *T megninii*, *T violaceum*, and *T. schoenleinii*. Many of these pathogens have geographically restricted ranges. *Trichophyton violaceum* is endemic in parts of Europe, Asia, Africa, and South America but is seldomly seen in the United States. *Trichophyton megninii* is found in parts of Africa and Europe, including Portugal, Sardinia, and Sicily. Africa and Eurasia are home to *T. schoenleinii*. In contrast, the range of *T. rubrum* is not restricted; hence the organism may cause disease worldwide (Demis, 1999).

CLINICAL PRESENTATIONS. The infecting pathogens are partially responsible for the two clinical presentations of tinea barbae. Zoophilic organisms, such as *T. mentagrophytes* and *T. verrucosum,* are more likely to produce the inflammatory pattern characterized by kerion formation with boggy, elevated nodules, draining pustules, and sinus tracts. Hair in infected areas may be broken, loose, or absent. The chin and neck are usually first involved and infection may spread to cover the entire beard area. However, the upper lip is rarely affected. This feature helps to distinguish tinea barbae from bacterial pyodermas, as these infections commonly involve the upper lip (Rippon, 1988). Other symptoms that may be seen with both conditions include prominent adenopathy, fever, and malaise.

The second clinical presentation of tinea barbae is the noninflammatory or sycosiform type, the more uncommon of the two varieties. This noninflammatory type often resembles bacterial folliculitis in that follicular pustules may be discrete. Other lesions may resemble tinea corporis. The hair within the affected areas may be very loose or broken, which helps to distinguish this presentation clinically from bacterial folliculitis. *Trichophyton violaceum* or *T. rubrum* are the most likely pathogens.

DIAGNOSIS. Clinical suspicion of tinea barbae should prompt a direct microscopic examination of infected hairs. Purulent debris may also contain fungal elements, but these may be difficult to find in the inflammatory presentation. Fungal cultures should be obtained to establish the diagnosis and identify the pathogen. Wood's light examination is usually nonproductive unless *M. canis* is the causative organism.

TABLE 24-4. *Oral Antimycotic Drugs for Tinea Barbae*

Drug	Dose	Duration of Therapy
Griseofulvin	Microsize 20 mg/kg/day Ultramicrosize 15 mg/kg/day	Minimum of 4 weeks. Generally, 6 weeks or longer required. Continue for at least 2 weeks after disease resolves.
Fluconazole	150 to 300 mg once weekly (preferred) 200 to 400 mg daily	4 to 6 weeks Up to 4 weeks
Itraconazole	400 mg/day 200 mg/day	1 week pulse. A second pulse may be required 3 weeks after the first is completed. 2 to 4 weeks
Terbinafine	250 mg/day	2 to 4 weeks

DIFFERENTIAL DIAGNOSIS. As discussed under Clinical Pres-entations, tinea barbae often resembles bacterial folliculitis (Ludwig, 1953). Tinea barbae must also be differentiated from acne vulgaris, actinomycosis, contact dermatitis, eczema herpeticum, herpes simplex, and herpes zoster.

TREATMENT. Left untreated, the inflammatory type of tinea barbae may resolve spontaneously, but alopecia and scar formation are common. The sycosiform variant is usually more chronic and spontaneous resolution is unlikely. For these reasons, treatment is recommended. Since the hair follicles are infected, oral antifungal medications are required (Drake et al, 1996b). Griseofulvin, fluconazole, itraconazole, and terbinafine may each be of some benefit. Treatment should be continued until the infection is cleared and new hair growth is apparent (Table 24-4).

Several adjunctive therapies may be helpful in tinea barbae. Warm saline or water compresses may be used to soften crusts and debris to aid in their removal. Topical 2% ketoconazole shampoo or 2.5% selenium sulfide lotion are helpful in removing the debris and may provide some antimycotic activity. Topical antibacterial agents such as mupirocin can aid in controlling secondary bacterial infections.

PREVENTION. The majority of tinea barbae infections are now zoophilic in origin. Contact with infected animals should be minimized. Infected animals should also be treated.

Tinea Cruris

DEFINITION. Tinea cruris is a dermatophytosis of the medial upper thighs and the inguinal, pubic, perineal, and perianal areas. Skin on the buttocks is also involved at times (Demis, 1999).

SYNONYMS. Eczema marginatum, gym itch, hobie itch, jock itch, ringworm of the groin, tinea inguinalis.

Incidence and Epidemiology. Although tinea cruris is more common in tropical climates, it has a worldwide distribution. Relatively high humidity and ambient temperature favor the growth of the causative organisms. Infections usually occur in postpubertal males but females can be affected. Epidemics have occurred as a result of crowded living conditions and/or shared bathing facilities as with members of armed forces, athletic teams, or prisoners. Sweating, tight clothing, such as shorts or athletic supporters, and wet bathing suits worn for a long period can predispose to infection. Other risk factors include obesity and diabetes mellitus. The causative pathogens may spread to the groin area from other dermatophytoses such as tinea pedis, tinea manuum, and tinea unguium.

The most commonly encountered pathogen is *T. rubrum*. Others commonly seen include *E. floccosum*, and *T. mentagrophytes*. *Epidermophyton floccosum* was once the major pathogen in tinea cruris and tinea cruris remains the only dermatophytosis in which *E. floccosum* plays a significant role (Rippon, 1988).

CLINICAL PRESENTATIONS. As with other dermatophytoses, the causative organisms often determine the clinical manifestations of the disease. Tinea cruris due to *T. rubrum* or *E. floccosum* is more likely to be chronic and relatively noninflammatory. There may be only slight erythema and an indistinct active margin. *Trichophyton mentagrophytes*, on the other hand, is usually associated with inflammatory disease. In acute cases, itching is often severe. There may be inflammation with vesicles at the edge of the lesions. Weeping and excoriations are sometimes present.

Both presentations are more likely to occur in men, possibly due to increased moisture in crural folds. Usually, the first area involved is the intertriginous fold near the scrotum (Rippon, 1988). The upper, medial thigh is the most commonly affected area. Infection may also involve the pubis, perineum, perianal area, and buttocks. Lesions may be unilateral or bilateral, symmetrical or asymmetrical. Although dermatophytes may colonize the scrotum, they typically do not infect scrotal skin. When redness or scaling are seen on the scrotum, the clinician should consider the possibility of other conditions such as candidiasis, secondary neurodermatitis, or contact dermatitis (Rippon, 1988; Elewski and Hazen, 1989).

DIAGNOSIS. The clinical suspicion of tinea cruris should be confirmed with KOH testing of scale from the lesion as well as fungal culture. Other causes of intertrigo in the groin, such as candidiasis, erythrasma, and psoriasis, should be ruled out.

DIFFERENTIAL DIAGNOSIS. Intertrigo is a nonspecific dermatitis characterized by erythema, burning, itching, maceration, and sometimes erosions involving the skin folds. Tinea cruris is only one cause of intertrigo seen in the groin. Other infectious causes include grampositive bacteria, such as *Staphylococcus aureus* and *Corynebacterium minutissiumum* (erythrasma). The deep red or coral fluorescence produced by the latter organism on examination with a Wood's lamp can be used to differentiate erythrasma from tinea cruris. Another difference is the absence of an active margin in erythrasma.

Candidiasis often resembles tinea cruris. Women are more likely to have candidal infections than men. Other risk factors that increase the likelihood of yeast infection include diabetes, obesity, systemic antibiotic therapy, and the use of oral contraceptives. These factors also increase the chance of concomitant dermatophyte and *Candida* infections. Scrotal involvement is much more likely in candidiasis. The presence of satellite pustules adjacent to the primary lesion helps to distinguish candidiasis (in which they are present) from tinea cruris.

Other conditions to be considered in the differential diagnosis include seborrheic dermatitis, psoriasis vulgaris (inverse type), irritant dermatitis, and contact dermatitis.

TREATMENT. Most topical antifungal agents are generally effective in the treatment of uncomplicated tinea cruris (Brodell and Elewski, 1997; Drake et al, 1996a). The spectra of the various medications should be kept in mind when making an empirical treatment choice. For example, tolnaftate has no effect on *Candida* and would not be a good initial choice unless candidiasis has been ruled out (Demis, 1999). Econazole nitrate has activity against *Candida* and some bacteria (Rupke, 2000) and could be beneficial when a secondary candidal or bacterial infection is suspected.

When topical agents prove ineffective, oral antimycotic drugs may be necessary. Other indications for systemic therapy include extensive disease, severe obesity,

and compromised immunity. For dermatophyte infection, ultramicrosized griseofulvin at a dose of 15 mg/kg/day can be given for 2–4 weeks: the microsized preparation requires a dose of 20 mg/kg/day for the same period (Lambert et al, 1989). Although griseofulvin is of little help in infections complicated by *Candida* species or bacteria, both fluconazole and itraconazole are effective against dermatophytes and *Candida* species. The adult dose of fluconazole is 150 mg/day for 2–3 weeks and the dose of itraconazole is 200 mg/day for 1 week or 100 mg/day for 2 weeks. Terbinafine at a dose of 250 mg/day for 1–2 weeks is also effective against dermatophytes (Lesher, 1999).

PREVENTION. The dermatophytes causing tinea cruris thrive in moist, warm environs. Measures that minimize exposure to these conditions can be preventive. Tight fitting, nonabsorbent clothing and prolonged exposure to wet clothing, such as bathing suits, should be avoided. Infected areas should be bathed daily and dried thoroughly, preferably with a hair drier. After the primary infection has resolved, absorbent powders containing an antimycotic such as miconazole or tolnaftate may prevent recurrence. Weight reduction may be beneficial in obese patients. Tinea pedis and pedal onychomycosis may serve as a reservoir for pathogens causing tinea cruris. Ideally, these infections must be eliminated in order to prevent reinfection of the groin. Suggesting to patients that they put on their socks before their undershorts may help stop spread of the organisms.

Tinea Pedis and Manuum

DEFINITION. Tinea pedis is a dermatophytosis of the plantar surface of the feet and toe webs. Similarly, tinea manuum is dermatophytosis of the palmar surface of the hands and interdigital spaces. Dermatophytoses of the dorsal hands and feet have a presentation, course, and prognosis more similar to that of tinea corporis and are excluded in the strict definition of this disease.

SYNONYMS. Athlete's foot, ringworm of the feet, ringworm of the hands (Demis, 1999).

INCIDENCE AND EPIDEMIOLOGY. Tinea pedis is the most common dermatophytosis. Approximately 70% of the population is estimated to have been infected at some time (Ganor et al, 1963; Rippon, 1988). Males are more likely to be infected, and incidence increases with age. Most patients are postpubescent. Tinea manuum is also a common malady associated with tinea pedis and the same pathogen causes the hand and foot infections. Chronic disease results and is often associated with tinea unguium (onychomycosis) of the finger and toenails.

Surprisingly, tinea pedis is relatively new to the Western world and its prevalence parallels the migration of *T. rubrum* throughout the globe. This common dermatophyte was originally endemic in three regions: Southeast Asia, portions of western Africa, and northern Australia. With worldwide travel, *T. rubrum* spread to Europe and the Americas in the later part of the nineteenth century. The first case of *T. rubrum* tinea pedis to be reported in the United States occurred in a Birmingham, Alabama WWI veteran in the early 1920s (Weidman, 1927). Today, *T. rubrum* is the most common dermatophyte worldwide (Rippon, 1988; Elewski and Hazen, 1989). Interestingly, it does not cause tinea pedis in the original endemic areas because no footwear is worn by the local people.

Tinea pedis and manuum are caused predominantly by *T. rubrum* and *T. mentagrophytes*, and less commonly by *E. floccosum* (Rippon, 1988). *Trichophyton rubrum* is viable outside the human host for only short periods of time. However, its prevalence and the presence of large numbers of arthroconidia in the environment combine to overcome this shortfall. The arthroconidia of *E. floccosum*, on the other hand, remain viable in the environment for years. Patients may acquire this organism from fomites, such as carpeting. *Trichophyton mentagrophytes* occurs as both zoophilic and anthropophilic varieties. The zoophilic variety is more likely to cause an inflammatory presentation. In children, *T. tonsurans* is often implicated in tinea pedis, especially in those with tinea capitis caused by this organism (Elewski, 1998a).

All of the above named pathogens produce infections that are generally limited to the stratum corneum, perhaps due to the antidermatophytic or fungistatic effect of human serum (Lorincz et al, 1958). *Trichophyton rubrum* usually causes a chronic, relatively noninflammatory disease. Sebaceous glands are thought to produce antimicrobial substances and their absence in palms and soles may account for the increased susceptibility of these areas to chronic infection. Mannan, a cell wall glycoprotein found in *T. rubrum*, has been observed to suppress in vitro cell-mediated immune function (Blake et al, 1991), and may also contribute to the chronicity of the clinical manifestations. The more inflammatory presentation associated with *T. mentagrophytes* may be a result of an allergic or hypersensitivity reaction. A dermatophytid reaction may also be associated and manifests as blister(s) on the sides of fingers and palms resembling dyshidrosis.

CLINICAL PRESENTATIONS. The infections produced by these pathogens generally fall within one of four clinical patterns of tinea pedis: moccasin, interdigital, inflammatory, and ulcerative. Moccasin tinea pedis is usually caused by *T. rubrum*. Dry, hyperkeratotic scale may involve the entire plantar surface, extending to the lateral foot. Erythema is mild and the condition may be asymptomatic. Occasionally, thick, hyperkeratotic scale with fissures may develop. One or both feet may be involved and toenail infection increases with duration of disease.

The interdigital presentation of tinea pedis consists of maceration, scaling, and fissuring of the toe webs. The skin between the fourth and fifth toe is most commonly affected. Adjacent areas may become involved but the dorsal skin usually remains clear. *Trichophyton rubrum* and *E. floccosum* are the common causes (Rippon, 1988). Hot, humid climates increase the symptoms and hyperhidrosis may increase the risk of infection. Other microorganisms, such as *Corynebacterium minutissimum* (erythrasma), other bacteria, and *Candida*, can also cause interdigital maceration and should be excluded. Secondary bacterial infections may contribute to the pathology, resulting in the so-called "dermatophytosis complex" (Leyden and Kligman, 1978). Bacterial byproducts preclude culture recovery of dermatophytes. Therapy must include antibacterial as well as antimycotic medications.

In inflammatory or vesicular tinea pedis, vesicles, bulla, and/or pustules are seen on the instep or mid-anterior plantar surface. These usually painful, pruritic lesions develop rapidly and are more likely to occur during summer months. They may also be accompanied by a vesicular hypersensitivity (dermatophytid or "id") reaction on the hands. Occasionally the inflammatory response is incapacitating and includes cellulitis, adenopathy, and lymphangitis. The zoophilic organism, *T. mentagrophytes* var. *mentagrophytes*, is more likely to cause such acute reactions.

Secondary bacterial infections may further increase inflammation and are thought to be responsible for the interdigital ulcers and erosions typically seen in ulcerative tinea pedis. Cellulitis, lymphangitis, fever, and malaise are frequent complications. *Trichophyton mentagrophytes* var. *mentagrophytes* is also the most common cause of ulcerative tinea pedis (Demis, 1999).

The presentation of tinea manuum is similar to that of moccasin tinea pedis. The palmar skin develops dry scale that can be quite hyperkeratotic. *Trichophyton rubrum* is the usual pathogen. About half of patients have only one palm involved, leading to the "one hand and two feet" presentation. This syndrome is common but the unilateral involvement of the hands has not been explained. Some, but not all, of the fingernails on the involved hand are also frequently infected. When present, the nail dystrophy is a clue that distinguishes tinea manuum from other palmar dermatoses.

DIAGNOSIS. Clinical suspicion supported by microscopic examination of scale mounted in KOH is sufficient to establish the diagnosis. A fungal culture serves to confirm the diagnosis and identify the pathogen.

DIFFERENTIAL DIAGNOSIS. Differential diagnoses vary depending on the clinical presentation. The dry scaling plaques of moccasin tinea pedis and tinea manuum resemble chronic contact dermatitis, psoriasis, eczema, and various keratodermas. Nail involvement, which may be seen in these two dermatophytoses, is a clinical clue. Candidiasis, hyperhidrosis, erythrasma, and other bacterial infections can produce lesions similar to those of interdigital tinea pedis. A coral–red fluorescence on Wood's light examination distinguishes erythrasma, and bacterial cultures may be required to differentiate the other bacterial causes. Inflammatory tinea pedis must be distinguished from dyshidrotic eczema, pustular psoriasis, primary blistering diseases and contact dermatitis.

TREATMENT. Topical and/or oral antifungal agents are used to treat tinea pedis, depending on the patient and the clinical presentation. Topical antifungals are generally effective for interdigital tinea pedis and tinea manuum not complicated by onychomycosis in immune competent hosts. Primary or secondary bacterial infections are often present in interdigital disease. Antifungal drugs with antibacterial activity, such as econazole or ciclopirox, are good first-line therapy (Rupke, 2000). Conversely, tolnaftate is not the best choice as it has little activity against *Candida* or bacteria (Drake et al, 1996a). Topical agents should be used as directed by the manufacturer for approximately 4 weeks, but terbinafine and butenafine may be effective with only 1 week of therapy (Villars and Jones, 1989; Bergstresser et al, 1993; Savin et al, 1994; Elewski et al, 1995a; Savin et al, 1997). Emollients containing lactic acid or urea (e.g., Lac Hydrin or Carmol 40) may be useful additions to therapy when extensive scaling or hyperkeratosis is present.

Oral antifungal drugs are generally required when treating moccasin and inflammatory tinea pedis, and tinea pedis or tinea manuum complicated by fungal nail involvement. Immunocompromised patients and those with peripheral vascular disease also require oral treatment. When nails are not involved, terbinafine (250 mg/day for 1–2 weeks), itraconazole (100 mg/day for 2 weeks or 400 mg/day for 1 week), or fluconazole (150–300 mg once a week for up to 8 weeks) may be effective (Lesher, 1999). Griseofulvin is often ineffective in tinea pedis (Moossavi, 2001).

When onychomycosis is present, the nail infection must be cleared to prevent recurrence of tinea pedis or tinea manuum. Treatment of onychomycosis requires 12 weeks of terbinafine 250 mg/day (Drake et al, 1997). Itraconazole is also effective and may be given either as a 200 mg/day dose for 12 weeks or 400 mg/day for 1 week per month for 3 to 4 consecutive months (Elewski et al, 1997b; Scher, 1999). A once-weekly 150–450 mg dose of fluconazole for 6 months is also effective (Scher, 1999) (Table 24–6).

PREVENTION. Avoidance of exposure to the infective agent and minimization of risk factors are critical in the prevention of both tinea pedis and tinea manuum. Protective footwear should be worn in public facilities such as hotels, gymnasiums, and locker rooms. To decrease the risk of recurrence, measures should be taken to reduce the amount of foot moisture. The patient should be instructed to thoroughly dry feet after baths and apply an antifungal powder or spray. Cotton socks changed frequently absorb sweat and reduce risk factors. Antifungal powder applied inside shoes may be helpful. Finally, prevention and effective treatment of tinea pedis are likely to prevent tinea manuum (Richardson and Elewski, 2000b).

Tinea Unguium (Onychomycosis)

DEFINITION. Tinea unguium is defined as infection of fingernails or toenails by dermatophyte fungi. Onychomycosis is a broader term that also encompasses nail infections by nondermatophyte moulds, yeasts, and occasionally bacteria.

INCIDENCE AND EPIDEMIOLOGY. Estimates of the prevalence of onychomycosis in the general population vary considerably from approximately 3% to over 13% (Heikkala and Stubbs, 1995; Elewski and Chaniff, 1997a). Prevalence increases with increasing age. One study showed that up to 28% of patients over 60 years of age had culture positive onychomycosis (Elewski and Chaniff, 1997a). Possible explanations include decreased immune function, poor peripheral circulation, prolonged exposure to the infective agents, and inability to maintain hygienic foot care (Drake et al, 1996c; Scher, 1996; Elewski and Chaniff, 1997a).

Dermatophytes are the cause of onychomycosis in over 90% of toenail infections and the majority of fingernail infections without paronychia (Ellis et al, 1997). The two most commonly isolated species in Europe and North America are *T. rubrum* and *T. mentagrophytes*. *Epidermophyton floccosum* is also seen, but less commonly (Summerbell, 1997). *Trichophyton tonsurans* may occur in children who have had or have been exposed to tinea capitis. Other pathogens include nondermatophyte moulds such as *Scytalidium* spp., *Scopulariopsis* spp., *Aspergillus* spp., and *Fusarium* spp. Secondary colonization of previously damaged nails accounts for other nondermatophytic infections. Yeasts such as *Candida albicans* may also be the infective fungal pathogens in fingernails.

TABLE 24–5. *Clinical Presentations of Tinea Unguium (Onychomycosis)*

Clinical Presentation	Appearance	Common Pathogen(s)	Other Pathogen(s)
DLSO	Onycholysis and subungual thickening. Yellowish-brown discoloration of nail plate.	*Trichophyton rubrum*	*T. mentagrophytes* *T. tonsurans* *E. floccosum*
WSO	Well-delineated opaque "white islands" on nail plate.	*Trichophyton mentagrophytes*	*Aspergillus terreus* *Acremonium potronii* *Fusarium oxysporum*
PSO and PWSO	Subungual hyperkeratosis. Proximal onycholysis. Leukonychia.	*Trichophyton rubrum*	
Total Dystrophic Onychomycosis	Nails are thickened and dystrophic.	May be end result of DLSO, WSO, or PSO	

DLSO, distal lateral subungual onychomycosis; WSO, white superficial onychomycosis; PSO, proximal subungual onychomycosis; PWSO, proximal white subungual onychomycosis.

CLINICAL PRESENTATIONS. Onychomycosis is classified into four clinical presentations and associated routes of invasion (Table 24–5). The most common form is distal lateral subungual onychomycosis (DLSO) in which the infectious agent invades the nail plate at the hyponychium or lateral nail groove and migrates proximally. The invasion is accompanied by a mild inflammatory response resulting in focal parakeratosis and subungual hyperkeratosis, leading to separation of the nail plate from the nail bed (onycholysis) and subungual thickening. Superinfection of the subungual space by bacteria or moulds often results in a yellowish-brown discoloration of the nail plate. Distal lateral subungual onychomycosis is most commonly seen in toenails, in part secondary to the greater incidence of tinea pedis as compared to tinea manuum. As in tinea pedis, *T. rubrum* is the most common cause of DLSO. *Trichophyton mentagrophytes, T. tonsurans*, and *E. floccosum* have also been associated with DLSO.

White superficial onychomycosis (WSO) occurs less frequently than DLSO and is caused by fungal invasion of the superficial nail plate. Characteristically, well delineated opaque "white islands" are seen on the nail (See Color Fig. 24–6 in separate color insert). These "white islands" grow radially and may coalesce to cover much of the nail. The infection may also move through the plate into the cornified layers of the nail bed and hyponychium. Eventually, the nail becomes rough, soft, and may crumble. As in DLSO, the toenails are more commonly involved. The most common pathogen is *T. mentagrophytes* (Elewski, 1998a). Nondermatophyte moulds, including *Aspergillus terreus, Acremonium potronii*, and *Fusarium oxysporum* have also been implicated (Zaias et al, 1996).

Proximal subungual onychomycosis (PSO) (and its variant, proximal white subungual onychomycosis [PWSO]), is the least common presentation in the immunocompetent population. However, PSO is more frequent in AIDS patients (Aly and Berger, 1996) and

in patients with peripheral vascular disease (Richardson and Elewski, 2000a). The pathogen invades the nail plate through the proximal nail fold and spreads distally from the lunula area. This results in subungual hyperkeratosis, proximal onycholysis, leukonychia, and eventual destruction of the proximal nail plate. *Trichophyton rubrum* is the most common etiologic agent and toenails are more often infected than fingernails.

Total dystrophic onychomycosis may be the result of all three of these primary presentations. The entire nail plate and bed are involved and the nail becomes thickened and dystrophic. Occasionally, dense creamy white subungual areas are seen. These are "dermatophytomas," which are composed of densely packed, somewhat abnormal hyphae, and relatively resistant to systemic antifungal therapy. Debridement of these lesions is necessary for optimal management (Richardson and Elewski, 2000a).

DIAGNOSIS. Subungual hyperkeratosis, onycholysis, and yellow–brown discoloration are characteristic features of onychomycosis. Risk factors include nail trauma, peripheral vascular disease, diabetes mellitus, immunosuppression, hyperhidrosis, and older age. The presence of tinea pedis, especially the moccasin type, is an important clinical clue to differentiate fungal nail pathology from inflammatory nail disorders. Only approximately 50% of nail dystrophy is due to fungal infections (Andre and Achten, 1987). Direct microscopy and fungal cultures are helpful in confirming the diagnosis.

DIFFERENTIAL DIAGNOSIS. Several conditions may present with nail dystrophy that clinically resembles onychomycosis. Psoriasis is probably the most common, and may cause onycholysis similar to that seen in DLSO. Characteristics that can distinguish psoriasis include fine surface pitting, salmon-colored "oil drops" and family or personal history. Although nails may be involved exclusively, cutaneous changes of psoriasis are generally present.

Lichen planus is a less common mimic of onychomycosis. Distinguishing characteristics of lichen planus are exaggerated longitudinal ridging (onychorrhexis) and the *angel wing deformity* in which the central nail is raised and the lateral areas are depressed (Elewski and Hay, 1996). Contact dermatitis can also resemble onychomycosis. The presence of contact dermatitis elsewhere on the body helps to differentiate this diagnosis. Onychomycosis rarely involves all 20 nails and 20-nail dystrophy (trachyonychia) is usually idiopathic. Nail products containing formaldehyde may cause yellowing and onycholysis in all exposed nails. Repeated trauma to nails may result in onycholysis with subsequent colonization with pigment-producing microorganisms. Clipping of the onycholytic nail in such cases will reveal a normal-appearing nail bed.

Other conditions in the differential diagnosis of onychomycosis include bacterial infections, idiopathic onycholysis, nail bed tumors, pachyonychia congenita, and yellow nail syndrome.

TREATMENT. Systemic antifungal agents are generally required for treatment of onychomycosis (Drake et al, 1996c). Griseofulvin and ketoconazole are both associated with low cure rates and hepatotoxicity. Fluconazole, itraconazole, and terbinafine are all effective, generally safe, and well tolerated (Table 24–6).

Fluconazole is not FDA approved for the treatment of onychomycosis, but it has been approved for this indication in other countries. Fluconazole is effective against both dermatophytes and *Candida* (Elewski, 1998b). One study showed an 80%–90% success rate in toenail onychomycosis with once weekly dosing of fluconazole over a 6- to 7-month treatment period (Scher et al, 1998; Scher, 1999). Due to its inhibition of the cytochrome P-450 enzyme system, fluconazole has some potentially significant drug interactions. Other serious adverse reactions include hepatotoxicity and Stevens-Johnson syndrome among others. These re-

actions are rare and liver function monitoring is not generally recommended. The most common adverse effects include nausea and headache but these rarely result in discontinuation of the drug.

Itraconazole does have an FDA-approved indication for the treatment of onychomycosis. Its effectiveness against dermatophytes has been supported by a number of studies (De Doncker et al, 1996; Odom et al, 1996; Havu et al, 1997; Elewski et al, 1997b; Scher, 1999). Itraconazole may also be effective against some nondermatophyte moulds and *Candida* (De Doncker et al, 1996). This drug, which is contraindicated in patients with congestive heart failure, inhibits CYP3A4 and has the potential for some significant drug interactions. Hepatotoxicity is also a possible serious adverse effect and hepatic enzyme tests should be monitored in patients with preexisting hepatic function abnormalities and in those taking the medication for more than 1 month (Moossavi, 2001).

Like fluconazole and itraconazole, terbinafine has proven effective in the treatment of onychomycosis due to dermatophytes and some moulds (Drake et al, 1997; Scher, 1999). However, it activity against yeasts is variable. Like the two azole drugs, terbinafine can be hepatotoxic. The manufacturers recommend that terbinafine not be given to anyone with preexisting liver disease, and also recommend obtaining serum ALT and AST levels before starting therapy and monthly during therapy.

Topical agents as therapy for onychomycosis are generally disappointing. A solution of 8% ciclopirox in a nail lacquer produced a complete cure after 48 weeks in only 5.5% of patients with toenail onychomycosis (Dermik Laboratories, 2000). Evaluations of other topical products are now ongoing.

PREVENTION. Measures to limit exposure to fungal pathogens are necessary to prevent primary nail infections and relapse. Patients should always wear protective footwear in public showers and hotel rooms. Manicure equipment should not be shared. Use of antifungal

TABLE 24–6. *Systemic Antimycotic Drugs for Treatment of Onychomycosis*

Drug	Dosage	Monitoring
Fluconazole	150–450 mg once weekly for 6 months for toenails or 3 months for fingernails	None
Itraconazole	*Intermittent Dosing* 200 mg bid (400 mg/day) for 1 week per month for 3 consecutive months for toenails and 2 months for fingernails	LFT's prior to initiation and periodically thereafter when therapy is continued for more than 1 month.
Itraconazole	*Fixed Dosing* 200 mg daily for 12 weeks for toenails and 8 weeks for fingernails	
Terbinafine	250 mg/day for 12 weeks for toenails and 6 weeks for fingernails	LFT's prior to initiation and monthly thereafter

LFT, liver function test.

powders containing miconazole, clotrimazole, and tolnaftate in shoes may help prevent recurrence of tinea pedis and tinea unguium.

Tinea Capitis

DEFINITION. Tinea capitis is a dermatophytosis of the scalp hair follicle, and is caused by species in the genera *Microsporum* and *Trichophyton*.

SYNONYMS. Ringworm of the scalp, microsporosis capitis (tinea capitis caused by *Microsporum* species), trichophytosis capitis (tinea capitis caused by *Trichophyton* species), and favus (tinea capitis caused by *Trichophyton schoenleinii*) (Demis, 1999).

INCIDENCE AND EPIDEMIOLOGY. Although the true incidence of tinea capitis is unknown, it continues to be a common disease with a worldwide distribution. Tinea capitis is seen most frequently in prepubescent children.

The most common etiologic agent worldwide is the zoophilic organism, *M. canis*. In the United States and Western Europe, *T. tonsurans* is the most frequently isolated pathogen (Richardson and Warnock, 1993; Elewski, 2000). The prominent causative role of *T. tonsurans* has not always been the case. *Microsporum audouinii* was the cause of the tinea capitis epidemics seen from the 1940s through the 1960s. Now, *M. audouinii* is very rarely seen in the United States. In some areas, other species are endemic. *Trichophyton violaceum*, for example, is found only in portions of Africa, Asia, and Europe, although isolated cases have been reported in nonendemic seaports. *Trichophyton soudanense, T. gourvilli*, and *T. yaoundei* are endemic to Africa. Although *T. schoenleinii* was responsible for sporadic outbreaks of favus in some mountainous areas of Arkansas and Kentucky in the past, these foci have been eradicated. *Trichophyton mentagrophytes, T. verrucosum, T. rubrum, T. megninii, and M. gypseum* may cause sporadic outbreaks of tinea capitis. Rarely, *M. vanbreuseghemii, M. distortum,* and *M. nanum* may be isolated.

All of these causative organisms may be classified according to the pattern of infections (Elewski, 2000). In ectothrix infections, arthroconidia form a sheath around the hair shaft. In contrast, arthroconidia are seen within the hair shaft in the endothrix pattern. Hairs with favic infections have hyphal fragments in linear chains along the longitudinal axis. Further classification schema are based on whether or not fluorescence is observed under a Wood's lamp.

Some causative agents of tinea capitis have specific geographic distributions, and this is particularly true with anthropophilic fungi. Tinea capitis due to some zoophilic fungi may be seen only in the range of the preferred host. Geophilic organisms are widely disbursed. They can cause disease worldwide.

The etiologic agent involved also influences the incidence of tinea capitis. For example, the incidence of *Trichophyton* infection in girls and boys is roughly equal, whereas *M. audouinii* infects boys five times more frequently than girls (Demis, 1999). *Microsporum canis* also favors boys although the ratio varies considerably. The male to female rate of infection changes after puberty. Women are much more likely to be infected by *Trichophyton* spp. However, *T. schoenleinii,* the causative agent of favus, infects men and women equally.

Tinea capitis is most often a disease seen in children, with the highest incidence occurring between the ages of 3 and 7 (Williams et al, 1995). *Microsporum* infections are rarely seen after puberty. In those persons with persistent infections, spontaneous cures often occur shortly after puberty, probably because of chemical changes in sebum. *Trichophyton* scalp infections also occur more often in children, but teenagers and adults may also be infected and develop a less severe presentation.

The incidence of *T. tonsurans* tinea capitis is highest among those of African or Hispanic descent. The reasons for this are not known, although some authors suggest a genetic predisposition and crowded living conditions among other possible explanations (Babel and Baughman, 1989). Factors other than race may be involved and include hair-care practices and cohabitation.

The factors that allow the spread of tinea capitis are also not known. The organisms can be easily isolated from the environment in areas where there is a high incidence of cases. However, most people living in this environment will not become infected. Even some persons with long, close contact with infected patients may not become infected. A *carrier state* in which the infectious organisms may be cultured from the scalp of clinically asymptomatic patients is known to exist in some people exposed to infected patients (Vargo and Cohen, 1993). This finding is more common in adults but may also be seen in children. Clearly, more than contact with the organism must be necessary for infection to occur.

CLINICAL PRESENTATIONS. The various dermatophytes involved in the etiology of tinea capitis often produce similar clinical manifestations. Lesions range from dry, scaly patches of alopecia to inflammatory pustules and kerions. Posterior cervical and postauricular lymphadenopathy, present in many patients with tinea capitis, is a helpful differentiating factor from other causes of alopecia. The clinical presentations offer a practical way of classifying the disease. Tinea capitis may be divided into four types: gray patch, black dot, inflammatory, and favus.

GRAY PATCH TINEA CAPITIS. Gray patch tinea capitis is sometimes called noninflammatory, although this is a misnomer in that there is an inflammatory response present that can be demonstrated histologically. Careful physical examination may also uncover some erythema. Nevertheless, the term is useful in that it distinguishes this type of tinea capitis from the more inflammatory type in which pustules, suppuration, and kerion formation may be seen.

The hallmark of gray patch tinea capitis is a round or oval, sharply demarcated patch of partial alopecia (Rippon, 1988). Within the patch, the hair is reduced to short stubble by the tendency of infected hairs to break off just above the skin. After starting as a papule, the lesion enlarges peripherally to form a patch with only mild inflammation. Scaling is most often seen in the early phases of the infection while the patch is still spreading. Some patients have a normal appearing scalp. Others have minimal amount of scale that may resemble dandruff. Rarely does a single patch occur. Patches seldom exceed 6–8 centimeters in diameter. Several patches may coalesce to form extensive areas of hair loss. However, it is unusual for the lesions to cover more than half of the total scalp surface. The locations of the primary lesions vary according to sex. In boys, the vertex of the scalp is the most frequent site. By contrast, girls are more likely to have lesions along areas where the hair is parted, perhaps because infectious arthroconidia have greater access to the scalp at these sites.

These gray patch lesions are common in tinea capitis due to *Microsporum* spp. Although *M. audouinii* is now very rarely seen, *M. canis* is still common worldwide and *M. ferrugineum* is common in parts of Africa and Asia. All three of these *Microsporum* spp. cause ectothrix infections and all usually produce a characteristic yellow–green fluorescence under Wood's light examination. The use of the Wood's lamp may reveal other less conspicuous areas of involvement or isolated infected hairs.

BLACK DOT TINEA CAPITIS. In this type of tinea capitis, endothrix infection of hair causes the shafts to break off at or below the surface of the scalp, leaving only arthroconidia-laden stubs visible. When the hairs are black, this results in the appearance of black dots. Other hair colors produce dots of the same color (Elewski, 2000). The number of dots may be minimal and scaling may conceal those that are present. For these reasons, black dots are not always seen in endothrix tinea capitis.

Trichophyton tonsurans is by far the most common pathogen seen in black dot tinea capitis; *T. violaceum* is sometimes the causative organism but *T. rubrum* is only rarely isolated. Other anthropophilic pathogens endemic to parts of Africa, including *T. soudanense*, *T. yaoundei*, and *T. gourvilii*, do not fluoresce under Wood's light examination.

The clinical presentation of black dot tinea capitis is variable. Lesions due to *T. tonsurans* tend to be smaller than those produced by *Microsporum* species in noninflammatory gray patch tinea capitis. There are often multiple, scattered, irregularly shaped patches of alopecia with indistinct borders. Scaling may be a prominent feature. In a pattern sometimes confused with refractory seborrheic dermatitis, *T. tonsurans* may produce mild to moderate scaling with minimal hair loss and erythema.

As with gray patch tinea capitis, black dot endothrix tinea capitis is seen more commonly in children, and only occasionally seen in adults, particularly women.

INFLAMMATORY TINEA CAPITIS. In addition to black dot tinea capitis, *T. tonsurans* infections may result in inflammatory disease. In fact, all dermatophytes capable of causing tinea capitis may also produce inflammatory lesions ranging from pustular folliculitis to kerions. This is especially true of zoophilic and geophilic organisms. Kerions are thought to arise secondary to a hypersensitivity reaction. Kerions, which usually occur as single lesions and may be tender and painful, begin as small furuncles, which over a short period, enlarge and become more inflamed. Follicular abscesses develop and pus may exude from multiple sites. Kerions may be sparsely covered with broken hairs. In the worst cases, kerions become a sharply delineated, indurated, granulomatous tumefaction, sometimes referred to as a "boggy mass." Secondary bacterial infections may occur but this is unusual. The active inflammation generally lasts from 5 weeks to 5 months. Afterwards, infected hairs are extruded and the scalp appears smooth with no further sign of infection. The hair may regrow completely. Occasionally there is a residual scarring alopecia (See Color Fig. 24–7 in separate color insert).

Several other signs and symptoms are sometimes associated with inflammatory tinea capitis. Systemic manifestations include adenopathy, fever, and malaise. A hypersensitivity reaction to the primary infection may result in skin-colored to violaceous papules or red papulovesicles; sites most often involved include the face, neck, trunk, and arms. When present, this "id" reaction helps to distinguish tinea capitis from bacterial furunculosis. Erythema nodosum has also been associated with kerions.

FAVUS. Another type of inflammatory tinea capitis is favus, which is caused almost exclusively by infection with *T. schoenleinii* and characterized by the formation of scutula. These cup-shaped, yellow crusts form within the hair follicles and are composed of hyphae, neutrophils, and epidermal cells. The scutula may be separate but may also coalesce to cover much of the scalp. The infected hairs, which have hyphae arranged in linear chains along the longitudinal axis, are usually lusterless and may be full-length or broken. Occasionally, these infected hairs produce a bluish-white fluorescence under Wood's light. Hairs arising within the affected follicles pierce the scutula and often become matted. A serous exudate and secondary bacterial infections may be present. In addition, a mousy odor may be noticeable, especially in the absence of good hygiene. The condition may progress to atrophy and scarring alopecia.

Classic favus is a chronic condition that may be acquired during childhood and persist throughout adult life. As stated previously, it has occurred in the United States in the past but is now very rare in developed countries. Favus is still prevalent in parts of Africa, Asia, and South America.

DIAGNOSIS. In the presence of scaling patches of alopecia with broken hairs, the clinical diagnosis of tinea capitis may seem obvious. However, a wide range of presentations can be observed. Inflammatory lesions, such as kerions, can easily be misdiagnosed as bacterial infections. Other conditions are also sometimes mistaken for tinea capitis or vice versa (see Differential Diagnosis below). In order to more accurately make the diagnosis, three simple procedures should be performed on any patient with unexplained hair loss or persistent scaling. These include *(1)* Wood's light examination, *(2)* direct microscopic examination of hair, and *(3)* fungal cultures.

Wood's light examination in a darkened room will produce fluorescence in hairs infected with certain dermatophyte species. *Trichophyton tonsurans* does not fluoresce. Occasionally, extensive infections will yield a silvery fluorescence that will light up the entire scalp. In contrast, *M. audouinii*, the pathogen seen during the epidemics of the mid-twentieth century, and selected other *Microsporum* species, produce a yellow–green fluorescence. Kerions rarely have fluorescent hairs. The fluorescence due to *M. canis*, which is still a common pathogen, may be present in early infections and disappear as inflammation develops. For these reasons, Wood's light examination is insufficient to diagnose tinea capitis when used alone, but may be helpful in delineating the infecting pathogen.

Direct microscopic examination of the hair can also be useful in confirming the diagnosis of tinea capitis and in characterizing the causative dermatophyte. To perform this procedure, several hairs are collected, preferably from noninflamed lesions. In some cases, a Wood's light can be used to help identify infected hairs. In black dot tinea capitis, hair stubs must be used, and

can be obtained by plucking with an epilating forceps or by prying them out with a needle or scalpel blade. Other methods include scraping the lesions with a microscope slide or scalpel blade or vigorous rubbing with a moistened gauze pad or cotton-tipped applicator. A toothbrush can also be combed over a lesion to collect hairs. The hairs are mounted in 10% to 40% KOH and examined immediately without heating in order to maintain the relationships of the fungal elements and hair shafts.

The presence of fungal elements infecting the KOH mounted hairs confirms the diagnosis. The pattern and site of invasion helps to speciate the pathogens. In general, *Microsporum* species cause ectothrix infections in which arthroconidia are found surrounding the hair shaft. *Trichophyton mentagrophytes* and *T. verrucosum* also result in ectothrix infections. *Trichophyton tonsurans* and *T. violaceum* produce endothrix infections in which the arthroconidia are seen within the hair shaft. *Trichophyton schoenleinii* invasion results in the longitudinal arrangement of hyphae within the hair shaft seen in the favic or favus-type pattern.

Due to the limitations of the above procedures, cultures are often required to establish the dermatophyte pathogen of scalp infections. Specimens may be collected in a number of ways. The simplest method is to press the surface of a suitable agar medium directly against the suspect lesion. When this is not possible, a sterile toothbrush can be used to scrape the affected areas. The bristles of the toothbrush are then pressed into the agar. Another possibility is to press the bristles of the patient's own hairbrush into the culture medium. Aspirates of pustular lesions may be cultured. The scutula lesions in favus type tinea capitis provide an abundant source for culture material.

DIFFERENTIAL DIAGNOSIS. Tinea capitis should be considered in the differential of any scaling patch of alopecia on the scalp. Other conditions that may have similar clinical presentations include: alopecia areata, discoid lupus erythematosus, dissecting cellulitis, folliculitis decalvans, impetigo, lichen planus, psoriasis, seborrheic dermatitis, and secondary syphilis.

TREATMENT. Tinea capitis requires systemic antifungal therapy (Drake et al, 1996b). Drugs, doses and duration of therapy are provided in Table 24–7. The "gold standard" and the only medication currently approved by the FDA for this indication is griseofulvin, which is available in a 125 mg/5 mL suspension of microsized particles, in 250 mg and 500 mg microsize tablets, and in ultramicrosize tablets ranging in strength from 125 mg to 330 mg. The ultramicrosized are better absorbed than the larger microsized particles, thus requiring a lower dose. Both formulations are better absorbed in

TABLE 24–7. *Treatment of Tinea Capitis*

Drug	Griseofulvin	Fluconazole*	Itraconazole*	Terbinafine*
Adult Dose	Microsize 20–25 mg/kg/day for 8 to 12 weeks Ultramicrosize 15 mg/kg/day for 8–12 weeks	200 mg/day for 3–6 weeks	5 mg/kg/day Usually 200 mg/day for 4 weeks *M. canis* may require 6 to 8 weeks	250 mg/day for 2–4 weeks *M. canis* may require 6 to 8 weeks
Pediatric Dose	As above Microsize suspension available in 125 mg/5 mL strength	6 mg/kg/day for 3–6 weeks Available in 10 mg and 40 mg/mL pleasant tasting suspension	5 mg/kg/day Most require 100 mg/day Very small children: 100 mg every other day Liquid formulation available	Weight 10–20 kg: 62.5 mg/day Weight 20–40 kg; 125 mg/day Weight > 40 kg: 250 mg/day Available only in 250 mg tablets.

*Not approved by FDA for use in tinea capitis.

the presence of fat and should be taken with meals. Griseofulvin, which is fungistatic, is deposited in keratin precursor cells and results in gradual replacement of infected keratin by healthy tissue. Treatment should be continued until the hair starts to regrow and fungal cultures are negative.

Alternative systemic drugs for tinea capitis include fluconazole, itraconazole, and terbinafine. These are useful when patients are allergic to, cannot tolerate, or fail griseofulvin therapy. Although the FDA has not approved any of these drugs for this indication, all three have been proven effective. Fluconazole, which is especially attractive for young children, is available in pleasant-tasting suspensions, has been approved for children 6 months of age and older for other indications, and can be taken without regard to meals. The dosing of itraconazole is more problematic. Itraconazole is available in 100 mg capsules and as a liquid solution, but the cyclodextrin vehicle of the solution can cause complications such as severe diarrhea. Itraconazole should be taken with food or a cola beverage to enhance absorption. Terbenafine is available only in 250 mg tablets. The dosage for children ranges from one-fourth tablet (62.5 mg) to a whole tablet, administered with or without food. While 2–4 weeks is the usual duration of therapy, longer duration (6–8 weeks) may be required for tinea capitis caused by *M. canis* (Moossavi, 2001).

Adjunctive therapy includes periodic usage of 1%–2% ketoconazole or 2.5% selenium sulfide shampoo to help reduce shedding of infected hairs and minimize spread. Some studies have shown upwards of 30% of adults exposed to *T. tonsurans* have positive fungal cultures and are thought to be asymptomatic carriers. Topical antifungal preparations applied to involved areas may also help reduce transfer of infection by stabilizing infectious particles.

The highly contagious nature of tinea capitis has made the decision on when an infected child may return to school somewhat controversial. By the time the child is seen by a physician for treatment, it is likely that he has already exposed many other children. In view of this, it seems unnecessary to stop a child from attending school if oral and topical antifungal treatments are used regularly. Most authorities permit return to school immediately after therapy is started.

PREVENTION. The prevention of anthropophilic tinea capitis involves both minimizing the risk of spread of the infection and prevention of reinfection. Fomites such as combs, brushes, and other hair accessories should be discarded. If applicable, the infected animal must be treated. Geophilic tinea capitis is generally so rare and benign that prevention is not an issue.

NONDERMATOPHYTE MOULDS

Definition

A few moulds have the ability to invade keratinized tissue and produce infections that clinically resemble dermatophytoses. Two of these, *Scytalidium dimidiatum* and *S. hyalinum*, can invade skin and nails (not hair). A third, *Scopulariopis brevicaulis*, causes only onychomycosis.

Etiology and Epidemiology

Scytalidium dimidiatum is a plant pathogen endemic to Africa, Asia, the Caribbean, Central, and South America, and several western U.S. states. Human infection is thought to result from contact with contaminated plants or soil. Most infections have occurred in endemic areas or on travelers to these areas. *Scytalidium hyalinum* is an albino, conidial, asexual variant of *S. dimidiatum* that has not been recovered from the environment.

Scopulariopis brevicaulis, a soil saprophyte with a worldwide distribution, only causes nail infections.

Pathogenesis

Like dermatophytes, *S. dimidiatum* and *S. hyalinum* are able to infect keratinized tissues of immunocompetent hosts. These moulds apparently produce keratinases that enable viability of the moulds in dry skin scrapings for up to 6 months (Hoeprich et al, 1994). Host response is noninflammatory, producing infections resembling those caused by anthropophilic dermatophytes.

Scopulariopsis brevicaulis is considered a primary pathogen of nails that may invade a damaged or traumatized nail in an opportunistic fashion. Toenails are more often infected by this common fungus than fingernails.

Clinical Presentations

The clinical presentations of infections by *S. dimidiatum* and *S. hyalinum* are indistinguishable from dermatophytosis. Infections of palms, soles, and nails occur, resembling interdigital tinea pedis, moccasin tinea pedis, tinea manuum, and distal subungual onychomycosis. The onychomycosis may also be a unique lateral onycholysis followed by nail plate infection. Lesions resembling candidal paronychia may also be seen.

Nail infection by *S. brevicaulis* is typically confined to a single toenail that may have been healthy or previously damaged. The first toenail is most often involved. It becomes thickened and yellow to brown in color, similar to the yellow to brown appearance of this mould in culture.

Diagnosis

As with the dermatophytoses, clinical suspicion should be confirmed with direct microscopic examination of KOH mounted scrapings as well as fungal cultures. *Scytalidium dimidiatum* and *S. hyalinum* are identical to one another and quite similar to dermatophytes on KOH preparations. Hyphae are seldomly pigmented and have a unique appearance that may help differentiate them from those of dermatophytes. *Scytalidium* hyphae may also be somewhat wider, although the width is variable. Since cultures must be done on cycloheximide-free media, it is helpful to advise the mycology laboratory of the possibility of this infection.

KOH preparations of nails revealing atypical hyphae may suggest infection by *S. brevicaulis*. Occasionally, lemon-shaped conidia may also be seen. Diagnosis should be confirmed by a fungal culture. Because this mould may also be a common contaminant, caution must be used in interpreting mycological results. The presence of atypical hyphae or conidia on KOH is very helpful.

Differential Diagnosis

Differential diagnoses for nondermatophyte mould cutaneous infections are the same as those of tinea pedis, tinea manuum, and onychomycosis and include psoriasis, eczema, keratoderma, and chronic contact dermatitis, among other conditions.

Treatment

There is no effective topical treatment for these nondermatophyte mould infections. Griseofulvin and ketoconazole are also ineffective (Gupta and Elewski, 1996). Itraconazole and terbinafine have demonstrated some efficacy against *S. brevicaulis* (Gupta et al, 2001).

Prevention

Preventive measures should focus on limiting exposure to the pathogens. Residents and travelers to endemic areas should wear protective footwear.

SUPERFICIAL CANDIDIASIS

Definition

Superficial candidiasis is defined as infection of cutaneous or mucosal epithelium by *Candida* species. These yeast fungi produce blastospores and pseudohyphae.

Etiology and Epidemiology

Candida species cause infections in all age groups but more commonly in newborns and the elderly. Other predisposing factors include underlying systemic disease such as diabetes, immunosuppression by disease or medication, antibiotic therapy, and disrupted epithelial barriers. Warm, moist environments favor *Candida* growth. *Candida albicans* is the most common cause of superficial candidiasis. Other species that may be involved include *C. tropicalis*, *C. parapsilosis*, *C. glabrata*, and *C. guilliermondii* (Scher, 1990).

Pathogenesis

Although part of the normal flora of the gastrointestinal and female genital tracts, *C. albicans* is usually not found on intact skin. Colonization and infection of the skin can be promoted by both host and yeast factors. *Candida albicans* can be isolated from the skin of immunocompetent adults, which has become macerated secondary to occlusion. Immunocompromised patients, particularly those with T-cell deficiencies such as HIV/AIDS, are particularly susceptible to oropharyngeal candidiasis. Factors that increase pathogenicity of the yeast include production of extracellular proteases, and increased epithelial and mucosal adherence (see Chapter 11).

Clinical Presentations

Cutaneous Candidiasis

CANDIDAL PARONYCHIA. Persons (such as dishwashers, food handlers, health-care workers, and children who suck their thumbs, etc.) who have prolonged exposure of their hands to moisture have an increased risk of developing candidal paronychia. Occasionally, manipulation of the cuticle by a manicurist may precede the infection. Initially, the proximal nail fold becomes red and edematous. Damage or loss of the cuticle and a purulent discharge from the nail fold soon follows. Chronic infections may result in nail dystrophy.

CANDIDAL ONYCHOMYCOSIS. This common form of candidal onychomycosis may follow candidal paronychia (Scher, 1990). *Candida* spp. first attacks the soft tissue around the nail and then invades the nail plate. Infection of the nail matrix may result in transverse depressions (Beau's lines), rough, irregular nail plates, and dystrophy (Andre and Achten, 1987). A second, much less common form of candidal onycholysis occurs in chronic mucocutaneous candidiasis. Here the organism invades the nail plate directly and may affect the entire thickness of the plate (Elewski et al, 1995b). A third variety of candidal onychomycosis resembles dermatophytic distal subungual onychomycosis, occurs more often on the hands, and is characterized by onycholysis and distal subungual hyperkeratosis.

CANDIDAL INTERTRIGO. Immunosuppression, diabetes, obesity, and prolonged antibiotic therapy predispose patients to candidal intertrigo (Hay, 1999). Moisture and heat trapping leading to maceration combine to make intertriginous areas more susceptible to *Candida* overgrowth and infection. Frequently infected areas include the axillae, groin, and skin under a pannus or under pendulous breasts. *Candida* is also often a cause of diaper dermatitis. Clinically, the skin becomes bright red and the epidermis may be denuded with a serous discharge. Satellite papules and pustules are often seen beyond a slightly scaly border. In contrast to tinea cruris, the scrotum may be involved (See Color Fig. 24–8 in separate color insert).

EROSIO INTERDIGITALIS BLASTOMYCETICA. Prolonged exposure of the hands to moisture and trapping of moisture under jewelry may lead to maceration and candidal infection of the interdigital web spaces. This infection occurs most often between the third and fourth fingers but occasionally affects the toes. Clinically, the interdigital skin appears macerated. Scale and superficial erosions or fissures may be present.

Mucosal Candidiasis

OROPHARYNGEAL CANDIDIASIS. Candidal infections of the oropharyngeal mucosa, tongue, and oral commissures are common in very young or old patients and in those immunocompromised by disease or medications. Susceptible patients include those with dentures, diabetes mellitus, HIV/AIDS, and on systemic antibiotics. Pseudomembranous candidiasis (thrush) is the most common candidal mucosal infection. White, curd like, friable plaques are seen on the tongue, buccal mucosa, gums, palate, and pharynx. Scraping easily removes the plaques to reveal shallow red ulcers. In acute atrophic candidiasis (candidal glossitis), painful, red, atrophic patches are seen on the dorsal tongue. Angular cheilitis (perleche) is candidiasis of the oral commissures and is characterized by maceration, erythema, and fissuring. Edentulous patients with redundant folds in the commissures leading to drooling and maceration are the most commonly affected. Persons who frequently lick their lips and children who suck their fingers are also at increased risk.

VAGINAL CANDIDIASIS AND CANDIDAL BALANITIS.. *Candida* species commonly colonize the vagina of immunocompetent adults. Overgrowth and infection produce pruritis, edema, erythema and a thick, creamy or cottage cheese-like vaginal discharge. The infection may spread from the vulva to the groin and upper thighs where it causes a candidal intertrigo. Although most patients have no apparent predisposition, diabetes mellitus, pregnancy, HIV/AIDS, and antibiotic therapy may be associated. Uncircumcised males may experience the same symptoms due to candidal balanitis (Sobel et al, 1998; Hay, 1999).

CHRONIC MUCOCUTANEOUS CANDIDIASIS. Although rare, chronic candidal infections of skin, mucous membranes and nails occur and are resistant to treatment. This condition, known as chronic mucocutaneous candidiasis, is often associated with underlying genetic, endocrine, or immunologic defects. Inheritance may be autosomal dominant or recessive. Hypoparathyroidism and hypoadrenalism are the most commonly associated endocrinopathies (Kirkpatrick et al, 1971). Immunologically, there are defects in T-lymphocyte function (Kirkpatrick, 1994). *Candida albicans* is the most common causative species. Clinical presentations range from persistent thrush, to red scaly plaques on the scalp and face, to generalized hyperkeratotic plaques. Nails may be minimally involved or can become thickened, friable, and dystrophic.

Diagnosis

The diagnosis of superficial candidiasis is often made from the typical appearance of the lesions and the presence of satellite vesicopustules. Clinical suspicion can be confirmed by examination of KOH-mounted scrapings and fungal culture.

Differential Diagnosis

The differential diagnoses vary depending on the clinical presentation. Paronychias associated with bacterial infections, hypoparathyroidism, Reiter's syndrome, and celiac disease, among others, should be differentiated from candidal paronychia. Onychomycosis may be caused by *Candida*, dermatophytes, or nondermatophyte moulds. Candidal intertrigo may be confused with tinea cruris, bacterial intertrigo, inverse psoriasis, erythrasma, Hailey Hailey disease, or seborrheic dermatitis. Erythema multiforme, pemphigus, lichen planus, leukoplakia, and secondary syphilis may present with oral lesions resembling those of the atrophic or ulcerative forms of oral candidiasis. Angular cheilitis due to *Candida* should be differentiated from that associated with riboflavin or iron deficiency, glucagonoma syndrome, and secondary syphilis. Finally, the lesions seen in chronic mucocutaneous candidiasis should be distinguished from tinea, bacterial pyoderma, acrodermatitis enteropathica, and halogenoderma.

Treatment

Generally, superficial candidiasis responds well to topical antifungal agents. However, candidal paronychia usually requires prolonged treatment. Imidazoles (miconazole and ketoconazole) and polyene (nystatin) antimycotic solutions, gels or lotions should be applied frequently. Sulfacetamide lotion and 4% thymol in chloroform have also been used (Hay, 1994). Fingers should be kept dry and warm. Oral fluconazole and itraconazole have been utilized but their effectiveness has not been adequately evaluated (Hay, 1999).

Candida onychomycosis confirmed by nail microscopy, biopsy, or culture often requires systemic therapy. Oral azoles such as fluconazole and itraconazole may be used. Itraconazole has been given in pulsed doses and fluconazole has been given once weekly, as in therapy of dermatophyte onychomycosis (Table 24–6).

In contrast, candidal intertrigo and interdigital candidiasis rarely require systemic therapy. Topical imidazoles, and allylamines are applied once or twice daily (Drake et al, 1996d). It is also necessary for patients to keep the affected areas dry, by using a blow dryer on intertriginous areas and applying an antifungal powder afterwards. Topical agents are also effective in the treatment of candidal diaper dermatitis.

Oropharyngeal candidiasis (thrush) responds well to topical nystatin suspension or lozenge and clotrimazole troches in immunocompetent patients. Immunocompromised patients, such as those with AIDS, often require treatment with oral fluconazole (50–200 mg/day) or itraconazole (100–200 mg/day) for 7 to 21 days depending on severity of disease, frequency of episodes, and state of immunocompromise of the patient.

Topical antifungal agents are usually effective in treatment of vaginal candidiasis. Nystatin or imidazole (miconazole, terconazole, etc.) creams, vaginal tablets, and suppositories are used for 1–7 days. Oral therapy with fluconazole (150 mg single dose or 100 mg daily for 5–7 days) and itraconazole (200 mg daily for 3–5 days) is also effective (Sobel et al, 1998; Hay, 1999).

Systemic anti-*Candida* therapy with fluconazole, itraconazole, or ketoconazole is usually necessary for the treatment of patients with chronic mucocutaneous candidiasis. Prolonged and repeated therapy is often required. Once a remission is induced, some authorities recommend that treatment be stopped in order to decrease the development of drug resistance (Kirkpatrick, 1994). For more detailed discussion on superficial candidiasis and its management, see Chapter 11.

Prevention

Reinfection with superficial candidiasis is a common problem. Efforts should be made to minimize those predisposing conditions that can be altered. Drying affected areas thoroughly to avoid maceration will help prevent recurrences in susceptible patients.

REFERENCES

Aly R, Berger T. Common superficial fungal infections in patients with AIDS. *Clin Infect Dis* 22(Suppl. 2): S128–S132, 1996.

Andre J, Achten G. Onychomycosis. *Int J Dermatol* 26:481–490, 1987.

Babel D E, Baughman S A. Evaluation of the adult carrier state in juvenile tinea capitis. *J Am Acad Dermatol* 21:1209–1212, 1989.

Back O, Faergeman J, Hornqvist R. Pityrosporum folliculitis; a common disease of the young and middle-aged. *J Am Acad Dermatol* 12:56–61, 1985.

Bergstresser P, Elewski B E, Hanifin J, Lesher J, Savin R, Shupack J, Stiller M, Tschen E, Zaias N, Birnbaum J E. Topical terbinafine and clotrimazole in interdigital tinea pedis: A multicenter comparison of cure and relapse rates with 1– and 4–week regimens. *J Am Acad Dermatol* 28:648–651, 1993.

Blake J S, Dahl M V, Herron M J, Nelson R D. An immunoinhibitory cell wall glycoprotein (mannan) from *Trichophyton rubrum*. *J Invest Dermatol* 96:651–661,1991.

Brodell R T, Elewski B E. Superficial fungal infections: errors to avoid in diagnosis and treatment. *Postgrad Med* 101:279–287, 1997.

Callaway J L. Dermatophytes as opportunistic organisms. *Lab Invest* 11:1132–1133, 1962.

Corte M, Jung K, Linker U, Martini H, Sapp-Boncelet I, Schulz H. Topical application of a 0.1% ciclopiroxolamine solution for the treatment of pityriasis versicolor. *Mycoses* 32:200–203, 1989.

De Doncker P, Decroix J, Pierard G E, Roelant D, Woestenborghs R, Jacqmin P, Odds F, Hermans A, Dockx P, Roseeuw D. Antifungal pulse therapy for onychomycosis: a pharmacokinetic and pharmacodynamic investigation of monthly cycles of 1–week pulse therapy with itraconazole. *Arch Dermatol* 132:34–41, 1996.

Delescluse R C J. Itraconazole in tinea versicolor; a review. *J Am Acad Dermatol* 23:551–554, 1990.

Demis D J (ed). Fungus infections. In: *Clinical Dermatology*. 26th ed. Philadelphia: Lippincott Williams and Wilkins, Section 17:1–23, 1999.

Dermik Laboratoies. Ciclopirox topical solution 8% package insert. Dermik Laboratoies, Berwyn, PA 2000.

Drake L A, Dinehart S M, Farmer E R, Goltz R W, Graham G F, Hordinsky M F, Lewis C W, Pariser D M, Skouge J W, Webster

S B, Whitaker D C, Butler B, Lowery B J, Elewski B E, Elgart M L, Jacobs P H, Lesher J L, Scher R K. Guidelines of care for superficial mycotic infections of the skin: tinea corporis, tinea cruris, tinea faciei, tinea manuum, and tinea pedis. Guideline/Outcomes Committee, American Academy of Dermatology. *J Am Acad Dermatol* 34:282–286, 1996a.

Drake L A, Dinehart S M, Farmer E R, Goltz R W, Graham G F, Hordinsky M F, Lewis CW, Pariser D M, Skouge J W, Webster S B, Whitaker D C, Butler B, Lowery B J, Elewski B E, Elgart M L, Jacobs P H, Lesher J L, Scher R K. Guidelines of care for superficial mycotic infections of the skin: tinea capitis and tinea barbae. Guidelines/Outcomes Committee, American Academy of Dermatology. *J Am Acad Dermatol* 34:290–294, 1996b.

Drake L A, Dinehart S M, Farmer ER, Goltz R W, Graham G F, Hordinsky M F, Lewis C W, Pariser D M, Skouge J W, Webster S B, Whitaker D C, Butler B, Lowery B J, Elewski B E, Elgart M L, Jacobs P H, Lesher J L, Scher R K. Guidelines of care for superficial mycotic infections of the skin: onychomycosis. Guidelines/Outcomes Committee, American Academy of Dermatology. *J Am Acad Dermatol* 34:116–121, 1996c.

Drake L A, Dinehart S M, Farmer ER, Goltz R W, Graham G F, Hordinsky M F, Lewis C W, Pariser D M, Skouge J W, Webster S B, Whitaker D C, Butler B, Lowery B J, Elewski B E, Elgart M L, Jacobs P H, Lesher J L, Scher R K. Guidelines of care for superficial mycotic infections of the skin: mucocutaneous candidiasis. Guidelines/Outcomes Committee, American Academy of Dermatology. *J Am Acad Dermatol* 34:110–115, 1996d.

Drake L A, Shear N H, Arlette J P, Cloutier R, Danby F W, Elewski B E, Garvis-Jones S, Giroux J M, Gratton D, Gulliver W, Hull P, Jones H E, Journet M, Krol A L, Leyden J J, Maddin S C, Ross J B, Savin R C, Scher R F, Sibbald G R, Tawfik N H, Zaias N, Tolpin M, Evans S, Birnbaum J E. Oral terbinafine in the treatment of of toenail onychomycosis: North American multicenter trial. *J Am Acad Dermatol* 37:740–745, 1997.

Elewski B E, Hazen P G. The superficial mycoses and the dermatophytes. *J Am Acad Dermatol* 21:655–673, 1989.

Elewski B E, Bergstresser P R, Hanifen J, Lesher J, Savin R, Shupack J, Stiller M, Tschen E, Zaias N, Birnbaum J E. Long-term outcome of patients with interdigital tinea pedis treated with terbinafine or clotrimazole. *J Am Acad Dermatol* 32:290–292, 1995a.

Elewski B E, Rinaldi M G, Weitzman I. *Diagnosis and Treatment of Onychomycosis. A Clinician's Handbook*. Califon, NJ: Gardiner-Caldwell SynerMed, 1995b.

Elewski B E, Hay R J. Update on the management of onychomycosis: highlights of the Third Annual International Summit on Cutaneous Antifungal Therapy. *Clin Infect Dis* 23:305–313, 1996.

Elewski B E Charif M A. Prevalence of onychomycosis in patients attending a dermatology clinic in northeastern Ohio for other conditions. *Arch Dermatol* 133:1172–1173, 1997a. (Letter).

Elewski B E, Scher R K, Aly R, Daniel R, Jones H E, Odom R B, Zaias N, Jacko M L. Double-blind, randomized conparison of itraconazole capsules vs. placebo in the treatment of toenail onychomycosis. *Cutis* 59:217–220, 1997b.

Elewski B E. *Cutaneous Fungal Infections*. 2nd ed. Malden, MA: Blackwell Science, p. 124, 1998a.

Elewski B E. Once-weekly fluconazole in the treatment of onychomycosis: introduction. *J Am Acad Dermatol* 38:73–76, 1998b.

Elewski B E. Tinea capitis: a current perspective. *J Am Acad Dermatol* 42:1–20, 2000.

Ellis D H, Marley J E, Watson A B, Williams T G. Non-dermatophytes in onychomycosis of the toenails. *Br J Dermatol* 136:490–493, 1997.

Faergemann J, Fredriksson T. An open trial of the effect of a zinc pyrithione shampoo in tinea versicolor. *Cutis* 25:667–669, 1980.

Faergemann J. Treatment of seborrhoeic dermatitis of the scalp with ketoconazole shampoo: a double-blind study. *Acta Derm Venerol* 70:171–172, 1990.

Ford G P, Ive F A, Midgley G. *Pityrosporum* folliculitis and ketoconazole. *Br J Dermatol* 107:691–695, 1982.

Ganor S, Perath M J, Raubitschek F. Tinea pedis in schoolchildren; an epidemiological study. *Dermatologica* 126:253–258, 1963.

Geary L K. Epidemiology of the dermatophytoses, sources of infection, modes of transmission and epidemicity. *Ann NY Acad Sci* 89:69–77, 1960.

Gemmer C M, DeAngelis Y M, Theelen B, Boekhout T, Dawson T L. Fast, non-invasive method for molecular detection and differentiation of *Malassezia* yeast species in human skin and application of the method to dandruff microbiology. *J Clin Microbiol* 40: 3350–3357, 2002.

Gupta A K, Elewski B E. Nondermatophyte causes of onychomycosis and superficial mycoses. *Curr Topics Med Mycol* 7:87–97, 1996.

Gupta A K, Gregurek-Novak T, Konnikov N, Lynde C W, Hofstader S, Summerbell R C. Itraconazole and terbinafine treatment of some nondermatophyte moulds causing onychomycosis of the toes and a review of the literature. *J Cut Med Surg* 5:206–210, 2001.

Havu V, Brandt H, Heikkila H, Hollmen A, Oksman R, Rantanen T, Saari S, Stubb S, Turjanmaa K, Piepponen T. A double-blind, randomized study comparing itraconazole pulse therapy with continuous dosing for the treatment of toe-nail onychomycosis. *Br J Dermatol* 136:230–234, 1997.

Hay R J, Midgley G. Short course ketoconazole therapy in pityriasis versicolor. *Clin Exp Dermatol* 9:542–545, 1984.

Hay R J. Antifungal therapy of yeast infections. *J Am Acad Dermatol* 31:S6–S9, 1994.

Hay R J. The management of superficial candidiasis. J Am Acad Dermatol 40:S35–S42, 1999.

Heikkila H, Stubbs S. The prevalence of onychomycosis in Finland. *Br J Dermatol* 133:699–701, 1995.

Hoeprich P D, Jordan M C, Ronald A R. Superficial fungal infections of the skin. In: *Infectious Diseases*. 5th ed. Philadelphia: J.B. Lippincott, 1029–1049, 1994.

Kane J, Summerbell R C. *Trichophyton, Microsporum, Epidermophyton*, and agents of superficial mycoses. In: *Manual of Clinical Microbiology*, 7th Ed., Murray P R, Baron E J, Pfaller M A, Tenover F C, Yolken R H, eds. Washington DC: ASM Press, 1275–1294, 1999.

Kirkpatrick C H, Rich R B, Bennett J E. Chronic mucocutaneous candidiasis: model building in cellular immunology. *Ann Intern Med* 74:955–978, 1971.

Kirkpatrick C H. Chronic mucocutaneous candidiasis. J Am Acad Dermatol 31:S14–S17, 1994.

Kwon-Chung K J, Bennett J E. Tinea Nigra. In: *Medical Mycology*. Philadelphia: Lea & Febiger, 191–197, 1992.

Lambert D R, Siegle R J, Camisa C. Griseofulvin and ketoconazole in the treatment of dermatophyte infections. *Int J Dermatol* 28:300–304, 1989.

Lesher J L Jr. Recent developments in antifungal therapy. *Dermatol Clin* 14:163–169, 1996.

Lesher J L Jr. Oral therapy of common superficial fungal infections of the skin. J Am Acad Dermatol 40:S31–S34, 1999.

Leyden J J, Kligman A M. Interdigital athelete's foot: the interaction of dermatophytes and resistant bacteria. *Arch Dermatolol* 114:1466–1472, 1978.

Lorincz A L, Priestley J O, Jacobs P H. Evidence for a humoral mechanism which prevents growth of dermatophytes. *J Invest Dermatol* 31:15–17, 1958.

Ludwig J S. Sycosis barbae due to *Trichophyton rubrum (purpureum)*. *Arch Dermatol Syph* 68:216–218, 1953.

Mandel E H. Current concepts of superficial fungus diseases. *NY State J Med* 61:1904–1912, 1961.

Marcon, M J, Powell D A. *Clin Micro Rev* 5:101–119, 1992.

Marks R, Pears AD, Walker AP. The effects of a shampoo containing zinc pyrithione on the control of dandruff. *Br J Dermatol* 112:415–422, 1985.

Moossavi M. Systemic antifungal therapy. Dermatol Clin 19:35–52, 2001.

Odom R, Daniel C R, III, Aly R. A double-blind, randomized comparison of itraconazole capsules and placebo in the treatment of onychomycosis of the toenail. *J Am Acad Dermatol* 35:110–111, 1996.

Powell F C, Muller S A. Kerion of the glabrous skin. *J Am Acad Dermatol* 7:490–494, 1982.

Richardson M D, Warnock D W. Dermatophytosis. In: *Fungal Infection: Diagnosis and Treatment*. Oxford: Blackwell Scientific Publications, 44–60, 1993.

Richardson M, Elewski B E. Tinea Unquium (Onychomycosis). In: *Superficial Fungal Infections*. Oxford: Health Press, 36–37, 2000a.

Richardson M, Elewski B E. Other Tinea Infections. In: *Superficial Fungal Infections*. Oxford: Health Press, 42–44, 2000b.

Rippon J W. *Medical Mycology: The Pathogenic Fungi and the Pathogenic Actinomycetes*, 3rd ed. Philadelphia: W B Saunders, 1988.

Rupke S J. Fungal skin disorders. *Prim Care* 27:407–421, 2000.

Savin R, Atton A V, Bergstresser P R, Elewski B E, Jones H E, Levine N, Leyden J, Monroe A, Pandya A, Shupack J. Efficacy of terbinafine 1% cream in the treatment of moccasin-type tinea pedis: results of placebo-controlled multicenter trials. *J Am Acad Dermatol* 30:663–667, 1994.

Savin R, De Villez R L, Elewski B E, Hong S, Jones T, Lowe N, Lucky A, Reynes B, Stewart D, Willis I. One-week therapy with twice-daily butenafine 1% cream versus vehicle in the treatment of tinea pedis: a multicenter, double-blind trial. *J Am Acad Dermatol* 35:S15–S19, 1997.

Scher R K. Diseases of the nails. In: Conn H, ed. *Current Therapy*. Philadelphia: W.B. Saunders, 736–742, 1990.

Scher R K. Onychomycosis: a significant medical disorder. *J Am Acad Dermatol* 35:S2–S5, 1996.

Scher R K, Breneman D, Rich P, Savin R C, Feingold D S, Konnikov N, Shupack J L, Pinnell S, Levine N, Lowe N J, Aly R, Odom R B, Greer D L, Mormon M R, Bucko A D, Tschen E H, Elewski B E, Smith E B. Once-weekly fluconazole (150, 300, or 450 mg) in the treatment of distal subungual onychomycosis of the toenail. *J Am Acad Dermatol* 38:S77–S86, 1998.

Scher RK. Onychomycosis: therapeutic update. J Am Acad Dermatol 40:S21–S26, 1999.

Shuster S. The aetiology of dandruff and the mode of action of therapeutic agents. *Br J Dermatol* 111:235–242, 1984.

Sobel J D, Faro S, Force R W, Foxman B, Ledger W J, Nyirjesy P R, Reed B D, Summers P R. Vulvovaginal candidiasis: epidemiologic, diagnostic, and therapeutic considerations. *Am J Obstet Gynecol* 178:203–211, 1998.

Summerbell RC. Epidemiology and ecology of onychomycosis. *Dermatology* 194(Suppl 1):32–36, 1997.

Vargo K, Cohen B A. Prevalence of undetected tinea capitis in household members of children with disease. *Pediatrics* 92:155–157, 1993.

Villars V, Jones T C. Clinical efficacy and tolerability of terbinafine (Lamisil)—a new topical and systemic fungicidal drug for treatment of dermatomycoses. *Clin Exp Dermatol* 14:124–127, 1989.

Weidman F D. Laboratory aspects of epidermophytosis. *Arch Dermatol* 15:415–450, 1927.

Williams J V, Honig P J, McGinley K J, Leyden J J. Semiquantitative study of tinea capitis and the asymptomatic carrier state in inner-city school children. *Pediatrics* 96:265–267,1995.

Wilson J W, Plunkett O A, Gregerson A. Nodular granulomatous perifolliculitis of the legs caused by *Trichophyton rubrum*. *Arch Dermatol Syph* 69:258–277, 1954.

Zaias N, Glick B, Rebell G. Diagnosing and treating onychomycosis. *J Fam Pract* 42:513–518, 1996.

25

Eumycetoma

BEATRIZ BUSTAMANTE AND PABLO E. CAMPOS

Mycetoma is a chronic subcutaneous infection that develops after one of the multiple etiologic microorganisms is inoculated into a site of skin trauma. Although mycetoma is primarily a subcutaneous disease, it can involve bone and lymph nodes by contiguous spread. Mycetoma show three clinical characteristics: tumor, sinuses, and grains. The tumor results as a consequence of a progressive and relatively painless swelling. Sinuses, which are very characteristic of the disorder but can be absent in early stages, drain pus and grains. Grains are colonies of the causative agent and may be black, white, or red. The etiological agents can be either a variety of fungal agents (eumycetoma) or filamentous, branching bacteria belonging to the aerobic actinomycetes (actinomycetoma).

Gill first described mycetoma while working in Madura, India in 1842, and this was subsequently documented by Godfrey in Madras (Godfrey, 1846). Gill reported this entity as *foot tumor*, and Colenbrook introduced the term *Madura foot* in 1846. Ballingal described the microscopic details of the disease for the first time in 1855; however, he did not define its etiology. In 1860, Carter described a fungal disease principally affecting the foot (Carter, 1860), and assigned a fungal origin to this disease in 1861. He also introduced the term mycetoma, meaning a fungus tumor, and extended the concept to include infections with grains that had colors other than black. During the second half of the nineteenth century, mycetomas were diagnosed around the world: in Europe in 1888, in Africa in 1894, and in the United States in 1896.

The hyphomycete isolated from a black grain was given the generic name *Madurella* by Brumpt (Brumpt, 1906). In 1913, Pinoy subclassified this disease into two categories: actinomycosis and true mycetoma, according to the type of etiological agent (Pinoy, 1913). In 1916, Chalmers and colleagues coined the term *maduromycoses* for the first time to refer to mycetomas of fungal etiology, rejecting the term Madura foot to include extrapedal localizations of this disease (Chalmers and Christopherson, 1916; Chalmers and Archibald, 1916).

Despite the acquisition of considerable new knowledge concerning this disease during the last century, there are still important gaps in information regarding several aspects of eumycetoma, mainly related to pathogenesis and management. The goal of this chapter is to review the epidemiological and clinical aspects of eumycetoma, also known as eumycotic mycetoma.

ETIOLOGY AND EPIDEMIOLOGY

More than 20 moulds, both hyaline and pigmented, can cause eumycetoma (Table 25–1). *Madurella mycetomatis* is the worldwide predominant pathogen, followed by *Scedosporium apiospermium*, which is the anamorph of *Pseudallescheria boydii, Leptosphaeria senegalensis*, and *Madurella grisea* (McGinnis and Fader, 1988). These four fungi account for approximately 95% of eumycetoma cases. Hereafter in this chapter, *S. apiospermum* will be used in place of *P. boydii*.

Although eumycetoma has been reported worldwide, most of the cases come from tropical and subtropical regions around the Tropic of Cancer, between 15 degrees south and 30 degrees north (Hay et al, 1992), with sporadic cases occurring in temperate zones. Most cases are reported from India, Sudan, Senegal, Somalia, Venezuela, Mexico, Yemen, and the Democratic Republic of Congo. Endemic regions are characteristically arid with a moderate rainy season (4–6 months), a rainfall of 50–1000 mm per year, and 30°C to 37°C of day temperature with small variation between day and night (Lavalle, 1992).

Temperature, rainfall, type of soil, and prevalent vegetation influence the prevalence of specific eumycetoma agents in a particular region (Boiron et al, 1998), with rainfall being the most influential factor. Black grain fungi cause mycetomas in arid regions, whereas white grain fungi cause mycetomas in regions with higher rainfall and without a significant dry season (Buot et al, 1987). *Madurella mycetomatis* prevails in hot and dry areas with low rainfall, and can be found in temperate zones, though it is rare in the equatorial zone

TABLE 25–1. *Eumycetoma Etiologic Agents and Their Geographical Distribution*

Etiologic Agents	Geographic Distribution
Black Grain Eumycetomas	
Corynespora cassicola	Africa
Curvularia geniculata	North America
Curvularia lunata	Africa, Asia
Exophiala jeanselmei	North, Central, and South America, Europe
Leptosphaeria senegalensis	Africa, Asia
Leptosphaeria tompkinsii	Africa, Asia
Madurella grisea	North, Central, and South America, Africa, Asia
Madurella mycetomatis	North, Central, and South America, Caribbean, Africa, Europe, Middle East, Asia
Phialophora verrucosa	Asia*
Pyrenochaeta mackinnonii	South America
Pyrenochaeta romeroi	Central and South America, Africa, Asia
White to Yellow Grain Eumycetomas	
Acremonium falciforme	North, Central, and South America, Asia, Europe, Oceania
Acremonium kiliense	Asia
Acremonium recifei	South America, Asia
Aspergillus nidulans	Africa
Aspergillus flavus	North America
Cylindrocarpon cyanescens	Asia
Cylindrocarpon destructans	Caribbean, West Africa
Fusarium moniliforme	Europe
Fusarium oxysporum	South America
Fusarium solani	South America, Caribbean, Africa, Asia
Neotestudina rosatii	West Africa
Polycytella hominis	Asia
Scedosporium apiospermum (*Pseudallescheria boydii*)	North, Central, and South America, Africa, Oceania, Europe, Asia

*Thai patients who traveled in Europe, Asia, and North America

(Mariat, 1963). *Scedosporium apiospermum* prevails in areas with hyperprecipitation (2000 mm/year) (Mahgoub, 1989; Hay et al, 1992), and has been reported sporadically in the northern temperate zone among sewage workers (Cooke and Kahler, 1955).

Most eumycetoma agents such as *M. mycetomatis*, *M. grisea*, *S. apiospermum*, and *N. rosatii* have been isolated from soil samples (Borelli, 1962; Thirumalachar and Padhye, 1968; Segretain and Mariat, 1968; Segretain and Mariat, 1971), and *M. mycetomatis* and *S. apiospermum* have also been isolated from termite mounds. *Leptosphaeria senegalensis* and *L. tompkinsii* are recovered from 50% of acacia dry thorns in the Senegal River region, but not from green thorns (Segretain and Mariat, 1968; Segretain and Mariat, 1971; Segretain, 1972), suggesting that thorns may play a role as mechanical vectors. Recently, the use of molecular techniques have facilitated the study of natural reservoirs of *M. mycetomatis*. Polymerase chain reaction-mediated detection followed by RFLP analysis have demonstrated the presence of the organism in 23% of soil samples from endemic areas of Sudan, and have successfully linked environmental and clinical isolates (Ahmed et al, 2002).

Reports of eumycetoma affecting animals are unusual. Cases due to *M. mycetomatis* have been reported in a horse (Van Amstel et al, 1984) and in dogs (Lambrechts et al, 1991). Cases due to *C. lunata* in dogs (Elad et al, 1991) and an unspecified organism in buffaloes have also been reported (Ramachandran 1968).

PATHOGENESIS

Disease usually develops as a result of minor trauma that inoculates contaminated material (usually soil) into the skin or subcutaneous tissue. A history of any trauma at the site of eumycetoma is uncommon, ranging from 0% to 34% of cases, with the higher figures reported from endemic areas of Sudan and India (Abbott, 1956; Yu et al, 1993). This observation suggests that either these fungi do not need deep inoculation, or that disease occurs after a prolonged incubation period (Lee et al, 1995).

After inoculation occurs, a poorly defined host response precludes the development of free fungal filaments in the infected tissue, and instead leads to the development of the characteristic grain. Neutrophil mediated–tissue reaction leads to partial grain disintegration, but most of it remains and perpetuates an inflammatory response. Macrophages and multinucleated giant cells clear dead neutrophils and grain fragments, and an epitheloid granuloma develops (Fahal et al, 1995).

Results of limited immunological studies performed among patients affected by mycetomas are scarce and conflicting. Mahgoub and coworkers found moderate compromise in the cell-mediated immune response (Mahgoub et al, 1977), while Bendl et al were not able to demonstrate any immunological alterations in 15 patients (Bendl et al, 1987).

CLINICAL ASPECTS

Eumycetoma principally affects immunocompetent men, living and working in rural areas. The male to female ratio ranges between 3:1 and 5:1. The age of onset of the disease ranges from 8 to 69 years, and the average duration of symptoms ranges between 7.7 and 9.8 years, varying from 1 month to 25 years (Green and Adams, 1964; Ravisse et al, 1992; Castro et al, 1993). Most patients with eumycetoma are not classically immunocompromised, although diabetes is a frequent comorbid illness. Indeed, 9 out of 26 mycetoma patients diagnosed over a 9-year period in the United

Kingdom had diabetes mellitus as an underlying disease (Hay et al, 1992). Eumycetoma has been reported in patients receiving immunosuppressive therapy for renal transplantation (Van Etta et al, 1983; Meis et al, 2000; O'Riordan et al, 2002) and myelogenous leukemia (Satta et al, 2000). Eumycetoma has also been reported in a man with idiopathic CD4 lymphopenia (Neumeister et al, 1995), but has not yet been reported in an HIV-infected patient.

Male predominance among eumycetoma patients can be explained by higher rates of exposure to the etiologic agents because of a higher tendency towards occupational cutaneous injury (e.g., farming), similar to the acquisition of other subcutaneous mycoses such as sporotrichosis and chromoblastomycosis. Male predominance could also be a consequence of higher susceptibility to this disease, an explanation based on an inhibitory effect of progesterone on the growth of *M. mycetomatis* and *Pyrenochaeta romeroi* in the laboratory (Mendez-Tovar et al, 1991).

The incubation period of eumycetoma is not well established, with most patients seeking care after long periods of disease and without recall of the inoculation event. Clinical characteristics and evolution of eumycetoma lesions are independent of the fungi involved; alterations of the clinical course occur depending on anatomic location, duration of lesions, and medical intervention. Lesions begin as small, firm, painless, indurated subcutaneous nodules or plaques that gradually increase in size. The clinical course is somewhat slower for eumycetoma than for actinomycetoma. Initially, the lesion is well demarcated and may be encapsulated, especially when *M. mycetomatis* is the etiological agent. The disease usually runs a chronic course from several years to decades, with lesions spreading slowly to adjacent structures by contiguous spread, and virtually never by hematogenous dissemination. The tumor develops as a result of the enlargement of nodules and formation of new ones; generally it is firm and round but may be soft and lobulated. Enlarged nodules open to the skin through sinus tracts, discharging sanguineous, seropurulent or purulent exudates that contain grains (See Color Figs. 25–1 and 25–2 in separate color insert). A history of sinus tracts discharging grains is present in up to 60% of the cases (Hazra et al, 1998).

Sinus tracts develop relatively early in the course of disease. At least one-third of patients have sinuses between 3 and 6 months of disease, and almost all patients after 1 year (Lynch, 1964). Established sinuses heal and recur, while new sinuses develop continually. Sinus tracts are very characteristic of mycetoma and helpful in support of the clinical diagnosis; however, other diagnoses must be considered.

Destruction of adjacent structures can be marked and is characteristic late in the course of the disease. When present, destructive lesions are relatively painless. Pain, fever, or other systemic symptoms are not characteristic of eumycetoma, and when present, suggest a secondary bacterial infection. Bacterial cellulitis should be ruled out when pain is present, especially when edema and increasing discharge are evident. Massive fibrosis occurs after healing of involved tissue, contributing to the tumor-like appearance and woody texture of the affected area.

Eumycetoma lesions are located most frequently in areas with a high frequency of repeated trauma, especially in the lower limbs. Feet, legs, and hands are the areas most commonly affected, accounting for approximately 90% of black grain mycetomas (Abbott, 1956) and 95% of *M. mycetomatis* mycetomas (Destombes et al, 1977). Involvement of the foot is more common in eumycetomas than in actinomycetomas, and occurs in 75% to 85% of cases (Abbott, 1956; Destombes et al, 1977). Extrapedal eumycetomas appear when repeated trauma over other parts of the human body occur, including areas such as the abdominal wall, where it is a common practice to carry organic products (e.g., vegetables, straw) without any skin protection (Lopez-Martinez et al, 1992). Rare anatomic sites described for eumycetoma include: intraspinal (Arbab et al, 1997), scalp (Abbott, 1956), neck (Gumma et al, 1986), mandible (Gumma et al, 1975a), eyelid (Aldrige and Kirk, 1940), perineum (Hay et al, 1992), testicle (Abbott, 1956), buttock (Soni et al, 2000; Ly et al, 2000), and thigh (Hay et al, 1992).

True multiple eumycetomas, those involving more than one anatomic site, are rare. The term *double eumycetomas*, as described in the literature, represents two lesions in the same anatomic region in most cases (Ravisse et al, 1992). Eumycetoma caused by more than one fungus is also a rare clinical occurrence. The coocurrence of *M. mycetomatis* and *M. grisea* in a foot lesion has been reported (Niño, 1962).

Lymphatic spread is uncommon with eumycetomas, occurring in 0.5% to fewer than 3% of the cases (Mahgoub, 1985). It appears to be more frequent in actinomycetomas, possibly because the grains are smaller in this condition (Camain, 1968). Among the agents of eumycetoma, *M. mycetomatis* has the lowest frequency of lymph node involvement; only 3 of 578 (0.5%) patients experienced this complication, possibly because of the extensive fibrous reaction that often accompanies this agent (El Hassan and Mahgoub, 1972).

Bone involvement occurs by contiguous spread, with changes occurring first in cortical bone (Sharif et al, 1991). Bone involvement is common, occurs in up to 76% of cases, and trends to greater bone involvement with longer duration of disease (Abbott, 1956; Castro et al, 1993). In addition, bone lesions are more frequent and occur sooner when they are located in body areas with thin subcutaneous tissue such as the feet, hands, and skull.

RADIOLOGY

The most frequent radiological findings in patients with eumycetomas are soft tissue swelling and osteolytic changes (See Color Figs. 25–3A and 25–3B), with loss of the cortical border and external erosion of the bone as the earliest osteolytic manifestations (Tomimori-Yamashita et al, 2001; McGinnis and Fader, 1988). Later, the medullary canal and epiphyses generally are affected, resulting in bone destruction followed by bone remodeling (McGinnis, 1996). Bone lesions can be manifest radiographically as demineralization, periosteal reaction, osteolysis, endosteal bone cavitation, sclerosis, and frank osteomyelitis (Castro et al, 1993). Osteolytic lesions associated with eumycetoma are usually few in number and small (Fig. 25–3A), measuring 2–10 mm in diameter, often with well-defined margins. Grossly, these lesions are filled with necrotic material and grains (McGinnis, 1996; Boiron et al, 1998). No particular pattern of bone involvement is associated with any specific eumycetoma agent. Moreover, it is not possible to differentiate between eumycetoma and actinomycetoma using plain X-rays, CT, MRI, or three-phase bone scans (Czechowski et al, 2001).

Computerized tomography and MRI typically demonstrate bone lesions earlier than plain X-rays. Computed tomography should be used to evaluate pedal mycetomas, whereas MRI is preferred for extrapedal lesions. In addition, CT has greater sensitivity to detect early bone involvement while MRI easily detects late manifestations as a coarse trabecular pattern, bone destruction, marrow infiltration, and sequestra (Sharif et al, 1991).

COMPLICATIONS

The most common complication among eumycetoma patients is secondary bacterial infection, which occurs in up to 66% of black grain eumycetoma cases (Ahmed and Abugroun, 1998). Massive bone destruction induced by eumycetomas can produce pathological fractures (Fahal et al, 1996a). Other complications are related mainly to the localized site of disease, e.g., deformity of the foot in tumoral pedal eumycetoma. Rare complications include cutaneo-pleuro-bronchial fistulae (Fahal et al, 1996b) and palatal abnormality (Fahal et al, 1996c).

DIFFERENTIAL DIAGNOSIS

The differential diagnosis of eumycetoma lesions at any stage of their evolution should always include actino-

mycetoma and botryomycosis. Aerobic filamentous actinomycetes produce the former, and nonfilamentous Gram-positive and Gram-negative bacteria produce the latter.

Exophytic verrucous eumycetoma lesions of the foot can mimic verrucous tuberculosis, blastomycosis, chromoblastomycosis, and sporotrichosis. More extensive tumoral pedal lesions without sinus tracts should be differentiated from elephantiasis of the foot, as well as benign and malignant tumors. When bone involvement is present, the differential diagnosis should include osteomyelitis, osseous tuberculosis, osteosarcoma, and other malignant bone tumors. Extrapedal lesions should be differentiated from dermatophytic pseudomycetoma when the scalp is affected. In addition, cutaneous tuberculosis, endemic fungal diseases such as blastomycosis and coccidioidomycosis, and cutaneous nocardiosis should be excluded.

DIAGNOSIS

When draining sinus tracts are present, these provide the optimum material for microscopic examination. Grains in discharged fluid are visible to the naked eye, and can be collected from dressings covering a draining sinus tract. If discharged grains are not available, a deep skin biopsy, taken from a small abscess or around a sinus tract, is necessary for both culture and histopathological studies.

Specimens should be submitted for macroscopic and microscopic examination and cultured appropriately. Grain color, size, shape, and consistency should be noted because these characteristics help to guide identification of the causative fungus. For example, *M. mycetomatis* grains are large, black, and hard; *L. senegalensis* grains are large, black, and firm to hard; *M. grisea* and *P. romeroii* grains are small, black, and soft to firm; and *S. apiospermum* and *A. nidulans* grains are large, white, and soft. After macroscopic exam, some grains should be placed in a drop of 10%–20% KOH on a slide, compressed between two slides, and examined under microscopy. This direct examination will differentiate the grains of eumycetomas from the grains of actinomycetomas. Eumycetoma grains contain intertwined, broad hyphae (2–5 μm), and may contain large swollen cells (15 μm or more) at the periphery.

Culture is essential for etiological diagnosis; however, culturing mycetoma specimens is laborious and complicated by a high rate of bacterial contamination. Prior to culture, grains should be washed several times with sterile saline solution to reduce bacterial and mould contamination, then crushed in sterile conditions and plated on Sabouraud dextrose agar media containing chloramphenicol 0.05 mg/ml. Medium containing cycloheximide should be avoided because it inhibits the growth of some eumycetoma agents, such as *S. apiospermum*, some *Fusarium* spp., and *Aspergillus* spp. Specimens should be incubated at room temperature and at 37°C for 6 to 8 weeks.

Species identification is based on both macroscopic and microscopic examination of colonies. Other tests may be helpful. For example, patterns of sugar assimilation and optimal growth temperature differentiate *M. mycetomatis* from *M. grisea*. The former can utilize glucose, galactose, lactose, and maltose, but not sucrose, and grows well at 37°C. On the other hand, *M. grisea* can utilize glucose, galactose, maltose, and sucrose, but not lactose, and grows well at 30°C (Satta et al, 2000).

HISTOPATHOLOGY

The basic histopathological picture of eumycetoma is chronic nonspecific granulomatous inflammation, with a central focus of acute inflammatory reaction surrounding one or more grains. A zone formed by histiocytes surrounds the central and abscessed focus, and a peripheral zone consists of new capillaries, isolated histiocytes, plasma cells, mast cells, and eosinophils. Lymphocytes characteristically are found infiltrating the fibrous tissue of the outer zone (Lavalle, 1992; Yu et al, 1993). The fungal hyphae, which constitute the main element of the grain, are more easily observed with the use of periodic acid Schiff or methenamine silver stains.

As shown in Table 25–2, histopathological characteristics on hematoxylin-eosin stain of black grain eumycetomas can be quite distinctive, and may allow for more specific presumptive diagnosis (Hay and Mackenzie, 1982; Hay, 2000). For example, *M. mycetomatis* grains, vesicular type, show a dense brown cement-like substance with hyphae and large chlamydospores in the periphery (See Color Figs. 25–4A and 25–B in separate color insert). By contrast, *E. jeanselmei* grains do not have cement-like substance. On the other hand, pale grain eumycetomas have similar histopathological findings, making their differentiation uncertain (Hay and Mackenzie, 1982). The use of immunofluorescent antibodies may facilitate the identification of the etiolog-

TABLE 25–2. *Appearance in Tissue Sections of Eumycetoma Grains for Selected Agents*

Causative Fungus	Grain Shape	Cement Characteristics	Hyphae Arrangement	Chlamydoconidia Characteristics
Black Grain Eumycetomas				
Exophiala jeanselmei	Round or oval with a hollow in the center	Cement absent	Hyphae located in the periphery	Located in the periphery
Leptosphaeria senegalensis	Round or lobulated	Black cement in periphery	Irregular network of hyphae in the center	Large and located in the periphery
Madurella grisea	Variable	Presence variable	Homogeneous network of hyphae in the center and dense network in the periphery	Located in the periphery
Madurella mycetomatis	Variable	Compact type: Homogeneous brown-cement throughout the grain	Hyphae throughout the grain	
		Vesicular type: Dense brown-cement in periphery	Hyphae located in the periphery	Large and located in the periphery
Pyrenochaeta romeroi	Variable	Presence variable	Central dense network of hyphae	Absent
White to Yellow Grain Eumycetomas				
Acremonium falciforme	Variable	Absent	Dense pattern of hyphae	Present
Fusarium spp.	Oval or lobulated	Absent	Dense pattern of interlaced hyphae	Rare
Neotestudina rosatii	Variable	Located in the periphery	Hyphae in the center and in the periphery. Presence of oval or rounded hyphal fragments	Located in the center
Scedosporium apiospermum	Polylobulated or oval	Absent	Dense network of interwoven hyphae	Large

ical agent in tissue sections. A specific fluorescent antibody conjugate for identification of *S. apiospermum* is available in some areas (Chandler et al, 1980).

SERODIAGNOSIS

There is no reliable serologic test available for diagnosis of eumycetoma. Lack of standardized preparation of the antigen(s) has hampered performance of such a test. In addition, many etiological agents of eumycetoma require independent testing with several antigens or the use of a polyvalent antigen preparation. Immunodiffusion (ID) and counterimmunoelectrophoresis (CIE) have been the most widely used tests for detection of antibodies in eumycetoma patients; both have provided inconsistent results (Murray and Mahgoub, 1968; Gumma and Mahgoub, 1975b; Hay and Mackenzie, 1983a). Serologic assays may play a role in the follow-up of patients on antifungal treatment, after the specific etiology is established. Enzyme linked immunosorbent assay (ELISA) is more sensitive and reproducible than ID and CIE (Wethered et al, 1988), but has the limitation that patients from endemic areas may also show elevated antibody titers by ELISA.

TREATMENT

No good evidence-based treatment recommendations are available for eumycetoma, since no large randomized treatment trials have been conducted. Moreover, the few clinical reports of the use of antifungal agents in the treatment of eumycetomas often involve a limited number of patients and fail to establish a definitive response status due to the limited period of follow-up.

Early surgery can be curative for a small, localized eumycetoma lesion amenable to total excision. For other lesions, patients should receive at least 6 months of antifungal therapy before surgical intervention (Welsh, 1991). Antifungal therapy may cure some lesions or reduce their size prior to surgery. Antifungal therapy may also reduce the recurrence rate when used following surgical debridement (Mahgoub and Gumma, 1984; Welsh, 1991). The course of chemotherapy is prolonged and should continue for months after apparent clinical cure.

In vitro and in vivo responses of antifungal drugs against eumycetoma agents are often conflicting. Although amphotericin B has in vitro activity against *M. mycetomatis*, *M. grisea*, and *E. jeanselmei*, in vivo responses are poor, and argue against a role for amphotericin B in the treatment of eumycetoma (Welsh, 1991; Restrepo, 1994). Liposomal amphotericin B has been used as treatment of two mycetomas caused by *M. grisea* and one by *Fusarium* spp. (3.4, 2.8, and 4.2 g total dose, respectively) with temporary remission followed by clinical relapses 6 months after therapy was

stopped in all three patients (Welsh et al, 1995). Black grain eumycetoma agents are sensitive to the older azoles in vitro, with itraconazole demonstrating the most activity, followed by ketoconazole, econazole, and miconazole (Venugopal et al, 1993). Clinical results have been variable (Welsh, 1991; Lee et al, 1995; Resnik and Burdick, 1995; Paugam et al, 1997; Degavre et al, 1998). In general, ketoconazole and itraconazole appear to perform better against black grain than white grain mycetomas (Poncio-Mendes et al, 2000). Fluconazole 400 mg per day is not effective for mycetoma caused by *M. mycetomatis*, *M.grisea*, and *S. apiospermum* (Diaz et al, 1992). Griseofulvin (a nonazole antifungal drug) appears to have little efficacy in the treatment of eumycetoma (Drohuet and Segretain, 1960; Mahgoub, 1976).

Ketoconazole is an effective agent for mycetoma associated with *M. mycetomatis* and has reported rates of success of at least 70% (Mahgoub and Gumma, 1984; Welsh, 1991; Hay et al, 1992; Welsh et al, 1995), especially when moderate doses and duration (400 mg per day for more than 6 months) are utilized (Poncio-Mendez et al, 2000). Ketoconazole is not an effective treatment for eumycetoma caused by *S. apiospermum* or *Acremoniun* species (Hay, 1983b). Although *M. grisea* responds in vitro only partially to either ketoconazole and itraconazole, these agents have resulted in clinical improvement and reduction in size, allowing for less extensive surgery (Severo et al, 1999; O'Riordan et al, 2002).

Management of *S. apiospermum* infections is challenging because this fungus has intrinsic resistance to some antifungal agents, including fluconazole and amphotericin B. Miconazole has the best in vitro activity among the first generation azoles against this fungus, but is no longer available in most areas. Ketoconazole alone or combined with surgery has been tried in the treatment of *S. apiospermum* mycetomas with varied outcomes (Symoens et al, 1980; Drouhet and Dupont, 1983; Hay, 1983b). Similarly, itraconazole alone or combined with surgery has been effective in some cases (Queiroz-Telles and Queiroz-Telles, 1988; Lexier and Walmsley, 1999).

The best therapeutic regimen for *Acremonium* eumycetoma is unknown due to the scarcity of reports concerning therapy of this disease. Some eumycetomas produced by *Acremonium* species have been treated successfully with itraconazole. One patient with eumycetoma caused by *A. falciforme* responded satisfactorily to itraconazole 200 mg/day for 10 weeks (Lee et al, 1995), and a patient with *A. kiliense* eumycetoma who had failed 3 years of ketoconazole 400 mg daily rapidly improved when treated with itraconazole 300 mg daily (Welsh, 1991). In addition, itraconazole is effective in the treatment of eumycetomas caused by *As-*

pergillus species, and *Arthrographis kalraei* (Degavre et al, 1997).

The new second generation triazoles, including voriconazole, posaconazole, and ravuconazole, hold great promise as potential agents for eumycetoma. Voriconazole has been approved recently as primary therapy of invasive aspergillosis and salvage therapy for both refractory scedosporiosis and fusariosis. Voriconazole, which demonstrates good in vitro fungicidal activity against *S. apiospermum* (McGinnis and Pasarell, 1998) and most *Aspergillus* species, has been used successfully to treat one patient with *S. apiospermum* meningoencephalitis and another with disseminated disease (Poza et al, 2000; Muñoz et al, 2000). To date there are few data involving the use of voriconazole in the treatment of eumycetoma. However, voriconazole, available in both oral and intravenous formulations, will likely become an important agent in the treatment of eumycetomas caused by *S. apiospermum,* some dematiaceous fungi and *Aspergillus* spp. and an oral alternative to existing therapy.

Posaconazole and ravuconazole, both investigational triazoles, also demonstrate good in vitro activity against many of the agents of eumycetoma. Preliminary results from the evaluation of posaconazole as salvage therapy of patients with various fungal infections including eumycetomas, resistant or refractory to standard treatment, are encouraging. Finally, there are promising results with the use of high-dose terbinafine (up to 1000 mg per day) for the treatment of eumycetoma (Hay, 1999).

Unsatisfactory response to drug therapy correlates with duration and extension of disease, susceptibility of the causative organism, and drug concentration at the affected tissues. The latter depends on drug pharmacokinetics and the local blood supply (Fahal et al, 1997). The absence of ischemic changes and necrosis in mycetoma lesions indicates that blood supply probably does not contribute significantly to the failure of medical treatment. Several eumycetoma fungal organisms produce extracellular cement, which prevents drugs, antibodies, and enzymes from reaching the fungus in tissue (Abbott, 1956; McGinnis, 1996). Also, it is possible that drugs cannot reach adequate concentrations in grains surrounded by fibrotic and abscessed tissue.

SURGERY

There is little doubt that surgery can be curative for small and well-delineated lesions of eumycetoma and removes the greater bulk of the lesion when used as an adjunct to antifungal treatment. Additional indications for surgery in the management of eumycetoma are less well defined. Use of surgery to drain sinuses and re-move grains, as a measure to reduce pain and swelling caused by inflammation, is generally discouraged. Current recommendations advocate delaying surgery until several months of antifungal chemotherapy and avoiding radical surgical procedures (McGinnis, 1996).

FOLLOW-UP

An accepted time of follow-up to define cure for eumycetoma has not been established. Some authors consider a patient cured only after 3 years without active disease (Bendl et al, 1987). Assessment of improvement, cure, or relapse is based on clinical parameters, such as decreasing discharge and swelling, healing of fistulae, and improvement on roentgenographic examination.

REFERENCES

Abbott P. Mycetoma in the Sudan. *Trans R Soc Trop Med Hyg* 50:11–24, 1956.
Ahmed A O, Abugroun E S. Unexpected high prevalence of secondary bacterial infection in patients with mycetoma. *J Clin Microbiol* 36:850–851, 1998.
Ahmed A, Adelmann D, Fahal A, Verbrugh H, van Belkum A, de Hoog S. Environmental occurrence of *Madurella mycetomatis*, the major agent of human eumycetoma in Sudan. *J Clin Microbiol* 40:1031–1036, 2002.
Aldrige J, Kirk R. Mycetoma of the eyelid. *Br J Ophthal* 24:211–212, 1940.
Arbab M A, el Hag I A, Abdul Gadir A F, Siddik H el-R. Intraspinal mycetoma: report of two cases. *Am J Trop Med Hyg* 56:27–29, 1997.
Bendl B J, Mackey D, Al-Saati F, Sheth K V, Ofole S N, Bailey T M. Mycetoma in Saudi Arabia. *J Trop Med Hyg* 90:51–59, 1987.
Boiron P, Locci R, Goodfellow M, Gumaa S A, Isik K, Kim B, McNeil M M, Salinas-Carmona M C, Shojaei H. Nocardia, nocardiosis and mycetoma. *Med Mycol* 36:26–37, 1998.
Borelli D. *Madurella mycetomi y Madurella grisea. Arch Venez Med Trop Parasit* 4:195–211, 1962.
Brumpt E. Les mycétomes. *Arch Parasitol* 10:489–564, 1906.
Buot G, Lavalle P, Mariat F, Suchil P. Étude épidémiologique des mycétomes au Mexique. *Bull Soc Pathol Exot* 80:329–339, 1987.
Camain R. Processus d'extension et de limitation des mycétomes africains. *Bull Soc Pathol Exot* 61:517–523, 1968.
Carter H V. On a new and striking form of fungus disease, principally affecting the foot, and prevailing endemically in many parts of India. *Trans Med Phys Soc Bombay* 6:104–142, 1860.
Castro L G, Belda Junior W, Salebian A, Cuce L C. Mycetoma: a retrospective study of 41 cases seen in Sao Paulo, Brazil, from 1978 to 1989. *Mycoses* 36:89–95, 1993.
Chandler F W, Kaplan W, Ajello L. *A color atlas and textbook of the histopathology of mycotic diseases*. London: Wolfe Medical Publication, 76–83, 222–239, 1980.
Chalmers A J, Archibald R G. A Sudanese maduromycosis. *Ann Trop Med Parasitol* 10:169–222, 1916.
Chalmers A J, Christopherson J B. A Sudanese actinomycosis. *Ann Trop Med Parasitol* 10:223–282, 1916.
Cooke W B, Kahler P W. Isolation of potentially pathogenic fungi from polluted water and sewage. *Public Health Rep* 70:689–694, 1955.

Czechowski J, Nork M, Haas D, Lestringant G, Ekelund L. MR and other imaging methods in the investigation of mycetomas. *Acta Radiol* 42:24–26, 2001.

Degavre B, Joujoux J M, Dandurand M, Guillot B. First report of mycetoma caused by *Arthrographis kalrae*: successful treatment with itraconazole. *J Am Acad Dermatol* 37:318–320, 1997.

Destombes P, Mariat L, Rosati G, Segretain G. Les mycétomes en Somalie—conclusions d'une enquête menée de 1959 à 1964. *Acta Tropica* 34:335–373, 1977.

Diaz M, Negroni R, Montero-Gei F, Castro L G, Sampaio S A, Borelli D, Restrepo A, Franco L, Bran J L, Arathoon E G, Stevens D A. A Pan-American 5-year study of fluconazole therapy for deep mycoses in the immunocompetent host. *Clin Infect Dis* 14:68–76, 1992.

Drohuet E, Segretain G. Sensibilité a la griséofulvine et a l'amphotericine B des agents des mycétomes fongiques. *Bull Soc Pathol Exot Filiales* 53:863–869, 1960.

Drohuet E, Dupont B. Laboratory and clinical assessment of ketoconazole in deep-seated mycosis. *Am J Med* 74:30, 1983.

Elad D, Orgal U, Yakobson B, Perl S, Golomb P, Trainin R, Tsur I, Shenkler S, Bor A. Eumycetoma caused by *Curvularia lunata* in a dog. *Mycopathologia* 116:113–118, 1991.

El Hassan A M, Mahgoub E S. Lymph node involvement in mycetoma. *Trans R Soc Trop Med Hyg* 66:165–169, 1972.

Fahal A H, el Toum E A, El Hassan A M, Mahgoub E S, Gumaa S A. The host tissue reaction to *Madurella mycetomatis*: new classification. *J Med Vet Mycol* 33:15–17, 1995.

Fahal A H, Sheik H E, El Hassan A M. Pathological fractures in mycetoma. *Trans R Soc Trop Med Hyg* 90:675–676, 1996a.

Fahal A H, Sharfi A R, Sheik H E, El Hassan A M, Mahgoub E S. Internal fistula formation: An unusual complication of mycetoma. *Trans R Soc Trop Med Hyg* 90:550–552, 1996b.

Fahal A H, Yagi H I, El Hassan A M. Mycetoma-induced palatal deficiency and pharyngeal plexus dysfuntion. *Trans R Soc Trop Med Hyg* 90:676–677, 1996c.

Fahal A H, el Hag I A, Gadir A F, el Lider A R, El Hassan A M, Baraka O Z, Mahgoub E S. Blood supply and vasculature of mycetoma. *J Med Vet Mycol* 35:101–106, 1997.

Godfrey J. Disease of the foot not hitherto described. *Lancet* 1:593–594, 1846.

Green W O Jr, Adams T E. Mycetoma in the United States: A review and report of seven additional cases. *Am J Clin Pathol* 42:75–91, 1964.

Gumma S A, Satir A A, Shehata A H, Mahgoub E S. Tumor of the mandible caused by *Madurella mycetomii*. *Am J Trop Med Hyg* 24:471–474, 1975a.

Gumma S A, Mahgoub E S. Counterimmunoelectrophoresis in the diagnosis of mycetoma and its sensitivity as compared to immunodiffusion. *Sabouraudia* 13:309–315, 1975b.

Gumma S A, Mahgoub E S, El Sid M A. Mycetoma of the head and neck. *Am J Trop Med Hyg* 35:594–600, 1986.

Hay R J, Mackenzie D W R. The histopathological features of pale grain eumycetoma. *Trans R Soc Trop Med Hyg* 76:839–844, 1982.

Hay R J, Mackenzie D W R. Mycetoma (madura foot) in the United Kingdom—A survey of forty-four cases. *Clin Exp Dermatol* 8:553–562, 1983a.

Hay R J. Ketoconazole in the treatment of fungal infection. Clinical and laboratory studies. *Am J Med* 74:16–19, 1983b.

Hay R J, Mahgoub E S, Leon G, Al-Sogair S, Welsh O. Mycetoma. *J Med Vet Mycol* 30:41–49, 1992.

Hay R J. Therapeutic potential of terbinafine in subcutaneous and systemic mycoses. *Br J Dermatol* 141:36–40, 1999.

Hay R J. Mycetoma (Maduromycosis). In: Strickland G T, ed. *Hunter's Tropical Medicine and Emerging Infectious Diseases*. 8th ed. Philadelphia: W.B. Saunders Company, 537–541, 2000.

Hazra B, Bandyopadhyay S, Saha S K, Banerjee D P, Dutta G. A study of mycetoma in eastern India. *J Commun Dis* 30:7–11, 1998.

Lambrechts N, Collett M G, Henton M. Black grain eumycetoma (*Madurella mycetomatis*) in the abdominal cavity of a dog. *J Med Vet Mycol* 29:211–214, 1991.

Lavalle P. Mycetoma. In: Canizares O, Harman R R M, ed. *Clinical Tropical Dermatology*. 2nd ed. Boston: Blackwell Scientific Publication, 41–60, 1992.

Lee M W, Kim J C, Choi J S, Kim K H, Greer D L. Mycetoma caused by *Acremonium falciforme*: successful treatment with itraconazole. *J Am Acad Dermatol* 32:897–900, 1995.

Lexier R, Walmsley S L. Successful treatment of Madura foot caused by *Pseudallescheria boydii* with *Escherichia coli* superinfection: a case report. *Can J Surg* 42:307–309, 1999.

Lopez-Martinez R, Mendez-Tovar L J, Lavalle P, Welsh O, Saul A, Macotela Ruiz E. Epidemiology of mycetoma in Mexico: study of 2105 cases. *Gac Med Mex* 128:477–481, 1992.

Ly F, Develoux M, Deme A, Dangou J M, Kane A, Ndiaye B, Toure P. Tumoral mycetoma of the buttock. *Ann Dermatol Venereol* 127:67–69, 2000.

Lynch J B. Mycetoma in the Sudan. *Ann R Coll Surg* 35:319–340, 1964.

Mahgoub E S. Medical management of eumycetoma. *Bull World Health Organ* 54:303–310, 1976.

Mahgoub E S, Gumma S A, El Hassan A M. Immunological status of mycetoma patients. *Bull Soc Pathol Exot Filiales* 70:48–54, 1977.

Mahgoub E S, Gumma S A. Ketoconazole in the treatment of eumycetoma due to *Madurella mycetomii*. *Trans R Soc Trop Med Hyg* 78:376–379, 1984.

Mahgoub E S. Mycetoma. *Semin Dermatol* 4:230, 1985.

Mahgoub E S. Mycetoma. In: Mahgoub E S, ed. *Tropical Mycoses*. Beerse-Belgium: Jansen Research Council 50–72, 1989.

Mariat F. Sur la distribution géographique et la répartition des agents de mycetomes. *Bull Soc Pathol Exot* 56:35–45, 1963.

McGinnis M R, Fader R C. Mycetoma: A contemporary concept. *Inf Dis Clin N Am* 2:939–954, 1988.

McGinnis M R. Mycetoma. *Dermatol Clin* 14:97–104, 1996.

McGinnis M R, Pasarell L. In vitro testing of susceptibilities of filamentous ascomycetes to voriconazole, itraconazole, and amphotericin B, with consideration of phylogenetic implications. *J Clin Microbiol* 36:2353–2355, 1998.

Meis J F, Schouten R A, Verweij P E, Dolmans W, Wetzels J F. Atypical presentation of *Madurella mycetomatis* mycetoma in a renal transplant patient. *Transpl Infect Dis* 2:96–98, 2000.

Mendez-Tovar L J, de Bièvre C, Lopez-Martinez R. Effets des hormones sexuelles humaines sur le development in vitro des agents d'eumycetoses. *J Mycol Med* 1:141–143, 1991.

Muñoz P, Marín M, Tornero P, Martín-Rabadán P, Rodríguez-Creixéms M, Bouza E. Successful outcome of *Scedesporium apiospermum* disseminated infection treated with voriconazole in a patient receiving corticosteroid teraphy. *Clin Infect Dis* 31:1499–1501, 2000.

Murray I G, Mahgoub E S. Further studies on the diagnosis of mycetoma by double diffusion in agar. *Sabouraudia* 6:106–110, 1968.

Neumeister B, Zollner T M, Krieger D, Sterry W, Marre R. Mycetoma due to *Exophiala jeanselmei* and *Mycobacterium chelonae* in a 73-year-old man with idiopathic CD4+ T lymphocytopenia. *Mycoses* 38:271–276, 1995.

Niño F L. Coexistencia de *Madurella mycetomi* y de *M. grisea* en una misma observacion de maduromicosis podal negra. *Mycopathologia* 16:323–332, 1962.

O'Riordan E, Denton J, Taylor P M, Kerr J, Short C D. Madura foot in the U.K.: fungal osteomyelitis after renal transplantation. *Transplantation* 73:151–153, 2002.

Paugam A, Torte-Schaefer C, Keita A, Chemla N, Chevrot A. Clicical cure of fungal madura foot with oral itraconazole. *Cutis* 60:191–193, 1997.

Pinoy E. Actinomycoses and mycetomas. *Bull Inst Pasteur* 11:929–938, 1913.

Poncio-Mendes R, Negroni R, Bonifaz A, Pappagianis D. New aspects of some endemic mycoses. *Med Mycol* 38:237–241, 2000.

Poza G, Montoya J, Redondo C, Ruiz J, Vila N, Rodriguez-Tudela J L, Cerón A, Simerro E. Meningitis caused by *Pseudallescheria boydii* treated with voriconazole. *Clin Infect Dis* 30:981–982, 2000.

Queiroz-Telles F, Queiroz-Telles J E. Treatment of paracoccidioidomycosis and *Pseudallescheria boydii* mycetoma with itraconazole: a preliminary report of two cases. *Rev Iberica Micología* 5:72, 1988.

Ramachandran P K. Mycetoma caused by an unknown fungus in Indian buffaloes (Bos bubalis). *Ceylan Vet J* 16:77–80, 1968.

Ravisse P, Huerre M, De Bièvre C, Philippon M, Larroque D, Avé P, Rouffaud M A. Les mycétomes en Mauritanie: Étude histologique de 150 cas. *J Mycol Med* 2:154–159, 1992.

Resnik B I, Burdick A E. Improvement of eumycetoma with itraconazole. *J Am Acad Dermatol* 33:917–919, 1995.

Restrepo A. Treatment of tropical mycoses. *J Am Acad Dermatol* 31:91–102, 1994.

Satta R, Sanna S, Cottoni F. *Madurella* infection in an immunocompromised host. *Int J Dermatol* 39:939–941, 2000.

Segretain G, Mariat F. Recherche sur la presence d' agents de mycètomes dans le sol et sur les épineux du Sénégal et de la Mauritanie. *Bull Soc Path Exot* 61:194–201, 1968.

Segretain G, Mariat F. Recherche sur l'écologie des agents de mycètomes fungiques au Sénégal. 5th Congress International Society Human and Animal Mycology, Paris, France, 153–154, 1971.

Segretain G. Epidémiologie des mycétomes. *Ann Soc Belge Med Trop* 52:277–286, 1972.

Severo L C, Vetoratto G, Oliveira Fde M, Londero A T. Eumycetoma by *Madurella grisea*. Report of the first case observed in the southern Brazilian region. *Rev Inst Med Trop Sao Paulo* 41:139–142, 1999.

Sharif H S, Clark D C, Aabed M Y, Aideyan O A, Mattsson T A, Haddad M C, Ohman S O, Joshi R K, Hasan H A, Haleem A. Mycetoma: comparison of MR imaging with CT. *Radiology* 178:865–870, 1991.

Soni N, Gupta A, Shekhawat N S. Mycetoma—an unusual site. *Surgery* 127:709–710, 2000.

Symoens J, Moens M, Dom J, Scheijgrond H, Dony J, Schuermans V, Legendre R, Finestine N. An evaluation of two years of clinical experience with ketoconazole. *Rev Infect Dis* 2:674–687, 1980.

Thirumalachar M J, Padhye A A. Isolation of *Madurella mycetomi* from soil in India. *Hindustan Antib Bull* 10:314–318, 1968.

Tomimori-Yamashita J, Ogawa M M, Hirata S H, Fischman O, Michalany N S, Yamashita H K, Alchorne M. Mycetoma caused by *Fusarium solani* with osteolytic lesions on the hand: case report. *Mycopathologia* 153:11–14, 2001.

Van Amstel S R, Ross M, Van Den Berg S S. Maduromycosis (*Madurella mycetomatis*) in a horse. *J South Afr Vet Assoc* 55:81–83, 1984.

Van Etta L L, Peterson L R, Gerding D N. *Acremonium falciforme* (*Cephalosporium falciforme*) mycetoma in a renal transplant patient. *Arch Dermatol* 119:707–708, 1983.

Venugopal P V, Venugopal T V, Ramakrishna E S, Ilavarasi S. Antimycotic susceptibility testing of agents of black grain eumycetoma. *J Med Vet Mycol* 31:161–164, 1993.

Yu A M, Zhao S, Nie L Y. Mycetomas in northern Yemen: identification of causative organisms and epidemiologic considerations. *Am J Trop Med Hyg* 48:812–817, 1993.

Welsh O. Mycetoma: Current concepts in treatment. *Int J Dermatol* 30:387–398, 1991.

Welsh O, Salinas M C, Rodriguez M A. Treatment of eumycetoma and actinomycetoma. *Curr Topics Med Mycol* 6:47–71, 1995.

Wethered D B, Markey M A, Hay R J, Mahgoub E S, Gumma S A. Humoral immune responses to mycetoma organisms: characterization of specific antibodies by the use of enzyme-linked immunosorbent assay and immunoblotting. *Trans R Soc Tro Med Hyg* 82:918–923, 1988.

26

Chromoblastomycosis

JOHN W. BADDLEY AND WILLIAM E. DISMUKES

Chromoblastomycosis is a chronic fungal infection of the skin and subcutaneous tissues characterized by the presence of nodular, verrucous lesions often of the lower extremities. Upon histopathologic examination of infected tissues, the characteristic finding is single or multiple sclerotic bodies, which are dark brown septate fungal cells that resemble yeast forms (See Color Fig. 26–1 in separate color insert). Sclerotic bodies often are referred to as muriform cells, with the term *muriform* designating the presence of vertical and horizontal septa of the cells. While chromoblastomycosis is caused by several species of dematiaceous, or pigmented, fungi, the most common causative organism is *Fonsecaea pedrosoi*. The disease is usually chronic, localized, and is rarely life-threatening. Surgical resection and cryotherapy are effective for small lesions, while antifungal agents, including itraconazole and flucytosine, are sometimes effective in more extensive disease.

For the purposes of this chapter, chromoblastomycosis is defined as a chronic infection of the skin or subcutaneous tissues caused by dematiaceous fungi and characterized by the presence of sclerotic bodies on histopathologic examination. Chromoblastomycosis is often referred to as *chromomycosis*, although these terms are not synonymous. The term chromomycosis has come to represent not only the classic definition of chromoblastomycosis, but also additional nonskin and subcutaneous infections due to dematiaceous fungi (Fader and McGinnis, 1988; Kwon-Chung and Bennett, 1992). Phaeohyphomycoses represent the broad group of fungal infections caused by dematiaceous fungi and are defined by the presence of yeast-like cells, hyphal forms, or pseudohyphae-like elements in tissue, but without the presence of sclerotic bodies as seen in chromoblastomycosis (Fader and McGinnis, 1988). Phaeohyphomycoses are distinct from chromoblastomycosis and are addressed in a separate chapter (See Chapter 17.).

MYCOLOGY

The organisms causing chromoblastomycosis are saprophytic fungi found in soil, wood, vegetation, pulp, and paper (Ridley, 1957; Gezuele et al, 1972). Several species of dematiaceous fungi cause chromoblastomycosis, and the similarity between organisms lies in the tissue appearance of sclerotic bodies (See Color Fig. 26–1 in separate color insert). Common etiologic agents include *Fonsecea pedrosoi*, *F. compacta*, *Phialophora verrucosa*, *Cladosporium carrioni*, *Rhinocladiella aquaspersa*, and *Botryomyces caespitosus*. Additional organisms reported as etiologic agents include *Exophiala spinifera*, *E. jeanselmei*, and *Aureobasidium pullulans* (Naka et al, 1986; Padhye and Ajello, 1987; Barba-Gomez et al, 1992; Padhye et al, 1996; Redondo-Bellon et al, 1997). A list of reported causative agents, with synonyms, is provided in Table 26–1.

Dematiaceous fungi causing chromoblastomycosis are slow growing and usually need to be incubated at least 4 weeks on standard fungal media, such as Sabouraud's dextrose agar. Most species form dark brown, green, or black velvety colonies upon incubation. Morphologic differences on media and microscopy are variable, and have led to placement of the causative organisms in many different genera. An example of the morphology of *Phialophora verrucosa* is shown in Color Figure 1–4 in Chapter 1. (See separate color insert.) The mycology and nomenclature of organisms that cause chromoblastomycosis have been reviewed extensively elsewhere (McGinnis, 1983; Fader and McGinnis, 1988; Kwon-Chung and Bennett, 1992).

EPIDEMIOLOGY

Chromoblastomycosis occurs worldwide, although the majority of reported cases are from tropical and subtropical regions of the Americas and Africa. Affected patients are frequently outdoor laborers, and the mode of acquisition of infection is traumatic inoculation of the fungus into exposed skin. Most patients do not recall a specific injury, but in a series of patients who remembered a traumatic inciting event, inoculation resulted from thorns, wood splinters, or minor cuts from tools (Minotto et al, 2001).

In certain parts of the world, different organisms are more likely than others to cause chromoblastomycosis.

TABLE 26–1. *Causative Agents of Chromoblastomycosis*

Organism (Synonyms)

Fonsecea pedrosoi (Hormodendrum pedrosoi, Phialophora pedrosoi, Rhinocladiella pedrosoi)
Fonsecea compacta (Hormodendrum compactum, Phialophora compacta, Rhinocladiella compacta)
Cladosporium carrionii (Cladophialophora ajelloi)
Rhinocladiella aquaspersa (Acrotheca aquaspersa)
Phialophora verrucosa
Botryomyces caespitosus
Exophiala jeanselmi
Exophiala spinifera
Aureobasidium pullulans

For example, in Brazil, Colombia, Japan, and humid parts of Venezuela, *F. pedrosoi* is the predominate causative agent (Campins and Scharyj, 1953; Velasquez et al, 1976; Fukushiro et al, 1983) while in Australia and arid parts of Venezuela, *C. carrionii* is the most common cause (Campins and Scharyj, 1953; Leslie and Beardmore, 1979). Site of involvement also seems to differ in patients from various geographic locations. In most countries, the lower extremities are the most frequently affected sites; the exceptions are Japan and Australia, where upper body sites predominate (Leslie and Beardmore, 1979; Fukushiro et al, 1983).

Most cases of chromoblastomycosis occur among males aged 30–60 years old; children are rarely affected. The male predominance probably represents increased exposure rates due to a preponderance of male outdoor workers in some countries. By contrast, in Japan, among a large series of cases the ratio of males to females was equal (Fukushiro, 1983).

CLINICAL MANIFESTATIONS

The cutaneous lesions of chromoblastomycosis are highly variable, and typically begin at the site of a traumatic inoculation of the fungal organism (McGinnis, 1983). Lesions grow slowly, and are asymptomatic in the majority of cases (Minotto et al, 2001). Symptoms, when present, include pruritus, and rarely, pain. Lesions are usually present months to years before patients seek medical attention and are diagnosed (Londero and Ramos, 1976; Queiroz-Telles et al, 1992; Rajendran et al, 1997; Minotto et al, 2001). In one series of 100 patients, the mean interval between first symptoms and diagnosis was 14 years (Minotto et al, 2001).

The most commonly involved anatomical sites are the lower extremities, particularly the foot, ankle, and lower leg. However, skin lesions can be present on virtually any part of the body, including the abdomen, chest, back, upper extremities, neck, face, and rarely, mucous membranes such as the nasal septum (Nakamura et al, 1972; Zaror et al, 1987; Bonifaz et al, 2001; Minotto et al, 2001). Although involvement of the subcutaneous tissues is common, invasion of muscle or bone is infrequent. Most skin lesions are localized, but disseminated disease has been reported in fewer than 5% of patients (Fukushiro, 1983; Minotto et al, 2001). Spread of lesions may occur by autoinoculation resulting from scratching, or lymphatic spread. Hematogenous dissemination is extremely rare, even among immunosuppressed patients, but has resulted in brain abscess and death in several cases (Fukushiro, 1983; Wackym, 1985; Takase et al, 1988).

The initial lesions of chromoblastomycosis are frequently small papules or nodules that become confluent to form irregular, verrucous plaques. In 1950, Carrion reported a series of agricultural workers with chromoblastomycosis and described five types of lesions seen during the progression of disease: nodular, tumorous, verrucous, plaque, and cicatricial lesions (Carrion, 1950). Nodular lesions are soft, pink growths that can be smooth, verrucous, or scaly. These lesions may continue to enlarge and form tumorous growths that appear papillomatous, lobulated, or may enlarge and resemble cauliflower (See Color Fig. 26–2 in separate color insert). Verrucous lesions, the most common type, have a wart-like appearance and are frequently present on the borders of the foot (Fader and McGinnis, 1988). Plaque lesions are slightly raised, pink to reddish in color, and are scaly (See Color Fig. 26–3 in separate color insert). Cicatricial lesions, often large and serpiginous, expand centrifugally while healing; atrophic scarring occurs in the center of the lesions (See Color Fig. 26–4 in separate color insert).

Complications of chromoblastomycosis include secondary bacterial infection, which may present with fever, pain, edema, and localized lymphadenopathy. For longstanding lesions, carcinomatous transformation, particularly to squamous cell cancer, has been described (Bayles, 1971; Foster and Harris, 1987; Minotto et al, 2001). Chronic lymphedema may also result in elephantiasis.

DIAGNOSIS AND PATHOLOGIC FINDINGS

The diagnosis of chromoblastomycosis is made on the basis of typical skin lesions and the presence of sclerotic bodies on histopathologic examination. Tissues, including skin scrapings, aspirated exudates, or biopsy specimens, can be visualized under the microscope and may demonstrate sclerotic bodies without special staining. Sclerotic bodies are seen in the dermis, while hyphal elements, when present, are confined to epidermal layers. Culture of the causative organism must be performed on fungal media containing antibiotics, such as Sabouraud's dextrose agar with chloramphenicol and cycloheximide, as bacterial contamination is common. Cultures should be incubated at 25°C to 30°C, and kept for 4–6 weeks (McGinnis, 1983; Fader and McGinnis, 1988; Kwon-Chung and Bennett, 1992).

Histopathologic examination of lesions of chromoblastomycosis reveals hyperkeratosis and pseudoepitheliomatous hyperplasia in the epidermis. In the dermis, a mixed pyogenic and granulomatous inflammatory process is seen: neutrophils, plasma cells, eosinophils, lymphocytes, and multinucleated giant cells. Fibrosis may be evident, particularly in older lesions (Uribe et al, 1989). Sclerotic bodies, also referred to as muriform cells, Medlar cells, or "copper pennies," are found in dermal tissue, and range in size from 5–15 μm in diameter (See Color Fig. 26–1 in separate color insert). The sclerotic bodies are dark brown in color, have thick walls, are septate, and may be single, in pairs, or in clusters. Sclerotic bodies may be found extracellularly among inflammatory cells, and intracellularly, in giant cells, and rarely, macrophages.

Transepithelial migration, or transepithelial elimination, is a pathologic finding in chromoblastomycosis. In this process, foreign matter, blood, damaged tissue, and sclerotic bodies are expelled through the epidermis as a healing process (Fader and McGinnis, 1988). Accordingly, transepthelial migration will manifest as black dots on the surface of lesions, which, upon slide microscopy with 10% or 20% KOH, reveal clotted blood and sclerotic bodies (Banks et al, 1985; Fader and McGinnis, 1988; Goette and Robertson, 1984).

TREATMENT

Chromoblastomycosis is a chronic disease that is difficult to treat. Spontaneous regression of lesions with complete resolution is extremely unusual (Howles et al, 1954). Therapy is usually sought for aesthetic or functional reasons, but therapy is also necessary to prevent associated complications. No single therapy is uniformly effective, and treatment modalities for chromoblastomycosis have been difficult to evaluate because of the small number of cases, and variability in extent of disease. Multiple therapeutic strategies, including surgical intervention, topical therapies (cryotherapy, applied heat), chemotherapy, or a combination of therapies have been used (Table 26–2). In a large retrospective review, Minotto and colleagues reported that disease was eradicated with therapy in 57% of patients (Minnoto et al, 2001). Over the period of this 30-year study, numerous therapies were used for different lengths of time, and therefore, an optimal therapy could not be determined. In another retrospective review of 51 cases, 31% of patients were cured, and 57% improved with various treatments (Bonifaz et al, 2001). The best results were achieved with cryosurgery for small lesions, and itraconazole for larger lesions.

For small or few lesions, surgical intervention is most effective (Conway and Berkeley, 1952; Bansal and Prabhakar, 1989), although adequate comparative studies are not available. Wide and deep resection to healthy tissue is necessary in order to prevent relapse, but as a result, skin grafting may be required. For larger, more extensive lesions, surgical resection is less

TABLE 26–2. *Methods of Treatment for Chromoblastomycosis*

Chemotherapy Drug	Dosage	Selected References
Flucyostine (p.o.)	50–150 mg/kg/day	Bopp, 1976; Lopes, 1981
Amphotericin B(i.v.)	0.5–1.0 mg/kg/day	Bopp, 1976; Astorga et al, 1981; Restrepo, 1994
Itraconazole (p.o.)	100–400 mg/day	Borelli, 1987; Restrepo et al, 1988; Queiroz-Telles et al, 1992; Bonifaz et al, 1997
Ketoconazole (p.o.)	200–400 mg/day	McBurney, 1982; Drouhet and Dupont, 1983
Fluconazole (p.o.)	200–800 mg/day	Diaz et al, 1992
Thiabendazole(p.o.)	25 mg/kg/day	Bayles, 1971
Terbinafine (p.o.)	500 mg/day	Esterre et al, 1996

Miscellaneous agents

Potassium iodide
Griseofulovin
Methotrexate
Vitamins

Other Therapies

Surgical resection	Conway and Berkeley, 1952; Bansal and Prabhakar, 1989
Cryotherapy	Pimentel et al, 1989; Bonifaz et al, 1997
Laser Therapy	Kultner and Siegle, 1986
Thermotherapy	Tagami et al, 1984; Hiruma et al, 1993
Electrosurgery and curettage	Restrepo, 1994

effective, and is often not possible for functional reasons (Bansal and Prabhakar, 1989).

Alternative procedures to surgical resection include minor interventions such as cryosurgery with liquid nitrogen, carbon dioxide laser therapy, and thermotherapy, all of which have been used with various degrees of success (Tagami et al, 1984; Kultner and Siegle, 1986; Pimentel et al, 1989; Hiruma et al, 1993; Bonifaz et al, 1997). For smaller lesions, cryotherapy is effective for lesions not in flexion areas, and may be beneficial in larger lesions as an adjunct to chemotherapy (Lubritz and Spence, 1978; Borelli, 1987; Kullavanijaya and Rojanavanich, 1995; Bonifaz et al, 1997; Bonifaz et al, 2001). Local heat therapy, which may be applied several times daily with pocket warmers, has been effective as single therapy in several cases, but may be more appropriate as an adjunct to chemotherapy or cryotherapy (Kinbara et al, 1982; Tagami et al, 1984; Borelli, 1987; Hiruma et al, 1993). Procedures such as curettage and desiccation are discouraged because of associated high recurrence rates and the potential for lymphatic dissemination (Fader and McGinnis, 1988; Bayles, 1992; Restrepo, 1994).

In general, chemotherapy for chromoblastomycosis has been minimally successful, and prolonged therapy is required. Chemotherapy is usually needed in cases of moderate or extensive disease, or when surgery is not possible. Chemotherapy may also be required for lesions in areas of flexion, where cryosurgery is contraindicated. The most commonly employed drugs are amphotericin B, flucytosine, and itraconazole, although there is experience with numerous antimicrobial agents (Table 26–2). Intravenous amphotericin B as single therapy appears to be minimally effective, and is often associated with adverse events after prolonged use (Bopp, 1976; Astorga et al, 1981; Fader and McGinnis, 1988; Restrepo, 1994; Rios-Fabra et al, 1994). Amphotericin B is used most commonly in combination with flucytosine for moderate or severe chromoblasomycosis (Bopp, 1976; Astorga, 1981; Fader and McGinnis, 1988; Restrepo, 1994). Treatment with amphotericin B orally, or by intralesional injection, has been used in several patients with limited success (Takahashi and Maie, 1981; Iijima et al, 1995).

Oral flucytosine, 50–150 mg/kg per day divided in 4 doses, has been used for up to 1 year with associated clinical improvement (Bopp, 1976; Lopes et al, 1978; Leslie and Beardmore, 1979; Uitto and Santa-Cruz, 1979; Lopes, 1981). However, when used as a single therapy, only partial response with progression of disease or relapse has occurred, suggesting clinical and microbiologic resistance (Oliviera et al, 1975). Subsequently, combination therapy with flucytosine and amphotericin B has been advocated and is sometimes ef-

fective (Bopp, 1976; Astorga et al, 1981; Restrepo, 1994).

Subsequently, other drugs used in combination with flucytosine include ketoconazole at 200 to 400 mg/day, or thiabendazole (Silber et al, 1983; Solano et al, 1983; Atukorala and Pothupitiya, 1985). Both regimens have been successful in several case reports, but no comparative trials have been performed. Two azole agents, including fluconazole and ketoconazole, have been used as single therapy to treat chromoblastomycosis in a small number of patients, but have not been very effective (Cuce et al, 1980; McBurney, 1982; Drouhet and Dupont, 1983; Diaz et al, 1992).

Itraconazole, a triazole, appears to be the most promising chemotherapeutic agent for the treatment of chromoblastomycosis; however, the appropriate dosage and duration of therapy are unknown. Antifungal susceptibility testing of itraconazole against Fonsecaea species and other agents of chromoblastomycosis shows good activity (Radford et al, 1997; deBedout et al, 1997; Johnson et al, 1998; McGinnis and Pasarell, 1998), and in one study, itraconazole showed better in vitro activity than either flucytosine or amphotericin B (deBedout et al, 1997). Clinical results with itraconazole have been variable, depending upon extent of disease, and length and dosage of therapy (Borelli, 1987; Lavalle, 1987; Restrepo et al, 1988; Queiroz-Telles et al, 1992; Bonifaz et al, 1997; Bonifaz et al, 2001). In an early open-label study of 14 patients with chromoblastomycosis, itraconazole was given at dosages of 100–400 mg daily for 4–8 months (Borelli, 1987). Among 9 patients with C. carrionii infection, cure was achieved in 8, and 1 improved; among 5 patients infected with F. pedrosoi, 2 were cured, and 3 improved. In the 2 cases of infection due to F. pedrosoi that were cured, itraconazole was given in combination with either flucytosine or local heat.

In a noncomparative open-label trial of 19 Brazilian patients with chromoblastomycosis due to F. pedrosoi, itraconazole at doses of 200–400 mg/day for 3–30.5 months was effective (Queiroz-Telles et al, 1992). Among 10 patients with mild to moderate disease, 8 achieved complete clinical and biologic cure. Among the remaining patients who had moderate or severe disease, all had clinical healing or improvement. Itraconazole was well tolerated, and no adverse events were reported that warranted discontinuation of therapy.

A recent trial evaluated combination therapy with itraconazole and cryosurgery, itraconazole alone, and cryosurgery alone in 12 patients with chromoblastomycosis due to F. pedrosoi (Bonifaz et al, 1997). Among patients with small lesions, cryotherapy appeared more effective than itraconazole alone at a dose of 300 mg/day. One group, comprised of patients with extensive disease, was treated with itraconazole until lesions maximally improved, followed by cryosurgery. Among these 4 patients, 2 were cured, and 2 improved. The authors suggest that cryosurgery may be a useful adjunct to chemotherapy for patients with extensive disease.

Newer agents that are potentially useful for the treatment of chromoblastomycosis include third-generation triazole agents, particulary voriconazole. Voriconazole has good in vitro activity against the dematiaceous fungi (McGinnis and Pasarell, 1998), and warrants further study. Terbinafine has been effective in the treatment of patients with chromoblastomycosis (Esterre et al, 1996; Tanuma et al, 2000). In an open-label pilot study of 43 patients, oral terbinafine at doses of 500 mg/day for 12 months gave very promising results, namely, mycologic cure in 82.5% of patients, and total cure in 47% of patients with lesions present longer than 10 years (Esterre et al, 1996).

Although promising new agents are available for the treatment of chromoblastomycosis, appropriate comparative trials to evaluate therapies remain difficult to perform due to the rarity of cases, variability of disease, and the need for prolonged therapy. Combination therapy with an antifungal drug plus surgical therapy or cryotherapy represents a potential advance in treatment and an important area for further study.

REFERENCES

Astorga B, Bonilla E, Martínez C, Mora W. Tratamiento de la cromomicosis con anfotericina B y 5-fluorocitosina. *Med Cut ILA* 9:125–128, 1981.

Atukorala D N, Pothupitiya G M. Treatment of chromomycosis with a combination of ketoconazole and 5-fluorocytosine. *Ceylon Med J* 30:193, 1985.

Banks I S, Palmier J R, Lanoie L, Connor D H, Meyers W M. Chromomycosis in Zaire. *Int J Dermatol* 24:302–307, 1985.

Bansal A S, Prabhakar P. Chromomycosis: a twenty-year-analysis of histolgocially confirmed cases in Jamaica. *Trop Geogr Med* 41:222–226, 1989.

Barba-Gomez J F, Mayorga J, McGinnis M R, Gonzalez-Mendoza A. Chromoblastomycosis caused by *Exophiala spinifera*. *J Am Acad Dermatol* 26:367–370, 1992.

Bayles M A H. Chromomycosis. *Arch Dermatol* 104:476–485, 1971.

Bayles M A H. Tropical mycoses. *Chemother* 38(Suppl 1):27–34, 1992.

Bonifaz A, Martínez-Soto E, Carrasco-Gerard E, Peniche J. Treatment of chromoblastomycosis with itraconazole, cryosurgery, and a combination of both. *Int J Dermatol* 35:542–547, 1997.

Bonifaz A, Carrasco-Gerard E, Saul A. Chromoblastomycosis: clinical and mycologic experience of 51 cases. *Mycoses* 44:1–7, 2001.

Bopp C. Cura de cromobladtomicose por novo tratamiento. *Med Cut ILA* 4:285–292, 1976.

Borelli D. A clinical trial of itraconazole in the treatment of deep mycoses and Leishmaniasis. *Rev Infect Dis* 9(Suppl 1):S57–S63, 1987.

Campins H, Scharyj M. Cromoblastomicosis: comentarios sobre 34 casos con estudio clinico, histologico I micologico. *Gac Med* (Caracas) 61:127–151, 1953.

Carrion A. Chromoblastomycosis. *Ann NY Acad Sci* 50:1255–1281, 1950.

Conway H, Berkeley W. Chromoblastomycosis (mycetoma form) treated by surgical excision. *AMA Arch Dermatol Syphil* 66:695–702, 1952.

Cucé L C, Wroclawski E L, Sampaio S A P. Treatment of paracoccidioidomycosis, candidiasis, chromomycosis, lobomycosis, and mycetoma with ketoconazole. *Int J Dermatol* 19:405–408, 1980.

De Bedout C, Gomez B L, Restrepo A. In vitro susceptibility testing of *Fonsecaea pedrosoi* to antifungals. *Rev Inst Med Trop S Paulo* 39:145–148, 1997.

Diaz M, Negroni R, Montero-Gei F, Castro L G M, Sampaio S A P, Borelli D, Restrepo A, Franco L, Bran J L, Arathoon E G. A Pan-American 5-year study of fluconazole therapy for deep mycosis in the immunocompetent host. *Clin Infect Dis* 14(Suppl):S568–S576 1992.

Drouhet E, Dupont B. Laboratory and clinical assessment of ketoconazole in deep-seated mycoses. *Am J Med* 74:30–47, 1983.

Esterre P, Inzan C K, Ramarcel E R, Andriantsimahavandy A, Ratsioharana M, Pecarrere J L, Roig P. Treatment of chromomycosis with terbinafine: preliminary results of an open pilot study. *Br J Dermatol* 134(Suppl 46):33–36; discussion 40, June 1996.

Fader R C, McGinnis M R. Infections caused by dematiaceous fungi: chromoblastomycosis and phaeohyphomycosis. *Infect Dis Clin of N Am* 2:925–938, 1988.

Foster H M, Harris T J. Malignant change (squamous carcinoma) in chronic chromoblastomycosis. *Aust N Z Surg* 57:775–777, 1987.

Fukushiro R. Chromomycosis in Japan. *Int J Dermatol* 22:221–229, 1983.

Gezuele E, Mackinnon J E, Conti-Diaz I A. The frequent isolation of *Phialophora verrucosa* and *Phialophora pedrosoi* from natural sources. *Sabouraudia* 10:266–273, 1972.

Goette D K, Robertson D. Transepithelial elimination in chromomycosis. *Arch Dermatol* 120:400–401, 1984.

Hiruma M, Kawada A, Yoshida M, Kouya M. Hyperthermic treatment of chromomycosis with disposable chemical pocket warmers. *Mycopathologia* 122:107–114, 1993.

Howles J K, Kennedy C B, Gavin W H, Brueck J W, Buddingh G J. Chromoblastomycosis. *AMA Arch Dermatol Syphil* 69:83–90, 1954.

Iijima S, Takase T, Otsuka F. Treatment of chromomycosis with oral high-dose amphotericin B. *Arch Dermatol* 131:399–401, 1995.

Johnson E M, Szekely A, Warnock D W. In-vitro activity of voriconazole, itraconazole and amphotericin B against filamentous fungi. *J Antimicrob Chemother* 42:741–745, 1998.

Kinbara T, Fukushiro R, Eryu Y. Chromomycosis—report of two cases successfully treated with local heat therapy. *Mykosen* 25:689–694, 1982.

Kullavanijaya P, Rojanavanich V. Successful treatment of chromoblastomycosis due to *Fonsecaea pedrosoi* by the combination of itraconazole and cryotherapy. *Int J Dermatol* 34:804–807, 1995.

Kultner B J, Siegle R J. Treatment of chromomycosis with CO$_2$ laser. *J Dermatol Surg Oncol* 12:965–968, 1986.

Kwon-Chung K J, Bennett J E. *Medical Mycology*. Philadelphia: Lea & Febiger, 1992.

Lavalle P, Suchil P, De Ovando F, Reynoso S. Itraconazole for deep mycoses: preliminary experience in Mexico. *Rev Infect Dis* 9:S64–S70, 1987.

Leslie D F, Beardmore G L. Chromoblastomycosis in Queensland: a retrospective study of 13 cases at the Royal Brisbane Hospital. *Aust J Dermatol* 20:23–30, 1979.

Londero A T, Ramos C D. Chromomycosis: a clinical and mycological study of thirty-five cases observed in the hinterland of Rio Grande do Sul, Brazil. *Am J Trop Med Hyg* 25:132–135, 1976.

Lopes C F, Alvarenga R J, Cisalpino E O, Resende M A, Oliveira L G. Six years' experience in treatment of chromomycosis with 5-fluorocytosine. *Int J Dermatol* 17:414–418, 1978.

Lopes C F. Recent developments in the therapy of chromoblastomycosis. *Bull Pan Am Health Organ* 15:58–64, 1981.

Lubritz R R, Spence J E. Chromoblastomycosis: cure by cryosurgery. *Int J Dermatol* 17:830–832, 1978.

McBurney E I. Chromoblastomycosis treatment with ketoconazole. *Cutis* 30:746–748, 1982.

McGinnis M R. Chromoblastomycosis and phaeohyphomycosis: new concepts, diagnosis and mycology. *J Am Acad Dermatol* 8:1–16, 1983.

McGinnis M R, Pasarell L. In vitro testing of susceptibilities of filamentous ascomycetes to voriconazole, intraconazole, and amphotericin B, with consideration of phylogenetic implications. *J Clin Microbiol* 36:2353–2355, 1998.

Minotto R, Bernardi C D V, Mallmann L F, Edelweiss M I A, Scroferneker M L. Chromoblastomycosis: A review of 100 cases in the state of Rio Grande do Sul, Brazil. *J Am Acad Dermatol* 44:585–592, 2001.

Naka W, Harada T, Nishikawa T, Fukushiro R. A case of chromoblastomycosis: with special reference to the mycology of the isolated *Exophiala jeanselmei*. *Mykosen* 29:445–452, 1986.

Nakamura T, Grant J A, Threlkeld R, Wible L. Primary chromoblastomycosis of the nasal septum. *Am J Clin Pathol* 58:365–370, 1972.

Oliveira, L G, Resende M A, Cisalpino E O, Figueiredo Y P, Lopes C F. *In vitro* sensitivity to 5-fluorocytosine of strains isolated from patients under treatment for chromomycosis. *Int J Dermatol* 141:141–143, 1975.

Padhye A A, Hampton A A, Hampton M T, Hutton N W, Proevost-Smith E, Davis M S. Chromoblastomycosis caused by *Exophiala spinifera*. *Clin Infect Dis* 22:331–335, 1996.

Pimentel E R, Castro L G, Cuce L C, Sampaio S A. Treatment of chromomycosis by cryosurgery with liquid nitrogen: a report of seven cases. *J Dermatolog Sur Oncol* 15:72–79, 1989.

Queiroz-Telles F, Purim K S, Fillus J N, Bordignon G F, Lameira R P, van Cutsem J, Cauwenbergh G. Itraconazole in the treatment of chromoblastomycosis fue to *Fonsecaea pedrosoi*. *Int J Dermatol* 31:805–812, 1992.

Radford S A, Johnson E M, Warnock D W. In vitro studies of activity of voriconazole (UK-109,496), a new triazole antifungal agent, against emerging and less-common mold pathogens. *Antimicrob Agents Chemother* 41:841–843, 1997.

Rajendran C, Ramesh V, Misra R S, Kandhari S, Upreti H B, Datta K K. Chromoblastomycosis in India. *Int J Dermatol* 36:29–33, 1997.

Redondo-Bellon P, Idoate M, Rubio M, Ignacio H J. Chromoblastomycosis produced by *Aureobasidium pullulans* in an immunosuppressed patient. *Arch Dermatol* 133:663–664, 1997.

Restrepo A, Gonzalez A, Gomez I, Arango M, DeBedout C. Treatment of chromoblastomycosis with itraconazole. *Ann NY Acad Sci* 544:504–516, 1988.

Restrepo A. Treatment of tropical mycoses. *J Am Acad Dermatol* 31:S91–S102, 1994.

Ridley M F, The natural habitat of *Cladosporium carrionii*, a cause of chromoblastomycosis in man. *Aust J Dermatol* 4:23–27, 1957.

Rios-Fabra A, Restrepo A, Isturiz R E. Fungal infection in Latin American countries. *Infect Dis Clin North Am* 8:129, 1994.

Silber J G, Gombert M E, Green K, Shalita A R. Treatment of chromomycosis with ketoconazole and 5-fluorocytosine. *J Am Acad Dermatol* 8:236–238, 1983.

Solano A, Hildago H, Castro C, Montero-Gei F. Cromomicosis. Tratamiento con la asociacion thiabendazole y 5-fluorocitosina, seis anos de seguimiento. *Med Cut ILA Lat Am* 11:413, 1983.

Tagami H, Ginoza M, Imaizumi S, Urano-Suehisa S. Successful treatment of chromoblastomycosis with topical heat therapy. *J Am Acad Dermatol* 10:615–619, 1984.

Takahashi S, Maie O. Cutaneous chromomycosis: therapy with intralesional amphotericin B injections. *Hautarzt* 32:567–570, 1981.

Takase T, Baba T, Ueno K. Chromomycosis. A case with a widespread rash, lymph node metastasis and multiple subcutaneous nodules. *Mycoses* 31:343–352, 1988.

Tanuma H, Hiramatsu M, Mukai H, Abe M, Kume, H, Nishiyama S, Katsuoka K. Case report. A case of chromoblastomycosis effectively treated with terbinafine. Characteristics of chromoblastomycosis in the Kitasato region, Japan. (Review). *Mycoses* 43:79–83, 2000.

Uitto J, Santa-Cruz D J. Chromomycosis. *J Cutan Pathol* 6:77–84, 1979.

Uribe F, Zuluga A I, Leon W, Restrepo A. Histopathology of chromoblastomycosis. *Mycopathologia* 105:1–6, 1989.

Velasquez L F, Restrepo A, Calle G. Cromomicosis: experiencia de doce anos. *Acta Med Colombiana* 1:165–171, 1976.

Wackym P A. Cutaneous chromomycosis in renal transplant recipients. *Arch Intern Med* 145:1036–1037, 1985.

Yanase K, Yamada M. "Pocket-warmer" therapy of chromomycosis. *Arch Dermatol* 114:1095, 1978.

Zaror L, Fischman O, Pereira C A, Felipe R G, Gregorio L C, Castelo A. A case of primary nasal chromomycosis. *Mykosen* 30:468–471, 1987.

VII

OTHER MYCOSES

27

Pneumocystosis

CATHERINE F. DECKER AND HENRY MASUR

Although considered an organism of low virulence, *Pneumocystis carinii* is an important cause of pneumonia in immunocompromised hosts, especially those with hematologic malignancies, organ transplants, HIV, certain congenital immunodeficiencies, and those receiving high-dose corticosteroids. Unfortunately, this pneumonia has continued to occur despite the recognition in the 1970s that chemoprophylaxis could greatly reduce the incidence of this disease in the immunocompromised host. A dramatic increase in incidence of *P. carinii* pneumonia occurred as the AIDS epidemic grew as did our knowledge of the initial manifestations, diagnosis, treatment and prevention of *P. carinii* pneumonia. Soon, thereafter, with the implementation of chemoprophylaxis in the late 1980s for the HIV-infected population, and with the widespread use of highly active antiretroviral therapy (HAART) in 1995, there has been a steady decline in cases (Kaplan, et al, 2000). However, *P. carinii* pneumonia will continue to occur in those who do not have access to medical care, those who are unaware they are infected, those who elect not to treat their HIV infection aggressively, or those who fail to respond to therapy.

MICROBIOLOGY

Pneumocystis was traditionally considered a protozoan since it was originally identified by Chagas in 1906. However, recent applications of molecular techniques demonstrated that the organism shares many characteristics with fungi, especially *Saccharomyces* (Edman et al, 1988; Stringer et al, 1989; Cailliez et al, 1996). However, *P. carinii* is unusual among fungi in that the organism lacks ergosterol in its plasma membranes and is insensitive to antifungal drugs that target ergosterol biosynthesis.

Based on its morphology, which is similar to that of protozoa, the life cycle of *P. carinii* has been divided into three stages: the trophozoite, found outside the cyst and believed to be intermediate between the sporozoite and the cyst; the cyst, a spherical or crescent-shaped form; and the sporozoite or intracystic bodies, found within the cysts (Barton et al, 1969). Since human *P. carinii* is not cultivatable in vitro, the life-cycle has not been fully elucidated. It has been suggested that the mode of replication occurs through binary fission and excystment (Hughes et al, 1977).

Advances in molecular biology have better delineated the metabolism of this organism. Sites of action and targets of some of the effective antimicrobial agents have been cloned, sequenced, and characterized. These include genes encoding dihydropteroate synthase (DHPS) and dihydrofolate reductase (DHFR), which are the targets of sulfamethoxazole and trimethoprim, respectively, and the cytochrome B locus, which is the site of action of atovaquone (Edman et al, 1989; Volpe et al, 1993).

EPIDEMIOLOGY

Serologic data in the United States indicate that most humans become subclinically infected with *P. carinii* during childhood and that this infection is usually well contained by an intact immune system (Pifer et al, 1978; Kovacs et al, 1988a; Peglow et al, 1990). Serological studies also have shown that *P. carinii* has a worldwide distribution. The mode of transmission in humans is likely through the respiratory route. Evidence supports that disease may be due to primary infection, reinfection, or reactivation. Reactivation of latent infection may occur if the host becomes immunosuppressed.

PATHOGENESIS/HOST DEFENSES

Based on the immunologic abnormalities found in patients who develop *P. carinii* pneumonia including patients with B cell defects, children with severe combined immunodeficiency disease, premature debilitated infants, and oncology patients receiving immunosuppressive drugs or organ transplant patients, (Hughes et al, 1975; Browne et al, 1986; Peters et al, 1987; Sepkowitz et al, 1992; Sugimoto et al, 1992; Tuan et al, 1992) both humoral and cell-mediated immunity are important host defenses against this infection (Roths and Sidman, 1993). However, cell-mediated immunity appears to occupy the pivotal role in the prevention and control of *P. carinii* infection. In addition, high-dose corticosteroid use for long time periods poses a great risk for the development of *P. carinii* pneumonia.

For patients with HIV infection, the degree of depletion of CD4+ lymphocytes correlates strongly with the likelihood of developing *P. carinii* pneumonia (Masur et al, 1989; Bozzette et al, 1990; Phair et al, 1990). Approximately 90% of *P. carinii* pneumonia cases in patients with HIV infection have been seen in HIV-1–infected patients with recent CD4 counts under 200 cells/mm^3. The majority of these cases occur at CD4 counts fewer than 100 cells/mm^3. Approximately 10%–15% of patients develop *P. carinii* pneumonia at CD4 cell counts greater than 200 cells/mm^3 (Chu et al, 1995). For patients with immunosuppressive disorders other then HIV, CD4 cell counts are less helpful.

For patients who have benefited from therapy with antiretroviral drugs in terms of a rise in CD4 count, considerable evidence supports the concept that CD4 cell counts continue to be an accurate indicator of susceptibility to *P. carinii* (Dworkin et al, 2001). The nadir of the CD4 cell count fall prior to the institution of HAART does not influence the predictive value of counts (Miller et al, 1999; Dworkin et al, 2000; Lyles et al, 2000).

Pneumocystis carinii is presumably inhaled, bypasses the defenses of the upper respiratory tract, and is deposited into the alveolar space. Individuals with intact immunity can control this primary infection, but the organism likely remains latent in the lungs. Disease occurs when cellular or humoral immunity becomes severely deficient. Organisms proliferate, evoking a mononuclear cell response. Alveoli become filled with proteinacous material. The principal histologic finding is the formation of a foamy vaculoated eosinophilic alveolar exudate. The alveolar-capillary permeability increases leading to impairment of gas exchange, not unlike that seen with adult respiratory distress syndrome. Physiologically, hypoxemia occurs with an increased alveolar-arterial oxygen gradient and respiratory alkalosis, impaired diffusion capacity along with alterations in lung compliance and total lung capacity. As the disease progresses in severity, there may also be hyaline membrane formation along with interstitial fibrosis and edema. Without treatment the disease will progress to respiratory failure and death.

PNEUMOCYSTIS CARINII PNEUMONIA

Presenting symptoms in patients with *P. carinii* pneumonia are usually nonspecific and include fever, nonproductive cough, dyspnea, substernal chest tightness, and shortness of breath (Engelberg et al, 1984; Kovacs et al, 1984). Cough may be similar to that seen with a viral infection, and the shortness of breath may be noticed only with exertion. Constitutional symptoms and prolonged prodromal illness may be present for months before presentation. AIDS patients tend to have a more indolent course with a longer duration of symptoms and less hypoxia than patients treated with cytoxic chemotherapy or corticosteroids (Kovacs et al, 1984).

Physical examination is often unrevealing, except for fever and tachypnea. Routine laboratory testing is also unremarkable except for nonspecific elevations of serum lactate dehydrogenase. The total white blood count may rise modestly. The radiologic findings are dictated by the stage of illness at the time the patient presents for evaluation. The typical chest radiograph is one of diffuse and symmetrical increased interstitial markings (Fig. 27–1). However, a substantial number of patients have atypical chest radiographs. Almost all types of infiltrates have been described with *P. carinii* pneumonia, from the classic diffuse infiltrates to cavities, upper lobe predominance, and lobar infiltrates. Some chest radiographs may be normal in HIV-infected and HIV-uninfected patients (Kovacs et al, 1984; Brenner et al, 1987; DeLorenzo et al, 1987). In patients with a normal chest radiograph, a high resolution (thin section) computed tomography scan of the chest will usually demonstrate a characteristic ground glass appearance (Gruden et al, 1997). Clinicians should be aware that the finding of a pneumothorax in an HIV-infected patient with no other precipitating cause should raise the possibility of *P. carinii* pneumonia.

Arterial blood gas abnormalities in patients with *P. carinii* pneumonia characteristically include hypoxemia, hypocarbia, and an increased alveolar–arterial (A–a) oxygen gradient. Normal arterial blood gases can be seen in up to 20% of patients who present with very mild disease, and this finding should not dissuade the

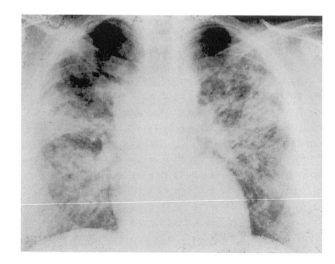

FIGURE 27–1. Chest radiograph showing symmetrical interstitial infiltrates typical of *Pneumocystis* pneumonia.

clinician from initiating an evaluation in patients with compatible symptoms and a CD4 cell count lower than 200 cells/mm^3.

EXTRAPULMONARY PNEUMOCYSTOSIS

Prior to the HIV epidemic, dissemination of *P. carinii* outside the lungs was considered to be a rare occurrence. Advances in detection by PCR analysis have affirmed the presence of *P. carinii* in blood (Lipschik et al, 1992). Extrapulmonary disease may be more common than once realized. When abdominal imaging studies are performed on patients with pneumocystis pneumonia, lesions in visceral organs can sometimes be recognized. These lesions, which often disappear during therapy, probably represent subclinical cases of disseminated pneumocystosis. However, no systematic evaluation of a series of patients has been done to determine the frequency of visceral hepatic, splenic, or renal lesions.

Extrapulmonary pneumocystosis occurs predominately in patients with advanced HIV infection and in those who are not taking prophylaxis or are receiving aerosolized pentamidine (Raviglione, 1990; Telzak et al, 1990). Extrapulmonary disease is generally not seen in patients receiving systemic prophylaxis with trimethoprim-sulfamethoxazole (TMP-SMX), dapsone, or atovaquone. Reported sites of dissemination include lymph nodes, liver, spleen, bone marrow, pleura, ear, choroid of the eye, thyroid, adrenal gland, intestines, and meninges (Raviglione, 1990; Telzak et al, 1990). Clinical manifestations of extrapulmonary disease may occur with or without lung involvement. *Pneumocystis carinii* can be detected by tissue biopsy or at autopsy. While extrapulmonary pneumocystosis is not invariably fatal, the mortality rate is difficult to estimate since extrapulmonary sites are rarely looked for unless extrapulmonary manifestions are clinically apparent.

LABORATORY DIAGNOSIS

The definitive diagnosis of *P. carinii* disease requires the demonstration of cysts or trophozoites within tissue or body fluids. Organisms are recognized via colorimetric or immunofluorescent stains since the organism cannot be cultured. Before the AIDS epidemic, the diagnosis of *P. carinii* pneumonia typically required an open lung biopsy, because of the low number of organisms and the lack of sputum production in infected patients. With the development of improved diagnostic techniques, diagnoses can now be established by less invasive methods. Virtually all patients can be diagnosed by careful analysis of bronchoalveolar lavage fluid (Meduri et al, 1991; Baughman, 1994). Induced sputum has been shown to be a sensitive, simple, and noninvasive means to diagnose *P. carinii* pneumonia and often precludes the need for bronchoscopy (Bigby et al, 1986; Kovacs et al, 1988b; Ng et al, 1990; Kirsch et al, 1992) with reported yields for recovery of the organism ranging from 70% to 95% at various institutions (Bigby et al, 1986; Pitchenik et al, 1986; Kovacs et al, 1988b).

The development of monoclonal antibodies has resulted in a rapid, sensitive and easy to perform immunofluorescence assay, which often is more efficient for detecting *P. carinii* in respiratory specimens than conventional colorimetric stains (Gill et al, 1987; Kovacs et al, 1988b; Kovacs et al, 1989; Ng et al, 1990).

More recently, molecular assays have been developed for detecting *P. carinii* in bronchoalveolar lavage (BAL) or induced sputum samples. Polymerase chain reaction (PCR) methods have used a variety of gene targets (Olsson et al, 1993; Sandhu et al, 1999), but those with the highest sensitivity use either a multicopy gene target (e.g., mitochondrial rRNA, major surface glycoprotein) (Wakefield et al, 1990; Huang et al, 1999) or a nested PCR assay requiring 2 amplification rounds (Lipschik et al, 1992; Lu et al, 1995).

Polymerase chain reaction has also allowed the detection of *P. carinii* in more easily obtained specimens such as oral washes or gargles (Helweg-Larsen et al, 1998; Fischer et al, 2001; Larsen et al, 2002). Such techniques are quite sensitive. Their specificity is reasonable, but several recent studies using PCR to detect *P. carinii* have found individuals who are positive by PCR but negative by stain. While some of these patients had clinical disease, others did not develop *P. carinii* pneumonia, suggesting asymptomatic colonization (Leigh et al, 1993; Sing et al, 2000). Quantitative PCR assays may allow distinction between colonization and disease.

TREATMENT

Trimethoprim-sulfamethoxazole and intravenous pentamidine are the most effective therapies for *Pneumocystis carinii* pneumonia. Both are efficacious in the treatment of *P. carinii* pneumonia: their efficacy depends on how hypoxemic patients are, and how immunosuppressed they are when therapy is started (Hughes et al, 1977; Brenner et al, 1987; Sattler et al, 1988; Masur, 1992). (Table 27–1).

Other effective regimens include trimethoprim-dapsone (Leoung et al, 1986; Medina et al, 1990; Safrin et al, 1996), primaquine-clindamycin (Ruf et al, 1991; Toma et al, 1993; Safrin et al, 1996), trimetrexate (Sattler et al, 1994), and atovaquone (Hughes et al, 1993).

Trimethoprim-sulfamethoxazole is the agent of choice for initial therapy of acute *P. carinii* pneumonia. While TMP-SMX is as potent as intravenous pen-

TABLE 27–1. *Drug Regimens for Treatment of* P. carinii *Pneumonia*

Agent	Dose	Interval	Route
Specific Therapy			
Trimethoprim/	5 mg/kg	6–8 hours	i.v. or p.o
sulfamethoxazole	25 mg/kg		
Pentamidine	4 mg/kg	24 hours	i.v.
Trimethoprim plus	5 mg/kg	8 hours	p.o
Dapsone	100 mg	24 hours	p.o
Clindamycin plus	600–900 mg	8 hours	p.o/i.v.
Primaquine	15–30 mg	24 hours	p.o
Atovaquone	750 mg	12 hours	p.o
Trimetrexate with	45 mg/m^2	24 hours	i.v.
Leucovorin	20 mg/m^2	6 hours	i.v.
Adjunctive Therapy			
Prednisone or Solumedrol (if room air PaO$_2$ < 70 mmHg within 72 hours of initiating therapy)	40 mg q 12 hours for 5 days then 40 mg q day for 5 days p.o. or i.v. then 20 mg qd for 11 days		

tamidine, it is less toxic. If a patient has mild disease (PaO$_2$ greater than 70 mmHg), and is able to tolerate oral medications, TMP-SMX may be given in the dosage of 2 double-strength tablets (160 mg TMP and 800 mg SMX) every 6–8 hours. The q 8-hour regimen is preferred by many clinicians since toxicity would be expected to be less than with q 6-hour dosing and there is no evidence that efficacy is improved with the higher dose. With more severe disease or if the patient is unable to tolerate oral medication, intravenous TMP-SMX (5 mg/kg TMP and 25 mg/kg sulfamethoxazole q 8 hours) should be given. Total duration of therapy is usually 21 days, but there is no concrete evidence that 21 days of therapy is more effective than 14 days (Catterell et al, 1985). Toxicity associated with TMP-SMX continues to hinder its use in many patients and occurs more frequently in HIV-infected patients than in patients without HIV infection. Toxicities include fever, rash, headache, nausea, vomiting, pancytopenia, hepatitis, and aseptic meningitis. Treatment-limiting toxicities usually occur between day 6 and day 10 of therapy. For AIDS patients, trials suggest that approximately 25% of patients are unable to tolerate a full course of TMP-SMX (Hardy et al, 1992; Schneider et al, 1992). Minor laboratory abnormalities should not be an indication to switch to a less effective alternative therapy.

Intravenous pentamidine is the most potent alternative agent to TMP-SMX as initial therapy in patients who are sulfonamide intolerant. The standard dose of pentamidine is 4 mg/kg/day, given intravenously over at least 1 hour for a minimum of 14–21 days. Small studies suggest that a lower dose of 3 mg/kg/day may be less toxic, but equally effective (Conte et al, 1987; Conte et al, 1990).

Dapsone, as a single agent, is not as effective as other alternatives in the treatment of *P. carinii* pneumonia.

Failure rates are approximately 40% in patients with HIV infection (Mills et al, 1988; Safrin et al, 1991). However, the combination of dapsone (100 mg/day) and trimethoprim (15 mg/kg/day) is comparable in efficacy to TMP-SMX (Leoung et al, 1986). Trimethoprim-dapsone is used as an alternative oral regimen in mild to moderate disease for patients intolerant of TMP-SMX. Approximately 50% of sulfonamide intolerant patients tolerate dapsone. This regimen can only be given orally and is therefore not suitable for patients with severe disease or gastrointestinal dysfunction. Because of the added complexity of taking dapsone and trimethoprim on different schedules, this regimen is not as easy to adhere to as TMP-SMX.

The combination of clindamycin and primaquine is another reasonable alternative for the treatment of *P. carinii* pneumonia (Ruf et al, 1991; Toma et al, 1993; Bozzette et al, 1995). Investigators report success rates of 75%–80% in open, noncomparative trials with patients who are intolerant to or failed standard treatment (Ruf et al, 1991; Toma et al, 1993). A randomized trial found the combination to be comparable in efficacy to TMP-SMX or TMP-dapsone in mild to moderate disease (Safrin et al, 1996). Clindamycin-primaquine has also been used as a salvage regimen in patients with pneumocystosis induced respiratory failure (Noskin et al, 1992), although many authorities are reluctant to use an oral agent (i.e., primaquine) in this setting. Primaquine base of 30 mg is the usual dose. Clindamycin is given either orally (300 mg to 450 mg every 6 to 8 hours) or intravenously (600 mg to 900 mg every 6 to 8 hours). Clindamycin alone is not effective in animal models unless primaquine is given concurrently.

Oral atovaquone is effective and well tolerated. However, atovaquone was associated with a higher rate of treatment failure and was less effective than TMP-

SMX in mild to moderate pneumocystosis (Hughes et al, 1993). In another study, oral atovaquone and intravenous pentamidine were found to have similar success rates in mild to moderate *P. carinii* pneumonia in AIDS patients who were intolerant to TMP-SMX. Atovaquone was better tolerated, but patients receiving atovaquone failed therapy more frequently and patients receiving pentamidine had more treatment-limiting adverse drug toxicities (Dohn et al, 1994). Low plasma atovaquone levels are associated with a poor response (Hughes et al, 1993). Low plasma levels have been in part due to the poor bioavailability of the drug. Even with the liquid formulation of atovaquone, absorption can be unpredictable and steady-state may not be reached for several days. Atovaquone absorption is improved by ingestion of a fatty meal. Atovaquone has a role as therapy for patients with mild, stable disease who have no evidence of gastrointestinal dysfunction. If neither TMP-SMX nor TMP-dapsone is tolerable and disease is mild, atovaquone is a reasonable option.

Trimetrexate in combination with leucovorin in patients with moderate to severe disease is also effective. However, trimetrexate is less effective and associated with more relapses than TMP-SMX, and is considered an alternative agent for patients who are intolerant of TMP-SMX and who cannot tolerate or do not respond to intravenous pentamidine (Sattler et al, 1994). Other agents with promising activity against *P. carinii* include analogs of primaquine, analogs of pentamidine, and echinocandins or pneumocandins.

Once the diagnosis of *P. carinii* is made, outpatient therapy with an oral agent, preferably TMP-SMX, is recommended for mild to moderately severe disease ($PaO_2 > 70$ mmHg). Other alternatives for oral outpatient therapy include TMP-dapsone, clindamycin-primaquine, and atovaquone. Patients who are more severely ill with moderate to severe disease or who cannot tolerate oral medications should be hospitalized and given intravenous TMP-SMX. In sulfonamide intolerant patients, intravenous pentamidine should be administered.

The use of corticosteroids in conjunction with antimicrobial agents has become the standard of care in the treatment of moderate–severe *P. carinii* pneumonia in AIDS patients (The National Institutes of Health, 1990). Three randomized controlled studies revealed that corticosteroids significantly decreased the frequency of early deterioration in oxygenation and improved survival in patients who had an initial room air $PO_2 < 70$ mmHg (Bozzette et al, 1990; Gagnon et al, 1990; Montaner et al, 1991). Corticosteroid therapy is not recommended unless the diagnosis of *P. carinii* is confirmed promptly (The National Institutes of Health, 1990). Corticosteroid therapy is logical to use in patients with disorders other than HIV and for all patients manifesting a slow response to therapy, although no prospective trials have documented this efficacy (Pareja et al, 1998).

Monitoring Therapy

Respiratory rate, arterial oxygenation, ventilation, temperature, and chest radiograph should be assessed to determine initial clinical status and then assessed serially to determine response to therapy. The median time to respond to therapy is 4–10 days. Laboratory tests should be done to recognize bone marrow, liver, pancreatic, or renal toxicity. Many HIV-infected patients will get worse with a decline in partial pressure of oxygen by 10–30 mmHg during the initial 2–5 days after initiation of specific therapy before clinical improvement is observed unless adjuvant corticosteroids are included in the regimen (Montaner et al, 1991). This decline has been attributed to dying organisms, which elicit an intense inflammatory response. The initial regimen should probably be continued for at least 5–10 days before lack of response or poor response dictate a change in therapy. Fluid status should be monitored carefully. Intravenous TMP-SMX is often given with a considerable volume load. In addition, *P. carinii* pneumonia may cause increased permeability of alveolar capillary membranes, which can lead to accumulation of interstitial and alveolar fluid and respiratory failure. Concomitant congestive heart failure due to processes unrelated to pneumocystosis may also occur. HIV-related or chemotherapy-related cardiomyopathy may not be evident until the patient is challenged with large volumes of fluids.

Survival from an episode of *P. carinii* pneumonia correlates with the pretreatment arterial–alveolar gradient (Brenner et al, 1987; Dohn et al, 1992). Other factors that influence outcome include: number of tachyzoites in bronchoalveolar lavage, degree of chest radiograph abnormality, level of LDH elevation, and (for patients with HIV infection low CD4 cell counts) (Kovacs et al, 1984; Brenner et al, 1987; Kales et al, 1987). For a patient with an initial PaO_2 of greater than 70 mmHg while breathing room air, expected response rates are 60% to 80% in non-AIDS patients and 80%–95% in patients with AIDS (Hughes et al, 1977; Brenner et al, 1987; Sattler et al, 1988). Evaluation of response to therapy should be based on clinical parameters (e.g., temperature, respiratory rate, oxygenation) and radiographic examination. The use of bronchoscopy to assess response to drug therapy is not helpful in the clinical setting using current quantitative techniques since cysts and trophozoites are difficult to quantitate accurately. In HIV-infected patients, *P. carinii* will be present in bronchoscopy specimens for many weeks after initiation of therapy, even in patients who rapidly improve (Shelhamer et al, 1984).

In a patient who appears to be failing therapy after 4 to 6 days, clinicians need to assess for other concurrent pulmonary processes. Cytomegalovirus, fungi, mycobacteria, respiratory viruses, or agents of atypical pneumonia may be present. Noninfectious causes such as congestive heart failure, embolic disease, or alveolar hemorrhage should be considered. A Swan-Ganz catheter may help evaluate for congestive heart failure. Empirical therapy for community-acquired pneumonia may be a reasonable strategy given the difficulty of diagnosing concurrent pneumonia. Prednisone should be added to the regimen if not already instituted. A change in therapy to a different agent is usually reserved until the patient has had 4 to 8 days of first line therapy and after other pulmonary processes have been investigated. Most authorities recommend a switch from TMP-SMX first to intravenous pentamidine and then to trimetrexate. If a patient is deteriorating or failing to improve on a regimen other than TMP-SMX, strong consideration should be given to using TMP-SMX, even if desensitization is required in the intensive care setting.

PREVENTION

Historically, the successful use of TMP-SMX in controlled trials for primary prevention of *P. carinii* pneumonia in pediatric oncology patients (Hughes et al, 1977) has been the model for the development of prophylactic strategies in other immunocompromised hosts at risk for *P. carinii* pneumonia (Fischl et al, 1988). Prophylaxis for *P. carinii* pneumonia has been shown most convincingly to decrease morbidity and mortality in patients with cancer and patients with HIV infection. Most authorities believe that it is prudent to institute primary prophylaxis for groups of patients felt to be at high risk including patients with organ transplants (especially lung or heart–lung transplants), lymphoreticular malignancies, HIV with low CD4 counts, and primary immunodeficiencies (Gryzan et al, 1988; Henson et al, 1991; Masur, 1992). Prophylaxis should be continued for as long as the immunosuppressive condition persists.

In patients with malignant neoplasms or organ transplants, observational studies provide data about when to initiate prophylaxis, and how long to continue it. The use of TMP-SMX for *P. carinii* pneumonia prophylaxis in bone marrow transplant patients has greatly reduced the incidence of pneumocystosis in this transplant population (Winston, 1993). Current guidelines for prophylaxis include all allogeneic hematopoietic stem cell transplant recipients or autologous recipients with underlying hematologic malignancies (e.g., lymphoma or leukemia) who are receiving intense conditioning regimens or graft manipulations or who have

recently received fludarabine or 2-chlorodeoxyadenosine. Prophylaxis should be administered from the time of engraftment for at least 6 months after transplant for all recipients. Prophylaxis should be continued for greater than 6 months after transplant for all persons who are receiving immunosuppressive therapy (e.g., prednisone or cyclosporine) or those who have chronic graft vs. host disease. Prophylaxis is usually begun 1–2 weeks before transplant (Centers for Disease Control, 2000).

Recommendations formulated to prevent *P. carinii* pneumonia in HIV-infected patients are based on large observational databases and controlled trials. Prophylactic agents should be initiated when an HIV-infected patient's absolute CD4 cell count falls below 200 cells/mm^3 (Masur et al, 2002) and for patients with oropharyngeal candidiasis regardless of CD4 cell count. Prior to the era of HAART, prophylaxis was recommended to be lifelong, once the patient's CD4 cell count fell below 200 cells/mm^3, the patient had oral candidiasis, or the patient had an episode of *P. carinii* pneumonia (Phair et al, 1990; Kovacs et al, 1992; Masur, 1992). Since HAART regimens have been used extensively, numerous studies have supported the cessation of primary or secondary prophylaxis in patients whose CD4 cell counts rise to > 200 cells/mm^3 as a consequence of HAART (Centers for Disease Control, 1999; Centers for Disease Control, 2001; Furrer et al, 1999; Furrer et al, 2001; Ledergerber et al, 2001; Masur et al, 2002). For some patients with CD4 counts > 200 cells/mm^3, it may be prudent, however, to continue prophylaxis in patients with high viral loads (i.e., > 50,000–100,000 copies/ml), rapidly declining CD4 cell counts, wasting, oral candidiasis, or a prior episode of *P. carinii* pneumonia at CD4 cell counts > 200 cell/mm^3.

Trimethoprim-sulfamethoxazole is the preferred chemoprophylactic agent in patients who can tolerate it. Trimethoprim-sulfamethoxazole is more effective than any other regimen (Table 27–2) (Hardy et al, 1992; Schneider et al, 1992; Bozzette et al, 1995; Podzamczer et al, 1995; Saah et al, 1995). The relative efficacy and toxicity of TMP-SMX as primary and secondary prophylaxis compared to other agents has been best assessed in randomized prospective trials involving patients with HIV infection. In European and American trials evaluating primary and secondary prophylaxis, either high dose (1 double strength [DS] per day) or low dose (1 single strength [SS] per day) TMP-SMX was found to be significantly more effective in preventing *P. carinii* than aerosolized pentamidine (Hardy et al, 1989; Schneider et al, 1992; Girard et al, 1993; Bozzette et al, 1995; Ioannidis et al, 1996). However, the rate of discontinuation of study drug because of

TABLE 27–2. *Drug Regimens for Prophylaxis for*
P. carinii *Pneumonia*

Agent	Total Daily Dose	Route	Interval
First Choice			
Trimethoprim/	160/800 mg (DS)	Oral	Daily
sulfamethoxazole	160/800 mg (DS)	Oral	Twice daily
	80/400 mg (SS)	Oral	Daily
Alternatives			
Pentamidine	300 mg	Aerosol	Monthly
Dapsone	100 mg	Oral	Daily
Pyrimethamine plus	75 mg	Oral	Weekly
dapsone plus	200 mg	Oral	Weekly
leucovorin	25 mg	Oral	Weekly
Atovaquone	1500 mg	Oral	Daily

DS, double strength; SS, single strength

toxicity was higher in the TMP-SMX groups than in the aerosolized pentamidine group. The incidence and types of adverse reactions were similar in both TMP-SMX groups, but the toxic effects occurred significantly sooner in the group receiving the higher dose. These adverse events appear to be partially dose-related (Schneider et al, 1992).

True breakthroughs of *P. carinii* pneumonia are unusual for patients who are adherent to the recommended regimens of TMP-SMX. There is no evidence that a single-strength TMP-SMX tablet daily is less effective than a double strength, although a study adequately powered to prove equivalence has not been done (Ioannidis et al, 1996). However, it is unclear whether regimens that employ fewer than 1 DS tablet daily provide as much efficacy for preventing toxoplasmosis or bacterial respiratory infections. There are data in patients with HIV infection to suggest that intermittent regimens (1 DS tablet thrice weekly) may be less effective than daily regimens. Lower doses of TMP-SMX are better tolerated than higher doses (El-Sadr et al, 1999). In children with malignant neoplasms, such differences were not observed (Hughes et al, 1987).

In a large trial (ACTG 081), 843 patients with HIV infection were randomized to TMP-SMX (1 DS tablet bid), dapsone (50 mg bid) or aerosolized pentamidine (300 mg once monthly). Fewer episodes of *P. carinii* pneumonia occurred among patients receiving TMP-SMX than in the other two arms when patients with CD4+ counts less than 100 cells/mm³ were considered but not when patients with higher CD4+ counts were assessed. In this trial, the efficacy of dapsone appeared to be better than aerosolized pentamidine. Dapsone given at doses of 50 mg per day or less was not as effective as 50 mg bid (Bozzette et al, 1995).

A secondary prophylaxis study in the United States involved 310 patients with HIV infection who were randomly assigned to aerosolized pentamidine by a Respirgard II nebulizer or 1 oral double-strength tablet of TMP-SMX daily (Hardy et al, 1992). By intent-to-treat analysis, the recurrence rate of *P. carinii* pneumonia was significantly higher among the patients assigned to aerosolized pentamidine (18%) than among those assigned to TMP-SMX (4%). As expected, patients who received TMP-SMX experienced considerable toxicity resulting in discontinuation of the agent.

Trimethoprim-sulfamethoxazole has advantages not provided by aerosolized pentamidine including low cost, oral formulation, and probable protective effect against disseminated pneumocystosis. In addition, because of TMP-SMX's broad spectrum of antimicrobial activity, it offers protection against toxoplasmosis and enteric pathogens. In addition, TMP-SMX confers protection against infection by *Haemophilus influenzae* and *Streptococcus pneumoniae* (Carr et al, 1992; Hardy et al, 1992).

Aerosolized pentamidine delivered by the Marqest ultrasonic nebulizer at a dose of 300 mg monthly has been the regimen evaluated in most trials. This regimen is effective, but it is not used as often as other regimens due to its inferior efficacy, cost, and concern about inducing cough that could disseminate other pathogens such as tuberculosis. Pentamidine delivered by the Fisons (Rochester, New York, USA) hand-held ultrasonic nebulizer at a dose of 60 mg every 2 weeks (after 5 loading doses) has also been shown to be highly effective for prophylaxis in a prospective, randomized trial (Montaner et al, 1991; Murphy et al, 1991). Other delivery systems have not been evaluated as extensively and cannot be recommended.

Aerosolized pentamidine is relatively well tolerated when delivered by the Respirgard II or the Fisons nebulizer in the indicated dosing regimens. Coughing or wheezing occurs in 30%–40% of patients, but this reaction may be diminished or prevented by the administration of beta-adrenergic agonist such as albuterol (Conte et al, 1986; Leoung et al, 1990; Montaner et al, 1991; Murphy et al, 1991). Bronchospasm rarely necessitates discontinuation of prophylaxis with aerosolized pentamidine treatment. Patients with reactive airway disease or bullous lung disease may not distribute aerosolized pentamidine effectively and thus may not obtain maximum protection. Disseminated pneumocystosis has been reported in patients receiving aerosolized pentamidine for prophylaxis (Hardy et al, 1989; Pareja et al, 1998), but it is not clear whether such cases are truly more frequent in patients receiving aerosolized pentamidine compared to those receiving other forms of prophylaxis or no prophylaxis.

Concern has been raised about potential outbreaks of tuberculosis among health-care workers and HIV-infected patients associated with the coughing induced by aerosol pentamidine. Before administering aerosolized pentamidine, all patients should be screened for tuberculosis and health-care workers should follow guidelines to minimize the risk of spread of TB to other patients and health-care workers (Centers for Disease Control, 1990; Blumberg et al, 1995). Ideally, aerosolized pentamidine should be administered in individual booths or rooms with negative pressure ventilation and direct exhaust to the outside. After the administration of aerosolized pentamidine, patients should not return to common waiting areas until coughing has subsided.

Dapsone, an attractive alternative to aerosolized pentamidine because it is oral, convenient, and inexpensive, is considered by some experts to be the best alternative for patients who cannot tolerate TMP-SMX (Bozzette et al, 1995; Ioannidis et al, 1996). Approximately 50%–80% of patients who are TMP-SMX intolerant will be able to tolerate dapsone (Holtzer et al, 1998). Dose reduction to improve tolerability is not recommended, because doses less than 100 mg qd are considerably less effective than the full-dose regimen.

Weekly doses of dapsone (200 mg) and pyrimethamine (75 mg) are well tolerated, but less efficacy than TMP-SMX (Lavelle et al, 1991). Dapsone-pyrimethamine has efficacy as a prophylactic regimen against *P. carinii* pneumonia that is similar to aerosol pentamidine but less effective than TMP-SMX. This drug combination has been assessed as a daily regimen (dapsone 50 mg p.o. qd plus pyrimethamine 75 mg weekly) or as a weekly regimen (dapsone 200 mg plus pyrimethamine 75 mg) (Girard et al, 1993; Opravil et al, 1995). It is not clear if pyrimethamine truly adds potency against *P. carinii* given the results of the ACTG 081 study mentioned previously (Bozzette et al, 1995). Dapsone alone has no antibacterial activity, and it is not clear if dapsone has adequate antitoxoplasma activity when used without pyrimethamine.

Two trials demonstrated that a daily atovaquone dose of 1500 mg of the liquid suspension has comparable prophylaxis efficacy to aerosolized pentamidine or oral dapsone (El-Sadr et al, 1998; Chan et al, 1999). Atovaquone does have activity against toxoplasma, but the relative efficacy of this regimen for preventing toxoplasmosis has not been adequately studied. Atovaqone has no antibacterial activity. Atovaquone is also much more expensive than other drug regimens.

Other potential prophylactic agents that have been used empirically or evaluated in small clinical trials include pyrimethamine-sulfadoxine, trimethoprim-dapsone, parenteral pentamidine and clindamycin-primaquine. Although these regimens probably have some efficacy, data evaluating these forms of prophylaxis are limited and not yet sufficient to warrant recommending any of them with confidence.

RECENT ADVANCES

Desensitization to Sulfonamides

The utility of TMP-SMX desensitization, or more appropriately gradual dose escalation has been controversial in terms of prophylaxis or therapy. In uncontrolled studies, some patients have been successfully desensitized to TMP-SMX in attempts to reduce the likelihood of adverse reactions from occurring in patients with a history of hypersensitivity-like reaction (Rubin et al, 1987; Carr et al, 1993; Absar et al, 1994; Gluckstein and Ruskin, 1995). Two randomized trials assessing desensitization as a method to improve long-term tolerance have been completed in patients with HIV infection. Both suggest that gradual dose escalation is useful when an endpoint of percent of patients still receiving TMP-SMX after several months is assessed (Para et al, 2000; Leoung et al, 2001).

Of concern are reports about severe systemic reactions in HIV-infected patients that resemble anaphylaxis or septic shock in patients who are rechallenged with TMP-SMX after experiencing toxicity within the previous 6–8 weeks. Although the mechanism remains unclear, the reaction has features of cytokine-mediated effects that are not related to IgE (Kelly et al, 1992; Martin et al, 1993). Clinicians should be aware that this syndrome may be due to TMP-SMX rather than some other process.

Sulfonamide Resistance/Dihydropteroate Synthase Mutations

Since *P. carinii* has been widely exposed to sulfonamide drugs (the most active component of the combination drug TMP-SMX), it is reasonable to expect that *P. carinii* might develop sulfonamide resistance. Both dapsone and TMP-SMX act by inhibiting folate biosynthesis enzyme dihydropteroate synthase (DHPS). Sulfonamide resistance results from point mutations in the DHPS gene. Since human *P. carinii* cannot be cultured and hence no sensitivities can be performed, resistance is elucidated by the indirect method of looking for *P. carinii* DHPS gene mutations (Lane et al, 1997). While the DHPS mutations have been found in patients taking low doses of TMP-SMX for *P. carinii* prophylaxis (Kazanjian et al, 1998; Mei et al, 1998), it is unclear if this mutation affects the response to therapeutic doses of TMP-SMX. While a Danish study reports that patients with mutant DHPS were less likely to survive *P. carinii* infections, two other trials recently found that there was no effect on survival or response to therapy in those who had mutant DHPS (Helweg-Larsen et al, 1999; Huang et al, 2000; Kanzanjian et al, 2000; Navin et al, 2001). Whether the presence of these mutations does, in fact, predict failure of prophylaxis or treatment courses remains controversial. Currently there is no compelling evidence to suggest that resistance testing is warranted for routine clinical indications.

REFERENCES

Absar N, Daneshvar H, Beall G. Desensitization to trimethoprim/sulfamethoxazole in HIV-infected patients. *J Allergy Clin Immunol* 93:1001–1005, 1994.

Barton E G J, Campbell W G J. *Pneumocystis carinii* in lungs of rats treated with cortisone acetate: Ultrastructural observations relating to the life cycle. *Am J Pathol* 54:209–236, 1969.

Baughman R P. Current methods of diagnosis. In: Walzer PD, ed. *Pneumocystis carinii* Pneumonia. New York: Marcel Dekker, 381–401, 1994.

Bigby T D, Margolskee D, Curtis J L, Michael P F, Sheppard D, Hadley W K, Hopewell P C. The usefulness of induced sputum in the diagnosis of *Pneumocystis carinii* pneumonia in patients with the acquired mmunodeficiency syndrome. *Am Rev Respir Dis* 133:515–518, 1986.

Blumberg H M, Watkins D L, Berschling J D, Antle A, Moore P, White N, Hunter M, Green B, Ray SM, McGowan JE. Preventing the nosocomial transmission of tuberculosis. *Ann Intern Med* 122:658–663, 1995.

Bozzette S A, Sattler F R, Chiu J, Wu A W, Gluckstein D, Kemper C, Bartok A, Niosi J, Abramson I, Coffman J, Hughlett C, Loya R, Cassens B, Akil B, Meng T C, Boylen C T, Nielsen D, Richman D D, Tilles J G, Leedom J, McCutchan J A. A controlled trial of early adjunctive treatment with corticosteroids for *pneumocystis carinii* pneumonia in the acquired immunodeficiency syndrome. *N Engl J Med* 323:1451–1457, 1990.

Bozzette S A, Finkelstein D M, Spector S A, Frame P, Powderly W G, He W, Phillips L, Craven D, van der Horst C, Feinberg J. A randomized trial of three antipneumocystis agents in patients with advanced human immunodeficiency virus infection. NIAID AIDS Clinical Trials Group. *N Engl J Med* 332:693–699, 1995.

Brenner M, Ognibene F P, Lack E E, Simmons J T, Suffredini A F, Lane H C, Fauci A S, Parrillo J E, Shelhamer J H, Masur H. Prognostic factors and life expectancy of patients with acquired immunodeficiency syndrome and *Pneumocystis carinii* pneumonia. *Am Rev Respir Dis* 136:1199–1206, 1987.

Browne M J, Hubbard S M, Longo D L, Fisher R, Wesley R, Ihde D C, Young R C, Pizzo P A. Excess prevalence of *Pneumocystis carinii* pneumonia in patients treated for lymphoma with combination chemotherapy. *Ann Intern Med* 104:338–344, 1986.

Cailliez J C, Seguy N, Denis C M, Aliouat E M, Mazars E, Polonelli L, Camus D, Dei-Cas E. *Pneumocystis carinii*: an atypical fungal micro-organism. *J Med Vet Mycol* 34:227–239, 1996.

Carr A, Tindall B, Brew B J, Marriott D J, Harkness J L, Penny R, Cooper D A. Low-dose trimethoprim-sulfamethoxazole prophylaxis for toxoplasmic encephalitis in patients with AIDS. *Ann Intern Med* 117:106–111, 1992.

Carr A, Penny R, Cooper D A. Efficacy and safety of rechallenge with low-dose trimethoprim-sulfamethoxazole in previously hypersensitive HIV-infected patients. *AIDS* 7:65–71, 1993.

Catterall J R, Potasman I, Remington J S. *Pneumocystis carinii* pneumonia in the patient with AIDS. *Chest* 88:758–762, 1985.

Centers for Disease Control. Guidelines for preventing the transmission of *Mycobacterium tuberculosis* in health-care settings, with special focus on HIV-related issues. *MMWR Morb Mortal Wkly Rep* 39:1–29, 1990.

Centers for Disease Control. 1999 USPHS/IDSA Guidelines for the prevention of opportunistic infections in persons infected with human immunodeficiency virus. *MMWR Morb Mortal Wkly Rep* 48:1–66, 1999.

Centers for Disease Control. Guidelines for preventing opportunistic infections among hematopoietic stem cell transplant recipients. *MMWR Morb Mortal Wkly Rep* 49:1–125, 2000.

Chan C, Montaner J, Lefebvre E A, Morey G, Dohn M, McIvor R A, Scott J, Marina R, Caldwell P. Atovaquone suspension compared with aerosolized pentamidine for prevention of *Pneumocystis carinii* pneumonia in human immunodeficiency virus-infected subjects intolerant of trimethoprim or sulfonamides. *J Infect Dis* 180:369–376, 1999.

Chu S Y, Hanson D L, Ciesielski C, Ward J W. Prophylaxis against *Pneumocystis carinii* pneumonia at higher CD4+ T-cell counts. *JAMA* 273:848, 1995.

Conte J E, Jr, Upton R A, Phelps R T, Wofsy C B, Zurlinden E, Lin E T. Use of a specific and sensitive assay to determine pentamidine pharmacokinetics in patients with AIDS. *J Infect Dis* 154:923–929, 1986.

Conte J E, Jr, Hollander H, Golden J A. Inhaled or reduced-dose intravenous pentamidine for *Pneumocystis carinii* pneumonia. A pilot study. *Ann Intern Med* 107:495–498, 1987.

Conte J E, Jr, Chernoff D, Feigal D W, Jr, Joseph P, McDonald C, Golden J A. Intravenous or inhaled pentamidine for treating *Pneumocystis carinii* pneumonia in AIDS. A randomized trial. *Ann Intern Med* 113:203–209, 1990.

DeLorenzo L J, Huang C T, Maguire G P, Stone D J. Roentgenographic patterns of *Pneumocystis carinii* pneumonia in 104 patients with AIDS. *Chest* 91:323–327, 1987.

Dohn M N, Baughman R P, Vigdorth E M, Frame D L. Equal survival rates for first, second, and third episodes of *Pneumocystis carinii* pneumonia in patients with acquired immunodeficiency syndrome. *Arch Intern Med* 152:2465–2470, 1992.

Dohn M N, Weinberg W G, Torres R A, Follansbee S E, Caldwell P T, Scott J D, Gathe J C, Haghighat D P, Sampson J H, Spotkov J, Deresinski S C, Meyer R D, Lancaster D J, Frame P T, Mohsenifar Z, Buckley R M, Cheung T, Hyland R, Chan C, Lang W, Mildvan D, Greenberg S B, Craven D, Hirsch M, Elsadr W, Joseph P, Hardy D, Brown N, Rogers M. Oral atovaquone compared with intravenous pentamidine for *Pneumocystis carinii* pneumonia in patients with AIDS. *Ann Intern Med* 121:174–180, 1994.

Dworkin M S, Hanson D L, Kaplan J E, Jones J L, Ward J W. Risk for preventable opportunistic infections in persons with AIDS after antiretroviral therapy increases CD4+ T lymphocyte counts above prophylaxis thresholds. *J Infect Dis* 182:611–615, 2000.

Dworkin M S, Hanson D L, Navin T R. Survival of patients with AIDS, after diagnosis of *Pneumocystis carinii* pneumonia, in the United States. *J Infect Dis* 183:1409–1412, 2001.

Edman J C, Kovacs J A, Masur H, Santi D V, Elwood H J, Sogin M L. Ribosomal RNA sequence shows *Pneumocystis carinii* to be a member of the fungi. *Nature* 334:519–522, 1988.

Edman J C, Edman U, Cao M, Lundgren B, Kovacs J A, Santi D V. Isolation and expression of the *Pneumocystis carinii* dihydrofolate reductase gene. *Proc Natl Acad Sci U S A* 86:8625–8629, 1989.

El-Sadr W M, Murphy R L, Yurik T M, Luskin-Hawk R, Cheung T W, Balfour H H, Jr., Eng R, Hooton T M, Kerkering T M, Schutz M, van der Horst C, Hafner R. Atovaquone compared with dapsone for the prevention of *Pneumocystis carinii* pneumonia in patients with HIV infection who cannot tolerate trimethoprim, sulfonamides, or both. Community Program for Clinical Research on AIDS and the AIDS Clinical Trials Group. *N Engl J Med* 339:1889–1895, 1998.

El-Sadr W M, Luskin-Hawk R, Yurik T M, Walker J, Abrams D, John S L, Sherer R, Crane L, Labriola A, Caras S, Pulling C, Hafner R. A randomized trial of daily and thrice-weekly trimethoprim-sulfamethoxazole for the prevention of *Pneumocystis carinii* pneumonia in human immunodeficiency virus-infected persons. Terry Beirn Community Programs for Clinical Research on AIDS (CPCRA). *Clin Infect Dis* 29:775–783, 1999.

Engelberg L A, Lerner C W, Tapper M L. Clinical features of *Pneumocystis* pneumonia in the acquired immune deficiency syndrome. *Am Rev Respir Dis* 130:689–694, 1984.

Fischer S, Gill V J, Kovacs J, Miele P, Keary J, Silcott V, Huang S, Borio L, Stock F, Fahle G, Brown D, Hahn B, Townley E, Lucey D, Masur H. The use of oral washes to diagnose *Pneumocystis carinii* pneumonia: a blinded prospective study using a polymerase chain reaction-based detection system. *J Infect Dis* 184:1485–1488, 2001.

Fischl M A, Dickinson G M, La Voie L. Safety and efficacy of sulfamethoxazole and trimethoprim chemoprophylaxis for *Pneumocystis carinii* pneumonia in AIDS. *Jama* 259:1185–1189, 1988.

Furrer H, Egger M, Opravil M, Bernasconi E, Hirschel B, Battegay M, Telenti A, Vernazza P L, Rickenbach M, Flepp M, Malinverni R. Discontinuation of primary prophylaxis against *Pneumocystis carinii* pneumonia in HIV-1-infected adults treated with combination antiretroviral therapy. Swiss HIV Cohort Study. *N Engl J Med* 340:1301–1306, 1999.

Furrer H, Opravil M, Rossi M, Bernasconi E, Telenti A, Bucher H, Schiffer V, Boggian K, Rickenbach M, Flepp M, Egger M. Discontinuation of primary prophylaxis in HIV-infected patients at high risk of *Pneumocystis carinii* pneumonia: prospective multicentre study. *AIDS* 15:501–507, 2001.

Gagnon S, Boota A M, Fischl M A, Baier H, Kirksey O W, La Voie L. Corticosteroids as adjunctive therapy for severe *Pneumocystis carinii* pneumonia in the acquired immunodeficiency syndrome. A double-blind, placebo-controlled trial. *N Engl J Med* 323:1444–1450, 1990.

Gill V J, Evans G, Stock F, Parrillo J E, Masur H, Kovacs J A. Detection of *Pneumocystis carinii* by fluorescent-antibody stain using a combination of three monoclonal antibodies. *J Clin Microbiol* 25:1837–1840, 1987.

Girard P M, Landman R, Gaudebout C, Olivares R, Saimot A G, Jelazko P, Certain A, Boue F, Bouvet E, Lecompte T, Coulaud J P. Dapsone pyrimethamine compared with aerosolized pentamidine as primary prophylaxis against *Pneumocystis carinii* pneumonia and toxoplasmosis in Hiv-infection. *N Engl J Med* 328:1514–1520, 1993.

Gluckstein D, Ruskin J. Rapid oral desensitization to trimethoprim-sulfamethoxazole (TMP-SMZ): use in prophylaxis for *Pneumocystis carinii* pneumonia in patients with AIDS who were previously intolerant to TMP-SMZ. *Clin Infect Dis* 20:849–853. 1995.

Gruden J F, Huang L, Turner J, Webb W R, Merrifield C, Stansell J D, Gamsu G, Hopewell P C. High-resolution CT in the evaluation of clinically suspected *Pneumocystis carinii* pneumonia in AIDS patients with normal, equivocal, or nonspecific radiographic findings. *Am J Roentgenol* 169:967–975, 1997.

Gryzan S, Paradis I L, Zeevi A, Duquesnoy R J, Dummer J S, Griffith B P, Hardesty R L, Trento A, Nalesnik M A, Dauber J H. Unexpectedly high incidence of *Pneumocystis carinii* infection after lung-heart transplantation. Implications for lung defense and allograft survival. *Am Rev Respir Dis* 137:1268–1274, 1988.

Hardy W D, Northfelt D W, Drake T A. Fatal, disseminated pneumocystosis in a patient with acquired immunodeficiency syndrome receiving prophylactic aerosolized pentamidine. *Am J Med* 87:329–331, 1989.

Hardy W D, Feinberg J, Finkelstein D M, Power M E, He W, Kaczka C, Frame P T, Holmes M, Waskin H, Fass R J, Powderly W G, Steigbigel R T, Zuger A, Holzman R S. A controlled trial of trimethoprim sulfamethoxazole or aerosolized pentamidine for secondary prophylaxis of *Pneumocystis carinii* pneumonia in patients with the acquired immunodeficiency syndrome—AIDS Clinical Trials Group Protocol 021. *N Engl J Med* 327:1842–1848, 1992.

Helweg-Larsen J, Jensen J S, Benfield T, Svendsen U G, Lundgren J D, Lundgren B. Diagnostic use of PCR for detection of *Pneumocystis carinii* in oral wash samples. *J Clin Microbiol* 36:2068–2072, 1998.

Helweg-Larsen J, Benfield T L, Eugen-Olsen J, Lundgren J D, Lundgren B. Effects of mutations in *Pneumocystis carinii* dihydropteroate synthase gene on outcome of AIDS-associated *P. carinii* pneumonia. *Lancet* 354:1347–1351, 1999.

Henson J W, Jalaj J K, Walker R W, Stover D E, Fels A O. *Pneumocystis carinii* pneumonia in patients with primary brain tumors. *Arch Neurol* 48:406–409, 1991.

Holtzer C D, Flaherty J F, Jr., Coleman R L. Cross-reactivity in HIV-infected patients switched from trimethoprim-sulfamethoxazole to dapsone. *Pharmacotherapy* 18:831–835, 1998.

Huang S N, Fischer S H, O'Shaughnessy E, Gill V J, Masur H, Kovacs J A. Development of a PCR assay for diagnosis of *Pneumocystis carinii* pneumonia based on amplification of the multicopy major surface glycoprotein gene family. *Diagn Microbiol Infect Dis* 35:27–32, 1999.

Huang L, Beard C B, Creasman J, Levy D, Duchin J S, Lee S, Pieniazek N, Carter J L, del Rio C, Rimland D, Navin T R. Sulfa or sulfone prophylaxis and geographic region predict mutations in the *Pneumocystis carinii* dihydropteroate synthase gene. *J Infect Dis* 182:1192–1198, 2000.

Hughes W T, Feldman S, Aur R J, Verzosa M S, Hustu H O, Simone J V. Intensity of immunosuppressive therapy and the incidence of *Pneumocystis carinii* pneumonitis. *Cancer* 36:2004–2009, 1975.

Hughes W T, Kuhn S, Chaudhary S, Feldman S, Verzosa M, Aur R J, Pratt C, George S L. Successful chemoprophylaxis for *Pneumocystis carinii* pneumonitis. *N Engl J Med* 297:1419–1426, 1977.

Hughes W T, Rivera G K, Schell M J, Thornton D, Lott L. Successful intermittent chemoprophylaxis for *Pneumocystis carinii* pneumonitis. *N Engl J Med* 316:1627–1632, 1650, 1987.

Hughes W, Leoung G, Kramer F, Bozzette S A, Safrin S, Frame P, Clumeck N, Masur H, Lancaster D, Chan C, Lavelle J, Rosenstock J, Falloon J, Feinberg J, Lafon S, Rogers M, Sattler F. Comparison of atovaquone (566c80) with trimethoprim-sulfamethoxazole to treat *Pneumocystis carinii* pneumonia in patients with AIDS. *N Engl J Med* 328:1521–1527, 1993.

Ioannidis J P, Cappelleri J C, Skolnik P R, Lau J, Sacks H S. A meta-analysis of the relative efficacy and toxicity of *Pneumocystis carinii* prophylactic regimens. *Arch Intern Med* 156:177–188, 1996.

Kales C P, Murren J R, Torres R A, Crocco J A. Early predictors of in-hospital mortality for *Pneumocystis carinii* pneumonia in the acquired immunodeficiency syndrome. *Arch Intern Med* 147:1413–1417, 1987.

Kaplan J E, Hanson D, Dworkin M S, Frederick T, Bertolli J, Lindegren M L, Holmberg S, Jones J L. Epidemiology of human immunodeficiency virus-associated opportunistic infections in the United States in the era of highly active antiretroviral therapy. *Clin Infect Dis* 30(Suppl 1):S5–S14, 2000.

Kazanjian P, Locke A B, Hossler P A, Lane B R, Bartlett M S, Smith J W, Cannon M, Meshnick S R. *Pneumocystis carinii* mutations associated with sulfa and sulfone prophylaxis failures in AIDS patients. *AIDS* 12:873–878, 1998.

Kazanjian P, Armstrong W, Hossler P A, Burman W, Richardson J, Lee C H, Crane L, Katz J, Meshnick S R. *Pneumocystis carinii* mutations are associated with duration of sulfa or sulfone prophylaxis exposure in AIDS patients. *J Infect Dis* 182:551–557, 2000.

Kelly J W, Dooley D P, Lattuada C P, Smith C E. A severe, unusual reaction to trimethoprim-sulfamethoxazole in patients infected with human immunodeficiency virus. *Clin Infect Dis* 14:1034–1039, 1992.

Kirsch C M, Jensen W A, Kagawa F T, Azzi R L. Analysis of induced sputum for the diagnosis of recurrent *Pneumocystis carinii* pneumonia. *Chest* 102:1152–1154, 1992.

Kovacs J A, Hiemenz J W, Macher A M, Stover D, Murray H W, Shelhamer J, Lane H C, Urmacher C, Honig C, Longo D L, Parker M M, Natanson C, Parrillo J E, Fauci A S, Pizzo P A, Masur H. *Pneumocystis carinii* pneumonia—a comparison between patients with the acquired immunodeficiency syndrome and patients with other immunodeficiencies. *Ann Intern Med* 100:663–671, 1984.

Kovacs J A, Halpern J L, Swan J C, Moss J, Parrillo J E, Masur H. Identification of antigens and antibodies specific for *Pneumocystis carinii*. *J Immunol* 140:2023–2031, 1988a.

Kovacs J A, Ng V L, Masur H, Leoung G, Hadley W K, Evans G, Lane H C, Ognibene F P, Shelhamer J, Parrillo J E, Gill V J. Diagnosis of *Pneumocystis carinii* pneumonia—improved detection in sputum with use of monoclonal antibodies. *N Engl J Med* 318:589–593, 1988b.

Kovacs J A, Halpern J L, Lundgren B, Swan J C, Parrillo J E, Masur H. Monoclonal antibodies to *Pneumocystis carinii*: identification of specific antigens and characterization of antigenic differences between rat and human isolates. *J Infect Dis* 159:60–70, 1989.

Kovacs J A, Masur H. Prophylaxis for *Pneumocystis carinii* pneumonia in patients infected with human immunodeficiency virus. *Clin Infect Dis* 14:1005–1009, 1992.

Lane B R, Ast J C, Hossler P A, Mindell D P, Bartlett M S, Smith J W, Meshnick S R. Dihydropteroate synthase polymorphisms in *Pneumocystis carinii*. *J Infect Dis* 175:482–485, 1997.

Larsen H H, Masur H, Kovacs J A, Gill V J, Silcott V A, Kogulan P, Maenza J, Smith M, Lucey D R, Fischer S H. Development and evaluation of a quantitative, touch-down, real-time PCR assay for diagnosing *Pneumocystis carinii* pneumonia. *J Clin Microbiol* 40:490–494, 2002.

Lavelle J P, Falloon J, Morgan A, Graziani A, Arakaki D, Byrne A, Pierce P, Masur H, MacGregor R. Weekly dapsone and dapsone/pyrimethamine for *Pneumocystis* pneumonia prophylaxis, VII International Conference on AIDS, Florence, 1991.

Ledergerber B, Mocroft A, Reiss P, Furrer H, Kirk O, Bickel M, Uberti-Foppa C, Pradier C, D'Arminio Monforte A, Schneider M M, Lundgren J D. Discontinuation of secondary prophylaxis against *Pneumocystis carinii* pneumonia in patients with HIV infection who have a response to antiretroviral therapy. Eight European Study Groups. *N Engl J Med* 344:168–174, 2001.

Leigh T R, Kangro H O, Gazzard B G, Jeffries D J, Collins J V. DNA amplification by the polymerase chain reaction to detect subclinical *Pneumocystis carinii* colonization in HIV-positive and HIV-negative male homosexuals with and without respiratory symptoms. *Respir Med* 87:525–529, 1993.

Leoung G S, Mills J, Hopewell P C, Hughes W, Wofsy C. Dapsone-trimethoprim for *Pneumocystis carinii* pneumonia in the acquired immunodeficiency syndrome. *Ann Intern Med* 105:45–48, 1986.

Leoung G S, Feigal D W, Montgomery A B, Corkery K, Wardlaw L, Adams M, Busch D, Gordon S, Jacobson M A, Volberding P A, Abrams D. Aerosolized pentamidine for prophylaxis against *Pneumocystis carinii* pneumonia—the San-Francisco Community Prophylaxis Trial. *N Engl J Med* 323:769–775, 1990.

Leoung G S, Stanford J F, Giordano M F, Stein A, Torres R A, Giffen C A, Wesley M, Sarracco T, Cooper E C, Dratter V, Smith J J, Frost K R. Trimethoprim-sulfamethoxazole (TMP-SMZ) dose escalation versus direct rechallenge for *Pneumocystis carinii* pneumonia prophylaxis in human immunodeficiency virus-infected patients with previous adverse reaction to TMP-SMZ. *J Infect Dis* 184:992–997, 2001.

Lipschik G Y, Gill V J, Lundgren J D, Andrawis V A, Nelson N A, Nielsen J O, Ognibene F P, Kovacs J A. Improved diagnosis of *Pneumocystis carinii* infection by polymerase chain reaction on induced sputum and blood. *Lancet* 340:203–206, 1992.

Lu J J, Chen C H, Bartlett M S, Smith J W, Lee C H. Comparison of six different PCR methods for detection of *Pneumocystis carinii*. *J Clin Microbiol* 33:2785–2788, 1995.

Lyles R H, Munoz A, Yamashita T E, Bazmi H, Detels R, Rinaldo C R, Margolick J B, Phair J P, Mellors J W. Natural history of human immunodeficiency virus type 1 viremia after seroconversion and proximal to AIDS in a large cohort of homosexual men. Multicenter AIDS Cohort Study. *J Infect Dis* 181:872–880, 2000.

Martin G J, Paparello S F, Decker C F. A severe systemic reaction to trimethoprim-sulfamethoxazole in a patient infected with the human immunodeficiency virus. *Clin Infect Dis* 16:175–176, 1993.

Masur H, Ognibene F P, Yarchoan R, Shelhamer J H, Baird B F, Travis W, Suffredini A F, Deyton L, Kovacs J A, Falloon J, Davey R, Polis M, Metcalf J, Baseler M, Wesley R, Gill V J, Fauci A S, Lane H C. CD4 counts as predictors of opportunistic pneumonias in human immunodeficiency virus (HIV) infection. *Ann Intern Med* 111:223–231, 1989.

Masur H. Prevention and treatment of *pneumocystis* pneumonia. *N Engl J Med* 327:1853–1860, 1992.

Masur H, Kaplan J E, Holmes K K. Recommendations of the U.S. Public Health Service and the Infectious Diseases Society of America. Guidelines for preventing opportunistic infections among HIV-infected persons—2002. *Ann Intern Med* 137:435–477, 2002.

Medina I, Mills J, Leoung G, Hopewell P C, Lee B, Modin G, Benowitz N, Wofsy C B. Oral therapy for *Pneumocystis carinii* pneumonia in the acquired immunodeficiency syndrome. A controlled trial of trimethoprim-sulfamethoxazole versus trimethoprim-dapsone. *N Engl J Med* 323:776–782, 1990.

Meduri G U, Stover D E, Greeno R A, Nash T, Zaman M B. Bilateral bronchoalveolar lavage in the diagnosis of opportunistic pulmonary infections. *Chest* 100:1272–1276, 1991.

Mei Q, Gurunathan S, Masur H, Kovacs J A. Failure of co-trimoxazole in *Pneumocystis carinii* infection and mutations in dihydropteroate synthase gene. *Lancet* 351:1631–1632, 1998.

Miller V, Mocroft A, Reiss P, Katlama C, Papadopoulos A I, Katzenstein T, van Lunzen J, Antunes F, Phillips A N, Lundgren J D. Relations among CD4 lymphocyte count nadir, antiretroviral therapy, and HIV-1 disease progression: results from the EuroSIDA study. *Ann Intern Med* 130:570–577, 1999.

Mills J, Leoung G, Medina I, Hopewell P C, Hughes W T, Wofsy C. Dapsone treatment of *Pneumocystis carinii* pneumonia in the acquired immunodeficiency syndrome. *Antimicrob Agents Chemother* 32:1057–1060, 1988.

Montaner J S G, Lawson L M, Gervais A, Hyland R H, Chan C K, Falutz J M, Renzi P M, Macfadden D, Rachlis A R, Fong I W, Garber G E, Simor A, Gilmore N, Fanning M, Taylor G D, Martel A Y, Schlech W F, Schechter M T. Aerosol pentamidine for secondary prophylaxis of AIDS-related *Pneumocystis carinii* pneumonia—a randomized, placebo-controlled study. *Ann Intern Med* 114:948–953, 1991.

Murphy R L, Lavelle J P, Allan J D, Gordin F M, Dupliss R, Boswell S L, Waskin H A, Davies S F, Graziano F M, Saag M S, Walter J B, Crane L R, Macdonell K B, Hodges T L, Pierce P F. Aerosol pentamidine prophylaxis following *Pneumocystis carinii* pneumonia in AIDS patients—results of a blinded dose comparison study using an ultrasonic nebulizer. *Amer J Med* 90:418–426, 1991.

Navin T R, Beard C B, Huang L, del Rio C, Lee S, Pieniazek N J, Carter J L, Le T, Hightower A, Rimland D. Effect of mutations in *Pneumocystis carinii* dihydropteroate synthase gene on outcome of *P. carinii* pneumonia in patients with HIV-1: a prospective study. *Lancet* 358:545–549, 2001.

Ng V L, Virani N A, Chaisson R E, Yajko D M, Sphar H T, Cabrian K, Rollins N, Charache P, Krieger M, Hadley W K, Hopewell

P C. Rapid detection of *Pneumocystis carinii* using a direct fluorescent monoclonal-antibody stain. *J Clin Microbiol* 28:2228–2233, 1990.

Noskin G A, Murphy R L, Black J R, Phair J P. Salvage therapy with clindamycin/primaquine for *Pneumocystis carinii* pneumonia. *Clin Infect Dis* 14:183–188, 1992.

Olsson M, Elvin K, Lofdahl S, Linder E. Detection of *Pneumocystis carinii* DNA in sputum and bronchoalveolar lavage samples by polymerase chain reaction. *J Clin Microbiol* 31:221–6, 1993.

Opravil M, Hirschel B, Lazzarin A, Heald A, Pechere M, Ruttimann S, Iten A, Vonoverbeck J, Oertle D, Praz G, Vuitton A, Mainini F, Luthy R. Once-weekly administration of dapsone pyrimethamine vs aerosolized pentamidine as combined prophylaxis for *Pneumocystis carinii* pneumonia and toxoplasmic encephalitis in human immunodeficiency virus-infected patients. *Clin Infect Dis* 20:531–541,1995.

Para M F, Finkelstein D, Becker S, Dohn M, Walawander A, Black J R. Reduced toxicity with gradual initiation of trimethoprim-sulfamethoxazole as primary prophylaxis for *Pneumocystis carinii* pneumonia: AIDS Clinical Trials Group 268. *J Acquir Immune Defic Syndr* 24:337–343, 2000.

Pareja JG, Garland R, Koziel H. Use of adjunctive corticosteroids in severe adult non-HIV *Pneumocystis carinii* pneumonia. *Chest* 113:1215–1224, 1998.

Peglow S L, Smulian A G, Linke M J, Pogue C L, Nurre S, Crisler J, Phair J, Gold J W, Armstrong D, Walzer P D. Serologic responses to *Pneumocystis carinii* antigens in health and disease. *J Infect Dis*; 161:296–306, 1990.

Peters S G, Prakash U B. *Pneumocystis carinii* pneumonia. Review of 53 cases. *Am J Med* 82:73–78, 1987.

Phair J, Munoz A, Detels R, Kaslow R, Rinaldo C, Saah A. The risk of *Pneumocystis carinii* pneumonia among men infected with human immunodeficiency virus type 1. Multicenter AIDS Cohort Study Group. *N Engl J Med* 322:161–165, 1990.

Pifer L L, Hughes W T, Stagno S, Woods D. *Pneumocystis carinii* infection: evidence for high prevalence in normal and immunosuppressed children. *Pediatrics* 61:35–41, 1978.

Pitchenik A E, Ganjei P, Torres A, Evans D A, Rubin E, Baier H. Sputum examination for the diagnosis of *Pneumocystis carinii* pneumonia in the acquired immunodeficiency syndrome. *Am Rev Respir Dis* 133:226–229,1986.

Podzamczer D, Salazar A, Jimenez J, Consiglio E, Santin M, Casanova A, Rufi G, Gudiol F. Intermittent trimethoprim-sulfamethoxazole compared with dapsone-pyrimethamine for the simultaneous primary prophylaxis of *Pneumocystis* pneumonia and toxoplasmosis in patients infected with HIV. *Ann Intern Med* 122:755–761, 1995.

Raviglione M C. Extrapulmonary pneumocystosis: The first 50 cases. *Rev Infect Dis* 12:1127–1138, 1990.

Roths J B, Sidman C L. Single and combined humoral and cell-mediated immunotherapy of *Pneumocystis carinii* pneumonia in immunodeficient SCID mice. *Infect Immun* 61:1641–1649, 1993.

Rubin R H, Iwamoto G K, Richerson H B, Flaherty J P. Trimethoprim-sulfamethoxazole desensitization in the acquired immunodeficiency syndrome [letter]. *Ann Intern Med* 16:355, 1987.

Ruf B, Rohde I, Pohle H D. Efficacy of clindamycin/primaquine versus trimethoprim/sulfamethoxazole in primary treatment of *Pneumocystis carinii* pneumonia. *Eur J Clin Microbiol Infect Dis* 10:207–210, 1991.

Saah A J, Hoover D R, Peng Y, Phair J P, Visscher B, Kingsley LA, Schrager LK. Predictors for failure of *Pneumocystis carinii* pneumonia prophylaxis. Multicenter AIDS Cohort Study. *Jama* 273:1197–1202, 1995.

Safrin S, Sattler F R, Lee B L, Young T, Bill R, Boylan C T, Mills J. Dapsone as a single agent is suboptimal therapy for *Pneumocystis carinii* pneumonia. *J Acquir Immune Defic Syndr* 4:244–249, 1991.

Safrin S, Finkelstein D M, Feinberg J, Frame P, Simpson G, Wu A, Cheung T, Soeiro R, Hojczyk P, Black J R. Comparison of three regimens for treatment of mild to moderate *Pneumocystis carinii* pneumonia in patients with AIDS. A double-blind, randomized, trial of oral trimethoprim-sulfamethoxazole, dapsone-trimethoprim, and clindamycin-primaquine. ACTG 108 Study Group. *Ann Intern Med* 124:792–802, 1996.

Sandhu G S, Kline B C, Espy M J, Stockman L, Smith T F, Limper A H. Laboratory diagnosis of *Pneumocystis carinii* infections by PCR directed to genes encoding for mitochondrial 5S and 28S ribosomal RNA. *Diagn Microbiol Infect Dis* 33:157–162, 1999.

Sattler F R, Cowan R, Nielsen D M, Ruskin J. Trimethoprim-sulfamethoxazole compared with pentamidine for treatment of *Pneumocystis carinii* pneumonia in the acquired immunodeficiency syndrome. A prospective, noncrossover study. *Ann Intern Med* 109:280–287, 1988.

Sattler F R, Frame P, Davis R, Nichols L, Shelton B, Akil B, Baughman R, Hughlett C, Weiss W, Boylen C T, Vanderhorst C, Black J, Powderly W, Steigbigel R T, Leedom J M, Masur H, Feinberg J, Benoit S, Eyster E, Gocke D, Beck K, Lederman M, Phair J, Reichman R, Sacks HS, Soiero R. Trimetrexate with leucovorin versus trimethoprim-sulfamethoxazole for moderate to severe episodes of *Pneumocystis carinii* pneumonia in patients with AIDS—a prospective, controlled multicenter investigation of the AIDS Clinical Trials Group Protocol-029/031. *J Infect Dis* 170:165–172, 1994.

Schneider M M, Hoepelman A I, Eeftinck Schattenkerk J K, Nielsen T L, van der Graaf Y, Frissen J P, van der Ende I M, Kolsters A F, Borleffs J C. A controlled trial of aerosolized pentamidine or trimethoprim-sulfamethoxazole as primary prophylaxis against *Pneumocystis carinii* pneumonia in patients with human immunodeficiency virus infection. The Dutch AIDS Treatment Group. *N Engl J Med* 327:1836–1841, 1992.

Sepkowitz K A, Brown A E, Telzak E E, Gottlieb S, Armstrong D. *Pneumocystis carinii* pneumonia among patients without AIDS at a cancer hospital. *JAMA* 267:832–837, 1992.

Shelhamer J H, Ognibene F P, Macher A M, Tuazon C, Steiss R, Longo D, Kovacs J A, Parker M M, Natanson C, Lane H C, Fauci A S, Parrillo J E, Masur H. Persistence of *Pneumocystis carinii* in lung tissue of acquired immunodeficiency syndrome patients treated for *Pneumocystis* pneumonia. *Am Rev Resp Dis* 130:1161–1165, 1984.

Sing A, Trebesius K, Roggenkamp A, Russmann H, Tybus K, Pfaff F, Bogner J R, Emminger C, Heesemann J. Evaluation of diagnostic value and epidemiological implications of PCR for *Pneumocystis carinii* in different immunosuppressed and immunocompetent patient groups. *J Clin Microbiol* 38:1461–1467, 2000.

Stringer S L, Hudson K, Blase M A, Walzer P D, Cushion M T, Stringer J R. Sequence from ribosomal RNA of *Pneumocystis carinii* compared to those of four fungi suggests an ascomycetous affinity. *J Protozool* 36:14S-16S, 1989.

Sugimoto H, Uchida H, Akiyama N, Nagao T, Tomikawa S, Mita K, Beck Y, Inoue S, Watanabe K, Nakayama Y, Sato K, Otsubo O. Improved survival of renal-allograft recipients with *Pneumocystis carinii* pneumonia by early diagnosis and treatment. *Transplantation Proceedings* 24:1556–1558, 1992.

Telzak E E, Cote R J, Gold J W M, Campbell S W, Armstrong D. Extrapulmonary *Pneumocystis carinii* infections. *Rev Infect Dis* 12:380–386, 1990.

The National Institutes of Health—University of California Expert Panel for Corticosteroids as Adjunctive Therapy for *Pneumocystis* Pneumonia. Consensus statement on the use of corticosteroids as adjunctive therapy for *Pneumocystis* pneumonia in the acquired immunodeficiency syndrome. *N Engl J Med* 323:1500–1504, 1990.

Toma E, Fournier S, Dumont M, Bolduc P, Deschamps H. Clindamycin/primaquine versus trimethoprim—sulfamethoxazole as primary therapy for *Pneumocystis carinii* pneumonia in AIDS: a randomized, double-blind pilot trial. *Clin Infect Dis* 17: 178–184, 1993.

Tuan I Z, Dennison D, Weisdorf D J. *Pneumocystis carinii* pneumonitis following bone marrow transplantation. *Bone Marr Transplant* 10:267–272, 1992.

Volpe F, Ballantine S P, Delves C J. The multifunctional folic acid synthesis fas gene of *Pneumocystis carinii* encodes dihydroneopterin aldolase, hydroxymethyldihydropterin pyrophosphokinase and dihydropteroate synthase. *Eur J Biochem*; 216:449–458, 1993.

Wakefield A E, Pixley F J, Banerji S, Sinclair K, Miller R F, Moxon E R, Hopkin J M. Amplification of mitochondrial ribosomal RNA sequences from *Pneumocystis carinii* DNA of rat and human origin. *Mol Biochem* Parasitol 43:69–76, 1990.

Winston D J. Prophylaxis and treatment of infection in the bone marrow transplant recipient. *Curr Clin Top Infect Dis* 13:293–321, 1993.

28

Miscellaneous Fungi

JOHN W. BADDLEY AND WILLIAM E. DISMUKES

Over the past decade, rare and unusual fungi, often common soil saprophytes, have been increasingly reported as causing invasive infections in humans. Possible reasons for an increased frequency of unusual fungal infections include increasing numbers of patients with immunosuppression, and increases in environmental exposures. This chapter focuses on unusual and rare yeast and mould organisms and their disease manifestations. Lobomycosis, a chronic skin infection caused by the yeast-like organism *Lacazia loboi*, is described, followed by infections due to basidiomycetes, and *Emmonsia parva*, the agent of adiaspiromycosis. Finally, rhinosporidiosis is discussed, although recent evidence indicates that the causative agent, *Rhinosporidium seeberi*, should no longer be classified as a fungus.

INFECTIONS DUE TO YEAST-LIKE ORGNAISMS

Lobomycosis

Lobomycosis is a chronic skin infection characterized by nodules, plaques, and verrucoid or ulcerated lesions. The agent of lobomycosis, now referred to as *Lacazia loboi* (Taborda et al, 1999), is a yeast-like organism in tissues, and is primarily a human pathogen. Dolphins (*Tursiops truncatus* and *Sotalia fluviatilis*) are the only nonhuman hosts that acquire natural infection (Migaki et al, 1971; Dudok van Heel, 1977; Cowan, 1993). Lobomycosis occurs in tropical and subtropical forests, and has been reported in South, Central, and North America, and in Europe (Rodriquez-Toro, 1993). The majority of cases are from the Brazilian and Colombian Amazonian regions; only recently has a case from the United States been described (Burns et al, 2000).

The natural habitat of *L. loboi* is unknown, and is difficult to investigate because the organism has never been isolated and cultured in vitro. Most infections occur on the skin in areas exposed to trauma, suggesting that the organism is present in soil or on vegetation (Rodriquez-Toro, 1993). An aquatic source is also likely, based on reported infections among dolphins (Migaki et al, 1971; Dudok van Heel, 1977; Cowan, 1993).

Lobomycosis was reported initially in 1930 by the dermatologist Jorge Lobo (Lobo, 1931), who described a native of the Amazon Valley who had numerous plaques and nodules in the lumbo-sacral region. His disease had slowly progressed for 19 years. Based on clinical and histologic findings of the case, Lobo believed that the etiologic fungus was similar to *Paracoccidioides brasiliensis*, and referred to the infection as keloidal blastomycosis.

Since the initial description of lobomycosis, greater than 300 human cases have been confirmed (Fuchs et al, 1990; Rodriguez-Toro, 1993). Lesions occur on cool, exposed areas such as the feet, legs, ears, arms, elbows, and less frequently the face. Lesions can be localized or disseminated throughout the skin, resulting from contiguous extension, autoinoculation, or lymphatic spread. A single case has been described which suggests visceral involvement (Monteiro-Gei, 1971). A patient with lobomycosis of the leg and knee for 47 years was found to have a presumed testicular tumor; however histopathology results showed granulomas with giant cells, and fungi consistent with lobomycosis.

Lobomycosis usually begins as a well-circumscribed, indurated papule, and as the cutaneous disease progresses, the lesions enlarge and new lesions appear. Nodular lesions are most frequent, although macules, papules, plaques, ulcers, and verrucous lesions may be present (See Color Fig. 28–1 in separate color insert) (Rodriques-Toro, 1993). Generally, the disease is insidious, and may progess over a period of 50 or more years (Pradinaud, 1998).

Diagnosis of lobomycosis is based on clinical features of the skin lesions and histologic examination with special stains of tissues; the organism has not yet been cultured in vitro. Microscopically, the dermis contains granulomas with foamy macrophages and multinucleated giant cells, without the presence of necrosis. Both macrophages and giant cells may ingest the fungi (Kwon-Chung and Bennett, 1992; Rodriguez-Toro, 1993). The fungus, between 5 and 12 μm in diameter, is yeast-like, lemon-shaped, and forms beads joined together by thin bridges (See Color Fig. 28–2 in separate color insert). Cells with multiple budding forms are seen frequently, and may resemble budding seen with

Paracoccidioides brasiliensis (Kwon-Chung and Bennett, 1992).

Therapy of lobomycosis is difficult, and treatment with amphotericin B, ketoconazole, trimethoprim, and flucytosine has been tried but is often of little benefit (Lawrence and Ajello, 1986; Caceres and Rodriguez-Toro, 1991). Miconazole is reported to have cured the lesions of a dolphin (Dudok van Heel, 1977). For small skin lesions, cryosurgery or electrosurgery may be curative. Clofazamine has been used with some success in addition to surgery (Talhari, 1981; Burns et al, 2000). For early lesions, surgical removal may be effective (Baruzzi et al, 1981), but in chronic cases relapse after surgery is frequent (Baruzzi et al, 1979; Caceres and Rodriguez-Toro, 1991).

INFECTIONS DUE TO MISCELLANEOUS MOULDS

Basidiomycosis

The basidiomycetes, comprising mushrooms and toadstools, are distributed widely in nature, with over 16,000 recognized species (Hawksworth et al, 1983). Basidiomycetes are common plant pathogens or soil saprophytes, but rarely cause invasive disease in humans (Greer, 1978). Although basidiomycetes are increasingly recognized as pathogens, their identification is problematic (Sigler and Abbott, 1997a). On examination of infected tissues, septate, hyaline hyphae are seen, and may be confused with those of *Aspergillus* species (Sigler et al, 1999). Frequently, cultures of tissue specimens show initial hyphal growth but are difficult to identify to the genus or species level (Sigler and Abbott, 1997a). Among basidiomycetes causing human infection, the most recognized species is *Filobasidella neoformans*, the teleomorph (sexual state) of *Cryptococcus neoformans*. Less common, but emerging, pathogens include *Schizophyllum commune*, *Coprinus* species, *Hormographiella aspergillata*, and *Ustilago* species.

Few cases of confirmed invasive infection due to basidiomyctes, other than those of *Filobasidella neoformans*, exist in the literature, but cases and identification of isolates as basidiomycetes appear to be increasing (Rihs et al, 1996). *Schizophyllum commune*, one of the more common pathogens, has been reported as causing a palatal ulcer that was treated successfully with amphotericin B (Restrepo et al, 1973). Other reports include several cases of invasive or allergic sinusitis (Kern and Uecker, 1986; Catalano et al, 1990; Rosenthal et al, 1992; Clark et al, 1996; Sigler et al, 1997b; Sigler et al. 1999), and a case of allergic bronchopulmonary mycosis (Kamei et al, 1994). Recently, a case of *S. commune* causing pulmonary disease and brain abscess was described in a patient receiving corticos-

teroid therapy for presumptive lymphoma (Rihs et al, 1996). The patient improved with amphotericin B and itraconazole, but later died of bacterial pneumonia and sepsis. *Coprinus cinereus* was the caustive agent in a well-documented case of aortic valve endocarditis (Speller and MacIver, 1971). No obvious source of infection was identified. Aortic valve tissue grew *C. cinereus*, but the patient died during valve replacement surgery and was not treated. A case of necrotizing bronchopneumonia in a leukemic patient was attributed to *Hormographiella aspergillata*, the anamorph of *C. cinereus* (Verweij et al, 1997). The patient failed to respond to therapy with amphotericin B and itraconazole, and died of respiratory failure. *Ustilago* species have been implicated as the cause of skin infection and a brain lesion (Greer, 1978); however, in neither case was identification confirmed with culture.

The ideal treatment for basidiomycete infections is unknown, and the paucity of cases does not allow for comparisons of outcomes with different antifungal agents. Amphotericin B has been effective in several cases, either as single therapy, or in combination with itraconazole (Greer and Bolanos, 1973; Restrepo et al, 1973; Rihs et al, 1996). Azole agents, particularly itraconazole and fluconazole, as single therapy have achieved mixed results (Marlier et al, 1993; Kamei et al, 1994). In four cases of sinusitis, surgical therapy alone was curative (Kern and Uecker, 1986; Catalano et al, 1990; Rosenthal et al, 1992). Recently, susceptibility data have been reported for approved and investigational antifungal drugs against a large number of basidiomycetes, several of which caused invasive infection (Gonzalez et al, 2001). For the species tested, 96-hour MICs for amphotericin B, itraconazole, voriconazole, and posaconazole were low (0.125–1 mcg/ml), whereas the MICs were somewhat higher for 5-flucytosine and fluconazole. Correlation between in vitro data and clinical efficacy is as yet unknown, but may become important as basidiomycete infections appear to be emerging.

Adiaspiromycosis

Adiaspiromycosis is an unusual pulmonary mycosis that affects man and animals, but is most common in rodents. Infection occurs after inhalation of dust-borne conidia of the mould *Emmonsia parva* (recently named *Chrysosporium parvum*). Two varieties of this organism have been shown to be pathogens: *E. parva* var. *crescens* causes disease in man and animals, and *E. parva* var. *parva* causes disease only in animals.

Adiaspiromycosis is a unique mycosis because the inhaled conidia enlarge but do not germinate or reproduce in the host tissues. The conidia form adiaspores, which resemble spherules, in tissue. Adiaspiromycosis is diagnosed by the characteristic finding of adiaspores, ranging in size from 50 to 500 μm, surrounded by granulomatous inflammation in tissue (See Color Fig. 28–3 in separate color insert).

The first human case of adiaspiromycosis, in which an adiaspore was found incidentally in a lung nodule from a patient with aspergillosis, was described in France (Doby-Dubois et al, 1964). Since the initial description, more than 40 human cases have been reported worldwide (England and Hochholzer, 1993). Pulmonary disease is most common, although adiaspiromycosis involving other organs, including peritoneum, skin, and bone, has been described (Kamalam and Thambiah, 1979; Echavarria et al, 1993; Turner et al, 1999).

A recent review describes the common features of infection in 11 cases of pulmonary adiaspiromycosis (England and Hochholzer, 1993). Lung infection can be localized (few adiaspores limited to a segment or lobe of lung), or disseminated (bilateral disease with multiple adiaspores). Because the inhaled conidia do not multiply but only enlarge in tissues, severity of disease and extent of infection may be related to the initial inoculum of inhaled conidia (Peres et al, 1992; England and Hochholzer, 1993).

In patients with localized lung disease, adiaspiromycosis is often an incidental finding in asymptomatic patients. In patients with disseminated lung disease, cough, dyspnea, asthenia, and fever are more frequently seen (Filho et al, 1990; England and Hochholzer, 1993). Physical examination is often normal, but may reveal basilar crackles on auscultation. In patients with disseminated disease, radiographic studies may reveal a reticulonodular pattern similar to that seen with miliary tuberculosis (England and Hochholzer, 1993).

Diagnosis of adiaspiromycosis is based on histopathologic examination of lung tissue. Culture of the organism is difficult, and sputum or bronchoalveolar lavage specimens are rarely culture positive in patients with disease (Filho et al, 1990; Turner et al, 1999). On gross examination of lung tissue, nodules, usually white to various shades of gray, can be seen. On microscopic exam, adiaspores (spherules) are found within the nodules (See Color Fig. 28–3 in separate color insert). In some instances the spherules may be confused with parasites such as *Dirofilaria* or *Strongyloides*, but can be easily distinguished from the characteristic spherules of *Coccidioides immitis*, which contain numerous endospores (Baird et al, 1988; Nicholson et al, 1992; England and Hochholzer, 1993).

Adiaspiromycosis often regresses and patients improve without any therapy. In contrast, a few patients have progressive disease that may contribute to fatal outcome (Peres et al, 1992; England and Hochholzer, 1993). Given the small number of reported cases of adiaspiromycosis, the utility of antifungal treatment in altering disease course is unknown. However, patients have improved when treated with various antimicrobial agents, including amphotericin B plus flucytosine, ketoconazole, and thiabendazole (Severo et al, 1989; Filho et al, 1990; Echavarria et al, 1993; Turner et al, 1999). In the rare cases of clinical progression, persistence of disease, or involvement of organs other than lung, surgical intervention may be required for cure (England and Hochholzer, 1993).

Rhinosporidiosis

Rhinosporidiosis is a chronic granulomatous infection of the mucous membranes characterized by the formation of friable, polypoid masses that most often involve the nose, nasopharynx, or conjunctiva. The etiologic agent is *Rhinosporidium seeberi*, which has traditionally been regarded as a fungus on the basis of morphologic and histochemical characteristics. Although recent evidence suggests that the organism may be a protistan parasite (Herr et al, 1999; Fredricks et al, 2000), rhinosporidiosis is considered here. Animal infections have occurred, as evidenced by a recent description of rhinosporidiosis in a domestic cat (Wallin et al, 2001). Rhinosporidiosis has a worldwide distribution, but most of the reported cases have occurred in India or Sri Lanka (Amesur, 1949; Karunaratne, 1964). Other geographic regions with a significant number of reported cases include areas of South America and Africa (Owor and Wamucota, 1978).

The first description of rhinosporidiosis was by Malbran in 1892, after examination of a nasal polyp revealed infection by a parasite. In 1900, Guillermo Seeber, for whom the organism is named, described the causative organism in a nasal polyp (Seeber, 1900). Since the initial description, approximately 2000 cases of rhinosporidiosis have been reported worldwide. Disease favors a male predominance (4:1), and usually affects those between 15 and 40 years of age. Nasal infection is twice as common as ocular infection (Karunaratne, 1964).

The precise mode of transmission of rhinosporidiosis is unknown, but trauma of the mucous membranes is probably necessary for most infections to occur (Ashworth, 1923). Increased prevalence of disease has been found among sand workers and divers (Noronha, 1933; Mandlick, 1937); moreover, in Sri Lanka, many cases involve rice paddy farmers, suggesting that water may transmit the organism. In dry areas, infections appear to increase after dust storms, which suggest that soil may also be a source of *R. seeberi* (Kaye, 1938).

Rhinosporidiosis typically involves the mucous membranes, with formation of red or purple pedunculated, polypoid masses. Lesions may range in size from small, discrete nodules, to extensive, lobulated masses. Lesions are friable, irregular, and frequently bleed. White dots are found on the outside of the lesions, which may give a strawberry-like appearance. The nasal mucosa is most frequently affected, but infection may also involve the nasopharynx, ocular tissue, urethra, and skin (Mahakrisnan et al, 1981; Sasidharan et al, 1987; van der Coer et al, 1992; Shrestha et al, 1998). Disseminated disease is rare (Agrawal and Sharma, 1959; Mahakrisnan et al, 1981). Patients with nasal mucosal involvement typically present with nasal obstruction or epistaxis. These symptoms may be accompanied by nasal drainage and pruritus, but seldom is there nasal pain. Ocular infection usually presents with tearing, bleeding, or foreign-body sensation (Roberson et al, 1985). The palpebral conjunctiva is most commonly affected, followed by the bulbar conjunctiva, corneal limbus, and lacrimal sac (Karunaratne, 1964).

Rhinosporidium seeberi has not been successfully cultured in the laboratory on fungal media, so the diagnosis of rhinosporidiosis is based on typical clinical features and histologic examination with special stains. Diagnosis of rhinosporidiosis can be made on histopathologic analysis of the excised lesion, but it can also be made after microspcopic analysis of nasal drainage (Fortin and Meisels, 1974; Chaudhary and Joshi, 1986). Examination of tissue reveals a variety of inflammatory cells including neutrophils, multinucleated giant cells, plasma cells, and lymphocytes. Vascularity of the tissue is prominent. On the epithelial surface of the lesion and in the submucosa, numerous sporangia are seen, ranging up to 300 μm in diameter (See Color Fig. 28–4 in separate color insert). Fungal stains, such as Gomori-methenamine silver, and periodic acid-Schiff, are useful to highlight the walls of the sporangia and small internal spores.

The best therapy for rhinosporidiosis is surgical excision of the lesions. Electrosurgery has been successful in many cases; however, recurrence of the lesions is not uncommon (Satyanarayana, 1960). Response to oral medications such as dapsone, amphotericin B, and griseofulvin is reported, although the effectiveness of medical therapy is unknown (Nair, 1979; Job et al, 1993).

REFERENCES

Agrawal S, Sharma K D. Generalized rhinosporidiosis with visceral involvement: report of a case. *Arch Dermatol* 80:22–26, 1959.

Amesur C A. Discussion on antibiotics and chemotherapy in the treatment of nasal sinusitis and its complications. In: Proceedings of the 40th International Congress of Otolaryngology. London, pp. 1–24, 1949.

Ashworth J H. On *Rhinosporidium seeberi* (Wernicke, 1903) with special reference to its sporulation and affinities. *Trans R Soc Edinburgh* 53:302–342, 1923.

Baird J K, Neafie R C, Connor D H. Parasitic infections. In: Dail D H, Hammar S P, eds. *Pulmonary Pathology*. New York: Springer-Verlag, 315–357, 1988.

Baruzzi R G, Lacaz de S, Souza P A A. Historia natural da doença de Jorge Lobo. Ocurrencia entre os indios Caiabi (Brasil Central). *Rev Inst Trop Med S Paulo* 21:302–338, 1979.

Baruzzi R G, Marcopito L F, Michalany N S, Livianu J, Pinto N R. Early diagnosis and prompt treatment by surgery in Jorge Lobo's disease (keloidal blastomycosis). *Mycopathol* 74:51–54, 1981.

Burns R A, Roy J S, Woods C, Padhye A A, Warnock D W. Report of the first human case of lobomycosis in the United States. *J Clin Microbiol* 38:1283–1285, 2000.

Cáceres S, Rodríquez-Toro G, Lobomicosis de 35 años de evolución. *Rev Soc Col Dermatol* 1:43–45, 1991.

Catalano P, Lawson W, Bottone E, Lebenger J. Basidiomycetous (mushroom) infection of the maxillary sinus. *Otolaryngol Head Neck Surg* 102:183–185, 1990.

Chaudhary S K, Joshi K R. Diagnosis of rhinosporidiosis by nasal smear examination. *J Indian Med Assoc* 84:274–276, 1986.

Clark S, Campbell C K, Sandison A, Choa D I. *Schizophyllum commune*: an unusual isolate from a patient with allergic fungal sinusitis. *J Infect* 32:147–150, 1996.

Cowan D F. Lobo's disease in a bottlenose dolphin (*Tursiops truncatus*) from Matagorda Bay, Texas. *J Wildl Dis* 29:488–489, 1993.

Doby-Dubois M, Chevrel M L, Doby J M, Louvet M. Premier cad humain d'adiaspiromycose par *Emmonsia crescens*, Emmons et Jellison, 1960. *Bull Soc Pathol Exot* 57:240–244, 1964.

Dudok van Heel W H. Successful treatment in a case of lobomycosis (Lobo's disease) in *Tursiops truncates* (Mont) at the Dolfinarium, Haderwijk. *Aquat Mammals* 5:8–15, 1997.

Echavarria E, Cano E L, Restrepo A. Disseminated adiaspiromycosis in a patient with AIDS. Case report. *J Med Veterin Mycol* 31:91–97, 1993.

England D M, Hochholzer L. Adiaspiromycosis: an unusual fungal infection of the lung. Report of 11 cases. *Am J Surg Pathol* 17:876–886, 1993.

Filho J V B, Amato M B P, Deheinzelin D. Respiratory failure caused by adiaspiromycosis. *Chest* 97:1171–1175, 1990.

Fortin R, Meisels A. Rhinosporidiosis. *Acta Cytol* 18:169–173, 1974.

Fredricks D N, Jolley J A, Leep P W, Kosek J C, Relman D A. *Rhinosporidium seeberi*: a human pathogen from a novel group of aquatic protistan parasites. *Emerg Infect Dis* 6:273–282, 2000.

Fuchs J, Milbradt R, Pecher S A. Lobomycosis (keloidal blastomycosis): case reports and overview. *Cutis* 46:227–234, 1990.

González G M, Sutton D A, Thompson E, Tijerina R, Rinaldi M G. In vitro activities of approved and investigational antifungal agents against 44 clinical isolates of basidiomycetous fungi. *Antimicrob Agents Chemother* 45:633–635, 2001.

Greer D L, Bolanos B. Pathogenic potential of *Schizophyllum commune* isolated from a human case. *Sabouraudia* 11:233–244, 1973.

Greer D L. Basidiomycetes as agents of human infections: a review. *Mycopathol* 65:133–139, 1978.

Hawksworth D L, Sutton B C, Ainsworth G C. *Ainsworth & Bisby's Dictionary of Fungi*, 7th ed. Kew, England: Commonwealth Mycological Institute, 1983.

Herr R A, Ajello L, Taylor J W, Arseculeratne J N, Mendoza L. Phylogenetic analysis of *Rhinosporidium seeberi's* 18S small subunit ribosomal DNA groups this pathogen among members of the protoctistan Mezomycetozoa clade. *J Clin Microbiol* 37:2750–2754, 1999.

Job A, Venkateswaran S, Mathan M, Krishnaswami H, Raman R. Medical therapy of rhinosporidiosis with dapsone. *J Laryngol Otol* 107:809–812, 1993.

Kamei K, Unno H, Nagao K, Kuriyama T, Nishimura K, Miyaji M. Allergic bronchopulmonary mycosis caused by the basidiomycetous fungus *Schizophyllum commune*. *Clin Infect Dis* 18:305–309, 1994.

Kamalam A, Thambiah A S. Adiaspiromycosis of human skin caused by *Emmonsia crescens*. *Sabouraudia* 17:377–381, 1979.

Karunaratne W A E. *Rhinosporidiosis in Man*. London: Athlone Press, 1964.

Kaye H. A case of rhinosporidiosis on the eye. *Br J Ophthalmol* 22:447–455, 1938.

Kern M E, Uecker F A. Maxillary sinus infection caused by the homobasidiomycetous fungus *Schizophyllum commune*. *J. Clin Microbiol* 23:1001–1005, 1986.

Kwon-Chung K J, Bennett J E. *Medical Mycology*. Philadelphia: Lea & Febiger, 1992.

Lawrence D N, Ajello L. Lobomycosis in Western Brazil: report of a clinical trial with ketoconazole. *Am J Trop Med Hyg* 35:162–166, 1986.

Lobo J. Um caso de lastomycose produzido por uma especie nova encontrado em Recife. *Rev Med Pernambuco* 1:763–765, 1931.

Mahakrisnan A, Rajasekaram V, Pandian P J. Disseminated cutaneous rhinosporidiosis treated with dapsone. *Trop Geo Med* 33:189–192, 1981.

Mandlick G S. A record of rhinosporidial polypi with some obvservatons on the mode of infection. *Indian Med Gaz* 72:143–147, 1937.

Marlier S, de Jaureguiberry J P, Aguilon E, Carloz J, Duval L, Jaubert D. Sinusite chronique due a *Schizophyllum commune au cours du SIDA*. *Presse Med* 22:1107, 1993.

Migaki G, Valerio M G, Irvine B, Garner F M. Lobo's disease in an Atlantic bottle-nosed dolphin. *J Am Vet Med Assoc* 159:578–582, 1971.

Montero-Gei. Blastomicosis queloidiana. In: *Memorias VII Congreso Iberolatinoamericano de Dermatologia*. Caracas, Venezuela: Sintesis Dosmil, 165, 1971.

Nair K K. Clinical trial of diaminodiphenylsulfone (DDS) in nasal and nasopharyngeal rhinosporidiosis. *Laryngoscope* 89:291–295, 1979.

Nicholson C P, Allen M S, Trastek V F, Tazelaar H D, Pairolero P C. *Dirofiliaria immitis*: a rare, increasing cause of pulmonary nodules. *Mayo Clin Proc* 67:646–650, 1992.

Noronha A J. A preliminary note on the prevalence of rhinosporidosis among sandworkers in Poona with a brief description of some histological features of the rhinosporidial polypus. *J Trop Med Hyg* 36:115–120, 1933,

Owor R, Wamucota W M. Rhinosporidiosis in Uganda: a review of 51 cases. *East Afr Med J* 55:582–586, 1978.

Peres L C, Figueieredo F, Peinado M, Soares F A: Fulminant disseminated pulmonary adiaspyromycosis in humans. *Am J Trop Med Hyg* 46:146–150, 1992.

Pradinaud R. *Loboa loboi*. In: vol. 4. Collier L, Balows A, Sussman M, eds. *Topley and Wilson's Microbiology and Microbial Infections*, New York: Oxford University Press, 585–594, 1998.

Restrepo A, Greer D L, Robledo M. Ulceraton of the palate caused by a basidiomycete *Schizophyllum commune*. *Sabouraudia* 11:201–204, 1973.

Rihs J D, Padhye A A, Good C B. Brain abscess caused by *Schizophyllum commune*: an emerging basidiomycete pathogen. *J Clin Microbiol* 34:1628–1632, 1996.

Roberson M C. Conjunctival rhinosporidiosis. *Ann Ophthalmol* 17:262–263, 1985.

Rodriguez-Toro G. Lobomycosis. *Int J Dermatol* 32:324–332, 1993.

Rosenthal J, Katz R, DuBois D B, Morrissey A, Machicao A. Chronic maxillary sinusitis associated with the mushroom *Schizophyllum commune* in a patient with AIDS. *Clin Infect Dis* 14:46–48, 1992.

Sasidharan K, Subramonia P, Moni V N, Aravindan K P, Chally R. Urethral rhinosporidiosis. Analysis of 27 cases. *Br J Urol* 59:66–69, 1987.

Satyanarayana C. Rhinosporidiosis: with a record of 255 cases. *Acta Otolaryngol* 51:348–366, 1960.

Seeber G. Un Nuevo esporozuario parasito del hombre: dos casos encontrades en polipos nasals. Thesis, Universidad nacional de Buenos Aires, 1900.

Severo L C, Geyer G R, Camargo J J, Porto N S. Adiaspiromycosis treated successfully with ketoconazole. *J Med Veterin Mycol* 27:265–268, 1989.

Shrestha S P, Hennig A, Parija S C. Prevalence of rhinosporidiosis of the eye and its adnexa in Nepal. *Am J Trop Med Hyg* 59:231–234, 1998.

Sigler L, Abbott S P. Characterizing and conserving diversity of filamentous basidiomycetes from human sources. *Microbiol Cult Collect* 13:21–27, 1997a.

Sigler L, Estrada S, Montealegre A, Jaramilo E, Arango E, de Bedoug C, Restrepo A. Maxillary sinusitis caused by *Schizophyllum commune* and experience with treatment. *J Med Vet Mycol* 35:365–370, 1997b.

Sigler L, Bartley J R, Parr D H, Morris A J. Maxillary sinusitis caused by medusoid form of *Schizophyllum commune*. *J Clin Microbiol* 37:3395–3398, 1999.

Speller D C E, MacIver A C, Endocarditis caused by a *Coprinus* species: a fungus of the toadstool group. *J Med Microbiol* 4:370–374, 1971.

Taborda P R, Taborda V A, McGinnis M R. *Lacazia loboi* gen. nov., comb. nov., the etiologic agent of lobomycosis. *J Clin Microbiol* 37:2031–2033, 1999.

Talhari S. Enfermedad de Jorge Lobo. *Arch Agent Dermatol* 31:23–26, 1981.

Turner D, Burke M, Bahse S, Blinder I, Yust. Pulmonary adiaspiromycosis in a patient with acquired immunodeficiency syndrome. *Eur J Clin Microbiol Infect Dis* 18:893–895, 1999.

van der Coer J M, Marres H A, Wielinga E W, Wong-Alcala L S. Rhinosporidiosis in Europe. *J Laryngol Otol* 106:440–443, 1992.

Verweij P E, van Kasteren M, van de Nes J, de Hoog G S, de Pauw B E, Meis J F G M. Fatal pulmonary infection caused by basidiomycete *Hormographiella aspergillata*. *J Clin Microbiol* 35:2675–2678, 1997.

Wallin L L, Coleman G D, Froeling J, Parker G A. Rhinosporidiosis in a domestic cat. *Med Mycol* 39:139–141, 2001.

VIII

SPECIAL PATIENT POPULATIONS

29

Fungal infections in neutropenic patients

JUAN GEA-BANACLOCHE, ANDREAS H. GROLL, AND THOMAS J. WALSH

Invasive fungal infections (IFIs) are a significant problem in neutropenic patients. They are common, difficult to diagnose, and associated with high mortality. This chapter is organized according to the clinical, diagnostic, and therapeutic approaches that are recommended for the management of neutropenic patients at risk for IFIs. Although any fungal pathogen may potentially cause infection in neutropenic patients (Walsh and Groll, 1999a), here the focus is on more common fungal infections with special emphasis on *Candida* spp., *Aspergillus* spp., *Fusarium* spp., *Scedosporium* spp., *Trichosporon* spp., and the Zygomycetes. The empirical treatment of persistent fever in the neutropenic patient is also reviewed.

MAGNITUDE AND SCOPE OF THE PROBLEM

The initial description of fungal infections in neutropenic patients was published more than 30 years ago (Bodey, 1966a). Bodey reviewed the records of all 454 patients with acute leukemia who died at the National Institutes of Health between 1954 and 1964 and found that 107 patients (24%) had a major fungal infection (excluding focal candidiasis). Despite the changes in clinical practice during the last 4 decades, more recent autopsy studies continue to show high frequencies of IFIs in leukemic patients: 25% overall in a study that included 12 hospitals in Europe, Canada, and Japan (Bodey et al, 1992), and a striking 58% in a more recent European report (Jandrlic et al, 1995). The frequencies are much lower for patients with solid tumors (1%–8%). These numbers must be interpreted with caution because of the selection bias inherent to autopsy studies, and the various definitions used in these series (Krick and Remington, 1976; Fraser et al, 1979; Wingard et al, 1979). The recent large trials of empirical antifungal therapy in neutropenic fever have documented relatively low frequencies of IFI (at the initiation of empirical therapy), ranging between 1.5% and 5.9% (Winston et al, 2000; Boogaerts et al, 2001) and similarly low frequencies of breakthrough infections during treatment, ranging between 2.6% and 5.5% (Boogaerts et al, 2001; Walsh et al, 2002). This broad

range of rates reflects in part methodological and definition issues, but also underscores that not all neutropenic patients are at the same risk (Walsh et al, 1994; Prentice et al, 2000).

The autopsy studies are also consistent on other points. A large percentage of fungal infections go undiagnosed during life. The general frequencies of pathogens are also fairly similar, with *Candida* comprising roughly 50% of all cases, *Aspergillus* 40% and the Zygomycetes, *Cryptococcus* and other pathogens accounting for the remainder. The current widespread use of azole prophylaxis is probably changing the epidemiology of IFI: *Candida albicans* is becoming less common, and other more resistant species (*C. glabrata*, *C. krusei*) are becoming more prevalent (Abbas et al, 2000; Bodey et al, 2002). At the same time, *Aspergillus* is emerging as the more common pathogen in some institutions, particularly in the setting of hematopoietic stem cell transplantation, where *Aspergillus* has replaced *Candida* as the most common fungal pathogen in a recent series (Martino et al, 2002).

DEFICITS IN HOST DEFENSE PREDISPOSING NEUTROPENIC PATIENTS TO INVASIVE FUNGAL INFECTIONS: IMPLICATIONS FOR MANAGEMENT

The difficulties in the diagnosis of IFIs have resulted in the development of management strategies that take into consideration the different risks of IFIs in different population groups (Walsh et al, 1994). Table 29–1 shows the most important contributing risk factors.

Protracted, profound myelosuppression has been recognized as a major risk factor for development of IFIs for more than 30 years (Bodey et al, 1966b). In fact, Gerson and coworkers found that granulocytopenia persisting for more than 21 days was the single most significant risk factor for invasive aspergillosis in patients with acute nonlymphocytic leukemia (Gerson et al, 1984). The importance of the duration of granulocytopenia as a major risk factor also has been demonstrated in more recent studies (Uzun et al, 2001; Rex et al, 2002). Other risk factors, including the use of broad spectrum antibacterial agents, corticosteroids,

TABLE 29–1. *Host Factors Related to Development of Invasive Fungal Infections*

Host Factors Associated with Increasing Development of Invasive Fungal Infections in Granulocytopenic Patients
Protracted Granulocytopenia
Corticosteroid therapy
Broad spectrum antibiotics
Relapsed neoplastic disease
Hematological neoplasias
Previous invasive pulmonary aspergillosis
Central venous catheters
Total body irradiation
Allogeneic bone marrow transplantation
T-cell depletion*
Graft vs. host disease*
Host Factors Associated with Possibly Reducing Development of Invasive Fungal Infections in Granulocytopenic Patients
Solid Tumors
Remission of neoplastic disease
Recovery from granulocytopenia related to
spontaneous recovery
recombinant hematopoietic cytokines**
stem cell reconstitution**
granulocyte transfusions**

    *Additional host factors further compromising the allogeneic bone marrow transplant recipient.
    **Investigational for reducing development of invasive fungal infections.

central venous catheters, the status of the patient's underlying disease, and the type of cytotoxic chemotherapy (especially agents that disrupt mucosal integrity) also contribute to the development of IFIs in patients with cancer (Bow et al, 1991).

Candida colonization has been shown to be an important risk factor for the development of superficial candidiasis and subsequent invasive infection (Guiot et al, 1994; Schwartz et al, 1984). Broad-spectrum antibiotics increase the risk of fungal colonization (Gualtieri et al, 1983), and in this way add to the risk of IFI. The type and status of the underlying neoplastic process contributes to the duration of granulocytopenia and hence the risk for infection. Patients with hematological malignancies have a much higher frequency of opportunistic mycoses than patients with solid tumors. In general, patients with acute myelogenous leukemia appear to be at higher risk than patients with acute lymphoblastic leukemia or lymphoma (Denning et al, 1998), but many confounding factors may be contributing to this association. Patients with relapsed vs. newly diagnosed neoplastic disease have an increased risk for infectious complications. The reasons are multifactorial, and include diminished bone marrow reserve and need for more intensive chemotherapy with increased mucosal disruption and opportunities for fungal colonization. Disruption of the mucosal barriers is an important factor in establishing disseminated candidiasis in animal models of granulocytopenia (Walsh and Pizzo, 1992). Similar findings have been

observed in patients receiving cytarabine for acute leukemia (Bow et al, 1991). Venous catheters also represent another portal of entry into the bloodstream for pathogenic yeasts.

Cancer therapies (radiation and chemotherapy) may increase the risk of IFIs by a variety of mechanisms. Corticosteroid use increases the risk of invasive aspergillosis, mainly through an inhibitory effect on phagocytosis (Schaffner and Schaffner, 1987). Their use also results in defective cell-mediated immunity. Duration and dose of glucocorticosteroids correlate strongly with the development of invasive aspergillosis during allogeneic stem cell transplantation (Ribaud et al, 1999). Many immunosuppressive agents have a less clear effect on fungal infections. As an example, fludarabine seems to be associated mainly with increased incidence of cryptococcosis (Chim et al, 2000). Radiation therapy also will decrease cell-mediated immunity and contribute to the disruption of mucosal barriers.

DIAGNOSIS OF INVASIVE FUNGAL INFECTIONS IN NEUTROPENIC PATIENTS

Clinical manifestations of IFIs in neutropenic patients are seldom specific and early laboratory detection of these infections remains difficult. The methods for detection of IFIs range from the conventional approaches of direct microscopic examination and culture of specimens to nonculture methods, many of which are under active investigation. These methods include the detection of pathogen-specific antigens, antibodies, metabolites, and nucleic acid sequences. While many of these methods are currently being developed, several have become standard laboratory tools (e.g., detection of cryptococcal capsular polysaccharide by latex agglutination or enzyme immunoassay).

Standard approaches to the laboratory diagnosis of IFIs depends upon *(1)* direct microscopic inspection of freshly obtained patient specimens for the presence of organisms, *(2)* recovery of fungi in cultures of blood, sterile body fluids, tissues, or other sites, and *(3)* histological identification of organisms morphologically consistent with certain species of fungi. Laboratory identification of *Candida* and *Aspergillus* isolates at the species level carries important implications for both prognosis and therapeutic choices. Investigative approaches to nonculture-based methods for rapid detection of deeply invasive mycoses may permit earlier initiation of effective antifungal therapy and therapeutic monitoring.

Clinical Manifestations

Invasive Candidiasis. Deeply invasive candidiasis is difficult to diagnose in neutropenic patients and is the cause of substantial morbidity and mortality in hospitalized patients. Bedside clinical evaluation is critical to assess a patient with possible invasive candidiasis. Recognition of the profile of subsets of patients at high risk for invasive candidiasis is essential. Acute disseminated candidiasis is characterized typically by fever, with or without sepsis syndrome. The physical exam is usually nonfocal, but may reveal vitreal opacities (a hallmark of *Candida* endophthalmitis in the nonneutropenic host), erythematous maculopapular cutaneous lesions and/or myalgias (Arena et al, 1981). Chronic disseminated candidiasis (hepatosplenic candidiasis) characteristically presents as new fever after recovery from neutropenia, with alkaline phosphatase elevation and tenderness in the upper abdomen (See Color Fig. 29–1 in separate color insert) (Kontoyiannis et al, 2000a). Radiological investigations are typically unrevealing in acute disseminated candidiasis, but are frequently the key diagnostic test in chronic disseminated candidiasis, where ultrasound, computed tomography (CT), and magnetic resonance imaging (MRI) may reveal characteristic "target-like" lesions in liver, spleen and kidneys (Thaler et al, 1988; Sallah et al, 1998; Kontoyiannis et al, 2000a) (Fig. 29–2).

Invasive Aspergillosis. The most common clinical presentation of invasive aspergillosis in the neutropenic patient is persistent or recurrent fever (Walsh and Dixon, 1989; Denning and Stevens, 1990). The respiratory tract is the most common portal of entry of *Aspergillus* spp. and the most common site of invasive aspergillosis. *Aspergillus* has a strong propensity for invasion of blood vessels resulting in vascular thrombosis, infarc-

tion, and tissue necrosis, which contribute to many of the clinical manifestations of pulmonary aspergillosis, namely, pleuritic pain, nonproductive cough, hemoptysis, and pleural rub (Gerson et al, 1985a; Gerson et al, 1985b). In the case of sinus aspergillosis, signs and symptoms include fever, orbital swelling, facial pain, and nasal congestion (Drakos et al, 1993). Angioinvasion by *Aspergillus* spp. may lead to cavernous sinus thrombosis. An ulcerated lesion on the hard palate or gingiva may also be present (Talbot et al, 1991).

Radiographic manifestations of invasive pulmonary aspergillosis include bronchopneumonia, lobar consolidation, segmental pneumonia, multiple nodular lesions resembling septic emboli, and cavitary lesions (Orr et al, 1978; Kuhlman et al, 1985; Hruban et al, 1987; Aquino et al, 1994; Caillot et al, 2001b) (See Color Fig. 29–3 in separate color insert). The chest roentgenogram may initially appear normal due to the paucity of inflammatory response. However, early use of CT may reveal a "halo sign," which is observed early in the majority of neutropenic patients with proven invasive pulmonary aspergillosis (Caillot et al, 2001b). The "halo sign" has been very well described (Kuhlman et al, 1985; Hruban et al, 1987; Caillot et al, 1997; Caillot et al, 2001b), and consists of a delicate infiltrate at the edges of the denser consolidation, possibly representing edema around the infarcted tissue. This edema constitutes a reversible injury to the lung tissue. With initiation of antifungal therapy, this process may be stabilized or reversed (Walsh et al, 1995b); after recovery from neutropenia, cavitation, and development of a "crescent sign" may occur (Caillot et al, 2001b).

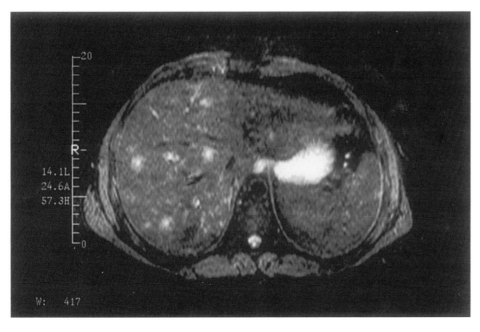

FIGURE 29–2. Computed tomography scan showing target-like lesions in liver of patient with chronic disseminated candidiasis.

The presence of such crescentic cavitary lesions in an immunocompromised patient with pulmonary infiltrates is most compatible with invasive pulmonary aspergillosis (Curtis et al, 1979; Slevin et al, 1982). Other early lesions visible on CT scan are peripheral or subpleural nodules contiguous with the pulmonary vascular tree. Early radiographic recognition of pulmonary lesions contributes to more prompt and appropriate antifungal therapy (Aisner et al, 1977; Kuhlman et al, 1985; Caillot et al, 1997). Investigators recently found that performing CT scans on all febrile neutropenic patients permitted earlier recognition of invasive aspergillosis, with improvement in time to detection of infiltrates from 7 to 1.9 days (Caillot et al, 1997).

Dissemination during invasive aspergillosis characteristically involves the central nervous system (CNS) and the skin; CNS involvement may be clinically silent, or can present dramatically as an embolic stroke (Walsh et al, 1985). Imaging (preferably by magnetic resonance) is indicated when the diagnosis of aspergillosis is made, even in the absence of symptoms. The neuroradiological findings are variable, as the pathological lesions may be infarction, hemorrhage, or abscess (De-Lone et al, 1999; Dietrich et al, 2001; Yamada et al, 2002). The CNS lesions may lack ring enhancement, particularly during neutropenia. Disseminated aspergillosis involving the skin is characterized by erythematous nodules with hemorrhagic infarctions. Septate hyphae with dichotomous branching are detected in the biopsy specimen (see Color Fig. 29–3D in separate color insert).

Fusariosis. *Fusarium* spp. may cause severe pulmonary, sinus, or disseminated infections in granulocytopenic patients undergoing intensive antileukemic chemotherapy or bone marrow transplantation (Anaissie et al, 1986; Anaissie et al, 1988; Martino et al, 1994a; Boutati and Anaissie, 1997; Segal et al, 1998). *Fusarium solani*, *F. oxysporum*, *F. moniliforme*, and *F. chlamydosporum* have been reported to cause disseminated infection in immunosuppressed patients. The portals of entry of *Fusarium* spp. include lungs, sinuses, catheters, and skin, particularly at periungual regions. *Fusarium* has become increasingly recognized as a cause of paronychia in neutropenic patients receiving broad-spectrum antibiotics. These portals of entry may lead to widespread dissemination, fungemia (blood cultures in disseminated fusariosis are positive in approximately one-half of cases), and occasionally, chronic hepatic infection upon recovery from neutropenia. Findings on physical examination include nodular cutaneous lesions as a reflection of disseminated infection (Nucci and Anaissie, 2002a) (See Color Fig. 29–4 in separate color insert). Biopsy of these lesions may reveal characteristic hyaline branching septate hyphae, which are not reliably distinguishable from those of *Aspergillus*, and extensive necrosis surrounding the fungal elements (Anaissie et al, 1988).

Scedosporiosis. *Scedosporium* species cause pneumonia and disseminated infections in neutropenic and other compromised hosts (Travis et al, 1985; Berenguer et al, 1989; Walsh et al, 1995c; Jabado et al, 1998; Walsh and Groll, 1999a; Groll and Walsh, 2001). Pneumonia due to *Scedosporium* spp. is clinically indistinguishable from that due to *Aspergillus* spp. As with pulmonary aspergillosis, dissemination complicating *Scedosporium* pneumonia often involves the central nervous system (Yoo et al, 1985; Berenguer et al, 1989; Nguyen, 2001) or may result in multiple cutaneous lesions. Diagnostic procedures and approaches, including chest CT scan, bronchoalveolar lavage (BAL), and lung biopsy, are similar to those for invasive pulmonary aspergillosis. *Scedosporium* spp. in tissue and direct smears resembles *Aspergillus* spp. as angular, septate, dichotomously branching hyphae. However, terminal annelloconidia may be observed histologically in some infected tissues. Definitive microbiological diagnosis is established by culture.

Zygomycosis. Zygomycetes constitute a class of organisms characterized by the presence of aseptate or sparsely septated, broad, ribbon-like hyphae in tissue. Recent case series from Europe and the United States have reported the characteristics of zygomycosis over the last decade (Pagano et al, 1997; Maertens et al, 1999a; Kontoyiannis et al, 2000b; Herbrecht et al, 2001). Rhinocerebral, pulmonary, and disseminated zygomycosis are the most frequently encountered conditions in immunocompromised patients. Rhinocerebral zygomycosis usually begins as an infection of the paranasal sinuses, especially the maxillary and ethmoid sinuses, and progresses to invade the orbit, retroorbital region, cavernous sinus, and brain. Angioinvasion with thrombosis causes ischemic necrosis. A black eschar on the palatal or nasal mucosa and drainage of a black discharge from the eye are clinical manifestations of infarction (Fig. 15–2).

Diagnosis of pulmonary zygomycosis requires a high degree of suspicion and an aggressive approach (Sugar, 1992; Pagano et al, 1997; Maertens et al, 1999a; Kontoyiannis et al, 2000b; Herbrecht et al, 2001). Careful evaluation of all patients with the pulmonary infarct syndrome and biopsy of suspicious skin lesions may improve diagnosis. Computed tomography of the chest can define the extent of disease and help determine the method of diagnosis. Bronchoscopy with transbronchial biopsy and bronchoalveolar lavage are the preferred methods of diagnosing pulmonary zygomycosis, but a fine needle aspiration or an open lung biopsy may sometimes be the only definitive diagnostic procedure for detection of this disease.

Rarely, primary cutaneous zygomycosis may develop in a neutropenic patient (Wirth et al, 1997), with risk of subsequent dissemination. Most of the Zygomycetes causing respiratory infections in immunocompromised or debilitated hosts have a high propensity for thrombotic invasion of blood vessels, and are associated with a rapidly evolving clinical course, high mortality, and relative resistance to antifungal therapy.

Trichosporonosis. *Trichosporon* spp. are pathogenic yeasts that cause fatal disseminated infection in immunocompromised patients, particularly those with neutropenia and mucosal disruption due to cytotoxic chemotherapy (Hoy et al, 1986; Walsh et al, 1986b). The portals of entry are the gastrointestinal tract and vascular catheters; however, investigators are increasingly recognizing that aspiration may lead to a disseminated trichosporonosis or bronchopneumonia. From these portals of entry, the organism can disseminate widely, resulting in a characteristic constellation of findings that include renal failure, pulmonary infiltrates, multiple cutaneous lesions, and chorioretinitis. This process, which can evolve into chronic hepatic trichosporonosis among patients who recover from neutropenia, typically follows persistent fungemia despite administration of amphotericin B.

Detection of Fungal Pathogens in the Neutropenic Host

Candida. Direct examination of a specimen provides information about the cellular composition of any inflammatory reaction, the relative amount of *Candida* spp. present, and the distinctive morphological features of the organism, such as the presence of budding yeast forms, pseudohyphae, and hyphae as well as the presence of other pathogens. Direct examination of urine may promptly identify *Candida* spp. as the cause of a urinary tract infection. The significance of candiduria depends upon the immune status of the host and the presence or absence of specific risk factors for disseminated candidiasis and must be interpreted accordingly (Goldberg et al, 1979; Lundstrom and Sobel, 2001). Febrile neutropenic patients with candiduria (in the absence of an urinary catheter) from a correctly collected urine specimen should be considered as having a high probability for invasive candidiasis. There is no lower limit for the concentration of *C. albicans* in the urine below which the diagnosis of upper urinary tract infection can be excluded (Navarro et al, 1997).

Yeasts other than *Candida* spp. may infect neutropenic patients, and differentiation from other genera is important. The presence of a capsule around initially cultured yeasts permits early consideration of *C. neoformans*, which can be further differentiated from *Candida* species by appropriate tests. *Trichosporon* may also be urease-positive (like *C. neoformans*) but is easily distinguishable by the presence of arthroconidia and different carbohydrate assimilation reactions. *Rhodotorula* species are urease-positive and have pink to orange–red colonies (Rusthoven et al, 1984; Samonis et al, 2001). *Malassezia furfur* is typically isolated only after incubation on a blood agar plate with a long-chain carbon source (e.g., olive oil) (Dankner et al, 1987).

Detection of *Candida* spp. in the bloodstream of any patient must be considered significant until proven otherwise. Indeed, even blood cultures growing *Candida* spp. from a vascular catheter are not to be considered as catheter colonization, since vascular catheters may be the target of fungemia from a distal site or the portal of entry of *Candida* spp. (Walsh et al, 1986a; Lecciones et al, 1992; Nucci and Anaissie, 2002b). Negative peripheral blood cultures do not reliably exclude the diagnosis of disseminated candidiasis. This question was addressed by determining the frequency with which lysis centrifugation blood cultures yielded *Candida* spp. in patients with autopsy-proven invasive candidiasis. Blood cultures were positive in 78% (7/9) of patients with > 3 organs infected by *Candida* compared to 28% (5/18) of patients with only 1 organ infected ($p = 0.024$) (Berenguer et al, 1993), demonstrating a direct relation between the tissue burden of *Candida* and the frequency of detection of fungemia by lysis centrifugation, and the relatively low sensitivity of the lysis centrifugation system in detection of fungemia in early deep candidiasis. Depending on the method used, blood cultures should be incubated for 5 to 7 days when there is suspicion of fungemia (Masterson and McGowan, 1988; Varettas et al, 2002). The BACTEC selective fungal medium has been shown to be equivalent to lysis centrifugation in detection of candidemia in some studies (Archibald et al, 2000). In addition, a recent comparison considered lysis centrifugation less useful because of a high proportion of false-positive results (Creger et al, 1998).

The limitations of clinical assessment, blood culture systems, and other conventional ancillary laboratory methods in early detection of invasive candidiasis warrant development of newer nonculture methods. Such methods are predicated upon the detection of antigens, antibodies, metabolites, cell wall elements, and nucleic acids. These methods should be considered investigational at this time (Walsh et al, 1995a).

Aspergillus. Although the genus *Aspergillus* consists of more than 600 species, only a few of these are pathogenic for humans (Rinaldi, 1983). The most common are *A. fumigatus* and *A. flavus*. Other species, such as *A. terreus*, *A. ustus*, and *A nidulans*, are also known pulmonary pathogens in humans. *Aspergillus niger* is commonly isolated in saprophytic conditions, such as chronic obstructive pulmonary disease and chronic sinusitis, but is seldom proven to be a cause of invasive pulmonary aspergillosis in cancer patients. *Aspergillus* spp. in tissue forms angular dichotomously branching septate hyphae, which may also be observed in invasive tissue infections, due to *Scedosporium* spp., *Fusarium* spp., and several less common fungi. Culture is the only way to distinguish these invasive fungi.

Aspergillus is an uncommon contaminant in most clinical microbiology laboratories. One should therefore evaluate carefully the significance of *Aspergillus* spp. isolated from a diagnostic specimen. Early studies found that positive nasal surveillance cultures of *A. flavus* during the midst of an outbreak of nosocomial aspergillosis in granulocytopenic patients correlated significantly with invasive pulmonary aspergillosis (Aisner et al, 1979). These findings have not been corroborated consistently in nonoutbreak settings. Certainly, the absence of a positive nasal surveillance culture in a persistently febrile granulocytopenic patient with a pulmonary infiltrate does not exclude a diagnosis of pulmonary aspergillosis. Conversely, isolation of *Aspergillus* spp. from the nares does not consistently predict the development of invasive aspergillosis.

By comparison, isolation of *Aspergillus* spp. from respiratory secretions from febrile granulocytopenic patients with pulmonary infiltrates is strongly associated with invasive aspergillosis. In a prospective study, Yu and colleagues found that isolation of *Aspergillus* spp. from respiratory secretions of high-risk patients was highly predictive of invasive pulmonary aspergillosis. Among 108 consecutive patients from whom *Aspergillus* spp. were isolated, 17 patients with granulocytopenia and/or leukemia had lung tissue examined; all had invasive pulmonary aspergillosis (Yu et al, 1986). Invasive aspergillosis was not found in nonimmunosuppressed patients or in nongranulocytopenic patients with solid tumors. Multivariate analysis demonstrated that granulocytopenia and absence of smoking were the most significant predictors of invasive aspergillosis in patients with respiratory tract cultures growing *Aspergillus* spp. A retrospective study also underscored the significance of isolation of *Aspergillus* spp. from respiratory secretions in high-risk populations (Treger et al, 1985). Thus, isolation of *Aspergillus* spp. from respiratory tract cultures of febrile granulocytopenic patients with pulmonary infiltrates should be considered a priori evidence of pulmonary aspergillosis.

Mucosal eschars may be observed by careful otolaryngological examination along the nasal turbinates or septum in patients with *Aspergillus* sinusitis. Biopsy and culture of these lesions may reveal invasive aspergillosis and allow prompt initiation of appropriate antifungal therapy. Similarly, if nasal lesions are not observed, a sinus aspirate may preclude the need for bronchoscopy if fungus is demonstrated in the aspirate. Although *Aspergillus* is the most common fungus isolated from the sinuses of immunocompromised patients, other fungi including the Zygomycetes, *Fusarium*, *Scedosporium*, *Curvularia*, and *Alternaria* may be recovered.

Bronchoalveolar lavage has been studied by several investigators and found to yield variable results in patients with tissue proven–invasive pulmonary aspergillosis—50% to 59% positivity (Albelda et al, 1984; Kahn et al, 1986; Verea-Hernando et al, 1989; Reichenberger et al, 1999). The combination of microbiologic culture with cytopathology increases the diagnostic yield. While the presence of *Aspergillus* spp. in BAL fluid in a febrile granulocytopenic patient with new pulmonary infiltrates is indicative of invasive aspergillosis, the absence of hyphal elements or positive culture by no means excludes the diagnosis. Indeed, as few as 30% of patients with invasive aspergillosis have had negative bronchoscopic studies in some series (Reichenberger et al, 1999). In the case of peripheral nodular lesions, a fine needle biopsy may have a better yield, even if morbidity is potentially higher (Tikkakoski et al, 1995; Jantunen et al, 2000; Jantunen et al, 2002). If the foregoing methods do not yield a microbiological diagnosis to explain new infiltrates in the recurrently febrile granulocytopenic patient, then open lung biopsy should be performed. The surgeon must biopsy both the peripheral as well as the central areas of abnormal lung, since the distribution of organisms may vary. The presence of hyphal elements in a tissue specimen must be interpreted cautiously due to the similar morphologic features of many pathogenic moulds. Culture is the only readily available diagnostic method that can reliably distinguish between these pathogens.

IMMUNODIAGNOSTIC METHODS FOR INVASIVE ASPERGILLOSIS. Although immunodiagnostic and molecular methods for early detection of invasive pulmonary aspergillosis remain investigational, the latest international consensus conference that provided definitions of IFIs in immunocompromised hosts for the first time included presence of *Aspergillus* antigen in the CSF, BAL fluid, or blood (two specimens) as one of the microbiological criteria for probable and possible aspergillosis (Ascioglu et al, 2002). These definitions are for clinical research purposes only, and in no way attempt to define clinical practice. Galactomannan has been described by various investigators to have great immunodiagnostic potential. Early studies reported the presence of galactomannan antigenemia by counter immunoelectropho-resis in experimental disseminated aspergillosis (Lehmann and Reiss, 1978; Reiss and Lehmann, 1979). Subsequently, galactomannan measured by radioim-munoassay and an enzyme-linked immunoassay was found in serum and urine in experimental disseminated aspergillosis and in invasive aspergillosis in patients (Dupont et al, 1987). Detection of galactomannan in urine was more sensitive than serum as a diagnostic source.

A more recently developed detection system em-ploying a direct sandwich ELISA appears to be more sensitive than the latex agglutination (LA) system. This system has been investigated in experimental as-pergillosis and in patients with proven or probable as-pergillosis. Verweij and colleagues compared results of this ELISA for detecting *Aspergillus* galactomannan with that of the Pastorex *Aspergillus* antigen LA test in 532 serum samples from 61 patients at risk for in-vasive aspergillosis (Verweij et al, 1995b). The ELISA gave positive results earlier in the course of infection than did the LA test, and the sensitivity and specificity were greater, 90% and 84% for the ELISA vs. 70% and 86% for LA. Several reports regarding the appli-cation of galactomannan in clinical practice have been published in the last few years (Denning, 2000). A re-cent prospective evaluation of the galactomannan sand-wich-ELISA assay in 186 hematological patients at risk for invasive aspergillosis measured galactomannan lev-els twice a week (Maertens et al, 1999b). A definitive diagnosis based on histopathology and culture was made in 71 patients; 27 had invasive aspergillosis and 44 did not have invasive aspergillosis. The sensitivity of the ELISA assay was 92.6% and the specificity was 95.4%. The positive and negative predictive values were also excellent (PPV = 93%, NPV = 95%). In a follow-up study, the same authors analyzed 362 con-secutive high-risk episodes, and were able to detect all proven cases of invasive aspergillosis using the ELISA methodology in neutropenic patients (Maertens et al, 2001).

Positive and negative predictive values depend on the prevalence of the disease. A test with sensitivity of 92.6% and specificity of 95.4%, when applied to a population where only 5% had invasive aspergillosis (prevalence 5% or pretest probability = 0.05), would result in a NPV of 99.5% but a PPV of only 51%. These estimates are relevant, because the prevalence of invasive aspergillosis varies in different clinical settings. Even in high-risk neutropenic populations, as described in some of the fever and neutropenia trials (Walsh et al, 2002), the prevalence of aspergillosis seldom reaches 10%. Under these circumstances, the ELISA test for galactomannan seems extremely useful to rule out in-vasive aspergillosis: a negative galactomannan makes

aspergillosis very unlikely. A positive result, on the other hand, has to be interpreted in the context of the rest of the clinical picture. Most diagnostic tests are less effective in clinical practice than in the research trials where they are tested. As an example, the sensitivity of galactomannan was lower in another European study that collected 3294 serum samples during 797 episodes that included adult and pediatric hematological patients in four groups: those with neutropenic fever, transplant patients undergoing weekly surveillance, patients with suspected pulmonary infection, and patients with suspected extrapulmonary infection (Herbrecht et al, 2002b).

Caillot and associates studied whether new noncul-ture strategies, consisting of early CT scanning coupled with antigen detection by ELISA, could improve diag-nosis and outcome in neutropenic patients (Caillot et al, 1997). Twenty-three histologically proven and 14 highly probable episodes of invasive pulmonary as-pergillosis in 37 hematologic, largely neutropenic, pa-tients were analyzed retrospectively. Bronchoalveolar lavage fluid was culture positive for *Aspergillus* spp. in 22 (69%) of 32 cases and the *Aspergillus* galactoman-nan antigen test on BAL was positive in 83% of cases. Other investigators have also studied the value of test-ing BAL fluid with the commercially available sand-wich-ELISA for galactomannan (Verweij et al, 1995a; Salonen et al, 2000; Seyfartg et al, 2001). The added utility of galactomannan detection in BAL remains to be resolved.

The detection of galactomannan by sandwich ELISA is obviously an important addition to the armamen-tarium of diagnostic tests that clinicians may use to de-tect invasive aspergillosis early. The best possible strat-egy for its use, either as a prospective screening test in patient populations at high risk for IFIs or as a diag-nostic test, may differ in different patient populations. Trials of different strategies with clinical outcomes as endpoints will be necessary before a firm recommen-dation can be made. In the meantime, those clinicians that are able to use this exciting technology should re-member the described causes of false-positive results (Gangneux et al, 2002) and the many opportunistic fungi other than *Aspergillus* that can cause severe in-vasive mould disease in the neutropenic host for whom the galactomannan test may be negative.

Molecular Diagnostic Methods for Invasive Aspergillo-sis. Polymerase chain reaction methods are being de-veloped that may also permit early detection of inva-sive aspergillosis in neutropenic patients (Tang et al, 1993; Hopfer et al, 1993). Initial studies suggested the utility of identifying A. *fumigatus* and A. *flavus* by PCR from BAL in 4 patients with proven or probable as-pergillosis, while detecting a positive PCR signal in only

6 (13%) of 46 BAL specimens from control patients (Tang et al, 1993). Einsele and colleagues have developed a PCR assay for the detection and identification of *Candida* and *Aspergillus* species (Einsele et al, 1997). The oligonucleotide primer pair consists of a consensus sequence for a variety of fungal pathogens and the species-specific probes used for species identification were derived from a comparison of the sequences of the 18S rRNA genes of *Candida* spp. and *Aspergillus* spp. While most PCR systems for detection of aspergillosis utilize whole blood or BAL as a source, serum as a test specimen for PCR detection has also been evaluated (Yamakami et al, 1996). Employing a nested PCR method, these investigators utilized two sets of oligonucleotide primers derived from the sequence of the variable regions V7 to V9 of the 18S rRNA genes of *A. fumigatus*. The DNA fragment of interest was detected in the serum of mice with disseminated aspergillosis and in patients with invasive aspergillosis. In a separate study, PCR in plasma was found to be less sensitive than whole blood in a small group of nine patients (Loeffler et al, 2000).

Fusarium. Fusarium species are frequently detected by advanced blood culture detection systems, such as lysis centrifugation. *Fusarium* spp. initially grow on solid media with hyphae exhibiting phialides and microconidia. The typical plantain-shaped macroconidia appear in more mature cultures. Consequently, initial culture reports from the clinical microbiology laboratory may erroneously report an *Acremonium* spp. Thus, any culture report from blood or tissue indicating *Acremonium* spp. from a neutropenic patient should be considered as possibly an early form of *Fusarium* spp. Unlike *Aspergillus* spp., many isolates of *Fusarium* spp. may be highly resistant in vitro and in vivo to amphotericin B and other available antifungal drugs. While current diagnostic approaches depend upon bedside evaluation, diagnostic imaging, tissue histopathology and culture, PCR methods also are being developed for detection of *Fusarium* spp. (Walsh et al, 1995a; Kappe et al, 1996).

Zygomycetes and *Trichosporon* spp. For a detailed discussion about diagnosis of infections by these and other opportunistic fungal pathogens, the reader is referred to the specific chapters that deal with these organisms. (See Chapter 13 [*Trichosporon*] and Chapter 15 [*Zygomycetes*].)

PREVENTION OF FUNGAL INFECTIONS DURING NEUTROPENIA

Established fungal infections have an extremely high mortality in persistently neutropenic patients and are difficult to diagnose early. As a result, current practice is to administer antifungal agents to patients who are at risk, even in the absence of proven infection. Ultimately, the goal is to prevent morbidity and mortality caused by IFIs. Different terms have been used to characterize the administration of antifungal agents in the absence of documented fungal infections. The most commonly used terms are prophylaxis, empirical treatment, and preemptive treatment. The administration of fluconazole to all patients undergoing conditioning chemotherapy is appropriately called *prophylaxis*, and the addition of an antifungal agent to the treatment regimen of a persistently febrile neutropenic patient is called *empirical therapy*. However, in both cases an antifungal agent is being administered to many patients who do not need the drug, in order to ensure that those patients who really need treatment receive treatment. In the first example, prospective studies have been shown that 10%–15% of patients undergoing bone marrow transplantation and given placebo will develop IFI compared with only 3.5% of patients given fluconazole as prophylaxis (Goodman et al, 1992; Slavin et al, 1995). Thus, the use of an agent with very little toxicity like fluconazole is easily justifiable. In the second example, "persistent fever during neutropenia" acts as a marker for risk and identifies a group of patients in whom the frequency of fungal infection is much higher. Although a fungal infection is documented in only approximately 3%–5% of these patients (up to 10% in high-risk subgroups), the administration of a potentially toxic antifungal agent seems justified because of the extremely high mortality of IFIs. Thus, empirical treatment has become accepted clinical practice (Hughes et al, 2002). By contrast, the term *preemptive therapy* has been used to describe the administration of antifungal agents to persistently febrile neutropenic patients with some clinical evidence of fungal infection other than undifferentiated fever (Walsh and Lee, 1993). The important general concept is that diverse approaches are used in an attempt to decrease the morbidity and mortality associated with IFIs during neutropenia. From this standpoint, all of these approaches are preventive strategies.

Prevention of Exposure: Environmental Control

Prevention of exposure is not possible for *Candida* infections, but is feasible (at least partially) for *Aspergillus*. A review of nosocomial aspergillosis found that the most common sources of clusters and outbreaks of nosocomial aspergillosis were *(1)* hospital construction and renovation and *(2)* defective and contaminated ventilation systems (Walsh and Dixon, 1989). Exposure of patients to *Aspergillus* conidia can be decreased significantly by the use of high-efficiency particulate air filtration (HEPA) filters and positive pressure rooms (Rhame, 1991). A recent report underscores the effectiveness of environmental control to significantly reduce the incidence of invasive aspergillosis (Oren et al, 2001). Aspergillosis developed in 50% of the patients treated during a 4-month period of extensive renovation of a hematology ward, and decreased to 0% after the installation of HEPA filters. In addition, the risk of aspergillosis in bone marrow transplantation patients who were not in HEPA-filtered rooms was 5.6 times higher in the classic study from the Fred Hutchinson Cancer Research Center (Wald et al, 1997). Other data from the International Bone Marrow Transplant Registry have confirmed that use of HEPA and/or laminar air flow (LAF) to prevent fungal infections decreases transplant-related mortality and increases survival after allogeneic bone marrow transplantation for leukemia (Passweg et al, 1998).

While use of HEPA filters has become more common, some patients continue to develop nosocomial pulmonary aspergillosis and other mould infections. There is growing evidence that contamination of the water distribution system with *Aspergillus* (Anaissie et al, 2002) and other filamentous moulds, e.g., *Fusarium* (Anaissie et al, 2001) plays a significant role in the epidemiology of hospital-acquired mould infection. Fatal infections caused by *Aspergillus terreus* from the soil of hospital plants have been reported (Lass-Florl et al, 2000). Although this type of event may be rare, exposure to wet soil should be avoided during profound neutropenia.

Primary Prophylaxis

Different strategies have been used in an attempt to reduce the frequency of IFIs. The studies that have used fluconazole and the studies with agents potentially active against moulds are considered separately.

Prophylaxis with Fluconazole. Since *Candida* is a common inhabitant of the human gastrointestinal tract, the majority of invasive *Candida* infections during neutropenia are postulated to originate after mucosal colonization evolves into superficial infection. Colonization of multiple sites with *Candida* as a significant risk factor for invasive candidiasis is in agreement with this theory. However, prevention of oropharyngeal candidiasis does not necessarily lead to prevention of deeply invasive candidiasis in cancer patients. Patients may have negative oropharyngeal cultures and stool cultures and yet still suffer from invasive candidiasis. Invasive candidiasis in granulocytopenic patients may be highly focal along the alimentary tract, allowing invasion into the GI tract without diffuse mucosal involvement (Walsh and Merz, 1986c). A common theme among studies of antifungal prophylaxis is the consistent reduction in superficial candidiasis without a concomitant reduction in invasive disease.

A consistent problem among the studies that have examined the potential usefulness of antifungal prophylaxis has been the relatively low incidence of IFI in neutropenic patients in general, which limits the power of the studies to detect a significant difference. As opposed to the studies of empirical therapy, where the presence of persistent fever identifies a subgroup of patients at high risk of IFI, most studies of prophylaxis have found a relatively low incidence of IFI and consequently have been underpowered. The studies in which the populations had substantial risk (e.g., allogeneic bone marrow transplantation) have clearly shown beneficial effects (Goodman et al, 1992; Slavin et al, 1995). In the study by Goodman and colleagues, fluconazole 400 mg/day or placebo was initiated on day 1 of marrow-ablative chemotherapy. Among 356 bone marrow transplant recipients, invasive candidiasis developed in 28 (15.7%) of 178 placebo patients and 5 (2.8%) of 179 fluconazole recipients ($p < 0.001$). Other benefits were noted. Fluconazole delayed the initiation of empiric amphotericin B therapy from day 17 to day 21 ($p < 0.004$). Infections due to *Candida krusei* were noted in both arms and their frequency was not significantly different. However, there was a significant reduction in fungal infection-attributable mortality, but no difference in overall mortality. Importantly, fluconazole was associated with minimal adverse effects in this setting. Another randomized, placebo-controlled trial reported by Slavin and coworkers compared fluconazole at 400 mg/day vs. placebo in 300 bone marrow transplant recipients (Slavin et al, 1995). Fluconazole was administered through the duration of granulocytopenia and until day +75 after transplantation. There was a significant reduction in number of fungal infections among fluconazole recipients (7%) compared with placebo recipients (18%) ($p = 0.004$). Survival was improved in fluconazole recipients; 31 deaths occurred up to day 110 after transplantation compared to 52 deaths in placebo recipients ($p = 0.004$). Long-term follow-up of these patients has confirmed the benefit in survival (Marr et al, 2000). In a Canadian multicenter study that included patients receiving intensive chemotherapy for acute leukemia or autologous bone marrow transplantation, fluconazole prophylaxis was beneficial in decreasing superficial fungal infections, definite and probable IFIs (6% vs. 24%, $p = 0.001$), and deaths attributable to fungal infection (6.6% vs. 37.5%, $p = 0.04$) (Rotstein et al, 1999). However, in this study there was no difference in the need for amphotericin B therapy or in overall mortality.

In contrast to the aforementioned studies, other prophylaxis trials have shown no significant difference in the incidence of IFI or the mortality attributable to fungal infection (Winston et al, 1993; Chandrasekar and Gatny, 1994; Schaffner and Schaffner, 1995; Kern et al, 1998). A multicenter, placebo-controlled trial of 257 adults undergoing chemotherapy for acute leukemia showed decreased fungal colonization and superficial infection, but no difference in IFIs between placebo-treated patients (7.5%) and fluconazole-treated patients (4%) (*p* = 0.3) (Winston et al, 1993). The lack of statistical significance in this large clinical trial may have been due to a low frequency of proven IFI and the early usage of empirical amphotericin B. A single-center trial in patients receiving chemotherapy for acute leukemias and lymphomas found no difference in IFI between the fluconazole and the placebo treatment groups (Schaffner and Schaffner, 1995). However, the time to starting amphotericin B was longer in the fluconazole group, and there was a trend toward reduced use of amphotericin B in this group (33% vs. 47%, *p* = 0.08). As in other studies, the incidence of oropharyngeal candidiasis was significantly reduced. Another small single-center study also showed reduced use of amphotericin B in the fluconazole group (Chandrasekar and Gatny, 1994). A more recent study failed to show any benefit of fluconazole over non-absorbable antifungal agents in 68 patients with refractory leukemia (Kern et al, 1998). Interestingly, this study suggested increases in bacterial infections and amphotericin B use in the fluconazole treated group.

More recently, Rex and coworkers have reported a retrospective analysis of the effect of systemic antifungal prophylaxis in 833 episodes of neutropenia among 322 patients with acute myelogenous leukemia treated between 1988 and 1992 (Rex et al, 2002). The authors chose this time period because it spanned the end of the era when prophylaxis was uncommon (only 38% of the patients treated between 1988 and 1990 received any systemic antifungal) and common (80% of the neutropenic episodes that occurred after January 1991 received prophylaxis). This comparison between episodes of neutropenia where prophylaxis (typically fluconazole 400 mg/day or amphotericin B 40 mg/day) was given and episodes of neutropenia where prophylaxis was not given has the advantages of size and power that many prospective randomized trials lack. The results show statistically significant reductions in favor of prophylaxis for IFIs (5% vs. 13%), empirical use of amphotericin B (26% vs. 34%), and death within 30 days of the first neutropenic episode (23% vs. 35%). As expected, the difference in IFIs was accounted for by a reduction in yeast infections (2% in prophylaxis group, 8% in no prophylaxis group). There was no difference in the frequency of mould infections (Rex et al, 2002).

In summary, the beneficial effects of prophylaxis with systemic antifungal agents are demonstrable in high-risk neutropenic patients (allogeneic hematopoietic stem cell transplants and acute myelogenous leukemia) but are difficult to demonstrate in lower risk neutropenic patients. When the risk is low, most studies are underpowered. Not surprisingly, a recent meta-analysis shows that the use of azole or systemic amphotericin B prophylaxis in oncologic patients with severe neutropenia is associated with significant benefit regarding four main endpoints: decreased need for therapeutic doses of parenteral antifungal agents, decreased superficial fungal infections, decreased IFIs, and decreased fungal-related mortality (Bow et al, 2002). The number of patients that require treatment to prevent one event for each one of these four endpoints are 10, 12, 22, and 52, respectively. In agreement with the studies highlighted above, the multivariate analysis identified hematopoietic stem cell transplantation (HSCT) and prolonged neutropenia as predictors of treatment effect. As in a previous metaanalysis (Gotzsche and Johansen, 1997), there was no difference in overall mortality and no effect on frequency of invasive aspergillosis.

Prophylaxis with Itraconazole. Fluconazole has no activity against moulds. Conversely, itraconazole has good activity against *Aspergillus* spp. and many dematiaceous moulds while maintaining the activity of fluconazole against yeasts. Several studies have compared itraconazole oral solution (in a formulation with hydroxypropyl-β-cyclodextrin [HDβCD]) with placebo (Menichetti et al, 1999), itraconazole with oral amphotericin B (Harousseau et al, 2000), and itraconazole with fluconazole, either as itraconazole capsules (Huijgens et al, 1999) or as oral solution (Morgenstern et al, 1999).

Itraconazole oral solution (2.5 mg/kg bid) was compared to placebo in a randomized, double-blind, multicenter study of 405 patients with hematological malignancies (not undergoing HSCT) (Menichetti et al, 1999). Itraconazole significantly reduced the frequency of proven and suspected fungal infections (24% in the itraconazole group vs. 33% in the placebo group). Interestingly, four cases of aspergillosis were detected in the itraconazole recipients and only one in the placebo group.

Itraconazole oral solution (2.5 mg/kg bid) was not statistically significantly better than oral amphotericin B in a double-blind, double-placebo, randomized, multicenter European trial among 557 patients (Harousseau et al, 2000), although trends favoring itraconazole were seen for proven IFIs (3.6% vs. 9.4%) and proven aspergillosis (1.8% vs. 3.3%). Of note, the median plasma concentration of itraconazole during the first week was < 0.5 μg/mL. Lower itraconazole levels have been associated with the occurrence of IFIs (Lamy et al, 1998; Glasmacher et al, 2000). Low levels of itraconazole may also have played a role in another trial that compared itraconazole capsules (100 mg bid) with fluconazole capsules (50 mg bid) in 213 adult patients with hematological malignancies (Huijgens et al, 1999). This study found no difference between fluconazole and itraconazole in any of the measured clinical endpoints.

A comparative trial of itraconazole oral solution (5 mg/kg/day) vs. fluconazole oral solution (100 mg/day) demonstrated fewer proven IFIs (0.3% vs. 1.4%) in the itraconazole-treated group. No cases of aspergillosis were documented in the itraconazole recipients compared to 4 cases in the fluconazole recipients. There were also fewer deaths caused by IFI in the itraconazole recipients (Morgenstern et al, 1999). However, the oral solution of itraconazole caused significantly more adverse effects than fluconazole, particularly gastrointestinal toxicity (nausea, vomiting, diarrhea) presumably due to HDβCD. The proportion of patients with serum levels of itraconazole > 250 µg/mL was 76% at week 1, and 84% and 86% at weeks 2 and 3, respectively.

Prophylaxis with Amphotericin B. Amphotericin B has been used as prophylaxis by the oral route, inhalation route, and the intravenous route (Bodey, 1969; Ezdinli et al, 1979; Menichetti et al, 1994; Harousseau et al, 2000).

Oral Prophylaxis. A study of fluconazole vs. high-dose oral amphotericin B (2 grams in four divided doses) in a large population of neutropenic patients showed equivalent effects of both regimens in preventing deeply invasive candidiasis (Menichetti et al, 1994). Fluconazole, however, was better tolerated. In our opinion, the lack of patient compliance with oral amphotericin B and the toxicity of amphotericin B preclude the use of this agent as a viable prophylactic compound. In addition, the oral formulation of amphotericin B is unavailable in many areas.

Inhaled Prophylaxis. Aerosolized amphotericin B was not effective in the prevention of invasive aspergillosis among neutropenic patients in a large prospective, randomized, multicenter trial (Schwartz et al, 1999). The frequency of proven, probable, or possible invasive aspergillosis was 4% (10/227) in patients who received aerosolized amphotericin B, not significantly better than the 7% (11/155) incidence in patients who received no inhalation prophylaxis.

Intravenous Prophylaxis. Systemic low dose amphotericin B has been used (Bodey et al, 1994), but has never shown more efficacy than fluconazole, and has proven significantly more toxic. Lipid formulations of amphotericin B as prophylaxis have also been attempted. Kelsey and coworkers performed a randomized, double-blind placebo-controlled study of liposomal amphotericin B, 2 mg/kg three times weekly in neutropenic patients. The lipid drug was well tolerated, but there was no significant reduction in proven or suspected IFIs, in part due to the very low incidence of proven IFIs in both the placebo group (3.4%), and the lipid-drug group (0%) (Kelsey et al, 1999).

In an interim analysis of a prospective study, investigators found that antifungal prophylaxis with liposomal amphotericin B was no more effective than no prophylaxis (Uhlenbrock et al, 2001). The study was motivated by the observation of decreased incidence of IFIs and fungal-related mortality on an oncology ward following the practice of administering liposomal amphotericin B 1–1.5 mg/kg/two or three times weekly as compared to historical controls. Interestingly, the investigators attributed the original observation to the more aggressive diagnostic workup that included fungal antigen monitoring by ELISA and frequent CT scans.

Prophylaxis with Echinocandins. Given that echinocandins have excellent activity against *Candida* spp. and significant activity against *Aspergillus* spp., echinocandins represent a very reasonable option for prophylaxis. A multicenter trial comparing micafungin, an investigational echinocandin, and fluconazole has recently been reported. In this double-blind study, 822 patients undergoing HSCT were randomized to receive micafungin 50 daily or fluconazole 400 mg daily. Prophylaxis was more successful with micafungin. Although both drugs prevented candidiasis, micafungin had a greater impact on prevention of invasive aspergillosis, $p = 0.07$ (van Burik et al, 2002).

Recommendations Regarding Primary Prophylaxis
Systemic antifungal drugs are effective as primary prophylaxis and should be used in groups at high risk. In the case of neutropenia, prophylaxis applies to patients with acute leukemia (particularly acute myelogenous leukemia) and recipients of allogeneic bone marrow or stem cell transplants. Prophylaxis is recommended in patients receiving autologous bone marrow transplants when prolonged neutropenia (> 10 days) is anticipated.

Fluconazole is the treatment of choice, as significant effectiveness has been shown in high-risk groups (Goodman et al, 1992; Slavin et al, 1995). Fluconazole-resistant *Candida albicans* seldom causes disseminated infection in neutropenic patients (Marr et al, 1997). The emergence of non-*albicans Candida* species, with decreased susceptibility or intrinsic resistance to triazoles, as occasional causes of breakthrough fungemia in patients receiving fluconazole is a cause of concern. Examples are *C. krusei* and *C. glabrata* (Abbas et al, 2000; Paterson et al, 2001; Bodey et al, 2002).

The role of itraconazole in prophylaxis in neutropenic patients is unclear. The main reason to choose itraconazole over fluconazole is itraconazole's activity against *Aspergillus* spp. Given the problems with absorption, tolerability of the liquid form, and drug interactions, itraconazole may soon be superseded by voriconazole and the echinocandins.

Voriconazole has not been tested as a purely prophylactic agent, but highly encouraging results of comparative trials with voriconazole vs. liposomal amphotericin B in high-risk patients with persistent febrile neutropenia (Walsh et al, 2002) and voriconazole vs. "standard treatment" for invasive aspergillosis (Herbrecht et al, 2002a) make voriconazole a very attractive option, However, the use of voriconazole as a prophylactic agent remains investigational. Carefully designed studies are necessary to assess its benefits in this setting.

Echinocandins, the newest class of antifungal drugs, offer great promise as prophylactic agents. They have excellent activity against fluconazole-susceptible and resistant *Candida* species (Villanueva et al, 2001) and also activity against *Aspergillus* (Maertens et al, 2002) and *Pneumocystis carinii* (Ito et al, 2000). The role of these agents in antifungal prophylaxis remains undefined at this point, although initial data are promising (van Burik et al, 2002).

Secondary Prophylaxis of Invasive Fungal Infections

A patient may be treated successfully for an IFI and still require further myelosuppressive chemotherapy or a stem cell transplant. The ultimate objective is to successfully treat the patient's neoplastic disease while preventing breakthrough fungal infection. For example, the feasibility of continued chemotherapy in the presence of chronic disseminated candidiasis (hepatosplenic candidiasis) is addressed below.

In the case of aspergillosis, Karp and coworkers demonstrated that aggressive antifungal therapy (during the neutropenia induced by subsequent courses of chemotherapy) prevented exacerbation or recurrence of invasive aspergillosis in patients with acute leukemia (Karp et al, 1988). Similar strategies have been used in HSCT (Richard et al, 1993; Martino et al, 1994b; Martino et al, 1997). Most patients have been treated with prophylactic antifungal agents, either itraconazole (Martino et al, 1994b) or amphotericin B. Surgical resection of remaining foci of disease prior to myeloablation has been used, but it does not seem to be indispensable (Michailov et al, 1996; Martino et al, 1997). The largest published systematic study (a retrospective case series) reported on 48 patients with documented or probable invasive aspergillosis prior to marrow transplantation (Offner et al, 1998). Twenty patients had undergone surgical resection. Sixteen of the 48 patients (33%) had a relapse, at a median of 15 days af-

ter the transplant (range 0–120 days). Patients receiving prophylaxis with an absorbable or intravenous antifungal drug had fewer relapses than those not receiving prophylaxis (28% vs. 57%, respectively). Given the collective experiences, the use of secondary antifungal prophylaxis is mandatory in the setting of aspergillosis and ongoing chemotherapy. Voriconazole should be considered the drug of choice in this situation based on the results of prophylactic and therapeutic trials with this agent (Herbrecht et al, 2002a; Walsh et al, 2002). Transplantation or a course of potentially curative antineoplastic therapy need not be postponed. In addition, surgical resection of an isolated pulmonary lesion may be highly beneficial.

EMPIRICAL ANTIFUNGAL THERAPY

The use of empirical antifungal therapy in the presence of persistent or recurrent fever during neutropenia is the last step in an attempt to prevent morbidity and mortality secondary to IFI before a definitive diagnosis is established (Table 29–2). While the majority of neutropenic patients with persistent fever do not have an occult fungal infection, the proportion of patients who do have an IFI increases steadily with duration of neutropenia (Gerson et al, 1984). At some point the risk of not administering effective antifungal therapy outweighs the risks associated with the toxicity of the drug. Empirical treatment should then be started. Hopefully, the availability of newer, less toxic agents should alter this balance and allow earlier intervention.

The evidence supporting the empirical addition of antifungal agents in persistently febrile neutropenic patients is less than optimal but reflects the state of the art of antifungal therapy at the time. Two randomized studies compared antifungal therapy against no therapy in the setting of persistent fever during neutropenia (Pizzo et al, 1982; EORTC, 1989). Both studies were performed when CT of the chest was used less frequently and before the widespread use of fluconazole prophylaxis and hematopoietic growth factor support. Both studies are limited by a small sample size. In the study by Pizzo and colleagues, 50 patients with persistent fever and neutropenia after 7 days of broad spectrum antibiotics were randomized to one of three treatments: discontinuing antibiotics and reevaluating, continuing the same regimen, or adding amphotericin B deoxycholate 0.5 mg/kg/day until resolution of fever and neutropenia. Several results of this study deserve emphasis. Deep-seated fungal infections or esophageal candidiasis were documented in 6% (1 of 18) of patients who received amphotericin B and 23% (7 of 32) of patients who did not. Two deaths caused by fungal infection occurred in patients who did not receive amphotericin B and one in the amphotericin B treated

TABLE 29–2. *Multicenter Randomized Trials of Empirical Antifungal Therapy in Persistently Febrile Neutropenic Patients*

Study	Viscoli et al, 1996	Prentice et al, 1997	White et al, 1998	Walsh et al, 1999b	Winston et al, 2000	Wingard et al, 2000	Boogaerts et al, 2001	Walsh et al, 2002
Compared	Fluconazole vs. AmphoB	L-AMB1 and L-AMB3 vs. AmphoB	ABCD vs. AmphoB	Ambisome vs. AmphoB	Fluconazole vs. AmphoB	Ambisome (L-AMB3 and L-AMB5) vs. AmphoB lipid complex	Itraconazole vs. AmphoB	Voriconazole vs. liposomal AmphoB
Endpoint(s)	Success: defervescence and survival 30 days from randomization in absence of modification of the antifungal/antibiotic regimen. Failure: death within 30 days, persistent fever, or any modification of treatment after randomization	1. Safety 2. Defervescence without breakthrough	Composite endpoint: Success is defined by all of: 1. Survival .7 days after ending Rx1. 2. No breakthrough fungal infection 3. No discontinuation of study drug 4. Lack of fever on the day of discontinuation of Rx	Composite endpoint: Success defined by all of: 1. No breakthrough fungal infection 2. Survival .7 days after ending Rx 3. No discontinuation of study drug 4. Resolution of fever during neutropenia 5. Successful Rx of baseline fungal infection	Composite endpoint: Unsatisfactory response defined if any of: 1. Persistent fever 2. New or progressive fungal infection 3. Change in anti-fungal 4. Discontinuation of the drug due to toxicity 5. Withdrawal 6. Death	Composite endpoint: Success defined by all of: 1. Fever resolution during neutropenia 2. Improvement/cure of baseline fungal infection 3. No breakthrough fungal infections 4. No death 5. No discontinuation of study drug due to toxicity 6. No administration of an alternative antifungal agent	Success: defervescence and recovery from neutropenia. Failure: break-through fungal infection, death, failure to defervesce, change in therapy Further outcome analysis using composite endpoint, similar result	Composite endpoint: Success defined by all of: 1. No breakthrough fungal infection 2. Survival .7 days after ending Rx 3. No discontinuation of study drug 4. Resolution of fever during neutropenia 5. Successful Rx of baseline fungal infection
Design	Open, randomized, multicenter	Open, randomized, multicenter	Randomized, double-blind, multicenter	Randomized, double-blind, multicenter equivalence study	Open label, randomized, multicenter	Randomized, double-blind, multicenter	Open-label, randomized, multicenter, equivalence trial	Randomized (stratified), open-label, multicenter equivalence study
Number of patients (n evaluable)	114 (112)	338 (335)	213 (193)	702 (687)	322 (317)	250 (244)	384 (360)	849 (837)
Duration of Neutropenia	Not reported	Not reported	Not reported		6 vs. 7.5		7 vs. 7 before study, 10 vs. 8 during study	19 vs. 18 (high risk) 13 vs. 12 (low risk)
Time of F&N before Rx	≥ 4 days	≥ 4 days	≥ 3 days	≥ 5 days	≥ 4 days	≥ 3 days	≥ 3 days	≥ 4 days

(continued)

TABLE 29–2. *Multicenter Randomized Trials of Empirical Antifungal Therapy in Persistently Febrile Neutropenic Patients (Continued)*

Study	Viscoli et al, 1996	Prentice et al, 1997	White et al, 1998	Walsh et al, 1999b	Winston et al, 2000	Wingard et al, 2000	Boogaerts et al, 2001	Walsh et al, 2002
Invasive Fungal Infection								
Initial		5 vs. 0	NR	11/343 vs. 11/344	10/158 vs. 9/159	1 vs. 0 vs. 1	2 vs. 4	13 vs. 6
Breakthrough	0	2 vs. 2		11/343 vs. 27/344	6/158 vs. 7/159	3 vs. 2 vs. 3	5 vs. 5	8 vs. 21
Total		7 vs. 2	14/98 14/95	22/343 vs. 38/344	16/158 vs. 16/159	4 vs. 2 vs. 4	7 vs. 9	21 vs. 27
Total deaths	3 vs. 2	5 vs. 5 vs. 14	16 vs. 13	25 vs. 36	27 (17%) vs. 34 (21%)	5 vs. 2 vs. 11	19 (11%) vs. 25 (14%)	33 vs. 25
Fungal deaths	0	0	1 vs. 1	4 vs. 1	7 vs. 7	1 vs. 0 vs. 3	2 vs. 4	1 vs. 2
Success	Fluconazole 75%, AmphoB 66%	64 vs. 58 vs. 49 (L-AMB3, L-AMB1, AmphoB)	50% vs. 43%	50% vs. 49%	68% vs. 69%	40% vs. 42% vs. 33.3%	47% vs. 38%	26% vs. 31%
Conclusion	Fluconazole is less toxic than amphotericin B, and may be equally effective in subgroups of patients	Superior safety profile of liposomal amphotericin B	No difference in efficacy, amphotericin B more nephrotoxic, ABCD more infusion-related toxicity	Equivalent in terms of "successful response"	No difference in efficacy, fluconazole much less toxic	Similar efficacy, L-AMB less toxic	Equivalent in terms of successful response, itraconazole much less toxic	Voriconazole almost equivalent to ambisome overall, but superior in preventing breakthrough fungal infections and in toxicity
Comment	Insufficient power to detect a difference in fungal infections	More efficacy only in the L-AMB3 group	Insufficient power to detect a difference in fungal infections	Ambisome had significantly less proven fungal infections (11 vs. 27) and less toxicity	Very low incidence of aspergillosis and fluconazole-resistant *Candida*	The study centered primarily on toxicity	Most failures in itraconazole group due to switch because of persistent fever	Lower success rate than in previous studies secondary to short duration of neutropenia, that precluded condition (4) of the composite endpoint

AmphoB, amphotericin B; L-AMB, liposomal amphotericin B; ABCD, amphotericin B colloidal dispersion; F&N, fever and neutropenia.

group. These differences were not statistically significant but suggested a trend and led to a subsequent randomized trial by the EORTC. This second study randomized 132 patients after 3 days of neutropenic fever to receive either 0.6 mg/kg of amphotericin B or continue antibacterial drugs alone. Six IFIs (6.6%) were documented in the group receiving antibiotics alone and only one IFI (1.5%) in the group that received amphotericin B. No fungal-related deaths occurred in the amphotericin B group vs. 4 deaths in the antibiotics alone group. The greatest benefits of empiric amphotericin B accrued to those who received no antifungal prophylaxis ($p = 0.04$), those who were severely neutropenic ($p = 0.06$), those with a clinically documented infection ($p = 0.03$), and those > 15 years old ($p = 0.06$) (EORTC, 1989). The EORTC investigators concluded that early amphotericin B in granulocytopenic patients with continued fever despite broad-spectrum antibiotics may be beneficial. Moreover, the authors emphasized this approach would be most beneficial for selected subgroups of persistently febrile neutropenic patients. This observation was prescient of subsequent studies that also have demonstrated the benefits of this approach in the highest risk patients with prolonged neutropenia.

It is reasonable to question whether results of these two studies constitute adequate proof that all neutropenic patients with persistent fever should receive antifungal therapy (Bennett, 2000). The recognition that differences exist between neutropenic groups of patients regarding risk of IFI is well established (Walsh et al, 1994; Prentice et al, 2000). High-risk patients with prolonged neutropenia derive the greatest benefit from empirical antifungal therapy, and the specific circumstances of each individual patient should be considered before starting antifungal therapy. Recent Guidelines from the Infectious Diseases Society of America (Hughes et al, 2002) suggest 5–7 days of persistent fever in the neutropenic patient as the time to start empiric amphotericin B.

Advances in the field suggest that the decision may become considerably simplified owing to (1) the use of newer agents with a much more favorable benefit: toxicity profile, and (2) new approaches to diagnosis. The main reason that empirical antifungal therapy has been controversial is the high risk of amphotericin-related toxicity. For example, in a retrospective analysis of 239 patients treated with amphotericin B for suspected or proven aspergillosis, Wingard and coworkers reported that the creatinine level doubled in 53% of patients and 14.5% of the patients required dialysis (Wingard et al, 1999). If newer drugs have less toxicity with similar efficacy, the decision to administer them will be easier. Conversely, if a group of patients with significantly higher risk of developing IFI can be identified, even potentially toxic interventions may be justified.

During the last decade several large studies have compared the use of amphotericin B with alternative antifungal agents (Table 29–2). These trials have included more than 2800 patients, and have demonstrated that several antifungal agents can be used successfully as empirical therapy during neutropenic fever. The clinician can choose depending on risk factors and toxicity.

Fluconazole vs. Amphotericin B. Two multicenter randomized trials have compared fluconazole with amphotericin B as empirical treatment of neutropenic fever. As shown in Table 29–2, the first study that compared fluconazole 6 mg/kg/day (up to 400 mg/day) with amphotericin B 0.8 mg/kg, was terminated after an interim analysis showed excess toxicity in the amphotericin B group (Viscoli et al, 1996). Importantly, patients with abnormal X-rays, history of aspergillosis, or colonization with *Aspergillus* spp. were not eligible. In addition, patients were allowed to receive nonabsorbable antifungal prophylaxis before enrollment. There were no documented fungal infections in this trial. This finding together with the small sample size make it difficult to draw any firm conclusions, other than amphotericin B is more toxic than fluconazole. The authors emphasized that the population of febrile neutropenic patients is heterogeneous, and that there are probably subgroups for whom fluconazole may be as effective as amphotericin B.

More recently, Winston and coinvestigators conducted an open-label trial in which neutropenic patients with persistent fever after 4 days of antibiotics were randomized to receive either fluconazole 800 mg on day 1, followed by 400 mg daily (n = 158), or amphotericin B 0.5 mg/kg/daily (n = 159) (Winston et al, 2000). Patients were not eligible if they had been receiving systemic antifungal agents or if they were colonized by *Aspergillus*. The study used a composite endpoint to define satisfactory or unsatisfactory response (Table 29–2). Both regimens were similar in terms of rate of satisfactory responses, 68 and 69% of fluconazole and amphotericin B recipients, respectively. The failures in the fluconazole group were typically related to persistent fever, whereas in the amphotericin B group, most failures were due to toxicity. Only 4% of the patients in each group developed new fungal infections during therapy, and there were no differences in mortality. Toxicity was less in the fluconazole arm. The authors concluded that fluconazole may be appropriate empirical therapy in persistently febrile neutropenic patients at low risk for invasive aspergillosis.

Lipid Formulations of Amphotericin B

AMPHOTERICIN B DOLLOIDAL DISPERSION VS. AMPHOTERICIN B. A double-blind, randomized controlled trial of amphotericin B colloidal dispersion (ABCD, 4 mg/kg/day) compared to amphotericin B (0.8 mg/kg/day) in 213 patients with febrile neutropenia for 3 or more days was the first large study involving a lipid formulation of amphotericin B in this population (White et al, 1998) (Table 29–2). More than half the patients were receiving cyclosporin A or tacrolimus following an allogeneic stem cell transplant. A successful treatment outcome included all of the following criteria: survival for 7 days after the last dose of study drug; lack of suspected or documented fungal infection during the study and within 7 days of the last dose of study drug; no discontinuation of study drug because of adverse events; and lack of fever on the day of discontinuation of therapy. There was no difference in the therapeutic response between the two groups: 50% of the ABCD recipients and 43.2% of amphotericin B recipients were treated successfully. The causes for discontinuation of the study drug between arms were not different. Although ABCD was associated with significantly less renal toxicity, ABCD was associated with more frequent infusion-related toxicities, particularly hypoxemia. This study lacked the power to detect a difference in frequency of breakthrough fungal infections.

LIPOSOMAL AMPHOTERICIN B VS. AMPHOTERICIN B DEOXYCHOLATE. The NIAID Mycoses Study Group compared liposomal amphotericin B (L-AMB) (3 mg/kg/day) to amphotericin B deoxycholate (0.6 mg/kg/day) in a double-blind randomized trial that enrolled 689 patients (Walsh et al, 1999b). This noninferiority study defined success as a composite of five criteria: survival for 7 days after initiation of study drug; resolution of fever during the period of neutropenia; successful treatment of any base-line fungal infection; absence of breakthrough fungal infections during administration of the study drug or within 7 days after the completion of treatment; and absence of premature discontinuation of the study drug because of toxicity or lack of efficacy (Table 29–2). Similar outcomes were observed in both treatment groups based on the primary endpoint of success (50% vs. 49%), although there were significantly fewer proven IFIs in patients receiving L-AMB (3.2%) vs. conventional amphotericin B 7.8%) ($p = 0.009$) in the secondary analysis. This difference was independent of risk category, age, and antifungal prophylaxis. There was also a trend for improved overall survival in the L-AMB group. Moreover, infusion-related toxicity and nephrotoxicity were significantly less for the L-AMB treated patients. This study unequivocally established L-AMB as a reasonable alternative to conventional amphotericin B for the empirical management of fever and neutropenia. The trial was double-blind and adequately powered, and both the overall outcome and each of the components of the composite endpoint showed equivalence. Every exploratory subgroup analysis showed similar results. Given the significantly lower toxicity of L-AMB, the only reason to choose amphotericin B after this trial was cost.

Other investigators compared two different dosages of liposomal amphotericin B (1 mg/kg/day and 3 mg/kg/day, L-AMB1 and L-AMB3, respectively) to amphotericin B deoxycholate (1 mg/kg/day) in 204 children and 134 adults with neutropenic fever. The primary endpoint was safety, with efficacy as a secondary endpoint. Response was defined as a composite of defervescence for 3 consecutive days and continued deferverescence until the end of the study (recovery of neutropenia), no addition of another antifungal agent, and no breakthrough fungal infection (Prentice et al, 1997) (Table 29–2). Toxicity was more frequent in the amphotericin B group (24% of patients doubled their serum creatinine, compared with 10% and 12% in the L-AMB1 and L-AMB3 arms, respectively). Among 335 patients evaluated for efficacy, success was noted in 49% of the patients receiving amphotericin B, in 58% of L-AMB1 patients, and 64% of L-AMB3 pateints.

LIPOSOMAL AMPHOTERICIN B VS. AMPHOTERICIN B LIPID COMPLEX. In a large multicenter, randomized double-blind study comparing the safety of liposomal amphotericin B (L-AMB) at doses of 3mg/kg/day (L-AMB3) or 5 mg/kg/day (L-AMB5) with amphotericin B lipid complex (ABLC) at a dose of 5 mg/kg/day was initiated in 244 persistently febrile neutropenic subjects (Wingard et al, 2000) (Table 29–2). The results of this study were internally consistent, and showed that L-AMB was significantly less toxic than ABLC, both in nephrotoxicity (42% of the patients on ABLC experienced doubling of the serum creatinine, compared with 14.1% to 14.8% of the L-AMB-treated patients) and in infusion-related reactions. The efficacy analysis showed no significant differences between the three study arms. Composite success rates were ABLC, 33.3%; L-AMB3, 40%; and L-AMB5, 42%. The reasons for failure were similar for both drugs, although more patients discontinued ABLC because of drug toxicity. Eight patients developed breakthrough IFIs.

ITRACONAZOLE VS. AMPHOTERICIN B DEOXYCHOLATE. In an open-label, multicenter, randomized trial comparing i.v. and p.o. itraconazole to amphotericin B deoxycholate, 384 patients were enrolled into this study that was powered to show equivalence (Boogaerts et al, 2001) (Table 29–2). Adult neutropenic patients with fever that persisted > 3 days while receiving broad-spectrum antibiotics were eligible. Allogeneic stem cell transplant recipients were excluded. Other exclusion criteria included strong suspicion of fungal infections during previous episodes of neutropenia and current treatment with drugs known to interact with itraconazole. Itraconazole was administered i.v. at a dose of 200 mg q 12 hours for the first 48 hours followed by 200 mg/day from day 3 to day 14. Oral itraconazole solution could be substituted after day 7. Amphotericin B deoxycholate was given at a dose of 0.7–1.0 mg/kg/day. Most patients had received previous antifungal prophylaxis. The primary efficacy analysis utilized criteria similar to those of earlier studies (Prentice et al, 1997; Walsh et al, 1999; Winston et al, 2000). However, patients were considered successful if they defervesced at any time within 28 days of study drug discontinuation. A significantly favorable response (defervescence and recovery from neutropenia) was documented in 47% of the patients in the itraconazole group, and 38% of the patients in the amphotericin B group. Breakthrough fungal infections and mortality rates in the two groups were similar. The causes of failure were different in the two groups. For instance, 38% of patients in the amphotericin B group vs. 19% in the itraconazole group failed because of intolerance to the study drug, leading to discontinuation. Furthermore, 20 and 10 patients receiving itraconazole and amphotericin B, respectively, failed because fever persisted after the resolution of neutropenia. An additional 19 and 1 patient (s) receiving itraconazole and amphotericin B, respectively, failed because of fever leading to a change in antifungal regimen (Boogaerts et al, 2001).

VORICONAZOLE VS. LIPOSOMAL AMPHOTERICIN B. In the most recent published trial, 849 patients were randomized to receive either liposomal amphotericin B (L-AMB) or voriconazole after 96 hours of fever and neutropenia. Voriconazole was given at a dose of 6 mg/kg q 12 hours × 2 (loading) followed by 4 mg/kg/12 hours (maintenance); L-AMB was given at the previously proven dose of 3 mg/kg/day. Patients were stratified according to risk, with allogeneic stem-cell transplant and chemotherapy for relapsed leukemia considered high risk factors (Walsh et al, 2002) (Table 29–2). The endpoint was success or failure defined according to a composite endpoint that had been validated in previous trials (Prentice et al, 1997; Walsh et al, 1999b; Winston et al, 2000; Boogaerts et al, 2001). However, the definition of resolution of fever was more stringent than in previous trials. The study was designed as a noninferiority trial. The overall success rate was 26% for the voriconazole group and 30.6% for those receiving L-AMB (32% and 30% in the high-risk group). The relatively low success rate can be explained by the inclusion of defervescence (defined as temperature < 38°C for 48 hours prior to recovery from neutropenia) as part of the composite endpoint. As the median time to recovery from neutropenia was only 5.4–5.5 days, there was very little time available for a patient

to become and remain afebrile for 48 hours. If defervescence is excluded from the composite endpoint, the success rates become 82% in the voriconazole group and 86% in the L-AMB group. Although voriconazole narrowly failed to fulfill the criteria for noninferiority, there was an impressive difference in breakthrough fungal infections in favor of voriconazole (1.9% vs. 5.0%, $p = 0.02$). This difference was even more marked in the high-risk category (1.4% vs. 9.2%, $p = 0.003$). The overall response in the high-risk population (n = 286) also showed comparability in all criteria. As in other open-label studies, many more patients discontinued voriconazole (22 patients) than L-AMB (5 patients) for persistent fever. There was no difference in the proportion of patients discontinuing the study drug because of adverse effects. Moderate nephrotoxicity (serum creatinine elevation to $\geq 1.5 \times$ normal) was more common with L-AMB, but the frequency of severe (serum creatinine $\geq 2 \times$ baseline) nephrotoxicity was similar. Visual hallucinations were more frequent in patients who received voriconazole (4.3% vs. 0.5%). In summary, this study showed voriconazole to be comparable to L-AMB in overall therapeutic success and superior in reducing documented breakthrough fungal infections, particularly in high-risk neutropenic patients (Walsh et al, 2002).

Recommendations Regarding Empirical Antifungal Therapy

Several antifungal agents have been shown in well-designed clinical trials to be effective for the management of persistently febrile neutropenic patients. This strategy is best utilized in high-risk patients (i.e., patients with prolonged neutropenia). Fluconazole should generally not be used, except in lower risk patients (Bodey, 2000). Lipid formulations of amphotericin B, and the two triazoles, itraconazole and voriconazole, have emerged as viable alternatives to standard amphotericin B deoxycholate with similar efficacy and less toxicity. Each of these agents may be preferable under different circumstances.

Lipid formulations of amphotericin B are at least as effective as amphotericin B (Prentice et al, 1997; Walsh et al, 1999b; Wingard et al, 2000). In addition, there is some evidence that the initial high acquisition cost of L-AMB is offset by the savings associated with the prevention of renal toxicity (Cagnoni et al, 2000). Apart from their equivalent efficacy to amphotericin B deoxycholate, lipid formulations may also be superior for the treatment of established fungal infections in humans (Leenders et al, 1997; Leenders et al, 1998; Johnson et al, 2002).

The availability of an intravenous preparation of itraconazole allows this compound to be considered a reasonable alternative in febrile neutropenic patients. Itraconazole may be less effective than amphotericin B in animal models of aspergillosis (Berenguer et al, 1994). The potential cardiotoxicity of itraconazole has been recently emphasized (Ahmad et al, 2001), but this complication has not been shown to be a frequent problem in oncology patients (Boogaerts and Maertens, 2001). Drug interactions with itraconazole require careful monitoring, particularly cyclosporin A. Itraconazole has not been studied for empirical therapy in HSCT recipients.

In the randomized trial comparing voriconazole to L-AMB, voriconazole was significantly better at preventing breakthrough fungal infections, particularly in the high-risk group (Walsh et al, 2002). Although voriconazole is less nephrotoxic than L-AMB, voriconazole is more frequently associated with transient visual disturbances and hallucinations. These findings are consistent with those of the randomized trial of voriconazole vs. amphotericin B, in which voriconazole demonstrated a survival advantage over conventional amphotericin B as treatment of invasive aspergillosis (Herbrecht et al, 2002a). Neither voriconazole nor itraconazole have activity against Zygomycetes.

In summary, both L-AMB and voriconazole now can be considered first-line agents for the empirical management of high-risk patients with persistent fever and neutropenia. Itraconazole is an alternative when drug interactions are not an issue, but this drug remains to be studied in allogeneic HSCT patients.

TREATMENT OF ESTABLISHED FUNGAL INFECTIONS

The critical elements of successful management of invasive fungal infections complicating neutropenia are:

1. Early diagnosis (this element of management is reviewed earlier in this chapter)
2. Initiation of aggressive pharmacological treatment
3. Reversal of immunosuppression (including recovery from neutropenia, discontinuation or reduction of immunosuppressive agents such as corticosteroids, and administration of cytokines or granulocyte transfusions)
4. Surgical resection of lesions where feasible

Pharmacological Treatment: What Drugs To Use
A full review of antifungal agents and treatment indications is beyond the scope of this chapter and the reader should see the appropriate other chapters. Here the focus is on selected topics in candidiaisis and invasive aspergillosis that pertain specifically to neutropenic hosts.

Candidiasis
Chronic Disseminated Candidiasis (Hepatosplenic Candidiasis). Among the different clinical presentations of candidiasis, chronic disseminated candidiasis (hepatosplenic candidiasis) deserves special attention. Although the clinical manifestations characteristically appear when neutropenia resolves, this disease is a specific complication of cancer chemotherapy. While most cases are caused by *Candida albicans*, *C. tropicalis*, *C. glabrata* and *C. krusei* have also been reported (Sallah et al, 1999; Quintini et al, 2001). Several antifungal agents may be effective therapy for this condition: amphotericin B deoxycholate (Thaler et al, 1988; Walsh et al, 1995d; Sallah et al, 1999; Pagano et al, 2002), lipid formulations of amphotericin B (Lopez-Berestein et al, 1987) and fluconazole (Anaissie et al, 1991; Kauffman et al, 1991). At least one case has been treated successfully with caspofungin (Pagano et al, 2002). In general, fluconazole is the agent of choice if the patient is clinically stable (Rex et al, 2000). Duration of therapy seems to be the most important variable related to successful treatment. In a recent series of 23 leukemic patients with hepatosplenic candidiasis, the median duration of antifungal therapy was 112 days (range 42–175 days) (Sallah et al, 1999). Very rarely, splenectomy may be required (Ratip et al, 2002). Due to the chronicity of this infection, a dilemma often occurs between treating the underlying neoplastic disease and the fungal infection. Immunosuppression could lead to progression of candidiasis or breakthrough candidemia. However, cancer chemotherapy can proceed despite the presence of active hepatosplenic candidiasis as long as continuous antifungal treatment and careful monitoring are performed (Anaissie et al, 1991; Katayama et al, 1994; Walsh et al, 1995d). For example, among 17 patients treated for chronic disseminated candidiasis, all but 2 were treated for their neoplastic process without progressive disease (Walsh et al, 1995d). Premature discontinuation of antifungal therapy during cancer chemotherapy was the likely cause of progressive candidiasis in these 2 patients.

Aspergillosis
Voriconazole should be considered the treatment of choice for invasive aspergillosis in neutropenic patients. The strongest evidence comes from a recent large, open-label, randomized, multicenter trial that compared voriconazole (6 mg/kg/12 hours on day 1 of treatment, followed by 4 mg/kg q12 hours i.v. for at least 7 days, after which time patients could switch to oral voriconazole, 200 mg twice daily) with intravenous amphotericin B deoxycholate (1.0 to 1.5 mg per kilogram once daily) (Herbrecht et al, 2002a). Patients with intolerance to study drug or no response could be switched to "other licensed antifungal therapy" and continue to

be evaluable. Only patients with probable or definite invasive aspergillosis (Ascioglu et al, 2002) were included. The results were the same whether the analysis included the whole intention-to-treat or the "modified intention-to-treat" population. The proportion of neutropenic patients (45%) was the same in both groups. Overall, voriconazole proved superior to amphotericin B (successful outcome 49.7% vs. 27.8%, respectively), as well as in almost every subgroup analysis, including neutropenia, definite aspergillosis, and extrapulmonary infection. In the neutropenic patients, the success rate was 50.8% for voriconazole and 31.7% for amphotericin B. In addition, voriconazole had better survival at 12 weeks (70.8% vs. 57.9%), as well as fewer adverse events and fewer severe adverse events. The most common voriconazole-associated adverse event was transient and reversible visual disturbances, which occurred in 45% of the patients. These were described as blurred vision, altered visual/color perception, or photophobia.

The results of this important trial are in agreement with a previously reported observational study that showed good responses in 48% (14% complete response, and 34% partial response) among 116 immunocompromised patients who were treated with voriconazole for invasive aspergillosis (Denning et al, 2002). Results of the Herbrecht et al study are also consistent with in vitro studies (Espinel-Ingroff, 2001), in vivo animal studies (Chandrasekar et al, 2000; Kirkpatrick et al, 2000), and the randomized clinical trial that compared voriconazole with L-AMB for empirical treatment of fever in neutropenic patients (Walsh et al, 2002). Although voriconazole is now considered the agent of choice against invasive aspergillosis in neutropenic patients, it must be emphasized that the overall satisfactory response rate is only approximately 50%. Clearly new strategies are needed for the treatment of this disease.

Until recently, amphotericin B had been considered the drug of choice for the treatment of aspergillosis in neutropenic patients. The disappointing 27.8% success rate of amphotericin B deoxycholate demonstrated in the aforementioned randomized trial (Herbrecht et al, 2002a) is within the range previously reported (Patterson et al, 2000). Although the lipid formulations of amphotericin B are less nephrotoxic than conventional amphotericin B deoxycholate, the value of these agents in improving the response rate or overall survival in neutropenic patients with invasive aspergillosis is unclear. Lipid formulations of amphotericin B have been shown to be at least as effective as conventional amphotericin B deoxycholate in pulmonary aspergillosis in persistently neutropenic rabbits (Allende et al, 1994; Francis et al, 1994), and clinical studies are consistent with these findings (Leenders et al, 1998). Lipid formulations of

amphotericin B have been useful in many cases as salvage therapy (Walsh et al, 1998) and are appropriate for neutropenic patients who are intolerant of or refractory to voriconazole. Itraconazole, an older triazole, has also been used to treat invasive aspergillosis, particularly since the recent development and availability of an intravenous formulation. Using a regimen of i.v. itraconazole for 2 weeks followed by oral itraconazole for 12 more weeks, Caillot and colleagues reported an overall response rate of 48.5% in 31 immunocompromised patients with pulmonary aspergillosis (Caillot et al, 2001a). Sixty percent were neutropenic A recent study of caspofungin demonstrated that this echinocandin was an effective alternative for salvage therapy in patients with refractory aspergillosis, including those with neutropenia (Maertens et al, 2002).

Surgical Management

Surgical intervention is frequently a critical component of the management of invasive fungal infections, particularly during neutropenia. Acute invasive fungal rhinosinusitis during neutropenia should be considered a surgical emergency and treated aggressively with extensive debridement and appropriate antifungal agents (Drakos et al, 1993; Rizk et al, 2000). Blood vessel invasion by moulds often causes vascular thrombosis, tissue ischemia, and infarction of adjacent tissue. Rhinocerebral zygomycosis usually begins as an infection of the maxillary and ethmoid sinuses. Involvement of the ethmoid sinus may progress to invade the orbit, retroorbital region, cavernous sinus, and brain. A similar clinical picture may be caused by *Aspergillus*, particularly *A. flavus*, and *Fusarium*. Of note, Zygomycetes are not susceptible to voriconazole. Thus, treatment of rhinosinusitis in neutropenic patients should include a high dose of a lipid formulation of amphotericin B pending definitive identification of the pathogen.

For pulmonary mould infections, surgery has been used with diagnostic or therapeutic intent. Several series over the last few years have reported excellent results with early resection of localized pulmonary fungal lesions (Bernard et al, 1997; Caillot et al, 1997; Reichenberger et al, 1998; Salerno et al, 1998; Pidhorecky et al, 2000). The goal of early surgery is to reduce the burden of disease and prevent life-threatening hemoptysis. The indications for surgery in one series from France, which described 19 patients, were prevention of hemoptysis, definitive diagnosis, or resection of a residual mass (Bernard et al, 1997). As a rule, the indications for surgery for invasive pulmonary aspergillosis include resection of a large lesion threatening the great vessels, pericardium, or other mediastinal structures, hemoptysis from a large cavitary lesion, intractable pleuritic pain, and invasion of ribs and other chest wall structures. Surgery may also be indicated in

Aspergillus osteomyelitis, central nervous system disease, and sinusitis, particularly involving ethmoid sinuses, and primary cutaneous ulcerative aspergillosis.

Massive hemoptysis typically occurs during the recovery phase after chemotherapy, when the neutropenia has resolved and the platelet count is rising, and is often fatal (Albelda et al, 1985; Panos et al, 1988; Pagano et al, 1995; Gorelik et al, 2000). One study found that aspergillosis was the most common cause of fatal hemoptysis in patients with acute leukemia (Panos et al, 1988). Caillot and colleagues perform emergency surgery to prevent massive hemorrhage when the CT scan shows a fungal lesion that abuts the pulmonary artery or its branches (Bernard et al, 1997; Caillot et al, 1997; Caillot et al, 2001c). In their studies, the presence of multiple lesions, thrombocytopenia or neutropenia are not contraindications for surgery. The most common procedure is lobectomy, plus segmentectomy and angioplasty if required. These same investigators have reported improved prognosis of their patients over the years after the introduction of this approach; 16 of 19 patients (84%) were considered cured in one of their studies (Bernard et al, 1997).

Other groups in Europe (Baron et al, 1998; Reichenberger et al, 1998) and the United States (Salerno et al, 1998; Pidhorecky et al, 2000) have reported their experiences with surgical management of fungal infections during neutropenia. Although the series are retrospective and relatively small, several conclusions can be drawn. First, surgery can be performed in compromised patients with invasive aspergillosis. Although significant surgical complications occurred, including bronchial dehiscence, pleural aspergillosis, and prolonged chest tube drainage, the perioperative mortality was low (11%–14%) and the overall survival rates compare favorably with a series based on medical management alone. Second, experience of the surgeon is essential. In one series, 5 of 18 patients had a nonfungal process (bacterial pneumonia or abscess). Third, there is no clear consensus on the indications for surgery.

When evaluating the surgical series that report high cure and survival rates, apparently better than average, one must be aware that the patients who undergo surgery are not representative of all patients with invasive aspergillosis. In fact, in an analysis of 87 cases of invasive aspergillosis seen between 1982 and 1995 at the Royal Free Hospital and School of Medicine in London, investigators found that the mere presence of at least 1 lesion with imaging features suggestive of aspergillosis was associated with a better prognosis, irrespective of surgery (Yeghen et al, 2000). However, the authors emphasized that survival at 2 years was 36% among 37 patients treated surgically, 20% for 12 patients with unresected pulmonary lesions, and 5%

for 21 patients diagnosed only by isolation of *Aspergillus* from respiratory secretions.

Granulocyte Transfusions

Granulocyte transfusions may be useful for the treatment of fungal infections in neutropenic patients under certain conditions. The effectiveness of granulocyte transfusions in bacterial and fungal infections in neutropenic animal models was shown 25–30 years ago (Dale et al, 1974; Debelak et al, 1974; Ruthe et al, 1978). Results of several studies in neutropenic patients with infection during treatment for acute leukemia appeared to support the use of this intervention, either prophylactically or therapeutically (Graw et al, 1972; Boggs, 1974; Higby et al, 1975; Alavi et al, 1977; Herzig et al, 1977; Clift et al, 1978). Subsequently, the use of granulocyte transfusions declined during the 1980s because of questionable overall efficacy (Strauss et al, 1981; Winston et al, 1982) and the occurrence of some cases of severe toxicity, especially acute respiratory distress syndrome. Wright and coworkers initially reported severe reactions with acute dyspnea, hypoxemia, and interstitial infiltrates in 14 of 22 courses of granulocyte transfusions when amphotericin B was administered at the same time as the granulocytes, but only in 2 of 35 courses when concurrent amphotericin B was not given (Wright et al, 1981). Some hypothesized that amphotericin B caused aggregation of neutrophils and enhanced pulmonary leukostasis (Berliner et al, 1985). These severe pulmonary reactions were not confirmed by other investigators (Dana et al, 1981), and, in retrospect, appear to be explained by a combination of diverse causes, predominantly alloimmunization and infection (Dutcher et al, 1989). Although these reactions to granulocyte transfusions have been observed seldomly in more recent reports, most investigators recommend separating in time the administration of granulocytes and amphotericin B.

Over the last decade, several critical reviews and metaanalyses of the initial reports of granulocyte transfusions have been performed (Strauss, 1993; Vamvakas and Pineda, 1996; Vamvakas and Pineda, 1997) and their conclusions are very similar: *(1)* granulocyte transfusions have demonstrated efficacy in the treatment of uncontrolled bacterial infections during persistent neutropenia; *(2)* the data on fungal infections are less conclusive, mainly because of a smaller number of patients treated as well as the presence of confounding factors; *(3)* no benefit could be demonstrated in patients receiving <4–5×10^{10} granulocytes. The technical advances of the last 15 years, in particular the use of granulocyte colony-stimulating factor (G-CSF) to mobilize the granulocytes and the use of continuous flow apheresis techniques for harvesting them, offer potential benefits. These include the promise of much larger neutrophil numbers, 4–8 × 10^{10} PMNs/unit, or 2 to 10 times more than the yield that was obtained with corticosteroids alone in the past (Liles et al, 1997; Strauss, 1998; Stroncek et al, 2001), and higher efficacy.

Reflecting the renewed interest in granulocyte transfusions, several case series or phase I/II clinical trials of neutropenic patients treated with G-CSF–mobilized granulocytes have been reported over the last 5 years (Dignani et al, 1997; Peters et al, 1999; Price et al, 2000; Lee et al, 2001; Illerhaus et al, 2002). As anticipated, the combination of G-CSF plus dexamethasone resulted in higher yields than G-CSF alone. The leucocyte concentrates used in these studies contained ≥ 1 × 10^{10} neutrophils. A measurable response of the patient's absolute neutrophil count (ANC) has been observed. In addition, transfused neutrophils have persisted in the circulation with sustained increase in the ANC after 24 hours, and a cumulative effect of repeated transfusions on the ANC has been documented. The correlation between the administered dose and the increase in ANC has been poor, although in general doses > 2 × 10^9/kg have been associated with increments of the ANC > 2 × 10^3/μL (Price et al, 2000).

There are several case reports where granulocyte transfusions seem to have been life-saving during fungal infection, both in neutropenic patients (Barrios et al, 1990; Helm et al, 1990; Catalano et al, 1997; Samadi et al, 2001) and in others with abnormal neutrophil function like chronic granulomatous disease (Bielorai et al, 2000). A small study of 15 neutropenic patients with refractory IFI showed very good results (11 favorable responses), probably due to the high dose of neutrophils that elicited a mean increase in the ANC of the recipients of 396/μL 24 hours after the transfusion (Dignani et al, 1997).

Granulocyte transfusions may be life-saving when given to the appropriate hosts. At the NIH Clinical Center, selective indications include fungal infection unresponsive to optimal medical therapy, neutropenia that is bound to persist for more than 4 or 5 days, and reasonable chance of ultimate bone marrow function recovery. Our only prophylactic indication is for patients with previously documented IFIs who are to undergo profound, prolonged neutropenia. As approximately 40% of our neutropenic patients exhibit some degree of respiratory compromise, careful monitoring and adjustment of the rates and doses of granulocytes are warranted.

Recombinant Human Cytokines in the Management of Established Fungal Infections in Neutropenic Patients

While the preceding discussion has emphasized the importance of neutrophil recovery to control IFIs in neutropenic patients, it is logical to recommend the use of agents that have been shown in controlled studies to decrease the duration of neutropenia, even if their documented effect on clinically significant outcomes is unclear. The American Society for Clinical Oncology recently updated its recommendations for the use of hematopoietic colony-stimulating factors (granulocyte—CSF and granulocyte-macrophage—CSF) (Ozer et al, 2000). Regarding the therapeutic use of G-CSF or GM-CSF, the weight of the evidence suggests that the outcome of febrile neutropenia in general is not improved. Consequently, the recommendation is that colony-stimulating factors "should not routinely be used," but they may be considered for high-risk patients, including those with ANC < 100 μL, uncontrolled primary disease, pneumonia, hypotension, sepsis syndrome and IFI. We would strongly recommend the administration of recombinant G-CSF or GM-CSF to persistently neutropenic patients who have a proven IFI and are not receiving a recombinant colony-stimulating factor.

For more detailed information on these growth factors and their potential use as adjuvant therapy of fungal infections in nonneutropenic hosts, see a recent review (Root and Dale, 1999). Both G-CSF and GM-CSF accelerate myelopoiesis and decrease the duration of neutropenia, but they are different cytokines with different targets and immunomodulatory effects. Both in vitro and ex vivo, G-CSF, GM-CSF and M-CSF have been shown to increase the fungicidal action of phagocytes against *Candida* and *Aspergillus* in a variety of experimental systems (Roilides et al, 1995a; Roilides et al, 1995b; Gaviria et al, 1999b). GM-CSF also prevents dexamethasone suppression of killing of *A. fumigatus* conidia by bronchoalveolar and peritoneal macrophages in mice (Roilides et al, 1995b; Brummer et al, 2001; Brummer et al, 2002). Interferon gamma may be superior at enhancing the antifungal activity of phagocytes (Roilides et al, 1995a; Gaviria et al, 1999a).

There is some evidence that Th1 immune responses may be necessary for the optimal control of fungal infections (Brieland et al, 2001; Centeno-Lima et al, 2002). In this regard, immune interventions to polarize the immune response toward a Th1 type may be beneficial. Two of the main cytokines involved in this kind of response are IL-12 and interferon gamma. Studies in animal models show that the administration of interferon gamma has some protective effect in BALB/c mice challenged with *Aspergillus* conidia (Nagai et al, 1995). Evidence of Th1/Th2 dysimmunoregulation in hepatosplenic candidiasis (Roilides et al, 1998) and invasive aspergillosis (Roilides et al, 2001), characterized by increased circulating levels of IL-10, has been demonstrated in humans. These patterns of cytokine dysregulation provide a rationale for use of GM-CSF and interferon gamma, alone or in combination, for adjunctive treatment of persistent or progressive IFIs. For a detailed discussion on adjunctive antifungal therapy, see Chapter 10.

REFERENCES

Abbas J, Bodey G P, Hanna H A, Mardani M, Girgawy E, Abi-Said D, Whimbey E, Hachem R, Raad I. *Candida krusei* fungemia. An escalating serious infection in immunocompromised patients. *Arch Intern Med* 160:2659–2664, 2000.

Ahmad S R, Singer S J, Leissa B G. Congestive heart failure associated with itraconazole. *Lancet* 357:1766–1767, 2001.

Aisner J, Wiernik P H, Schimpff S C. Treatment of invasive aspergillosis: relation of early diagnosis and treatment to response. *Ann Intern Med* 86:539–543, 1977.

Aisner J, Murillo J, Schimpff S C, Steere A C. Invasive aspergillosis in acute leukemia: correlation with nose cultures and antibiotic use. *Ann Intern Med* 90:4–9, 1979.

Alavi J B, Root R K, Djerassi I, Evans A E, Gluckman S J, MacGregor R R, Guerry D, Schreiber A D, Shaw J M, Koch P, Cooper R A. A randomized clinical trial of granulocyte transfusions for infection in acute leukemia. *N Engl J Med* 296:706–711, 1977.

Albelda S M, Talbot G H, Gerson S L, Miller W T, Cassileth P A. Role of fiberoptic bronchoscopy in the diagnosis of invasive pulmonary aspergillosis in patients with acute leukemia. *Am J Med* 76:1027–1034, 1984.

Albelda S M, Talbot G H, Gerson S L, Miller W T, Cassileth P A. Pulmonary cavitation and massive hemoptysis in invasive pulmonary aspergillosis. Influence of bone marrow recovery in patients with acute leukemia. *Am Rev Respir Dis* 131:115–120, 1985.

Allende M C, Lee J W, Francis P, Garrett, K, Dollenberg H, Berenguer J, Lyman C A, Pizzo P A, Walsh, T J. Dose-dependent antifungal activity and nephrotoxicity of amphotericin B colloidal dispersion in experimental pulmonary aspergillosis. *Antimicrob Agents Chemother* 38:518–522, 1994.

Anaissie E, Kantarjian H, Jones P, Barlogie B, Luna M, Lopez-Berestein G, Bodey G P. *Fusarium*. A newly recognized fungal pathogen in immunosuppressed patients. *Cancer* 57:2141–2145, 1986.

Anaissie E, Kantarjian H, Ro J, Hopfer R, Rolston K, Fainstein V, Bodey G. The emerging role of *Fusarium* infections in patients with cancer. *Medicine (Baltimore)* 67:77–83, 1988.

Anaissie E, Bodey G P, Kantarjian H, David C, Barnett K, Bow E, Defelice R, Downs N, File T, Karam G, et al. Fluconazole therapy for chronic disseminated candidiasis in patients with leukemia and prior amphotericin B therapy. *Am J Med* 91:142–150, 1991.

Anaissie E J, Kuchar R T, Rex J H, Francesconi A, Kasai M, Muller F M, Lozano-Chiu M, Summerbell R C, Dignani M C, Chanock S J, Walsh T J. Fusariosis associated with pathogenic *Fusarium* species colonization of a hospital water system: a new paradigm for the epidemiology of opportunistic mold infections. *Clin Infect Dis* 33:1871–1878, 2001.

Anaissie E J, Stratton S L, Dignani M C, Summerbell R C, Rex J H, Monson T P, Spencer T, Kasai M, Francesconi A, Walsh T J. Pathogenic *Aspergillus* species recovered from a hospital water system: a 3-year prospective study. *Clin Infect Dis* 34:780–789, 2002.

Aquino S L, Kee S T, Warnock M L, Gamsu G. Pulmonary aspergillosis: imaging findings with pathologic correlation. *Am J Roentgenol* 163:811–815, 1994.

Archibald L K, McDonald L C, Addison R M, McKnight C, Byrne T, Dobbie H, Nwanyanwu O Kazembe P, Reller L B, Jarvis W R. Comparison of BACTEC MYCO/F LYTIC and WAMPOLE

ISOLATOR 10 (lysis-centrifugation) systems for detection of bacteremia, mycobacteremia, and fungemia in a developing country. *J Clin Microbiol* 38:2994–2997, 2000.

Arena F P, Perlin M, Brahman H, Weiser B, Armstrong D. Fever, rash, and myalgias of disseminated candidiasis during antifungal therapy. *Arch Intern Med* 141:1233, 1981.

Ascioglu S, Rex J H, de Pauw B, Bennett J E, Bille J, Crokaert F, Denning D W, Donnelly J P, Edwards J E, Erjavec Z, Fiere D, Lortholary O, Maertens J, Meis J F, Patterson T F, Ritter J, Selleslag D, Shah P M, Stevens D A, Walsh T J. Defining opportunistic invasive fungal infections in immunocompromised patients with cancer and hematopoietic stem cell transplants: an international consensus. *Clin Infect Dis* 34:7–14, 2002.

Baron O, Guillaume B, Moreau P, Germaud P, Despins P, De Lajartre A Y, Michaud J L. Aggressive surgical management in localized pulmonary mycotic and nonmycotic infections for neutropenic patients with acute leukemia: report of eighteen cases. *J Thorac Cardiovasc Surg* 115:63–68; discussion 68–69, 1998.

Barrios N J, Kirkpatrick D V, Murciano A, Stine K, Van Dyke R B, Humbert J R. Successful treatment of disseminated *Fusarium* infection in an immunocompromised child. *Am J Pediatr Hematol Oncol* 12:319–324, 1990.

Bennett J. Editorial response: choosing amphotericin B formulations—between a rock and a hard place. *Clin Infect Dis* 31:1164–1165, 2000.

Berenguer J, Diaz-Mediavilla J, Urra D, Munoz P. Central nervous system infection caused by *Pseudallescheria boydii*: case report and review. *Rev Infect Dis* 11:890–896, 1989.

Berenguer J, Buck M, Witebsky F, Stock F, Pizzo PA, Walsh T J. Lysis-centrifugation blood cultures in the detection of tissue-proven invasive candidiasis. Disseminated versus single-organ infection. *Diagn Microbiol Infect Dis* 17:103–109, 1993.

Berenguer J, Ali N M, Allende M C, Lee J, Garrett K, Battaglia S, Piscitelli S C, Rinaldi M G, Pizzo P A, Walsh T J. Itraconazole for experimental pulmonary aspergillosis: comparison with amphotericin B, interaction with cyclosporin A, and correlation between therapeutic response and itraconazole concentrations in plasma. *Antimicrob Agents Chemother* 38:1303–1308, 1994.

Berliner S, Weinberger M, Ben-Bassat M, Lavie G, Weinberger A, Giller S, Pinkhas J. Amphotericin B causes aggregation of neutrophils and enhances pulmonary leukostasis. *Am Rev Respir Dis* 132:602–605, 1985.

Bernard A, Caillot D, Couaillier J F, Casasnovas O, Guy H, Favre J P. Surgical management of invasive pulmonary aspergillosis in neutropenic patients. *Ann Thorac Surg* 64:1441–1447, 1997.

Bielorai B, Toren A, Wolach B, Mandel M, Golan H, Neumann Y, Kaplinisky C, Weintraub M, Keller N, Amariglio N, Paswell J, Rechavi G. Successful treatment of invasive aspergillosis in chronic granulomatous disease by granulocyte transfusions followed by peripheral blood stem cell transplantation. *Bone Marrow Transplant* 26:1025–1028, 2000.

Bodey G P. Fungal infections complicating acute leukemia. *J Chronic Dis* 19:667–687, 1966a.

Bodey G P, Buckley M, Sathe Y S, Freireich E J. Quantitative relationships between circulating leukocytes and infection in patients with acute leukemia. *Ann Intern Med* 64:328–340, 1966b.

Bodey G P. The effect of amphotericin B on the fungal flora in feces. *Clin Pharmacol Ther* 10:675–680, 1969.

Bodey G, Bueltmann B, Duguid W, Gibbs D, Hanak H, Hotchi M, Mall G, Martino P, Meunier F, Milliken S. Fungal infections in cancer patients: an international autopsy survey. *Eur J Clin Microbiol Infect Dis* 11:99–109, 1992.

Bodey G P, Anaissie E J, Elting L S, Estey E, O'Brien S, Kantarjian H. Antifungal prophylaxis during remission induction therapy for acute leukemia: fluconazole versus intravenous amphotericin B. *Cancer* 73:2099–2106, 1994.

Bodey G P. Management of persistent fever in the neutropenic patient. *Am J Med* 108:343–345, 2000.

Bodey G P, Mardani M, Hanna H A, Boktour M, Abbas J, Girgawy E, Hachem R Y, Kontoyiannis D P, Raad I I. The epidemiology of *Candida glabrata* and *Candida albicans* fungemia in immunocompromised patients with cancer. *Am J Med* 112:380–385, 2002.

Boggs D R. Transfusion of neutrophils as prevention or treatment of infection in patients with neutropenia. *N Engl J Med* 290:1055–1062, 1974.

Boogaerts M, Maertens J. Clinical experience with itraconazole in systemic fungal infections. *Drugs* 61(Suppl 1):39–47, 2001.

Boogaerts M, Winston D J, Bow E J, Garber G, Reboli A C, Schwarer A P, Novitzky N, Boehme A, Chwetzoff E, De Beule K. Intravenous and oral itraconazole versus intravenous amphotericin B deoxycholate as empirical antifungal therapy for persistent fever in neutropenic patients with cancer who are receiving broad-spectrum antibacterial therapy. A randomized, controlled trial. *Ann Intern Med* 135:412–422, 2001.

Boutati E I, Anaissie E J. *Fusarium*, a significant emerging pathogen in patients with hematologic malignancy: ten years' experience at a cancer center and implications for management. *Blood* 90:999–1008, 1997.

Bow E J, Shore T B, Kilpatrick M G, Scott B A, Schacter B. Relationship of invasive fungal disease and high-dose cytarabine plus etoposide containing remission-induction regimens for acute myeloid leukemia. *Blood* 78 (suppl):55A, 1991.

Bow E J, Laverdiere M, Lussier N, Rotstein C, Cheang M S, Ioannou S. Antifungal prophylaxis for severely neutropenic chemotherapy recipients: a meta analysis of randomized-controlled clinical trials. *Cancer* 94:3230–3246, 2002.

Brieland J K, Jackson C, Menzel F, Loebenberg D, Cacciapuoti A, Halpern J, Hurst S, Muchamuel T, Debets R, Kastelein R, Churakova T, Abrams J, Hare R, O'Garra A. Cytokine networking in lungs of immunocompetent mice in response to inhaled *Aspergillus fumigatus*. *Infect Immun* 69:1554–1560, 2001.

Brummer E, Maqbool A, Stevens D A. In vivo GM-CSF prevents dexamethasone suppression of killing of *Aspergillus fumigatus* conidia by bronchoalveolar macrophages. *J Leukoc Biol* 70:868–872, 2001.

Brummer E, Maqbool A, Stevens D A. Protection of peritoneal macrophages by granulocyte/macrophage colony-stimulating factor (GM-CSF) against dexamethasone suppression of killing of *Aspergillus*, and the effect of human GM-CSF. *Microbes Infect* 4:133–138, 2002.

Cagnoni P J, Walsh T J, Prendergast M M, Bodensteiner D, Hiemenz S Greenberg R N, Arndt C A, Schuster M, Seibel N, Yeldandi V, Tong K B. Pharmacoeconomic analysis of liposomal amphotericin B versus conventional amphotericin B in the empirical treatment of persistently febrile neutropenic patients. *J Clin Oncol* 18:2476–2483, 2000.

Caillot D, Casasnovas O, Bernard A, Couaillier J F, Durand C, Cuisenier B, Solary E, Piard F, Petrella T, Bonnin A, Couillault G, Dumas M, Guy H. Improved management of invasive pulmonary aspergillosis in neutropenic patients using early thoracic computed tomographic scan and surgery. *J Clin Oncol* 15:139–147, 1997.

Caillot D, Bassaris H, McGeer A, Arthur C, Prentice H G, Seifert W, De Beule K. Intravenous itraconazole followed by oral itraconazole in the treatment of invasive pulmonary aspergillosis in patients with hematologic malignancies, chronic granulomatous disease, or AIDS. *Clin Infect Dis* 33:e83–90, 2001a.

Caillot D, Couaillier J F, Bernard A, Casasnovas O, Denning D W, Mannone L, Lopez J, Couillault G, Piard F, Vagner O, Guy H. Increasing volume and changing characteristics of invasive pulmonary aspergillosis on sequential thoracic computed tomogra-

phy scans in patients with neutropenia. *J Clin Oncol* 19:253–259, 2001b.

Caillot D, Mannone L, Cuisenier B, Couaillier J F. Role of early diagnosis and aggressive surgery in the management of invasive pulmonary aspergillosis in neutropenic patients. *Clin Microbiol Infect* 7(Suppl 2):54–61, 2001c.

Catalano L, Fontana R, Scarpato N, Picardi M, Rocco S, Rotoli B. Combined treatment with amphotericin-B and granulocyte transfusion from G-CSF-stimulated donors in an aplastic patient with invasive aspergillosis undergoing bone marrow transplantation. *Haematologica* 82:71–72, 1997.

Centeno-Lima S, Silveira H, Casimiro C, Aguiar P, do Rosario V E. Kinetics of cytokine expression in mice with invasive aspergillosis: lethal infection and protection. *FEMS Immunol Med Microbiol* 32:167–173, 2002.

Chandrasekar P H, Gatny C M. Effect of fluconazole prophylaxis on fever and use of amphotericin in neutropenic cancer patients. Bone Marrow Transplantation Team. *Chemotherapy* 40:136–143, 1994.

Chandrasekar P H, Cutright J, Manavathu E. Efficacy of voriconazole against invasive pulmonary aspergillosis in a guinea-pig model. *J Antimicrob Chemother* 45:673–676, 2000.

Chim C S, Liang R, Wong S S, Yuen K Y. Cryptococcal infection associated with fludarabine therapy. *Am J Med* 108:523–524, 2000.

Clift R A, Sanders J E, Thomas E D, Williams B, Buckner C D. Granulocyte transfusions for the prevention of infection in patients receiving bone-marrow transplants. *N Engl J Med* 298:1052–1057, 1978.

Creger R J, Weeman K E, Jacobs M R, Morrissey A, Parker P, Fox R M, Lazarus H M. Lack of utility of the lysis-centrifugation blood culture method for detection of fungemia in immunocompromised cancer patients. *J Clin Microbiol* 36:290–293, 1998.

Curtis A M, Smith G J, Ravin C E. Air crescent sign of invasive aspergillosis. *Radiology* 133:17–21,1979.

Dale D C, Reynolds H Y, Pennington J E, Elin R J, Pitts T W, Graw R G Jr. Granulocyte transfusion therapy of experimental *Pseudomonas* pneumonia. *J Clin Invest* 54:664–671, 1974.

Dana B W, Durie B G, White R F, Huestis D W. Concomitant administration of granulocyte transfusions and amphotericin B in neutropenic patients: absence of significant pulmonary toxicity. *Blood* 57:90–94, 1981.

Dankner W M, Spector S A, Fierer J, Davis C E. *Malassezia* fungemia in neonates and adults: complication of hyperalimentation. *Rev Infect Dis* 9:743–753, 1987.

Debelak K M, Epstein R B, Andersen B R. Granulocyte transfusions in leukopenic dogs: in vivo and in vitro function of granulocytes obtained by continuous-flow filtration leukopheresis. *Blood* 43:757–766, 1974.

DeLone D R, Goldstein R A, Petermann G, Salamat M S, Miles J M, Knechtle S J, Brown W D. Disseminated aspergillosis involving the brain: distribution and imaging characteristics. *Am J Neuroradiol* 20:1597–1604, 1999.

Denning D W, Stevens D A. Antifungal and surgical treatment of invasive aspergillosis: review of 2,121 published cases. *Rev Infect Dis* 12:1147–1201, 1990.

Denning D W, Marinus A, Cohen J, Spence D, Herbrecht R, Pagano L, Kibbler C, Kcrmery V, Offner F, Cordonnier C, Jehn U, Ellis M, Collette L, Sylvester R. An EORTC multicentre prospective survey of invasive aspergillosis in haematological patients: diagnosis and therapeutic outcome. EORTC Invasive Fungal Infections Cooperative Group. *J Infect* 37:173–180, 1998.

Denning D W. Early diagnosis of invasive aspergillosis. *Lancet* 355:423–424, 2000.

Denning D W, Ribaud P, Milpied N, Caillot D, Herbrecht R, Thiel E, Haas A, Ruhnke M, Lode H. Efficacy and safety of voriconazole in the treatment of acute invasive aspergillosis. *Clin Infect Dis* 34:563–571, 2002.

Dietrich U, Hettmann M, Maschke M, Doerfler A, Schwechheimer K, Forsting M. Cerebral aspergillosis: comparison of radiological and neuropathologic findings in patients with bone marrow transplantation. *Eur Radiol* 11:1242–1249, 2001.

Dignani M C, Anaissie E J, Hester J P, O'Brien S, Vartivarian S E, Rex J H, Kantarjian H, Jendiroba D B, Lichtiger B, Andersson B S, Freireich E J. Treatment of neutropenia-related fungal infections with granulocyte colony-stimulating factor-elicited white blood cell transfusions: a pilot study. *Leukemia* 11:1621–1630, 1997.

Drakos P E, Nagler A, Or R, Naparstek E, Kapelushnik J, Engelhard D, Rahav G, Ne'emean D, Slavin S. Invasive fungal sinusitis in patients undergoing bone marrow transplantation. *Bone Marrow Transplant* 12:203–208, 1993.

Dupont B, Huber M, Kim S J, Bennett J E. Galactomannan antigenemia and antigenuria in aspergillosis: studies in patients and experimentally infected rabbits. *J Infect Dis* 155: 1–11, 1987.

Dutcher J P, Kendall J, Norris D, Schiffer C, Aisner J, Wiernik P H. Granulocyte transfusion therapy and amphotericin B: adverse reactions? *Am J Hematol* 31:102–108, 1989.

Einsele H, Hebart H, Roller G, Loffler J, Rothenhofer I, Muller C A, Bowden R A, van Burik J, Engelhard D, Kanz L, Schumacher U. Detection and identification of fungal pathogens in blood by using molecular probes. *J Clin Microbiol* 35:1353–1360, 1997.

EORTC International Antimicrobial Therapy Cooperative Group. Empiric antifungal therapy in febrile granulocytopenic patients. *Am J Med* 86:668–672, 1989.

Espinel-Ingroff A. In vitro fungicidal activities of voriconazole, itraconazole, and amphotericin B against opportunistic moniliaceous and dematiaceous fungi. *J Clin Microbiol* 39:954–958, 2001.

Ezdinli E Z, O'Sullivan D D, Wasser L P, Kim U, Stutzman L. Oral amphotericin for candidiasis in patients with hematologic neoplasms. An autopsy study. *JAMA* 242:258–260, 1979.

Francis P, Lee J W, Hoffman A, Peter J, Francesconi A, Bacher J, Shelhamer J, Pizzo P A, Walsh T J. Efficacy of unilamellar liposomal amphotericin B in treatment of pulmonary aspergillosis in persistently granulocytopenic rabbits: the potential role of bronchoalveolar D-mannitol and serum galactomannan as markers of infection. *J Infect Dis* 169:356–368, 1994.

Fraser D W, Ward J I, Ajello L, Plikaytis B D. Aspergillosis and other systemic mycoses. The growing problem. *JAMA* 242:1631–1635, 1979.

Gangneux J P, Lavarde D, Bretagne S, Guiguen C, Gandemer V. Transient *Aspergillus* antigenaemia: think of milk. *Lancet* 359: 1251, 2002.

Gaviria J M, van Burik J A, Dale D C, Root R K, Liles W C. Comparison of interferon-gamma, granulocyte colony-stimulating factor, and granulocyte-macrophage colony-stimulating factor for priming leukocyte-mediated hyphal damage of opportunistic fungal pathogens. *J Infect Dis* 179:1038–1041, 1999a.

Gaviria J M, van Burik J A, Dale D C, Root R K, Liles W C. Modulation of neutrophil-mediated activity against the pseudohyphal form of *Candida albicans* by granulocyte colony-stimulating factor (G-CSF) administered in vivo. *J Infect Dis* 179: 1301–1304, 1999b.

Gerson S L, Talbot G H, Hurwitz S, Strom B L, Lusk E J, Cassileth P A. Prolonged granulocytopenia: the major risk factor for invasive pulmonary aspergillosis in patients with acute leukemia. *Ann Intern Med* 100:345–351, 1984.

Gerson S L, Talbot G H, Hurwitz S, Lusk E J, Strom B L, Cassileth P A. Discriminant scorecard for diagnosis of invasive pulmonary aspergillosis in patients with acute leukemia. *Am J Med* 79:57–64, 1985a.

Gerson S L, Talbot G H, Lusk E, Hurwitz S, Strom B L, Cassileth

P A. Invasive pulmonary aspergillosis in adult acute leukemia: clinical clues to its diagnosis. *J Clin Oncol* 3:1109–1116, 1985b.

Glasmacher A, Hahn C, Molitor E, Sauerbruch T, Marklein G, Schmidt-Wolf I G H. Definition of itraconazole target concentration for antifungal prophylaxis. 40th Interscience Conference on Antimicrobial Agents and Chemotherapy, Toronto, Ontario. American Society for Microbiology, Abstr. 700, 2000.

Goldberg P K, Kozinn P J, Wise G J, Nouri N, Brooks R B. Incidence and significance of candiduria. *JAMA* 241:582–584, 1979.

Goodman J L, Winston D J, Greenfield R A, Chandrasekar P H, Fox B Kaizer H, Shadduck R K, Shea T C, Stiff P, Friedman D J, et al. A controlled trial of fluconazole to prevent fungal infections in patients undergoing bone marrow transplantation. *N Engl J Med* 326:845–851, 1992.

Gorelik O, Cohen N, Shpirer I, Almoznino-Sarafian D, Alon I, Koopfer M, Yona R, Modai D. Fatal haemoptysis induced by invasive pulmonary aspergillosis in patients with acute leukaemia during bone marrow and clinical remission: report of two cases and review of the literature. *J Infect* 41:277–282, 2000.

Gotzsche P C, Johansen H K. Meta-analysis of prophylactic or empirical antifungal treatment versus placebo or no treatment in patients with cancer complicated by neutropenia. *BMJ* 314:1238–1244, 1997.

Graw R G Jr, Herzig G, Perry S, Henderson E S. Normal granulocyte transfusion therapy: treatment of septicemia due to gram-negative bacteria. *N Engl J Med* 287:367–371, 1972.

Groll A H, Walsh T J. Uncommon opportunistic fungi: new nosocomial threats. *Clin Microbiol Infect* 7(Suppl 2):8–24, 2001.

Gualtieri R J, Donowitz G R, Kaiser D L, Hess C E, Sande M A. Double-blind randomized study of prophylactic trimethoprim/sulfamethoxazole in granulocytopenic patients with hematologic malignancies. *Am J Med* 74:934–940, 1983.

Guiot H F, Fibbe W E, van 't Wout J W. Risk factors for fungal infection in patients with malignant hematologic disorders: implications for empirical therapy and prophylaxis. *Clin Infect Dis* 18:525–532, 1994.

Harousseau J L, Dekker A W, Stamatoullas-Bastard A, Fassas A, Linkesch W, Gouveia J, De Bock R, Rovira M, Seifert W F, Joosen H, Peeters M, De Beule K. Itraconazole oral solution for primary prophylaxis of fungal infections in patients with hematological malignancy and profound neutropenia: a randomized, double-blind, double-placebo, multicenter trial comparing itraconazole and amphotericin B. *Antimicrob Agents Chemother* 44:1887–1893, 2000.

Helm T N, Longworth D L, Hall G S, Bolwell B J, Fernandez B, Tomecki K J. Case report and review of resolved fusariosis. *J Am Acad Dermatol* 23:393–398, 1990.

Herbrecht R, Letscher-Bru V, Bowden R A, Kusne S, Anaissie E J, Graybill J R, Noskin G A, Oppenheim Andres E, Pietrelli L A. Treatment of 21 cases of invasive mucormycosis with amphotericin B colloidal dispersion. *Eur J Clin Microbiol Infect Dis* 20:460–466, 2001.

Herbrecht R, Denning D W, Patterson T F, Bennett J E, Greene R E, Oestmann J W, Kern W V, Marr K A, Ribaud P, Lortholary O, Sylvester R, Rubin R H, Wingard J R, Stark P, Durand C, Caillot D, Thiel E, Chandrasekar P H, Hodges M R, Schlamm H T, Troke P F, de Pauw B. Voriconazole versus amphotericin B for primary therapy of invasive aspergillosis. *N Engl J Med* 347:408–415, 2002a.

Herbrecht R, Letscher-Bru V, Oprea C, Lioure B, Waller J, Campos F, Villard O, Liu K L, Natarajan-Ame S, Lutz P, Dufour P, Bergerat J P, Candolfi E. *Aspergillus* galactomannan detection in the diagnosis of invasive aspergillosis in cancer patients. *J Clin Oncol* 20:1898–1906, 2002b.

Herzig R H, Herzig G P, Graw R G Jr, Bull M I, Ray K K. Successful granulocyte transfusion therapy for gram-negative septicemia. A prospectively randomized controlled study. *N Engl J Med* 296:701–705, 1977.

Higby D J, Yates J W, Henderson E S, Holland J F. Filtration leukapheresis for granulocyte transfusion therapy. Clinical and laboratory studies. *N Engl J Med* 292:761–766, 1975.

Hopfer R L, Walden P, Setterquist S, Highsmith W E. Detection and differentiation of fungi in clinical specimens using polymerase chain reaction (PCR) amplification and restriction enzyme analysis. *J Med Vet Mycol* 31:65–75, 1993.

Hoy J, Hsu K C, Rolston K, Hopfer R L, Luna M, Bodey G P. *Trichosporon beigelii* infection: a review. *Rev Infect Dis* 8:959–967, 1986.

Hruban R H, Meziane M A, Zerhouni E A, Wheeler P S, Dumler J S, Hutchins G M. Radiologic-pathologic correlation of the CT halo sign in invasive pulmonary aspergillosis. *J Comput Assist Tomogr* 11:534–536, 1987.

Hughes W T, Armstrong D, Bodey G P, Bow E J, Brown A E, Calandra T, Feld R, Pizzo P A, Rolston K V, Shenep J L, Young L S. 2002 guidelines for the use of antimicrobial agents in neutropenic patients with cancer. *Clin Infect Dis* 34:730–751, 2002.

Huijgens P C, Simoons-Smit A M, van Loenen A C, Prooy E, van Tinteren H, Ossenkoppele G J, Jonkhoff A R. Fluconazole versus itraconazole for the prevention of fungal infections in haemato-oncology. *J Clin Pathol* 52:376–380, 1999.

Illerhaus G, Wirth K, Dwenger A, Waller C F, Garbe A, Brass V, Lang H, Lange W. Treatment and prophylaxis of severe infections in neutropenic patients by granulocyte transfusions. *Ann Hematol* 81:273–281, 2002.

Ito M, Nozu R, Kuramochi T, Eguchi N, Suzuki S, Hioki K, Itoh T, Ikeda F. Prophylactic effect of FK463, a novel antifungal lipopeptide, against *Pneumocystis carinii* infection in mice. *Antimicrob Agents Chemother* 44:2259–2262, 2000.

Jabado N, Casanova J L, Haddad E, Dulieu F, Fournet J C, Dupont B Fischer A, Hennequin C, Blanche S. Invasive pulmonary infection due to *Scedosporium apiospermum* in two children with chronic granulomatous disease. *Clin Infect Dis* 27: 1437–1441, 1998.

Jandrlic M, Kalenic S, Labar B, Nemet D, Jakic-Razumovic J, Mrsic M, Plecko V, Bogdanic V. An autopsy study of systemic fungal infections in patients with hematologic malignancies. *Eur J Clin Microbiol Infect Dis* 14:768–774, 1995.

Jantunen E, Piilonen A, Volin L, Parkkali T, Koukila-Kahkola P, Ruutu T, Ruutu P. Diagnostic aspects of invasive *Aspergillus* infections in allogeneic BMT recipients. *Bone Marrow Transplant* 25:867–871, 2000.

Jantunen E, Piilonen A, Volin L, Ruutu P, Parkkali T, Koukila-Kahkola P, Ruutu T. Radiologically guided fine needle lung biopsies in the evaluation of focal pulmonary lesions in allogeneic stem cell transplant recipients. *Bone Marrow Transplant* 29:353–356, 2002.

Johnson P C, Wheat L J, Cloud G A, Goldman M, Lancaster D, Bamberger D M, Powderly W G, Hafner R, Kauffman C A, Dismukes W E. Safety and efficacy of liposomal amphotericin B compared with conventional amphotericin B for induction therapy of histoplasmosis in patients with AIDS. *Ann Intern Med* 137:105–109, 2002.

Kahn F W, Jones J M, England D M. The role of bronchoalveolar lavage in the diagnosis of invasive pulmonary aspergillosis. *Am J Clin Pathol* 86:518–523, 1986.

Kappe R, Fauser C, Okeke C N, Maiwald M. Universal fungus-specific primer systems and group-specific hybridization oligonucleotides for 18S rDNA. *Mycoses* 39:25–30, 1996.

Karp J E, Burch P A, Merz W G. An approach to intensive antileukemia therapy in patients with previous invasive aspergillosis. *Am J Med* 85:203–206, 1988.

Katayama K, Koizumi S, Yamagami M, Tamaru Y, Ichihara T, Konishi M, Maekawa S, Seki H, Taniguchi N. Successful peritransplant therapy in children with active hepatosplenic candidiasis. *Int J Hematol* 59:125–130, 1994.

Kauffman C A, Bradley S F, Ross S C, Weber D R. Hepatosplenic candidiasis: successful treatment with fluconazole. *Am J Med* 91:137–141, 1991.

Kelsey S M, Goldman J M, McCann S, Newland A C, Scarffe J H, Oppenheim B A, Mufti G J. Liposomal amphotericin (AmBisome) in the prophylaxis of fungal infections in neutropenic patients: a randomised, double-blind, placebo-controlled study. *Bone Marrow Transplant* 23:163–168, 1999.

Kern W, Behre G, Rudolf T, Kerkhoff A, Grote-Metke A, Eimermacher H, Kubica U, Wormann B, Buchner T, Hiddemann W. Failure of fluconazole prophylaxis to reduce mortality or the requirement of systemic amphotericin B therapy during treatment for refractory acute myeloid leukemia: results of a prospective randomized phase III study. German AML Cooperative Group. *Cancer* 83:291–301, 1998.

Kirkpatrick W R, McAtee R K, Fothergill A W, Rinaldi M G, Patterson T F. Efficacy of voriconazole in a guinea pig model of disseminated invasive aspergillosis. *Antimicrob Agents Chemother* 44:2865–2868, 2000.

Kontoyiannis D P, Luna M A, Samuels B I, Bodey G P. Hepatosplenic candidiasis. A manifestation of chronic disseminated candidiasis. *Infect Dis Clin North Am* 14:721–739, 2000a.

Kontoyiannis D P, Wessel V C, Bodey G P, Rolston K V. Zygomycosis in the 1990s in a tertiary-care cancer center. *Clin Infect Dis* 30:851–856, 2000b.

Krick J A, Remington J S. Opportunistic invasive fungal infections in patients with leukaemia lymphoma. *Clin Haematol* 5:249–310, 1976.

Kuhlman J E, Fishman E K, Siegelman S S. Invasive pulmonary aspergillosis in acute leukemia: characteristic findings on CT, the CT halo sign, and the role of CT in early diagnosis. *Radiology* 157:611–614, 1985.

Lamy T, Bernard M, Courtois A, Jacquelinet C, Chevrier S, Dauriac C, Grulois J, Guiguen C, Le Prise P Y. Prophylactic use of itraconazole for the prevention of invasive pulmonary aspergillosis in high risk neutropenic patients. *Leuk Lymphoma* 30:163–174, 1998.

Lass-Florl C, Rath, P, Niederwieser D, Kofler G, Wurzner R, Krezy A, Dierich M P. *Aspergillus terreus* infections in haematological malignancies: molecular epidemiology suggests association with in-hospital plants. *J Hosp Infect* 46:31–35, 2000.

Lecciones J A, Lee J W, Navarro E E, Witebsky F G, Marshall D, Steinberg S M, Pizzo P A, Walsh T J. Vascular catheter-associated fungemia in patients with cancer: analysis of 155 episodes. *Clin Infect Dis* 14:875–883, 1992.

Lee J J, Chung I J, Park M R, Kook H, Hwang T J, Ryang D W, Kim H J. Clinical efficacy of granulocyte transfusion therapy in patients with neutropenia-related infections. *Leukemia* 15:203–207, 2001.

Leenders A C, Reiss P, Portegies P, Clezy K, Hop W C, Hoy J, Borleffs J C, Allworth T, Kauffmann R H, Jones P, Kroon F P, Verbrugh H A, de Marie S. Liposomal amphotericin B (AmBisome) compared with amphotericin B both followed by oral fluconazole in the treatment of AIDS-associated cryptococcal meningitis. *AIDS* 11:1463–1471, 1997.

Leenders A C, Daenen S, Jansen R L, Hop W C, Lowenberg B, Wijermans P W, Cornelissen J, Herbrecht R, van der Lelie H, Hoogsteden H C, Verbrugh H A, de Marie S. Liposomal amphotericin B compared with amphotericin B deoxycholate in the treatment of documented and suspected neutropenia-associated invasive fungal infections. *Br J Haematol* 103:205–212, 1998.

Lehmann P F, Reiss E. Invasive aspergillosis: antiserum for circulating antigen produced after immunization with serum from infected rabbits. *Infect Immun* 20:570–572, 1978.

Liles W C, Huang J E, van Burik J A, Bowden R A, Dale D C. Granulocyte colony-stimulating factor administered in vivo augments neutrophil-mediated activity against opportunistic fungal pathogens. *J Infect Dis* 175:1012–1015, 1997.

Loeffler J, Hebart H, Brauchle U, Schumacher U, Einsele H. Comparison between plasma and whole blood specimens for detection of *Aspergillus* DNA by PCR. *J Clin Microbiol* 38:3830–3833, 2000.

Lopez-Berestein G, Bodey G P, Frankel L S, Mehta K. Treatment of hepatosplenic candidiasis with liposomal-amphotericin B. *J Clin Oncol* 5:310–317, 1987.

Lundstrom T, Sobel J. Nosocomial candiduria: a review. *Clin Infect Dis* 32:1602–1607, 2001.

Maertens J, Demuynck H, Verbeken E K, Zachee P, Verhoef G E, Vandenberghe P, Boogaerts M A. Mucormycosis in allogeneic bone marrow transplant recipients: report of five cases and review of the role of iron overload in the pathogenesis. *Bone Marrow Transplant* 24:307–312, 1999a.

Maertens J, Verhaegen J, Demuynck H, Brock P, Verhoef G, Vandenberghe P, Van Eldere J, Verbist L, Boogaerts M. Autopsy-controlled prospective evaluation of serial screening for circulating galactomannan by a sandwich enzyme-linked immunosorbent assay for hematological patients at risk for invasive aspergillosis. *J Clin Microbiol* 37:3223–3228, 1999b.

Maertens J, Verhaegen J, Lagrou K, Van Eldere J, Boogaerts M. Screening for circulating galactomannan as a noninvasive diagnostic tool for invasive aspergillosis in prolonged neutropenic patients and stem cell transplantation recipients: a prospective validation. *Blood* 97:1604–1610, 2001.

Maertens J, Raad I, Petrikkos G, Selleslag D, Petersen B, Sable C, Kartsonis N, Ngai A, Taylor A, Patterson T, Denning D, and Walsh T. Update of the multicenter, noncomparative study of caspofungin in adults with invasive aspergillosis refractory or intolerant to other antifungal agents. Abstracts of the 42nd Interscience Conference on Antimicrobial Agents and Chemotherapy, San Diego, CA. American Society for Microbiology. Abstr. M-868; p. 388; 2002.

Marr K A, White T C, van Burik J A, Bowden R A. Development of fluconazole resistance in *Candida albicans* causing disseminated infection in a patient undergoing marrow transplantation. *Clin Infect Dis* 25:908–910, 1997.

Marr K A, Seidel K, Slavin M A, Bowden R A, Schoch H G, Flowers M E, Corey L, Boeckh M. Prolonged fluconazole prophylaxis is associated with persistent protection against candidiasis-related death in allogeneic marrow transplant recipients: long-term follow-up of a randomized, placebo-controlled trial. *Blood* 96:2055–2061, 2000.

Martino P, Gastaldi R, Raccah R, Girmenia C. Clinical patterns of *Fusarium* infections in immunocompromised patients. *J Infect* 28(Suppl 1):7–15, 1994a.

Martino R, Nomdedeu J, Altes A, Sureda A, Brunet S, Martinez C, Domingo-Albos A. Successful bone marrow transplantation in patients with previous invasive fungal infections: report of four cases. *Bone Marrow Transplant* 13:265–269, 1994b.

Martino R, Lopez R, Sureda A, Brunet S, Domingo-Albos A. Risk of reactivation of a recent invasive fungal infection in patients with hematological malignancies undergoing further intensive chemo-radiotherapy. A single-center experience and review of the literature. *Haematologica* 82:297–304, 1997.

Martino R, Subira M, Rovira M, Solano C, Vazquez L, Sanz G F, Urbano-Ispizua A, Brunet S, De la Camara R. Invasive fungal infections after allogeneic peripheral blood stem cell transplantation: incidence and risk factors in 395 patients. *Br J Haematol* 116:475–482, 2002.

Masterson K C, McGowan J E Jr. Detection of positive blood cultures by the Bactec NR660. The clinical importance of five versus seven days of testing. *Am J Clin Pathol* 90:91–94, 1988.

Menichetti F, Del Favero A, Martino P, Bucaneve G, Micozzi A, D'Antonio D, Ricci P, Carotenuto M, Liso V, Nosari A M. Preventing fungal infection in neutropenic patients with acute leukemia: fluconazole compared with oral amphotericin B. The GIMEMA Infection Program. *Ann Intern Med* 120:913–918, 1994.

Menichetti F, Del Favero A, Martino P, Bucaneve G, Micozzi A, Girmenia C, Barbabietola G, Pagano L, Leoni P, Specchia G, Caiozzo A, Raimondi R, Mandelli F. Itraconazole oral solution as prophylaxis for fungal infections in neutropenic patients with hematologic malignancies: a randomized, placebo-controlled, double-blind, multicenter trial. GIMEMA Infection Program. Gruppo Italiano Malattie Ematologiche dell' Adulto. *Clin Infect Dis* 28:250–255, 1999.

Michailov G, Laporte J P, Lesage S, Fouillard L, Isnard F, Noel-Walter M P, Jouet J P, Najman A, Gorin N C. Autologous bone marrow transplantation is feasible in patients with a prior history of invasive pulmonary aspergillosis. *Bone Marrow Transplant* 17:569–572, 1996.

Morgenstern G R, Prentice A G, Prentice H G, Ropner J E, Schey S A, Warnock D W. A randomized controlled trial of itraconazole versus fluconazole for the prevention of fungal infections in patients with haematological malignancies. U.K. Multicentre Antifungal Prophylaxis Study Group. *Br J Haematol* 105:901–911, 1999.

Nagai H, Guo J, Choi H, Kurup V. Interferon-gamma and tumor necrosis factor-alpha protect mice from invasive aspergillosis. *J Infect Dis* 172:1554–1560, 1995.

Navarro E E, Almario J S, Schaufele R L, Bacher J, Walsh T J. Quantitative urine cultures do not reliably detect renal candidiasis in rabbits. *J Clin Microbiol* 35:3292–3297, 1997.

Nguyen B D. Pseudallescheriasis of the lung and central nervous system: multimodality imaging. *Am J Roentgenol* 176:257–258, 2001.

Nucci M, Anaissie E. Cutaneous infection by *Fusarium* species in healthy and immunocompromised hosts: implications for diagnosis and management. *Clin Infect Dis* 35:909–920, 2002a.

Nucci M, Anaissie E. Should vascular catheters be removed from all patients with candidemia? An evidence-based review. *Clin Infect Dis* 34:591–599, 2002b.

Offner F, Cordonnier C, Ljungman P, Prentice H G, Engelhard D, De Bacquer D, Meunier F, De Pauw B. Impact of previous aspergillosis on the outcome of bone marrow transplantation. *Clin Infect Dis* 26:1098–1103, 1998.

Oren I, Haddad N, Finkelstein R, Rowe J M. Invasive pulmonary aspergillosis in neutropenic patients during hospital construction: before and after chemoprophylaxis and institution of HEPA filters. *Am J Hematol* 66:257–262, 2001.

Orr D P, Myerowitz R L, Dubois P J. Patho-radiologic correlation of invasive pulmonary aspergillosis in the compromised host. *Cancer* 41:2028–2039, 1978.

Ozer H, Armitage J O, Bennett C L, Crawford J, Demetri G D, Pizzo P A, Schiffer C A, Smith T J, Somlo G, Wade J C, Wade J L 3rd, Winn R J, Wozniak A J, Somerfield M R. 2000 update of recommendations for the use of hematopoietic colony-stimulating factors: evidence-based, clinical practice guidelines. American Society of Clinical Oncology Growth Factors Expert Panel. *J Clin Oncol* 18:3558–3585, 2000.

Pagano L, Ricci P, Nosari A, Tonso A, Buelli M, Montillo M, Cudillo L, Cenacchi A, Savignana C, Melillo L. Fatal haemoptysis in pulmonary filamentous mycosis: an underevaluated cause of death in patients with acute leukaemia in haematological complete remission. A retrospective study and review of the literature. Gimema Infection Program (Gruppo Italiano Malattie Ematologiche dell'Adulto). *Br J Haematol* 89:500–505, 1995.

Pagano L, Ricci P, Tonso A, Nosari A, Cudillo L, Montillo M, Cenacchi A, Pacilli L, Fabbiano F, Del Favero A. Mucormycosis in patients with haematological malignancies: a retrospective clinical study of 37 cases. GIMEMA Infection Program (Gruppo Italiano Malattie Ematologiche Maligne dell'Adulto). *Br J Haematol* 99:331–336, 1997.

Pagano L, Mele L, Fianchi L, Melillo L, Martino B, D'Antonio D, Tosti M E, Posteraro B, Sanguinetti M, Trape G, Equitani F, Carotenuto M, Leone G. Chronic disseminated candidiasis in patients with hematologic malignancies. Clinical features and outcome of 29 episodes. *Haematologica* 87:535–541, 2002.

Panos R J, Barr L F, Walsh T J, Silverman H J. Factors associated with fatal hemoptysis in cancer patients. *Chest* 94:1008–1013, 1988.

Passweg J R, Rowlings P A, Atkinson K A, Barrett A J, Gale R P, Gratwohl A, Jacobsen N, Klein J P, Ljungman P, Russell J A, Schaefer U W, Sobocinski K A, Vossen J M, Zhang M J, Horowitz M M. Influence of protective isolation on outcome of allogeneic bone marrow transplantation for leukemia. *Bone Marrow Transplant* 21:1231–1238, 1998.

Paterson P J, McWhinney P H, Potter M, Kibbler C C, Prentice H G. The combination of oral amphotericin B with azoles prevents the emergence of resistant *Candida* species in neutropenic patients. *Br J Haematol* 112:175–180, 2001.

Patterson T F, Kirkpatrick W R, White M, Hiemenz J W, Wingard J R, Dupont B, Rinaldi M G, Stevens D A, Graybill J R. Invasive aspergillosis. Disease spectrum, treatment practices, and outcomes. I3 Aspergillus Study Group. *Medicine (Baltimore)* 79:250–260, 2000.

Peters C, Minkov M, Matthes-Martin S, Potschger U, Witt V, Mann G, Hocker P, Worel N, Stary J, Klingebiel T, Gadner H. Leucocyte transfusions from rhG-CSF or prednisolone stimulated donors for treatment of severe infections in immunocompromised neutropenic patients. *Br J Haematol* 106:689–696, 1999.

Pidhorecky I, Urschel J, Anderson T. Resection of invasive pulmonary aspergillosis in immunocompromised patients. *Ann Surg Oncol* 7:312–317, 2000.

Pizzo P A, Robichaud K J, Gill F A, Witebsky F G. Empiric antibiotic and antifungal therapy for cancer patients with prolonged fever and granulocytopenia. *Am J Med* 72:101–111, 1982.

Prentice H G, Hann I M, Herbrecht R, Aoun M, Kvaloy S, Catovsky D, Pinkerton C R, Schey S A, Jacobs F, Oakhill A, Stevens R F, Darbyshire P J, Gibson B E. A randomized comparison of liposomal versus conventional amphotericin B for the treatment of pyrexia of unknown origin in neutropenic patients. *Br J Haematol* 98:711–718, 1997.

Prentice H G, Kibbler C C, Prentice A G. Towards a targeted, risk-based, antifungal strategy in neutropenic patients. *Br J Haematol* 110:273–284, 2000.

Price T H, Bowden R A, Boeckh M, Bux J, Nelson K, Liles W C, Dale D C. Phase I/II trial of neutrophil transfusions from donors stimulated with G-CSF and dexamethasone for treatment of patients with infections in hematopoietic stem cell transplantation. *Blood* 95:3302–3309, 2000.

Quintini G, Barbera V, Gambino R, Spadola V, Minardi V, Mariani G. Successful treatment of hepatosplenic candidiasis in an elderly patient with acute myeloid leukemia using liposomal daunorubicin and fluconazole. *Haematologica* 86:E18, 2001.

Ratip S, Odabasi Z, Karti S, Cetiner M, Yegen C, Cerikcioglu N, Bayik M, Korten V. Clinical microbiological case: chronic disseminated candidiasis unresponsive to treatment. *Clin Microbiol Infect* 8:442–444, 2002.

Reichenberger F, Habicht J, Kaim A, Dalquen P, Bernet F, Schlapfer R, Stulz P, Perruchoud A P, Tichelli A, Gratwohl A, Tamm M. Lung resection for invasive pulmonary aspergillosis in neutropenic patients with hematologic diseases. *Am J Respir Crit Care Med* 158:885–890, 1998.

Reichenberger F, Habicht J, Matt P, Frei R, Soler M, Bolliger C T,

Dalquen P, Gratwohl A, Tamm M. Diagnostic yield of bronchoscopy in histologically proven invasive pulmonary aspergillosis. *Bone Marrow Transplant* 24:1195–1199, 1999.

Reiss E, Lehmann P F. Galactomannan antigenemia in invasive aspergillosis. *Infect Immun* 25:357–365, 1979.

Rex J H, Walsh T J, Sobel J D, Filler S G, Pappas P G, Dismukes W E, Edwards J E. Practice guidelines for the treatment of candidiasis. Infectious Diseases Society of America. *Clin Infect Dis* 30:662–678, 2000.

Rex J H, Anaissie E J, Boutati E, Estey E, Kantarjian H. Systemic antifungal prophylaxis reduces invasive fungal in acute myelogenous leukemia: a retrospective review of 833 episodes of neutropenia in 322 adults. *Leukemia* 16:1197–1199, 2002.

Rhame F S. Prevention of nosocomial aspergillosis. *J Hosp Infect* 18(Suppl A):466–472, 1991.

Ribaud P, Chastang C, Latge J P, Baffroy-Lafitte L, Parquet N, Devergie A, Esperou H, Selimi F, Rocha V, Derouin F, Socie G, Gluckman E. Survival and prognostic factors of invasive aspergillosis after allogeneic bone marrow transplantation. *Clin Infect Dis* 28:322–330, 1999.

Richard C, Romon I, Baro J, Insunza A, Loyola I, Zurbano F, Tapia M, Iriondo A, Conde E, Zubizarreta A. Invasive pulmonary aspergillosis prior to BMT in acute leukemia patients does not predict a poor outcome. *Bone Marrow Transplant* 12:237–241, 1993.

Rinaldi M G. Invasive aspergillosis. *Rev Infect Dis* 5:1061–1077, 1983.

Rizk S S, Kraus D H, Gerresheim G, Mudan S. Aggressive combination treatment for invasive fungal sinusitis in immunocompromised patients. *Ear Nose Throat J*, 79, 278–280, 282, 284–275, 2000.

Roilides E, Holmes A, Blake C, Pizzo P A, Walsh T J. Effects of granulocyte colony-stimulating factor and interferon-gamma on antifungal activity of human polymorphonuclear neutrophils against pseudohyphae of different medically important *Candida* species. *J Leukoc Biol* 57:651–656, 1995a.

Roilides E, Sein T, Holmes A, Chanock S, Blake C, Pizzo P A, Walsh T J. Effects of macrophage colony-stimulating factor on antifungal activity of mononuclear phagocytes against *Aspergillus fumigatus*. *J Infect Dis* 172:1028–1034, 1995b.

Roilides E, Sein T, Schaufele R, Chanock S J, Walsh T J. Increased serum concentrations of interleukin-10 in patients with hepatosplenic candidiasis. *J Infect Dis* 178:589–592, 1998.

Roilides E, Sein T, Roden M, Schaufele R L, Walsh T J. Elevated serum concentrations of interleukin-10 in nonneutropenic patients with invasive aspergillosis. *J Infect Dis* 183:518–520, 2001.

Root R K, Dale D C. Granulocyte colony-stimulating factor and granulocyte-macrophage colony-stimulating factor: comparisons and potential for use in the treatment of infections in nonneutropenic patients. *J Infect Dis* 179(Suppl 2):S342–352, 1999.

Rotstein C, Bow E J, Laverdiere M, Ioannou S, Carr D, Moghaddam N. Randomized placebo-controlled trial of fluconazole prophylaxis for neutropenic cancer patients: benefit based on purpose and intensity of cytotoxic therapy. The Canadian Fluconazole Prophylaxis Study Group. *Clin Infect Dis* 28: 331–340, 1999.

Rusthoven J J, Feld R, Tuffnell P G. Systemic infection by *Rhodotorula* spp. in the immunocompromised host. *J Infect* 8:241–246, 1984.

Ruthe R C, Andersen B R, Cunningham B L, Epstein R B. Efficacy of granulocyte transfusions in the control of systemic candidiasis in the leukopenic host. *Blood* 52:493–498, 1978.

Salerno C T, Ouyang D W, Pederson T S, Larson D M, Shake J P, Johnson E M, Maddaus M A. Surgical therapy for pulmonary aspergillosis in immunocompromised patients. *Ann Thorac Surg* 65:1415–1419, 1998.

Sallah S, Semelka R, Kelekis N, Worawattanakul S, Sallah W. Diagnosis and monitoring response to treatment of hepatosplenic candidiasis in patients with acute leukemia using magnetic resonance imaging. *Acta Haematol* 100:77–81, 1998.

Sallah S, Semelka R C, Wehbie R, Sallah W, Nguyen N P, Vos P. Hepatosplenic candidiasis in patients with acute leukaemia. *Br J Haematol* 106:697–701, 1999.

Salonen J, Lehtonen O P, Terasjarvi M R, Nikoskelainen J. *Aspergillus* antigen in serum, urine and bronchoalveolar lavage specimens of neutropenic patients in relation to clinical outcome. *Scand J Infect Dis* 32:485–490, 2000.

Samadi D S, Goldberg A N, Orlandi R R. Granulocyte transfusion in the management of fulminant invasive fungal rhinosinusitis. *Am J Rhinol* 15:263–265, 2001.

Samonis G, Anatoliotaki M, Apostolakou H, Maraki S, Mavroudis D, Georgoulias V. Transient fungemia due to *Rhodotorula rubra* in a cancer patient: case report and review of the literature. *Infection* 29:173–176, 2001.

Schaffner A, Schaffner T. Glucocorticoid-induced impairment of macrophage antimicrobial activity: mechanisms and dependence on the state of activation. *Rev Infect Dis* 9(Suppl 5):S620–629, 1987.

Schaffner A, Schaffner M. Effect of prophylactic fluconazole on the frequency of fungal infections, amphotericin B use, and health care costs in patients undergoing intensive chemotherapy for hematologic neoplasias. *J Infect Dis* 172:1035–1041, 1995.

Schwartz R S, Mackintosh F R, Schrier S L, Greenberg P L. Multivariate analysis of factors associated with invasive fungal disease during remission induction therapy for acute myelogenous leukemia. *Cancer* 53:411–419, 1984.

Schwartz S, Behre G, Heinemann V, Wandt H, Schilling E, Arning M, Trittin A, Kern W V, Boenisch O, Bosse D, Lenz K, Ludwig W D, Hiddemann W, Siegert W, Beyer J. Aerosolized amphotericin B inhalations as prophylaxis of invasive *Aspergillus* infections during prolonged neutropenia: results of a prospective randomized multicenter trial. *Blood* 93:3654–3661, 1999.

Segal B H, Walsh T J, Liu J M, Wilson J D, Kwon-Chung K J. Invasive infection with *Fusarium chlamydosporum* in a patient with aplastic anemia. *J Clin Microbiol* 36:1772–1776, 1998.

Seyfartrg H J, Nenoff P, Winkler J, Krahl R, Haustein U F, Schauer J. *Aspergillus* detection in bronchoscopically acquired material. Significance and interpretation. *Mycoses* 44:356–360, 2001.

Slavin M A, Osborne B, Adams R, Levenstein M J, Schoch H G, Feldman A R, Meyers J D, Bowden R A. Efficacy and safety of fluconazole prophylaxis for fungal infections after marrow transplantation—a prospective, randomized, double-blind study. *J Infect Dis* 171:1545–1552, 1995.

Slevin M L, Knowles G K, Phillips M J, Stansfeld A G, Lister T A. The air crescent sign of invasive pulmonary aspergillosis in acute leukaemia. *Thorax* 37:554–555, 1982.

Strauss R G, Connett J E, Gale R P, Bloomfield C D, Herzig G P, McCullough J, Maguire L C, Winston D J, Ho W, Stump D C, Miller W V, Koepke J A. A controlled trial of prophylactic granulocyte transfusions during initial induction chemotherapy for acute myelogenous leukemia. *N Engl J Med* 305:597–603, 1981.

Strauss R G. Therapeutic granulocyte transfusions in 1993. *Blood* 81:1675–1678, 1993.

Strauss R G. Neutrophil (granulocyte) transfusions in the new millennium. *Transfusion* 38:710–712, 1998.

Stroncek D F, Yau Y Y, Oblitas J, Leitman S F. Administration of G—CSF plus dexamethasone produces greater granulocyte concentrate yields while causing no more donor toxicity than G—CSF alone. *Transfusion* 41:1037–1044, 2001.

Sugar A M. Mucormycosis. *Clin Infect Dis* 14(Suppl 1):S126–129, 1992.

Talbot G H, Huang A, Provencher M. Invasive *Aspergillus* rhinosinusitis in patients with acute leukemia. *Rev Infect Dis* 13:219–232, 1991.

Tang C M, Holden D W, Aufauvre-Brown A, Cohen J. The detection of *Aspergillus* spp. by the polymerase chain reaction and its evaluation in bronchoalveolar lavage fluid. *Am Rev Respir Dis* 148:1313–1317, 1993.

Thaler M, Pastakia B, Shawker T H, O'Leary T, Pizzo P A. Hepatic candidiasis in cancer patients: the evolving picture of the syndrome. *Ann Intern Med* 108:88–100, 1988.

Tikkakoski T, Lohela P, Paivansalo M, Kerola T. Pleuro-pulmonary aspergillosis. US and US-guided biopsy as an aid to diagnosis. *Acta Radiol* 36:122–126, 1995.

Travis L B, Roberts G D, Wilson W R. Clinical significance of *Pseudallescheria boydii*: a review of 10 years' experience. *Mayo Clin Proc* 60:531–537, 1985.

Treger T R, Visscher D W, Bartlett M S, Smith J W. Diagnosis of pulmonary infection caused by *Aspergillus*: usefulness of respiratory cultures. *J Infect Dis* 152:572–576, 1985.

Uhlenbrock S, Zimmermann M, Fegeler W, Jurgens H, Ritter J. Liposomal amphotericin B for prophylaxis of invasive fungal infections in high-risk paediatric patients with chemotherapy-related neutropenia: interim analysis of a prospective study. *Mycoses* 44:455–463, 2001.

Uzun O, Ascioglu S, Anaissie E J, Rex J H. Risk factors and predictors of outcome in patients with cancer and breakthrough candidemia. *Clin Infect Dis* 32:1713–1717, 2001.

Vamvakas E C, Pineda A A. Meta-analysis of clinical studies of the efficacy of granulocyte transfusions in the treatment of bacterial sepsis. *J Clin Apheresis* 11:1–9, 1996.

Vamvakas E C, Pineda A A. Determinants of the efficacy of prophylactic granulocyte transfusions: a meta-analysis. *J Clin Apheresis* 12:74–81, 1997.

van Burik J, Ratanatharathorn V, Lipton J, Miller C B, Bunin N, Walsh T J. Randomized, double-blind trial of micafungin (MI) versus fluconazole (FL) for prophylaxis of invasive fungal infections in patients (pts) undergoing hematopoietic stem cell transplant (HSCT), NIAID/BAMSG Protocol 46. 42nd Interscience Conference on Antimicrobial Agents and Chemotherapy, San Diego, CA. American Society for Microbiology, Abstract: M-1238, p. 1401, 2002.

Varettas K, Taylor P C, Mukerjee C. Determination of the optimum incubation period of continuously monitored blood cultures from patients with suspected endocarditis or fungaemia. *Pathology* 34:167–169, 2002.

Verea-Hernando H, Martin-Egana M T, Montero-Martinez C, Fontan-Bueso J. Bronchoscopy findings in invasive pulmonary aspergillosis. *Thorax* 44:822–823, 1989.

Verweij P E, Latge J P, Rijs A J, Melchers W J, De Pauw B E, Hoogkamp-Korstanje J A, Meis J F. Comparison of antigen detection and PCR assay using bronchoalveolar lavage fluid for diagnosing invasive pulmonary aspergillosis in patients receiving treatment for hematological malignancies. *J Clin Microbiol* 33: 3150–3153, 1995a.

Verweij P E, Stynen D, Rijs A J, de Pauw B E, Hoogkamp-Korstanje J A, Meis J F. Sandwich enzyme-linked immunosorbent assay compared with Pastorex latex agglutination test for diagnosing invasive aspergillosis in immunocompromised patients. *J Clin Microbiol* 33:1912–1914, 1995b.

Villanueva A, Arathoon E G, Gotuzzo E, Berman R S, DiNubile M J, Sable C A. A randomized double-blind study of caspofungin versus amphotericin for the treatment of candidal esophagitis. *Clin Infect Dis*, 33, 1529–1535, 2001.

Viscoli C, Castagnola E, Van Lint M T, Moroni C, Garaventa A, Rossi M R, Fanci R, Menichetti F, Caselli D, Giacchino M, Congiu M. Fluconazole versus amphotericin B as empirical antifungal therapy of unexplained fever in granulocytopenic cancer patients: a pragmatic, multicentre, prospective and randomised clinical trial. *Eur J Cancer* 32A:814–820, 1996.

Wald A, Leisenring W, van Burik J A, Bowden R A. Epidemiology of *Aspergillus* infections in a large cohort of patients undergoing bone marrow transplantation. *J Infect Dis* 175:1459–1466, 1997.

Walsh T J, Hier D B, Caplan L R. Fungal infections of the central nervous system: comparative analysis of risk factors and clinical signs in 57 patients. *Neurology* 35:1654–1657, 1985.

Walsh T J, Bustamente C I, Vlahov D, Standiford H C. Candidal suppurative peripheral thrombophlebitis: recognition, prevention, and management. *Infect Control* 7:16–22, 1986a.

Walsh T J, Newman K R, Moody M, Wharton R C, Wade J C. Trichosporonosis in patients with neoplastic disease. *Medicine (Baltimore)* 65:68–279, 1986b.

Walsh T J, Merz W G. Pathologic features in the human alimentary tract associated with invasiveness of *Candida tropicalis*. *Am J Clin Pathol* 85:498–502, 1986c.

Walsh T J, Dixon D M. Nosocomial aspergillosis: environmental microbiology, hospital epidemiology, diagnosis and treatment. *Eur J Epidemiol* 5:131–142, 1989.

Walsh T J, Pizzo P A. Experimental gastrointestinal and disseminated candidiasis in immunocompromised animals. *Eur J Epidemiol* 8:477–483, 1992.

Walsh T J, Lee J W. Prevention of invasive fungal infections in patients with neoplastic disease. *Clin Infect Dis* 17(Suppl 2):S468–S480, 1993.

Walsh T J, Hiemenz J, Pizzo P A. Evolving risk factors for invasive fungal infections—all neutropenic patients are not the same. *Clin Infect Dis* 18:793–798, 1994.

Walsh T J, Francesconi A, Kasai M, Chanock S J. PCR and single-strand conformational polymorphism for recognition of medically important opportunistic fungi. *J Clin Microbiol* 33:3216–3220, 1995a.

Walsh T J, Garrett K, Feurerstein E, Girton M, Allende M, Bacher J, Francesconi A, Schaufele R, Pizzo P A. Therapeutic monitoring of experimental invasive pulmonary aspergillosis by ultrafast computerized tomography, a novel, noninvasive method for measuring responses to antifungal therapy. *Antimicrob Agents Chemother* 39:1065–1069, 1995b.

Walsh T J, Peter J, McGough D A, Fothergill A W, Rinaldi M G, Pizzo P A. Activities of amphotericin B and antifungal azoles alone and in combination against *Pseudallescheria boydii*. *Antimicrob Agents Chemother* 39:361–1364, 1995c.

Walsh T J, Whitcomb P O, Revankar S G, Pizzo P A. Successful treatment of hepatosplenic candidiasis through repeated cycles of chemotherapy and neutropenia. *Cancer* 76:2357–2362, 1995d.

Walsh T J, Hiemenz J W, Seibel N L, Perfect J R, Horwith G, Lee L, Silber J L, DiNubile M J, Reboli A, Bow E, Lister J, Anaissie, E J. Amphotericin B lipid complex for invasive fungal infections: analysis of safety and efficacy in 556 cases. *Clin Infect Dis* 26:383–1396, 1998.

Walsh T J, Groll A H. Emerging fungal pathogens: evolving challenges to immunocompromised patients for the twenty-first century. *Transpl Infect Dis* 1:247–261, 1999a.

Walsh T J, Finberg R W, Arndt C, Hiemenz J, Schwartz C, Bodensteiner D, Pappas P, Seibel N, Greenberg R N, Dummer S, Schuster M, Holcenberg J S. Liposomal amphotericin B for empirical therapy in patients with persistent fever and neutropenia. National Institute of Allergy and Infectious Diseases Mycoses Study Group. *N Engl J Med* 340:764–771, 1999b.

Walsh T J, Pappas P, Winston D J, Lazarus H M, Petersen F, Raffalli J, Yanovich S, Stiff P, Greenberg R, Donowitz G, Schuster M, Reboli A, Wingard J, Arndt C, Reinhardt J, Hadley S, Finberg R, Laverdiere M, Perfect J, Garber G, Fioritoni G, Anaissie E, Lee J. Voriconazole compared with liposomal amphotericin B for empirical antifungal therapy in patients with neutropenia and persistent fever. *N Engl J Med* 346:225–234, 2002.

White M H, Bowden R A, Sandler E S, Graham M L, Noskin G A, Wingard J R, Goldman M, van Burik J A, McCabe A, Lin J S, Gurwith M, Miller C B. Randomized, double-blind clinical trial of amphotericin B colloidal dispersion vs amphotericin B in the empirical treatment of fever and neutropenia. *Clin Infect Dis* 27:796–302, 1998.

Wingard J R, Merz W G, Saral R. *Candida tropicalis*: a major pathogen in immunocompromised patients. *Ann Intern Med* 91:539–543, 1979.

Wingard J R, Kubilis P, Lee L, Yee G, White M, Walshe L, Bowden R, Anaissie E, Hiemenz J, Lister J. Clinical significance of nephrotoxicity in patients treated with amphotericin B for suspected or proven aspergillosis. *Clin Infect Dis* 29:1402–1407, 1999.

Wingard J R, White, M H, Anaissie E, Raffalli J, Goodman J, Arrieta A. A randomized, double-blind comparative trial evaluating the safety of liposomal amphotericin B versus amphotericin B lipid complex in the empirical treatment of febrile neutropenia. L Amph/ABLC Collaborative Study Group. *Clin Infect Dis* 31:155–1163, 2000.

Winston D J, Ho W G, Gale R P. Therapeutic granulocyte transfusions for documented infections. A controlled trial in ninety-five infectious granulocytopenic episodes. *Ann Intern Med* 97:509–515, 1982.

Winston D J, Chandrasekar P H, Lazarus H M, Goodman J L, Silber J L, Horowitz H, Shadduck R K, Rosenfeld C S, Ho W G, Islam M Z. Fluconazole prophylaxis of fungal infections in patients with acute leukemia. Results of a randomized placebo-controlled, double-blind, multicenter trial. *Ann Intern Med* 118:495–503, 1993.

Winston D J, Hathorn J W, Schuster M G, Schiller G J, Territo M C. A multicenter, randomized trial of fluconazole versus amphotericin B for empiric antifungal therapy of febrile neutropenic patients with cancer. *Am J Med* 108:282–289, 2000.

Wirth F, Perry R, Eskenazi A, Schwalbe R, Kao G. Cutaneous mucormycosis with subsequent visceral dissemination in a child with neutropenia: a case report and review of the pediatric literature. *J Am Acad Dermatol* 36:336–341,1997.

Wright D G, Robichaud K J, Pizzo P A, Deisseroth A B. Lethal pulmonary reactions associated with the combined use of amphotericin B and leukocyte transfusions. *N Engl J Med* 304:1185–1189, 1981.

Yamada K, Shrier D A, Rubio A, Shan Y, Zoarski G H, Yoshiura T, Iwanaga S, Nishimura T, Numaguchi Y. Imaging findings in intracranial aspergillosis. *Acad Radiol* 9:163–171, 2002.

Yamakami Y, Hashimoto A, Tokimatsu I, Nasu M. PCR detection of DNA specific for *Aspergillus* species in serum of patients with invasive aspergillosis. *J Clin Microbiol* 34:2464–2468, 1996.

Yeghen T, Kibbler C C, Prentice H G, Berger L A, Wallesby R K, McWhinney P H, Lampe F C, Gillespie, S. Management of invasive pulmonary aspergillosis in hematology patients: a review of 87 consecutive cases at a single institution. *Clin Infect Dis* 31:859–868, 2000.

Yoo D, Lee W H, Kwon-Chung K J. Brain abscesses due to *Pseudallescheria boydii* associated with primary non-Hodgkin's lymphoma of the central nervous system: a case report and literature review. *Rev Infect Dis* 7:272–277, 1985.

Yu V L, Muder R R, Poorsattar A. Significance of isolation of *Aspergillus* from the respiratory tract in diagnosis of invasive pulmonary aspergillosis. Results from a three-year prospective study. *Am J Med* 81:249–254, 1986.

30

Fungal infections in blood or marrow transplant recipients

KIEREN A. MARR

Blood or marrow transplantation (BMT) has been used increasingly for therapy of hematological and non-hematological malignancies. Our understanding of the basic mechanisms by which transplantation of donor stem cells yields effective therapy of malignancies has evolved over the last few decades, with resultant changes in conditioning regimens and stem cell products influencing the risks for infectious complications. Perhaps one of the most important recent changes impacting infectious risks involves the introduction of nonmyeloablative, or toxicity-reduced transplant regimens. These regimens, which to date have been investigated primarily in people who are ineligible for standard myeloablative BMT because of medical conditions or age, employ lower doses of myeloablative conditioning therapy, with some regimens yielding very little neutropenia or gastrointestinal mucositis (Childs et al, 2000; Garban et al, 2001; Junghanss and Marr, 2002a; Junghanss et al, 2002b). Although the depth and duration of neutropenia may be dramatically reduced, these patients may have a protracted period of graft-vs.-host disease (GVHD). Graft-vs. host (GVH) effects result from infused donor-derived immune cells recognizing host cells, resulting in potentially beneficial antitumor effects and detrimental organ toxicities (GVHD). Thus, a certain degree of GVH may be desired in order to achieve graft vs. tumor effects. The major risk periods for fungal infections can thus occur both early and late after BMT—early risks are associated with myelosuppression and organ toxicities, and late risks are associated with GVHD and its therapies.

Recent studies have reported a trend toward late infections in both myeloablative and nonmyeloablative BMT recipients (Jantunen et al, 1997; Wald et al, 1997; Williamson et al, 1999; Baddley et al, 2001; Martino et al, 2001; Grow et al, 2002; Junghanss et al, 2002b; Marr et al, 2002c). Fungal infections, especially those caused by filamentous organisms, now occur predominantly during the GVHD period. The results of case-series and one case-control study published to date suggest that patients who undergo nonmyeloablative BMT

have fewer early bacterial infections associated with shorter periods of neutropenia, but retain significant risks for aspergillosis and candidal infections late after transplant, in association with late CMV infection and GVHD (Martino et al, 2001; Junghanss and Marr, 2002a; Junghanss et al, 2002b).

Time until engraftment, and severity of GVHD, both important factors influencing fungal infection risks, are predictable based on the stem cell product. Recipients of cord blood have higher risks for early fungal infections compared to recipients of marrow from HLA-matched related donors, largely because of low doses of stem cells and a prolonged period of myelosuppression (Marr et al, 2002b). Likewise, there have been reports that CD34-selection, a process performed with a goal of reducing relapse of malignancy, leads to increased risks for CMV and fungal infections in autologous BMT patients (Holmberg et al, 1999; Crippa et al, 2002). The severity of risks according to type of BMT is shown in Figure 30–1.

Infection risks are not stable, but are dynamic variables that evolve according to the time line of immune reconstitution and development of other posttransplant complications. Figure 30–2 diagrams risks for specific fungal infections according to time after transplant. Neutropenia and organ toxicities contribute to risks during the early time period, especially in recipients of myeloablative BMT (not shown on the diagram). Development of GVHD and delayed immune reconstitution dictate the severity of risks during the late time periods.

Table 30–1 lists the risk factors that have been associated with the development of candidal infections and filamentous fungal infections in BMT recipients. These risks may be related to the BMT recipient, type of BMT, or to complications that arise subsequent to transplant. Transplantation at an older age increases the risks for disseminated candidiasis (Goodrich et al, 1991) and aspergillosis (Morrison et al, 1993; Wald et al, 1997; Marr et al, 2002b). Type of stem cells transfused impacts the risks for early disease which appears to be primarily due to variable engraftment parameters

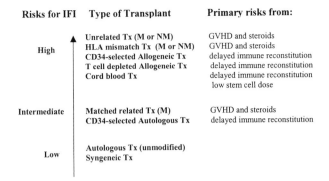

Risks for IFI	Type of Transplant	Primary risks from:
High	Unrelated Tx (M or NM) HLA mismatch Tx (M or NM) CD34-selected Allogeneic Tx T cell depleted Allogeneic Tx Cord blood Tx	GVHD and steroids GVHD and steroids delayed immune reconstitution delayed immune reconstitution delayed immune reconstitution low stem cell dose
Intermediate	Matched related Tx (M) CD34-selected Autologous Tx	GVHD and steroids delayed immune reconstitution
Low	Autologous Tx (unmodified) Syngeneic Tx	

FIGURE 30–1. Severity of risks for fungal infections according to type of BMT conditioning and stem cell product (Tx, transplant; M, myeloablative; NM, nonmyeloablative), (courtesy of M. Boeckh, Fred Hutchinson Cancer Research Center).

(Marr et al, 2002c). Other posttransplant complications, such as CMV infection and disease have been associated with high risks for subsequent candidiasis and aspergillosis (Marr et al, 2000c; Marr et al, 2002c). The results of most recent studies evaluating risks using multivariable modeling emphasize that the impact of many of these variables may be primarily due to receipt of high doses of corticosteroids (Baddley et al, 2001; Grow et al, 2002). Whether viral infections confer independent risks for subsequent fungal infection, or serve as a marker for severe immune suppression is currently unclear. Clearly the risks for fungal infections, both candidiasis and those caused by filamentous fungi, are not only increased by absolute neutropenia, but are impacted by lymphocyte-mediated immunity as well. Reconstitution of CD4+ T cells has been implicated in high risks for CMV and Epstein Barr virus (EBV) infections, and slow recovery at least partly explains the high risks observed in adult recipients of T-cell depleted

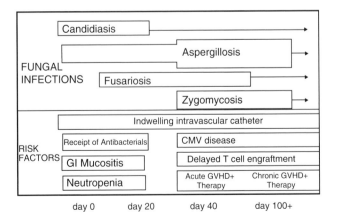

FIGURE 30–2. Time line of fungal infections and major corresponding risk periods and factors after myeloablative BMT. Day 0 is day of receipt of stem cell product.

stem cell transplants compared to children (Small et al, 1999). More recently, animal models have demonstrated that T cell immunity is important for regulating risks and outcomes of both candidiasis and aspergillosis (Cenci et al, 1997a; Cenci et al, 1997b; Cenci et al, 1998; Cenci et al, 1999; Cenci et al, 2000; Mencacci et al, 2001; Cenci et al, 2002). Accordingly, lymphocytopenia confers an increased risk for aspergillosis after non-T cell depleted BMT (Marr et al, 2002c), and full haplotype-mismatched BMT recipients may have increased risks for fungal infections (Williamson et al, 1999). One recent study of Aspergillus-specific T-cell responses in patients with invasive aspergillosis noted that favorable outcomes correlated with reconstitution of Th-1-type cellular immune responses (Hebart et al, 2002).

Finally, donor variables, such as CMV seropositivity, may impact risks for infection (Marr et al, 2002c; Nichols et al, 2002). Recent, unpublished studies have shown associations between donor polymorphisms within innate immune response genes and candidiasis post-BMT. Fungal infection risks are thus impacted by a composite of donor, host, and posttransplant complication variables. As larger cohorts of patients with infections are characterized, it may be possible to uncover the biological factors underlying each of these associations.

Recent data suggest that there may be different risks for different types of filamentous fungal infections. The observation that Zygomycete infections are most common late after BMT in people with severe GVHD might represent the propensity of these organisms to cause disease in people who have a history of prolonged corticosteroid use (Ribes et al, 2000). Risks for specific fungal infections are most certainly impacted by the host factors outlined, as well as microbial exposure and the propensity of each of these organisms to cause disease in a specific milieu. For this reason, elucidation of virulence properties of pathogenic fungi is a topic of increasing medical importance.

FUNGAL INFECTIONS: PATHOGENESIS AND THERAPY

As mentioned above, fungal infections in BMT patients are caused predominantly by Candida species and moulds; infections with other yeasts, such as Cryptococcus neoformans and dimorphic fungi, e.g., Histoplasma capsulatum, are notably infrequent, even in hyperendemic regions (Vail et al, 2002). Whether the low incidence is representative of type or chronicity of immune dysfunction or receipt of prophylactic antifungal drugs is unknown. The following section describes clinical manifestations and pathogenesis and focuses pri-

TABLE 30–1. *Factors Described to Either Increase (↑) or Decrease (↓) the Risk for Fungal Infections in Bone Marrow Transplant Patients*

Factor	Candida	Aspergillus	Fusarium	Zygomycetes
Older age*	↑	↑		
Underlying disease				
CML-chronic phase		↓		
Hematologic malignancy in non-first remission		↑		
Aplastic anemia		↑		
Myelodysplastic syndrome		↑		↑
Multiple myeloma		↑	↑	
Type of BMT				
Autologous		↓		
CD34-selection		↑		
HLA-MM/UR allogeneic	↑	↑	↑	
Stem cell product**				
HLA-matched PBSC		↓ (early)		
Cord blood		↑		
Receipt of total body irradiation	↑			
Transplant in LAF		↓		
Season of transplant		↑		
Construction		↑		
CMV seropositivity (recipient)		↑		
CMV infection or disease	↑	↑		
Respiratory virus infection		↑		
Prolonged neutrophil engraftment	↑	↑		
2° neutropenia after engraftment	↑	↑		
Acute GVHD	↑	↑		↑
Chronic GVHD		↑		
Receipt of corticosteroids		↑		
Prior bacteremia	↑			
Receipt of antibacterial drugs	↑			
Microbial colonization	↑	↑		

*Age $\geq$ 18 and $\geq$ 40 years have been shown to increase risk for infection compared to age < 18.

**Stem cell products were compared to bone marrow.

CML, chronic myelogenous leukemia; BMT, bone marrow transplant; HLA-MM, human lymphocyte antigen-mismatched; UR, unrelated donor, PBSC, peripheral blood stem cell; LAF, laminar airflow; CMV, cytomegalovirus; GVHD, graft-vs.-host disease.

Only factors significantly associated with risks in multivariable models are shown.

Sources: Morrison et al, 1993; Jantunen et al, 1997; Wald et al, 1997; Marr et al, 2000b,c; Baddley et al, 2001; Grow et al, 2002; Marr et al, 2002b; Marr et al, 2002c.

marily on the two major pathogens of importance in BMT recipients, *Candida* species and *Aspergillus* species. Discussion of the less frequent filamentous fungal pathogens follows, preceding a detailed section focused on therapy.

Manifestations, Pathogenesis, and Diagnosis

Candidiasis. Infections caused by *Candida* species can be called acute or chronic, terms that describe differences in both clinical presentation and pathogenesis. Acute candidiasis refers to bloodstream infection, or acute deep tissue infection caused by hematogenous seeding. Acute infection frequently manifests as fever and sepsis, with positive blood cultures. One recent study performed in cancer patients showed that the most common clinical presentation is fever, which occurred in 99% of patients sampled (Viscoli et al, 1999). The severity of presentation and frequency of complications are dependent upon the immune status of the host and the relative virulence of the *Candida* species.

Dissemination to specific organs (kidneys, skin, eyes, heart, central nervous system, and lungs) may result from hematogenous spread, especially in neutropenic patients with bloodstream infection with *C. albicans*.

In BMT recipients, the most frequent mode of acquisition of *Candida* species is GI tract invasion during periods of severe mucositis. The results of several studies have suggested that certain species are more able to invade the GI tract mucosal barrier (Cole et al, 1996; Mellado et al, 2000). *Candida albicans* and *C. tropicalis*, the most frequent causes of candidiasis among BMT recipients not receiving any antifungal prophylactic therapy, appear to have a unique ability to invade tissues. One recent study, which examined the ability of genetically manipulated *C. albicans* to invade through mucosal tissues in a murine model, observed that invasion is tightly linked to the ability of the organism to form hyphae (Andrutis et al, 2000). Although other species, notably *C. glabrata* and *C. krusei*, are not able to form hyphae, these organisms can also gain entrance into the bloodstream through the GI tract, especially in neutropenic patients who are colonized during periods of mucositis.

Although BMT recipients are at high risk for developing invasive candidiasis via the GI tract, acquisition through intravascular catheters is common. *Candida parapsilosis* is an organism most frequently acquired through this route. Older reports focused on the epidemic nature of *C. parapsilosis* infections, with several nosocomial outbreaks identifying contamination of intravascular infusates as a potential source (Plouffe et al, 1977). Recent risk factor analyses performed in neonates have verified that colonization on the hands of health-care workers is associated with infection in this population (Saiman et al, 2000). The precise source of candidal infection is rarely identified; preventive measures for controlling infection must include basic infection control practices such as adherence to strict hand-washing policies.

Chronic candidiasis is a term frequently used to signify hepatosplenic disease. As opposed to candidemia, patients with chronic candidiasis may present with clinical manifestations long after initial infection. *Candida* species, which invade the portal vasculature during neutropenia and GI mucositis, seed the liver and/or spleen; symptoms and signs of abdominal pain, fever, and tenderness, plus increased alkaline phosphatase levels, become apparent only after engraftment, concurrent with a relative degree of immune reconstitution, and inflammation of hepatic lesions (Thaler et al, 1988; Kontoyiannis et al, 2000a). Pathologic examination of hepatic candidal lesions typically reveals chronic inflammation. Bodey and colleagues described the histopathological distinction between chronic lesions with granulomatous inflammation and hepatic candidal abscess formation, comprised predominantly of coagulative necrosis (Bodey and Luna, 1998). As with acute candidiasis, chronic disease is most frequently caused by *C. albicans*, although non-*albicans* species have been identified as potential causes of disease in an autopsy study of patients who received azole antifungal prophylaxis (van Burik et al, 1998).

Diagnosis of candidemia relies on identification of the organism in blood culture. Multiple advances in blood culture techniques have occurred over the last decade, and include the lysis centrifugation blood culture system (Wampole Laboratories, Cranbury, NJ) and the BacT/Alert Microbial Detection System (Organon Teknika Corporation, Durham, NC), which have increased the sensitivity and rapidity of detection of candidemia (Kiehn et al, 1983; Wilson et al, 1992). Yield remains somewhat variable, in part because the frequency of detection of *Candida* species depends upon fungal burden, which varies among patients studied. Efforts are underway to develop culture-independ-

ent methodologies, such as antigen detection and PCR for identification of organisms as the cause of bloodstream and/or tissue disease (Walsh and Chanock, 1998). These methods, and the yield of radiography to diagnose hepatosplenic candidiasis, are discussed in more detail in Chapter 11.

Aspergillosis. Infections caused by *Aspergillus* species typically manifest in the sinopulmonary tract. Most frequently, acquisition occurs by inhalation of conidia; in the absence of effective macrophage-mediated conidial killing, these cells can germinate into potentially invasive hyphae (Latge, 1999). Hyphal growth occurs unchecked in the absence of a sufficient neutrophilic response, potentially resulting in vascular invasion and hematogenous dissemination.

Although disease is frequently recognized and presumed to be established in the respiratory tract, case reports and larger series have documented that *Aspergillus* species may invade the GI tract. The GI tract can serve as a portal of entry, resulting in isolated colitis, and in some cases, hepatic lesions in the absence of apparent pulmonary disease (Catalano et al, 1997). Filamentous fungi, as well as *Candida* species, have been implicated as a cause of neutropenic colitis, or typhlitis, in immunocompromised patients (Ortiz et al, 2000). Retrospective studies have shown that identification of *Aspergillus* species as colonizing organisms in either respiratory samples or stool of BMT recipients connotes a high positive predictive value for subsequent invasive disease (Wald et al, 1997). The exception is *A. niger* isolated from stool, which is not associated with subsequent invasive disease. Whether the risk associated with *Aspergillus* species in stool is indicative of a portal of entry or merely represents the likelihood of prior sinopulmonary exposure is unknown. Regardless, isolation of a potentially pathogenic organism from nonsterile sites in patients at risk should initiate a thorough evaluation for other signs of disease, and consideration of preemptive antifungal therapy.

Aspergillus species can cause multiple sinopulmonary syndromes, ranging from allergic sinusitis to invasive sinusitis with extrapulmonary spread to distant organs. Bone marrow transplant recipients are at risk for the most severe invasive manifestations. In the most recent cohort studies, 11% of infections caused by *Aspergillus* species were limited to invasive sinusitis; in the vast majority of patients, these organisms are found to be the cause of pneumonia, with or without recognized sinus disease (Marr et al, 2002b). Infections caused by *A. flavus* and *A. niger* are more frequently limited to the sinuses possibly because these species have larger conidia that get trapped in upper airways more frequently than *A. fumigatus*, which can reach the depths of alveolar spaces. The pathogenesis of disease, and differences between *Aspergillus* species are discussed in more detail in Chapter 14.

The clinical manifestations of diseases caused by *Aspergillus* species are the combined result of microbial tissue invasion and the host inflammatory responses elicited to keep the organism in check. Hence, the radiographic presentation of invasive pulmonary infection can vary from one or more isolated small nodules (Fig. 30–3a), to cavitary lesions (Fig. 30–3b), to extensive, unilateral or bilateral infiltrates (Figs. 30–3c, 30–3d). Ground-glass infiltrates are not uncommon and appear to occur more frequently in BMT recipients compared to other neutropenic patients. One study found that diffuse infiltrates caused by *Aspergillus* species were most common in BMT patients who developed disease postengraftment during GVHD (Marr et al, 2000a). The results of animal models suggest that these unusual manifestations may result from "dysregulated" or delayed clearance of mononuclear inflammation, or hemorrhage (Berenguer et al, 1995). More studies are necessary to determine the pathogenesis of this broad spectrum of disease manifestations. In the meantime, clinicians should be aware that even though certain radiographic presentations may be typical for invasive pulmonary aspergillosis (i.e., nodular or cavitary lesions), disease may be manifest with a spectrum of radiographic findings.

Currently, the definitive diagnosis of aspergillosis relies upon histopathologic and/or microbiologic identification of the organism in tissue. As several studies have documented that the yield of culture of both tissue biopsies and bronchoalveolar lavage fluid (BALF) is low, and therapy of proven disease is associated with the worst outcomes, efforts have been directed towards establishing methods to more rapidly diagnose infection (Levy et al 1992; Patterson et al, 2000; Lin et al, 2001; Denning et al, 2002). Multiple diagnostic tests that rely on detection of circulating antigens are in use in Europe and Japan. These assays, which can detect cell wall components such as galactomannan and β-glucan, appear to have good sensitivity and specificity for diagnosis of aspergillosis in BMT recipients (Miyazaki et al, 1995; Maertens et al, 2001). One study performed in BMT recipients found that both sensitivity and specificity of the Platelia galactomannan double-sandwich enzyme-linked immunoassay (EIA) was at least 90% (Maertens et al, 2001). Despite the high positive and negative predictive values, the duration of time between positive assays and clinical manifestation of infection may be variable. In the Maertens' study, 6 days was the median number of days in which a positive assay preceded initiation of antifungal therapy based on clinical signs. It may be that the performance of the assay could be improved by using lower cut-offs for positivity, especially in this population, given the

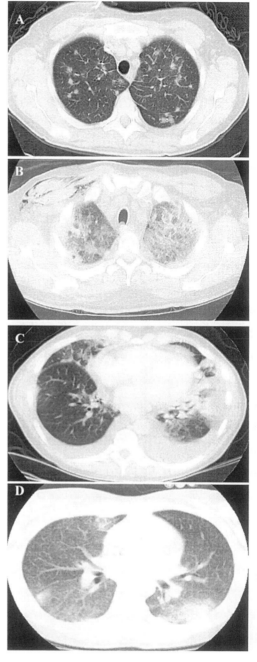

FIGURE 30–3. Radiographic presentations of aspergillosis in allogeneic BMT recipients. Appearance can vary from isolated pulmonary lesions (*a*), to cavitary lesions (*b*), to infiltrates (*c* and *d*). Infiltrates are frequently pleural based (*c* and *d*), but ground-glass infiltrates can appear either surrounding nodular lesions (*a*), or as isolated findings (*d*).

high prevalence of aspergillosis and the frequent use of prophylactic and empiric antifungal therapy. More studies will be necessary to optimize performance characteristics of these assays in other hosts, especially in children, who appear to have frequent false-positive results during GI mucositis and neutropenia (Sulahian et al, 2001). Other diagnostic assays that have been developed in multiple centers rely on PCR detection of circulating nucleic acids (Einsele et al, 1997). These and other assays currently under investigation are discussed in more detail in Chapter 14.

Infections Caused By Other Fungi. Other fungi are much less commonly associated with invasive disease among BMT recipients. The most common of these pathogens include the filamentous fungi, *Fusarium* spp. and the Zygomycetes. Infections with other fungi such as *Scedosporium* spp., *Trichosporon* spp., *Cryptococcus neoformans*, and dematiaceous moulds, (e.g., *Alternaria* spp. and *Bipolaris* spp.) do occur in BMT patients. However, these infections are relatively infrequent and are not reviewed here (Perfect and Schell, 1996; Walsh and Groll, 1999a; Marr et al, 2002b).

Fusarium species are the second most common filamentous fungal pathogen in BMT recipients, and *F. solani* is the most common species (Boutati and Anaissie, 1997; Marr et al, 2002b). Clinical presentation of disseminated fusariosis is similar to that of aspergillosis. Acquisition is usually through the sinopulmonary tract, but these organisms can also cause isolated onychomycosis and gain entry through cellulitis involving the extremities (Boutati and Anaissie, 1997). Frequent recovery of these organisms from blood and tissue, and the propensity to cause disseminated disease is thought to be due to the ability of *Fusarium* spp. to produce adventitious unicellular propagules in vivo (Schell, 1995). Only a few fungi are capable of producing adventitious forms or conidia in vivo, and infection with organisms that have this capability (*Fusarium* spp., *Aspergillus terreus*, *Acremonium* spp., and *Paecilomyces* spp.) is characterized by frequent hematogenous dissemination with skin lesions, growth of the organism in blood culture, and a relative resistance to therapy with amphotericin B products (Perfect and Schell, 1996). Risk factors for fusariosis include neutropenia and GVHD (Boutati and Anaissie, 1997; Marr et al, 2002b). Patients who receive BMT from HLA-mismatched or unrelated donors, as well as people with an underlying diagnosis of multiple myeloma, appear to be at particularly high risk (Marr et al, 2002b).

Infections caused by the Zygomycetes such as *Rhizopus* spp. and *Mucor* spp., also appear to be increasing in frequency in BMT recipients (Marr et al, 2002b). These moulds can be acquired through the sinopulmonary tract, or less frequently through mucosal breaks in the GI tract, leading to sinusitis, pneumonia, or lesions in the liver or GI tract (Oliver et al, 1996; Ribes et al, 2000; Kontoyiannis et al, 2000b). Recent studies report that the rate of hematogenous dissemination of Zygomycetes in BMT recipients is roughly equivalent to that of *Aspergillus* species, with disseminated lesions recognized in approximately 25% of proven or probable infections associated with both pathogens (Marr et al, 2002b). Zygomycosis tends to occur later after receipt of allogeneic BMT, with GVHD as the most important risk factor. In one study, the underlying diagnosis of myelodysplastic syndrome was associated with significantly higher risk of zygomycosis in a multivariable risk factor analysis, possibly related to severity of GVHD in this patient population (Marr et al, 2002b).

THERAPEUTIC APPROACH

Therapy of invasive fungal infections entails both preventive strategies as well as treatment of established infection. In BMT recipients, prevention of infection is critical. It can be argued that the most important therapeutic advances in the supportive care of BMT recipients within the last decade have occurred due to the effective measures to prevent gram-negative bacterial infections, CMV disease, and candidiasis. One recent multivariable analysis of outcomes among unrelated donor BMT recipients with chronic myelogenous leukemia found that two important predictors of overall survival were receipt of ganciclovir for prevention of CMV infection, and fluconazole for prevention of candidiasis (Hansen et al, 1998).

Prevention: Prophylaxis
Strategies to prevent fungal infections may rely on administration of antifungals "prophylactically" in high-risk patients, "empirically" in patients with fever during neutropenia, and "preemptively" in patients in whom a more specific indicator of fungal infection is detected. There are advantages and disadvantages to each of these strategies.

Prophylactic administration of azole antifungal drugs has become common practice in BMT recipients, due to several randomized trials performed in the early 1990s that showed efficacy in preventing candidiasis (Goodman et al, 1992; Slavin et al, 1995). The first large randomized trial comparing fluconazole with placebo until neutrophil engraftment in both autologous and allogeneic BMT recipients showed that fluconazole was associated with decreased fungal infection and fungal infection-related death, although there was no difference in overall survival (Goodman et al, 1992). A second trial compared fluconazole with placebo, both administered for a longer period of time during GVHD in allograft recipients (Slavin et al, 1995). The results of this trial, and a subsequent long-term follow up study of the same randomized cohort, verified that fluconazole decreases infection, infection-related death, and the overall mortality of allograft recipients (Marr et al, 2000b). Another study documented that the prophylactic use of fluconazole decreases the incidence of hepatosplenic candidiasis in BMT recipients (van Burik et al, 1998). Optimal doses and durations of fluconazole administration continue to be a matter of debate.

Unfortunately, the successful prevention of fungal infections has been dampened due to the emergence of azole-resistant *Candida* species and moulds. Most reports suggest that liberal azole use is associated with selection of resistant *Candida* species, namely *C. glabrata* and *C. krusei* (Bodey et al, 2002; Marr et al, 2000c). Perhaps more importantly, the incidence of aspergillosis has increased in many centers, with this organism surpassing yeasts as the cause of infection-related mortality. The estimated incidence of invasive aspergillosis approximates 10%–15% in most BMT centers, with the majority of infections diagnosed late after engraftment, during GVHD (Wald et al, 1997; Williamson et al, 1999; Grow et al, 2002). Figure 30–4 shows the one year cumulative incidence of proven or probable invasive aspergillosis in the largest cohort of allogeneic BMT patients described to date (Marr et al, 2002c).

Due to this shift in epidemiology, efforts have turned towards establishing a preventive strategy that will encompass moulds as well as yeasts. Several studies have been performed to determine if itraconazole is better than placebo (Menichetti et al, 1999), amphotericin B (Harousseau et al, 2000), or fluconazole (Morgenstern et al, 1999) for prevention of infection in neutropenic patients. Although the results of these studies suggested promise with regards to prevention of aspergillosis, the studies were not performed in high-risk BMT recipients. A trial that compared outcomes of BMT patients who received either itraconazole or fluconazole for 100 days after transplant has been completed recently, and preliminary results suggest that itraconazole may be better than fluconazole in preventing *Aspergillus* infec-

tions (Winston et al, 2001). However, other reports have suggested that long-term administration of itraconazole may be limited by a significant amount of nausea and vomiting, especially in children (Foot et al, 1999). Multiple trials are currently evaluating the utility of newer mould-active triazole antifungal drugs, such as voriconazole and posaconazole, and echinocandins for antifungal prophylaxis in BMT recipients.

Prevention: Empirical Therapy

One approach to prevention of fungal infections is to administer antifungal agents to neutropenic patients with fever that persists despite antibiotics. This practice was established in the 1980s, with the performance of two randomized trials that compared outcomes of febrile neutropenic patients who received either no antifungal therapy or amphotericin B deoxycholate (Pizzo et al, 1982; EORTC, 1989). Both trials showed that amphotericin B was associated with fewer fungal infections. Which antifungal is best for treatment of fever during neutropenia has been the subject of multiple studies performed subsequently. Most of these studies did not enroll enough BMT patients to compare efficacy of preventing infection, especially in people already receiving some type of systemically absorbed antifungal drug as prophylaxis (Marr, 2002a). Evaluation of toxicity endpoints and composite variables showed efficacy, but fewer toxicities of empirical therapy with fluconazole, itraconazole, and lipid formulations of amphotericin B compared to amphotericin B deoxycholate (Marr, 2002a). Whether the toxicity concerns are great enough to warrant the use of the more expensive formulations is a matter of continued debate. Expense has limited their widespread adoption in many large cancer centers. Either mould-active triazole antifungal drugs such as voriconazole (Walsh et al, 2002) or lipid amphotericin B formulations (Walsh et al, 1999b) may be appropriate for treatment of fever during neutropenia in BMT recipients who are receiving

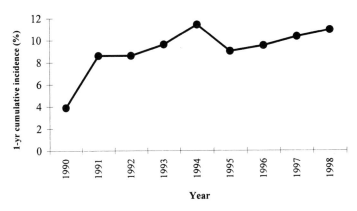

FIGURE 30–4. The annual incidence of proven or probable aspergillosis among a cohort of allogeneic BMT recipients at the Fred Hutchinson Cancer Research Center. (Modified from Marr et al, 2002b).

fluconazole prophylactically. However, fever during neutropenia is not frequently caused by fungal infections in patients who are receiving prophylaxis. Recent studies have found that < 5% of high-risk BMT patients who are febrile while receiving systemically absorbed antifungal prophylaxis actually had fungal infections as a cause of their fevers (Walsh et al, 2002). Whether empirical therapy is necessary in these patients is not clear. It may be that some of the newer diagnostic assays may allow for the development of preemptive strategies in order to avoid high toxicities and costs associated with empirical antifungal use.

Prevention: Preemptive Therapy

Preemptive is a term used to describe therapy administered early during the course of infection, in some settings preempting the development of disease. For CMV, strategies using pp65-antigenemia and PCR to identify infection in BMT recipients have been very successful at preventing CMV disease and attributable mortality (Boeckh, 1999). The development of new diagnostic assays for fungal infections may allow for the similar development of preventive strategies. To date, studies have focused on the use of serial CT-scanning to initiate early antifungal therapy. Although one small study noted that screening with sensitive radiographic tests may lead to decreased Aspergillus-associated mortality compared to historic controls (Caillot et al, 1997), the costs and inability to routinely screen for long durations after BMT have limited the applicability of this approach. Other studies have reported that screening with PCR or antigenemia assays may allow for the establishment of earlier diagnoses of aspergillosis (Walsh and Chanock, 1998a). Large, randomized studies are needed to determine the utility of these assays for preventive strategies in BMT recipients.

Prevention: Other Methods

Aside from prophylactic or preemptive antifungal administration, other methods to prevent fungal infections in BMT recipients include avoidance of exposure, and minimizing the severity or duration of risk. Aspergillus and other moulds are most frequently acquired from the hospital or external environment, although a certain number of BMT patients who develop disease early after transplant appear to have reactivation from a previously acquired infection. Efforts to minimize exposure to Aspergillus species during the periods of risk have focused on air filtration, either through laminar airflow (LAF), or high-efficiency particulate air filtration (HEPA). No randomized trials have been performed to measure the utility of these measures; however, several multivariable models to define risk factors for aspergillosis have shown that both may be useful to prevent infection early after transplant (Sherertz et al, 1987; Wald et al, 1997; Cornet et al,

1999). The important limitation to the use of containment practices is that they are only useful during the period of time during which they are employed. Many experienced clinicians have recently questioned the utility of LAF at a time when disease is most frequently acquired outside of the hospital, late after transplant.

The environmental source of Aspergillus species has also been called into question with the results of several recent studies suggesting that moulds may be a common contaminant in hospital water supplies (Anaissie et al, 2001b; Anaissie and Costa, 2001a; Warris et al, 2001; Anaissie et al, 2002; Warris et al, 2002). The findings of Aspergillus species (including A. fumigatus) and Fusarium species in hospital water supplies, with high amounts of spores recovered in and around patient bathrooms, has led some clinicians to suggest that it may be prudent to avoid aerosolization of water through showering during the period of high risk. Other studies have reported outbreaks of hospital-acquired A. terreus infections with apparent association with vegetation (plants) within the hospital (Lass-Florl et al, 2000). Although the exact environmental source of moulds is rarely determined, even during periods of outbreaks, most centers have instituted infection-control practices that focus on air monitoring, patient avoidance of vegetation and food known to have high mould content (i.e., pepper), and patient avoidance of activities that are associated with aerosolization of conidia (i.e., mowing the lawn, gardening, vacuuming, etc). More studies are necessary to determine whether other infection-control practices can minimize infection late after BMT.

It may also be possible to prevent infection by minimizing the severity and the duration of risks. Efforts to prevent fungal infections have focused on the roles of immune modulators to decrease neutropenia. Few placebo-controlled randomized studies employing hematopoietic growth factors or granulocyte infusions to prevent infection have been performed; however, the results of small randomized trials and risk-factor analyses suggest that minimizing the period of neutropenia is associated with fewer Candida and Aspergillus infections (Wingard, 1998). Optimizing risk reduction during the GVHD period is important, and recent risk factor analyses have shown that factors other than neutropenia, namely corticosteroid exposure, viral (CMV) infections, and lymphopenia may be the strongest predictors of postengraftment aspergillosis (Grow et al, 2002; Marr et al, 2002c). Minimizing the use of corticosteroids for GVHD is prudent, when possible.

Therapy of Documented Infection

For a long time, clinicians have balanced the need for establishing a microbial diagnosis of fungal infections with the desire to minimize complications associated with invasive procedures. Mould infections are especially difficult to diagnose with certainty without performance of some type of invasive procedure, e.g., bronchoalveolar lavage (BAL) or lung biopsy. Although complications are rare subsequent to BAL, lung biopsy may elicit hemorrhage and infection in neutropenic, thrombocytopenic patients (Hoffer et al, 2001). One may treat patients with suggestive radiographic lesions presumptively with antifungal agents; however, without a definitive diagnosis, there is a substantial risk of administering misdirected therapy. Establishing a microbial diagnosis has become especially important now that multiple effective antifungal drugs other than deoxycholate amphotericin B are available for use.

Treatment of Candidiasis

Therapy of infections caused by *Candida* is dependent on the causative species. While fluconazole has been shown to be equivalent with amphotericin B for treatment of candidemia in nonneutropenic patients, candidiasis in neutropenic patients and BMT recipients is frequently caused by azole-resistant organisms, such as *C. glabrata* or *C. krusei* (Viscoli et al, 1999; Marr et al, 2000c). In these patients, even *C. albicans* may become resistant to fluconazole through continued exposure during prophylactic therapy (Marr et al, 1997; Marr et al, 2001). For this reason, and because azole drugs, especially fluconazole and itraconazole, have not been evaluated extensively for therapy of invasive infection in severely immunosuppressed patients, standard therapy of bloodstream infection should include an amphotericin B formulation, or possibly alternative therapy with an echinocandin. High doses (≥ 0.8 mg/kg/day) of amphotericin B deoxycholate or a lipid formulation of amphotericin B may be best therapy of infections caused by *C. glabrata* or *C. krusei*, as there is some indication that these organisms are relatively resistant to amphotericin B (Rex et al, 2000). Use of newer agents that have good activity against *Candida* species, such as echinocandins, should be acceptable given their in vitro activity (Espinel-Ingroff, 1998). Although experience with these compounds is not yet extensive, a large, double-blind study comparing caspofungin with amphotericin B for treatment of invasive candidiasis has been completed (Mora-Duarte et al, 2002). Results of this study suggest comparable efficacy, and fewer toxicities associated with caspofungin therapy. Duration of therapy for candidemia should continue for at least 2 weeks after the last positive blood culture in order to minimize the likelihood of metastatic sequelae such as chorioretinitis and endocarditis (Rex et al, 2000).

Multiple antifungal drugs have been shown to be effective for treatment of hepatosplenic candidiasis, including fluconazole, as most infections are caused by susceptible *C. albicans*. Although no randomized stud-

ies have been performed to identify the best antifungal for treatment, most clinicians favor the use of an amphotericin B formulation as initial therapy, followed by maintenance therapy with an azole antifungal until resolution of lesions (Kontoyiannis et al, 2000a). Anecdotal success has been reported using echinocandin antifungals for therapy of hepatosplenic candidiasis as well, which is consistent with the distribution of these drugs to the liver (Groll and Walsh, 2001). The reader is referred to a detailed discussion of treatment for *Candida* infections in Chapter 11.

Treatment of Mould Infections

Historically, the only effective therapy for mould infections was amphotericin B. The introduction of new triazoles and echinocandins has now challenged this "gold standard," with recent evidence that alternative therapy may be indicated for non-*Aspergillus* mould infections, and for treatment of infection that does not initially respond to amphotericin B formulations. No randomized studies have compared therapy with amphotericin B deoxycholate to lipid formulations of amphotericin B, although the latter formulations have fewer nephrotoxicities and infusion-related toxicities, both of which may occur at high frequency in BMT recipients (Walsh et al, 1998b; Wingard et al, 2000).

Differentiating infections with *Aspergillus* species and other mould pathogens has become critical, as optimal therapy for each may differ. While amphotericin B remains the current therapy of choice for zygomycosis, several retrospective open-label studies suggest that the best outcomes result from therapy with high doses of lipid amphotericin B formulations, in conjunction with aggressive surgical debridement of involved tissue and granulocyte-stimulation or replacement (Herbrecht et al, 2001; Kontoyiannis et al, 2000b). Emerging data indicate that optimal therapy for *Fusarium* spp. and *Scedosporium* spp. may be a new mould-active triazole antifungal drug. Reports of outcomes using voriconazole and posaconazole have been encouraging, leading some experienced clinicians to suggest that these drugs should now be considered first-line therapy for these opportunistic filamentous mould infections.

The standard algorithm for treating invasive aspergillosis has been to administer amphotericin B deoxycholate as initial (primary) therapy and then to switch to either a mould-active triazole, an echinocandin, or a lipid formulation of amphotericin B should the patient develop serious toxicities or fail to respond to initial therapy. Only one randomized, double-blind study has been performed to evaluate the use of a lipid formulation of amphotericin B as primary therapy for invasive aspergillosis. In this study, amphotericin B colloidal dispersion (ABCD) at a dose of 6 mg/kg/day was equivalent in efficacy to amphotericin B deoxycholate, 1.0–1.5 mg/kg/day, but was associated with significantly less nephrotoxicity (Bowden et al, 2002). Despite the lack of data to support superior efficacy, the lipid formulations are favored by many clinicians because of their potential to deliver high doses of amphotericin B to target tissues without an increase in toxicities. Salvage studies have shown that voriconazole, posaconazole, and caspofungin are associated with successful therapy when used as a second-line agent in approximately 40% of patients (Denning et al, 2002).

Recently, the algorithm for standard therapy for invasive aspergillosis has been challenged with trials that compared amphotericin B with voriconazole. Although the response rates of aspergillosis in allogeneic BMT recipients using amphotericin B formulations only approximated 10%–15% (Ribaud et al, 1999; Patterson et al, 2000; Lin et al, 2001; Denning et al, 2002), responses were noted in 26% of allogeneic BMT patients who received voriconazole either as primary or secondary therapy (Denning et al, 2002). More convincing evidence that voriconazole may be an effective therapy comes from a recent open label–randomized trial that compared voriconazole as primary therapy with the standard algorithm of amphotericin B followed by the investigator's choice of other licensed antifungal therapy. The results of this trial indicate that clinical outcomes and overall survival are improved with voriconazole used as primary therapy (Herbrecht et al, 2002). In vitro and in vivo studies suggest that combination antifungal therapy, employing an echinocandin with either a mould-active triazole or an amphotericin B formulation for invasive aspergillosis, may be even more efficacious. Clinical studies evaluating the safety and efficacy of the various combinations are in the planning stage.

Common practice is to continue antifungal therapy for the duration of time that the patient is receiving immunosuppressive drugs. Allogeneic BMT recipients with pulmonary mould infections should receive prolonged antifungal therapy, at least as long as patients are receiving high doses of corticosteroid therapy for GVHD. The cumulative dose and duration of corticosteroids exposure are closely associated with negative outcomes of antifungal therapy; consequently, every effort should be made to minimize exposure to corticosteroids (Ribaud et al, 1999).

Adjunctive Therapy

The utility of adjunctive therapy using immune modulating agents, such as hematopoietic growth factors or granulocyte transfusions, continues to be a matter of debate. No definitive randomized studies have been performed. Up to now, studies have only justified the safety of immunomodulating therapy, with anec-

dotes suggesting efficacy. Granulocyte colony-stimulating factor (G-CSF) and granulocyte-macrophage colony-stimulating factor (GM-CSF) are used frequently in patients who are neutropenic and have invasive fungal infections. Adjunctive immunotherapy may be especially important for treatment of mould infections characterized by a large circulating fungal burden and relative resistance to antifungal drugs, as with disseminated fusariosis. In addition, other reports emphasize that outcomes of therapy for zygomycosis are improved with rapid resolution of neutropenia (Kontoyiannis et al, 2000b). The potential utility of neutrophil transfusions as adjunctive therapy has been rejuvenated with the development of G-CSF primed community donor transfusions (Hubel et al, 2001). Studies evaluating the safety and efficacy of such transfusions, and the use of interferon-gamma for adjunctive therapy of aspergillosis in neutropenic patients are either ongoing or in development.

The role of surgical debridement of pulmonary fungal lesions is also a matter of debate, as no randomized studies have been performed, and noncontrolled studies are impacted by selection bias. Anecdotal reports and case series suggest that there is a definite role for surgical resection in patients who present with severe hemoptysis and fungal lesions abutting large vessels, and in patients in whom further myelosuppressive therapy is intended (Offner et al, 1998). In many centers, patients who present pretransplant with isolated pulmonary fungal lesions undergo resection when possible. This practice is justified by the results of case series that suggest that recurrent fungal infection occurs less frequently in patients who have undergone surgical resection before myeloablative therapy. As mentioned above, surgical resection of infection caused by Zygomycetes appears to be strongly associated with successful therapy.

SUMMARY

The risks and time of occurrence of fungal infections have evolved with new BMT techniques and supportive care strategies; however, patients who are immunosuppressed for long durations of time during GVHD continue to have prolonged risks for fungal infections. In this setting, mould infections have emerged as the primary concern. Preventive strategies that employ mould-active antifungal drugs for prophylactic and preemptive administration are being explored. These new agents have been shown to yield some benefits for therapy of documented infection, especially when used early after definitive diagnosis. It is possible that the availability of these less toxic antifungal agents, combined with new nonmyeloablative BMT procedures, will curb fungal infection-related mortality in years to come. Meanwhile, more innovative approaches are necessary to tailor preventive and therapeutic strategies.

REFERENCES

Anaissie E J, Costa S F. Nosocomial aspergillosis is waterborne. *Clin Infect Dis* 33:1546–1548, 2001a.

Anaissie E J, Kuchar R T, Rex J H, Francesconi A, Kasai M, Muller F M, Lozano-Chiu M, Summerbell R C, Dignani M C, Chanock S J, Walsh T J. Fusariosis associated with pathogenic *Fusarium* species colonization of a hospital water system: a new paradigm for the epidemiology of opportunistic mold infections. *Clin Infect Dis* 33:1871–1878, 2001b.

Anaissie E J, Stratton S L, Dignani M C, Summerbell R C, Rex J H, Monson T P, Spencer T, Kasai M, Francesconi A, Walsh T J. Pathogenic *Aspergillus* species recovered from a hospital water system: a 3-year prospective study. *Clin Infect Dis* 34:780–789, 2002.

Andrutis K, Riggle P, Kumamoto C, Tzipori S. Intestinal lesions associated with disseminated candidiasis in an experimental animal model. *J Clin Microbiol* 38:2317–2323,2000.

Baddley J, Stroud T, Salzman D, Pappas P. Invasive mold infections in allogeneic bone marrow transplant recipients. *Clin Infect Dis* 32:1319–1324, 2001.

Berenguer J, Allende M C, Lee J W, Garrett K, Lyman C, Ali N M, Bacher J, Pizzo P A, Walsh T J. Pathogenesis of pulmonary aspergillosis. Granulocytopenia versus cyclosporine and methylprednisolone-induced immunosuppression. *Am J Respir Crit Care Med* 152:1079–1086, 1995.

Bodey G, Luna M. Disseminated candidiasis in patients with acute leukemia: two diseases? *Clin Infect Dis* 27:238, 1998.

Bodey G P, Mardani M, Hanna, H A, Boktour M, Abbas J, Girgawy E, Achem R Y, Kontoyiannis D P, Raad I I. The epidemiology of *Candida glabrata* and *Candida albicans* fungemia in immunocompromised patients with cancer. *Am J Med* 112:380–385, 2002.

Boeckh M. Current antiviral strategies for controlling cytomegalovirus in hematopoietic stem cell transplant recipients: prevention and therapy. *Transplant Infect Dis* 1:165–178, 1999.

Boutati E, Anaissie E. *Fusarium*, a significant emerging pathogen in patients with hematologic malignancy: ten years' experience at a cancer center and implications for management. *Blood* 90:999–1008, 1997.

Bowden R, Chandrasekar P, White M H, Li X, Pietrelli L, Gurwith M, van Burik J A, Laverdiere M, Safrin S, Wingard J R. A double-blind, randomized, controlled trial of amphotericin B colloidal dispersion versus amphotericin B for treatment of invasive aspergillosis in immunocompromised patients. *Clin Infect Dis* 35:359–366, 2002.

Caillot D, Casasnovas O, Bernard A, Couaillier J-F, Durand C, Cuisenier B, Solary E, Piard F, Petrella T, Bonnin A, Couillault G, Dumas M, Guy H. Improved management of invasive aspergillosis in neutropenic patients using early thoracic computed tomographic scan and surgery. *J Clin Oncol* 15:139–147, 1997.

Catalano L, Picardi M, Anzivino D, Insabato L, Notaro R, Rotoli B. Small bowel infarction by *Aspergillus*. *Haematologica* 82:182–183, 1997.

Cenci E, Mencacci A, Del Sero G, Bistoni F, Romani L. Induction of protective Th1 responses to *Candida albicans* by antifungal therapy alone or in combination with an interleukin-4 antagonist. *J Infect Dis* 76:217–226, 1997a.

Cenci E, Perito S, Enssle K, Mosci P, Latge J, Romani L, Bistoni F. Th1 and Th2 cytokines in mice with invasive aspergillosis. *Infect Immun* 65:564–570, 1997b.

Cenci E, Mencacci A, Fe d'Ostiani C, Del Sero G, Mosci P, Montagnoli C, Bacci A, Romani L. Cytokine- and T helper-dependent lung mucosal immunity in mice with invasive pulmonary aspergillosis. *J Infect Dis* 178:1750–1760, 1998.

Cenci E, Mencacci A, Del Sero G, Bacci A, Montagnoli C, d'Ostiani C F, Mosci P, Bachmann M, Bistoni F, Kopf M, Romani L. Interleukin-4 causes susceptibility to invasive pulmonary aspergillosis through suppression of protective type I responses. *J Infect Dis* 180:1957–1968, 1999.

Cenci E, Mencacci A, Bacci A, Bistoni F, Kurup V P, Romani L. T cell vaccination in mice with invasive pulmonary aspergillosis. *J Immunol* 165:381–388, 2000.

Cenci E, Mencacci A, Spreca A, Montagnoli C, Bacci A, Perruccio K, Velardi A, Magliani W, Conti S, Polonelli L, Romani L. Protection of killer antiidiotypic antibodies against early invasive aspergillosis in a murine model of allogeneic T-cell-depleted bone marrow transplantation. *Infect Immun* 70:2375–2382, 2002.

Childs R, Chernoff A, Contentin N, Bahceci E, Schrump D, Leitman S,Read E J, Tisdale J, Dunbar C, Linehan W M, Young N S, Barrett A J. Regression of metastatic renal-cell carcinoma after nonmyeloablative allogeneic peripheral blood stem cell transplantation. *N Eng J Med* 343:750–758, 2000.

Cole G T, Halawa A A, Anaissie E J. The role of the gastrointestinal tract in hematogenous candidiasis from the laboratory to the bedside. *Clin Infect Dis* 22:S73–S88, 1996.

Cornet M, Levy V, Fleury L, Lortholary J, Barquins S, Coureul M H, Deliere E, Zittoun R, Brucker G, Bouvet A. Efficacy of prevention by high-efficiency particulate air filtration or laminar airflow against *Aspergillus* airborne contamination during hospital renovation. *Infect Control Hosp Epidemiol* 20:508–513, 1999.

Crippa F, Holmberg L, Carter R, Hooper H, Marr K, Bensinger W, Chauncey T, Corey L, Boeckh M. Infectious complications after autologous CD34 selected peripheral blood stem cell transplantation. *Biol Blood Marr Transplant* 8:281–289, 2002.

Denning D W, Ribaud P, Milpied N, Caillot D, Herbrecht R, Thiel E, Haas A, Ruhnke M, Lode H. Efficacy and safety of voriconazole in the treatment of acute invasive aspergillosis. *Clin Infect Dis* 34:563–571, 2002.

Einsele H, Hebart H, Roller G, Loffler J, Rothenhofer I, Muller C A, Bowden R A, vanBurik J A, Engelhard D, Kanz L, Schumacher U. Detection and identification of fungal pathogens in blood by using molecular probes. *J Clin Microbiol* 35:1353–1360, 1997.

EORTC International Antimicrobial Therapy Cooperative Group. Empiric antifungal therapy in febrile granulocytopenic patients. *Am J Med*, 86:668–672, 1989.

Espinel-Ingroff A. Comparison of in vitro activities of the new triazole SCH56592 and the echinocandins MK-0991 (L-743,872) and LY303366 against opportunistic filamentous and dimorphic fungi and yeasts. *J Clin Microbiol* 36:2950–2956, 1998.

Foot A B, Veys P A, Gibson B E. Itraconazole oral solution as antifungal prophylaxis in children undergoing stem cell transplantation or intensive chemotherapy for haematological disorders. *Bone Marr Transplant* 24:1089–1093, 1999.

Garban F, Attal M, Rossi J, Payen C, Fegueux N, Sotto J. Immunotherapy by non-myeloablative allogeneic stem cell transplantation in multiple myeloma: results of a pilot study as salvage therapy after autologous transplantation. *Leukemia* 15:642–646, 2001.

Goodman J L, Winston D J, Greenfield R A, Chandrasekar P H, Fox B, Kaizer H, Shadduck R K, Shea T C, Stiff P, Friedman D J, Powderly W G, Silber J L, Horowitz H, Lichtin A, Wolff S N, Mangan S F, Silver S M, Weisdorf D, Ho W G, Gilbert G, Buell D. A controlled trial of fluconazole to prevent fungal infections in patients undergoing bone marrow transplantation. *N Engl J Med* 326:845–851, 1992.

Goodrich J M, Reed C, Mori M, Fisher L D, Skerrett S, Dandliker P S, Klis B, Counts G W, Myers J D. Clinical features and analysis of risk factors for invasive candidal infection after marrow transplantation. *J Infect Dis* 164:731–740, 1991.

Groll A H, Walsh T J. Caspofungin: pharmacology, safety and therapeutic potential in superficial and invasive fungal infections. *Expert Opin Investig Drugs* 10:1545–1558, 2001.

Grow W, Moreb J, Roque D, Manion K, Leather H, Reddy V, Khan S, Finiewicz K, Nguyen H, Clancy C, Mehta P, Wingard J. Late onset of invasive aspergillus infection in bone marrow transplant patients at a university hospital. *Bone Marr Transplant* 29:15–19, 2002.

Hansen J A, Gooley T A, Martin P J, Appelbaum F, Chancey T R, Clift R A, Petersdorf E W, Radich J, Sanders J E, Storb R F, Sullivan K M, Anasetti C. Bone marrow transplants from unrelated donors for patients with chronic myeloid leukemia. *N Engl J Med* 338:962–968, 1998.

Harousseau J, Dekker A, Stamatoullas-Bastard A, Fassa A, Linkesch W, Gouveia J, Bock R D, Rovira M, Seifert W, Joosen H, Peeters M, Beule K D. Itraconazole oral solution for primary prophylaxis of fungal infections in patients with hematologic malignancy and profound neutropenia: a randomized, double-blind, double-placebo, multicenter trial comparing itraconazole and amphotericin B. *Antimicrob Agents Chemother* 44:1887–1893, 2000.

Hebart H, Bollinger C, Fisch P, Sarfati J, Meisner C, Baur M, Loeffler J, Monod M, Latge J P, and Einsele H. Analysis of T-cell responses to *Aspergillus fumigatus* antigens in healthy individuals and patients with hematologic malignancies. *Blood* 100:4521–4528, 2002.

Herbrecht R, Letscher-Bru V, Bowden R A, Kusne S, Anaissie E J, Graybill J R, Noskin G A, Oppenheim A E, Pietrelli L A. Treatment of 21 cases of invasive mucormycosis with amphotericin B colloidal dispersion. *Eur J Clin Microbiol Infect Dis* 20:460–466, 2001.

Herbrecht R, Denning D W, Patterson T F, Bennett J E, Greene R E, Oestmann J-W, Kern W V, Marr K A, Ribaud P, Lortholary O, Sylvester R, Rubin R H, Wingard J R, Stark P, Durand C, Caillot D, Thiel E, Chandrasekar P H, Hodges M R, Schlamm H T, Troke P F, de Pauw B. Randomized comparison of voriconazole and amphotericin B for primary therapy of invasive aspergillosis. *N Engl J Med* 347:408–415, 2002.

Hoffer F A, Gow K, Flynn P M, Davidoff A. Accuracy of percutaneous lung biopsy for invasive pulmonary aspergillosis. *Pediatr Radiol* 31:144–152, 2001.

Holmberg L, Boeckh M, Hooper H, Leisenring W, Rowley S, Heimfeld S, Press O, Maloney D, McSweeney P, Corey, L, Maziarz R, Appelbaum F, Bensinger W. Increased incidence of cytomegalovirus disease after autologous CD34-selected peripheral blood stem cell transplantation. *Blood* 94:4029–4035, 1999.

Hubel K, Dale D C, Liles W C. Granulocyte transfusion therapy: update on potential clinical applications. *Curr Opin Hematol* 8:161–164, 2001.

Jantunen E, Ruutu P, Niskanen L, Volin L, Parkkali T, Koukila-Kahkola P, Ruutu T. Incidence and risk factors for invasive fungal infections in allogeneic BMT recipients. *Bone Marrow Transplant* 19:801–808, 1997.

Junghanss C, Marr K. Infectious risks and outcomes after stem cell transplantation: are non-myeloablative transplants changing the picture? *Curr Opin Infect Dis* 15:347–353, 2002a.

Junghanss C, Marr K, Carter R A, Sandmaier B M, Maris M B, Maloney D G, Chauncey T, McSweeney P A, Storb R. Incidence of bacterial and fungal infections after nonmyeloablative compared to myeloablative allogeneic stem cell transplantation (HSCT). *Biol Blood Marr Transplant* 8:512–520, 2002b.

Kiehn T, Wong B, Edward F, Armstrong D. Comparative recovery of bacteria and yeasts from lysis-centrifugation and a conventional blood culture system. *J Clin Microbiol* 18:300–304, 1983.

Kontoyiannis D, Luna M, Samuels B, Bodey G. Hepatosplenic candidiasis. A manifestation of chronic disseminated candidiasis. *Infect Dis Clin N Amer* 14:721–739, 2000a.

Kontoyiannis D, Wessel V, Bodey G, Rolston K. Zygomycosis in the 1990s in a tertiary care center. *Clin Infect Dis* 30:851–856, 2000b.

Lass-Florl C, Rath P, Niederwieser D, Kofler G, Wurzner R, Krezy A, Dierich M P. *Aspergillus terreus* infections in haematological malignancies: molecular epidemiology suggests association with in-hospital plants. *J Hosp Infect* 46:31–35, 2000.

Latge J P. *Aspergillus fumigatus* and aspergillosis. *Clin Microbiol Rev* 12:310–350, 1999.

Levy H, Horak, D A, Tegtmeier B R, Yokota S B, Forman S J. The value of bronchoalveolar lavage and bronchial washings in the diagnosis of invasive pulmonary aspergillosis. *Respir Med* 86: 243–248, 1992.

Lin S, Schranz J, Teutsch S. Aspergillosis case-fatality rate: systematic review of the literature. *Clin Infect Dis* 32:358–366, 2001.

Maertens J, Verhaegen J, Lagrou K, Van Eldere J, Boogaerts M. Screening for circulating galactomannan as a noninvasive diagnostic tool for invasive aspergillosis in prolonged neutropenic patients and stem cell transplantation recipients: a prospective validation. *Blood* 97:1604–1610, 2001.

Marr K A, White T C, van Burik J A H, Bowden R A. Development of fluconazole resistance in *Candida albicans* causing disseminated infection in a patient undergoing marrow transplantation. *Clin Infect Dis* 25:908–910, 1997.

Marr K, Carter R, Myerson D, Boeckh M, Corey L. Aspergillosis in HSCT recipients: evidence for two distinct pathophysiologic conditions associated with engraftment status. In *American Society of Hematology 42nd Annual Meeting*, San Francisco, CA, abstract #3403, 2000a.

Marr K, Seidel K, Slavin M, Bowden R, Schoch H, Flowers M, Corey L, Boeckh M. Prolonged fluconazole prophylaxis is associated with persistent protection against candidiasis-related death in allogeneic marrow transplant recipients: long-term follow-up of a randomized, placebo-controlled trial. *Blood* 96:2055–2061, 2000b.

Marr K A, Seidel K, White T C, Bowden R A. Candidemia in allogeneic blood and marrow transplant recipients: evolution of risk factors after the adoption of prophylactic fluconazole. *J Infect Dis* 181:309–316, 2000c.

Marr K A, Lyons C N, Ha K, Rustad T R, White T C. Inducible azole resistance associated with a heterogeneous phenotype in *Candida albicans*. *Antimicrob Agents Chemother* 45:52–59, 2001.

Marr K A. Empirical antifungal therapy—new options, new tradeoffs. *N Engl J Med* 346:278–280, 2002a.

Marr K, Carter R, Crippa F, Wald A, Corey L. Epidemiology and outcome of mould infections in hematopoietic stem cell transplant recipients. *Clin Infect Dis* 34:909–917, 2002b.

Marr K, Carter R, Boeckh M, Corey L. Invasive aspergillosis in stem cell transplant recipients: changing epidemiology and risk factors. Blood. 100:4358–4366, 2002c.

Martino R, Caballero M D, Canals C, San Miguel J, Sierra J, Rovira M, Solano C, Bargay J, Perez-Simon J, Leon A, Sarra J, Brunet S, de la Camara R. Reduced-intensity conditioning reduces the risk of severe infections after allogeneic peripheral blood stem cell transplantation. *Bone Marr Transplant* 28:341–347, 2001.

Mellado E, Cuenca-Estrella M, Regadera J, Gonzalez M, Diaz-Guerra T M, Rodriguez-Tudela J L. Sustained gastrointestinal colonization and systemic dissemination by *Candida albicans*, *Candida tropicalis* and *Candida parapsilosis* in adult mice. *Diagn Microbiol Infect Dis* 38:21–28, 2000.

Mencacci A, Perruccio K, Bacci A, Cenci E, Benedetti R, Martelli

M F, Bistoni F, Coffman R, Velardi A, Romani, L. Defective antifungal T-helper 1 (TH1) immunity in a murine model of allogeneic T-cell-depleted bone marrow transplantation and its restoration by treatment with TH2 cytokine antagonists. *Blood* 97:1483–1490, 2001.

Menichetti F, DelFavero A, Martino P, Bucaneve G, Micozzi A, Girmenia C, Barbabietola G, Pagano L, Leoni P, Specchia G, Caiozzo A, Raimondi R, Mandelli F, Program G I. Itraconazole oral solution as prophylaxis for fungal infections in neutropenic patients with hematologic malignancies: A randomized, placebo-controlled, double-blind, multicenter trial. *Clin Infect Dis* 28:250–255, 1999.

Miyazaki T, Kohno S, Mitsutake K, Maesaki S, Tanaka K, Ishikawa N, Hara K. Plasma (1,3)-beta-D-glucan and fungal antigenemia in patients with candidemia, aspergillosis, and cryptococcosis. *J Clin Microbiol* 33:3115–3118, 1995.

Mora-Duarte J, Betts R, Rotstein C, Colombo A L, Thompson-Moya L, Smietana J, Lupinacci R, Sable C, Kartsonis N, Perfect J. Caspofungin Invasive Candidiasis Study Group. Comparison of caspofungin and amphotericin B for invasive candidiasis. *N Engl J Med* 347:2020–2029, 2002.

Morgenstern G, Prentice A, Prentice H, Ropner J, Schey S, Warnock, D. A randomized controlled trial of itraconazole versus fluconazole for the prevention of fungal infections in patients with hematological malignancies. *Brit J Haematol* 105:901–911, 1999.

Morrison V, Haake R, Weisdorf D. Non-*Candida* fungal infections after bone marrow transplantation: risk factors and outcome. *Amer J Med* 96:497–503, 1993.

Nichols W G, Corey L, Gooley T, Davis C, Boeckh M. High risk of death due to bacterial and fungal infection among cytomegalovirus (CMV) seroponegative recipients of stem cell transplantations from seropositive donors: evidence for indirect effects of primary CMV infection. *J Infect Dis* 185:273–282, 2002.

Offner F, Cordonnier C, Ljungman P, Prentice H, Engelhard D, DeBacquer D, Meunier F, DePauw B. Impact of previous aspergillosis on the outcome of bone marrow transplantation. *Clin Infect Dis* 26:1098–1103, 1998.

Oliver M, Voorhis W V, Boeckh M, Mattson D, Bowden R. Hepatic mucormycosis in a bone marrow transplant recipient who ingested naturopathic medicine. *Clin Infect Dis* 22:521–524, 1996.

Ortiz J, Gonzalez San-Martin F, Abad M, Geigo F, Garcia-Macias M C, Bullon A. Necrotizing enterocolitis caused by *Aspergillus* in immunodepressed patient. *Rev Esp Enferm Dig* 92:826, 2000.

Patterson T F, Kirkpatrick W R, White M, Hiemenz J W, Wingard J R, Dupont B, Rinaldi M G, Stevens D A, Graybill J R. Invasive aspergillosis. Disease spectrum, treatment practices, and outcomes. I3 *Aspergillus* Study Group. *Medicine (Baltimore)* 79:250–260, 2000.

Perfect J, Schell W. The new fungal opportunists are coming. *Clin Infect Dis* 22:S112–S118, 1996.

Pizzo P A, Robichaud K J, Gill F A, Witebsky F G. Empiric antibiotic and antifungal therapy for cancer patients with prolonged fever and granulocytopenia. *Am J Med* 72:101–111, 1982.

Plouffe J F, Brown D G, Silva J, Jr., Eck T, Stricof R L, Fekety F R, Jr. Nosocomial outbreak of *Candida parapsilosis* fungemia related to intravenous infusions. *Arch Intern Med* 137:1686–1689, 1977.

Rex J, Walsh T, Sobel J, Filler S, Pappas P, Dismukes W, Edwards J. Practice guidelines for the treatment of candidiasis. *Clin Infect Dis* 30:662–678, 2000.

Ribaud P, Chastang C, Latge J., Baffroy-Lafitte L., Parquet N, Devergie A, Esperou H, Selimi F, Rocha V, Derouin F, Socie G, Gluckman E. Survival and prognostic factors of invasive aspergillosis after allogeneic bone marrow transplantation. *Clin Infect Dis* 28:322–330, 1999.

Ribes J, Vanover-Sams C, Baker D. Zygomycetes in human disease. *Clin Microbiol Rev* 13:236–301, 2000.

Saiman L, Ludington E, Pfaller M, Rangel-Frausto S, Wiblin R T, Dawson J, Blumberg H M, Patterson J E, Rinaldi M, Edwards J E, Wenzel R P, Jarvis W. Risk factors for candidemia in Neonatal Intensive Care Unit patients. The National Epidemiology of Mycosis Survey Study Group. *Pediatr Infect Dis J* 19:319–324, 2000.

Schell W A. New aspects of emerging fungal pathogens. A multifaceted challenge. *Clin Lab Med* 15:365–387, 1995.

Sherertz R J, Belani A, Kramer B S, Elfenbein G J, Weiner R S, Sullivan M L, Thomas R G, Samsa G P. Impact of air filtration on nosocomial *Aspergillus* infections. Unique risk of bone marrow transplant recipients. *Am J Med* 83:709–718, 1987.

Slavin M A, Osborne B, Adams R, Levenstein M J, Schoch H G, Feldman A R, Meyers J D, Bowden R A. Efficacy and safety of fluconazole prophylaxis for fungal infections after marrow transplantation—a prospective, randomized, double-blind study. *J Infect Dis* 171:1545–1552, 1995.

Small, T N, Papadopoulos E B, Boulad F, Black P, Castro-Malaspina H, Childs B H, Collins N, Gillio A, George D, Jakubowski A, Heller G, Fazzari M, Kernan N, MacKinnon S, Szabolcs P, Young J W, O'Reilly R J. Comparison of immune reconstitution after unrelated and related T-cell-depleted bone marrow transplantation: effect of patient age and donor leukocyte infusions. *Blood* 93:467–480, 1999.

Stevens D A, Kan V L, Judson M A, Morrison V A, Dummer S, Denning D W, Bennett J E, Walsh T J, Patterson T F, Pankey G A. Practice guidelines for diseases caused by *Aspergillus*. *Clin Infect Dis* 30:696–709, 2000.

Sulahian A, Boutboul F, Ribaud P, Leblanc T, Lacroix C, Derouin F. Value of antigen detection using an enzyme immunoassay in the diagnosis and prediction of invasive aspergillosis in two adult and pediatric hematology units during a 4-year prospective study. *Cancer* 91:311–318, 2001.

Thaler M, Pastakia B, Shawker T H, O'Leary T, Pizzo P A. Hepatic candidiasis in cancer patients: the evolving picture of the syndrome. *Ann Intern Med* 108:88–100, 1988.

Vail G, Young R, Wheat L, Filo R, Cornetta K, Goldman M. Incidence of histoplasmosis following allogeneic bone marrow transplantation or solid organ transplant in a hyperendemic area. *Transplant Infect Dis*, 4:148–151, 2002.

van Burik J H, Leisenring W, Myerson D, Hackman R C, Shulman H M, Sale G E, Bowden R A, McDonald G B. The effect of prophylactic fluconazole on the clinical spectrum of fungal diseases in bone marrow transplant recipients with special attention to hepatic candidiasis. *Medicine* 77:246–254, 1998.

Viscoli C, Girmenia C, Marinus A, Collette L, Martino P, Vandercam B, Doyen C, Lebeau B, Spence D, Krcmery V, De Pauw B, Meunier F. Candidemia in cancer patients: a prospective, multicenter surveillance study by the Invasive Fungal Infection Group (IFIG) of the European Organization for Research and Treatment of Cancer (EORTC). *Clin Infect Dis* 28:1071–1019, 1999.

Wald A, Leisenring W, van Burik J H, Bowden R A. Epidemiology of *Aspergillus* infections in a large cohort of patients undergoing bone marrow transplantation. *J Infect Dis* 175:1459–1466, 1997.

Walsh T, Chanock S. Diagnosis of invasive fungal infections in transplant recipients. In: Bowden R, Ljungman P, Paya C, eds. *Transplant Infections*. Philadelphia: Lippincott-Raven Publishers, 79–103, 1998a.

Walsh T, Hiemenz J, Seibel N, Perfect J, Horwith G, Lee L, Silber J, DiNubile M, Reboli A, Bow E, Lister J, Anaissie E. Amphotericin B lipid complex for invasive fungal infections: analysis of safety and efficacy in 556 cases. *Clin Infect Dis* 26:1383–1396, 1998b.

Walsh T, Groll A. Emerging fungal pathogens: evolving challenges to immunocompromised patients for the twenty-first century. *Trans Infect Dis* 1:257–261, 1999a.

Walsh T, Finberg R, Arndt C, Hiemenz J, Schwartz C, Bodensteiner D, Pappas P, Seibel N, Greenberg R, Dummer S, Schuster M, Holcenberg J, for the National Institute of Allergy and Infectious Disease Mycoses Study Group. Liposomal amphotericin B for empiric therapy in patients with persistent fever and neutropenia. *N Engl J Med* 340:764–771, 1999b.

Walsh T, Pappas P, Winston D, Lazarus H, Petersen F, Raffalli J, Yanovich S, Stiff P, Greenberg R, Donowitz G, Lee J for the National Institute of Allergy and Infectious Disease Mycoses Study Group. Voriconazole compared with liposomal amphotericin B for empirical antifungal therapy in patients with neutropenia and persistent fever. *N Engl J Med* 346:225–334, 2002.

Warris A, Gaustad P, Meis J F, Voss A, Verweij P E, Abrahamsen TG. Recovery of filamentous fungi from water in a paediatric bone marrow transplantation unit. *J Hosp Infect* 47:143–148, 2001.

Warris A, Voss A, Abrahamsen T G, Verweij P E. Contamination of hospital water with *Aspergillus fumigatus* and other molds. *Clin Infect Dis* 34:1159–1160, 2002.

Williamson E, Millar M, Steward C., Cornish J, Foot A, Oakhill A, Pamphilion D, Reeves B, Caul E, Warnock D, Marks D. Infections in adults undergoing unrelated donor bone marrow transplantation. *Brit J Haematol* 104:560–568, 1999.

Wilson M, Weinstein M, Reimer L, Mirrett S, Reller L. Controlled comparison of the BacT/Alert and BACTEC 660/730 nonradiometric blood culture systems. *J Clin Microbiol* 30:323–329, 1992.

Wingard J. Growth factors and other immunomodulators. In: Bowden R, Ljungman P, Paya, C, eds. *Transplant Infections*. Philadelphia: Lippincott-Raven, 367–378, 1998.

Wingard J R, White M, Anaissie E, Raffalli J, Goodman J, Arrieta A, and the LAmph/ABLC Collaborative Study Group. A randomized double-blind comparative trial evaluating the safety of liposomal amphotericin B versus amphotericin B lipid complex in the empirical treatment of febrile neutropenia. *Clin Infect Dis* 31:1155–1163, 2000.

Winston D, Maziarz R, Chandrasekar P, Lazarus H, Goldman M, Leitz G, Territo M. Long-term antifungal prophylaxis in allogeneic bone marrow transplant patients: a multicenter, randomized trial of intravenous/oral itraconazole vs. intravenous/oral fluconazole. American Society for Microbiology, 43rd Annual Meeting, Orlando, FL. Abstract #2002, 2001.

31

Fungal infections in solid organ transplant recipients

PETER G. PAPPAS

Solid organ transplantation has become an effective life-sparing modality for thousands of patients with organ failure syndromes. In spite of important advances in surgical technique and immunosuppressive regimens that have made solid organ transplantation a safer procedure today when compared to previous decades, there remain substantial risks of infection and other complications related to the procedure. Among the infectious complications of organ transplantation, none is associated with a greater impact on morbidity and mortality than invasive fungal infections (IFI) (Paya, 1993; Hibberd and Rubin 1994; Hadley and Karchmer, 1995a; Dictar et al, 2000). Fungal infections in organ transplant recipients (OTRs) vary in frequency, etiology, and pathogenesis according to the type of organ transplant procedure. Variations in immunosuppressive regimens, surgical technique, infection control, and exposure history further complicate evaluation of these patients. Moreover, the incidence of IFIs among this group of patients varies considerably from center to center, and an understanding of the overall burden of these infections according to type of organ transplant is lacking.

Thus, the clinician is faced with a number of challenges in assessing the OTR with possible IFI. First, there is a lack of sensitive and specific diagnostic assays that might lead to earlier intervention. Second, once a diagnosis of proven or suspected fungal infection is established, therapy is frequently toxic, which may be dose-limiting. Third, significant potential for drug–drug interactions exists between existing antifungal agents and immunosuppressive agents. Fourth, only limited data are available that facilitate early identification of patients who are at the highest risk for IFI within each transplant group. This chapter describes risk factors for developing IFIs among OTRs, reviews the specific fungal pathogens, and discusses an approach to the diagnosis, therapy, and prevention of these potentially devastating infections.

DETERMINING THE "NET STATE OF IMMUNOSUPPRESSION"

As advanced by Rubin (Rubin, 1994), the concept of "net state of immunosuppression" is a useful, albeit vague assessment of the overall risk of infection in the OTR. Quantitation of this risk in a reliable and reproducible manner is difficult. Assessing the net state of immunosuppression encompasses a number of host and environmental factors, each of which can impact host defense (Table 31–1). Included among these factors are dose, duration, and temporal sequence of specific immunosuppressive agents; underlying immune deficiency such as autoimmune disease and other functional immune deficits; integrity of the mucocutaneous barrier; anatomic abnormalities such as devitalized tissue and fluid collections; neutropenia and lymphopenia; underlying metabolic conditions such as renal insufficiency, malnutrition, diabetes mellitus, hepatic failure; and infection with immunomodulating viruses such as cytomegalovirus (CMV), Epstein Barr virus (EBV), hepatitis B and C viruses, human herpes virus (HHV-6), and human immunodeficiency virus (Fishman and Rubin, 1998).

While this approach is a useful guide to the assessment of risk for infection in OTRs, it does not take into account specific risk factors related either to different organ transplants or to surgical technique. A gross estimate of overall immunologic impairment can be made, but it does not provide a specific means by which the physician might more accurately determine the risk of IFI.

SPECIFIC FACTORS ASSOCIATED WITH INVASIVE FUNGAL INFECTION IN ORGAN TRANSPLANT RECIPIENTS

The development of IFI following solid organ transplantation is influenced by a number of different vari-

TABLE 31–1. *Factors Influencing the "Net State of Immunosuppression" in Solid Organ Transplant Recipients*

Immunosuppressive therapy

Dose and duration of individual agents
Recent rejection episodes
Use of antithymocyte globulin, total nodal irritation

Underlying immune disorders

Autoimmune disease
Antibody deficiency, complement deficiency, and other functional
   immune defects

Integrity of mucocutaneous barrier

Devitalized tissue, undrained fluid collections, hematomas

Neutropenia, lymphopenia

Metabolic conditions

Acute or chronic renal failure
Hepatic failure
Malnutrition
Diabetes mellitus
Alcoholism
Metabolic acidosis

Chronic viral infections

Cytomegalovirus
Epstein-Barr virus
Hepatitis B and C viruses
Human herpes virus 6
Human immunodeficiency virus types 1 and 2
Human T-cell lymphotrophic virus type 1

Adapted from Fishman and Rubin, 1998.

ables. These include the type and timing of the organ transplant; the specific immunosuppressive regimen including the timing and frequency of rejection episodes; donor transmitted infections; comorbid conditions and coinfections in the recipient, especially viral infections; perioperative fungal colonization; and other factors including previous exposure and recent epidemiology. Each of these variables is discussed below.

Type of Solid Organ Transplant

The risk of IFI varies depending on the organ transplanted. Moreover, distribution of causative organisms also varies with the type of transplant. Some risk factors are common to all OTRs such as retransplantation, prolonged ICU stay with mechanical ventilation, requirement for surgical reexploration, primary graft nonfunction, and active CMV infection. Other risk factors are specific to the type of transplant, and may relate to the type of anastomosis, differences in intensity of immunosuppression, or other variables.

Kidney. Kidney transplantation is associated with the least risk of IFI. The cumulative incidence of IFI following renal transplantation varies between 2% and 14% (Patel and Paya, 1997; Patel, 2001), and the most common fungi causing infection are *Candida* spp., followed by *Aspergillus* spp., and *Cryptococcus neoformans* (Howard et al, 1978; Paya, 1993; Abbott et al, 2001). In geographic regions where *Histoplasma capsulatum* and *Coccidioides immitis* are endemic, these organisms can also be important pathogens in the posttransplant period. For instance, histoplasmosis was seen among renal allograft recipients in two large urban outbreaks in Indianapolis (Wheat et al, 1983), and coccidioidomycosis was found to be the most common IFI among renal transplant recipients in Arizona (Cohen et al, 1982). Sporadic reports of other fungi causing significant infection include *Fusarium* spp. and other hyalohyphomycetes (Heinz et al, 1996), the zygomycetes (Chkhotua et al, 2001), *Trichosporon asahii* and other pathogenic yeasts (Lussier et al, 2000), and the phaeohyphomycotic agents (Revankar et al, 2002).

Candida infection may be mucocutaneous, urinary, or deeply invasive. Factors predisposing to urinary tract infection include bladder catheterization, structural abnormalities or disruption of urinary flow, corticosteroids, and diabetes mellitus (Gallis et al, 1975). Asymptomatic urinary tract colonization with *Candida* spp. is particularly common in this OTR group and can be associated with significant consequences. Most commonly, renal parenchymal disease may result from ascending infection from the bladder (Peterson et al 1982; Nampoory et al, 1996; Patel 2001). Rarely, urinary tract colonization can be associated with the development of a ureteral fungus ball, leading to obstruction of urinary flow and threatening allograft survival (Gallis et al 1975). Nosocomial candidemia in renal transplant recipients is most commonly associated with recognized risk factors for invasive candidiasis among nontransplanted patients such as indwelling venous catheter, and can occasionally lead to secondary involvement of the allograft from hematogenous spread (Hadley and Karchmer, 1995a; Patel, 2001).

Risk factors for the development of invasive aspergillosis are less well established in renal transplant patients. Underlying diabetes mellitus, cadaveric allograft, increased corticosteroid usage, retransplantation, and recent CMV infection have been associated with invasive aspergillosis (Paterson and Singh, 1999; Patterson et al, 2000). Involvement of the lungs or disseminated multiorgan disease is most common, but focal extrapulmonary disease, e.g., cerebral abscess (Carlini et al, 1998; Garcia et al, 1998), endocarditis (Marin et al, 1999; Viertel et al, 1999), tuboovarian abscess (Kim et al, 2001), and focal prostatic or ureteral involvement (Shirwany et al, 1998; Kaplan-Pavlovic et al, 1999) have been reported.

Among the other fungal pathogens reported among renal transplant recipients, *C. neoformans* is the most common, occurring in approximately 2% of patients (Husain et al 2001). Zygomycoses, phaeohyphomycoses, and hyalohyphomycoses are less commonly reported. Risk factors for the development of these infections are poorly defined, but most occur beyond 4 to 6 months posttransplantation and are often associated with chronic allograft rejection and higher dose immunosuppression (Hibberd and Rubin, 1994; Hadley and Karchmer, 1995a).

Pancreas and Kidney–Pancreas. Invasive fungal infections among pancreas and kidney–pancreas transplant recipients occur much more frequently than among renal transplant recipients. The cumulative incidence of IFIs in this group ranges between 6% and 38%, with the predominance of these infections due to *Candida* spp. (Paya, 1993; Lumbreras et al, 1995; Benedetti et al, 1996). A much smaller proportion is due to *Aspergillus* spp. and other filamentous moulds (Lumbreras et al, 1995; Smets et al, 1997; Patel and Paya, 1997).

The increased risk of IFI in this group largely relates to surgical and technical issues. Specifically, the type of surgical anastomosis can be associated with local complications and *Candida* superinfection (Hesse et al, 1985; Benedetti et al, 1996; Pirsch et al, 1998). Bladder drained pancreas transplants are associated with a much higher incidence of urinary tract infections due to all causes, but especially due to *Candida* spp. In contrast, enterically drained pancreatic transplants are much more likely to develop enteric leaks leading to polymicrobial intraabdominal infections in which *Candida* is an important pathogen (Pirsch et al, 1998). Experts disagree as to which of these two anastomotic and drainage procedures leads to fewer postoperative fungal infections, as the published data vary according to center.

As with other OTRs, the risk of IFI is significantly greater among patients with recent CMV infection, graft rejection or failure, surgical reoperation, higher dose immunosuppression (especially corticosteroids), and bacterial coinfection.

Liver. Historically, liver transplantation has been associated with the highest risk of IFI among solid organ transplant recipients with an incidence as high as 42% (Wajszczuk et al, 1985). This rate has dropped in recent years to approximately 10%–20% (Viviani et al, 1992; Hadley et al, 1995b; Patel et al, 1996). Changes in surgical technique, immunosuppressive regimens, and improved patient selection have led to this signif-

icant decrease in IFI rates. The vast majority of IFIs in liver transplant recipients are caused by *Candida* spp. and usually occur within the first month posttransplant (Castaldo et al, 1991; Collins et al, 1994; Wade et al, 1995). *Aspergillus* spp. and the agents of zygomycosis are much less frequent in this population (Kusne et al, 1988; Hadley et al, 1995b; Patel et al, 1996).

Risk factors for the development of IFI have been well defined in the liver transplant population. In an elegant study by Collins and colleagues, several important and independent variables were related to increased risk of fungal infection in the posttransplant period (Collins et al, 1994). These included baseline creatinine ≥ 3 mg/dL, operative time ≥ 11 hours, retransplantation, active CMV infection, and an intraoperative requirement of > 50 units of blood products. The risk of fungal infection was < 1% without any risk factor, compared to 67% among patients with two or more of these risk factors (Collins et al, 1994). In addition, choledochojejunostomy anastomosis and early colonization with a fungal pathogen were strongly associated with the development of IFI in this study. Others have identified similar trends among liver transplant recipients and have consistently related prolonged intraoperative time, requirement for a large number of blood products, CMV infection, and choledochojejunostomy anastomosis to an increased risk of developing IFI (Castaldo et al, 1991; Patel et al, 1996; Kusne et al, 1998).

Heart. There is a moderate risk of IFI following heart transplantation. The reported rate occurrence ranges from 4% to 35% (Waser et al, 1994; Kramer et al, 1993), although more recent reports suggest an overall rate of less than 10% (Miller et al, 1994; Grossi et al, 2000). *Candida* spp. account for at least two-thirds of the fungal infections with most infections occurring within the first 2 months posttransplant. Invasive aspergillosis is somewhat more common in cardiac compared to liver and kidney transplant recipients for reasons possibly related to the degree of immunosuppression (Hofflin et al, 1987). Recent data among these patients suggest that the risk of death due to IFI is significantly higher (36% vs. 12%), $p < 0.0001$) than infections due to either bacterial or viral pathogens (Miller et al, 1994). Invasive aspergillosis is an especially important cause of death in heart transplant patients, accounting for almost 25% of deaths in European studies (Grossi et al, 1992).

Invasive *Candida* infections among heart transplant recipients are usually limited to candidemia and its complications. In addition, preexisting colonization with *Candida* spp. of ventricular assist devices is an established risk factor for the subsequent development of invasive *Candida* infection (Goldstein et al, 1995; Argenziano et al, 1997). Mediastinitis due to *Candida* is another important postoperative complication (Hofflin et al, 1987). Active CMV infection, the use of anti-lymphocyte antibodies, and treatment for rejection are the most common risk factors associated with IFI in heart transplant recipients.

Lung and Heart–Lung. In most transplant centers, the rate of IFI among lung and heart–lung transplant recipients is greater than among recipients of heart transplants alone (Dummer et al, 1986, Kramer et al, 1993, Gordon and Avery, 2001). The cumulative incidence among this group of transplant recipients ranges between 10% and 36% with most recent figures suggesting a rate of approximately 15% (Mehrad et al, 2001). Recent data suggest that *Aspergillus* spp. have emerged as the dominant pathogens in this population (Yeldandi et al, 1995). At one institution, among 28 episodes of IFI, 14 (50%) were due to *Aspergillus* spp., 12 (43%) due to *Candida* spp., and 1 each due to *C. neoformans* and *C. immitis* (Kramer et al, 1993).

Invasive aspergillosis occurs in between 3.3% and 16% of lung and heart–lung recipients (Yeldandi et al, 1995; Westney et al, 1996; Cahill et al, 1997; Husni et al, 1998; Gordon and Avery, 2001). The enhanced risk of developing invasive aspergillosis among lung transplant recipients relates to several factors: prior airway colonization with *Aspergillus* spp. (Cahill et al, 1997); CMV infection (Husni et al, 1998); environmental exposure through routine daily activities; and hypogammoglobulinemia. The latter has been identified as a potential risk factor, although this observation has not been confirmed by other investigators (Goldfarb et al, 2000). In addition, smoking substances such as marijuana is an additional risk among this group of patients (Marks et al, 1996). Furthermore, patients with single lung transplants appear to have a greater risk of invasive aspergillosis than double lung transplants, a risk that is likely due to colonization with *Aspergillus* spp. in the remaining native lung (Westney et al, 1996). Interestingly, preexisting *Aspergillus* spp. and *Scedosporium* colonization among patients with cystic fibrosis is not associated with a significantly increased risk of IFI due to these organisms posttransplantation (Nunley et al, 1998; Cimon et al, 2000). In fact, among all lung transplant recipients, those with cystic fibrosis appear to be at a somewhat lesser risk of invasive mould disease than other lung transplant recipients.

In addition to nosocomial candidemia, *Candida* infections complicating lung transplantation include mycotic aneurysm involving the aortic anastomosis, mediastinal wound infection, and necrotizing bronchitis at the tracheal anastomotic site (Brooks et al, 1985; Dauber et al, 1990; Kramer et al, 1993; Kanj et al, 1996).

Pneumocystis carinii pneumonia (PCP) occurs more commonly in heart–lung and lung transplant recipients than in any other solid organ transplant group (Dummer et al, 1986). In a prospective study of heart–lung recipients not receiving TMP/SMX prophylaxis, *P. carinii* was identified in 88% of patients utilizing serial BAL specimens. Thirty-five percent of these patients were symptomatic, 24% subclinical, and 41% asymptomatic (Gryzan et al, 1988). *Pneumocystis carinii* pneumonia is now very uncommon with the widespread use of TMP/SMX prophylaxis.

Small Bowel. There is considerable risk of IFI following small bowel transplantation, ranging between 33% and 59% (Reyes et al, 1992; Kusne et al 1996). In addition to risk factors common to other OTRs, intraoperative complications include small bowel anastomotic leak as the unique risk factor associated with this type of transplantation. Not surprisingly, *Candida* spp. constitute the majority of fungal pathogens in small bowel transplant recipients, with *Aspergillus* and other moulds playing a lesser role. Prospective data among small bowel transplant patients are limited given the relative rarity of this transplant procedure, which has largely been limited to children with congenital small bowel disorders and highly selected adult patients (Reyes et al, 1998).

Timing of Invasive Fungal Infection in Organ Transplant Recipients

Despite the differences in frequency and distribution of pathogens among the various transplant groups, the timing of these infections following organ transplantation is similar. As such, the posttransplant period can be divided into three intervals when assessing the risk and type of IFI: 0–1 month, 1–6 months, and beyond 6 months posttransplant (Fig. 31–1). Understanding the temporal relatedness of the posttransplant interval to the risk and type of IFI can be very useful to the clinician in formulating a specific diagnosis and guiding empiric therapy. It also highlights the differences in pathogenesis for IFI during these intervals (Rubin, 1994; Patel and Paya, 1997; Fishman and Rubin, 1998; Patel, 2001).

Infections in the first month posttransplant are dominated by *Candida* spp. and are usually related to technical and surgical problems in addition to traditional nosocomial risk factors. Thus, anastomotic leaks, early graft failure, reoperations, central venous catheter-associated fungemia, and catheter-associated urinary tract infections are common. In one study among liver transplant recipients, over 50% of IFIs occurred within the first 10 days posttransplant, almost all of them caused by *Candida* spp. (Collins et al, 1994). In the absence of early graft failure, retransplantation, signifi-

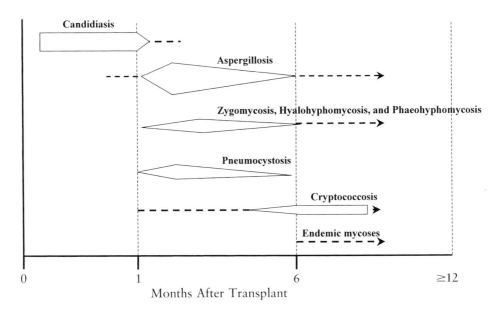

FIGURE 31–1. Timeline of fungal infections in solid organ transplant recipients.

cant pretransplant immunosuppression, or other mitigating circumstances, mould infections, especially those due to *Aspergillus* spp., are uncommon during this period. Donor-related infections, especially those due to *Candida* spp. and *Aspergillus* spp., often present during this first interval, 0–1 months posttransplantation.

During the second interval, 1–6 months posttransplantation, the effects of intense immunosuppression become manifest as the impact of nosocomial and surgical-related infections diminish. This second phase is dominated by mould infections, especially aspergillosis, zygomycosis, scedosporiosis, and less common mould diseases. *Pneumocystis carinii* pneumonia is also common during this period among patients not receiving TMP/SMX prophylaxis. The peak incidence of aspergillosis is between 1 and 4 months, but there continues to be small risk of invasive aspergillosis throughout the posttransplant period (Hibberd and Rubin, 1994; Hadley and Karchmer, 1995a; Husain et al 2001). The development of IFI during this time interval often follows evidence of active disease with an immunomodulating virus such as CMV, HHV-6, EBV, or hepatitis B and C.

The interval beyond 6 months posttransplantation is generally considered to be the period during which IFI is least likely to occur. Nonetheless, especially among patients with chronic rejection, graft dysfunction, late CMV infection, and other transplant-associated viral infections, IFI may occur. The late posttransplant period is dominated by fungal infections due to *C. neoformans*, regionally endemic mycoses, and some of the more unusual pathogens including the phaeohyphomycotic agents. However, mould infections due to *Aspergillus* spp. and the agents of zygomycoses may occur at any time in the posttransplant period (Peddi et al, 1996; Singh et al, 1997b; Husain et al, 2001).

Immunosuppressive Regimen

The most important factor effecting the risk of IFI after the first month of transplantation is the intensity and duration of immunosuppression produced by the agents used to prevent organ rejection. Most OTRs currently receive either a cyclosporine or tacrolimus-based immunosuppressive regimen. This is perhaps the most important change in immunotherapy over the last several years, and allows clinicians to reduce the level of glucocorticosteroid exposure. Reduction in overall glucocorticosteroid exposure has had a significant impact on decreasing the overall incidence of IFI among OTRs.

Immunosuppression is initiated at high levels in the immediate posttransplant period when the risk of graft rejection is greatest. Currently, such regimens employ the use of cyclosporine or tacrolimus in combination with mycophenolate mofetil or azathioprine and glucocorticosteroids in most patients. Typically, these regimens are continued at higher doses in the early posttransplant period, and gradually tapered to a chronic maintenance regimen within 6 months in the absence of significant rejection (Denton et al, 1999). In selected patients, antithymocyte globulin (e.g., OKT$_3$, ATG) is administered during the early posttransplant period to prevent acute rejection. The administration of these agents increases the risk of CMV infection and subsequently IFI. No doubt this approach to immunotherapy in OTRs will continue to evolve as safer and more effective agents are developed.

Studies among liver transplant recipients comparing cyclosporine and tacrolimus have not demonstrated any clear difference with respect to incidence of IFI (Kusne et al, 1992; The U.S. Multicenter FK506 Study Group, 1994; Hadley et al, 1995b). Similarly, studies among renal transplant recipients comparing regimens utilizing mycophenolate mofetil or azathioprine have not demonstrated any significant difference in rate of IFIs (Bernabeu-Wittel et al, 2002). Moreover, recent data suggest that use of the calcineurin inhibitors (cyclosporine, tacrolimus, and sirolimus) has led to decreased rates and severity of IFI because of their modest in vitro antifungal activity. Thus, the recent reduction in IFIs associated with the calcineurin inhibitors may not only relate to a glucocorticosteroid-sparing effect, but also to modest antifungal activity.

Some of the more convincing data concerning the relationship between the use of cyclosporine and decrease in observed frequency of IFIs come from the Stanford Cardiac Transplantation Group in a study involving 110 patients. In this study, 26% of patients who received primarily corticosteroids vs. 14% of patients on cyclosporine-based regimens developed IFI (Hofflin et al, 1987). Other groups have made similar observations, and the general consensus has emerged that there has been a marked decrease in the overall burden of fungal disease among OTRs maintained on calcineurin-based immunosuppressive regimens.

The timing and frequency of rejection episodes as it relates to intensification of immunosuppressive regimens is also an important factor associated with IFIs in OTRs. Pulse-dose glucocorticosteroids are commonly administered in this setting, usually coupled with an overall intensification of immunosuppressive therapy. In addition, specific antilymphocyte therapy is often administered in this setting. Together, these interventions invariably lead to a higher rate of CMV reactivation and a concomitant increased risk of IFI.

Donor-Related Fungal Infections

The vast majority of donor-related transplant infections are viral in origin. Well-documented donor-related infections are CMV, EBV, hepatitis B, hepatitis C, and HIV. Donor-related fungal infections are much less common; often the source of the pathogen is suspected to be the donor, but convincing proof is lacking. Nonetheless, several very well-documented cases of donor-transmitted fungal infections have been reported, including cases of histoplasmosis (Wong and Allen, 1992; Limaye et al, 2000), coccidioidomycosis (Wright et al, 2001; Tripathy et al, 2002), cryptococcosis (Kanj et al, 1996), candidiasis (Battaglia et al, 2000), and aspergillosis (Keating et al, 1996).

Among donors from areas that are endemic for histoplasmosis and coccidioidomycosis, a suspicion for la-

tent disease must be maintained. However, transmission of the two pathogens, *H. capsulatum* and *C. immitis*, has been very uncommon. Of more concern is the risk of donor associated *Aspergillus* infection among lung transplant recipients, where colonization of the donor lung with *Aspergillus* spp. is common (Cahill et al, 1997). Similarly, there is significant potential for lung donor–related cryptococcosis among donors who have unrecognized asymptomatic pulmonary nodules or granulomatous disease.

Comorbid Conditions and Infections in the Recipient

Underlying diseases in the host contribute to the "net state of immunosuppression," and no doubt influence the risk of IFI. Factors that have most commonly been associated with an increased risk include renal dysfunction and the need for peritoneal or hemodialysis, diabetes mellitus, neutropenia, malnutrition, mechanical ventilation, admission to an intensive care unit, and recipients of chronic immunosuppressive therapy pretransplant (Fishman and Rubin, 1998). The degree to which these factors individually influence risk has been difficult to discern.

Among viral infections that increase the risk of IFI, CMV is clearly the most common. Ample evidence from large retrospective studies relate active CMV disease to increased risk of fungal infection in OTRs (Collins et al, 1994; Hadley et al, 1995b; Patel et al, 1996; Husni et al, 1998). Additional data suggest active hepatitis C infection is an important risk factor for IFI. Recently, Rogers and colleagues demonstrated an association between HHV-6 seropositivity and a significantly increased risk of IFI by a multivariate analysis. In this study, 32% percent of HHV-6 culture-positive liver transplant recipients vs. 4% of HHV-6 culture-negative transplant recipients developed IFI ($p = 0.0009$) (Rogers et al, 2000).

SPECIFIC FUNGAL PATHOGENS

Candida species

Candida spp. are by far the commonest invasive fungal pathogens among OTRs. Virtually all of the common *Candida* spp., including *C. albicans, C. glabrata, C. tropicalis, C. parapsilosis, C. krusei, C. lusitaniae, C. rugosa, C. kefyr,* and *C. gulliermondii* have been reported in this population. *Candida albicans* is the commonest species, accounting for approximately 50% of invasive infections. *Candida glabrata, C. tropicalis,* and *C. parapsilosis* are the next most frequent species. In contrast to hematopoetic stem cell transplant recipients, *Candida krusei* is a relatively uncommon pathogen in OTRs. The emergence of the non*albicans* species as pathogens among OTRs is not entirely understood, but appears to parallel their emergence in the nontransplant setting. Clearly, the broad use of prophylactic and empiric antifungal therapy, particularly with the azoles, has played an important role in the transition from predominantly *C. albicans* to a significant proportion of non-*albicans Candida* isolates. Factors leading to candidemia are similar among OTRs and nontransplant patients, but the rate of complicated infection as evidenced by disseminated disease appears to be greater among OTRs than among non-transplanted patients (Meunier et al, 1992; Rubin, 1994).

Intraabdominal infections secondary to *Candida* infections are significantly more common among liver, pancreas, and small bowel transplant recipients compared to other OTRs. The former patients undergo disruption of the normal anatomy of the small bowel, common bile duct, and/or pancreatic duct with the potential for intraabdominal anastomotic leakage. Intraabdominal infectious complications usually occur within the first month posttransplant and are frequently polymicrobial. Sternal wound infections among heart and heart–lung transplants due to *Candida* spp. have been reported, and can be associated with significant morbidity and mortality (Brooks et al, 1985; Hofflin et al, 1987; Dauber et al, 1990). Among lung transplants, anastomotic infections secondary to *Candida* spp. have been reported (Kanj et al, 1996).

Urinary tract infections due to *Candida* are common among OTRs owing to the need for bladder catheterization during the period of hospitalization, particularly in the immediate postoperative period. Candiduria is a particularly worrisome complication among renal transplant recipients where it can be a harbinger of complicated upper tract disease. Thus, candiduria is usually regarded as a significant urinary infection or as an important predictor of increased risk of invasive candidiasis (Collins et al, 1994; Patel et al, 1996). An unusual complication of *Candida* urinary tract infection in OTRs is the development of a ureteral fungus ball due to *Candida* spp, (Gallis et al, 1975). While this complication is most often seen in renal transplant recipients, it can be seen in any OTR, and may clinically mimic fungus ball due to less common urinary pathogens such as *Aspergillus* spp.

Another important syndrome due to *Candida* spp. relates to vascular anastomotic infections. True "mycotic" aneurysms occurring at the site of the vascular anastomosis due to *Candida* spp. have been reported among pancreatic (Ciancio et al, 1996), renal (Potti et al, 1998), and heart–lung transplant recipients (Dowling et al, 1990). Although rare, these represent a very significant and highly lethal postoperative complication. Less common complications of *Candida* infection include septic arthritis, chronic meningitis, endocardi-

tis, and rarely, pneumonia (Ralph and Hussain, 1996; Choi et al, 2000).

Aspergillus

Invasive aspergillosis is reported among all transplant groups; however, lung transplant recipients seem to be uniquely predisposed to infections with *Aspergillus* spp. As many as 10% of lung transplant recipients will develop significant infection with *Aspergillus* and another 10% develop *Aspergillus* colonization posttransplantation (Paterson and Singh, 1999). Among other OTRs, the risk of invasive aspergillosis is substantially less including heart (6% to 7%), liver (2% to 3%), and renal transplant recipients. *Aspergillus fumigatus* is the most common causative species; however, infections due to *A. flavus, A. niger, A. terreus, A. nidulans, A. glaucus, A. ustus, A. versicolor,* and other less common species have been reported. Moreover, multiple species may be isolated from the same patient.

Aspergillus spores are ubiquitous in the environment, and infection often begins as a result of inhalation, resulting in lower respiratory tract colonization. Disease may be confined to the lungs or may disseminate to virtually any organ, but most commonly the skin, central nervous system, heart, and the endocrine glands, especially the thyroid (Denning, 1998; Patterson et al, 2000). Disseminated disease is associated with a mortality of greater than 80% (Lin et al, 2001).

Ulcerative tracheobronchitis due to *Aspergillus* is a recently described syndrome among lung transplant recipients (Kramer et al 1991). This disease is characterized by superficial invasion of the tracheobronchial tree, typically at the site of an anastomosis, but may occur virtually anywhere within the proximal airway. The disease has been reported among other transplant groups (Sayiner et al, 1999), but is distinctly uncommon outside of lung transplant recipients. Patients with this form of aspergillosis are usually either asymptomatic or minimally symptomatic with chronic nonproductive cough. Bronchoscopy reveals single or multiple ulcerative lesions, usually at the anastomotic site.

Aspergillus spp. frequently colonize the upper airways, which makes it difficult to distinguish between invasive disease and asymptomatic colonization among certain patients. However, the detection of significant *Aspergillus* colonization in the upper airways is strongly predictive of invasive disease in most OTRs with a positive predictive value of at least 60% (Horvath and Dummer, 1996; Brown et al, 1996; Cahill et al, 1997; Perfect et al, 2002). Thus, a preemptive approach to therapy among colonized, high-risk patients may be warranted.

Other manifestations of invasive aspergillosis in OTRs include sinusitis, thoracic empyema, and angioinvasion at virtually any site (Paterson and Singh,

1999; Patterson et al, 2000). Furthermore, *Aspergillus* has been reported as a cause of urinary tract fungus ball and prostate abscess in renal and liver transplant recipients (Shirwany et al, 1998; Kaplan-Pavlovcic et al, 1999).

Invasive aspergillosis usually occurs between 1 to 4 months posttransplantation, but may occur several years following transplantation, especially among patients undergoing intensification of immunosuppressive therapy or receiving higher dose corticosteroids for allograft rejection. Additional risk factors for invasive aspergillosis include CMV infection and early graft failure (Peterson et al, 1982; Husni et al, 1998). Among lung transplant recipients, those who receive single lungs are at greater risk of developing invasive aspergillosis than double lung recipients (Gordon and Avery, 2001).

The source of *Aspergillus* infection can be difficult to discern. Recent studies have suggested that nosocomial transmission occurs, although the frequency of this event is unclear (Patterson, 1999; Patterson et al, 2000). Also, the recipient may serve as his own reservoir for *Aspergillus*, especially among single lung transplant recipients (Westney et al, 1996). Community-acquired infection occurs, but its relative importance compared to nosocomial acquisition remains unknown. Donor-related infection has been reported, but its relative importance compared to other sources of infection is not known (Keating et al, 1996).

Cryptococcus

Cryptococcus is the third most common IFI in OTRs, and usually occurs in the late posttransplant period (Husain et al, 2001). Disease is most commonly due to *C. neoformans var. neoformans*, although disease due to *C. neoformans var. gattii*, *C. albidus*, and *C. laurentii* has been reported. Manifestations of cryptococcal disease are similar among OTRs and HIV-infected individuals. Primary infection usually occurs following inhalation (Kapoor et al, 1999), although there are sporadic reports of direct primary cutaneous disease possibly resulting from direct inoculation (Hunger et al, 2000; Nosanchuk et al, 2000). Most patients present with nonspecific respiratory symptoms, unexplained fever, or an asymptomatic nodule on chest roentgenogram. Asymptomatic infection with *C. neoformans* is common; thus, it is unclear how often extrapulmonary dissemination occurs in OTRs. The central nervous system is the most common extrapulmonary site of cryptococcal disease in OTRs, followed by involvement of the skin and subcutaneous tissue, bones, and prostate. Cutaneous involvement is more common in OTRs than among nonimmunocompromised patients. Atypical cellulitis is the most common cutaneous manifestation in this population, and must be distinguished from cel-

lulitis due to common bacterial and mycobacterial pathogens (Anderson et al, 1992). Among OTRs, liver transplant recipients appear to be at a somewhat greater risk of developing cryptococcosis with an overall incidence of 1% to 3.5% (Kusne et al, 1988; Wade et al, 1995; Singh et al, 1997a). Cryptococcemia is especially common in this group and is generally associated with a worse clinical outcome (Dromer et al, 1996; Pappas et al, 2001).

Donor transmission of *C. neoformans* has been suggested in rare instances. A recent report in a lung transplant recipient from whom *C. neoformans* was isolated from a bronchial washing obtained 2 days postoperative strongly suggests a donor source of infection (Kanj et al, 1996).

Recent experience among OTRs with cryptococcosis suggest that outcomes are at least as good as among patients who are otherwise normal hosts (Dromer et al, 1996; Pappas et al, 2001). This paradox is not well understood, but could relate to the intensity with which patients are followed after organ transplantation and the ability to make a diagnosis earlier in the course of infection. Corticosteroids may have an ameliorating effect early in the course of cryptococcosis, particularly when the central nervous system is involved. Lastly, the use of the calcineurin inhibitors, especially tacrolimus, which possess not only modest in vitro antifungal activity, but also excellent CNS penetration, may have a beneficial effect on the natural history and severity of CNS cryptococcosis in OTRs. Investigators also suggest that a relative increase in cutaneous expression of disease may be the result of poor antifungal activity of tacrolimus at lower temperatures found in cutaneous tissue (Husain et al, 2001).

Zygomycetes

Zygomycetes has been reported in all organ transplant recipients. Disease may be due to several Zygomycetes including, but not limited to, *Rhizopus* spp., *Mucor* spp., *Cunninghamella bertholletiae*, *Absidia* spp., and *Conidiobolus coronatus*. Risk factors for invasive Zygomycosis include neutropenia, ketoacidosis, renal failure, and treatment of chronic rejection, especially with high-dose steroids. Clinical disease often involves the paranasal sinuses leading to destructive lesions and central nervous system involvement by direct extension. Thus, the classical presentation of rhinocerebral zygomycosis involvement is the most readily recognized disease manifestation among OTRs. The lungs are also a commonly involved site, although virtually any organ can be involved (Singh et al, 1995; Demirag et al, 2000; Lee et al, 2001; Jimenez et al, 2002). Multiple organ involvement consistent with hematogenous dissemination is reported, but is less common than that due to invasive aspergillosis, even though the pathogenesis of both disorders involves angioinvasion. *Conidiobolus coronatus, a* Zygomycete effecting patients living in tropical areas, has been reported as a cause of disseminated disease (Walker et al, 1992).

The typical clinical finding associated with zygomycosis is a necrotizing, locally invasive process. Necrotizing wound infections have been associated with Zygomycetes (Jimenez et al, 2002), and infection of a renal allograft has also been reported (Chkhotua et al, 2001). In addition, localized gastrointestinal zygomycosis characterized by giant gastric and/or colonic ulcers have been reported (Sheu, 1998; Ju et al, 2001; Timmoth et al, 2001).

Phaeohyphomycoses

The agents of phaeohyphomycosis consist of over 100 pigmented moulds and a growing number of these species have been reported to cause disease among OTRs (Singh et al, 1997b; Revankar et al, 2002). The clinical spectrum of these infections includes invasive sinusitis, pneumonia, endophthalmitis, skin and musculoskeletal involvement, CNS disease, gastrointestinal involvement, and disseminated disease. Disease due to *Exophiala* spp., *Dactylaria constricta, Alternaria* spp., *Bipolaris spicifera, Curvularia spp., Cladophialophora bantiana, Colletotrichum crassipes, Phaeocremonium parasiticum* and *Fonsecaea pedrosoi* has been reported (Gold et al, 1994; Salama et al, 1997; von Eiff et al, 1997; Mesa et al, 1999; Malani et al, 2000; Castro et al, 2001; Magina et al, 2001; Halaby et al, 2001). In a recent review of disseminated phaeohyphomycosis in OTRs, Revankar and colleagues noted that only 16% of patients survived despite therapy (Revankar et al, 2002). In another review of the same disease, Singh and colleagues noted that cutaneous and synovial involvement was usually caused by *Exophiala* spp., whereas systemic infections including CNS involvement were caused by less common organisms such as *Ochroconis gallopavum* and *Cladophialophora bantiana* (Singh et al, 1997b). Phaeohyphomycotic infections are usually late-occurring, and specific risk factors for development have not been clearly delineated.

Endemic Fungi

Infections due to *C. immitis* and *H. capsulatum* are not uncommon among OTRs who have lived in endemic areas. The true incidence of these infections is unknown, but estimates range between 0.3% and 6% with most cases occurring within the first year posttransplant (Davies et al, 1979; Wheat et al, 1983; Holt et al, 1997). A history of prior infection without evidence of active disease does not exclude potential donors or recipients at most centers. Nonetheless, the potential for donor-related transmission with either of these organisms remains a concern in endemic areas.

One recent report clearly documenting donor-related *H. capsulatum* transmission to two kidney recipients residing in geographically diverse nonendemic areas underscores this point (Limaye et al, 2000). Another report of two donor-related cases of coccidioidomycosis in one liver and one renal transplant recipient without evidence of prior exposure further emphasizes the need to ascertain evidence of disease activity among donor patients with a previous history of coccidioidomycosis or histoplasmosis (Wright et al, 2001).

Histoplasmosis is the most commonly reported endemic mycosis among OTRs. The majority of reports have been described among renal transplant recipients although histoplasmosis has also been described in liver, heart, and lung recipients (Peddi et al, 1996; Shallott et al, 1997; Vinayek et al, 1998; Jha et al, 1999; Bacal et al, 2001). Transmission from the donor organ has been documented in several of these cases (Hood et al, 1965; Watanabe et al, 1988; Wong and Allen, 1992; Botterel et al, 1999; Limaye et al, 2000). Histoplasmosis in OTRs usually presents as disseminated disease although focal involvement of the central nervous system (Karalakulasingam et al, 1976; Livas et al, 1995), skin (Farr et al, 1981), renal papilla (Superdock et al, 1994), and gastrointestinal tract has been described. In addition, cecal and ileal perforation associated with gastrointestinal histoplasmosis has been described (Zainudin et al, 1992; Brett, 1988).

Coccidioidomycosis following organ transplantation has been reported in up to 6% of OTRs living in the endemic area of the desert in the southwest United States (Cohen et al, 1982). Disease is probably due to either recent environmental exposure or to reactivation of a latent infection, as there is less documentation of donor-related transmission. Clinical features of coccidioidomycosis in this population vary from pneumonia to disseminated disease involving skin, musculoskeletal structures, and the central nervous system (Cohen et al, 1982; Holt et al, 1997). The majority of cases of posttransplant coccidioidomycosis have been reported among renal, heart, and liver transplant recipients.

In contrast to histoplasmosis and coccidioidomycosis, blastomycosis is distinctly uncommon among OTRs, even among patients residing in endemic areas. There has been no evidence to suggest donor-related transmission of *B. dermatitidis*, and fewer than 15 cases of transplant-associated blastomycosis have been reported (Serody et al, 1993; Pappas 1997). Disease manifestations in this group tend to parallel those of the normal host; however, disseminated disease including involvement of the central nervous system is more commonly observed. Overall, mortality among OTRs and other immunocompromised hosts with blastomycosis has been significantly higher than among otherwise normal patients (Pappas et al, 1994).

Sporotrichosis due to *Sporothrix schenckii* and *S. cyanensis* has been reported sporadically among OTRs (Agarwal et al, 1994; Grossi et al, 2000). There is no evidence to suggest donor-transmitted infections, and most cases have been reported in conjunction with recognized environmental exposure. Disease has been limited to the skin and subcutaneous tissue in most cases, although pulmonary and disseminated disease have been reported (Gullberg et al, 1987).

Other Fungi

Disease due to other pathogenic yeasts and moulds has been reported sporadically among OTRs. Fusariosis due to *F. solani*, *F. oxysporum*, *F. moniliforme*, and *F. sacchari* has been reported (Heinz et al, 1996; Guarro et al, 2000; Sampathkumar and Paya, 2001). Infection due to *Fusarium* spp. is often associated with prolonged periods of neutropenia, although fusariosis can present among OTRs without neutropenia. Unlike aspergillosis, patients with fusariosis are frequently fungemic (Boutati and Anaissie, 1997). Localized infection involving the sinuses, lungs, skin, and soft tissue, as well as disseminated disease are reported. Another ubiquitous hyalohyphomycete, *Paecilomyces lilacinus*, is a rare cause of cutaneous and sinus disease in OTRs (Clark, 1999; Blackwell et al, 2000; Hilmarsdottir, et al, 2000).

Trichosporonosis due to *T. asahii* (formerly *T. beiglii*), a pathogenic yeast often associated with intravenous catheter-related infections, may cause disseminated disease in OTRs. In addition, funguria due to *T. asahii* has been reported among OTRs (Lussier et al, 2000). Fatal fungemia due to *Trichoderma harzianum* has also been observed (Guarro et al, 1999).

Pneumocystis carinii

Infection due to *Pneumocystis carinii* is reported in all organ transplant recipients, although it is most common among lung and heart–lung transplant recipients (Gryzan et al, 1988; Janner et al, 1996; Gordon et al, 1999). The incidence of *P. carinii* pneumonia (PCP) is greatest within the first year after transplantation. Gordon and colleagues suggested an eightfold higher incidence of PCP in the first year following transplant compared to the combined incidence in all subsequent years among OTRs at one institution (Gordon et al, 1999). For patients with PCP associated with transplantation, recent receipt of antithymocyte globulin, CMV infection, and therapy for organ rejection are considered important risk factors (Hardy et al, 1984). In the absence of antimicrobial prophylaxis, up to 17% of solid organ transplant recipients may develop PCP (Gordon et al, 1999). The lungs are the primary target of *P. carinii*, although extrapulmonary disease similar to that seen among patients with AIDS can occur. The widespread use of antimicrobial prophylaxis with TMP/SMX, sulfadoxime/pyrimethamine, or other antipneumocystis agents in the first few months posttransplantation has led to dramatic decrease in the incidence of documented PCP disease (Torre-Cisneros et al, 1999).

APPROACH TO DIAGNOSIS

A diagnosis of IFI is often elusive in OTRs, relating in part to the relative paucity and nonspecificity of the signs and symptoms associated with IFI in immunocompromised patients generally, and in OTRs specifically. Thus, a high index of suspicion and an aggressive approach to diagnosis is warranted in clinically compatible situations. The basis of a diagnosis of IFI depends on: *(1)* the isolation of a pathogenic organism from a properly obtained clinical specimen, usually associated with clinical or radiographic evidence of disease; *(2)* the demonstration of fungal organisms in cytologic or histopathologic studies; or *(3)* serologic detection of a specific antibody or fungal antigen from blood, serum, urine, cerebrospinal fluid, or bronchoalveolar lavage fluid.

Culture of certain fungi from any site virtually always suggests disease, even in the absence of clinical signs and symptoms. Examples include *H. capsulatum*, *C. immitis*, *B. dermatitidis*, *S. schenckii*, and *P. brasiliensis*. Isolation of *C. neoformans* from specimens other than sputum is almost always indicative of invasive disease. In rare circumstances, isolation of *C. neoformans* from the sputum can represent colonization only, but the recovery of this organism from respiratory secretions in an OTR must always be accompanied by an aggressive diagnostic approach (chest CT and/or bronchoscopy) directed at evaluating the possibility of parenchymal lung disease.

Isolation of *Candida* spp. from the blood should always be considered a true infection, even in the absence of clinical signs and symptoms (Rex et al, 2000). Controversy persists over the relative value of positive blood cultures obtained from a peripheral vein vs. those obtained through a central venous catheter, although most experts agree that any positive blood culture for *Candida* spp., regardless of the site from which it was obtained, should be regarded as a true positive. Isolates of *Candida* from other normally sterile sources should similarly be regarded as indicative of invasive disease. *Candida* spp. isolated from drains, urinary catheters, sputum, and other nonsterile sites often represent colonization only, and must be interpreted in the clinical context of the individual patient. The main value of isolation of *Candida* from a nonsterile site is in helping to predict the future development of invasive candidiasis, and guiding empiric therapy in patients who are perceived to be at high risk.

Isolation of *Aspergillus* spp. from blood cultures is uncommon, although disease due to *Fusarium* spp., *Paecilomyces lilacinus*, and other rare moulds may be associated with fungemia. The isolation of a mould from other clinical specimens such as sputum, BAL, or tissue biopsy are best interpreted with clinical, radiographic, and histopathologic correlation. Nonetheless, a positive culture for *Aspergillus* spp. from respiratory secretions is associated with a 60% to 80% positive predictive value of invasive disease among transplant recipients (Horvath and Dummer, 1996; Cahill et al, 1997; Mehrad et al, 2001; Perfect et al, 2001).

Direct visualization of an organism on a histopathologic specimen is an indispensable means of establishing tissue invasion. The demonstration on biopsy of fungal elements invading tissue often distinguishes a proven from a possible or probable case of invasive mould disease in an immunocompromised patient. Special stains such as Gomori methanamine silver (GMS), periodic acid Schiff (PAS), and Fontana-Masson can help to demonstrate fungal organisms in tissue.

Varieties of serologic tests have been used successfully in the early detection of fungal infections. Among the approved tests, detection of cryptococcal antigen in serum or cerebrospinal fluid remains the most reliable of these serologic assays, maintaining a high sensitivity and specificity. The measurement of *Histoplasma* antigen in serum and urine has also been useful in the diagnosis of histoplasmosis in immunocompromised patients (Wheat et al, 2000). The urine *Histoplasma* antigen assay has a sensitivity of at least 90% among immunocompromised patients with disseminated disease. In addition, among AIDS patients with disseminated histoplasmosis, serial urine *Histoplasma* antigens have been utilized to follow response to therapy and to predict relapse (Wheat, 1994). Among the other endemic fungi, reliable serologic testing is available for *C. immitis*. The detection of antibodies by complement-fixation or ELISA is a sensitive and specific marker of coccidioidomycosis (Galgiani et al, 2000).

New serologic assays directed at detecting early evidence of invasive candidiasis and invasive aspergillosis are under development (Verweij et al, 2000; Odabasi et al, 2002). Tests to detect fungal-associated 1-3 beta-D-glucan in serum have been advocated for detection of invasive candidiasis, although at present, this assay is investigational (Odabasi et al, 2002). Several assays to detect *Aspergillus* galactomannan antigen as evidence of invasive aspergillosis are currently used in Europe, but none are currently approved in the United States (Verweij, 2000). While the use of these assays and the interpretation of test results in the clinical setting remain controversial, it is likely that at least one of these assays will be widely available in the near future.

ANTIFUNGAL THERAPY

Approaches to the prevention and treatment of IFIs in OTRs continue to evolve. Not only are there several new agents for which a specific role in organ transplantation has yet to be defined, but there are also new ways of administering older agents (e.g., inhaled lipid formulations of amphotericin B for the prevention of fungal pneumonia in lung transplant recipients). A detailed approach to specific therapy for each fungal pathogen is not discussed in this section, and the reader is referred to the treatment sections in the specific chapters dealing with each pathogen. A general approach to therapy for established disease, preemptive antifungal therapy, and antifungal prophylaxis is discussed below.

Proven and Suspected Disease

Invasive Candidiasis. Among patients with life-threatening invasive candidiasis including patients with complicated intravenous catheter-associated infections, amphotericin B deoxycholate at doses of 0.6 to 1.0 mg/kg/day is advised (Rex et al, 2000). The lipid formulations of amphotericin B are all less nephrotoxic than the parent compound and have been adopted as primary therapy for invasive candidiasis in some medical centers. These lipid agents are particularly attractive alternatives among patients who are receiving other nephrotoxic agents such as cyclosporine or tacrolimus. Among patients requiring parenteral antifungal therapy, the echinocandins, e.g., caspofungin, hold promise as effective agents in this clinical setting. Recent data among patients with invasive candidiasis indicate equivalence of caspofungin and conventional amphotericin B for treatment of this disorder (Mora-Duarte et al, 2002), suggesting that caspofungin will be an effective alternative to amphotericin B for invasive *Candida* infections. This approach would be particularly attractive among OTRs because the echinocandins are relatively nontoxic, lacking any significant nephrotoxicity, and can be given concomitantly with the calcineurin inhibitors and other immunosuppressive agents.

Fluconazole remains a mainstay of antifungal therapy for nonlife-threatening invasive *Candida* infections for which there is little concern about antifungal resistance. Fluconazole is well tolerated parenterally and orally, but has significant drug–drug interactions with cyclosporine, tacrolimus, and sirolimus, leading to increased levels of these immunosuppressive agents. Among the expanded-spectrum triazoles including voriconazole, posaconazole, and ravuconazole, only voriconazole is currently approved. This azole has yet to be evaluated extensively for the treatment of invasive candidiasis in OTRs.

Length of therapy with any of the above agents for invasive *Candida* infection should be dictated by specific clinical circumstances including clinical response. Generally, therapy lasting no less than 14 days beyond the last positive culture and resolution of related symptoms is warranted, consistent with recently published guidelines (Rex et al, 2000).

Invasive Aspergillosis. Historically, amphotericin B deoxycholate, 1.0–1.5 mg/kg/day, has been regarded as the "gold standard" for treatment of invasive aspergillosis and the role of the lipid formulations of amphotericin B has been relegated to salvage therapy. However, at many centers, the lipid agents have become the drugs of choice for proven or suspected invasive aspergillosis because of their reduced nephrotoxicity. Convincing data to suggest superior efficacy have not been demonstrated. Among patients with invasive aspergillosis, doses of the lipid formulations between 4 and 6 mg/kg/day have been advocated (see Chapter 14).

Voriconazole has excellent activity against most *Apergillus* spp., is considered fungicidal against *Aspergillus* spp., and is an effective first line agent for patients with invasive disease. In a recently completed study, voriconazole was superior to amphotericin B deoxycholate and other licensed antifungal therapy among patients with proven or suspected invasive aspergillosis, including a significant number of OTRs (Herbrecht et al, 2002). Caspofungin also has demonstrated promising activity as salvage therapy for patients with invasive aspergillosis. The more interesting use of the echinocandins may relate to their potential as combination agents with either an expanded spectrum triazole (voriconazole, posaconazole, or ravuconazole) or a lipid formulation of amphotericin B. Data evaluating combination therapy in vitro and in animal models have been conflicting, but the theoretical advantage of combination over monotherapy has led to preliminary use of this therapeutic approach in some patients with proven and probable invasive aspergillosis.

Cryptococcosis. The treatment of cryptococcosis in solid OTRs varies little from that in other immunocompromised patients including those with AIDS. For patients with central nervous system disease, at least 2 weeks of induction therapy with an amphotericin B formulation, with or without flucytosine, followed by consolidation therapy with oral fluconazole at a dose of at least 400 mg daily is preferred by many authorities (Saag et al, 2000). The duration of maintenance therapy with fluconazole is debated, with some investigators suggesting discontinuation within 6 months following negative cerebrospinal fluid cultures and clinical recovery from infection as opposed to chronic lifetime suppressive therapy (Pappas et al, 2001). Neither ap-

proach has been studied in a prospective manner, but it is clear that clinical and mycologic relapses following 6 months of successful therapy have been very uncommon in OTRs. The optimal treatment of extra-neural cryptococcosis is not clearly defined. For many patients, an initial course of an amphotericin B preparation is advised to gain control of the disease, followed by fluconazole, at least 400 mg/day, for several months. Among clinically stable patients who are not cryptococcemic, initial therapy with fluconazole is acceptable. The role of the newer expanded spectrum triazoles remains unclear as there are only limited published data on treatment of cryptococcosis with these agents.

Endemic Mycoses. The treatment of histoplasmosis, coccidioidomycosis, and blastomycosis have recently been reviewed and guidelines have been established for management of these infections (Wheat et al, 2000; Chapman et al, 2000; Galgiani et al, 2000). Among OTRs, a more aggressive initial approach with an amphotericin B preparation as "induction" therapy followed by itraconazole is advocated by most experts. Fluconazole plays a lesser role in treatment of these endemic mycoses with the exception of patients with coccidioidal meningitis.

Pneumocystosis. Trimethoprim/sulfamethoxazole is the agent of choice for treatment of PCP and extrapulmonary pneumocystosis. Therapy is administered at 15–20 mg/kg/day of trimethoprim and 75–100 mg/kg/day of sulfamathoxazole divided into 3 or 4 daily doses. Pentamidine is the preferred alternative among patients who cannot tolerate TMP/SMX or in whom this combination is contraindicated. Pentamidine is given at a dose of 3–4 mg/kg/day. Other alternative regimens include atovaquone 750 mg two times daily, and combination therapy with clindamycin 600 to 900 mg every 6 to 8 hours and primaquine 15–30 mg daily. Corticosteroids as adjunctive therapy among patients with PCP have not been evaluated prospectively in OTRs, and their role in this setting has been questioned (Fishman, 1995).

Other Fungi. Published guidelines for the treatment of less common IFIs in transplant recipients are not available. Therapy of these infections in OTRs should reflect accepted therapy for these infections in other immunocompromised patients.

Preemptive Antifungal Therapy

Preemptive antifungal therapy is defined as therapy initiated among patients who are at very high risk of developing IFI based on an assessment of individual risk factors, which may include fungal colonization, type of surgical anastomosis, renal failure, retransplantation, extended intraoperative time, early graft failure, and other conditions. With the exception of liver transplant recipients, there are limited studies in other OTRs. In an observational study of 33 patients with renal insufficiency undergoing liver transplantation, 36% of patients who did not receive preemptive antifungal therapy vs. 7% of patients who received preemptive therapy with a lipid formulation of amphotericin B developed an IFI (Singh et al, 2001). A recently completed but unpublished study evaluating the effectiveness of fluconazole 400 mg/day or lower dose liposomal amphotericin (2 mg/kg/day) as preemptive therapy in high-risk liver transplant recipients should more accurately address the appropriateness of this approach in a well-defined population.

Some authors have advocated preemptive therapy in discreet clinical situations that include pulmonary colonization with *Aspergillus* spp. shortly after transplantation, following excision of focal pulmonary nodules due to *C. neoformans* or *H. capsulatum* without evidence of other disease, and asymptomatic candiduria in the renal transplant recipient (Hibberd and Rubin, 1994). In a prospective, nonrandomized and open-label study of preemptive antifungal therapy, 26 lung transplant recipients with fungal colonization of the tracheobronchial tree were given either fluconazole or itraconazole until the surgical anastomoses appeared normal and cultures were consistently negative. Only 2(8%) of 26 patients in this study developed *Aspergillus* tracheobronchitis (Hamacker et al, 1999).

Prophylactic Antifungal Therapy
Antifungal prophylaxis is widely practiced but inadequately studied in liver, pancreas, lung, and heart–lung transplant recipients (Mora et al, 1991; Villacian and Paya, 1999). The largest study to date compared fluconazole 400 mg daily to placebo given for the first 70 days posttransplant among 212 liver transplant recipients in a randomized, double-blind study. In this study, 6% vs. 23% of fluconazole and placebo recipients, respectively, developed IFI, but neither regimen reduced mortality (Winston et al, 1999). In a small, randomized, double-blind study of 86 liver transplant patients, 0% vs. 16% ($p < 0.01$) of recipients of a lipid formulation of amphotericin B vs. placebo, respectively, developed IFI in the first month posttransplant (Tollemar et al, 1995). More recently, in an observational study of 200 low-risk liver transplant recipients who did not receive antifungal prophylaxis, the incidence of IFI was 3.6% during the first 100 days posttransplant, suggesting that antifungal prophylaxis in a low-risk population is unnecessary (Karchmer et al, 2002).

Recent studies among lung transplant recipients have examined the use of inhaled amphotericin B preparations for primary prophylaxis of invasive fungal pneumonia and bronchitis. These uncontrolled studies demonstrate the safety of a nebulized lipid agent and amphotericin B deoxycholate and efficacy in preventing IFI in the early postoperative period (Reichenspurner et al, 1997; Palmer et al, 2001; Monforte et al, 2001). Aside from these recent studies, there are few data that address the best approach to antifungal prophylaxis in OTRs. As such, antifungal prophylaxis is largely practiced in a center-to-center approach based on local experience, epidemiology, and perceived risk of IFI.

SUMMARY

Despite advances in surgical technique and refinements in immunosuppressive regimens, fungal infections continue to be a significant cause of morbidity and mortality among OTRs. It is important to establish the risk of IFI following transplantation based on the knowledge of the type and timing of transplant, immunosuppressive regimen, rejection episodes, donor history, recipient comorbidities and coinfections, and recent epidemiology. Invasive candidiasis, aspergillosis, cryptococcosis, zygomycosis, and pneumocystosis constitute the majority of IFIs in this population, and a high index of suspicion must be maintained in order to establish early diagnosis. Newer antifungal drugs, especially the broad spectrum triazoles and the echinocandins, offer promise for the treatment of IFIs. However, targeted prophylaxis for high-risk individuals and early diagnosis offer the best hope to these OTRs who are uniquely susceptible to serious complications from IFI.

REFERENCES

Abbott K C, Hypolite I, Poropatich R K, Hshieh P, Cruess D, Hawkes C A, Agodoa L Y, Keller R A. Hospitalizations for fungal infections after renal transplantation in the United States. *Transplant Infect Dis* 3:203–211, 2001.

Agarwal S K, Tiwari S C, Dash S C, Mehta S N, Saxena S, Banerjee U, Kumar R, Bhunyan U N. Urinary sporotrichosis in a renal allograft recipient. *Nephron* 66:485, 1994.

Anderson D J, Schmidt C, Goodman J, Pomeroy C. Cryptococcal disease presenting as cellulitis. *Clin Infect Dis* 14:666–672, 1992.

Argenziano M, Catanese K A, Moazami N, Gardocki M T, Weinberg A D, Clavenna M W, Rose E A, Scully B E, Levin H R, Oz M C. The influence of infection on survival and successful transplantation in patients with left ventricular assist devices. *J Heart Lung Transplant* 16:822–831, 1997.

Bacal F, Andrade A C, Migueletto B C, Bocchi E A, Stolf N A, Fiorelli A I, Strabelli T M, Benvenuti L A, Brandao C M, Bellotti G, Ramires J A. Histoplasmosis as a late infectious complication following heart transplantation in a patient with Chagas' disease. *Arquivos Brasileiros de Cardiologia* 76:403–408, 2001.

Battaglia M, Ditonno P, Fiore T, De Ceglie G, Regina G, Selvaggi F P. True mycotic arteritis by *Candida albicans* in 2 kidney transplant recipients from the same donor. *J Urol* 163:1236–1237, 2000.

Benedetti E, Gruessner A C, Troppmann C, Papalois B E, Sutherland D E, Dunn D L, Gruessner R W. Intra-abdominal fungal infections after pancreatic transplantation: incidence, treatment, and outcome. *J Am Coll Surg* 183:307–316, 1996.

Bernabeu-Wittel M, Naranjo M, Cisneros J M, Canas E, Gentil M A, Algarra G, Pereira P, Gonzalez-Roncero F J, de Alarcon A, Pachon J. Infections in renal transplant recipients receiving mycophenolate versus azathioprine-based immunosuppression. *Eur J Clin Microbiol Infect Dis* 21:173–180, 2002.

Blackwell W, Ahmed K, O'Docherty C, Hay R J. Cutaneous hyalohyphomycosis caused by *Paecilomyces lilacinus* in a renal transplant patient. *Br J Dermatol* 143:873–875, 2000.

Botterel F, Romand S, Saliba F, Reynes M, Bismuth H, Samuel D, Bouree P. A case of disseminated histoplasmosis likely due to infection from a liver allograft. *Eur J Clin Microbiol Infect Dis* 18:662–664, 1999.

Boutati E I, Anaissie E J. *Fusarium*, a significant emerging pathogen in patients with hematologic malignancy: ten years' experience at a cancer center and implications for management. *Blood* 90: 999–1008, 1997.

Brett M T, Kwan J T, Bending M R. Caecal perforation in a renal transplant patient with disseminated histoplasmosis. *J Clin Pathol* 41:992–995, 1988.

Brooks R G, Hofflin J M, Jamieson S W, Stinson E B, Remington J S. Infectious complications in heart-lung transplant recipients. *Am J Med* 79:413–422, 1985.

Brown R S, Lake J R, Katzman B A, Ascher N L, Somberg KA, Emond J C, Roberts J P. Incidence of significance of *Aspergillus* cultures following liver and kidney transplantation. *Transplant* 61:666–669, 1996.

Cahill B C, Hibbs J R, Savik K, Juni B A, Dosland B M, Edin-Stibbe C, Hertz M I. *Aspergillus* airway colonization and invasive disease after lung transplantation. *Chest* 112:1160–64, 1997.

Carlini A, Angelini D, Burrows L, DeQuirico G, Antonelli A. Cerebral aspergillosis: long term efficacy and safety of liposomal amphotericin B in kidney transplant. *Nephrol Dial Transplant* 13: 2659–2661, 1998.

Castaldo P, Stratta R J, Wood P, Markin R S, Patil KD, Shaefer M S, Langnan A N, Reed E C, Shujun L, Pillen T J, Shaw B W. Clinical spectrum of fungal infections after orthotopic liver transplantation. *Arch Surg* 126:149–156, 1991.

Castro L G, da Silva Lacaz C, Guarro J, Gene J, Heins-Vaccari E M, de Freitas Leite R S, Arriagada G L, Regueera M M, Ito E M, Valente NY, Nunes R. Phaeohyphomycotic cyst caused by *Colletotrichum crassipes*. *J Clin Microbiol* 39:2321–2324, 2001.

Chapman S W, Bradsher R W, Campbell G D, Pappas P G, Kauffman C A. Practice guidelines for the management of patients with blastomycosis. *Clin Infect Dis* 30:679–683, 2000.

Chkhotua A, Yussim A, Tovar A, Weinberger M, Sobolev V, Bar-Nathan N, Shaharabani E, Shapira Z, Mor E. Mucormycosis of the renal allograft: case report and review of the literature. *Transplant Int* 14:438–441, 2001.

Choi I S, Kim S J, Kim B Y, Joh J W, KM Y I, Lee S K, Huh W S, Oh H Y, Kim D J, Kim Y G, Kim M K, Ko Y H, Lee B B. *Candida* polyarthritis in a renal transplant patient: case report of a patient successfully treated with amphotericin B. *Transplant Proc* 32:1963–1964, 2000.

Ciancio G, Burke G W, Viciana A L, Ruiz P, Ginzburg E, Dowdy L, Roth D, Miller J. Destructive allograft fungal arteritis following simultaneous pancreas-kidney transplantation. *Transplant* 61: 1172–1175, 1996.

Cimon B, Carrere J, Vinatier J F, Chazalette J P, Chabasse D, Bouchara J P. Clinical significance to *Scedosporium apiospermum* in patients with cystic fibrosis. *Eur J Clin Microbiol Infect Dis* 19:53–56, 2000.

Clark N M. *Paecillomyces lilacinus* infection in a heart transplant

recipient and successful treatment with terbinafine. *Clin Infect Dis* 28:1169–1170, 1999.

Cohen I M, Galgini J N, Potter D, Ogden D A. Coccidioidomycosis in renal transplant replacement therapy. *Arch Intern Med* 142: 489–494, 1982.

Collins L A, Samore M H, Roberts M S, Luzzati R, Jenkins R L, Lewis W D, Karchmer A W. Risk factors for invasive fungal infections complicating orthotopic liver transplantation. *J Infect Dis* 170:644–652, 1994.

Dauber H J, Paradis I L, Dummer J S. Infectious complications in pulmonary allograft recipients. *Clin Chest Med* 11:291–308, 1990.

Davies S F, Sarosi G A, Peterson P K, Khan M, Howard RJ, Simmons R L, Najarian J S. Disseminated histoplasmosis in renal transplant recipients. *Am J Surg* 137:686–691, 1979.

Denning D W. Invasive aspergillosis. *Clin Infect Dis* 26:781–805, 1998.

Denton M K, Magee C C, Sayegh M H. Immunosuppressive strategies in transplantation. *Lancet* 353:1083–1091, 1999.

Dictar M O, Maiolo E, Alexander B, Jacob N, Veron M T. Mycoses in the transplanted patient. *Med Mycol* 38:251–258, 2000.

Demirag A, Elkhammas E A, Henry M L, Davies E A, Pelletier R P, Bumgardner G L, Dorner B, Ferguson R M. Pulmonary *Rhizopus* infection in a diabetic renal transplant recipient. *Clin Transplant* 14:8–10, 2000.

Dowling R D, Baladi N, Zenati M, Dummer J S, Kormos R L, Armitage J M, Yousem S A, Hardesty R L, Griffith B P. Disruption of the aortic anastomosis after heart-lung transplantation. *Ann Thorac Surg* 49:118–122, 1990.

Dromer F, Mathouin S, Dupont B, Brugiere O, Letenneur L, and the French Cryptococcosis Study Study Group. *Clin Infect Dis* 22(Suppl 2):S154–S160, 1996.

Dummer S J, Montero C G, Griffith B P, Hardesty R L, Paradis I L, Ho M. Infections in heart-lung transplant recipients. *Transplant* 41:725–729, 1986.

Farr B, Beacham B E, Atuk N O. Cutaneous histoplasmosis after renal transplantation. *So Med J* 74:635–637, 1981.

Fishman J A. *Pneumocystis carinii* and parasitic infections in transplantation. *Infec Dis Clin N Amer* 9:1005–1044, 1995.

Fishman J A, Rubin R H. Infection in organ-transplant recipients. *N Engl J Med* 338:1741–1751, 1998.

Galgiani J N, Ampel N M, Catanzaro A, Johnson R H, Stevens D A, Williams P L. Practice guidelines for the treatment of coccidioidomycosis. *Clin Infect Dis* 30:658–661, 2000.

Gallis H A, Berman R A, Cate T R, Hamilton J D, Gunnels J C, Stickel D L. Fungal infections following renal transplantation. *Arch Intern Med* 135:1163–1172, 1975.

Garcia A, Mazuecos A, Flayo A, Perez-Requena J, Mangas A, Alonso F, Ceballos M, Rivero M. Isolated cerebral aspergillosis without a portal of entry-complete recovery after liposomal amphotericin B and surgical treatment. *Nephrol Dialysis Transplant* 9:2385–2387, 1998.

Gold W L, Vellend H, Salit I E, Campabell I, Summerbell R, Rinaldi M, Simor A E. Successful treatment of systemic and local infections due to *Exophiala* spp. *Clin Infect Dis* 19:339–341, 1994.

Goldfarb N S, Avery R K, Goormastic M, Mehta A C, Schilz R, Smedira N, Pien L, Haug M T, Gordon S M, Hague L K, Dresing J M, Evans-Walker T, Maurer J R. Hypogammaglobulinemia in lung transplant recipients. *Transplant* 71:242–246, 2001.

Goldstein D J, El-Amir N G, Ashton R C, Catanese K, Rose E A, Levin H R, Oz M C. Fungal infections in left ventricular assist device recipients: incidence, prophylaxis, and treatment. *ASAIO J* 41:873–875, 1995.

Gordon S M, LaRosa S P, Kalmadi S, Arroliga A C, Avery R K, Truesdell-LaRosa L, Longworth D L. Should prophylaxis for *Pneumocystis carinii* pneumonia in solid organ transplant recipients ever be discontinued? *Clin Infect Dis* 28:240–246, 1999.

Gordon S M, Avery R K. Aspergillosis in lung transplantation: incidence, risk factors, and prophylactic strategies. *Transplant Infect Dis* 3:161–167, 2001.

Grossi P, De Maria R, Caroki A, Zaina MS, Minoli L. Infections in heart transplant recipients: the experience of the Italian heart transplantation program. *J Heart Lung Transplant* 11:847–866, 1992.

Grossi P, Glaudio F, Fiocchi R, Dalla Gasperina D. Prevalence and outcome of invasive fungal infections in 1,963 thoracic organ transplant recipients. *Transplant* 70:112–116, 2000.

Gryzan S, Paradis I L, Zeevi A, Duquesnoy R J, Dummer J S, Griffith B P, Hardesty R L, Trento A, Nalesnik M A, Dauber J H. Unexpectedly high incidence of *Pneumocystis carinii* infection after heart-lung transplantation: implications for lung defense and allograft survival. *Am Rev Respir Dis* 137:1268–1274, 1988).

Guarro J, Antolin Ayala M I, Gene J, Gutierrez-Calzada J, Nieves-Diez C, Ortoneda M. Fatal case of *Trichoderma harzianum* infection in a renal transplant recipient. *J Clin Microbiol* 37:3751–3755, 1999.

Guarro J, Nucci M, Akiti T, Gene J, Barreiro M D, Goncalves R T. Fungemia due to *Fusarium sacchari* in an immunosuppressed patient. *J Clin Microbiol* 38:419–421, 2000.

Gullberg R M, Quintanilla A, Levin M L, Williams J, Phair J P. Sporotrichosis: recurrent cutaneous, articular, and central nervous system infection in a renal transplant recipient. *Rev Infect Dis* 9:369–375, 1987.

Hadley S, Karchmer A W. Fungal infections in solid organ transplant recipients. *Infect Dis Clin N Am* 9:1045–1074, 1995a.

Hadley S, Samore M H, Lewis W D, Jenkins R L, Karchmer A W, Hammer S M. Major infectious complications after orthotopic liver transplantation and comparison of outcomes in patients receiving cyclosporine or FK506 as primary immunosuppression. *Transplant* 59:851–859, 1995b.

Halaby T, Boots H, Vermeulen A, van der Ven A, Geguin H, van Hooff H, Jacobs J. Phaeohyphomycosis caused by alternaria infectoria in a renal transplant recipient. *J Clin Microbiol* 39:1952–1955, 2001.

Hamacher J, Spiliopoulos A, Kurt A M, Nicod L P, and the Geneva Lung Transplantation Group. Pre-emptive therapy with azoles in lung transplant patients. *Eur Respir J* 13:180–186, 1999.

Hardy A M, Wajszczuk C P, Suffredini A F, Hakala T R, Ho M. *Pneumocystis carinii* pneumonia in renal-transplant recipients treated with cyclosporine and steroids. *J Infect Dis* 149:143–147, 1984.

Heinz T, Perfect J, Schell W, Ditter E, Ruff G, Serafin D. Soft tissue fungal infections: surgical management of 12 immunocompromised patients. *Plast Reconstr Surg* 97:1391–1399, 1996.

Herbrecht R, Denning D W, Patterson T F, Bennett J E, Greene R E, Oestmann J W, Kern W V, Marr K A, Ribaud P, Lortholary O, Sylvester R, Rubin R H, Wingard J R, Stark P, Durand C, Caillott D, Thiel E, Chandrasekar P H, Hodges M R, Schlamm H T, Troke P F, de Pauw B, and the Invasive Fungal Infections Group of the European Organization for Research and Treatment of Cancer and the Global Aspergillus Study Group. Voriconazole versus amphotericin B for primary therapy of invasive aspergillosis. *N Engl J Med* 347:408–415, 2002.

Hesse U J, Sutherland D E R, Najarian J S, Simmons R L. Intraabdominal infections in pancreas transplant recipients. *Ann Surg* 203:153–162, 1986.

Hibberd P L, Rubin R H. Clinic aspects of fungal infection in organ transplant recipients. *Clin Infect Dis* 19(Suppl 1):S33–S40, 1994.

Hilmarsdottir I, Thorsteinsson S B, Asmundsson P, Bodvarsson M, Arnadottir M. Cutaneous infection caused by *Paecilomyces lilac-*

inus in a renal transplant patient: treatment with voriconazole. *Scand J Infect Dis* 32:331–332, 2000.

Hofflin J M, Potasman I, Baldwin J C, Oyer P E, Stinson E B, Remington J S. Infectious complications in heart transplant recipients receiving cyclosporine and corticosteroids. *Ann Intern Med* 106:209–216, 1987.

Holt C D, Winston D J, Kubak B, Imagawa D K, Martin P, Goldstein L, Olthoff K, Millis J M, Shaked A, Shackleton C R, Busuttil R W. Coccidioidomycosis in liver transplant patients. *Clin Infect Dis* 24:216–221, 1997.

Hood A B, Inglis F G, Lowenstein L, Dossetor J B, MacLean L D. Histoplasmosis and thrombycytopenic purpura: transmission by renal homotransplantations. *Can Med Assoc J* 93:587–592, 1965.

Horvath J A, Dummer S. The use of respiratory-tract cultures in the diagnosis of invasive pulmonary aspergillosis. *Am J Med* 100:171–178, 1996.

Howard R J, Simmons R L, Najarian J S. Fungal infections in renal transplant recipients. *Ann Surg* 188:598–605, 1978.

Hunger R E, Paredes B E, Quattroppani C, Krahenbuhl S, Braathen L R. Primary cutaneous cryptococcosis in a patient with systemic immunosuppression after liver transplantation. *Dermatol* 200:352–355, 2000.

Husain S, Wagener M M, Singh N. *Cryptococcus neoformans* infection in organ transplant recipients: variables influencing clinical characteristics and outcome. *Emerg Infect Dis* 7:1–14, 2001.

Husni R N, Gordon S M, Longworth D L, Arroliga A, Stillwell P C, Avery R K, Maurer J R, Mehta A, Kirby T. Cytomegalovirus infection is a risk factor for invasive aspergillosis in lung transplant recipients. *Clin Infect Dis* 26:753–755, 1998.

Janner D, Bork J, Baum M, Chinnock R. *Pneumocystis carinii* pneumonia in infants after heart transplantation. *J Heart Lung Transplant* 15:758–763, 1996.

Jha V, Sree Kiishna V, Varma N, Varma S, Chakrabarti A, Kohlo H S, Sud K, Gupta K L, Sakhuja V. Disseminated histoplasmosis 19 years after renal transplantation. *Clin Nephrol* 51:373–378, 1999.

Jimenez C, Lumbreras C, Aguado J M, Loinaz C, Paseiro G, Andres A, Morales J M, Sanchez G, Garcia I, Del Palacio A, Moreno E. Successful treatment of *Mucor* infection after liver or pancreas-kidney transplantation. *Transplant* 73:476–480, 2002.

Ju J H, Park H S, Shin M J, Yang C W, Kim Y S, Choi Y J, Song H J, Kim S W, Chung I S, Bang B K. Successful treatment of massive lower gastrointestinal bleeding caused by mixed infection of cytomegalovirus and mucormycosis in a renal transplant recipient. *Am J Nephrol* 21:232–236, 2001.

Kanj S S, Welty-Wolf K, Madden J, Tapson V, Baz M A, Davis D, Perfect J R. Fungal infections in lung and heart transplant recipients: report of 9 cases and review of the literature. *Medicine* 75:142–156, 1996.

Kaplan-Pavlovcic S, Masera A, Ovcak Z, Kmetec A. Prostatic aspergillosis in a renal transplant recipient. *Nephrol Dialysis Transplant* 14:1778–1780, 1999.

Kapoor A, Flechner S M, O'Malley K, Paolone D, File T M, Cutrona A F. Cryptococcal meningitis in renal transplant patients associated with environmental exposure. *Transplant Infect Dis* 1:213–217, 1999.

Karalakulasingam R, Arora K K, Adams G, Serratoni F, Martin DG. Meningoencephalitis caused by *Histoplasma capsulatum*: occurrence in a renal transplant recipient and a review of the literature. *Arch Intern Med* 136:217–220, 1976.

Karchmer A W, Pappas P, Merion R, Cloud G, Hadley S, Rabkin J, Schuster M, Andes D, Kauffman C, Delaney J, Daly J, Kusne S, Alexander B. Invasive fungal infection in liver transplant recipients considered at low risk. Abstracts of the Infectious Diseases

Society of America 40th Annual Meeting, Chicago, IL, p. 47; Abstract 16; 2002.

Keating M R, Guerrero M A, Daly R C, Walker R C, Davies S F. Transmission of invasive aspergillosis from a subcliically infected donor to three different organ transplant recipients. *Chest* 109: 1119–1124, 1996.

Kim S W, Nah M Y, Ueum C H, Kim N H, Choi H S, Juhng S W, Choi K C. Pelvic aspergillosis with tubo-ovarian abscess in a renal transplant recipient. *J Infect* 42:215–217, 2001.

Kramer M R, Denning D W, Marshall S E, Ross D J, Berry G, Lewiston N J, Stevens D A, Theodore J. Ulcerative tracheobronchitis after lung transplantation: a new form of invasive aspergillosis. *Am Rev Respir Dis* 144:552–558, 1991.

Kramer M R, Marshal S E, Starnes V A, Gamberg P, Amitai Z, Theodore J. Infectious complications in heart-lung transplantation analysis of 200 episodes. *Arch Intern Med* 153:2010–2016, 1993.

Kusne S, Dummer S, Singh N, Iwatsuki S, Makowka L, Esquivel C, Tzakis A G, Starzi T E, Ho M. Infections after liver transplantation: an analysis of 101 consecutive cases. *Medicine* 67:132–143, 1988.

Kusne S, Fung J, Alessiani M, Martin M, Torre-Cisneros J, Irish W, Ondick L, Jain A, Abu-Elmagd K, Takaya S. Infections during a randomized trial comparing cyclosporine to FK 506 immunosuppression in liver transplantation. *Transplant Proc* 24:429–430, 1992.

Kusne S, Furukawa H, Abu-Elmagd K, Irish W, Rakela J, Fung J, Starzl T E, Todo S. Infectious complications after small bowel transplantation in adults: an update. *Transplant Pro* 28:2761–2762, 1996.

Lee E, Vershvovsky Y, Miller F, Waltzer W, Suh H, Nord E P. Combined medical surgical therapy for pulmonary mucormycosis in a diabetic renal allograft recipient. *Am J Kid Dis* 38:E37, 2001.

Limaye A P, Connolly P A, Sagar M, Fritsche T R, Cookson B T, Wheat J, Stamm W E. Transmission of *Histoplasma capsulatum* by organ transplantation. *N Engl J Med* 343:1163–1166, 2000.

Lin S J, Schranz J, Teutsch S M. Aspergillosis case-fatality rate: systemic review of the literature. *Clin Infect Dis* 32:658–666, 2001.

Livas I C, Nechay P S, Nauseef W M. Clinical evidence of spinal and cerebral histoplasmosis twenty years after renal transplantation. *Clin Infect Dis* 20:692–695, 1995.

Lumbreras C, Fernandez I, Velosa J, Munn S, Sterioff S, Paya C V. Infectious complications following pancreatic transplantation: incidence, microbiological and clinical characteristics, and outcome. *Clin Infect Dis* 20:514–520, 1995.

Lussier N, Laverdiere M, Delorme J, Weiss K, Dandavino R. *Trichosporon beigelii* funguria in renal transplant recipients. *Clin Infect Dis* 31:1299–1301, 2000.

Magina S, Libosa C, Santos P, Oliveira G, Lopes J, Rocho A, Mesquita-Guimaraes J. Cutaneous alternariosis by *Alternaria chartarum* in a renal transplanted patient. *Br J Dermatol* 142: 1261–1262, 2000.

Malani P N, Bleicher J J, Kauffman C A, Davenport D S. Disseminated *Dactylaria constricta* infection in a renal transplant recipient. *Transplant Infect Dis* 3:40–43, 2001.

Marin P, Garcia-Martos P, Carcia-Doncel A, Garcia-Tapia A, Aznar E, Perez R J, Valverde S. Endocarditis by *Aspergillus fumigatus* in a renal transplant. *Mycopathologia* 145:127–129, 1999.

Marks W H, Florence L, Lieberman J, Chapman P, Howard D, Roberts P, Perkinson D. Successfully treated invasive pulmonary aspergillosis associated with smoking marijuana in a renal transplant recipient. *Transplant* 61:1771–1783, 1996.

Mehrad B, Giusppe P, Martinez F J, Clark T, Iannettoni M D, Lynch J P. Spectrum of *Aspergillus* infection in lung transplant recipients. *Chest* 119:169–175, 2001.

Mesa A, Henao J, Gil M, Durango G. Phaeohyphomycosis in kidney transplant patients. *Clin Transplant* 13:273–276, 1999.

Meunier F, Aoun M, Bitar N. Candidemia in immunocompromised patients. *Clin Infect Dis* 14:S120–S125, 1992.

Miller L W, Naftel D C, Bourge R C, Kirklin J K, Brozena S C, Jarcho J, Hobbs R E, Mills R M, and the Cardiac Transplant Research Database Group. Infection after heart transplantation: a multi-institutional study. *J Heart Lung Transplant* 13:381–393, 1994.

Monforte V, Roman A, Gavalda J, Bravo C, Tenorio L, Ferrer A, Maestre J, Morell F. Nebulized amphotericin B prophylaxis for *Aspergillus* infection in lung transplantation: study of risk factors. *J Heart Lung Transplant* 20:1274–1281, 2001.

Mora-Duarte J, Betts R, Rotstein C, Colombo A L, Thompson-Moya L, Smietana J, Lupinacci R, Sable C, Kartsonis N, Perfect J. Caspofungin Invasive Candidiasis Study Group. Comparison of caspofungin and amphotericin B for invasive candidiasis. *N Engl J Med* 347:2020–2029, 2002.

Mora N P, Cofer J B, Solomon H, Goldstein R M, Gonwa T A, Husberg B S, Klintmalm G B. Analysis of severe infections (INF) after 180 consecutive liver transplants: the impact of amphotericin B prophylaxis for reducing the incidence and severity of fungal infections. *Transplant Proc* 23:1528–1530, 1991.

Nampoory M R, Khan Z U, Johny K V, Constandi J N, Gupta I, Al-Muzairi I, Samhan M, Mozavi M, Chugh T D. Invasive fungal infections in renal transplant recipients. *J Infect* 33:95–101, 1996.

Nosanchuk J D, Shoham S, Fries B C, Shapiro S, Levitz S M, Casadevall A. Evidence of zoonotic transmission of *Cryptococcus neoformans* from a pet cockatoo to an immunocompromised patient. *Ann Intern Med* 132:205–208, 2000.

Nunley D R, Ohori N P, Grgurich W F, Tacono A T, Williams P A, Keenan R J, Dauber J H. Pulmonary aspergillosis in cystic fibrosis lung transplant recipients. *Chest* 114:1321–1329, 1998.

Odabasi Z, Mattiuzzi G, Ostrosky-Zeichner L, Estey E, Kantarjian H, Rex J H. Detection of (1-3)-β-D-glucan (BG) in the serum of leukemia patients (pts) with invasive fungal infections (IFI). Abstracts of the 42nd Interscience Conference on Antimicrobial Agents and Chemotherapy, San Diego, CA, p. 396; Abstract M-902, 2002.

Palmer S M, Drew R H, Whitehouse J D, Tapson V F, Davis R D, McConnell R R, Kanj S S, Perfect J R. Safety of aerosolized amphotericin B lipid complex in lung transplant recipients. *Transplant* 72:545–548, 2001.

Pappas P G, Threlkeld M G, Bedsole G D, Cleveland K O, Gelfand M S, Dismukes W E. Blastomycosis in immunocompromised patients. *Medicine*, 72:311–325, 1994.

Pappas P G. Blastomycosis in the immunocompromised patient. *Sem Respir Infect* 12:243–251, 1997.

Pappas P G, Perfect J R, Cloud G A, Larsen R A, Pankey G A, Lancaster D J, Henderson H, Kauffman C A, Haas D W, Saccente M, Hamill R J, Holloway M S, Warren R M, Dismukes W E. Cryptococcosis in human immunodeficiency virus-negative patients in the era of effective azole therapy. *Clin Infect Dis* 33:690–699, 2001.

Patel R, Portela D, Badley A D, Harmsen W S, Larson-Keller J, Ilstrup D M, Keating M R, Wiesner R H, Krom R A, Paya C V. Risk factors of invasive *Candida* or non-*Candida* fungal infections after liver transplantation. *Transplant* 62:926–934, 1996.

Patel R, Paya C V. Infections in solid organ transplant recipients. *Clin Microbiol Rev* 10:86–124, 1997.

Patel R. Infections in recipients of kidney transplants. *Infect Dis Clin N Am* 15:901–951, 2001.

Paterson D L, Singh N. Invasive aspergillosis in transplant recipients. *Medicine* 78:123–138, 1999.

Patterson J E. Epidemiology of fungal infections in solid organ transplant patients. *Transplant Infect Dis* 1:229–236, 1999.

Patterson J E, Peters J, Calhoon J H, Levine S, Anzueto A, Al-Abdely H, Sanchez H, Patterson R, Rech T F, Jorgensen J H, Rinaldi M G, Sako E, Johnson S, Speeg V, Halff G A, Trinkle J K. Investigation and control of aspergillosis and other filamentous fungal infections in solid organ transplant recipients. *Transplant Infect Dis* 2:22–28, 2000.

Patterson T F, Kirkpatrick W R, White M, Hiemenz J W, Wingard J R, Dupont B, Rinaldi G, Stevens D A, Graybill J R. Invasive aspergillosis: disease spectrum, treatment, practice, and outcomes. *Medicine* 79:250–260, 2000.

Paya C V. Fungal infections in solid-organ transplantation. *Clin Infect Dis* 16:677–688, 1993.

Peddi V R, Hariharan S, First M R. Disseminated histoplasmosis in renal allograft recipients. *Clin Transplant* 10:160–165, 1996.

Perfect J R, Cox G M, Lee J Y, Kauffman C A, de Repentigny L, Chapman S W, Morrison V A, Pappas P, Hiemenz J W, Stevens D A, and the Mycoses Study Group. The impact of culture isolation of *Aspergillus* species: a hospital-based survey of aspergillosis. *Clin Infect Dis* 33:1824–1833, 2001.

Peterson P K, Ferguson R, Fryd D S, Balfour H H, Rynasiewicz J, Simmons R L. Infectious diseases in hospitalized renal transplant recipients: a prospective study of a complex and evolving problem. *Medicine* 61:360–371, 1982.

Pirsch J D, Odorico J S, D'Alessandro A M, Knechtle S J, Becker B N, Sollinger H W. Post-transplant infections in enteric versus bladder-drained simultaneous pancreas-kidney transplant recipients. *Transplant* 66:1746–1750, 1998.

Potti A, Danielson B, Sen K. "True" mycotic aneurysm of a renal artery allograft. *Am J Kid Dis* 31:E3, 1998.

Ralph E D, Hussain Z. Chronic meningitis caused by *Candida albicans* in a liver transplant recipient: usefulness of the polymerase chain reaction for diagnosis and for monitoring treatment. *Clin Infect Dis* 23:191–192, 1996.

Reichenspurner H, Gamberg P, Nitschke M, Valantine H, Hunt S, Oyer P E, Reitz B A. Significant reduction in the number of fungal infections after lung, heart-lung, and heart transplantation using aerosolized amphotericin B prophylaxis. *Transplant* 29:627–628, 1997.

Revankar S G, Patterson J E, Sutton D A, Pullen R, Rinaldi M G. Disseminated phaeohyphomycosis: review of an emerging mycosis. *Clin Infect Dis* 34:467–476, 2002.

Rex J H, Walsh T J, Sobel J D, Filler S G, Pappas P G, Dismukes W E, Edwards J E. Practice guidelines for the treatment for candidiasis. *Clin Infect Dis* 30:662–678, 2000.

Reyes J, Abu-Elmagd K, Tzakis A, Nour B, Casavilla A, Kusne S, Green M, Alessiani M, Jain A, Fung J J, Todo S, Starzl T E. Infectious complications after human small bowel transplantation. *Transplant* 24:1249–1250, 1992.

Reyes J, Bueno J, Kocoshis S, Green M, Abu-Elmagd K, Furukawa H, Barksdale E M, Strom S, Fung J J, Todo S, Irish W, Starzl T E. Current status of intestinal transplantation in children. *J Pediatr Surg* 33:243–254, 1998.

Rogers J, Rohal S, Carrigan D R, Kusne S, Knox K K, Gayowski T, Wagener M M, Fung J J, Singh N. Human herpesvirus-6 in liver transplant recipients. *Transplant* 69:2566–2573, 2000.

Rubin R H. Infection in the organ transplant recipient. In: Rubin R H, Young L S, eds. *Clinical Approach to Infections in the Compromised Host.* 3rd ed. New York: Plenum Publishing, 629–705, 1994.

Saag M S, Graybill R J, Larsen R A, Pappas P G, Perfect J R, Powderly W G, Sobel J D, Dismukes W E. Practice guidelines for the management of cryptococcal disease. *Clin Infect Dis* 30:710–718, 2000.

Salama A D, Rogers T, Lord G M, Lechler R I, Mason P D. Multiple *Cladosporium* brain abscesses in a renal transplant patient: aggressive management improves outcome. *Transplant* 63:160–162, 1997.

Sampathkumar P, Paya C V. *Fusarium* infection after solid-organ transplantation. *Clin Infect Dis* 32:1237–1240, 2001.

Sayiner A, Kursat S, Toz H, Duman S, Onal B, Tumbay E. Pseudomembranous necrotizing bronchial aspergillosis in a renal transplant recipient. *Nephro Dialysis Transplant* 14:1784–1785, 1999.

Serody J S, Mill M R, Detterbeck F C, Harris D T, Cohen M S. Blastomycosis in transplant recipients: report of a case and review. *Clin Infect Dis* 16:54–58, 1993.

Shallot J, Pursell K J, Bartolone C, Williamson P, Benedetti E, Layden T J, Wiley T E. Disseminated histoplasmosis after orthotopic liver transplantation. *Liver Transplant Surg* 3:433–434, 1997.

Sheu B S, Lee P C, Yang H B. A giant gastric ulcer caused by mucormycosis infection in a patient with renal transplantation. *Endoscopy* 30:S60–S61, 1998.

Shirwany A, Sargent S J, Dmochowski R R, Bronze M S. Urinary tract aspergillosis in a renal transplant recipient. *Clin Infect Dis* 27:1336, 1998.

Singh N, Gayowski T, Singh J, Yu V L. Invasive gastrointestinal zygomycosis in a liver transplant recipient: case report and review of zygomycosis in solid-organ transplant recipients. *Clin Infect Dis* 20:617–620, 1995.

Singh N, Gayowski T, Wagener M, Doyle H, Marino I R. Invasive fungal infections in liver transplant recipients receiving tacrolimus as the primary immunosuppressive agent. *Clin Infect Dis* 24:179–184, 1997a.

Singh N, Chang F Y, Gayowski T, Marino I R. Infections due to dematiaceous fungi in organ transplant recipients: case report and review. *Clin Infect Dis* 24:369–374, 1997b.

Singh N, Paterson D L, Gayowski T, Wagener M M, Marino I R. Preemptive prophylaxis with a lipid preparation of amphotericin B for invasive fungal infections in liver transplant recipients requiring renal replacement therapy. *Transplant* 71:910–913, 2001.

Smets Y F, van der Pijl J W, van Dissel J T, Ringers F J, de Fijter J W, Lemkes H H. Infectious disease complications of simultaneous pancreas kidney transplantation. *Nephrol Dialysis Transplant* 12:764–771, 1997.

Superdock K R, Dummer J S, Koch M O, Gilliam D M, Van Buren D H, Nylander W A, Richie R E, MacDonell R C, Johnson H K, Helderman J H. Disseminated histoplasmosis presenting as urinary tract obstruction in a renal transplant recipient. *Am J Kid Dis* 23:600–604, 1994.

The U.S. Multicenter FK506 Liver Study Group. A comparison of tacrolimus (FK 506) and cyclosporine for immunosuppresion in liver transplantation. *N Engl J Med* 331:1110–1115, 1994.

Timmouth J, Baker J, Gardiner G. Gastrointestinal mucormycosis in a renal transplant patient. *Canadian J Gastro* 15:269–271, 2001.

Tollemar J, Hockerstedt K, Ericzon B G, Jalanko H, Ringden O. Liposomal amphotericin B prevents invasive fungal infections in liver transplant recipients. *Transplant* 59:45–50, 1995.

Torre-Cisneros J, De la Mata M, Pozo J C, Serrano P, Briceno J, Solorzano G, Mino G, Pera C, Sanchez-Guijo. Randomized trial of weekly sulfadoxine/pyrimethamine versus daily low-dose treimethoprim-sulfamethoxazole for the prophylaxis of *Pneumocystis carinii* pneumonia after liver transplantation. *Clin Infect Dis* 29:771–774, 1999.

Tripathy U, Yung G L, Kriett J M, Thistlewaite P A, Kapelanski D P, Jamieson S W. Donor transfer of pulmonary coccidioidomycosis in lung transplantation. *Ann Thoracic Surg* 73:306–308, 2002.

Verweij P E, Meis J F. Microbiological diagnosis of invasive fungal infections in transplant recipients. *Transplant Infect Dis* 2:80–87, 2000.

Viertel A, Ditting T, Pistorius K, Geiger H, Scheuermann E H, Just-Nubling G. An unusual case of *Aspergillus* endocarditis in a kidney transplant recipient. *Transplant* 68:1812–1813, 1999.

Villacian J S, Paya C V. Prevention of infections in solid organ transplant recipients. *Transplant Infect Dis* 1:50–64, 1999.

Vinayek R, Balan V, Pinna A, Linden P K, Kusne S. Disseminated histoplasmosis in a patient after orthotopic liver transplantation. *Clin Transplant* 12:274–277, 1998.

Viviani M A, Tortorano A M, Malaspina C, Colledan M, Paone G, Rossi G, Bordone G, Pagano A. Surveillance and treatment of liver transplant recipients for candidiasis and aspergillosis. *Eur J Epidemiol* 8:433–436, 1992.

von Eiff C, Bettin D, Proctor R A, Rolauffs B, Lindner N, Winkelmann W, Peters G. *Phaeocremonium parasiticum* infective endocarditis following liver transplantation. *Clin Infect Dis* 25:1251–1253, 1997.

Wade J J, Rolando N, Hayllar K, Philpott-Howard J, Casewell M W, Williams R. Bacerial and fungal infections after liver transplantation: an analysis of 284 patients. *Hepatol* 21:1328–1336, 1995.

Wajsczczuk C P, Dummer J S, Ho M, Van Thiel D H, Starzi T E, Iwatsuki S, Shaw B. Fungal infections in liver transplant recipients. *Transplant* 40:347–353, 1985.

Walker S D, Clark R V, King C T, Humphries J E, Lytle L S, Butkus D E. Fatal disseminated *Conidiobolus coronatus* infection in a renal transplant patient. Review. *Am J Clin Path* 98:559–564, 1992.

Wantanabe M, Hotchi M, Nagasaki M. An autopsy case of disseminated histoplasmosis probably due to infection form a renal allograft. *Acta Pathologica Jap* 38:769–780, 1988.

Waser M, Maggiorini M, Luthy A, Laske A, von Segesser L, Mohacsi P, Opravil M, Turina M, Follath F, Gallino A. Infectious complications in 100 consecutive heart transplant recipients. *Eur J Clin Microbiol Infect Dis* 13:12–18, 1994.

Westney G E, Kesten S, de Hoyos A, Chapparro C, Winton T, Maurer J R. *Aspergillus* infection in single and double lung transplant recipients. *Transplant* 61:915–919, 1996.

Wheat L J, Smith E J, Sathapatayavongs B, Batteiger B, Filo R S, Leapman S B, French M V. Histoplasmosis in renal allograft recipients: two large urban outbreaks. *Arch Intern Med* 143:703–707, 1983.

Wheat J. Histoplasmosis: recognition and treatment. *Clin Infect Dis* 19(Suppl 1):S19–27, 1994.

Wheat J, Sarosi G, McKinsey D, Hamill R, Bradsher R, Johnson P, Loyd J, Kauffman C. Practice guidelines for the management of patients with histoplasmosis. *Clin Infect Dis* 30:688–695, 2000.

Winston D J, Pakrasi A, Busuttil R W. Prophylactic fluconazole in liver transplant recipients: a randomized, double-blind, placebo-controlled trial. *Ann Intern Med* 131:729–737, 1999.

Wong S Y, Allen D M. Transmission of disseminated histoplasmosis via cadaveric renal transplantation: case report. *Clin Infect Dis* 14:232–234, 1992.

Wright P, Pappagianis D, Davis C A, Taylor J, Moser S A, Louro A, Wilson M, Pappas P G. Transmission of *Coccidioides immitis* from donor organs :a description of two fatal cases of disseminated coccidioidomycosis. Abstracts of the Infectious Diseases Society of America 39th Annual Meeting, San Francisco, CA, pg 145; Abstract 619; 2001.

Yeldandi V, Laghi F, McCabe M A, Larson R, O'Keefe P, Husain A, Montoya A, Garrity E R. *Aspergillus* and lung transplantation. *J Heart Lung Transplant* 14:883–890, 1995.

Zainudin B M, Kassim F, Annuar N M, Lim C S, Ghazali A K, Murad Z. Disseminated histoplasmosis presenting with ileal perforation in a renal transplant recipient. *J Trop Med Hygiene* 95:276–279, 1992.

32

Fungal infections among patients with AIDS

BERTRAND DUPONT, PETER G. PAPPAS, AND WILLIAM E. DISMUKES

Fungal infections are the most frequent opportunistic diseases during the course of HIV infection. Those mycoses, which are usually controlled by cellular immunity, are most commonly observed. However, in patients with AIDS, the immune deficit is complex (Spellberg and Edwards, 2001) and worsens with time in nontreated patients, allowing uncommon mycotic diseases to develop (Cunliffe and Denning, 1995; Perfect et al, 1993). *Pneumocystis carinii* (recently classified as a fungus), *Candida albicans*, responsible for mucosal candidiasis, and *Cryptococcus neoformans*, the most frequent cause of meningitis, are the three major fungal pathogens in patients with AIDS. In endemic areas, infections due to dimorphic fungi also represent an important group. *Histoplasma capsulatum, Coccidioides immitis*, and *Penicillium marneffei* are the most important endemic pathogens. In some AIDS patients, mycotic disease is often the consequence of a reactivation several years after a primary infection (Wheat, 1995).

The time of occurrence of opportunistic fungal infections parallels the intensity of the immune deficit. Fungal infections can be the initial sign of HIV infection, are a good marker of the severity of the immune deficit, and often have prognostic value. Some fungal infections are relatively benign such as oropharyngeal candidiasis while others are severe and have a poor prognosis such as cryptococcal meningitis or invasive aspergillosis. Since 1996 the use of highly active antiretroviral therapy (HAART) has markedly reduced the incidence and the severity of opportunistic fungal infections in patients living in countries that can afford the high costs of HAART. Several helpful reviews are devoted to fungal infections in patients with AIDS (Diamond, 1991; Wheat, 1995; Ampel, 1996; Dupont et al, 2000).

PNEUMOCYSTOSIS

This chapter does not address *Pneumocystis carinii* infections in AIDS patients. For a detailed discussion on this topic, see Chapter 27.

CANDIDIASIS

Mucosal candidiasis is the most prevalent infection in HIV-positive patients, and nearly all AIDS patients will develop some clinical manifestations of candidiasis during the course of their illness (Klein et al, 1984). Among *Candida* species, *C. albicans* is almost exclusively responsible for clinical disease. Other species such as *C. glabrata, C. tropicalis, C krusei*, or *C. parapsilosis* may be associated with *C. albicans* in culture; however these non-*albicans* species are often present in low number and their pathogenic role is doubtful and rarely proven. *Candida dubliniensis* may be mistaken for *C. albicans*; the former has been isolated from the oral cavity particularly in patients suffering from recurrent episodes of infection (Sullivan and Coleman, 1998). Beside impairment of cellular immunity and of Th1 type response, a lack of integrity of host tissue and an alteration in equilibrium of the oral flora predispose to oropharyngeal candidiasis. Antimicrobial drugs given for a bacterial or a parasitic infection may represent an additional predisposing factor. An increase in colonization preceeds infection. HIV-positive patients can be heavily colonized without clinical signs or symptoms.

Clinical Manifestations and Treatment

Oropharyngeal candidiasis (OPC) is the most common disease and will occur in ≥ 90% of HIV-infected patients if they do not receive HAART. The lower the CD4 cell count, the higher the risk of developing OPC, although OPC can occur in patients with CD4 counts of 200–400 cells/mm^3. Thrush, or acute pseudomembranous candidiasis, is the most common clinical form of OPC, and characterized by the presence of white patches on an erythematous mucosa. Patches can become confluent, with white pseudomembranes generally spread throughout the oral cavity, involving the dorsal and ventral parts of the tongue, gums, cheeks, and hard and soft palate. The membranes are adherent to the underlying mucosa and can be removed by scraping, revealing a raw erythematous base. Symptoms vary from patient to patient and may not be proportional to the intensity of the intraoral disease. Some patients are symptomless, while others will complain of a furrowed tongue, mouth pain, odynophagia, dysphagia, or burning. Mycologic examination in wet preparations of scraping or swabbed specimens shows numerous blastospores and pseudohyphae with few polymorphonuclear leukocytes. Heavy growth of *Candida* species is obtained by culture in 2 days.

Any patient with thrush must be tested for HIV infection. Presence of thrush allows classification of the patient into clinical group B (symptomatic HIV disease) of the Centers for Diseases Control (CDC) classification (CDC, 1993). Other clinical forms of OPC include atrophic erythematous candidiasis, which involves the tongue and/or palatal mucosa, is less frequent than thrush, possibly underdiagnosed, and can precede the appearance of typical thrush. Angular cheleitis is generally associated with thrush present on the adjacent buccal mucosa. A sabbural tongue, also called "dirty tongue," may be difficult to differentiate from thrush and mycological sampling of the mouth is useless as HIV-positive patients are often heavily colonized with *Candida* in the absence of disease. From a clinical viewpoint, thrush is rarely exclusively localized to the tongue. Hairy leucoplakia due to EBV and often associated with thrush is characterized by white parallel vertical stria localized on both sides of the tongue. Sabbural tongue and hairy leukoplakia do not disappear with antifungal treatment.

Treatment of the first episode of oral thrush or other forms of OPC may be with topical antifungal agents, formulated so as to allow prolonged contact with the affected mucosa. Topical medications should be given 4–6 times a day, administered apart from meals, swallowed after several minutes contact with the lesions, and continued for 2 to 3 weeks. Suitable topical drugs include the polyenes—amphotericin B and nystatin, and the azoles—clotrimazole and miconazole. Numerous commercial formulations are available in different countries as suspensions, powders, oral gels, and tablets for chewing or sucking. In cases of relapsing or chronic OPC, topical treatment is less likely to be effective and may in fact be refused by the patient. Oral ketoconazole is a suitable alternative; however, poor gastrointestinal absorption and liver toxicity are concerns. The treatment of choice is oral fluconazole, 50–100 mg per day for 7 to 14 days. The oral solution of itraconazole, 100–200 mg per day, is an effective alternative. In patients with inadequate response, the daily dose of fluconazole or itraconazole can be raised. While chronic suppressive therapy with fluconazole is effective in the prevention of relapse, emergence of azole resistance is a concern (Rex et al, 2000). See below for discussion of management of OPC refractory to azole therapy.

Esophageal candidiasis, typically observed in patients with more advanced immunosuppression than is OPC,

classifies the patient into group C, AIDS indicator conditions (CDC, 1993). While oral thrush is almost always present in patients with esophagitis, this may not be true in patients treated with a topical oral agent. Esophagitis may be latent and discovered by an endoscopic examination performed for a nonspecific gastric disturbance. The most suggestive symptom of esophageal candidiasis is dysphagia. Some patients complain of nausea or vomiting, especially with esophageal bleeding. Patients may have fever, odynophagia, and occasionally posterior thoracic pain. Endoscopic examination of the esophagus reveals characteristic confluent white plaques adherent to the erythematous mucosa, sometimes covering the entire mucosal surface. A stratification of severity can be established, based on extension of lesions, presence of ulcerations, and narrowing of the lumen. In a patient with oral thrush and retrosternal dysphagia, an endoscopic examination of the esophagus is not mandatory to prove the diagnosis of esophageal candidiasis. Following failure of systemic antifungal therapy, endoscopic examination is useful to rule out azole resistance and other etiologies such as herpes simplex virus, cytomegalovirus, atypical mycobacterial ulceration, or idiopathic ulcer (Wilcox, 1992).

Systemic therapy is required to effectively treat esophageal candidiasis. Oral fluconazole 100–400 mg per day for 2–3 weeks is the drug of choice (Rex et al, 2000). Itraconazole, caspofungin or voriconazole are alternative therapies and less toxic than iv amphotericin B. In cases of failure due to resistance to fluconazole, these therapies may be especially effective (Ally et al, 2001; Villanueva et al, 2001).

Other forms of candidiasis in HIV-infected/AIDS patients are less frequent. Laryngitis should be suspected in a patient with thrush and hoarseness and is sometimes diagnosed during a bronchoscopy. Symptomatic vulvovaginitis is much less frequent than OPC. Anitis or balanitis is uncommon. *Candida* intertrigo and paronychia are more frequent than in HIV-negative persons. *Candida* does not seem to play an etiologic role in diarrhea in HIV-infected patients. However, *Candida* OPC and/or esophagitis may contribute to malnutrition in symptomatic patients who decrease their alimentation. Systemic candidiasis in AIDS patients is rare. Candidemia may occur in some patients and while possibly due to functional defects of polymorphonuclear leukocytes (Szele et al, 1992; Pitrak et al, 1993) is more likely due to the presence of an infected intravenous catheter. However, candidemia is still a rare event in HIV/AIDS patients (Launay et al, 1998). Anecdotal reports have been published describing cholecystitis, prostatitis, or osteitis due to *Candida*.

Oropharyngeal candidiasis and esophagitis have a tendency to recur in patients with a low CD4 count. Consequently, these patients are often treated with protracted or repeated courses of systemic antifungal agents. Cases refractory to fluconazole were reported in up to 15% of patients with advanced AIDS before the era of HAART. Low CD4 count (< 50/mm^3), frequent courses of azole therapy, and prolonged treatment have been shown to predispose to clinical resistance (Maenza et al, 1996; Walmsley et al, 2001). Fluconazole MICs $\geq$ 16–32 μg/l are often correlated with clinical failure (Redding et al, 1994; Revanker et al, 1998). Clinical resistance has been reported in patients not previously exposed to fluconazole but who were sexual partners of patients who were receiving this antifungal agent and harboring *Candida* strains with a high MIC (Dromer et al, 1997). Molecular biology studies indicate that a majority of patients carry the same clone of *Candida* for many years (Redding et al, 1994). The main mechanism of resistance to fluconazole is an efflux of the drug from the yeast cell through the activation of efflux pumps, which are selective for fluconazole or the azole class (responsible for cross resistance to all azole drugs). Since the advent of HAART there has been a marked decrease in all forms of candidiasis in HIV-infected patients. Resistance of *Candida* to antifungal drugs in AIDS patients appears to be less common than in the early to mid-1990s.

For more detailed discussion of candidiasis, see Chapter 11.

CRYPTOCOCCOSIS

Traditionally, the encapsulated yeast *Cryptococcus neoformans* has had two varieties: *C. neoformans* variety *neoformans* with two serotypes, A and D, and *C. neoformans* variety *gattii* with two serotypes, B and C. Serotype A has been recently associated with a new variety, *C. neoformans* variety *grubii*, which is ubiquitous in temperate and tropical climates and is present in soil particularly when enriched with bird droppings (Franzot et al, 1999). Serotype D is present in Europe and to a lesser degree in North America (Dromer et al, 1996). Serotype B and C are present in tropical and subtropical areas. Serotype B has been isolated in the vicinity of *Eucalyptus* trees: *E. camaldulensis* and *E. tereticornis* particularly in Australia, California, and Florida (Speed and Dunt, 1995). The ecological niche of serotype C, only rarely isolated from patients and from almond trees in Columbia, is still unknown.

Virtually all cryptococcal infections in HIV-positive patients are caused by *C. neoformans* var. *neoformans*; this is true even in areas where both varieties *C. neoformans* and *C. gattii* are equally prevalent (Kwon-Chung et al, 1990). By contrast, in Sao Paulo, Brazil, non-HIV-associated cryptococcosis is equally due to var. *neoformans* and var. *gattii*. However, almost all HIV-associated cases are due to var. *neoformans*. There are strong arguments to indicate that clinical cryptococcosis results from reactivation of a previous primary infection; however, disease may follow recent primary infection in some patients. Alveolar macrophages, cellular immunity and Th1 type immune response are the main lines of defense against *Cryptococcus*. In the 1980s, HIV infection became the leading predisposing factor for cryptococcosis, occurring with an incidence of 6% to 12% in the United States, 3% to 8% in Europe and 15% to 35% in Central and South Africa or South East Asia (Mitchell and Perfect, 1995). In France from 1985 to 1993, 83% of 1013 reported cases of cryptococcosis occurred in HIV-positive patients (Dromer et al, 1996). Since 1996 with the introduction of HAART, there has been a decrease of approximately 70% in the number of cases. Cryptococcosis, an AIDS-defining opportunistic infection (CDC, 1993), generally occurs in persons with a CD4 count below 50/mm^3.

Clinical Manifestations

The most common site of *C. neoformans* infection at the time of diagnosis is the meninges. Moreover, *C. neoformans* is the principal cause of meningitis in AIDS patients (Zuger et al, 1986; Chuck and Sande, 1989; Clark et al, 1990; Dismukes, 1998). Cryptococcal meningitis or meningoencephalitis, which may be associated with lung disease, disseminated disease, or be the only site of clinical disease, carries a poor prognosis with a 20% to 25% death rate despite appropriate treatment. Symptoms of meningitis are typically subacute, occasionally acute, with fever and headache as the most common manifestations, followed by nausea, vomiting, and malaise. Neck stiffness is not common. Delay between first symptom and diagnosis is often several weeks. With time, more symptoms are manifest. The presence of fever and altered mental status or cranial nerve palsy is more suggestive of meningoencephalitis. Paresis of limbs or seizures are less frequent. The patient can present with change of mood, personality changes, memory loss, visual and auditory dysfunction, obtundation, or coma.

Pulmonary symptoms are present in 40% to 50% of AIDS patients with cryptococcosis and can precede the occurrence of meningeal symptoms. The lung is the site of the initial infection with *C. neoformans*. Pulmonary symptoms vary from asymptomatic to dyspnea, productive cough, and sometimes respiratory distress. There is no specific picture on chest radiograph; findings include segmental or lobar infiltrates, nodules, and enhanced interstitial markings (Cameron et al, 1990). In some patients a mixed infection is present, for example, pneumocystosis and cryptococcosis. The diagnosis of cryptococcal lung disease can be confirmed by isolation of the typical encapsulated yeasts in sputum or more frequently in bronchoalveolar lavage (BAL). The use of selective medium is useful to recognize a few colonies of *Cryptococcus* among a large number of *Candida* colonies present in sputum or in BAL. Detection of cryptococcal polysaccharide antigen in BAL or serum is diagnostic.

Aside from lung and CNS disease, cryptococcosis can involve many other organs (Zuger et al, 1986; Chuck and Sande, 1989; Clark et al, 1990). Approximately 10% of patients have skin lesions, which are protean, may mimick Molluscum contagiosum umbilicated papulonodules, or present as an ulceration or acneiform rash. Any recent suspicious cutaneous lesion in a patient with HIV or AIDS must be biopsied for culture and/or histology to check for *C. neoformans*. Adenopathy, splenomegaly, or hepatomegaly can be present. Urinary tract infection, typically prostatitis, is generally latent. Fever may be the only symptom of cryptococcal disease and occasionally a patient may present as fever of unknown origin; in such case, the detection of cryptococcal antigen in serum may be the only marker of infection. In this setting, a positive blood or urine culture is diagnostic.

A diagnosis of cryptococcosis makes sampling of CSF mandatory even in the absence of any neurological symptoms. Other studies in a patient with suspected cryptococcosis should include: blood culture, chest radiography, skin examination, and testing for cryptococcal antigen in blood and CSF. The CSF opening pressure should always be recorded before removal of CSF, and has important prognostic value. An opening pressure more than 25 ml of water necessitates lowering of pressure via decompression with repeated lumbar punctures or other approaches (Graybill et al, 2000). Cerebrospinal fluid is usually clear and may have normal or mildly abnormal values (white blood cell count, protein, and glucose) reflecting a minimal inflammatory response. Hypoglycorrhachia, if present, is highly compatible with cryptococcal meningitis. Examination of CSF with India ink shows the typical encapsulated yeasts in 68%–88% of cases. Culture of CSF will be positive within 3 to 7 days in 95%–100% of cases. Antigen detection is present in almost 100% of AIDS-associated cases, sometimes with very high titers (> 1/10000). Moreover, the result is immediate. (Mitchell and Perfect, 1995). In case of meningitis, serum antigen detection is positive in more than 90% of cases and represents a screening test for the diagnosis of cryptococcosis in patients with unexplained fever or recent headache. Although the detection of cryptococcal antigen in urine or BAL is not well validated, a positive result should alert the practitioner to the possibility of cryptococcosis. The typical encapsulated yeast of *C. neoformans* can be seen in fluids (BAL, urine) or in tissue (skin, lymph node, or bone marrow).

Computed tomography scan of the brain is usually normal and is useful to rule out other central nervous system opportunistic diseases such as toxoplasmosis or lymphoma, which cause ring-enhancing mass lesions. Cryptococcal brain abscesses (cryptococcomas) are rare and less frequent than in HIV-negative patients. However, *C. neoformans* var. *gattii*, serotype C, although unusual in AIDS, has a propensity to produce chronic mass lesions in brain or lung (Speed and Dunt, 1995).

Treatment

The results of several comparative trials with a large number of patients facilitate a general consensus on the treatment of cryptococcal meningitis. The regimen of choice is induction therapy with combination iv amphotericin B 0.7–1.0 mg/kg/day and oral flucytosine 100 mg/kg/day given for at least 2 weeks. In patients stable or improving, a switch to consolidation therapy with oral fluconazole 400 mg/day for an additional 8–10 weeks is recommended (van der Horst et al, 1997). A lumbar puncture for a CSF sample is useful at week 2 and week 10, the end of this primary treatment. A negative CSF culture at week 2 has good prognostic value. The relatively high dose of amphotericin B (0.7–1.0 mg/kg/day) has aided in reducing the early mortality reported with lower amphotericin B dose (0.3–0.4 mg/kg/day) (Saag et al, 1992). Induction therapy utilizing flucytosine at a dose of 100 mg/kg/day is well tolerated and appears to reduce the relapse rate during subsequent maintenance therapy (Saag et al, 1999). Itraconazole can replace fluconazole during the consolidation phase of therapy; however, the erratic absorption of itraconazole and more frequent itraconazole-drug interactions make fluconazole easier to use.

Following successful primary induction and consolidation therapy, maintenance therapy with 200 mg fluconazole daily is necessary to avoid relapse (Saag et al, 1999). Fluconazole is superior to itraconazole and to iv amphotericin B as maintenance therapy (Powderly et al, 1992). Maintenance treatment is prescribed lifelong; without such therapy the relapse rate is > 50%, indicating that cure is not obtained despite clearance of yeasts. In patients who are treated successfully with HAART, it may be possible to stop the maintenance therapy without adverse consequences (Masur et al, 2002). Limited data support this approach (Aberg et al, 2002; Mussini et al, 2001).

The same treatment approach as described above for cryptococcal meningitis can be used for extra CNS cryptococcosis. Alternative regimens as primary treatment include fluconazole 400–800 mg daily with or without flucytosine 100–150 mg/kg/day. Lipid formulations of amphotericin B can be used in patients intolerant of conventional amphotericin B (Coker et al, 1993; Leenders et al, 1997). In vitro resistance to amphotericin B is extremely rare. High MICs to fluconazole are common but there is no good correlation between in vitro susceptibility and clinical results. Serial clonal isolates in relapse patients treated with fluconazole may exhibit a progressive increase in MICs. In such cases it seems logical to increase the dose of fluconazole to 800–1000 mg daily and/or to add flucytosine or to switch to itraconazole plus flucytosine. However, experience with such regimens is limited and anecdotal. There are no data from large studies with new antifungal drugs or new formulations of existing drugs regarding therapy of cryptococcosis.

An elevated CSF opening pressure ≥ 25 cm of water is an indication to withdraw 30 ml CSF daily or two or three times a week until improvement (Graybill et al, 2000). In refractory cases, a lumbar or ventricular shunting procedure is necessary. Treatment with corticosteroids appears deleterious in this setting. Persistent or late intracranial hypertension due to impaired resorption of CSF or obstruction to circulation of CSF may benefit from a ventriculoperitoneal shunt (Liliang et al, 2002). There is no specific treatment for visual loss or deafness aside from palliative measures to reduce intracranial hypertension.

Primary prophylaxis with 200 mg fluconazole daily in HIV-infected/AIDS patients can reduce the incidence of cryptococcosis; however, this approach is expensive, predisposes to the emergence of resistance in opportunistic yeasts, *Candida* and *Cryptococcus*, and does not improve survival (Powderly, 2000). The incidence of cryptococcosis in the United States or Europe does not justify prophylaxis with fluconazole. However, the incidence is much higher in tropical countries including Africa (Dupont et al, 2000). Data from Thailand indicate that itraconazole, 200 mg daily, reduces the incidence of penicilliosis, cryptococcosis, and histoplasmosis (Chariyalertsak et al, 2002).

For more detailed discussion of cryptococcosis, see Chapter 12.

COMMON DIMORPHIC FUNGAL INFECTIONS

Among fungal infections due to dimorphic fungi, only three are frequent in AIDS patients: histoplasmosis, coccidioidomycosis, and penicilliosis (Wheat et al, 1990; Supparatpinyo et al, 1994; Ampel, 1996; Warnock et al, 1998).

Histoplasmosis
Histoplasmosis due to *Histoplasma capsulatum* is endemic in the eastern and central United States and Central and South America. In HIV-positive patients living in endemic areas such as Indianapolis, Indiana in North America, the incidence of histoplasmosis varies from 1% to 25% (Wheat et al, 1990; McKinsey et al, 1997).

Disease can be due to primary infection following an exposure event, or reactivation of a latent infection. Outside endemic areas, disease usually represents reactivation occurring several years after the primary infection, particularly the case in Europe (McKinsey et al, 1997; Warnock et al, 1998; Dupont et al, 2000). It is important to obtain a travel history including brief trip in tropical countries, caves or other geographic areas endemic for histoplasmosis. Histoplasmosis, which generally occurs in patients with a low CD4 counts, usually less than 100 cells/mm^3, is an AIDS-defining illness in its disseminated form (McKinsey et al, 1997).

Clinical Manifestations
The disease is often disseminated and fever is frequent (75%), accompanied by weight loss, fatigue, and sweats. Pneumonia is present in 50%–60% of cases, and hepatomegaly, spleno-megaly, or lymphadenopathy in 25% of cases. Central nervous system involvement occurs in approximately 15% of patients, either as meningitis or a space-occupying lesion (Wheat et al, 1990). Signs and symptoms of septic shock or respiratory failure are seen in 10% of cases and are associated with a poor prognosis (Wheat et al, 2000a). Pancytopenia is found in 20% of patients at presentation. Various cutaneous lesions are seen including maculopapular rashes, pustules, papules, and skin or oral ulcers. These lesions are nonspecific, but provide easy access to tissue for biopsy and diagnosis. Histoplasmosis-associated mediastinal fibrosis and chronic fibrocavitary lung disease are unusual in this population. Gastrointestinal masses, chorioretinitis, endocarditis, and pleural effusion have been reported.

The chest radiograph demonstrates patchy infiltrates or diffuse interstitial pneumonia in severe cases. Blood, bone marrow aspirate, urine, BAL fluid, and CSF cultures may yield *Histoplasma*. The typical yeasts can be seen in these samples and in smear of buffy coat or whole blood in patients with disseminated disease. Histopathology of skin, lymph node, lung, or bone marrow can provide presumptive evidence of histoplasmosis. Serodiagnostic tests by immunodiffusion or complement fixation are often negative but may be helpful when positive. *Histoplasma* antigen detection in blood, urine, or CSF is a specific and sensitive test, particularly among patients with disseminated disease. Antigenuria correlates well with response to therapy and is useful to detect relapsing histoplasmosis (Wheat et al, 1990).

Histoplasmosis due to *Histoplasma capsulatum* variety *duboisii* does not occur frequently in AIDS patients. This form of histoplamosis is seen exclusively among patients living in or who have travelled to Central and West Africa. Histoplasmosis due to *H. duboisii* is probably underdiagnosed in its endemic area.

Treatment

Amphotericin B and itraconazole are effective against both *H. capsulatum* and *H. duboisii* (Wheat et al, 1990; Wheat et al, 2000b). Among patients with severe disease including diffuse pneumonia, septic shock, or any life-threatening complication, first line treatment is amphotericin B 0.7–1.0 mg/kg/day. In stable and improved patients after 10–14 days, this regimen can be switched to oral itraconazole 400 mg/day for 12 weeks (Lortholary et al, 1999). Mild forms of histoplasmosis can be treated initially with itraconazole with a loading dose of 300 mg twice daily for 3 days then 400 mg daily for 12 weeks. Fluconazole is less effective than itraconazole at similar doses; however, fluconazole is a reasonable therapy at 400–800 mg/day in selected patients. Maintenance therapy is necessary to avoid relapses in AIDS patients (Wheat et al, 2000b). Itraconazole at 200 mg/day lifelong is the drug of choice, and is superior to amphotericin B (1 mg/kg) once or twice a week. Ketoconazole is less effective than amphotericin B. Recently available data support that stopping maintenance therapy is appropriate in patients treated effectively with HAART (Dupont et al, 2000; Masur et al, 2002). Primary prophylaxis should be considered in areas where the incidence of histoplasmosis is highest (McKinsey et al, 1999).

For more detailed discussion of histoplasmosis, see Chapter 18.

Coccidioidomycosis

This disease, which is endemic in the southwestern United States and in parts of Mexico, Central, and South America, is acquired by inhalation of arthroconidia present in the soil. The lung is the primary target organ. In highly endemic areas such as Arizona, the annual rate of infection is as high as 27% among patients with AIDS vs. fewer than 4% in non-AIDS patients (Bronnimann et al, 1987). In the majority of cases, disease probably occurs following reactivation rather than as a primary infection. Extrathoracic coccidioidomycosis involving sites other than lungs and hilar or cervical lymph nodes is an AIDS-defining illness (CDC, 1993).

Clinical Manifestations

The most common symptoms of coccidioidomycosis in AIDS patients are fever, cough, and weight loss. Chest radiography reveals a variety of abnormalities in more than 60% of patients including focal pulmonary alveolar infiltrates, discrete nodules, hilar lymphadenopathy, and pleural effusions. In 40% of patients, a diffuse reticulonodular infiltrate is present. Approximately 12% of patients develop meningitis and 5% present with cutaneous disease and concomitant pulmonary involvement. Subcutaneous abscesses have been especially associated with AIDS patients. Nine percent of patients present with localized extrathoracic lymph node or liver involvement. Fungemia, thyroiditis, peritonitis, and adrenal, bone, joint, and prostate disease have been reported (Bronnimann et al, 1987; Fish et al, 1990; Galgiani and Ampel, 1990).

The CD4 cell count is usually below 200 cells/mm^3 and often below 50 cells/mm^3. Definitive diagnosis relies on *(1)* visualization of the typical spherules containing numerous endospores in clinical specimens, and *(2)* isolation of *C. immitis* in culture. Because of the risk of laboratory contamination, this fungus should be handled with caution, in accordance with safety regulations. Serology with complement fixation testing of serum and CSF may remain negative in 25% of AIDS patients with active coccidioidal disease. Cerebrospinal fluid analysis typically shows leukocytic pleocytosis, decreased glucose, and increased protein. Culture for *C. immitis* in CSF is positive in $\geq$ 50% of cases (Fish et al, 1990).

Treatment

The drug of choice for severe life-threatening coccidioidal infection, including diffuse reticulonodular lung involvement, is iv amphotericin B at $\geq$ 1 mg/kg/day. When the disease is controlled, generally after 2 or 3 weeks, switching to an oral triazole drug should be considered. Fluconazole 400–800 mg/day is a good alternative, particularly in patients with meningitis; itraconazole 400 mg/day has also given good results, especially in patients with skeletal disease (Fish et al, 1990; Galgiani et al, 2000a; Galgiani et al, 2000b). For patients with meningitis, intrathecal amphotericin B may be added to parenteral amphotericin B. Fluconazole is the currently preferred treatment of coccidioidal meningitis (Galgiani et al, 2000b). Lifelong maintenance therapy with a triazole (fluconazole 400 mg/day or itraconazole 400 mg/day) is necessary to avoid relapse in AIDS patients (Masur et al, 2002). The impact of HAART is beneficial with regard to the incidence of new cases but has had little impact on the overall management of coccidioidomycosis (Dupont et al, 2000).

For more detailed discussion of coccidioidomycosis, see Chapter 20.

Penicilliosis

Penicillium marneffei is a dimorphic fungus present in soil in Southeast Asia, including northern Thailand, south China, Laos, Cambodia, and Vietnam. A few cases of penicilliosis have also been reported in Hong Kong, India, and Indonesia. A probable autochthonous case was reported in Africa. *Penicillium marneffei* is associated with several species of bamboo rats; however, contact with soil seems the most important risk factor regarding exposure to this fungus. In northern Thailand, penicilliosis has become the third most common AIDS-defining opportunistic disease, following tuberculosis and cryptococcosis (Deng et al, 1988; Drouhet, 1993; Supparatpinyo et al, 1994; Sobottka et al, 1996). Penicilliosis probably occurs as a silent primary infection and only becomes clinically apparent following reactivation years later when cellular immunity is profoundly depressed due to advanced HIV disease.

Clinical Manifestations

The portal of entry is the lung in most reported cases. As with histoplasmosis, disseminated penicilliosis is very common at presentation and CD4 counts are uniformly very low, usually below 50 cells/mm^3. In one study of 92 patients with disseminated penicilliosis seen at Chiang Mai University Hospital in Thailand, 86 (93%) were HIV infected (Supparatpinyo et al, 1994). The clinical characteristics of these patients included fever (93%), anemia (78%), pronounced weight loss (76%), skin lesions (68%), generalized lymphadenopathy (58%), hepatomegaly (51%), cough (49%), diarrhea (31%), splenomegaly (16%), and jaundice (8%). Skin lesions, especially a generalized papular rash, are very suggestive of the diagnosis of penicilliosis in patients at risk. Some of the papules with central umbilication mimick lesions caused by Molluscum contagiosum. Subcutaneous nodules, acne-like lesions and folliculitis may also be present. Genital ulcers (6%) or palatal papules have been reported. The mean duration of illness before patients presented for care in this study was 4 weeks (range 1 day to 3 years); most patients were young men. Several AIDS patients had other simultaneous opportunistic infections including oral candidiasis, tuberculosis, cryptococcosis, and cerebral toxoplasmosis. Chest radiography is abnormal in almost 30% of patients with disseminated penicilliosis. Diffuse reticulonodular opacities and localized alveolar opacities are most common. Diffuse alveolar infiltrates and pleural effusion are less common (Deng et al, 1988; Drouhet, 1993).

Imported cases of penicilliosis are generally diagnosed earlier in the course of disease. Fever, with or without pancytopenia, skin and/or lung lesions should also suggest a diagnosis of leishmaniasis or disseminated histoplasmosis. For any HIV-positive patient, a history of living in or previous travel to Southeast Asia is the first clue towards considering a diagnosis of penicilliosis (Warnock et al, 1998; Dupont et al, 2000).

In the Chiang Mai series, diagnosis of penicilliosis was made by culture of the fungus in blood (76%), skin lesions (90%), bone marrow aspirate (100%), sputum (34%) and other sites including CSF, pharynx, and pleural fluid (Supparatpinyo et al, 1994). The culture at 25°C shows a filamentous fungus growing in 2 days. The organism belongs to the *Penicillium* genus, has a symmetric or asymmetric biverticillium structure, and produces a red pigment that diffuses into the surface and depth of the culture medium. The organism grows as a yeast when incubated at 35°C–37°C. The galactomannan test for detection of *Aspergillus* antigen cross-reacts with *P. marneffei*; however, the diseases are clinically different and direct examination of culture easily distinguishes between the two organisms. Presumptive diagnosis of penicilliosis can be made by histopathologic examination of sputum, bone marrow, skin or lymph node, and finding the typical oval or elongated, nonbudding *P. marneffei* yeasts, 3–8 μm in length, with a characteristic septation.

Treatment

At present, itraconazole and amphotericin B are the mainstays of therapy for penicilliosis in all patients, regardless of their immune status. A combination regimen of induction treatment with amphotericin B 0.6 mg/kg/day for approximately 2 weeks followed by consolidation treatment with itraconazole 400 mg/day for 10 weeks is highly effective in > 95% of patients (Sirisanthana et al, 1998). This combination regimen clears fungal cultures more rapidly than a course of itraconazole alone. Chronic maintenance (suppressive) therapy is recommended for all patients with persistent immunocompromise. Itraconazole 200 mg/day is the drug of choice (Supparatpinyo et al, 1998). In geographic areas where *P. marneffei* and other opportunistic fungal pathogens are endemic, primary prophylaxis with itraconazole 200 mg/day is also recommended to prevent penicilliosis, histoplasmosis, and cryptococcosis (Chariyalertsak et al, 2002).

For more detailed discussion of penicilliosis, see Chapter 23.

ASPERGILLOSIS

Invasive aspergillosis is usually seen among neutropenic cancer patients and patients treated with corticosteroids. AIDS is not considered a major risk factor because the cellular defect in HIV-infected patients mainly impacts T lymphocytes and less so neutrophils or macrophages, the main defense against *Aspergillus* spp. Nevertheless, since 1990 invasive aspergillosis has been reported among patients with advanced HIV disease, especially in patients with CD4 cell counts below 50/mm^3 (Denning et al, 1991; Lortholary et al, 1993; Khoo and Denning, 1994). The classical risk factors for invasive aspergillosis, namely, neutropenia and corticosteroid therapy, are absent in approximately 50% of reported *Aspergillus* infected AIDS cases.

Clinical Manifestations

The lungs are the most common site of infection. In a study of 33 AIDS patients with invasive aspergillosis, mainly pulmonary disease, fever was always present, with a median temperature of 39°C; cough and dyspnea were present in 97% and 80% of cases, respectively, and chest pain and hemoptysis in 20% and 17%, respectively (Lortholary et al, 1993). Radiographically, nodular lesions or cavitary infiltrates were common and suggestive of aspergillosis although not specific. Bilateral interstitial infiltrates were also noted. Invasive necrotizing tracheobronchitis manifested by acute dyspnea and wheezing is a clinical form of aspergillosis also seen in AIDS patients (Lortholary et al, 1993). Bronchoscopy reveals necrotic ulceration of the trachea with pseudomembranes (Kemper et al, 1993). Obstructing bronchial aspergillosis with chest pain, hemoptysis, and dyspnea may precede necrotizing tracheobronchitis (Denning et al, 1991). A majority of patients have a history of prior pulmonary infection and preexisting cystic pulmonary lesions or bullae may represent a risk factor for invasive pulmonary aspergillosis among patients with AIDS. Extrapulmonary metastatic *Aspergillus* disease occurs and the CNS and heart are most often involved. *Aspergillus* endocarditis and sinusitis have been reported among patients with AIDS.

There is a good correlation between a positive BAL culture for *Aspergillus* and histologically proven diagnosis in immunocompromised patients, including AIDS patients. The *Aspergillus* spp. most often implicated in disease are *A. fumigatus*, *A. flavus*, *A. niger*, and *A. terreus*. Detection of galactomannan antigen and/or PCR for *Aspergillus* may help to establish diagnosis; however, their roles remain unclear. Prognosis of invasive aspergillosis in AIDS patients is poor with a mean survival < 2–4 months despite antifungal treatment. This opportunistic infection is very unusual among patients receiving and responding to HAART.

Treatment

Therapy consists of amphotericin B ≥ 1.0 mg/kg/day, one of the lipid formulations of amphotericin B 3–6 mg/kg/day, or oral itraconazole 400–600 mg/day. However, the disease is rapidly progressive among most AIDS patients despite systemic antifungal therapy. Although no large body of data supports use of newer antifungal agents for invasive aspergillosis in patients with AIDS, it is reasonable to assume that voriconazole and the echinocandins, as well as immunomodulating agents, may have a role in this clinical setting. No prophylaxis approach is applicable (Stevens et al, 2000).

For more detailed discussion of aspergillosis, see Chapter 14.

OTHER FUNGAL INFECTIONS

Paracoccidioidomycosis, Blastomycosis, and Sporotrichosis

These mycoses that are felt to be contained by T cell-mediated host defenses have been described in AIDS patients, but their reported incidence has not increased in parallel with the other mycoses (Wheat 1995; Dupont et al, 2000). The scarcity of reported cases of paracoccidioidomycosis in AIDS patients in Latin America remains unexplained. In a review of 27 cases (Goldani and Sugar, 1995), paracoccidioidomycosis occurred mainly in patients with advanced AIDS who were not receiving prophylaxis with trimethoprim-sulfamethoxazole for *Pneumocystis carinii*. In areas endemic for *P. brasiliensis*, HIV positivity has been limited mostly to larger towns and paracoccidioidomycosis limited to more rural areas. Almost all reported cases of AIDS-associated paracoccidioidomycosis have occurred in Brazil, with only one case reported from Venezuela. In the series reported by Goldani and Sugar, the overall male to female ratio was 3.5:1, which is lower than the sex ratio of 13:1 observed in the HIV-negative population. Reactivation of latent disease probably accounts for most cases, but among patients living in rural areas primary infection cannot be excluded (Benard and Duarte, 2000). Most of the reported patients had advanced AIDS with CD4 cell counts well below 200/mm^3.

In 70% of AIDS patients with paracoccidioidomycosis, disease is widely disseminated. About two-thirds of patients have lung involvement with often severe cough and dyspnea. Chest radiography is usually nonspecific, revealing diffuse interstitial infiltrates in most patients. Approximately 50% of patients have skin lesions that include a disseminated maculopapular rash and nodular or ulcerative lesions. Adenopathy is present in approximately one-third of patients. Prolonged fever, weight loss, hepatomegaly, and splenomegaly are common. Meningitis is rare (Goldani and Sugar, 1995; Wheat, 1995).

The diagnosis of paracoccidioidomycosis is usually made by direct microscopic examination and culture of clinical specimens, most commonly skin and lymph nodes. Cultures of blood, bone marrow, and CSF may also be positive. Antibody detection is positive in a small number of patients. An assay for *P. brasiliensis* antigen and PCR for *P. brasiliensis* DNA are promising diagnostic tools in these patients. Histopathologic findings are characterized by a granulomatous reaction with macrophages, lymphocytes, and giant cells.

Although there is no consensus regarding the optimal treatment, aggressive therapy may likely reduce the high overall mortality. Therapeutic options include sulfonamides, amphotericin B, and the azole drugs—ketoconazole, and itraconazole, as primary treatment followed by lifelong maintenance therapy with trimethoprim-sulfamethoxazole, ketoconazole, or itraconazole (Mendez et al, 1994).

Blastomycosis, a relatively common endemic mycosis in immunocompetent persons, is an uncommon disorder among HIV-positive patients (Pappas, 1992;

Wheat, 1995). Over 30 cases of blastomycosis have been reported in patients with AIDS, and most have CD4 cell counts well below 200/mm^3. Pulmonary infection, asymptomatic or symptomatic, develops following inhalation of infectious spores. Reactivation disease also occurs as evidenced among patients with AIDS and other patients who have been out of the endemic area for several years. Localized pleuropulmonary disease is present in approximately 50% of cases; extrapulmonary dissemination is equally common, including spread to the skin and the central nervous system. Disseminated disease is associated with a high early mortality.

Amphotericin B is considered the initial treatment of choice, particularly for patients with severe disease. For patients who are improved or stable after 2–4 weeks of amphotericin B, it is reasonable to switch to oral itraconazole 200–400 mg/day and maintain chronic suppressive therapy with itraconazole indefinitely in those patients who remain severely immunosuppressed (Pappas et al, 1992; Chapman et al, 2000). The risk of CNS relapse must be considered among patients receiving chronic therapy with itraconazole, given its poor CNS penetration.

Sporotrichosis usually manifests as a localized lymphocutaneous disease in the immunocompetent host. Disseminated disease occurs most frequently in severely immunocompromised individuals. In a review of 16 cases of disseminated sporotrichosis among HIV-infected patients, all patients presented with diffuse ulcerative skin lesions (Al-Tawfiq and Wools, 1998). Other sites of disease included the CNS, joints, eyes, spleen, and bone marrow. *Sporothrix schenckii* fungemia was noted in two patients. Fifteen of the 16 patients were men. The mean CD4 cell count was 73/mm^3. Six of these patients died despite therapy. A second series of cases of sporotrichosis in AIDS patients has recently been reported (Rocha et al, 2001). Histopathology and culture of cutaneous lesions, synovial fluid, sputum, or CSF usually leads to the diagnosis. Examination of purulence from involved areas may demonstrate typical cigar-shaped yeast forms; however, the organism may appear atypical with large round elements reaching 8 μm in diameter, simulating *C. neoformans* (Rocha et al, 2001).

The optimal therapy for disseminated sporotrichosis in HIV-positive patients has not been determined. Parenteral amphotericin B for the most severe cases followed by itraconazole appears to be the most reasonable approach to therapy. Itraconazole should be considered for long-term maintenance therapy among those patients with severe disease manifestations and who remain significantly immunosuppressed (Kauffman et al, 2000).

For more detailed discussion of paracoccidioidomy-cosis, blastomycosis, and sporotrichosis, see Chapters 21, 19, and 22, respectively.

UNCOMMON FUNGAL DISEASES

A variety of uncommon fungi also cause invasive mycoses in AIDS patients. Among many of these patients, risk factors other than HIV/AIDS include intravenous drug use, alcoholism, chronic hepatitis, catheter-associated infections, neutropenia, and trauma (Perfect et al, 1993; Cunliffe and Denning, 1995).

Zygomycosis is usually encountered among AIDS patients with other risk factors including diabetic ketoacidosis, neutropenia, hemodialysis, and intravenous drug use. Three cases of zygomycosis with isolated renal infections in AIDS patients occurred in two intravenous drug users (Smith et al, 1989; Santos et al, 1994), and another patient had a massive renal infarction (Vesa et al, 1992). In three cases of cerebral zygomycosis, basal ganglia masses were reported (Hopkins et al, 1994). Other cases of zygomycosis in AIDS patients include three patients with brain abscesses (Micozzi and Wetli, 1985; Cuadrado et al, 1988); and single patients with rhinocerebral disease (Blatt et al, 1991); cutaneous disease (Hopwood et al, 1992); posttraumatic cutaneous and knee joint infection (Mostaza et al, 1989); pharyngeal ulceration (Chavanet et al, 1990); and gastric infection (Brullet et al, 1993). The causative organisms of zygomycosis in AIDS patients have included *Absidia corymbifera*, *Cunninghamella bertholletiae*, and *Rhizopus arrhizus*.

For more detailed discussion of zygomycoses, see Chapter 15.

AIDS patients with infections due to *Scedosporium apiospermum* (*Pseudallescheria boydii*) have been described with pneumonia (Cunliffe and Denning, 1995; Rollot et al, 2000); renal and pulmonary infection (Scherr et al, 1992); endocarditis (Raffanti et al, 1990); meningitis and brain abscess (Montero et al, 1998); and sinusitis (Eckburg et al, 1999). *Scedosporium prolificans* was responsible for a case of cutaneous and pulmonary disease (Cunliffe and Denning, 1995).

For more detailed discussion of scedosporiosis, see Chapter 16.

Five cases of infection due to *Saccharomyces cerevisiae* in AIDS patients have been reported including three with pulmonary disease (Al-Tawfik et al, 1989, Perfect et al 1993; Cunliffe and Denning, 1995). In addition, three cases caused by *Trichosporon* spp. have been reported in AIDS patients with catheters, including two with central venous catheter-associated fungemia and one with peritonitis and a peritoneal catheter. Outcome was favorable in each case with antifungal treatment and withdrawal of the catheter (Leaf and Simberkoff, 1989, Parsonnet, 1989, Barchiesi et al, 1993).

For more detailed discussion of *Saccharomyces* and *Trichosporon* infections, see Chapter 13.

As is shown in the following list, rare cases of fungal disease in AIDS patients have also been attributed to very uncommon fungal pathogens:

- invasive alternariosis (Wiest et al, 1987)
- hepatic abscesses caused by *Aureobasidium pullulans* (Yarrish et al, 1991)
- disseminated adiaspiromycosis (Echavaria et al, 1993) and pulmonary adiaspiromycosis (Turner et al, 1999)
- disseminated cutaneous *Emmonsia pasteuriana* infection (Gori et al, 1998)
- invasive *Fusarium* infections involving lung (Del Palacio-Hernanz et al, 1989a), sinuses (Bossi et al, 1995), and oral cavity (Paugam et al, 1999)
- systemic infection caused by *Penicillium decumbens* (Alvarez, 1990)
- CNS infection caused by *Rhinocladiella atrovirens* (Del Palacio-Hernanz et al, 1989b)
- fungemia and catheter infection due to *Rhodotorula rubra* (Lui et al, 1998)
- *Sporobolomyces* infection (Morris et al 1991)
- chronic sinusitis due to *Schizophyllum commune* (Rosenthal et al, 1992; Marlier et al, 1993)
- *Scytalidium dimidiatum* cutaneous infection (Marriott et al, 1997)
- suppurative lymphadenitis and chronic sinusitis due to *Lecythophora hoffmannii* (Marriott et al, 1997).

IMPACT OF HIGHLY ACTIVE ANTIRETROVIRAL THERAPY ON FUNGAL INFECTIONS

Highly active antiretroviral therapy has had a triple impact on the natural course of opportunistic infections in AIDS patients: *(1)* led to a marked decrease in the number of infections; *(2)* made it possible to stop the primary prophylaxis for many fungal infections; and *(3)* made it possible to stop chronic maintenance therapy of established fungal infections (Detels et al, 2001). The routine use of HAART has resulted in dramatic declines in morbidity and mortality among HIV-infected patients with advanced immune dysfunction (Palella et al, 1998). In effectively treated patients, the incidence of opportunistic infections has decreased at least 50% to 70%. Highly active antiretroviral therapy has had an especially important impact on the incidence of *P. carinii* pneumonia, *M. avium* complex disease, cytomegalovirus infection, mucosal candidiasis, cryptococcosis, dimorphic fungal infections, and invasive aspergillosis. Highly active antiretroviral therapy asso-

ciated immune reconstitution has made it possible to withdraw primary prophylaxis against *P. carinii* and to stop the chronic maintenance therapy for relapsing mucosal candidiasis and other fungal diseases (Soriano et al, 2000). Clinical resistance to fluconazole in patients with OPC and esophageal candidiasis has almost disappeared in patients responding to HAART.

A successful response to HAART is characterized by a marked reduction in viral load and a subsequent increase in CD4 cell count. However, the partial restoration of cell-mediated immunity and possibly other immune effectors (Sempowski and Haynes, 2002) may facilitate the development of an inflammatory reaction at the site of previous infection, which can mimic reactivation of the opportunistic disease. This paradoxical effect has been reported in AIDS patients with CMV retinitis, atypical *Mycobacterium* infections, cryptococcosis, and histoplasmosis (Blanche et al, 1998; Woods et al, 1998; DeSimonne et al, 2000; Cheng et al, 2000; Memain et al, 2000). Such immune reconstitution reactions raise the diagnostic challenge of a relapse of the initial opportunistic infection vs. a new opportunistic disease and raise the issue of timing of the initiation of HAART following initial treatment of an acute opportunistic infection. In cases of immune restoration, treatment with an antiinflammatory drug, including corticosteroids, may be effective without necessitating a change in HAART or the antiinfective treatment.

REFERENCES

Aberg J A, Price R W, Heeren D M, Bredt B. A pilot study of the discontinuation of antifungal therapy for disseminated cryptococcal disease in patients with acquired immunodeficiency syndrome, following immunologic response to antiretroviral therapy. *J Infect Dis* 185:1179–1182, 2002.

Ally R, Schürmann, Kreisel W, Carisu G, Aguirrebengoa K, Dupont B, Hodges M, Troke P, Romero A J. A randomized, double-blind, double dummy, multicenter trial of voriconazole and fluconazole in the treatment of esophageal candidiasis in immunocompromised patients. *Clin Infect Dis* 33:1447–1454, 2001.

Al-Tawfik O W, Papasian C J, Dixon A Y, Potter L M. *Saccharomyces cerevisiae* pneumonia in a patient with acquired immune deficiency syndrome. *J Clin Microb* 27:1689–1691, 1989.

Al-Tawfiq J A, Wools K K. Disseminated sporotrichosis and *Sporothrix schenckii* fungemia as the initial presentation of human immunodeficiency virus infectection. *Clin Infect Dis* 26:1403–1406, 1998.

Alvarez S. Systemic infection caused by *Penicillium decumbens* in a patient with acquired immunodeficiency syndrome. *J Infect Dis* 162:283, 1990.

Ampel N M. Emerging disease issues and fungal pathogens associated with HIV infection. *Emerging Infect Dis* 2:109–116, 1996.

Barchiesi F, Morbiducci V, Ancarani F, Arzeni D, Scalise G. *Trichosporon beigelii* fungaemia in an AIDS patient. *AIDS* 7:139–140, 1993.

Benard G, Duarte A J S. Paracoccidioidomycosis: a model for evaluation of the effects of human immunodeficiency virus infection on the natural history of endemic tropical diseases. *Clin Infect Dis* 31:1032–1039, 2000.

Blanche P H, Gombert B, Ginsburg C H, Passeron A, Stubei I, Salmon D, Sicard D. HIV combination therapy: immune restitution causing cryptococcal lymphadenitis dramatically improved by anti-inflammatory therapy. *Scand J Infect Dis* 30:615–616, 1998.

Blatt S P, Lucey D R, De Hoff D, Zellmer R B. Rhinocerebral zygomycosis in a patient with AIDS. *J Infect Dis* 164:215–216, 1991.

Bossi P, Mortier E, Michon C, Gaudin H, Simonpoli A M, Pouchot J, Vinceneux P. Sinusite à *Fusarium solani* chez un patient atteint de SIDA. *J Mycologie Medicale* 5:56–57, 1995.

Bronnimann D A, Adam R D, Galgiani J N, Habib M P, Petersen E A, Porter B, Bloom J W. Coccidioidomycosis in the acquired immunodeficiency syndrome. *Ann Intern Med* 106:372–379, 1987.

Brullet E, Andreu X, Elias J, Roig J, Cervantes M. Gastric mucormycosis in a patient with acquired immunodeficiency syndrome. *Gastrointest Endos* 39:106–107, 1993.

Cameron M L, Bartlett J A, Gallis H A, Waskin H A. Manifestations of pulmonary cryptococcosis in patients with acquired immunodeficiency syndrome. *Rev Infect Dis* 12:768–777, 1990.

Centers for Disease Control and Prevention. 1993 revised classification system for HIV infection and expanded surveillance case definition for AIDS among adolescents and adults. *MMWR Morb Mortal Wkly Rep* 41:1–19, 1993.

Chapman S W, Bradsher R W, Jr., Campbell G D, Pappas P G, Kauffman, C A. Practice guidelines for management of patients with blastomycosis. *Clin Infect Dis* 30:679–683, 2000.

Chariyalertsak S, Supparatpinyo K, Sirisanthana T, Nelson K E. A controlled trial of itraconazole as primary prophylaxis for systemic fungal infections in patients with advanced human immunodeficiency virus infection in Thailand. *Clin Infect Dis* 34:277–284, 2002.

Chavanet P, Lefranc T, Bonnin A, Waldner A, Portier H. Unusual cause of pharyngeal ulcerations in AIDS. *Lancet* 336:383–384, 1990.

Cheng V C C, Yuen K-Y, Chan W-M, Wong S S Y, Ma E S K, Chan R M T. Immunorestitution disease involving the innate and adaptive response. *Clin Infect Dis* 30:882–892, 2000.

Chuck S L, Sande MA. Infections with *Cryptococcus neoformans* in the acquired immunodeficiency syndrome. *N Engl J Med* 321:794–799, 1989.

Clark R A, Greer D, Atkinson W, Valainis G T, Hyslop N. Spectrum of *Cryptococcus neoformans* infection in 68 patients infected with human immunodeficiency virus. *Rev Infect Dis* 12:768–777, 1990.

Coker R J, Viviani M, Gazzard B G, Dupont B, Pohle H D, Murphy S M, Atouguia J, Champalimaud J L, Harris J R W. Treatment of cryptococcosis with liposomal amphotericin B (AmBisome) in 23 patients with AIDS. *AIDS* 7:829–835, 1993.

Cuadrado L M, Guerrero A, Garcia Asenjo J A L, Martin F, Palau E, Urra DG. Cerebral mucormycosis in two cases of acquired immunodeficiency syndrome. *Arch Neurol* 45:109–111, 1988.

Cunliffe N A, Denning D W. Uncommon invasive mycoses in AIDS. *AIDS* 9:411–420, 1995.

Del Palacio-Hernanz A, Casado V A, Lopez F P, Quiros H O, Palancar M P. Infeccion oportunista pulmonar por *Fusarium moniliforme* en paciente con SIDA. *Revista Iberica de Micologia* 6:144–147, 1989a.

Del Palacio-Hernanz A, Moore M K, Campbell C K, Del Palacio-Perez-Medel A, Del Castillo-Cantero R. Infection of the central nervous system by *Rhinocladiella atrovirens* in a patient with acquired immunodeficiency syndrome. *J Med Vet Mycol* 27:127–130, 1989b.

Deng Z, Ribas J L, Gibson D W, Connor D H. Infection caused by *Penicillium marneffei* in China and Southeast Asia: review of eighteen published cases and report of four more Chinese cases. *Rev Infect Dis* 10:640–652, 1988.

Denning D W, Follansbee S E, Scolaro M, Norris S, Edelstein H, Stevens D A. Pulmonary aspergillosis in the acquired immunodeficiency syndrome. *N Engl J Med* 324:654–662, 1991.

DeSimonne J A, Roger J, Pomerantz, Babinchak T J. Inflammatory reactions in HIV1-infected persons after initiation of active antiretroviral therapy. *Ann Intern Med* 133:447–454, 2000.

Detels R, Tarwater P, Phair J P, Margolick J, Riddler S A, Munoz A. Effectiveness of potent antiretroviral therapies on the incidence of opportunistic infections before and after AIDS diagnosis. *AIDS* 15:347–355, 2001.

Diamond R D. The growing problem of mycoses in patients infected with the human immunodeficiency virus. *Rev Infect Dis* 13:480–486, 1991.

Dismukes W E. Cryptococcal meningitis in patients with AIDS. *J Infect Dis* 157:624–628, 1998.

Dromer F, Mathoulin S, Dupont B, Laporte A. Epidemiology of cryptococcosis in France: 9-year survey (1985–1993). *Clin Infect Dis* 23:82–90, 1996.

Dromer F, Improvisi L, Dupont B, Eliaszewicz M, Pialoux G, Fournier S. Oral transmission of *Candida albicans* isolates between partners in HIV-infected couples could contribute to dissemination of fluconazole-resistant isolates. *AIDS* 11:1095–1101, 1997.

Drouhet E. Penicilliosis due to *Penicillium marneffei*: a new emerging systemic mycosis in AIDS patients travelling or living in Southeast Asia. Review of 44 cases reported in HIV infected patients during the last 5 years compared to 44 cases of non AIDS patients reported over 20 years. *J Mycolog e Medicale* 4:195–224, 1993.

Dupont B, Graybill J R, Armstrong D, Laroche R, Touze J E, Wheat L J. Fungal infections in AIDS patients. *J Med Vet Mycol* 30:19–28, 1992.

Dupont B, Crewe Brown H H, Westermann K, Martins M D, Rex J H, Lortholary O, Kauffmann C A. Mycoses in AIDS. *Med Mycol* 38:259–267, 2000.

Echavarria E, Cano E L, Restrepo A. Disseminated adiaspiromycosis in a patient with AIDS. *J Med Vet Mycol* 31:91–97, 1993.

Eckburg P B, Zolopa A R, Montoya J G. Invasive fungal sinusitis due to *Scedosporium apiospermum* in a patient with AIDS. *Clin Infect Dis* 29:212–213, 1999.

Fish D G, Ampel N M, Galgiani J N, Dols C L, Kelly P C, Johnson C H, Pappagianis D, Edwards J E, Wasserman R B, Clark R J. *Coccidioides immitis* in patients with human immunodeficiency virus infections: a review of 77 patients. *Medicine* (Baltimore) 69:384–391, 1990.

Franzot S P, Salkin I F, Casadevall A. *Cryptococus neoformans* var. *grubii*: separate varietal status for *Crytpococcus neoformans* serotype A isolates. *J Clin Micro* 37:838–840, 1999.

Galgiani J N, Ampel N M. *Coccidioides immitis* in patients with human immunodeficiency virus infections. *Semin Respir Infect* 5:151–154, 1990.

Galgiani J N, Catanzaro A, Cloud G A, Johnson R H, Williams P L, Mirels L F, Nassar F, Lutz J, Stevens D A, Sharkey P K, Singh V R, Larsen R A, Delgado K L, Flanagan C, Rinaldi M G, and the NIAID Mycoses Study Group. Comparison of oral fluconazole and itraconazole for progressive non-meningeal coccidioidomycosis. *Ann Intern Med* 133:676–686, 2000a.

Galgiani J N, Ampel N M, Catanzaro A, Johnson R H, Stevens DA, Williams P L. Practice guidelines for the treatment of coccidioidomycosis. *Clin Infect Dis* 30:658–661, 2000b.

Goldani L Z, Sugar A M. Paracoccidioidomycosis in AIDS: an overview. *Clin Infect Dis* 21:1275–1281, 1995.

Gori S, Drouhet E, Gueho E, Huerre M, Lofaro A, Parenti M, Dupont B. Cutaneous disseminated mycosis in a patient with AIDS due to a new dimorphic fungus. *J Mycologie Medicale* 8:57–63, 1998.

Graybill J R, Sobel J, Saag M, Van Der Horst C, Powderly W, Cloud G, Riser L, Hamill R, Dismukes W. Diagnosis and management of increased intracranial pressure in patients with AIDS and cryptococcal meningitis. *Clin Infect Dis* 30:47–54, 2000.

Hopkins R J, Rothman M, Fiore A, Goldblum S E. Cerebral mucormycosis associated with intravenous drug use: three case reports and review. *Clin Infect Dis* 19: 1133–1137, 1994.

Hopwood V, Hicks D A, Thomas S, Evans E G V. Primary cutaneous zygomycosis due to *Absidia corymbifera* in a patient with AIDS. *J Med Vet Mycol* 30:399–402, 1992.

Kauffman C A, Hajjeh R, Chapman S for the Mycoses Study Group. Practice guidelines for the management of patients with sporotrichosis. *Clin Infect Dis* 30:684–687, 2000.

Kemper C A, Hostetler J S, Follansbee S, Ruane P, Covington D, Leong S S, Deresinski S C, Stevens D A. Ulcerative and plaque-like tracheobronchitis due to infection with *Aspergillus* in patients with AIDS. *Clin Infect Dis* 17:344–352, 1993.

Khoo S, Denning D W. *Aspergillus* infection in the acquired immune deficiency syndrome. *Clin Infect Dis.* 19:541–548, 1994.

Klein R S, Harris C A, Butkus Small C, Moll B, Lesser M, Friedland G H. Oral candidiasis in high risk patients as the initial manifestation of the acquired immunodeficiency syndrome. *N Engl J Med* 311:354–358, 1984.

Kwon-Chung K J, Varma A, Howard D H. Ecology of *Cryptococcus neoformans* and prevalence of its two varieties in AIDS and non-AIDS associated cryptococcosis. In: Vanden Bossche H, MacKenzie D W R, Cauwenbergh G, Van Cutsem J, Drouhet E, Dupont B, eds. *Mycoses in AIDS Patients.* New York: Plenum Press, 103–113, 1990.

Launay O, Lortholary O, Bourges Michel C, Jarrousse B, Bentata M, Guillevin L. Candidemia: A nosocomial complication in adults with late-stage AIDS. *Clin Infect Dis* 26:1134–1141, 1998.

Leaf H L, Simberkoff M S. Invasive trichosporonosis in a patient with a acquired immunodeficiency syndrome. *J Infect Dis* 160: 356–357, 1989.

Leenders A C, Reiss P, Portegies P, Clezy K, Hop W C J, Hoy J, Borleffs J C C, Allworth T, Kauffman R H, Jones P, Kroon F P, Verbrugh H A, de Marie S. Liposomal amphotericin B (Am-Bisome) compard with amphotericin B followed by oral fluconazole in the treatment of AIDS-associated cryptococcal meningitis. *AIDS* 11:1463–1471, 1997.

Liliang P-C, Liang C-L, Chang W-N, Lu K, Lu C-H. Use of ventriculoperitoneal shunts to treat uncontrollable intracranial hypertension in patients who have cryptococcal meningitis without hydrocephalus. *Clin Infect Dis* 34:e64–e68, 2002.

Lortholary O, Denning D W, Dupont B. Endemic mycoses: a treatment update. *J Antimicrob Chemother* 43:321–331, 1999.

Lortholary O, Meyohas M C, Dupont B, Cadranel J, Salmon-Ceron D, Peyramond D, Simonin D. Invasive aspergillosis in patients with acquired immunodeficiency syndrome: report of 33 cases. *Am J Med* 95:177–187, 1993.

Lui A Y, Turett G S, Karter D L, Bellman P C, Kislak J W. Amphotericin B lipid complex therapy in AIDS patient with *Rhodotorula rubra* fungemia. *Clin Infect Dis* 27:892–893, 1998.

McKinsey D, Spiegel R A, Hutwagner L, Stanford J, Driks M R, Brewer J, Gupta M R, Smith D L, O'Connor M C, Dall L. Prospective study of histoplasmosis patients infected with human immunodeficiency virus: incidence, risk factors, and pathophysiology. *Clin Infect Dis* 24:1195–1203, 1997.

McKinsey D S, Wheat L J, Cloud G A, Pierce M, Black J R, Bamberger D M, Goldman M, Thomas C J, Gutsch H M, Moskovitz B, Dismukes W E, Kauffman C A and the NIAID Mycoses Study Group. Itraconazole prophylaxis for fungal infections in patients with advanced human immunodeficiency virus infection: randomized, placebo-controlled, double-blind study. *Clin Infect Dis* 28:1049–1056, 1999.

Maenza J R, Keruly J C, Moore R D, Chaisson R E, Merz W G, Gallant J E. Risk factors for fluconazole-resistant candidiasis in human immunodeficiency virus-infected patients. *J Infect Dis* 173:219–225, 1996.

Marlier S, De-Jaureguiberry J P, Aguilon P, Carloz E, Duval J L, Jaubert D. Sinusite chronique due à *Schizophyllum commune* au cours du SIDA. *Presse Medicale* 22:1107, 1993.

Marriott D J E, Wong K H, Aznar E, Harkness J L, Cooper D A, Muir D. *Scytalidium dimidiatum* and *Lecythophora hoffmannii*: unusual causes of fungal infections in a patient with AIDS. *J Clin Microbiol* 35:2949–2952, 1997.

Masur H, Kaplan J E, Holmes K K. Recommendations of the U.S. Public Health Service and the Infectious Diseases Society of America. Guidelines for preventing opportunistic infections among HIV-infected persons—2002. *Ann Intern Med* 137:435–477, 2002.

Memain N, Blanche P, Benveniste O, Salmon O, Breton G, Salmon D, Dromer F, Lortholary O. Paradoxical reactions due to immune restoration during *Cryptococcus neoformans* infection in AIDS. 41st Intersicence Conference on Antimicrobial Agents and Chemotherapy, American Society for Microbiology, Chicago, IL. Abstract J. 674. p 376, 2001.

Mendez R P, Negroni R, Arechavala A. Treatment and control of cure. In: Franco M, Lacaz C S, Restrepo A, Del Negro G, eds. *Paracoccidioidomycosis*, 1st ed. Boca Raton, FL: CRC Press, 373–392, 1994.

Micozzi M S, Wetli C V. Intravenous amphetamine abuse, primary cerebral mucormycosis, and acquired immunodeficiency. *J Forensic Sciences* 30:504–510, 1985.

Mitchell T G, Perfect J R. Cryptococcosis in the era of AIDS—100 years after the discovery of *Cryptococcus neoformans*. *Clin Microbiol Rev* 8:515–548, 1995.

Montero A, Cohen J E, Fernandez M A, Mazzolini G, Gomez C R, Perugini J. Cerebral pseudallescheriasis due to *Pseudallescheria boydii* as the first manifestation in AIDS. *Clin Infect Dis* 26:1476–1477, 1998.

Morris J T, Beckius M, Mc Allister CK. *Sporobolomyces* infection in an AIDS patient. *J Infect Dis* 11:316–318, 1991.

Mostaza J M, Barbado F J, Fernandez-Martin J, Pena-Yanez J, Vasquez-Rodriguez J J. Cutaneoarticular mucormucosis due to *Cunninghamella bertholletiae* in a patient with AIDS. *Rev Infect Dis* 11:316–318, 1989.

Mussini C, Cossarizza A, Pezzotti P, Antinori A, De Luca A, Ortolani P, Rizzardini G, Mongiardo N, Esposito R. Discontinuation or continuation of maintenance therapy for cryptococcal meningitis in patients with AIDS treated with HAART. 8th Conference on Retroviruses and Opportunisitic Infections, Chicago, IL. Abstract 546, 2001.

Palella F J Jr., Delaney K M, Moorman A C, Loveless M O, Fuhrer J, Satten G A, Aschman D J, Holmberg S D. Declining morbidity and mortality among patients with advanced human immunodeficiency virus infection. *N Engl J Med* 338:853–860, 1998.

Pappas P G, Pottage J C, Powderly G, Fraser V J, Stratton C W, McKenzie S, Tapper M L, Chmel H, Bonebrake F C, Blum R, Shafer R W, King C, Dismukes W E. Blastomycosis in patients with the acquired immunodeficiency syndrome. *Ann Intern Med* 116:847–853, 1992.

Parsonnet J. *Trichosporon beigelii* peritonitis. *So Med J* 82:1062–1063, 1989.

Paugam A, Baixench M T, Frank N, Bossi P, de Pinieux G, Tourte-Schaefer C, Dupouy-Comet J. Localized oral *Fusarium* in an AIDS patient with malignant lymphoma. *J Infect* 39:153–154, 1999.

Perfect J R, Schell W A, Rinaldi M G. Uncommon invasive fungal pathogens in the acquired immunodeficiency syndrome. *J Med Vet Mycol* 31:175–179, 1993.

Pitrak D L, Bak P M, De Marais P, Novak R M, Andersen B R. Depressed neutrophil superoxide production in human immunodeficiency virus infection. *J Infect Dis* 167:1406–1410, 1993.

Powderly W G. Prophylaxis for opportunistic infections in an era of effective antiretroviral therapy. *Clin Infect Dis* 31:597–601, 2000.

Powderly W G, Saag M S, Cloud G A, Robinson P, Meyer R D, Jacobson J M, Graybill J R, Sugar A M, McAuliffe V J, Follansbee S E, Tuazon C U, Stern J J, Feinberg J, Hafner R, Dismukes W E, the NIAID AIDS Clinical Trials Group and the NIAID Mycoses Study Group. A controlled trial of fluconazole or amphotericin B to prevent relapse of cryptococcal meningitis in patients with the acquired immunodeficiency syndrome. *N Engl J Med* 326:793–798, 1992.

Raffanti S P, Fyfe B, Carreiro S, Sharp S E, Hyma B A, Ratzan K R. Native valve endocarditis due to *Pseudallescheria boydii* in a patient with AIDS: case report and review. *Rev Infect Dis* 12:993–996, 1990.

Redding S, Smith J, Farinacci G, Rinaldi M, Fothergill A, Chalberg-Rhine J, Pfaller M. Resistance of *Candida albicans* to fluconazole during treatment of oropharyngeal candidiasis in a patient with AIDS: documentation by in vitro susceptibility testing and DNA subtype analysis. *Clin Infect Dis* 18:240–242, 1994.

Revankar S G, Dib O P, Kirkpatrick W R, McAtee R K, Fothergill A W, Rinaldi M G, Redding S W, Patterson T F. Clinical evaluation and microbiology of oropharyngeal infection due to fluconazole-resistant *Candida* in human immunodeficiency virus-infected patients. *Clin Infect Dis* 26:960–963, 1998.

Rex J H, Walsh T J, Sobel J D, Filler S G, Pappas P G, Dismukes W E, Edwards J E. Practice guidelines for treatment of candidiasis. Infectious Diseases Society of America. *Clin Infect Dis* 30:662–678, 2000.

Rocha M M, Dassin T, Lira R, Lima E L, Severo L C, Londero A T. Sporotrichosis in patients with AIDS: report of case and review. *Rev Iber Micol* 18:133–136, 2001.

Rollot F, Blanche P, Richaud-Thiriez B, Le Pimbec-Barthes F, Riquet M, Dusser D, Salmon D, Sicard D. Pneumonia due to *Scedosporium apiospermum* in a patient with HIV infection. *Scand J Infect Dis* 32:439, 2000.

Rosenthal J, Katz R, Dubois D B, Morrissey A, Machicao A. Chronic maxillary sinusitis associated with the mushroom *Schizophyllum commune* in a patient with AIDS. *Clin Infect Dis* 14:46–48, 1992.

Saag M S, Powderly W G, Cloud G A, Robinson P, Grieco M H, Sharkey P, Thompson S E, Sugar A M, Tuazon C A, Fisher J F, Hyslop N, Jacobson J M, Hafner R, Dismukes W E, the NIAID Mycoses Study Group, and the AIDS Clinical Trials Group. Comparison of amphotericin B with fluconazole in the treatment of acute AIDS-associated cryptococcal meningitis. *N Engl J Med* 326:83–89, 1992.

Saag M S, Cloud G A, Graybill J R, Sobel J D, Tuazon C U, Johnson P C, Fessel W J, Moskovitz B L, Wiesinger B, Cosmatos D, Riser L, Thomas C, Hafner R, Dismukes W E, and the NIAID Mycoses Study Group. A comparison of itraconazole versus fluconazole as maintenance therapy for AIDS-associated cryptococcal meningitis. *Clin Infect Dis* 28:291–296, 1999.

Santos J, Espigado P, Romero C, Andreu J, Rivero A, Pineda J A. Isolated renal mucormycosis in two AIDS patients. *Eur J Clin Microbiol Infect Dis* 13:430–432, 1994.

Scherr G R, Evans S G, Kiyabu M T, Klatt E C. *Pseudallescheria boydii* infection in the acquired immunodeficiency syndrome. *Arch Path Lab Med* 116:535–536, 1992.

Sempowski G D, Haynes B F. Immune reconstitution in patients with HIV infection. *Ann Rev Med* 53:269–284, 2002.

Sirisanthana T, Supparatpinyo K, Periens T, Nelson K E. Amphotericin B and itraconazole for treatment of disseminated *Penicillium marneffei* infection in human immunodeficiency virus-infected patients. *Clin Infect Dis* 26:1107–1110, 1998.

Smith A G, Bustamante C I, Gilmor G D. Zygomycosis (absidiomycosis) in an AIDS patient. *Mycopathologia* 105:7–10, 1989.

Sobottka I, Albrecht H, Mack D, Stellbrink H J, Van Luzen J, Tintelnot K, Laufs R. Systemic *Penicillium marneffei* infection in a German AIDS patient. *Eur J Clin Microbiol Infect Dis* 15:256–269, 1996.

Soriano V, Dona C, Rodriguez-Rosado R, Barreiro P, Gonzalez-Lahoz J. Discontinuation of secondary prophylaxis for opportunistic infections in HIV-infected patients receiving highly active antiretroviral therapy. *AIDS* 14:383–386, 2000.

Speed B, Dunt D. Clinical and host differences between infections with the two varieties of *Cryptococcus neoformans*. *Clin Infect Dis* 21:28–34, 1995.

Spellberg B, Edwards J E, Jr. Type 1/Type 2 immunity in infectious diseases. *Clin Infect Dis* 32:76–102, 2001.

Stevens D A, Kan V L, Judson M A, Morrison V A, Dummer S, Denning D W, Bennett J E, Walsh T J, Patterson T F, Pankey G A. Practice guidelines for diseases caused by *Aspergillus*. *Clin Infect Dis* 30:696–709, 2000.

Sullivan D, Coleman D *Candida dubliniensis*: characteristics and identification. *J Clin Microb* 36:329–334, 1998.

Supparatpinyo K, Khamwan C, Baosoung V, Nelson K E, Sirisanthana T. Disseminated *Penicillium marneffei* infection in Southeast Asia. *Lancet* 334:110–113, 1994.

Supparatpinyo K, Perriens J, Nelson K E, Srisanthana T. A controlled trial of itraconazole to prevent relapse of *Penicillium marneffei* infection in patients infected with the human immunodeficiency virus. *N Engl J Med* 339:1739–1743, 1998.

Szelc C M, Mitcheltree C, Roberts R L, Stiehm E R. Deficient polymorphonuclear cell and mononuclear cell antibody-dependent cellular cytotoxicity in pediatric and adult human immunodeficiency virus infection. *J Infect Dis.* 166:486–493, 1992.

Turner D, Burke M, Bashe E, Blinder S, Yust I. Pulmonary adiaspiromycosis in a patient with acquired immunodeficiency syndrome. *Eur J Clin Microbiol Infect Dis* 18:893–895,1999.

van der Horst C M, Saag M S, Cloud G A, Hamill R J, Graybill J R, Sobel J D, Johnson P C, Tuazon C U, Kerkering T, Moskovitz B L, Powderly W G, Dismukes W E, and the NIAID Mycoses Study Group and the AIDS Clinical Trials Group. Treatment of cryptococcal meningitis associated with the acquired immunodeficiency syndrome. *N Engl J Med* 337:15–21, 1997.

Vesa J, Bielsa O, Arango O, Liado C, Gelabert A. Massive renal infarction due to mycormycosis in an AIDS patient. *Infection* 20:234–236, 1992.

Villanueva A, Arathoon E G, Gotuzzo E, Berman R S, DiNubile M J, Sable C A. A randomized double-blind study of caspofungin versus amphotericin B for the treatment of candidal esophagitis. *Clin Infect Dis* 33:1529–1535, 2001.

Walmsley S, King S, McGeer A, Ye Y, Richardson S. Oropharyngeal candidiasis in patients with human immunodeficiency virus: correlation of clinical outcome with in vitro resistance, serum azole levels, and immunosuppression. *Clin Infect Dis* 32:1554–1561, 2001.

Warnock D W, Dupont B, Kauffman C A, Sirisanthana T. Imported mycoses in Europe. *Med Mycol* 36:87–94, 1998.

Wheat L J, Connolly-Stringfield P A, Baker R L, Curfman M F, Eads M E, Israel K S, Norris S A, Webb D H, Zeckel M L. Disseminated histoplasmosis in the acquired immune deficiency syndrome: clinical findings, diagnosis and treatment, and review of the literature. *Medicine* (Baltimore) 69:361–374, 1990.

Wheat J. Endemic mycoses in AIDS: a clinical review. *Clin Microbiol Rev* 8:146–159, 1995.

Wheat J, Chetchotisakd P, Williams B, Connolly P, Shutt K, Hajjeh R. Factors associated with severe manifestations of histoplasmosis in AIDS. *Clin Infect Dis* 30:877–881, 2000a.

Wheat J, Sarosi G, McKinsey D, Hamil R, Bradsher R, Johnson P, Loyd J, Kauffman C. Practice guidelines for the management of patients with histoplasmosis. *Clin Infect Dis* 30:688–695, 2000b.

Wiest P M, Wiese K, Jacobs M R, Morrissey A B, Abelson T I, Witt W, Lederman M M. *Alternaria* infection in a patient with acquired immunodeficiency syndrome: case report and review of invasive *Alternaria* infections. *Rev Infect Dis* 9:799–803, 1987.

Wilcox C M. Esophageal disease in the acquired immunodeficiency syndrome: etiology, diagnosis, and management. *Am J Med* 92:412–421, 1992.

Woods II M L, MacGinly R, Eisen D P, Allworth A M. HIV combination therapy partial immune restitution unmasking latent cryptococcal infection. *AIDS* 12:1491–1494, 1998.

Yarrish R, Sepulveda J, Tores R, Britton D. Invasive *Aureobasidium* infection in a patient with the acquired immunodeficiency syndrome. *7th International Conference on AIDS,* Florence, Italy, Abstract MB *2214,* 1991.

Zuger A, Louie E, Holzman R S, Simberkoff M S, Rahal J J. Cryptococcal disease in patients with the acquired immunodeficiency syndrome: diagnostic features and outcome of treatment. *Ann Intern Med.* 104:234–240, 1986.

Index

Note: Page numbers followed by f and t refer to figures and tables, respectively.

ABC-transporter genes, azole resistance and, 114–16, 115f
Abscess
  brain
    in aspergillosis, 229, 229f
    in candidiasis, 158, 173–74
    in fusariosis, 254–55
    in mucormycosis, 244, 246
    in phaeohyphomycosis, 275, 276t, Color Figure 17–2
    tubo-ovarian, blastomycotic, 304
Absidia corymbifera, 241
Acquired immunodeficiency syndrome (AIDS). *See* HIV/AIDS
Acremonium eumycetoma, 391t, 394t, 395–96
Acremonium spp., 256t, 261–62
  clinical manifestations, 262
  diagnosis, 262
  epidemiology, 261–62
  susceptibility data, 262
  treatment, 262
Adiaspiromycosis, 421–22, 497, Color Figure 28–3
Adjunctive antifungal therapy, 125–35
  after blood or marrow transplantation, 465
  for cryptococcal meningitis, in HIV-AIDS, 201
  hematopoietic growth factors and other cytokines as, 125–32, 126f, 126t, 127t, 128f, 129t
  intravenous immunoglobulin as, 134
  monoclonal antibodies as, 134
  in neutropenic patients, 127–29, 128f, 129t, 446–48
  for phagocyte dysfunction, 128f, 130–31
  white blood cell transfusions as, 132–34, 133t
Adrenal dysfunction
  amphotericin B–induced, 38
  in histoplasmosis, 291, 291f
  in paracoccidioidomycosis, 336
Adult respiratory distress syndrome, blastomycotic, 303, 303f
African Americans, coccidioidomycosis in, 320, Color Figure 20–8

African histoplasmosis, 285, 286–87, 292, 294, 296, 492, Color Figure 18–15
Agar disc diffusion, 17
AIDS. *See* HIV/AIDS
Air contamination, aspergillosis from, 25, 463
"Air crescent" sign, in pulmonary aspergillosis, 228, 228f, 231, 429–30
Air filtration, 28, 224
  after blood or marrow transplantation, 463
  during neutropenia, 434–35
Allergic bronchopulmonary aspergillosis, 224, 225–26
Alopecia
  differential diagnosis, 383
  from fluconazole, 73
  partial, in gray patch tinea capitis, 382
  scarring, in inflammatory tinea capitis, 382, Color Figure 24–7
Alternaria spp., 275, 276t, 497
Amphotericin B, 33–45
  in children, 37
  colloidal dispersion. *See* Amphotericin B colloidal dispersion (ABCD)
  and flucytosine, for cryptococcal meningitis, 39–40, 60, 491
  immunodulatory effects, 34
  indications
    for *Acremonium* spp. infection, 262
    for aspergillosis, 232–33, 232t, 438–45, 439t, 440t, 495
    for aspergillosis, after organ transplantation, 481
    for blastomycosis, 306–07, 308
    for *Blastoschizomyces capitatus*, 214
    for candidiasis, 40, 74–75, 75t, 165–67, 166t, 169–74
      after blood or marrow transplantation, 464
      after organ transplantation, 480
      in neutropenic patients, 438–44, 439t, 440t
    for chromoblastomycosis, 401t, 402
    for coccidioidomycosis, 321–23, 493

    for cryptococcosis, 195–201, 196t, 199t, 481, 491–92
    for entomophthoramycosis, 249
    for eumycetoma, 395
    for fusariosis, 256t, 257
    for histoplasmosis, 294–96, 493
    for *Malassezia* infections, 211
    for mucormycosis, 246–47
    for neutropenic fever, 438–45, 439t–40t
    for *Paecilomyces* spp. infection, 264
    for paracoccidioidomycosis, 340, 340t
    for penicilliosis, 361–62, 494
    for phaeohyphomycoses, 278–79
    for *Scedosporium apiospermum* infection, 256t, 260
    for *Scopulariopsis* spp. infection, 256t, 263
    for sporotrichosis, 352
    for trichosporonosis, 212–13
  intraarticular, 42
  intrabladder, 42
  intraocular, 41–42, 171
  intraperitoneal, 42
  intrathecal, 41
  intraventricular, 41
  lipid complex. *See* Amphotericin B lipid complex (ABLC).
  lipid preparations, 42–46
    adverse effects, 44
    chemistry, 36t, 42–43
    comparative trials, 44–45
    costs, 45
    dosage and administration, 45
    indications
      for aspergillosis, 45, 232–33, 232t
        after blood or marrow transplantation, 464–65
        after organ transplantation, 481
        in neutropenic patients, 444–45
      for candidiasis
        after blood or marrow transplantation, 464
        after organ transplantation, 480
      for cryptococcosis, 45, 200, 490–91
      for mucormycosis, 246–47

Amphotericin B (*Continued*)
  for neutropenic fever, 44–45, 439t–40t, 441–44
  pharmacodynamics, 43–44
  pharmacology and pharmacokinetics, 36t, 43
  prophylactic, after organ transplantation, 482
  therapeutic index, 43
  therapeutic indications, 43
  liposomal, 36t, 42–46. *See* Liposomal amphotericin B (L-AmB)
  mechanisms of action, 33–34, 111–12
  nebulized, 42
  pediatric dosing, 165
  prophylaxis, in neutropenic patients, 437
  resistance to, 34–35, 113
  spectrum of activity, 34–35
  structure, 34f
  structure, compared to nystatin, 50–51, 50f
  susceptibility data, 34–35, 53, 53t, 112t, 113, 236t
  topical, 41
  treatment failures, 33
Amphotericin B colloidal dispersion (ABCD), 36t, 42–45, Color Figure 3–2
  for aspergillosis, 232–33, 232t
  for neutropenic fever, 439t–40t, 441–42
Amphotericin B deoxycholate, 33–42
  adverse effects, 37–38
  chemistry, 33, 34f
  in children, 37
  combination therapy, 39–40
  dosage and administration, 36t, 40–42, 41t
  drug interactions, 39
  indications. *See* Amphotericin B
  mechanisms of action, 33–34
  pharmacodynamics, 37
  pharmacology and pharmacokinetics, 35, 36t, 37
  in pregnancy, 42
  sodium loading prior to use, 38
  spectrum of activity, 34–35
Amphotericin B in lipid emulsion (ABLE), 36t, 42
Amphotericin B lipid complex (ABLC), 36t, 42–45
  for aspergillosis, 232–33, 232t
  for cryptococcosis, 200
  for neutropenic fever, 439t–40t, 442
Anamorphic fungi
  classification, 4–5
  definition, 3
Aneurysm, mycotic, *Candida*, 157
Angular cheilitis, 148, 386, 489, Color Figure 11–1
Anidulafungin, 88–90, 89f, 90–92
  antifungal activity in vitro, 90, 90t, 91t, 112t, 119
  antimicrobial interactions, 91
  clinical efficacy, 92
  drug interactions, 92

efficacy in animal models, 91
pharmacokinetics, 91–92, 91t
safety and tolerance, 92
status of clinical development, 92
structure, 89f
Annular plaque, in tinea corporis, 373, Color Figure 24–4
Antibiotic medium 3 (AM3), 16
Antibodies
  detection procedures, 12–14. *See also* Serologic testing *for specific diseases*
  monoclonal, for invasive fungal infections, 134
Antifungal drug(s). *See also specific antifungal drugs*
  adjunctive therapy. *See* Adjunctive therapy
  chemoprophylaxis, 28
    after blood or marrow transplantation, 461–62, 462f
    after organ transplantation, 482
    in neutropenic patients
      primary, 435–38
      secondary, 438
  empirical therapy
    after blood or marrow transplantation, 462–63
    in neutropenic patients, 438–44, 439t–40t
  preemptive therapy
    after blood or marrow transplantation, 463
    after organ transplantation, 481–82
  presumptive therapy, in febrile neutropenic patients, 170–71
  susceptibility testing, 15–18, 111, 112t. *See also* Resistance
    agar disc diffusion, 17
    Etest, 17
    interpretation, 17–18, 71, 164, 164t
    M27-A reference method, 15–17, 71, 163–64
    M38-A reference method, 17
Antigen detection procedures, 12–14. *See also* Serologic testing *for each disease*
Antiretroviral therapy, highly active (HAART)
  opportunistic fungal infections and, 497
  for refractory oropharyngeal candidiasis, 167
Apophysomyces elegans, 241
D-Arabinitol assay, 163
Arthritis
  blastomycotic, 304
  Candida, 162, 173
Arthrographis kalrae, 264
Articular disease. *See* Joint disease
Ascomycota, 4
Aspergillosis, 221–35, 494–95
  amphotericin B for, 45, 232–33, 232t, 481
  azoles for, 79, 232t, 233
  caspofungin for, 95, 232t, 234
  clinical syndromes, 225–30, 494–95

saprophytic/superficial
  aspergilloma, lung, 225
  fungus ball, sinuses, 225
  onychomycosis, 225
  otomycosis, 225
allergic manifestations
  allergic bronchopulmonary, 225–26
  allergic sinusitis, 226
invasive
  cerebral, 229, 229f, 430
  cutaneous, 229, 430
  disseminated, 229, 430
  osteomyelitis, 229–30
  pulmonary, 227–28, 227f, 228f, 429–30, 494–95, Color Figure 29–3
  sinusitis, 228–29
  tracheobronchitis, 228–29, 495
  unusual, 230
contaminated water, 224–25
diagnosis, 230–32, 431–34
environmental control measures, 28, 434–35
epidemiology, 25, 224–25
flucytosine for, 60
HEPA filtration for contaminated air, 224
historical review, 221
host defenses, 223–24
invasive, 226–30, 432–33
  after blood or marrow transplantation, 224–25
  clinical manifestations and pathogenesis, 459–60, 460f
  diagnosis, 230–32, 460–61
  galactomannan antigen 13, 231, 432–33, 481, 495
  incidence, 462, 462f
  risk factors, 456–57, 458t
  surgical treatment, 445–46, 465
  treatment, 232–34, 232t, 464–65, 495
  after organ transplantation, 474, 476–77, 481
  antifungal drug chemoprophylaxis for, 28, 234
  exposure and transmission, 25, 224–25
  in HIV-AIDS, 494–95
  in lung and heart-lung transplant recipients, 225, 473, 476
  mortality rates, 227, 227t
  in neutropenic patients, 223–24
    antifungal therapy, 232–34, 332t, 444–45
    clinical manifestations, 429–30, Color Figure 29–3
    detection of pathogen, 431–34
    secondary prophylaxis, 438
    surgical management, 445–46
  organisms causing, 222–23, 222t
  prevention, 235
  in renal transplant recipients, 471–72
  treatment
    adjunctive therapy, 125–35, 234, 446–48, 465

antifungal agents, 232–34, 232t, 444–45, 464–65
 factors affecting, 226–27, 226t
 guidelines, 234
 surgery, 445–46, 465
liposomal nystatin for, animal models, 55–56
micafungin for, 97
pathogenesis, 223–24
serologic testing, 13, 231, 432–33, 460–61, 481, 495
terbinafine for, 108
Aspergillus flavus, 222–23, Color Figures 14–1B and 14–2B
 susceptibility data, 70t, 91t, 93t, 96t
Aspergillus fumigatus, 222, Color Figures 14–1A and 14–2A
 susceptibility data, 18, 70t, 91t, 96t, 105t, 111, 112t
Aspergillus niger, 223, Color Figures 14–1D and 14–2D
 susceptibility data, 91t, 93t, 96t,
Aspergillus spp.
 causing invasive infections, 222, 222t
 identification, 431–34, 480
 mycology, 222–23, 222t, Color Figures 14–1 and 14–2
 mycotoxins, 223
 susceptibility data, 70t, 91t, 93t, 96t, 111, 112t, 230, 430
  Etest method, 17
  interpretation, 17–18
  M38-A method, 17
Aspergillus terreus, 223, Color Figures 14–1C and 14–2C
 susceptibility data, 70t, 91t, 93t, 96t, 430
Atovaquone, for pneumocystosis, 410–11, 410t
ATP binding cassette (ABC)-transporter genes, azole resistance and, 114–16, 115f
Aureobasidium pullulans, 497
Azoles, 64–80
 adverse effects, 72–73, 72t. *See also specific azole drugs*
 chemistry, 64–65, 65f
 classification, 114
 combination therapy, with amphotericin B, 39
 drug interactions, 67–69, 68t
 indications, 73–80, 73t, 75t, 77t
  for aspergillosis, 79, 232–34, 232t, 444–45, 465
  for blastomycosis, 76–77, 77t, 307–08
  for candidiasis, 73–75, 73t, 75t, 165–74, 166t, 168t, 444, 464
  for chromoblastomycosis, 402–03
  for chronic mucocutaneous candidiasis, 169
  for coccidioidomycosis, 77–78, 77t, 321–23
  for cryptococcosis, 75–76, 195–201, 196t, 199t
  for endemic mycoses, 76–79, 77t
  for eumycetoma, 395–96

  for fusariosis, 80, 256
  for histoplasmosis, 77t, 78, 294–96
  for malasseziosis, 211
  for mucormycosis, 79, 247
  for *Paecilomyces* infections, 263
  for paracoccidioidomycosis, 77t, 78, 340–41, 340t
  for penicilliosis, 79, 361–62
  for phaeohyphomycosis, 79, 279
  for scedosporiosis, 79–80, 260
  for sporotrichosis, 77t, 78–79, 351
  for trichosporonosis, 213
 mechanism of action, 65–66
 pharmacokinetics, 66–67, 66t
 prophylaxis, 80
  after blood or marrow transplantation, 461–62
 resistance to, 71–72, 114–19, 115f
  by alterations in ergosterol biosynthetic pathway, 117–18
  by alterations of cellular target, 117
  by altered drug transport, 114–17
  alternative mechanisms, 118–19
  genome approaches, 119
  high-frequency, 116
  multiple mechanisms, 118
  reversibility, 115–16
 spectrum of activity, 69–71, 70t, 112t, 114
 susceptibility testing, 15–18, 71, 111, 163–64, 164t

BACTEC selective medium, 431, 459
Bamboo rats, *Penicillium marneffei* infection in, 356–57, 356t
Barbiturates, azoles and, 68
Basidiobolomycosis, 247–49
Basidiobolus ranarum, 247
Basidiomycosis, 421
 clinical manifestations, 421
 pathogens, 421
 treatment, 421
Basidiomycota, 4
Beauveria bassiana, 264
Bezoars. *See* Fungal balls
Biofilms, azole resistance and, 118–19
Bipolaris spp., 276t, 277
Black dot tinea capitis, 382
Black grain eumycetoma, 391t, 394, 394t. *See also* Eumycetoma
Black piedra, 273, 367, 368, 369
Bladder, hyperemia of, in candiduria, 161, Color Figure 11–10
Blastomyces dermatitidis, 299, 300f, 305–6. *See also* Blastomycosis
Blastomycetes, 4–5
Blastomycosis, 299–308, 495–96
 after organ transplantation, 478, 481
 articular, 304
 azoles for, 76–77, 77t, 307–8
 central nervous system, 304
 clinical manifestations, 301–5
  unusual, 304–5
 conditions associated with, 305
 cutaneous, 303, Color Figures 19–7 to 19–12

 diagnosis, 305–6
 epidemiology, 300–02
  blastomycin skin testing, 306
 genitourinary, 304
 in HIV-AIDS, 305, 495–96
 immunity, 300–01
 in immunocompromised population, 305
 ocular, 304–5
 organism, 299, 300f
  mycelial phase, 299
  yeast phase, 299, 300f
 osseous, 303
 pathogenesis, 301
 in pregnancy, 305
 prevention, 308
 pulmonary, 302–3, 302f, 303f
  adult respiratory distress syndrome, 303
 terbinafine for, 107
 treatment, 76–77, 77t, 306–8, 495
Blastoschizomyces capitatus (*Trichosporon capitatum*), 207t, 213–14
 clinical manifestations, 214
 diagnosis, 214
 epidemiology, 213
 organism, 213
 susceptibility data, 207t, 213–14
 treatment, 214
Blood culture methods, 8
Blood or marrow transplantation
 aspergillosis after, 223–25, 459–61
  clinical manifestations and pathogenesis, 227–30, 459–60, 460f
  diagnosis, 230–32, 431–34, 460–61
  incidence, 462, 462f
  prevention, 434–38, 461–63
  risk factors, 456–57, 457f, 458t
  surgical treatment, 445–46, 465
  treatment, 232–34, 444–45, 464–65
 candidiasis after, 458–59
  clinical manifestations and pathogenesis, 153–55, 157, 429, 458–59
  diagnosis, 163, 431, 459
  prophylaxis, 174, 434–38
  risk factors, 456–57, 457f, 458t
  treatment, 169–71, 444, 464
 fungal infections after, 456–66
  adjunctive therapy, 125–35, 446–48, 465
  antifungal therapy
   documented infection, 463–65
   empirical, 462–63
   preemptive, 463
   prophylaxis, 461–62,
  clinical manifestations and pathogenesis, 457–61
  environmental control measures, 463
  risk factors, 456–57, 457f, 458t
  surgical treatment, 445–46, 465
  therapeutic approach, 461–65
  timing, 456, 457f
  type of transplantation and, 456, 457f

Blood or marrow transplantation (*Continued*)
  fusariosis after, 457f, 458t, 461, 464
  graft vs. host disease (GVHD), 456–57, 457f, 460–63, 465
  phaeohyphomycosis after, 273
  Pneumocystis carinii pneumonia after, 412
  zygomycosis after, 457, 457f, 458t, 461, 464
Bone lesions
  in aspergillosis, 229–30
  in blastomycosis, 303
  in candidiasis, 162, 173
  in coccidioidomycosis, 319, 319f
  in cryptococcosis, 194
  in eumycetoma, 392–93, Color Figure 25–3
  in mucormycosis, 245
  in paracoccidioidomycosis, 337
  in sporotrichosis, 348–49
Bone marrow toxicity, flucytosine, 61
Bone marrow transplantation. *See* Blood or marrow transplantation
Brain abscess
  in aspergillosis, 229, 229f
  in candidiasis, 158, 173–74
  in phaeohyphomycosis, 275, 276t, Color Figure 17–2
Bronchoalveolar lavage, in neutropenic patients, 432
Bronchopulmonary aspergillosis, allergic, 224, 225–26
Burn infections
  Aspergillus-associated, 229
  Candida-associated, 162–63
"Burning mouth" syndrome, *Candida*, 148

Calcineurin inhibitors, after organ transplantation, fungal infections and, 475
Calcofluor white stain, 6
Calcofluor-KOH procedure, in phaeohyphomycosis, 278
CaMDR1 multidrug transporter gene, azole resistance and, 114–16, 115f, 119
Candida albicans, 143–75. See also Candidiasis, individual *Candida* spp
  diagnosis, 163
  epidemiology and pathogenesis, 146–47
    DNA typing of spp., 146–47
    hospital acquired, 146
    sources of organism, 146
  identification, 143, 163
    in neutropenic host, 431
    in organ transplant recipient, 479
  resistance, 113–21
    amphotericin B, 163–65, 164t
    azoles, 71–72, 114–19
    current situation, 120–21
    flucytosine, 163–65, 164t
    susceptibility data, 69–71, 111, 112t, 163–65, 164t

amphotericin B, 34–35, 112t, 163–64, 164t
azoles, 69–71, 70t, 112t, 163–64, 164t
echinocandins, 90t, 92t, 96t, 112t, 164t
Etest method, 17
flucytosine, 112t, 164t
interpretation, 17–18, 111, 113t, 164, 164t
liposomal nystatin, 53–54, 53t
M27-A2 method, 15–17, 71, 164, 164t
terbinafine, 105t
virulence factors, 144–46
Candida bloodstream infections. *See* Candidiasis, candidemia.
Candida dubliniensis, 144, 163, 488
  resistance, 114, 115, 118
  susceptibility data, 53t, 54
Candida glabrata, 143, 163–64, 164t
  candidemia, 153
  resistance to, 71–72, 114–17, 120–21
  susceptibility data, 53t, 70t, 90t, 92t, 96t, 105t, 112t, 163–64, 164t, 170
  vulvovaginal candidiasis, 168
Candida guilliermondii, 144
  susceptibility data, 53t, 90t, 92t, 96t, 105t
Candida keyfer, 144
  susceptibility data, 53t, 70t, 105t
Candida krusei, 144, 163–64, 164t
  resistance to, 71–72, 114, 120–21
  susceptibility data, 53t, 70t, 90t, 92t, 96t, 105t, 112t, 163–64, 164t, 170
Candida lusitaniae, 144, 163–64, 164t
  resistance to amphotericin B, 53t, 70t, 164–65, 164t
  susceptibility data, 53t, 70t, 90t, 92t, 163–64, 164t
Candida parapsilosis, 43, 163–64, 164t
  candidemia, neonates, 154
  susceptibility data, 53t, 70t, 90t, 92t, 96t, 105t, 112t, 163–64, 164t
Candida spp., uncommon non-*Albicans*, 145t
Candida stellatoidea, 144
Candida tropicalis, 144, 163–64, 164t
  candidemia, 154
  resistance to, 114, 115
  susceptibility data, 53t, 70t, 90t, 92t, 96t, 105t, 112t, 163–64, 164t
Candidiasis, 143–75, 488–90
  arthritis, 162
    clinical manifestations, 162
    treatment, 173
  abdominal (gastrointestinal), 149, 161–62
    biliary, 162
      cholecystitis, 162
    clinical manifestations, 149, 161–62
    diarrhea, 149
    enterocolitis, 149
    gastric, 149

hepatic. *See* chronic systemic (hepatosplenic)
  peritonitis, 161
  treatment, 172–73
  azoles for, 73–75, 73t, 75t, 165–74
  candidemia, 153–55. See *Candida* bloodstream infections, disseminated candidiasis
    asymptomatic, 154
    blood cultures, 154
    clinical manifestations, 154, 428–29
      cutaneous, 429, 458, Color Figure 29–1
      hepatosplenic, 157, 429, 429f, 459
      ocular, 155, 429, Color Figure 11–7
    diagnosis, 163, 431, 459, 479–80
    epidemiology, 153–54
      risk factors, 153–54, 458–59, 458t, 471, 473–74, 489
      sources, 154
      mortality rates, 154–55
    treatment, 40, 74–75, 75t, 169–70, 464, 480–81
  cardiac and endovascular, 155–57, 172
    clinical manifestations, 155–57
    endocarditis, 155–56
    endarteritis, 156–57
    myocarditis, 155
    pericarditis, 155
    suppurative thrombophlebitis, 156–57
    treatment, 172
  caspofungin for, 94–95, 167, 464, 480
  central nervous system, 158
    abscess, 158
    clinical manifestations, 158
    meningitis, 158
      acute, 158
      chronic, 158
    shunt infection, 158
    treatment, 173–74
  chronic systemic (hepatosplenic), 157, 428–29
    clinical manifestations, 157, 157f, 428–29, 429f, 459
    diagnosis, 157, 157f
    treatment, 171, 444
  cutaneous, 149–51, 385–87
    erosio interdigitalis blastomycetica, 150, 386
    chronic mucocutaneous, 150–51, 386–87, Color Figure 11–3
      groups I-VII, 150
      antigen specific defects, 150
      clinical manifestations, 151
      endocrinopathies associated with, 150–51
      evaluation of patients, 151
    folliculitis, 150
    generalized, 149
    intertrigo, 150, 386, 489
    neonatal (congenital cutaneous), 158
    onychomycosis, 73t, 74, 150, 386, 387
    paronychia, 150, 385–86, 489
    treatment, 169, 387

diagnosis, 163, 431, 459, 479
  blood cultures, 163, 431, 459, 479
  CAND-TEC detection system, 14, 163
  polymerase chain reaction, 163, 431, 459
  serologic testing, 163, 431
  speciation, 163
    CHROMager media, 7, 163
    fermentation and assimilation assays, 163
disseminated, 154. *See also* candidemia, chronic systemic (hepatosplenic)
epidemiology, 23–24, 25–26, 146–47, 153–54, 428, 428t, 456–58, 457f, 458t, 470–75, 474f
esophageal, 148–49, 489–90
  classification, 148
  clinical manifestations, 148–49, 489, Color Figure 11–2
  diagnosis, 149
  differential diagnosis, 149
  prevention, 174
  refractory, antifungal, 167, 489–90
  risk factors, 148
  treatment, 73t, 74, 166–67, 166t, 489–90
flucytosine for, 40, 165, 172, 173–74
in burn patients, 162–63
in HIV/AIDS , 147–49, 152t, 165–68, 488–90
in intensive care patients, 174–75
in neutropenic patients, 174, 428–29, 431, 444, 457–58, 458t, 464
in solid organ transplant patients, 471–74, 474t, 475–76, 480–81
mediastinitis, treatment, 173
micafungin for, 97
neonatal, 157–58
  congenital cutaneous, 158
  prevention, 175
  systemic, 157–58
  treatment, 171
nystatin, liposomal, for, 55–56
ocular, 155
  chorioretinitis, 155, Color Figure 11–7
  endophthalmitis, 155
  treatment, 171–72
oropharyngeal, 147–48, 386, 488–89
  acute pseudomembranous, 147, 488–89, Color Fig 11–1
  angular cheilitis (perleche), 148, 489, Color Figure 11–1
  chronic atrophic stomatitis, 147–48
  chronic hyperplastic, 148
  clinical manifestations, 147–48, 488–89
  midline glossitis (median rhomboid glossitis), 148
  prevention, 174
  refractory, antifungal, 167, 489–90
  sabbural tongue, 489
  treatment, 73–74, 73t, 165–66, 166t, 167, 387, 489–90

osteomyelitis, 162
  secondary to candidemia, 162
  secondary to contiguous spread, 162
  treatment, 173
pathogenesis, 146–47, 428, 428t, 457–58, 458t, 470
pediatric dosing of drugs, 165
prophylaxis, 174–75
  for oropharyngeal candidiasis, 174
  for esophageal candidiasis, 174
  for intensive care unit patients, 174–75
  for neonatal candidiasis, 175
  for neutropenic patients, 174, 435–38
  for recurrent vulvovaginal candidiasis, 174
pulmonary, 159
  secondary to bronchogenic spread, 159, 159f
  secondary to candidemia, 159
systemic. See also candidemia, chronic systemic (hepatosplenic)
urinary, 159–161. *See also* Candiduria.
  asymptomatic candiduria, 159–61
  balanitis, penile, 169, 386, 489
  clinical manifestations, 161, 386
  cystitis, 161, 476, Color Figure 11–10
  diagnosis, 160–61
  epidemiology, 159–60, 475–76
  fungus ball, 160, 476
  renal, 160
  species, 160
  treatment, 73t, 74, 171
vulvovaginitis, 151–53, 386–87
  acute symptomatic, 151, 152t, 153, 489
  asymptomatic colonization, 151, 152t
  clinical manifestations, 153, 386, Color Figure 11–5
  diagnosis, 153
  in HIV-AIDS, 152, 152f, 168
  pathogenesis, 151–53, 152t
  recurrent, 152, 152t, 153
    prevention, 174
    sexual transmission theory, 152
    vaginal relapse theory, 152–53
  treatment, 73t, 74, 167–69, 168t, 387
Candiduria, 159–61, Color Figure 11–10
CAND-TEC test for candidiasis, 14, 163
Carbamazepine, azoles and, 68
Case definition, in outbreak investigations, 27
Caspofungin, 88–90, 89f, 92–95
  antifungal activity in vitro, 92–93, 92t, 93t, 112t, 119, 164t
  antimicrobial interactions, 93
  for aspergillosis, 95, 234, 481
  for candidiasis, 94–95, 167, 170
    after blood or marrow transplantation, 464
    after organ transplantation, 480
  clinical efficacy, 94–95
  drug interactions, 95
  efficacy in animal models, 93

pharmacokinetics, 93–94, 94t
  resistance to, 119–20
  safety and tolerance, 95
  status of clinical development, 95
  structure, 89f
CDR genes, azole resistance and, 114–17, 119
Cell wall, 3
Cell wall synthesis inhibitors
  echinocandins, 88–98
  nikkomycins, 98–99
Cellulitis, cryptococcal, 194, Color Figure 12–8
Central nervous system infection
  in aspergillosis, 229, 229f, 430
  in blastomycosis, 304
  in candidiasis, 158
  in coccidioidomycosis, 319
  in cryptococcosis. See Cryptococcal meningitis
  in histoplasmosis, 291–92, 292f, 295–96
  in mucormycosis, 245
  in paracoccidioidomycosis, 337
  in phaeohyphomycosis, 275
  Rhodutorula, 207
  in sporotrichosis, 349
CgCDR genes, azole resistance and, 114–16
Cheilitis, angular, 148, 386, 489, Color Figure 11–1
Chemoprophylaxis, antifungal drug. *See* Antifungal drug(s), chemoprophylaxis
Chest radiography
  in blastomycosis, 302–3, 302f, 303f
  in coccidioidomycosis, 316–18, 317f, 318f
  in histoplasmosis, 288, 288f–89f
  in paracoccidioidomycosis, 335, 335f
  in *Pneumocystis carinii* pneumonia, 408–9, 408f
  in pulmonary aspergillosis, 227, 227f, 231, 429–30, 459–60, 460f
  in pulmonary cryptococcosis, 191–92, 192f–93f
  in sporotrichosis, 349, 349f
Children
  amphotericin B in, 37
  antifungal drug dosing, 165
  candidiasis in. *See* Neonatal candidiasis
  flucytosine in, 61
  sporotrichosis in, 349
Chitin-synthesis inhibitors, 98–99. *See also* Nikkomycins
Chorioretinitis
  Candida, 155, Color Figure 11–7
  Trichosporon, 212
CHROMagar Candida media, 7, 163
Chromoblastomycosis (chromomycosis), 275, 399–403
  clinical manifestations, 400, Color Figures 26–2 to 26–4
  definition, 399
  diagnosis, 400–01
  epidemiology, 399–400

Chromoblastomycosis (chromomycosis) (*Continued*)
  flucytosine for, 60
  mycology, 399, 400t
    causative agents, 399, 400t
    sclerotic bodies in, 400–1, Color Figure 26–1
  terbinafine for, 107
  treatment, 401–3, 401t
Chromomycosis, 399
Chrysosporium spp., 264, 421, Color Figure 28–3
Chytridiomycota, 4
Cicatricial skin lesions, in chromoblastomycosis, 400, Color Figure 26–4
Cisapride, azoles and, 67–68
Cladophialophora bantiana, 277, Color Figure 17–3
Cladophialophora spp., 276t, 277, Color Figure 17–3
Cladosporium spp., 276t, 277
Clindamycin, plus primaquine, for pneumocystosis, 410, 410t
Clinical specimens
  collection, 5–6, 370
  direct microscopic examination, 6, Color Figures 1–1 and 1–2
Clotrimazole, for candidiasis, 73t, 165, 166t, 168t
Coccidioides immitis, 311, 312f, 313
  life cycle, 312f
  susceptibility data, liposomal nystatin, 53t, 54
  taxonomy, 312–13
Coccidioides posadasii, 312–13
Coccidioides spp.
  ecology, 312
  life-cycle, 311, 312f
  taxonomy, 312–13
Coccidioidin skin test reactivity
  prevalence, 313–14, 314f
  relation to disease, 316
Coccidioidomycosis, 311–23, 493
  in African Americans, 320, Color Figure 20–8
  after organ transplantation, 319–20, 478
  azoles for, 77–78, 77t, 321–23
  clinical manifestations, 316–19, 493
  diagnosis, 320–21, Color Figure 20–9
  disseminated, 318–19, 319f, 322–23
    articular disease, 319
    meningitis, 319
    osseous disease, 319
  epidemiology, 313–15, 314f, 493
  erythema multiforme, 316–17, Color Figure 20–3
  erythema nodosum, 317, Color Figure 20–3
  in HIV-AIDS, 319, 493
  immune response, 318
  in immunocompromised population, 319–20
  occupational factors, 314–15
  pathology, 315–16
  in pregnancy, 320

prevention, 323
  pulmonary, 316–18, 317f–18f, 322
    sequelae, 317–18, 318f
  serologic testing, 13, 320–21
  treatment, 77–78, 77t, 321–23, 493
    options, 321–22
    strategies, 322–23, 493
  vaccine candidates, 316, 323
Coelomycetes, 4
Cokeromyces recurvatus, 241
Colletotrichum gloeosporioides, 264
Complement fixation test, 12
  in coccidioidomycosis, 13, 321
  in histoplasmosis, 12, 293
  in sporotrichosis, 350
Computed tomography
  in hepatosplenic candidiasis, 157, 157f
  in mediastinal granuloma, 289, 290f
  in pulmonary aspergillosis, 227–28, 228f, 231, 429–30, Color Figure 29–3
Conidiobolomycosis, 247–49
Conidiobolus coronatus, 247
Conidiobolus incongruous, 247
Contact dermatitis, vs. onychomycosis, 380
Coprinus cinereus, 421
Corticosteroids
  for allergic bronchopulmonary aspergillosis, 226
  amphotericin B and, 39
  fungal infections and, 429
    post-transplant, 457, 474–75
  for histoplasmosis, 294
  phaeohyphomycosis and, 273
  for pneumocystosis, 410t, 411
"Crescent" sign, in pulmonary aspergillosis, 228, 228f, 231, 429–30
Cryotherapy, for chromoblastomycosis, 402
Cryptococcosis, 188–201
  antigen testing, 195
  after organ transplantation, 474, 477, 481
  azoles for, 75–76, 195–201, 196t, 199t
  central nervous system. *See* meningitis
  clinical manifestations, 191–94, 192f–93f, 490
  diagnosis, 194–95, 491, Color Figures 12–9 and 12–10
  epidemiology, 189–90, 190f, 490
  flucytosine for, 196t, 197, 198–200, 199t
  in HIV-AIDS, 190, 192–94, 198–201, 199t, 490–92
  laboratory findings, 194–95, Color Figures 12–9 and 12–10
  meningitis
    amphotericin B and flucytosine for, 39–40, 60, 195–200, 196t, 199t, 491
    azoles for, 75–76, 195–201, 196t, 199t
    clinical manifestations, 192–94, 490

increased intracranial pressure, 193, 201
  in HIV-AIDS, 192–94, 490, 491
    adjunctive therapy, 201, 492
    initial therapy, 39–40, 198–200, 199t, 491–92
    maintenance therapy, 199t, 200–01, 491
  in HIV-negative patient, 196t, 197–98
  prognostic factors, 193–94
  terbinafine for, 108
  organism, 188–89, 490
  pathogenesis, 190–91
  prevention, 201
  pulmonary, 191–92, 192f–93f, 490–91
    in HIV-AIDS, 191–92, 192f, 198, 199t, 490–91
    in HIV-negative patient, 191–92, 196–97, 196t
  risk factors, 189–90, 190f
  serologic testing, 14, 195
  skeletal infections, 194
  skin infection, 194, 491, Color Figures 12–7 and 12–8
  treatment, 195–201, 491–92
    in HIV-AIDS, 198–201, 199t, 491–92
    in HIV-negative patient, 196–98, 196t
Cryptococcus albidus, 188
Cryptococcus laurentii, 188
Cryptococcus neoformans
  antibodies to, 134
  ecology, 189
  identification, 188, 195
  microbiology, 188
  susceptibility data, 15–17, 111, 112t, 195
  variety *gattii*, 188–89, 490
  variety *grubii*, 188, 490
  variety *neoformans*, 188–89, 490
  virulence factors, 190–91
CT. *See* Computed tomography
Culture
  limitations, 8
  methods, 7–8
Culture media
  antibacterial antibiotics added to, 7
  antifungal drug susceptibility testing, 16, 17
  with colorimetric indicator, 16–17
  types, 7
Cunninghamella bertholletiae, 241
Curvularia spp., 276t, 277
Cutaneous fungal infections, 367–87. *See also* Skin lesions
  candidal. *See* cutaneous candidiasis
  dermatophyte. *See* Dermatophytoses
  nondermatophyte moulds, 384–85
  superficial mycoses, 367–69
Cyclophosphamide, amphotericin B and, 39
Cyclosporin A, fluconazole with, 69, 120
Cyclosporine
  after organ transplantation, fungal infections and, 475
  azoles and, 69, 120

CYP450 enzymes, azoles and, 69
Cytokines, 125–32, 447–48
    in aspergillosis, 125, 126f
    biologic properties, 125–27
    clinically relevant, 125, 126t
    dosage and administration, 131–32
    for invasive fungal infections, 127–31,
        128f, 129t
        in neutropenic patients, 447–48
    pharmacology, 131–32
    toxicity, 131–32
Cytomegalovirus infection, post-transplant
    fungal infections and, 475
Cytosine arabinoside, flucytosine and, 61

Dapsone, prophylaxis, for *Pneumocystis
    carinii* pneumonia, 413t, 414
Deferoxamine therapy, mucormycosis
    and, 243
Dematiaceous fungi, 271–79, 276t. *See
    also* Phaeohyphomycoses
Denture stomatitis, 147–48, Color Figure
    11–1
Dermatophytes
    characteristics, 371–72, 371f, Color
        Figure 24–3
    classification, 370
    susceptibility data, terbinafine, 104,
        105t
Dermatophytoses, 370–84. *See also* Tinea
    entries
    clinical manifestations, 372–84
    culture methods, 370
    epidemiology, 370
    etiologic agents, 371–72, 371f, Color
        Figure 24–3
    microscopic examination, 370
    mycology, 370
    pathogenesis, 372
    specimen collection and transport, 370
    terbinafine for, 106–7
    treatment 373–74, 373t, 374t, 375,
        375t, 376, 378, 380, 380t,
        383–84, 384t
Desert rheumatism coccidioidomycosis,
    317
Diabetes mellitus
    eumycetoma and, 391–92
    vulvovaginal candidiasis and, 151–52
Diabetic ketoacidosis, mucormycosis and,
    243, 244, Color Figure 15–2
Dialysis, peritoneal, *Candida* peritonitis
    complicating, 161, 172
Digitalis glycosides, amphotericin B and,
    39
Digoxin, azoles and, 69
Dihydropteroate synthase mutations,
    414–15
Dimorphic fungi
    organisms
        Blastomyces dermatitidis, 299–308
        Coccidioides immitis, 311–23
        Histoplasma capsulatum, 285–96
        Paracoccidioides brasiliensis, 328–41
        Penicillium marneffei, 355–62
        Sporothrix schenckii, 346–52

phenotypic identification, 8
susceptibility in vitro
    to amphotericin B, 34
    to azoles, 69–70, 70t, 71
    to caspofungin, 92–93
    to liposomal nystatin, 53t, 54
    to terbinafine, 105, 106t
Distal lateral subungual onychomycosis,
    379, 379t
DNA fingerprinting methods, 11–12
DNA-based identification, 9–11
Dofetilide, azoles and, 68
Doxorubicin, amphotericin B and, 39

Echinocandins, 88–98. *See also specific
    drugs*
    antifungal activity in vitro, 88, 90, 90t,
        91t, 92–93, 92t, 93t, 95–96, 96t,
        112t, 119
    animal models, 91, 93, 96
    for aspergillosis, 95, 233–34, 481
    for candidiasis, 94–95, 165
        after blood or marrow
            transplantation, 464
        after organ transplantation, 480
    drug interactions, 92, 95, 98
    mechanism of action, 88, 89f
    pharmacokinetics, 90, 91–92, 93–94, 97
    prophylaxis, in neutropenic patients,
        437, 438
    resistance to, 90, 119–20
    safety and tolerance, 90, 92, 95, 98
    structure, 88, 89f
Electrophoretic karyotyping, for DNA
    fingerprinting analysis, 12
Emmonsia parva, 421, Color Figure 28–3
Emmonsia pasteuriana, 497
Empirical antifungal therapy
    after blood or marrow transplantation,
        462–63
    in neutropenic patients, 438–44,
        439t–40t
Endemic mycoses. *See also* Dimorphic
    fungi
    after organ transplantation, 478–79,
        481
    azoles for, 76–79, 77t
    terbinafine for, 107
Endocarditis
    Aspergillus, 230
    Candida, 155–56, 172
    Histoplasma, 291, 295
    Rhodutorula, 207
    S. cerevisiae, 209
Endocrine disturbances
    azole-induced, 72t, 73
    in blastomycosis, 304
    chronic mucocutaneous candidiasis and,
        150–51
Endophthalmitis
    Acremonium, 262
    Candida, 155, 171–72, Color Figure
        11–7
    in fusariosis, 254
    in phaeohyphomycoses, 276t
    in sporotrichosis, 349

Endoscopy, in esophageal candidiasis, 149
Enolase antigen assay, *Candida*, 163
Entomophthorales, 241, 242f, 247
Entomophthoramycosis
    clinical manifestations, 248
    diagnosis, 248–49
    ecology and epidemiology, 247–48
    etiology, 247
    treatment, 249
Environmental control measures, 28
    after blood or marrow transplantation,
        463
    during neutropenia, 434–35
Enzyme linked immunosorbent assay
    (ELISA), 12
    in aspergillosis, 13, 231, 433
    in coccidioidomycosis, 13
    in histoplasmosis, 13
Eosinophilia, in coccidioidomycosis, 315
Epidemiology of systemic fungal diseases,
    23–28
    exposure and transmission, 24–26
    outbreak investigations, 26–27
    prevention, 27–28
    surveillance, 23–24
Epidermophyton floccosum, 371, 371f,
    Color Figure 24–3
ERG11 gene, azole resistance and, 114,
    115f, 117
Ergosterol biosynthetic pathway
    alterations, azole resistance and,
    117–18
Ergot alkaloids, azoles and, 68
Erosio interdigitalis blastomycetica, 150,
    386
Erythema multiforme, in
    coccidioidomycosis, 317, Color
    Figure 20–3
Erythema nodosum, in coccidioidomycosis,
    317, Color Figure 20–3
Esophageal candidiasis
    antifungal refractory, management, 167,
        489–90
    azoles for, 73t, 74
    classification, 148
    clinical manifestations, 148–49, Color
        Figure 11–2
    in HIV-AIDS, 148, 489
    prevention, 174
    treatment, 73t, 74, 166–67, 166t,
        489–90
Estrogen, vulvovaginal candidiasis and,
    151
Etest, 17
Eucalyptus trees, *Cryptococcus
    neoformans* var *gattii* and, 189,
    490
Eumycetoma, 271, 276t, 390–96
    clinical aspects, 391–93, Color Figures
        25–1 and 25–2
    complications, 393
    diagnosis, 393–94
    differential diagnosis, 393
    double, 392
    epidemiology, 390–91, 391t
    etiology, 390–91, 391t

Eumycetoma (*Continued*)
    follow-up, 396
    histopathology, 394–95, 394t, Color
        Figure 25–4
    pathogenesis, 391
    radiology, 393, Color Figure 25–3
    serologic testing, 395
    surgical management, 396
    terbinafine for, 107
    treatment, 395–96
Exophiala eumycetoma, 391t, 394t, 395
Exophiala jeanselmei, 276t, 277, Color
        Figure 17–1
Eye. *See* Ocular *entries*

Favus, 382–83
Febrile neutropenia, 171, 427–44. *See also*
        Fungal infections in neutropenic
        patients
Fibrosing mediastinitis, in histoplasmosis,
        290, 294
Filobasidella neoformans, 421
Fluconazole, 64–80
    adverse effects, 72–73, 72t
    chemistry, 64–65, 65f
    with cyclosporin A, 120
    drug interactions, 67–69, 68t
    indications
        for *Acremonium* endophthalmitis,
            262
        for blastomycosis, 76, 77t, 307
        for candidiasis, 73–75, 73t, 75t, 165,
            166, 166t, 168, 169–70, 171–72,
            173
            after organ transplantation, 480
            in HIV-AIDS, 489
            in neutropenic patients, 444
        for coccidioidomycosis, 77–78, 77t,
            321–23, 493
        for cryptococcosis, 76, 196–200,
            196t, 199t, 481, 491
        for eumycetoma, 395
        for histoplasmosis, 77t, 78, 295, 493
        for malassezioses, 211, 369, 369t
        for neutropenic fever, 439t–40t, 441
        for onychomycosis, 380, 380t
        for paracoccidioidomycosis, 77t, 78,
            340, 340t, 341
        for sporotrichosis, 77t, 78, 351
        for tinea barbae, 375t
        for tinea capitis, 384, 384t
        for tinea corporis, 374t
        for tinea cruris, 376
        for tinea pedis and manuum, 378
        for trichosporonosis, 213
    mechanism of action, 65–66
    pediatric dosing, 165
    pharmacokinetics, 66–67, 66t
    prophylaxis, 28, 80
        after blood or marrow
            transplantation, 461–62
        after solid organ transplantation, 482
        for candidiasis, 174–75
        in HIV-AIDS, 492
        in intensive care unit patients,
            174–75

    in neutropenic patients, 174, 435–36,
        437
    resistance to
        in HIV-AIDS, 167, 489–90
        in vitro, 71–72, 114, 119
    spectrum of activity, 69–71, 70t, 112t
    susceptibility testing, 70t, 71, 112t
        for *Candida* spp., 111, 113t, 164,
            164t
Flucytosine, 59–61
    adverse effects, 60–61
    in children, 61
    combination therapy with amphotericin
        B, 39–40, 60, 401, 491
    dosage and administration, 60
    drug interactions, 61
    indications, 60
        for candidiasis 40, 60, 165, 173
        for chromoblastomycosis, 401t, 402
        for cryptococcosis, 39–40, 60, 197t,
            197–99, 199t, 200, 491
        for phaeohyphomycosis, 279
    mechanism of action, 59, 113
    pediatric dosing, 165
    pharmacology, 59–60
    precautions, 61
    in pregnancy, 61
    renal function monitoring with, 59–60
    resistance to, 60, 113–14
    susceptibility testing, 112t, 113, 164,
        164t
FKS genes, echinocandin resistance, 119–20
Fonsecaea pedrosoi, 276t, 277
Fontana-Masson stain, in
        phaeohyphomycosis, 272
Foreign body phaeohyphomycosis, 274
Fungal balls
    Aspergillus, 225
    Candida, 160, 161, 476
    in phaeohyphomycosis, 274
Fungal infections. *See also specific*
        diseases
    after blood or marrow transplantation,
        456–66. *See also* Blood or
        marrow transplantation
    after organ transplantation, 470–82. *See*
        also Organ transplantation
    cutaneous, 367–87. *See also* Skin
        lesions
    diagnosis, 5–18. *See also* Laboratory
        diagnostic procedures
    exposure and transmission, 24–26
    in HIV-AIDS, 23, 28, 488–97. *See also*
        HIV-AIDS
    in neutropenic patients, 427–48. *See*
        also Neutropenic patients
    nomenclature, 5
    outbreak investigations, 26–27
    prevention, 27–28. *See also* Antifungal
        drug(s), chemoprophylaxis;
        Environmental control measures
    surveillance, 23–24
    systemic, epidemiology, 23–28
Fungi
    anamorphic, 3, 4–5
    classification, 3–4

    dimorphic. *See* Dimorphic fungi
    distinctive characteristics, 3
    identification, 8–11
    nomenclature, 5
    reproduction, 3–4
    structure, 3
    subtyping, 11–12
Fusariosis
    after blood or marrow transplantation,
        461, 464
    after organ transplantation, 479
    clinical manifestations, 254–55, 254t,
        Color Figure 16–1, Color Figure
        29–4
    diagnosis, 255–56, Color Figure 16–2
    disseminated, 254–55
    epidemiology, 252–53
    in HIV-AIDS, 497
    in neutropenic patients, 430, Color
        Figure 29–4
    pathogenesis, 253
    treatment, 257–58, 257t
        adjunctive, 258
        azoles for, 80
Fusarium eumycetoma, 391t, 394t, 395
Fusarium onychomycosis, 254t, 258
Fusarium paronychia, 254
Fusarium spp.
    identification, 255–56, 434, Color
        Figure 16–2
    mycotoxins, 253
    susceptibility data, 256–57, 256t

Galactomannan assay, in aspergillosis, 13,
        231, 432–33, 460–61, 481, 495
Gastrointestinal toxicity
    azoles, 72, 72t
    flucytosine, 60–61
GenBank database, 9–11
Genetic relatedness, assessment, 11–12
Genitourinary tract
    aspergillosis of, 230
    blastomycosis of, 304
    candidiasis of, 159–61
    histoplasmosis of, 292
    paracoccidioidomycosis of, 337
    S. cerevisiae infections of, 209
Genome approaches, to azole resistance,
        119
Gentian violet, for candidiasis, 165, 166t
Geotrichum candidum, 264
Giemsa stain, 6
Gilchrist's disease (blastomycosis), 299
Glucan-synthesis inhibitors. *See*
        Echinocandins
Glucatell assay for candidiasis, 163
Grains, in eumycetoma, 391t, 391–94,
        394t, Color Figures 25–1 and
        25–2
Gram stain, 6
Granulocyte transfusions. *See* White blood
        cell transfusions
Granulocyte colony-stimulating factor
    biologic properties, 125
    dosage and administration, 131
    for fusariosis, 258

for invasive fungal infections, 129, 129t, 130, 131, 447
for stimulation of white blood cell transfusions and, for invasive fungal infections, 132–34, 133t, 447
toxicity, 132
Granulocyte-macrophage colony-stimulating factor
biologic properties, 125–26
dosage and administration, 131–32
for fusariosis, 258
for invasive fungal infections, 128–29, 128f, 129t, 130, 131, 447
toxicity, 132
Granuloma
Candida, 150
mediastinal, in histoplasmosis, 289–90, 290f, 294
in paracoccidioidomycosis, 331
Granulomatous tenosynovitis, in sporotrichosis, 348–49
Gray patch tinea capitis, 382
Griseofulvin
for tinea barbae, 375t
for tinea capitis, 383–84, 384t
for tinea corporis, 374t
for tinea cruris, 376
Growth factors. See Hematopoietic growth factors

HAART. See Antiretroviral therapy, highly active (HAART)
Hair, microscopic examination, 383
Hairy leukoplakia, in HIV-AIDS, 489
"Halo" sign, in pulmonary aspergillosis, 227–28, 228f, 231, 429, Color Figure 29–3
Hand washing, guidelines, 28
Heart failure, from itraconazole, 73
Heart transplantation, fungal infections after, 472–73
Heart-lung transplantation, fungal infections after, 473
Hematopoietic growth factors
in aspergillosis, 125, 126f
biologic properties, 125–26
clinically relevant, 125, 126t
for invasive fungal infections, 128–29, 128f, 129t, 130, 131, 447
pharmacology, 131–32
Hematopoietic stem cell transplantation. See Blood or marrow transplantation
HEPA filters. See High energy particulate air filtration
Hepatitis C infection, post-transplant fungal infections and, 475
Hepatosplenic candidiasis, 157, 157f, 171, 429, 429f, 444
after blood or marrow transplantation, 459
Hepatotoxicity
azoles, 72, 72t
flucytosine, 61
Heterotroph, 3

HHV-6, post-transplant fungal infections and, 475
High-efficiency particulate air filtration (HEPA) filters, 28
after blood or marrow transplantation, 463
during neutropenia, 434–35
Histopathologic studies, 6–7
Histoplasma capsulatum (Histoplasma capsulatum var. capsulatum)
antibodies to, 293
antigen detection, 293
characteristics, 358, 358t
culture, 292–93
ecology, 286
organism
mycelial phase, 285, 286f
yeast phase, 285, 294, Color Figure 18–2
Histoplasma capsulatum var. farciminosum, 285
Histoplasma duboisii (Histoplasma capsulatum var. duboisii) infection
clinical manifestations, 292, 492, Color Figure 18–15
diagnosis, 294
ecology, 286–87
organism, 285, 358, 358t, Color Figure 18–2
treatment, 296, 493
Histoplasmosis, 285–96, 492–93
African, 292, 296, Color Figure 18–15
after organ transplantation, 478
antigen detection, 293
false positive reactions, 293
azoles for, 77t, 78
broncholithiasis in, 290
central nervous system, 291–92, 292f, 295–96
clinical manifestations, 287–92, 287t, 492
culture methods, 292–93
diagnosis, 292–94
disseminated, 290–92
acute, 290–91
adrenal enlargement in, 291, 291f
chronic, 291
endocarditis in, 291, 295
in immunocompromised patients, 290–91
skin lesions in, 291, 492, Color Figures 18–11 and 18–12
treatment, 295
ecology and epidemiology, 286–87, 286f, 492
environmental control measures, 28
epidemic, 288, 288f, 289f, 294
fibrosing mediastinitis in, 290, 294
gastrointestinal, 292
genitourinary tract, 292
histopathological examination, 293–94, Color Figure 18–16
in HIV-AIDS, 290–91, 492–93
mediastinal granuloma in, 289–90, 290f, 294

ocular, presumed, 292
organism, 285, 286f, Color Figure 18–2
osteoarticular, 292
pathogenesis, 287
pericarditis in, 290, 290f, 294–95
prevention, 296
pulmonary
acute, 287–89, 288f–89f, 294, 492
chronic, 289, 289f, 294, 492
complications, 289–90, 290f, 294–95
treatment, 294–95
serologic testing, 12–13, 293
skin tests, 294
terbinafine for, 107
treatment, 77t, 78, 294–96, 493
HIV-AIDS, fungal infections in, 488–97
aspergillosis in, 494–95
blastomycosis in, 305, 495–96
candidiasis in, 147–50, 165–68, 488–90
coccidioidomycosis in, 319, 493
cryptococcosis in, 190, 192–95, 198–201, 199t, 490–92
meningeal, 193, 198–201, 199t, 490–92
pulmonary, 191–92, 192f, 198, 199t, 490–92
HAART for
opportunistic fungal infections and, 497
for refractory oropharyngeal candidiasis, 167
histoplasmosis in, 286, 290–91, 492–93
immune reconstitution reaction, 497
miscellaneous fungal diseases in, 497
opportunistic fungal infections in, 488–97
epidemiology, 23
prevention, 28
uncommon pathogens, 496–97
paracoccidioidomycosis in, 337, 495
penicilliosis in, 355–56, 357, 358–59, 360–62, 493–94
pneumocystosis in, 408, 412, 488. See also Pneumocystis carinii pneumonia
Saccharomyces cerevisiae infection in, 496–97
scedosporiosis in, 496
sporotrichosis in, 496
trichosporonosis in, 496–97
zygomycosis in, 496
Homographiella aspergillata, 421
Hortea werneckii (Phaeoannellomyces werneckii, Exophiala werneckii), 273, 367, 368
Hospital water supplies, contamination, aspergillosis from, 25, 463
Human immunodeficiency virus infection. See HIV/AIDS
Hyalohyphomycosis. See also Aspergillosis; Penicilliosis
characteristics of agents, 253t
specific agents, 5, 252–65, 253t
specific diseases
caused by Acremonium spp., 261–62
caused by Chrysosporium spp., 264

Hyalohyphomycosis (*Continued*)
    caused by *Paecilomyces* spp., 263–64
    caused by *Scopulariopsis* spp.,
        262–63
    caused by *Trichoderma* spp., 264–65
    fusariosis, 252–58, 257t
    scedosporiosis, 258–61
    susceptibility data, 256t
Hydrocortisone, amphotericin B and, 39
Hyperbaric oxygen, for mucormycosis,
    247
Hyperthermia
    for chromoblastomycosis, 402
    for sporotrichosis, 351
Hyphae, 3
Hyphomycetes, 4
Hypoglycemic agents, oral, azoles and, 69

Immune response
    in aspergillosis, 125, 126f, 223–24
    in coccidioidomycosis, 318
    in cryptococcosis, 191
    in histoplasmosis, 287
    to medically relevant fungi, 125, 127t
    in paracoccidioidomycosis, 332–33,
        Color Figure 21–3
Immunochemical staining, 6
Immunodiffusion test
    in aspergillosis, 13
    in histoplasmosis, 12–13, 293
Immunodiffusion tube precipitin (IDTP)
        test, in coccidioidomycosis, 13,
        320
Immunoglobulin, intravenous, for invasive
        fungal infections, 134
Immunosuppressive regimen, after organ
        transplantation, fungal infections
        and, 474–75
Immunosuppressive net state, after organ
        transplantation, factors affecting,
        470, 471t
India ink stain, 6
    for cryptococcosis, 194, Color Figure
        12–9
Inflammatory tinea capitis, 382, Color
        Figure 24–7
Intensive care unit, candidiasis
        prophylaxis in, 174–75
Interferon-γ
    biologic properties, 126, 126t
    dosing and administration, 131–32
    for invasive fungal infections, 128t,
        130–31, 447–48
    toxicity, 132
Interleukin-4, 127, 126t
Interleukin-10, 127
Interleukin-12, 126–27, 126t
Interleukin-15, 127
Intertrigo, *Candida*, 150, 386, 387, Color
        Figure 24–8
Intracranial pressure, in cryptococcal
        meningitis, 193, 201, 492
Iron, serum, mucormycosis and, 243–44
Itraconazole, 64–80
    adverse effects, 72–73, 72t
    chemistry, 64, 65f

drug interactions, 67–69, 68t
indications
    for aspergillosis, 79, 226, 233, 445
    for blastomycosis, 76–77, 77t, 307,
        308
    for candidiasis, 73–74, 73t, 75t, 165,
        166, 166t, 169, 489
    for chromoblastomycosis, 401t,
        402–03
    for coccidioidomycosis, 77–78, 77t,
        321, 322, 493
    for cryptococcosis, 75–76, 196–201,
        196t, 199t, 491–92
    for eumycetoma, 395–96
    for histoplasmosis, 77t, 78, 294, 295,
        493
    for malasseziosis, 369, 369t
    for mucormycosis, 247
    for neutropenic fever, 439t–40t,
        442–43
    for onychomycosis, 73t, 74, 380,
        380t
    for *Paecilomyces* infections, 264
    for paracoccidioidomycosis, 77t, 78,
        340, 340t, 341
    for penicilliosis, 79, 362, 494
    for phaeohyphomycosis, 79, 279
    for scedosporiosis, 79, 260
    for *Scopulariopsis* spp. infection, 263
    for sporotrichosis, 77t, 78–79, 351
    for tinea barbae, 375t
    for tinea capitis, 384, 384t
    for tinea corporis, 374t
    for tinea cruris, 376
    for tinea pedis and manuum, 378
    for trichosporonosis, 213
mechanism of action, 65–66
pharmacokinetics, 66–67, 66t
prophylaxis, 28, 80
    after blood or marrow
        transplantation, 462
    for histoplasmosis, 296
    in neutropenic patients, 436–37
    for penicilliosis, 362
resistance to, in vitro, 71–72
    mechanisms of resistance, 114–19
spectrum of activity, 69–71, 70t, 112t
susceptibility testing, 70t, 71, 112t
    for *Candida* spp., 111, 113t, 164, 164t

Joint disease
    in blastomycosis, 304
    in candidiasis, 162
    in coccidioidomycosis, 319
    in cryptococcosis, 194
    in histoplasmosis, 292
    in paracoccidioidomycosis, 337
    in sporotrichosis, 348–49

Karyotyping, for DNA fingerprinting
        analysis, 12
Keratitis
    Fusarium, 254, 258
    in phaeohyphomycoses, 274
Kerion, production, in inflammatory tinea
        capitis, 382

Ketoconazole, 64–80
    adverse effects, 72–73, 72t
    chemistry, 64, 65f
    drug interactions, 67–69, 68t
    indications
        for blastomycosis, 76–77, 77t, 307
        for candidiasis, 165, 166, 166t
        for chromoblastomycosis, 401t, 402
        for coccidioidomycosis, 77–78, 77t,
            321
        for entomophthoramycosis, 249
        for eumycetoma, 395
        for histoplasmosis, 77t, 78, 294
        for malasseziosis, 369, 369t
        for paracoccidioidomycosis, 77t, 78,
            340–41, 340t
    mechanism of action, 65–66
    pharmacokinetics, 66–67, 66t
    resistance to, in vitro, 71–72
    spectrum of activity, 69–71, 70t
    susceptibility testing, 71
Kidney transplantation, fungal infections
        after, 471–72
Kidney-pancreas transplantation, fungal
        infections after, 472
KOH preparation, 6, Color Figures 1–1
        and 1–2

Laboratory diagnostic procedures, 5–18
    blood culture, 8
    culture, 7–9
    direct microscopic examination, 6,
        Color Figures 1–1 and 1–2
    histopathologic studies, 6–7
    molecular diagnostics, 14–15
    molecular identification, 9–11
    molecular subtyping, 11–12
    phenotypic identification, 8–9, Color
        Figures 1–3 and 1–4
    serologic testing, 12–14
    specimen collection, 5–6, 370
    susceptibility testing, 15–18, 71
Lacazia loboi, 420–21, Color Figures
        28–1 and 28–2
Laminar airflow, after blood or marrow
        transplantation, 463
Latex agglutination test, 12
    in aspergillosis, 13
    in coccidioidomycosis, 13, 320–21
    in cryptococcosis, 14, 195, 491
Lecythophora hoffmannii, 397
Lecythophora mutabilis, 264
Leptosphaeria senegalensis, 390–91, 391t,
        393, 394t
Leukocyte infusions, amphotericin B and,
        39
Lipid preparations of amphotericin B. *See*
        Amphotericin B
Lipopeptides, echinocandin. *See*
        Echinocandins
Liposomal amphotericin B (L-AmB). *See*
        Amphotericin B, liposomal
    for aspergillosis, 232–33, 232t
    for cryptococcosis, 45, 200, 490–91
    for eumycetoma, 395
    for histoplasmosis, 295

for neutropenic fever, 439t, 440t, 442
for mucormycosis, 246–47
Liposomal nystatin. *See* Nystatin,
    liposomal
Liver transplantation, fungal infections
    after, 472
Lobomycosis, 420–21, Color Figures 28–1
    and 28–2
Lovastatin, azoles and, 68
Lung. *See also* Pulmonary *entries*
Lymphocutaneous sporotrichosis, 348,
    Color Figures 22–1 to 22–4
Lymphocytopenia, post-transplant fungal
    infections and, 457
Lysis-centrifugation method for blood
    cultures, 8

M27-A reference method, for
    susceptibility testing, 15–17, 71,
    163–64
M38-A reference method, for
    susceptibility testing, 17
Macrophage, in paracoccidioidomycosis,
    333, Color Figure 21–3
Macrophage colony-stimulating factor
    administration, 131
    biologic properties, 126
    for invasive fungal infections, 128t,
        129, 129t, 130, 131
Madurella grisea, 390–91, 391t, 392, 393,
    394, 394t
Madurella mycetomatis, 390–91, 391t,
    393, 394, 394t, 395, Color
    Figure 25–4
Majocchi's granuloma, in tinea corporis,
    373, Color Figure 24–5
Malassezia furfur
    characteristics, 209–10, 367
    susceptibility data, 207t, 210
Malassezia furfur–complex, 368
Malassezia pachydermatis, 210, 368
Malassezia spp., 209–10, 367–68
Malasseziosis, 209–11, 367–68, 369,
    369t, Color Figure 24–1
    clinical manifestations, 210, 367
        cutaneous, 367–68, 369, 369t, Color
            Figure 24–1
    diagnosis, 210–11, 368
    epidemiology, 210
    organism, 209–10, 367
    treatment, 211, 369, 369t
Mannan antigen assay for candidiasis,
    163
Marrow transplantation. *See* Blood or
    marrow transplantation
Mediastinal granuloma, in histoplasmosis,
    289–90, 290f, 294
Mediastinal lymphadenopathy, in
    histoplasmosis, 288, 288f
Mediastinitis
    Candida, 173
    fibrosing, in histoplasmosis, 290, 294
Melanin production
    in *Cryptococcus neoformans*, 190–91
    by dematiaceous moulds, 271, 272
    as virulence factor, 190–91, 272

Meningitis
    blastomycotic, 304
    Candida, 158, 173–74
    coccidioidal, 319, 323
    cryptococcal. *See* Cryptococcal
        meningitis
    Histoplasma, 291–92, 292f, 295
    in paracoccidioidomycosis, 337
    in phaeohyphomycoses, 275, 276t
        Color Figure 17–2
    Rhodotorula, 207
    in sporotrichosis, 349–50
Methenamine-silver stain, 6
Micafungin, 88–90, 89f, 95–98
    antifungal activity in vitro, 95–96, 96t,
        112t, 119
    antimicrobial interactions, 96
    clinical efficacy, 97–98
    drug interactions, 98
    efficacy in animal models, 96
    pharmacokinetics, 97, 97t
    prophylaxis, 98
        after blood or marrow
            transplantation, 437
        in neutropenic patients, 437
    safety and tolerance, 98
    status of clinical development, 98
    structure, 89f
Microsatellite regions, as DNA
    fingerprinting probes, 12
Microscopic examination, 6, Color
    Figures 1–1 and 1–2
Microsporum audouinii, 371
Microsporum canis, 371, 371f, Color
    Figure 24–3
Microsporum spp., characteristics, 371,
    371f, Color Figure 24–3
Midazolam, azoles and, 68
Minimum inhibitory concentration
    (MIC)
    interpretation, 17–18, 71, 163–64
    methods for determining, 15–17, 71,
        163–64
Molecular diagnostics, 14–15
Molecular identification, 9–11
Molecular subtyping, 11–12
Monoclonal antibodies, for invasive
    fungal infections, 134
Mortierella spp., 241
Moulds
    characteristics, 3
    dermatophyte. *See* Dermatophytoses
    nondermatophyte, 384–85
    phenotypic identification, 8, Color
        Figures 1–3 and 1–4
    susceptibility in vitro
        to amphotericin B, 34
        to anidulafungin, 90, 91t
        to azoles, 70–71, 70t
        to caspofungin, 92, 93t
        Etest method, 17
        interpretation, 18
        to liposomal nystatin, 53, 53t, 54
        M38-A method, 17
        to micafungin, 96, 96t
        to terbinafine, 104, 105t

Mucicarmine stain, 6
    for cryptococcosis, 194, Color Figure
        12–10
Mucocutaneous candidiasis, chronic,
    150–51, 169, 386–87
Mucor spp., 241
Mucorales, 241, 242f
Mucormycosis, 241–47
    clinical manifestations, 244–45
        cutaneous, 245, Color Figure 15–3
        disseminated, 245, 246
        gastrointestinal, 245
        miscellaneous forms, 245
        pulmonary, 244–45, 246
        rhinocerebral, 244, 246, 430, Color
            Figure 15–2
    diagnosis, 245–46, Color Figure 15–4
    ecology and epidemiology, 241–42
    etiology, 241, 242f
    pathogenesis, 242–44
        corticosteroids, role in, 242–43
        diabetes mellitus, 243
        iron, role in, 243–44
        phagocytes, role in, 242–43
        neutrophils, role in, 242–43
    survival rate, 247
    treatment, 246–47
Mulberry-like stomatitis, in
    paracoccidioidomycosis, 336,
    336f
Multidrug transporter genes, azole
    resistance and, 114–17, 115f
Multilocus enzyme electrophoresis (MEE),
    for DNA fingerprinting analysis,
    11
Mycelium, 3
Mycetoma, fungal. *See* Eumycetoma
Mycotic aneurysm, *Candida*, 157
Myriodontium keratinophilum, 264

Natamycin, for *Fusarium* keratitis, 258
National Nosocomial Infections
    Surveillance (NNIS) system, 24
NEMIS surveillance program, 23–24
Neonatal candidiasis, 157–58, 157f
    congenital cutaneous, 158
    prevention, 175
    systemic, 158
    treatment, 171
Neuromuscular blocking agents,
    amphotericin B and, 39
Neutropenic patients
    adjunctive antifungal therapy for,
        127–29, 128t, 129t, 446–48
    amphotericin B empiric therapy for,
        44–45, 438–44, 439t, 440t
    aspergillosis in, 223–35, 429–46
        antifungal therapy, 79, 232–34, 232t,
            444–45
        clinical manifestations and diagnosis,
            227–30, 429–30, Color Figure
            29–3
        detection of pathogen, 230–32,
            431–34
        empirical therapy, 438–44, 439t, 440t
        primary prophylaxis, 235, 435–38

Neutropenic patients (*Continued*)
  secondary prophylaxis, 438
  surgical management, 445–46, 465
azoles for, 80, 439t, 440t, 444–45
candidiasis in 74–75, 75t, 153–55, 174,
      428–29, 431, 435–44, 439t, 440t
  antifungal therapy, 74–75, 75t,
      169–70, 444
  clinical manifestations, 154–62,
      428–29
  detection of pathogen, 163, 431
  empirical therapy, 438–44, 439t,
      440t
  primary prophylaxis, 435–38
febrile
  empirical therapy, 44–45, 438–44,
      439t–40t
  presumptive therapy, 170–71
fusariosis in, 80, 254–55, 254t, 257–58,
      257t, 430, 434, Color Figure
      29–4
G-CSF-stimulated white blood cell
      transfusions for, 132–34, 133t,
      447
invasive fungal infections in, 427–48
  clinical manifestations, 428–31, 429t
  detection of fungal pathogens,
      431–34
    Aspergillus, 431–34
    Candida, 431
    Fusarium, 434
  diagnosis, 428–34
    aspergillosis, 429–30
    candidiasis, 428–29
    fusariosis, 430
    scedosporiosis, 430
    trichosporonosis, 431
    zygomycosis, 430–31
  host factors predisposing to, 427–28,
      428t
  magnitude and scope of problem, 427
  prevention, 434–44
    empirical antifungal therapy,
      438–44, 439t, 440t
    prevention of exposure, 434–35
    primary prophylaxis, 435–38
    secondary prophylaxis, 438
  scedosporiosis in, 80, 259–61, 276t,
      277–78, 260, 261, 279, 430
  treatment, 444–48
    cytokines, 447–48
    granulocyte transfusions, 446–47
    pharmacological, 444–45
    surgical, 445–46
    white blood cell transfusions for,
      446–47
  trichosporonosis in, 212–13, 431
  zygomycosis in, 244–47, 430–31
Nikkomycin Z, 99, 99f
  antifungal activity in vitro, 99
  synergistic activity, 99
Nikkomycins, 98–99
  mechanism of action, 98–99
Nodules
  cutaneous, in chromoblastomycosis,
      400, Color Figure 26–2

pulmonary, coccidioidal, 317, 318f
subcutaneous, in blastomycosis, 303,
      Color Figure 19–12
Nonsteroidal antiinflammatory drugs,
      amphotericin B and, 39
Nucleic acid sequence-based amplification
      (NASBA) assay, in aspergillosis,
      14–15
Nystatin, 49–56
  antifungal activity in vitro, 53, 53t
  for candidiasis, 165, 166t
  chemistry, 49–50, 50f
  development, 49
  liposomal
    adverse effects, 52–53
    animal models of infection, 55–56
    antifungal activity in vitro, 53–54,
      53t
    chemistry, 50
    combination therapy, 54
    development, 49
    human clinical studies, 56
    mechanism of action, 50–51
    pharmacokinetics, 51–52, 51t
  mechanism of action, 50–51
  postantifungal effect, 54–55
  resistance to, 54–55
  structure, 50–51, 50f

Occupational factors
  in blastomycosis, 300–1
  in coccidioidomycosis, 314–15
  in paracoccidioidomycosis, 331
  in sporotrichosis, 347–48
Ocular blastomycosis, 304–5
Ocular candidiasis, 155, 171–72, Color
      Figure 11–7
Ocular histoplasmosis, presumed, 292
Ocular phaeohyphomycosis, 274
Onychomycosis, 378–81
  Aspergillus, 225
  Candida, 73t, 74, 150, 169, 386, 387
  clinical presentations, 379, 379t
    distal lateral subungual, 379, 379t
    proximal subungual, 379, 379t
    proximal white subungual, 379,
      379t
    white superficial, 379, 379t, Color
      Figure 24–6
    total dystrophic, 379, 379t
  definition, 378
  diagnosis, 379
  differential diagnosis, 379–80
  epidemiology, 378
  Fusarium, 254, 258
  prevention, 380–81
  Scopulariopsis brevicaulis, 384, 385
  specimen collection and transport, 370
  terbinafine for, 106–7
  treatment, 380, 380t
Organ transplantation, solid
  aspergillosis after, 474, 476–77, 480,
      481,
  blastomycosis after, 478, 481
  candidiasis after, 473–74, 475–76, 479,
      480–81

coccidioidomycosis after, 319–20, 475,
      478, 480
cryptococcosis after, 474, 475, 477,
      480–81
endemic mycoses after, 478–79, 481
fungal infections (invasive) after,
      470–82
  antifungal therapy, 480–82
    documented/suspected infection,
      480–81
    preemptive, 481–82
    prophylactic, 482
  comorbid conditions and, 475
  diagnostic approach, 479–80
  donor-related, 475
  immunosuppressive regimen and,
      474–75
  risk factors, 470–79
  timing, 473–74, 474f
  type of transplant and, 471–73
    heart, 472
    kidney, 471–72
    lung and heart-lung, 473
    liver, 472
    pancreas and kidney-pancreas, 472
    small bowel, 473
fusariosis after, 479
histoplasmosis after, 478
immunosuppressive net state after,
      factors affecting, 470, 471t
phaeohyphomycosis after, 273, 478
Pneumocystis carinii pneumonia after,
      412, 479, 481
sporotrichosis after, 479
trichosporonosis after, 479
zygomycosis after, 474, 477–78
Oropharyngeal candidiasis, 147–48, 386,
      387, 488–89
  antifungal refractory, 167
  azoles for, 73–74, 73t
  clinical manifestations, 147–48, 386,
      489, Color Figure 11–1
  in HIV-AIDS, 148, 488–89
  prevention, 174
  sabbural tongue, 489
  treatment, 73–74, 73t, 165–66, 166t,
      167, 387, 489–90
Oropharyngeal paracoccidioidomycosis,
      336, 336f
Oropharyngeal ulcers, in histoplasmosis,
      291, Color Figure 18–12
Osseous lesions. *See* Bone lesions
Otomycosis, *Aspergillus*, 225
Outbreak investigations, 26–27
Oxygen, hyperbaric, for mucormycosis,
      247

Paecilomyces spp., 256t, 263–64
  clinical manifestations, 263
  diagnosis, 263
  epidemiology, 263
  susceptibility data, 256t, 263–64
  treatment, 264
Pancreas transplantation, fungal infections
      after, 472
Pancreatitis, *Candida* superinfections, 173

Papanicolaou stain, 6
Paracoccidioides brasiliensis
    antibodies to, 332–33, 338–39
    antigen detection, 338–39
    estradiol-binding protein, 329
    identification, 338–39, Color Figure
        21–10
    microbiology, 328–29, 338, Color
        Figures 21–1 and 21–2
Paracoccidioidomycosis, 328–41, 495
    adrenal dysfunction in, 336
    azoles for, 77t, 78, 340–41, 340t, 495
    bone and joint lesions, 337
    central nervous system, 337
    clinical forms, 332, 332t
    clinical manifestations, 332t, 334–38,
        495
    cutaneous, 336, 336f, 495
    demographic data, 331, 495
    diagnosis, 338–39, 495
        cultures, 338
        direct examination, 338
        histopathology, 331–32, Color Figure
            21–3
        serologic testing, 338–39
    differential diagnosis, 337–38
    ecology, 330
    epidemiology, 329–31
    gastrointestinal, 337
    genitourinary tract, 337
    geographic distribution, 329–30, 495
    in HIV-AIDS, 337, 495
    immune response
        cell-mediated, 333, Color Figure 21–3
        humoral, 332–33
    lymph node involvement, 331–32, 336,
        337f
    molecular probes in, 329, 339, 495
    mucous membrane lesions, 336, 336f
    natural history, 334f
    pathogenesis, 332–33, 332t
    prevention, 341
    pulmonary, 331, 334–35, 335f, 495
    sequelae, 337
    treatment, 339–41, 340t, 495
        amphotericin B, 340, 340t
        azoles, 77t, 78, 340–41, 340t
        sulfonamides, 339–40, 340t
Paracoccidioidin skin test, 330, 339
Paronychia
    Candida, 150, 169, 385–86
    Fusarium, 254
PCR. *See* Polymerase chain reaction
        (PCR) amplification
Penicilliosis, 355–62, 493–94
    azoles for, 79, 362
    bamboo rats, role in transmission,
        356–57, 356t
    clinical manifestations, 358–59, 359t
        unusual, 359
    diagnosis, 359–61, 360t
    disseminated
        signs and symptoms, 358–59, 359t,
            494, Color Figures 23–3 to 23–5
        treatment, 361–62, 362t
    epidemiology, 356–57, 356t, 493

history, 355–56
    in HIV-AIDS, 355–56, 357, 358–59,
        360–62, 493–94
    in HIV-negative patients, 359
    pathology and pathogenesis, 357–58,
        358t
    prevention, 362, 494
    susceptibility data, 361, 362t
    treatment, 79, 361–62, 362t
        initial, 361–62
        maintenance, 362
Penicillium decumbens, 497
Penicillium marneffei
    antibodies to, 360–61
    antigen detection, 361
    characteristics, 358, 358t
    history, 355
    identification, 359–61, 360t, Color
        Figures 23–1 and 23–6
    mycology, 357, Color Figures 23–1 and
        23–2
    susceptibility data, 361, 362t
Pentamidine, for pneumocystosis, 410,
        410t
    after organ transplantation, 481
    prophylaxis, 413–14, 413t
Pericarditis
    in aspergillosis, 230
    in candidiasis, 155, 172
    in histoplasmosis, 290, 290f, 294–95
Periodic acid-Schiff staining, 6
Peritoneal dialysis, *Candida* peritonitis
        complicating, 161, 172
Peritonitis
    Candida, 161, 172
    Rhodutorula, 207
    S. cerevisiae, 209
Perleche, 148, 386, 489, Color Figure
        11–1
Phaeoannellomyces werneckii (*Hortaea
        werneckii, Exophiala werneckii*),
        273, 367, 368,
Phaeohyphomycoses, 5, 271–79. *See also*
        Chromoblastomycosis;
        Eumycetoma
    after blood or marrow transplantation,
        273
    after organ transplantation, 273, 478
    azoles for, 79, 279
    clinical manifestations, 273–75
    culture, 272
    cutaneous, 274
    definition, 271, 399
    diagnosis, 278
    etiological agents, 275–78, 276t
        Alternaria spp., 275, 276t
        Bipolaris spp., 277, 276t
        Cladophialophora spp., 277, 276t
        Cladosporium spp., 277, 276t
        Curvularia spp., 277, 276t
        Fonsecaea spp., 277, 276t
        Phialophora spp., 277, 276t
        Rhinocladiella spp., 277, 276t
        Scedosporium spp., 277–78, 276t
        Wangiella spp., 278, 276t
    foreign body, 274

histopathology, 272
    in HIV-AIDS, 497
    keratitis in, 274
    laboratory studies, 278
    management, 278–79
    ocular, 274
    pathophysiology, 272–73
    risk factors, 273, 273t
    sinusitis in, 274, 278
    subcutaneous, 274, Color Figure 17–1
    superficial, 273
    systemic, 274–75, Color Figure 17–2
    taxonomy/ecology, 271–72
Phagocyte dysfunction, adjunctive
        antifungal therapy for, 128f,
        130–31
Phenotypic identification, 8–9, Color
        Figures 1–3 and 1–4
Phenytoin, azoles and, 69
Phialophora spp., 276t, 277
Phialophora verrucosa, 399, Color Figure
        1–4
Phospholipases, candidal, 144
Piedra
    black, 273, 367, 368, 369
    white, 211, 367, 368, 369
Piedraia hortae, 273, 367, 368, 369
Pigeon droppings, *Cryptococcus
        neoformans* and, 189
Pimozide, azoles and, 68
Pityriasis versicolor, 367–69, 369t, Color
        Figure 24–1
Plaque skin lesions
    in chromoblastomycosis, 400, Color
        Figure 26–3
    in sporotrichosis, 348, Color Figure
        22–1
    in tinea corporis, 373, Color Figure
        24–4
Pneumocystis carinii. *See* P. carinii
        pneumonia and pneumocystosis
Pneumocystis carinii pneumonia
    after blood or marrow transplantation,
        412
    after organ transplantation, 412, 479,
        481
    identification of organism, 409
    in HIV-AIDS, 408, 412
    in lung and heart-lung transplant
        recipients, 473
    prophylaxis, 412–14, 413t
    radiology, 408
    symptoms and signs, 408–9, 408f
    treatment, 409–12, 410t
Pneumocystosis, 407–15
    epidemiology, 407, 479
    extrapulmonary, 409, 479
    host defenses, 407–8
    laboratory diagnosis, 409
    microbiology, 407
    monitoring therapy, 411–12
    pathogenesis, 407–8
    prevention, 412–14, 413t
    pulmonary, 408–9, 408f. *See also*
        Pneumocystis carinii pneumonia
    sulfonamide desensitization, 414

Pneumocystosis (*Continued*)
  sulfonamide resistance/dihydropteroate
    synthase mutations, 414–15
  treatment, 409–12, 410t, 479
Polymerase chain reaction (PCR)
    amplification, 9–10
  in aspergillosis, 14–15, 231–32, 433–34
  in candidiasis, 15
  in fusariosis, 255–56
  nested, 10
  panfungal, 14–15
  in paracoccidioidomycosis, 339
  in pneumocystosis, 409
Polysaccharide capsule, *Cryptococcus
    neoformans*, 190–91
Posaconazole
  chemistry, 64, 65f
  drug interactions, 67–69, 68t
  indications
    for aspergillosis, 233
    for eumycetoma, 396
    for fusariosis, 258
    for mucomycosis, 79, 247
    for phaeohyphomycoses, 279
    for trichosporonosis, 215
  pharmacokinetics, 66–67, 66t
  spectrum of activity, 69–71, 70t, 112t
  susceptibility testing, 71, 112t
Potassium iodide
  for entomophthoramycosis, 249
  for sporotrichosis, 350–51
Prednisone, for pneumocystosis, 410t,
    411
Preemptive antifungal therapy
  after blood or marrow transplantation,
    463
  after organ transplantation, 481–82
Pregnancy
  amphotericin B deoxycholate in, 42
  blastomycosis in, 305
  coccidioidomycosis in, 320
  flucytosine in, 61
Progesterone, dermatophytoses and, 372
Prosthetic valve endocarditis, *Candida*,
    156
Proximal subungual onychomycosis, 379,
    379t
Proximal white subungual onychomycosis,
    379, 379t
*Pseudallescheria boydii (Scedosporium
    apiospermum)*, 256t, 258–60,
    276t, 277–78, 279, 496
  eumycetoma, 391, 391t, 393, 394t,
    395
Pseudohypha, 3
Pseudomembranous candidiasis, acute,
    147, Color Figure 11–1
Pulmonary aspergilloma, 225
Pulmonary aspergillosis, invasive, 227–28,
    227f, 228f, 429–30, 460, 460f,
    494–95, Color Figure 29–3
Pulmonary blastomycosis, 302–3, 302f,
    303f
Pulmonary candidiasis, 159, 159f
Pulmonary coccidioidomycosis, 316–18,
    317f–18f, 322

Pulmonary cryptococcosis, 191–92,
    192f–93f
  in HIV-AIDS, 191–92, 192f, 198, 199t,
    490–91
  in HIV-negative patient, 196–97, 196t
Pulmonary fusariosis, 254
Pulmonary histoplasmosis
  acute, 287–89, 288f–89f, 294
  chronic, 289, 289f, 294
  complications, 289–90, 290f, 294–95
  treatment, 294–95
Pulmonary mucormycosis, 244–45, 246
  in neutropenic patients, 430–31
Pulmonary paracoccidioidomycosis, 331,
    334–35, 335f
Pulmonary pneumocystosis, 408–9, 408f.
    See also Pneumocystis carinii
    pneumonia
Pulmonary sporotrichosis, 349, 349f
Pulmonary toxicity, amphotericin B, 44
Pulmonary trichosporonosis, 212
Pyrimethamine, prophylaxis for
    Pneumocystis carinii pneumonia,
    413t, 414

Quinidine, azoles and, 68

Radiography, chest
  in blastomycosis, 303–04, 302f, 303f
  in candidiasis, 159, 159f
  in coccidioidomycosis, 317–18, 317f,
    318f
  in histoplasmosis, 288, 288f–89f
  in paracoccidioidomycosis, 335, 335f
  in *Pneumocystis carinii* pneumonia,
    408–9, 408f
  in pulmonary aspergillosis, 227, 227f,
    228f, 231, 429–30, 460, 460f,
    Color Figure 29–3
  in pulmonary cryptococcosis, 191–92,
    192f–93f
  in sporotrichosis, 349, 349f
Radioimmunoassay, 12
  in histoplasmosis, 13
Ramichloridium spp., 276t, 277
Randomly amplified polymorphic DNA
    (RAPD) analysis, 10
  for DNA fingerprinting analysis, 12
Rash, azole-induced, 72–73, 72t
Ravuconazole
  for aspergillosis, 233
  chemistry, 65, 65f
  for eumycetoma, 396
  mechanism of action, 65–66
  for mucormycosis, 79, 247
  pharmacokinetics, 66–67, 66t
  for phaeohyphomycosis, 279
  spectrum of activity, 69–71, 70t, 112t
  susceptibility testing, 71, 112t
  for trichosporonosis, 213
Repetitive element or complex probe, for
    DNA fingerprinting analysis,
    11–12
Reproduction of fungi
  classification based on, 3–4
  types, 3

Resistance to antifungal drugs, 111–21
  to amphotericin B, 34–35, 113
  to azoles, 71–72, 114–19, 115f
    by altered drug transport, 114–17
    alternative mechanisms, 118–19
    genome approaches, 119
    involving alterations in ergosterol
      biosynthetic pathway, 117–18
    involving alterations of cellular
      target, 117
    multiple mechanisms, 118
  current situation, 120–21
  to echinocandins, 90, 119–20
  to fluconazole
    in HIV-AIDS, 490
    in vitro, 71–72, 114
  to flucytosine, 60, 113–14
  interpretive breakpoint values against
    Candida spp., 111, 113t
  to liposomal nystatin, 54
  surviving in presence of, 120
  to voriconazole, 71–72
  vs. susceptibility, 111
Restriction fragment length polymorphism
    (RFLP) procedure, 9, 11
Reticuloendothelial system, in
    paracoccidioidomycosis, 336,
    337f
Rheumatism, desert, coccidioidomycosis,
    317
Rhinocerebral mucormycosis, 244, 246,
    Color Figure 15–2
Rhinocladiella spp., 276t, 277, 497
Rhinosinusitis
  Aspergillus, 228
  in mucomycosis, 244
  in neutropenic patients, surgical
    management, 445
Rhinosporidiosis *(Rhinosporidium
    seeberi)*, 422–23, Color Figure
    28–4
Rhizopus oryzae (Rhizopus arrhizus), 241
Rhizopus spp., 241
Rhodotorulosis, 206–8
  clinical manifestations, 207
  diagnosis, 207–8
  epidemiology, 206
  in HIV-AIDS, 497
  species, 206
  susceptibility data, 206, 206t
  treatment, 208
Rhodotorula rubra, 206, 207t, 497
Rifabutin, azoles and, 68
Rifampin, azoles and, 68
RPMI-1640 broth, 15, 16

Sabbural tongue, in HIV-AIDS, 489
Saccharomyces, 208–9
  clinical manifestations, 208–9
    endocarditis, 209
    fungemia, 209
    genitourinary, 209
    peritonitis, 209
    respiratory, 209
  diagnosis, 209
  treatment, 209

Saccharomyces cerevisiae
organism, 208
in HIV-AIDS, 496–97
resistance, to liposomal nystatin, 54
susceptibility data, 207t, 209
Saksenaea vasiformis, 241
Scalp infections, specimen collection and
transport, 370, 383
Scedosporiosis (pseudallescheriasis),
258–61
after blood or marrow transplantation,
464
azoles for, 79–80
clinical manifestations, 259, 260–61,
276t, 277–78
diagnosis, 259, 261
epidemiology, 258–59, 260
in HIV-AIDS, 496
in neutropenic patients, 430
susceptibility data, 256t, 259–60, 261
treatment, 260, 261, 279
*Scedosporium apiospermum
(Pseudallescheria boydii)*, 256t,
258–60, 276t, 277–78, 279, 496
eumycetoma, 391, 391t, 393, 394t, 395
Scedosporium prolificans, 256t, 260–61,
276t, 278, 279, 496
Schizophyllum commune, 421, 497
Sclerotic bodies, in chromoblastomycosis,
401, Color Figure 26–1
SCOPE surveillance program, 23–24
Scopulariopsis brevicaulis, 262, 384, 385
Scopulariopsis spp., 256t, 262–63
clinical manifestations, 262–63
susceptibility data, 256t, 263
treatment, 263
Scutula, in favus, 382–83
Scytalidium dimidiatum, 384–85, 497
Scytalidium hyalinum, 384–85
Seborrheic dermatitis, 367, 368, 369, 369t
Sentinel surveillance systems, 23–24
SENTRY antimicrobial surveillance
program, 23–24
Serologic testing, 12–14
for aspergillosis, 13, 231, 432–33, 460–61
for blastomycosis, 305–6
for candidiasis, 13–14, 163, 431, 459,
480
for coccidioidomycosis, 13, 320–21
for cryptococcosis, 14, 195, 491
for eumycetoma, 395
for histoplasmosis, 12–13, 293, 492
in organ transplant recipient, 480
for paracoccidioidomycosis, 338–39
for penicilliosis, 360–61
for sporotrichosis, 350
Simvastatin, azoles and, 68
Sinus tracts, in eumycetoma, 392, Color
Figures 25–1 and 25–2
Sinusitis
in asperigillosis
allergic, 226
invasive, 228–29
in conidiobolomycosis, 248
in mucormycosis, 244
in phaeohyphomycoses, 274, 276t, 278

Sirolimus, azoles and, 68
Skeletal lesions. *See* Bone lesions
Skeletal muscle relaxants, amphotericin B
and, 39
Skin lesions
in aspergillosis, 229, 430
in blastomycosis, 303, Color Figures
19–7 to 19–12
in candidiasis, 149–51, 385–86, Color
Figures 11–3, 11–6, and 24–8
in chromoblastomycosis, 400, Color
Figures 26–2 to 26–4
in coccidioidomycosis, 318–19, Color
Figures 20–3 and 20–8
in cryptococcosis, 194, Color Figures
12–7 and 12–8
in eumycetoma, 391–93, Color Figures
25–1, 25–2, and 25–3
in fusariosis, 254, 255, Color Figures
16–1 and 29–4
in histoplasmosis, 291, Color Figures
18–11, 18–12, and 18–15
in malasseziosis, 367–68, 369, 369t,
Color Figure 24–1
in mucormycosis, 245, 431, Color
Figure 15–3
in paracoccidioidomycosis, 336, 336f
in penicilliosis, 359, Color Figures 23–3
to 23–5
in phaeohyphomycosis, 274, Color
Figure 17–1
specimen collection and transport, 370
in sporotrichosis, 348, Color Figures
22–1 to 22–4
in tinea corporis, 373, Color Figures
24–4 and 24–5
in timea versicolor, 367–68, Color
Figure 24–1
in trichosporonosis, 212
Skin test
coccidioidin, 313–14, 314f, 316
histoplasmin, 286t, 294
paracoccidioidin, 330, 339
sporotrichin, 350
Small bowel transplantation, fungal
infections after, 473
Solid organ transplantation. *See* Organ
transplantation
Spherules
adiaspiromycosis, 422, Color Figure
28–3
coccidioidal, 320, Color Figure 20–9
Spores
asexual, 3
sexual, 3
Sporobolomyces, 207t, 214, 497
Sporothrix schenckii
identification, 346–47
histopathology, 350, Color Figure
22–6
mycology, 346–47
virulence factors, 347
Sporotrichin skin test, 350
Sporotrichosis, 346–52, 496
after organ transplantation, 479
amphotericin B for, 352, 496

asteroid body, 350, Color Figure 22–6
azoles for, 77t, 78–79, 351, 496
central nervous system, 349
in children, 349
clinical manifestations, 348–50
diagnosis, 350, 496
disseminated, 349, 496
epidemiology, 347–48
outbreaks, 348
in HIV-AIDS, 349, 496
hyperthermia for, 351
in immunocompromised population,
349–50
lymphocutaneous, 348, 496, Color
Figures 22–1 to 22–4
osteoarticular, 348–49
potassium iodide for, 350–51
prevention, 352
pulmonary, 349, 349f
surgery for, 352
tenosynovitis, 348–49
terbinafine for, 107, 351
treatment, 350–52, 496
Sporulation, visualization, 8, Color
Figures 1–1 to 1–4
Staining procedures, 6–7
Stem cell transplantation. *See* Blood or
marrow transplantation
Stomatitis
atrophic, in candidiasis
acute, 148
chronic, 147–48, Color Figure 11–1
mulberry-like, in
paracoccidioidomycosis, 336,
336f
Subcutaneous phaeohyphomycosis, 274,
Color Figure 17–1
Subungual onychomycosis
distal lateral, 379, 379t
proximal, 379, 379t
Sulfadiazine, for paracoccidioidomycosis,
339, 340t
Sulfamethoxypyridazine, for
paracoccidioidomycosis, 339,
340t
Sulfonamides. *See* Trimethoprim-
sulfamethoxazole
desensitization, 414
for paracoccidioidomycosis, 339–40,
340t
resistance to, 414–15
Superficial mycoses, 367–69
clinical presentations, 367–68
black piedra, 367–69
malasseziosis, 367–69
tinea nigra, 367–69
white piedra, 367–69
definition, 367
diagnosis, 368
differential diagnosis, 368–69
etiology and epidemiology, 367
pathogenesis, 367
prevention, 369
treatment, 369, 369t
Superficial onychomycosis, white, 379,
379t, Color Figure 24–6

Superficial phaeohyphomycosis, 273
Surveillance, epidemiologic, 23–24
Susceptibility testing, 15–18, 111, 112t.
        See also Resistance; *specific
        antifungal drugs*
    agar disc diffusion, 17
    Etest, 17, 113
    interpretation, 17–18, 111, 113t
    M27-A reference method, 15–17, 113,
        163–64
    M38-A reference method, 17
Syncephalastrum spp., 241

T-cell defect
    in chronic mucocutaneous candidiasis,
        150–51, 386
Teleomorph, 3
Tenosynovitis, granulomatous, in
        sporotrichosis, 348–49
Terbinafine, 104–8
    adverse effects, 108
    antifungal activity in vitro, 104–5, 105t,
        106t
    combination therapy, 108
    dosage and administration, 106
    drug interactions, 108
    indications
        for chromoblastomycosis, 107, 403
        for eumycetoma, 107, 396
        for onychomycosis, 106–7, 380, 380t
        for *Scopulariopsis* spp. infection, 263
        for sporotrichosis, 107, 351
        for tinea barbae, 375t
        for tinea capitis, 107, 384, 384t
        for tinea corporis, 107, 374t
        for tinea cruris, 107, 376
        for tinea pedis and manuum, 107,
            378
    mechanism of action, 104
    oral, 105–6
    pharmacodynamics, 104–5
    pharmacokinetics, 105–6
    topical, 106
Thiabendazole, for chromoblastomycosis,
        401t, 402
Thrush. *See also* Oropharyngeal
        candidiasis
    in HIV-AIDS, 147, 488–89
Thymus transplantation, for chronic
        mucocutaneous candidiasis, 169
Tinea barbae, 374–75, 375t
    clinical manifestations, 374
    diagnosis, 374–75
    epidemiology, 374
    treatment, 374, 374t
Tinea capitis, 381–84
    clinical presentations, 381–83
        black dot, 382
        favus, 382–83
        gray patch, 382
        inflammatory, 382, Color Figure 24–7
    diagnosis, 383
    epidemiology, 381
    terbinafine for, 107
    treatment, 383–84, 384t

Tinea corporis, 372–74
    clinical presentations, 373, Color
        Figures 24–4 and 24–5
    diagnosis, 373
    epidemiology, 372–73
    prevention, 374
    treatment, 373–74, 373t, 374t
Tinea cruris, 375–76
    clinical manifestations, 375–76
    diagnosis, 376
    epidemiology, 375
    prevention, 376
    treatment, 376
Tinea manuum, 376–78
    clinical manifestations, 377
    diagnosis, 377–78
    epidemiology, 376–77
    prevention, 378
    treatment, 378
Tinea nigra, 273, 367, 368, 369
Tinea pedis, 376–78
    clinical manifestations, 377
        inflammatory (vesicular), 377
        interdigital, 377
        moccasin, 377
        ulcerative, 377
    diagnosis, 377–78
    epidemiology, 376–77
    prevention, 378
    treatment, 378
Tinea profunda, 373
Tinea unguium. *See also* Onychomycosis,
        378–81
    clinical manifestations, 379, 379t
        distal lateral sublungual,
            379–379t
        white superficial, 379, 379t
        proximal subungual, 379–379t
        total dystrophic, 379, 379t
    definition, 378
    diagnosis, 378–80
    epidemiology, 378
    prevention, 380–81
    treatment, 380, 380t
Tinea versicolor, 367, 368, 369, 369t,
        Color Figure 24–1
Tongue, sabbural, in HIV-AIDS, 489
Topical therapy
    for candidiasis, 73t, 165–69, 166t,
        168t, 387
    for malassezioses, 369, 369t
    for onychomycosis, 380
    for piedras, 369
    for tinea capitis, 384
    for tinea corporis, 373–74, 373t
    for tinea nigra, 369
    for tinea pedis and manuum, 378
Total dystrophic onychomycosis, 379,
        379t
Triazolam, azoles and, 68
Trichoderma spp., 256t, 264–65
    clinical manifestations, 264
    susceptibility data, 256t, 264–65
    treatment, 265
Trichophyton concentricum, 372

Trichophyton mentagrophytes complex,
        371f, 372, Color Figure 24–3
Trichophyton rubrum, 371, 371f, Color
        Figure 24–3
Trichophyton schoenleinii, 372
Trichophyton spp., characteristics,
        371–72, 371f, Color Figure 24–3
Trichophyton tonsurans, 371f, 372, Color
        Figure 24–3
Trichophyton violaceum, 372
Trichosporon asahii, 207t, 213
    characteristics, 211
    susceptibility data, 207t
Trichosporon spp.
    characteristics, 211
    white piedra from, 211, 367, 368, 369
Trichosporonosis, 211–13
    after organ transplantation, 479
    clinical manifestations, 212
    diagnosis, 212
    epidemiology, 211–12
    in HIV-AIDS, 496–97
    in neutropenic patients, 431
    organism, 211
    treatment, 212–13
Trimethoprim, plus dapsone, for
        pneumocystosis, 410, 410t
Trimethoprim-sulfamethoxazole
    desensitization, 414
    for entomophthoramycosis, 249
    for paracoccidioidomycosis, 339–40,
        340t
    for pneumocystosis, 409–10, 410t
        after organ transplantation, 481
        prophylaxis, 412–13, 413t
    resistance to, 414–15
        dihydropteroate synthase mutations,
            414–15
    toxicity, 410
Trimetrexate, plus leucovorin, for
        pneumocystosis, 410t, 411
Tubo-ovarian abscess, blastomycotic,
        304
Tumor necrosis factor-α, biologic
        properties, 127, 126t

Ulcers, mucous membrane/skin
    in blastomycosis, 303, Color Figures
        19–10 and 19–11
    oropharyngeal, in histoplasmosis, 291,
        Color Figure 18–12
    in paracoccidioidomycosis, 336, 336f
    in phaeohyphomycoses, 274, 276t
    in tinea pedis, 377
Urinary tract infections. *See also*
        Genitourinary tract
    Candida, 159–61, Color Figure 11–10
        after organ transplantation, 476
        treatment, 171
    S. cerevisiae, 209
Ustilago spp., 421

Vaginal discharge, in vulvovaginal
        candidiasis, 153, Color Figure
        11–5

Vaginitis
    Candida. See Vulvovaginal candidiasis
    S. cerevisiae, 209
Ventriculoperitoneal shunt, for
        cryptococcal meningitis, 201,
        492
Verrucous skin lesions
    in blastomycosis, 303, Color Figures
        19-7 to 19-9
    in chromoblastomycosis, 400, Color
        Figure 26-2
Vertebral osteomyelitis, in coccidioido-
        mycosis, 319, 319f, Color
        Figure 20-8
Vincristine, azoles and, 69
Viral infections, post-transplant fungal
        infections and, 457
Visual disturbances, from voriconazole,
        73
Vitrectomy, for *Candida* endophthalmitis,
        171
Voriconazole, 64-80
    adverse effects, 72-73, 72t
    chemistry, 64-65, 65f
    drug interactions, 67-69, 68t
    indications
        for aspergillosis, 79, 233
            after blood or marrow
                transplantation, 465
            after organ transplantation, 481
            in neutropenic patients, 444-45
        for blastomycosis, 76-77
        for candidiasis, 74, 167
        for cerebral aspergillosis, 229
        for chromoblastomycosis, 403
        for coccidioidomycosis, 78, 323
        for empirical therapy, febrile
            neutropenic patients, 438-41,
            439t, 440t, 443

        for eumycetoma, 396
        for fusariosis, 80, 257-58
        for neutropenic fever, 439t-40t,
            442-43, 444
        for paracoccidioidomycosis, 78
        for scedosporiosis, 80, 260
        for trichosporonosis, 213
    mechanism of action, 65-66
    pharmacokinetics, 66-67, 66t
    prophylaxis, 80
        in neutropenic patients, 438
    resistance to, 71-72
    spectrum of activity, 69-71, 70t, 112t
    susceptibility testing, 71, 112t
Vulvovaginal candidiasis, 151-53, 386,
        387
    azoles for, 73t, 74
    in HIV-AIDS, 168
    pathogenesis, 151-53, 152f
    recurrent, 152-53, 169
        prevention, 174
        sexual transmission theory, 152
        treatment, 169
        vaginal relapse theory, 152-53
    symptoms, 153, Color Figure 11-5
    treatment, 73t, 74, 167-69, 168t

Wangiella dermatitidis, 276t, 278
Warfarin, azoles and, 69
Water contamination, aspergillosis from,
        25, 463
White blood cell transfusions
    for chronic mucocutaneous candidiasis,
        169
    complications, 39, 134, 446
    G-CSF–stimulated, in neutropenic
        patients, 132-34, 133t, 446-47,
        447, 465
    indications, 134, 446-47

White piedra, 211, 367, 368, 369
White superficial onychomycosis, 379,
        379t, Color Figure 24-6
White to yellow grain eumycetoma, 391t,
        394, 394t. *See also* Eumycetoma
Wood's light examination, in tinea capitis,
        383
Wright's stain, 6

Yeast-like organisms, infections due to,
        206-14, 420-21
Yeasts
    characteristics, 3
    phenotypic identification, 8-9
    susceptibility in vitro
        to amphotericin B, 34, 112t
        to anidulafungin, 90, 90t, 112t
        to azoles, 70, 70t, 71, 112t
        to caspofungin, 92, 92t, 112t
        to flucytosine, 60, 112t
        to liposomal nystatin, 53-54, 53t
        M27-A2 refence method, 15-17
        to micafungin, 95-96, 96t, 112t
        to terbinafine, 104-5, 105t

Zygomycetes, class
    Mucorales, 241
    Entomophthorales, 241
    taxonomy, 241, 242t
Zygomycoses, 241-49
    after blood or marrow transplantation,
        461, 464
    after organ transplantation, 474, 477-78
    entomophthoramycosis, 247-49
    in HIV-AIDS, 496
    mucormycosis, 241-47
    in neutropenic patients, 430-31
    treatment, 246-24, 249
Zygomycota, 4